DM Entrance Examination
CARDIOLOGY–3

Fourth Edition

DAVINDER PAL SINGH
DM Resident (Cardiology)
Indira Gandhi Medical College, Shimla (HP)
Presently working as Cardiologist, NMC DIP, Dubai (UAE)

PEEPEE PUBLISHERS AND DISTRIBUTORS (P) LTD.®

DM Entrance Examination Cardiology–3

Published by
Pawaninder P. Vij and Anupam Vij

Peepee Publishers and Distributors (P) Ltd.
Head Office: 160, Shakti Vihar, Pitam Pura, Delhi-110 034 (India)

Correspondence Address:
7/31, First Floor, Ansari Road, Daryaganj
New Delhi-110 002 (India)
Ph: 41512412, 23246245, 9811156083
e-mail: peepee160@yahoo.co.in
e-mail: peepee160@gmail.com
www.peepeepub.com
join us on facebook.com/pp.publishers

First Edition: 2015

Fourth Edition: 2021

ISBN: 978-81-8445-280-8

PREFACE

Super specialisation in cardiology has gained new peak of interest in recent years. Every aspirant want to join cardiology in a good institution. I tried to fulfill the expectations of those students by writing this book. This book offers a collection of questions of various DM Cardiology Entrance Examinations from all over India.

From the feedback of students, I have compiled all questions chapterwise for better and easy to understand.

I would like to thank my teachers and my colleagues (past and present) who directly and indirectly influenced me in writing this book.

Last of all, I am deeply indebted to my wife and daughter, who accepted with understanding the inconvenience associated with my long preoccupation with the book.

Davinder Pal Singh

ACKNOWLEDGEMENTS

Prof PC Negi (HOD, IGMC, Shimla)

Prof R Bhardwaj (IGMC, Shimla)

Dr Arvind Kandoria (IGMC, Shimla)

Dr Sanjeev Asotra (IGMC, Shimla)

Dr Neeraj Ganju (IGMC, Shimla)

Dr Rajeev Merwaha (IGMC, Shimla)

Dr Mandeep Garg (Fortis Escort, New Delhi)

Dr Jyoti Prakash (GB Pant, New Delhi)

Dr Nirmal Kolte (IGMC, Shimla)

Dr Ravi Kumar (IGMC, Shimla)

Dr Rajesh (IGMC, Shimla)

Dr Vivek Rana (IGMC, Shimla)

Dr Sharath Babu (CMC, Vellore)

Dr Ambudhar (IGMC, Shimla)

Dr Kunal Mahajan (IGMC, Shimla)

Dr Prince (IGMC, Shimla)

CONTENTS

CHAPTER ONE

ISCHEMIC HEART DISEASE

1. **Diabetic patient with aVR elevation on ECG most likely:**
(a) Left man stenosis
(b) Unable to localize in NSTEM
(c) CSA
(d) All

2. **Male with MI–pH showing alkalosis:**
PO_2 – 55 PCO_2–30
HCO_3–23 Not true
(a) A-a gradient is (N)
(b) Respiratory alkalosis
(c) Alveolar hyperventilation
(d) Adequate compensated

3. **Most sensitive test for significant stenosis in 60% stenosis with atypical chest pain:**
(a) IVUS (b) FFR
(c) OCT (d) NIRS

4. **FFR which is true:**
(a) < 0.9 is significant stenosis
(b) Nitroglycerine high dose in place of adenosine in lung disease
(c) Depends on HR/SBP
(d) Depends on viable area of ischemic myocardium

5. **Indication for PCI in class II stable angina with DVD:**
(a) Rx asymptomatic ischemia
(b) Prevention of MI
(c) Prevention of SCD
(d) Rx symptomatic ischemia

6. **Rotational atherectomy may not be done:**
(a) SVG graft (b) Bifurcation
(c) Ostial (d) DM

7. **A 44 years female with chest pain/SOB BP 90/48 and HR 120, RR 40, pH 7.48, pCO_2 18, HCO_3 10, pO_2 66 next is:**
(a) Trop I with aspirin
(b) PTE-CT angio
(c) ECHO for LV dysfunction
(d) HCO_3

8. **Patient with CAD which is not CI?**
(a) Interferon A (b) Cisplatin
(c) Imatinib (d) FU

9. **Least atherosclerotic CAD risk in:**
(a) Cushing's syndrome (b) Acromegaly
(c) Hypothyroidism (d) SLE

10. **Rotational atherectomy–all are contraindications *except:***
(a) Extreme tortuosity of artery
(b) Ostial stenosis
(c) Post balloon dilatation
(d) High thrombus burden

11. **Study used for 'Risk calculator' in cardiovascular diseases:**
(a) Cross-sectional study (b) Cohort study
(c) RCT (d) Nested case control study

12. **Postoperative MI–most common in:**
(a) 24-48 hours (b) 7 days
(c) Immediately (d) 12 hours

13. **Following occlusion of myocardial blood flow without collaterals. All are true *except:***
(a) Viability starts to decrease after 2 hours
(b) Fall in ATP in 2 sec
(c) Decreased LV function in 2 minutes
(d) Necrosis is complete with 6 hours

14. **Intention to treat analysis, CABG V/S medical therapy. But most patients of surgery underwent medical therapy. They should be:**
(a) Excluded from trial

(b) Regarded as medical therapy arm
(c) Regarded as surgical therapy

15. Elderly with T wave inversion in V_1-V_4:
(a) Proximal LAD disease
(b) Mid LAD
(c) Distal LAD
(d) Proximal RCA

16. IABP tracings true is:
(a) Increases C.O. by 1.5 L – 2L
(b) Trials show no utility
(c) Excellent bridge to transplantation
(d) Also useful in respiratory failure

17. Nocturnal angina – A/E:
(a) It occurs in NREM
(b) Not associated with unstable angina
(c) Wall–stress ↑
(d) ↑ Sympathetic activity

18. Recent trials all T/E:
(a) Mediterranean diet ↓ MACE
(b) IABP has no mortality benefit at 30 days
(c) Percutaneous occlusion for AA benefit in young but not in old
(d) In NSTEMI in medical management prasugrel improves mortality compared to clopidogrel

19. Match the following–All T/E:
(a) First cardiac catheterization–Forssmann
(b) First angiography–Sones
(c) First stenting–Andreas Gruentzig
(d) Philip Reed–ICD

20. Acute pulmonary edema with MI A/E:
(a) Sublingual captopril
(b) Intermittent TV Isosorbide bolus
(c) NIV
(d) Milrinone

21. Most common time for perioperative MI:
(a) Intraoperatively (b) < 4 hours
(c) 3 days (d) 7 days

22. Fibrinolysis–absolute C/I–all *except:*
(a) Major surgrey–3 weeks back
(b) ICH
(c) AD
(d) A malignant intracranial drug tumor

23. First to occur in AMI:
(a) Metabolic changes (b) Wall motion absent
(c) ECG changes

24. 43-year-old woman, 3 months from MI, NYHA-II, EF-43% RWMA, next done–premature PVC with baseline ST-T:
(a) Treadmill→if positive angio
(b) Medical stabilization
(c) CT angio→CAG
(d) Directly CAG

25. A 62 years old post menopausal/atypical chest pain, pre test prob. of CAD:
(a) Low (b) Very Low
(c) Intermediate (d) High

26. Least effective in treatment of refractory angina:
(a) Cardiac transplant
(b) External counter pulsation
(c) Spinal nerve stimulator
(d) Chelation therapy

27. Chronic stable angina–elective PCI–benefit:
(a) Prevent infarct
(b) Prevent mortality
(c) Prevent both infarct and mortality
(d) Not infarct and mortality

28. Immediate intervention in NSTEMI A/E:
(a) HF (b) Sustained VT/VF
(c) New MR murmur (d) Grace score > 140

29. Urgent invasive in NSTEMI:
(a) BP < 100 (b) VT/VF
(c) Troponin positive

30. High risk in USA A/E:
(a) Age–79 (b) ST deviation–0.6 mm
(c) Q wave in ECG (d) Trop positive

31. Cause of ST elevation A/E:
(a) Hypokalemia (b) Hypothermia
(c) ICH (d) Pericarditis

32. True about STK:
(a) Most fibrin specific (b) 90% TIMI-III
(c) Enzyme (d) Allergic reaction – 25%

33. Post MI pericardiac drug not given:
(a) Narcotic analgesic (b) NSAID
(c) Aspirin (d) Colchicine

34. **Prinzmetal's angina A/E:**
(a) 1/3rd obstructive CAD on CAG
(b) Smoking not RF
(c) Beta blocker can be detrimental
(d) Can occur without classic RF

STEMI with Wasp Sting (T/F) (35-38)

35. **Konis Surgery:**

36. **Capacitabine–cause:**

37. **Morphine given for pain:**

38. **Glucagon better than adrenaline:**

39. **Guiding wire thickness:**
(a) 0.035 inches (b) 0.35 inches
(c) 0.014 inches (d) 0.32 inches

40. **LIMA to LAD (visualizing anastomotic site)**
(a) Left lateral (b) LAO cranial
(c) RAO cranial (d) PA candal

41. **Rational atherectomy true is:**
(a) With abciximab – 5 times CKMB elevation
(b) Compared to balloon angioplasty MACE is less
(c) Procedural success in angiographic success without in hospital complication

42. **Dose modification not required in renal patients:**
(a) Abciximab (b) Tirofiban
(c) Eptifibatide (d) Ximelagatran

43. **ACC/AHA class I indication:**
(a) Thrombolysis only
(b) Facilitated PCI
(c) Thrombolysis and rescue PCI
(d) Pharmaco invasive therapy

44. **Direct II a inhibitor:**
(a) Rivaroxaban (b) Apixaban
(c) Dabigatran (d) Enoxaparin

45. **Anti IIa: Xa factor highest:**
(a) Enoxaparin (b) Tinzaparin
(c) Dalteparin (d) Donaproid

46. **LMCA isolated stenosis ESC 2010 indication (for PCI):**
(a) I (b) IIa
(c) IIb (d) III

47. **Trials of Prasugrel A/E:**
(a) PLAZO (b) Principle TIME
(c) Triton TIME (d) SWAP

48. **Collagen plug for vascular protection:**
(a) Angioseal
(b) Collastage
(c) Fenostat

49. **True:**
(a) Angiographic success stenosis > 75% and DES < 25%
(b) Clinical success stenosis < 78%
(c) CKMB
(d) Procedural success–angiography within hospital complication

50. **All are risk factors for stent thrombosis *except:***
(a) Hypersensitivity to stent polygon
(b) HTN
(c) DM
(d) Renal failure

51. **RCA involvement suggested by:**
(a) ST ↑ II > III (b) Predominant S in V1
(c) ST elevation in III (d) ST ↓ V1 > aVL

52. **IABP–true A/E:**
(a) May be used in AR
(b) May be used in AS
(c) May be used in VSD
(d) May be used in MR

53. **High risk in UA A/E:**
(a) S3
(b) Pulmonary edema
(c) Age 75
(d) T wave inversion > 0.2 mm

54. **Morphine C/I:**
(a) STEMI (b) NSTEMI
(c) Pulmonary edema (d) TOF

55. **CIN risk increases ______ <GFR.**
(a) 40 (b) 60
(c) 30 (d) 45

56. **CIN A/E:**
(a) NaCl not useful
(b) Hydration helpful
(c) Less contrast helpful

57. CIN prevention GFR < 60 ml/min:
(a) 1-2 ml/kg NS can 24 hours pre procedure
(b) Post procedure 150 ml/hour NS
(c) Sodium bicarb > saline
(d) Loop diuretics useful

58. FFR useful for:
(a) Vasospasm
(b) Intermediate coronary lesion
(c) MI

59. FFR true:
(a) Not reliable in the presence of collaterals
(b) Good accuracy
(c) Used in MI

60. STE in aVR true:
(a) LAD (b) TVD
(c) LCX (d) RCA

61. Instant thrombosis A/E:
(a) Definite thrombosis–proven thrombus @ autopsy/angio
(b) Probable thrombosis–within 30 days of index procedure
(c) Possible thrombosis–beyond 30 days
(d) Very late – > 6 months

62. Advantage of stents over balloon angioplasty:
(a) ↓ target vessels revascularization
(b) ↓ long term mortality
(c) ↓ long term MI risk

63. All are true *except:*
(a) Prasugrel no mortality benefit beyond clopidogrel
(b) Prasugrel recommended in NSTEMI managed medically
(c) Once daily dosing
(d) 60 mg loading

64. Type A coronary lesion is:
(a) No or little calcium
(b) Tubular > 10 mm
(c) Thrombus present
(d) Total occlusion less than 2 months

65. MI in elderly less frequent is:
(a) Chest pain (b) Heart failure
(c) Killip > 2 (d) LBBB

66. SHOCK 2 trial in acute myocardial infarction patients with cardiogenic shock concludes:
(a) Use of IABP counter pulsation did not significantly reduce the 30 days mortality
(b) Use of IABP counter pulsation significantly reduced the 30 days mortality
(c) Use of IABP counter pulsation did not significantly reduce the 1 year mortality
(d) Use of IABP counter pulsation significantly reduced the 1 year mortality

67. The indirect index of measuring the driving pressure for microcirculatory flow distal to the stenosis relative to the coronary driving pressure in the absence of stenosis is:
(a) Absolute flow reserve
(b) Relative flow reserve
(c) Fractional flow reserve
(d) Coronary flow reserve

68. Largest trial of aspirin in STEMI patients which provided the single strongest evidence of mortality benefit of aspirin:
(a) ISIS 2 (b) CLARITY TIMI
(c) HORIZONS AMI (d) TRITON TIMI 38

69. All are used in provocative test for prinzmetal angina *except:*
(a) Hyperventilation
(b) Intracoronary acetyl choline
(c) Intracoronary ergonovine
(d) Intracoronary adrenaline

70. A 60-year-old male patient who underwent CABG 3 days back develops hypotension. Clinical examination revealed elevated JVR. ECG was normal, PCWP was low. His Echo is likely to show:
(a) Akinesia of LV anterior wall
(b) RV infarction
(c) Severe MR
(d) Localized pericardial clot on RA side

71. Cystic medial necrosis is found in the following *except:*
(a) Atherosclerosis
(b) Marfan syndrome
(c) Loeys-Dietz syndrome
(d) Ehlers-Danlos syndrome type IV

72. Coronary blood flow:
(a) 500 ml/min–at rest
(b) Ceases at systole
(c) Can't be measured by echo

(d) Autoregulation
(e) Directly affected by vagal act

73. **Chest pain:**
(a) Anterior chest pain with back radiation S/O–AD
(b) Spodick sign–specific for pericarditis
(c) GERD–retrosternal chest pain–bending
(d) Pleuritic chest pain hypotension–massive PE
(e) Chest pain with RVHF–anterior wall MI

74. **HIT: (T/F)**
(a) Usually in 24 hours
(b) LMWH > UFH
(c) Warfarin ↑ – TOC
(d) Serotonin release assay–for diagnosis
(e) Ab against PF4–plalelet–seen

75. **STEMI: (T/F)**
(a) < 6 hours chest pain Normal Trop I R/O MI
(b) EMRAS, REACT for pharmacoinvasive strategy
(c) Rescue PCI class I
(d) As per 2013 1 month DAPT in DES
(e) Mortality benefit with thrombolysis > 24 hours

76. **ECG findings of acute MI: (T/F)**
(a) STE in aVR indicates proximal LAD lesion before first septal artery
(b) STE in inferior leads in presence of anterior MI suggests mid-LAD disease
(c) aRBBB suggests lesion after first septal
(d) STE in lead II> lead III suggests LCx occlusion
(e) STE in V_4R in IWMI indicates RVMI

77. **Investigation for atherosclerosis: (T/F)**
(a) Palpography measures temperature of the lesion
(b) IVUS–best to detect in stent restenosis
(c) NIRS is based on the absorption of light by organic molecules
(d) Polarization sensitive OCT, which provides assessment of plaque collagen content
(e) Angioscopy allows direct visualization of the plaque surface and luminal thrombus

78. **How many fold coronary flow can increase due to vasodilation?**
(a) 23 times (b) 12 times
(c) 45 times (d) 67 times

79. **Troponin level does not increase in following condition:**
(a) STEMI (b) Myocarditis
(c) Renal disease (d) Liver disease

80. **Plaque fissuring/disruption is less common in:**
(a) Lipid burden in atheroma 70%
(b) Thin cap atheroma
(c) Thick cap atheroma
(d) Luminal area of stenotic area, 4.0 mm square

81. **Following is true for atrial infarction incidence in patients with STEMI:**
(a) 10% (b) 5%
(c) 15% (d) 25%

82. **Infarct expansion is less in following condition:**
(a) Diabetes mellitus
(b) Hypertrophied myocardium
(c) Multivessel disease
(d) Gout

83. **Following criteria favours myocardial infarction in presence of LBBB *except:***
(a) ST segment elevation greater than 1 mm and concordant with QRS complex
(b) ST segment depression greater than 1 mm in V1, V2, V3
(c) ST segment depression greater than 1 mm in II, III, AVF
(d) ST segment elevation greater than 5 mm and discordant with QRS complex

84. **Which one of the following is not true for MRI in acute myocardial infarction?**
(a) It assesses perfusion in infarcted and non-infarcted myocardium
(b) Repurfused myocardium
(c) Assess coronary anatomy precisely
(d) Identifies myocardial fibrosis, wall thinning

85. **Which one of the following thrombolytic agents is more fibrin specific?**
(a) Streptokinase (b) Teneclaplase
(c) Alteplase (d) Reteplase

86. **Which one of the following is not true in classification of TIMI flow grade?**
(a) TIMI grade 1 (b) TIMI grade 2
(c) TIMI grade 3 (d) TIMI grade 4

87. **What minimum level of damage to left ventricular myocardium is required in patients with STEMI for cardiogenic shock?**

(a) 50% (b) 60%
(c) 70% (d) 80%

88. Which one of the following is not true for right ventricular infarction?
(a) Hypotension
(b) Kussmaul sign
(c) Elevated JVP
(d) Basal crepitations in lungs

89. Which one of the following is not true for pseudo-aneurysm of LV after infarction?
(a) It lacks any elements of myocardial wall
(b) It is made up of organised thrombus and pericardium
(c) It communicates with LV cavity through a narrow neck
(d) It communicates with LV cavity through a wide neck

90. Which one of the following is not true for Ranolazine?
(a) It inhibits late inward sodium current
(b) It is used in angina
(c) It prolongs QT interval
(d) It decreases heart rate

91. Which one of the following is not true for bivalirudin?
(a) It is direct thrombin inhibitor
(b) It has half life of 3 hours
(c) It does not cause thrombocytopenia
(d) It is used in percutaneous coronary interventions

92. Which one of the following drugs is not used for provocative testing for vasospastic angina?
(a) Hyperventilation
(b) Intracoronary acetylcholine
(c) Intracoronary ergonovine
(d) Intracoronary phenyl epinephrine

93. Coronary calcification on computerised tomography is helpful in predicting obstructive CAD. Which one of the following is true?
(a) Sensitivity 90% (b) Sensitivity 50%
(c) Sensitivity 60% (d) Sensitivity 80%

94. Which one of the following is not true for nicorandil?
(a) It is potassium channel activator
(b) It can produce ulcerations in gastrointestinal tract
(c) It has negative chronotropic effect
(d) It is venodilator and coronary dilator

95. Which one of the following drugs is not used in drug eluting stent?
(a) Zotarolimus (b) Cyclosporine
(c) Sirolimus (d) Paclitaxel

96. Incidence of acute MI due to aortic dissection is:
(a) 5% to 10% (b) 1% to 2%
(c) 20% to 30% (d) 40% to 50%

97. In TRITONTIMI 38 trial clopidogrel was compared with:
(a) Cangrelor (b) Prasugrel
(c) Ticagrelor (d) Vorapaxar

98. What fold risk of infarction increases with use of cocaine (in first 60 minutes after cocaine use)?
(a) 2 fold (b) 5 fold
(c) 10 fold (d) 24 fold

99. Which is not a correct match for the characteristics of type A, B and C coronary lesions as per ACC/AHA classification?
(a) Type B–Tubular
(b) Type C–Ostial
(c) Type A–Concentric
(d) Type C–Total occlusion more than 3 months old

100. Obligatory ischemia is a feature of which of the following coronary anomalies?
(a) Ectopic RCA from right cusp
(b) Coronary artery fistulas
(c) Anomalous left coronary artery from pulmonary artery
(d) Anomalous left coronary artery from opposite sinus

101. The third universal definition of MI defines MI associated with PCI as elevation of cardiac troponin values of:
(a) > 3 × 99th percentile URL in patients with normal baseline values
(b) > 5 × 99th percentile URL in patients with normal baseline values
(c) > 10 × 99th percentile URL in patients with normal baseline values
(d) > 20 × 99th percentile URL in patients with normal baseline values

102. Which randomized trial compared outcomes of optimal medical therapy versus percutaneous coronary intervention in patients with known significant CAD and objective evidence of myocardial ischemia?

(a) Freedom trial (b) Courage trial
(c) Fame trial (d) Syntax trial

103. Absolute contraindications to fibrinolytic therapy include all *except:*

(a) Previous intracranial hemorrhage or stroke of unknown origin at any time
(b) Pregnancy or within 1 week postpartum
(c) Ischemic stroke in the preceding 6 months
(d) Aortic dissection

104. Dose adjustment is needed for all of the following antithrombotic agents in patients with chronic kidney disease (estimated creatinine clearance < 60 mL/min):

(a) Eptifibatide (b) Tirofiban
(c) Clopidogrel (d) Bivalirudin

105. What is false regarding ticagrelor?

(a) 180 mg loading dose followed by 90 mg BD maintenance dose
(b) Concurrent aspirin dose is 150 mg OD
(c) Plato trial concluded that ticagrelor as compared with clopidogrel significantly reduced major adverse cardiovascular events without an increase in the rate of overall major bleeding
(d) Onset offset trial concluded that ticagrelor achieved more rapid and greater platelet inhibition than high-loading-dose clopidogreal

106. Which of the following substances action is not endothelium dependent?

(a) Adenosine (b) Histamine
(c) Endothelin (d) Acetylcholine

107. Time to reperfusion therapy is the most important determinator of outcomes in acute MI. In this context, which of the following is a recommended treatment goal?

(a) First medical contact (FMC) to ECG and diagnosis 60 minutes
(b) First medical contact to fibrinolysis (FMC to needle time) 60 minutes
(c) First medical contact to primary PCI (FMC to balloon time) 90 minutes
(d) None of the above

108. Not a branch of right coronary artery:

(a) Obtuse marginal
(b) Acute marginal
(c) Posterior descending artery
(d) Conal branch

109. Rotational artherectomy is not done in:

(a) Ostial lesions
(b) Calcified lesions
(c) Instant restenosis
(d) Degenerated vein grafts

110. Myocardial bridges are most common in:

(a) LAD (b) RCA
(c) Major OM (d) Diagonal

111. Select the true statement:

(a) Levels of abciximab may remain detectable upto 2 weeks after discontinuation
(b) The correlation of anti Xa/anti IIa for low molecular weight heparin is a good predictor of potency
(c) Dalteparin has the highest IIa: Xa ratio
(d) Lepirudin is reversible inhibitor of thrombin

112. It is reasonable to use IVUS for which of the following coronary interventions, procedures?

(a) Assessment of angiographically in determinant left main CAD
(b) One year after cardiac transplantation to exclude donor CAD
(c) Determine the mechanism of stent restenosis
(d) All of the above

113. P2 ↑/12 inhibitor – no liver activation required:

(a) Ticagrelor (b) Clopidogrel
(c) Ticlopidine (d) Prosegrel

114. Shortest acting antiplatelet:

(a) Clopidogrel (b) Aspirin
(c) Congrelor (d) Prosegrel

115. Patient treated for CAD develops skin rashes, leucopenia thrombocytopenia – drug responsible:

(a) Clopidogrel (b) Ticagrelar
(c) Ticlopidine (d) Enalapril

116. GP263a inhibitors useful in:

(a) UA (b) PTCA
(c) STEMI (d) All

117. Dabigatran:

(a) Activated X inhibitor (b) Activated II inhibitor
(c) XII inhibitor (d) Fibrin inhibitor

118. LMWH in acute CAD A/E:

(a) Better than heparin in acute MI
(b) Better results with aspirin
(c) Easy infusion
(d) Better to continue after discharge

119. Main hemodynamic effect of IABP:

(a) ↓ Preload (b) ↓ Afterload
(c) ↑ Co (d) ↓ Contractility
(e) All

120. Most common cause of unstable angina:

(a) Plaque rupture with thrombosis
(b) Secondary
(c) Thrombus embolism
(d) Spasm

121. In CoPD patient, for stress test used is:

(a) Adenosine (b) Dobutamine
(c) Dopamine (d) Diltiazem

122. DES better over BMS with respect to:

(a) Restenosis (b) Cost
(c) Thrombosis (d) Procedure

123. DES preferred in A/E:

(a) >4 mm (b) 2.5-3.5 m
(c) Length > 3.5 m

124. Procedure of choice in ACS patient who requires noncardiac surgery I in 1 month is:

(a) DES (b) Balloon angioplasty
(c) BMS (d) CABG

125. NSTEMI – A/E:

(a) Nitrate (b) Anticoagulants
(c) Thrombolytics (d) Morphine

126. Dipyridamole scan showing ↓ severe than normal:

(a) LBBB (b) 99% stenosis RCA
(c) Bradycardia (d) LMCA stenosis

127. Silent MI A/E:

(a) Common in DM
(b) Follows circadian rhythm
(c) Mainly due to spasm
(d) Occurrence 2.5%

128. Plaque rupture is diagnostically characterized by:

(a) IVUS (b) Angiography
(c) MRI (d) Angioscopy

129. Myocardial stunning A/E:

(a) Free radial injury (b) ↓ Energy requirement

130. Following statements are true about surgical ventricular reconstruction *except:*

(a) Endoventricular patch plasty is also known as Dor procedure
(b) A purse-string suture is placed between the infarcted and normal myocardium. Endoventricular Dacron path is used to exclude the infarcted segment
(c) RV dysfunction is a contraindication to Dor procedure
(d) Ideally, the operation was designed to reduce end systolic volume by at least 50% irrespective of LV size

131. Anatomic variables associated with stent thrombosis are all *except:*

(a) Long lesions (b) Multivessel disease
(c) Left main disease (d) Bifurcation lesion

132. All are true about plaque characteristics on IVUS and OCT *except:*

(a) Both are good at identifying calcium in plaque, and less so at identifying fibrous and lipid tissue
(b) In IVUS images, calcium appears as a bright echogenic signal with a corresponding shadow on the far side of the calcium
(c) In OCT images, calcium appears as an area of increased signal intensity with well demarcated border
(d) Fibrous tissue appears as an area of heterogenous signal intensity beneath the media on both IVUS and OCT images

133. Diphasic response on dobutamine stress echo indicates all *except:*

(a) Low dose dobutamine infusion – ↑ wall thickening
High dose dobutamine infusion – ↓ wall thickening
(b) Low dose dobutamine infusion – ↓ wall thickening
High dose dobutamine infusion – ↑ wall thickening
(c) Most specific sign of myocardial viability
(d) Any improvement in RWMA by at least one grade in two or more segments during stress signify viability

134. Which of the following pairs is not correctly matched?

(a) Elinogrel–reversible, direct-acting P2Y12-receptor inhibitor
(b) Vorapaxar–selective, PAR-1 inhibitor that blocks thrombin-mediated platelet activation

(c) Terutroban–thromboxane A2 synthase inhibitor
(d) Ridogrel–dual inhibitor of thromboxane A2 synthase and thromboxane-receptor

135. Which of the following is a correct statement?
(a) Arteriogenesis is the process by which new capillaries develop from the preexisting vasculature
(b) Angiogenesis is the process of collateral vessel enlargement, caused by remodeling or growth of preexisting arteriolar collateral connections
(c) Vasculogenesis, is defined as the de novo formation of a primitive vascular network from differentiating precursor mesodermal cells, such as endothelial progenitor cells, in the absence of preexisting vasculature
(d) Bevacizumab causes angiogenesis through VEGF

136. All are seen best in the views *except:*
(a) LMCA–AP caudal view
(b) Origin of PDA–RAO view
(c) MID LAD–LAO cranial view
(d) Ostium of RCA–LAO caudal view

137. All are true about adenosine *except:*
(a) Adenosine dilates coronary arteries through activation of A 2 receptors
(b) Adenosine mediated vasodilation is enhanced by lowering LDL levels
(c) It has a differential sensitivity for the microcirculation
(d) None of the above

138. Atrial infarction is characterized by all *except:*
(a) It occurs in upto 10% patients with STEMI if PR-segment displacement is used as criteria
(b) It occurs more commonly in right atrium
(c) It occurs more frequently in atrial appendage
(d) It has been linked to elevated atrial natriuretic peptide levels

139. A 54-year-old female presents with chronic stable angina, normal ECG, type 2 diabetes mellitus and critical lower limb ischemia due to peripheral arterial disease of right common iliac artery. False statement regarding management of this patient is:
(a) Should undergo pharmacologic stress testing/imaging for risk stratification
(b) Aspirin and ACEI: both decrease MI and death
(c) CAG should be done to plan revascularization, if stress test shows inducible multiple perfusion defects of small size
(d) If CAG reveals significant stenosis in >1 coronary artery, CABG or PCI have similar recommendation to improve unacceptable angina despite maximum medical therapy

140. A 55-year-old patient with history of MI (LVEF 35%) on optimal medical treatment for the last 6 months, now presented with exertional dyspnea NYI1A class II. Patient's survival expectancy is good. True statement regarding:
(a) Should receive subcutaneous ICD to reduce all cause mortality
(b) Should receive CRT to reduce SCO only (if LBBB > 150 ms with normal sinus rhythm)
(c) Should receive CRT-D to reduce SCD only (if LBBB > 120 ms with normal sinus rhythm)
(d) Should receive ICD to reduce SCD only

141. Which among the following is most suitable for pre discharge risk stratification by exercise stress testing in STEMI:
(a) A 75-year-old male who received fibrinolysis 48 hours ago is now chest pain free without ST elevation on his ECG
(b) A 65-year-old female who received a PCI to her LAD artery 4 days ago and had no other stenosis > 50% on coronary angiogram
(c) A 52-year-old male who received fibrinolysis 6 days ago and has pulmonary rales and a third heart sound on physical examination
(d) A 68-year-old female who received thrombolysis for an inferior STEMI 4 days ago and has had intermittent atrial fibrillation

142. A 40-year male presented in emergency with NSTEMI, on examination BP is 90/70, basal crepts+, what is the status for use of beta blocker?
(a) Beta blockers are contraindicated
(b) Only bisoprolol can be used
(c) Reassess need for beta blocker after 24 hours
(d) Metoprolol tartrate is better than metoprolol succinate in this situation

143. Which is not true about prinzmetal variant angina?
(a) Patients with associated severe fixed obstruction lend paradoxically to have a more benign course
(b) Approximately one third of patients exhibit severe fixed coronary obstruction
(c) Elevated serum its CRP supports contribution of inflammation to the condition
(d) Polymorphism of $\alpha 2$ presynaptic and $\beta 2$ post synaptic receptors may be associated

144. A 50-year-old male with a history of hypertension, diabetes and persistent atrial fibrillation, for which he was receiving warfarin, underwent stenting to proximal LAD using drug eluting stent. Patient comes under low hemorrhagic risk. The best combination of drugs following his interventions will be:

(a) Aspirin, clopidogrel and warfarin for 1 month; then warfarin and clopidogrel for 12 months followed by warfarin alone
(b) Aspirin, clopidogrel and warfarin for 6 months; then warfarin and clopidogrel/Aspirin for 6 months followed by warfarin alone
(c) Aspirin, clopidogrel and warfarin for 12 months; then warfarin alone
(d) Aspirin and warfarin for 12 months; then clopidogrel alone

145. Which of the following statements is true regarding non-ST elevation acute coronary syndromes (NSTE-ACS) compared with ST elevation myocardial infarctions (STEMI)?

(a) Initial mortality of NSTE-ACS is higher
(b) Six-month mortality of STEMI is higher
(c) Long term mortality of NSTE-ACS is equal to or higher than STEMI
(d) STEMI patients are older with more comorbidity

146. Lead aVR ST↓ S/O all *except:*

(a) MVD (b) Prox. LAD
(c) LMCA (d) RCA

147. Patient with 180/105, chest pain, wide mediastinum, inf. leads T^-, next investigation:

(a) TEE (b) CT
(c) TTE (d) MRI

148. SV graft stenosis at discharge in:

(a) 5% (b) 10%
(c) 20% (d) 30%

149. Odd's ratio–fibrinolysis 300 died out of 33000 and PCI 200/3300:

(a) 0.65 (b) 1.2
(c) 0.065 (d) 1.65

150. False is:

(a) R_1 no stenosis has negligible contribution
(b) $R_2 > R_3 > R_1$
(c) R_3 in stenosis subepicardial > subendocardial

151. Late stent thrombosis:

(a) 1 day (b) 1-30 days
(c) 30 days–1 year (d) > 1 year

152. Not successful thrombolysis next step:

(a) PCI (b) Double dose
(c) Wait watch (d) CABG

153. False:

(a) Dabigatran useful in mech. valve
(b) NOAC in AF with MVP
(c) Xarelto in DVT
(d) All

154. Flase:

(a) Rely–Dabigatran
(b) Aristotle–Apixaban
(c) Rodut AF–Rivaroxaban
(d) Avarose–Edoxaban

155. TRITON–TMI trial for:

(a) Prasugrel (b) Clopidogrel
(c) Ticagrelor

156. Thinopyredines A/E:

(a) Clopidogrel (b) Prasugrel
(c) Ticagrelor (d) Ticlopidine

157. Discrete and ostial S/O:

(a) < 5 mm and < 3 mm (b) < 10 mm and < 3 mm
(c) 10-20 mm and < 2 mm

158. LBBB with AMI S/O:

(a) ST ↑ 1 mm concordant
(b) ST ↓ 2 mm V_1, V_2, V_3
(c) ST ↑ 3 mm discordant

159. SVG grafts–False:

(a) 20% at 1 year
(b) 2% per year from 1-5 years
(c) 8% per year from 6-10 years

160. MI patient with EF < 20% what to do?

(a) ICD now (b) Wait 40 days then ICD
(c) CRT (d) Transplant

161. Hemodynamically not significant lesion in FFR:

(a) > 0.8 (b) < 0.8
(c) 0.75–0.80 (d) 0.9–1

162. Trial not shown benefit of thrombus aspiration:

(a) TAPAS (b) AIMI
(c) EXPIRA (d) EXPORT

163. Anticoagulant on Factor X all *except:*
(a) Dabigatran (b) Apixaban
(c) Riveroxaban (d) Edoxaban

164. Class I Indication for PCI in STEMI–A/E:
(a) Ischemia <12 hours (b) Ischemia 12-24 hours
(c) Cardiogenic shock (d) Failed thrombolysis

165. DAPT in patient with fibrinolysis after STEMI for:
(a) 14 days (b) 1 month
(c) 6 months (d) 1 year

166. SYNTAX score of upto ________ is class 2nd for PCI.
(a) 22 (b) 18
(c) 26 (d) 32

167. Aspirin false:
(a) Efficiency ↓ with other NSAIDs
(b) Irreversible COS inhibitor
(c) Half life 7-10 days
(d) Chewable asp. onset of action 15 min

168. Clopidogrel resistance:
(a) CYP 2C19 (b) APOB
(c) PCSKI (d) PLT 243

169. Maximum afterload reduction with improved coronary flow:
(a) IABP (b) Impella
(c) Abiomed

170. True about ticagrelor:
(a) Dyspnoea is due to obstruction of airways
(b) Increased efficacy with aspirin 325 mg
(c) No dose modification above age of 75 years
(d) Dose reduction needed in renal failure

171. Which of the following not useful when added with thrombolytic therapy:
(a) Aspirin (b) Clopidogrel
(c) Eptifibatide (d) Enoxaparin

172. True regarding PCI:
(a) PCI is treatment of choice in elderly presenting 3 hour after onset of symptoms
(b) Primary PCI to be done at least 2 hours after thrombolysis due to high risk of bleeding
(c) Thrombus extraction reduces infarct size in patient with MI
(d) PCI of non infarct related artery useful in patient without cardiogenic shock

173. False regarding coronary flow:
(a) Coronary veins have constant flow systole and diastolic
(b) Coronary arteries have phasic flow increasing during diastole
(c) Maximum myocardial compression at subendocardial level as compared to subepicardial level

174. IABP true statement:
(a) Causes decreases in systolic BP
(b) Deflated in mid systole
(c) Cannot be used in dual chamber pacemaker patients
(d) Subepicardial flow increased more as compared to subendocardial flow

175. In patient of MI, ABG showing Ph = 7.55, PO_2 58 mm Hg, PCO_2 = 30 mm Hg, Base excess = 0, true statement A/E:
(a) Due to morphine overdose
(b) Basic abnormality is respiratory alkalosis
(c) Due to pulmonary edema
(d) Alveolar hyperventilation

176. All can be done in beating heart without CABG *except:*
(a) Closed valve valvotomy
(b) Pericardiectomy
(c) Aortic arch repair
(d) CABG

177. Post MI pericarditis all true *except:*
(a) DOC is steroids
(b) Aspirin is useful for symptomatic relief
(c) Antibody mediated

178. All true about FFR *except:*
(a) Gives estimate of microcirculatory flow
(b) Absolute flow reserve ratio of max flow to resting flow
(c) Relative flow reserve ratio of flow in stenotic segment to normal segment

179. FREEDOM trial:
(a) PCI decrease mortality vs CABG
(b) CABG increase stroke
(c) Everolimus Eluting stent increase mortality
(d) Off pump CABG (most patient included)

180. Past MI-SAM and MR all given *except:*
(a) BB (b) Pure alpha agonist
(c) IV fluids (d) NTG

181. Linked angina A/E:
(a) Forward bending
(b) Esophageal stimulation by acid mimic
(c) Normal coronary artery
(d) Aggravated by food

182. Most effective mortality benefit (Primary prevention):
(a) PSA < 50 years
(b) Quit smoking in 35 years
(c) PAP – 18-65 years
(d) TMT– > 50 years, asymptomatic

183. Side effect antianginal A/E:
(a) Ranolazine–increase QT
(b) Trimetazidine–fatty acid inhibitor with increase in blood sugar in diabetics
(c) Perhexiline–inhibit FA oxidation
(d) Ivabridine–disturbance in night vision

184. High sensitivity troponin A/E:
(a) Increases after sternous exercise
(b) Positive in 95 % normal individual
(c) Can detect 0.005 ng/ml
(d) More specific than conventional

185. ECG:
(a) Pan artries (b) Prox LAD occlusion
(c) LCX (d) Distal LAD

186. High risk CAD A/E:
(a) CAC > 150
(b) On perfusion scan > 10% ischemic myocardium
(c) CT – multivessel disease
(d) ST depression > 2 mm on TMT at stage 2 – Duke protocol

187. 6 years old male with class II angina pretest probability:
(a) Very low risk (b) Low risk
(c) Intermediate risk (d) High risk

188. FFR true A/E:
(a) Adenosine 12 mg I/V is used
(b) Used in tandem lesions
(c) Can be calculated by coronary angiogram
(d) Decreased in acute MI

189. CABG (urgent) all true *except:*
(a) Stop ticagrelor 24 hours before
(b) Stop clopidogrel 24 hours before
(c) Stop aspirin 24 hours before
(d) Stop tirofiban 2-4 hours before

190. Spironolactone in MI A/E:
(a) EF < 40%
(b) DM
(c) LV systolic dysfunction
(d) All

191. CABG indication A/E:
(a) DM + TVD with EF > 50%
(b) MVD with LMCA with EF < 50%
(c) LAD calcification
(d) All

192. Acute MI A/E:
(a) Pre-hospital fibrinolysis have no survival benefit
(b) Shift to PCI in high risk after fibrinolysis
(c) Recent trial have shown benefit in PCI to non affected vessel in primary PCI

193. TMT ST ↑ in precordial leads with baseline q waves indicates all *except:*
(a) AWMI (b) Ischemia
(c) RWMA (d) Poor prognosis

194. True all *except:*
(a) Sones–coronary angiography
(b) Forssman–first catheterization
(c) ICD–Kriklin
(d) Stent–J.F.S. Esser

195. Linked angina all *except:*
(a) Ppt. by GERD acid reflux
(b) ↑ by bending forward
(c) Normal coronaries
(d) ↑ after fatty food

196. Freedom trial true:
(a) CABG ↑ stroke
(b) Off pump used
(c) Everolimus used

197. High sensitive troponin T all *except:*
(a) Detects upto 0.005 ng/ml
(b) 95% reference population + ve
(c) In HF, the prevalence of detectable troponin is high

198. Ticagrelor true *except:*

(a) Uricosuric
(b) Increase serum creatinine
(c) Contraindicated in AV block/sick sinus syndrome patients
(d) Increases bleeding complications when used with ketaconazole

199. Cardiovascular effects of adenosine all *except:*

(a) Depression of automaticity
(b) Negative dromotropic
(c) Renal vasodilatation
(d) Coronary steal phenomenon

200. Coronary angiogram in human first done by:

(a) Mason Sones (b) Werner Forrsman
(c) William Cournard (d) Charles Dotter

201. 55 years old with naïve HTN with BP=158/95 mm Hg, aortogram shows mild narrowing of right coronary artery abnormality and right renal artery thrombi, first line of management:

(a) Aspirin
(b) Atorvastatin
(c) Renal artery stenting
(d) Amlodipine

202. Ranolazine all *except:*

(a) Inhibits late Na+
(b) No hemodynamics effect on HR/BP
(c) ↑ ses Hb A1C
(d) Prevents arrhythmias

203. EP changes of ischemia:

(a) ↑ ed APD
(b) Membrane fragility k^+ effusion
(c) Ca influx
(d) Vmax and amplitude ↓

204. STICH trial all *except:*

(a) Included patients with CHF
(b) EF<35%
(c) Better outcomes with ventricular aneurysm
(d) No effect on mortality

205. IABP all *except:*

(a) Deflated at peak R wave
(b) Inflates at peak T wave
(c) ↑ ed CO
(d) ↑ ed mean BP

206. Rotational atherectomy all C/I *except:*

(a) High plaque burden
(b) High thrombus burden
(c) Extreme tortuosity
(d) Ostial site

207. High sensitivity troponin assay all/*except:*

(a) High PPV
(b) 100 times analytic sensitivity
(c) ↑ ed severe PAH
(d) ↑ ed with severe physical exercise

208. Patients with MI with RBBB of within 2 hours, management:

(a) Thrombolysis (b) Angioplasty
(c) TPI

209. Inf. Leads–ST ↑ Signficant, Asymmetric BP:

(a) USG doppler-UL (b) CT angio
(c) MR angio (d) Cardiac cath

210. Cocaine induced MI all *except:*

(a) MI 4-6 hours later
(b) Cause sympathetic stimulation and coronary Vc
(c) Less complication than other MI
(d) Occurrence MI unrelated to route and dose

211. True about microvascular angina in metabolic syndrome X *except:*

(a) IVUS may show coronary atherosclerosis
(b) B blockers C/I
(c) Coronary reactivity study gold standard
(d) High risk of CAD complication

212. Earliest change in coronary artery occlusion:

(a) Regional dyskinesia (b) ↑ LVEDP
(c) Angina (d) ECG changes

213. Acute MI with pulmonary edema all given *except:*

(a) S/L captopril
(b) Multiple doses of isosorbide dinitrate
(c) Milrinone
(d) CPAP

214. Coronary ischemia not caused by:

(a) ALCAPA
(b) Myocardial bridging
(c) Abnormal RCA from left sinus
(d) ALCAOS

215. Proximal LAD 60% block, FFR -0.75, what to do next?
(a) Stress thallium
(b) Repeat with nicorandil
(c) Repeat CAG+FFR after 6 months
(d) Stent implantation

216. DEB, drug used:
(a) Sirolimus (b) Zatorolimus
(c) Paclitaxel (d) Everolimus

217. Wrong match:
(a) Acetylcholine require intact endothelium for vasoconstriction
(b) Adenosine can cause coronary vasodilation independent of endothelium
(c) Hypoxia–systemic vasodilation
(d) ↓ CO_2–cerebral vasodilation

218. MI complicated by HIT during PCI:
(a) Low dose heparin (b) Abciximab
(c) LMWH (d) Bivalirudin

219. Accelerated atherosclerosis all *except:*
(a) Marfan (b) Progeria
(c) Werner (d) Homocystinuria

220. MI 5 hours treatment:
(a) PAMI
(b) STK
(c) tPA
(d) ½ does tPA + GP II b IIIa

221. TIMI risk score all *except:*
(a) > 65 years (b) Male
(c) >2 angina in 24 hours (d) Aspirin > 7 days

222. False +ve Trop –I all *except:*
(a) Fibrin clot (b) Creatinine
(c) Heterophile Ab (d) R factor

223. Primary PCI require all *except:*
(a) Hospital > 200 PCI/year
(b) On site cardiac surgery
(c) Operator > 75/year
(d) Door to balloon < 90 min

224. RVMI all *except:*
(a) AV sequential pacing hazardous
(b) ST ↑ in V1-V4 may occur
(c) Resolution of ST ↑ in V4R in 48 hours
(d) Rapid y descent

225. AIVR all *except:*
(a) Functional re-entry
(b) Variable morphology
(c) Benign
(d) Independent to type on infarction location and size

226. Prevalence of CHD in population:
(a) < 1/100 (b) 6-8/1000
(c) 20/1000 (d) 50/1000

227. Cardiac surgery:
(a) Hamman sign on auscultation
(b) Post cardiac surgery
(c) Atherosclerosis
(d) Small VSD

228. Massive AWMI killip-III, thrombolysed → hemodynamically stable, next line of management:
(a) Stabilization for 7 days → TMT
(b) Transfer to PCI facility
(c) Stabilization for 7 days → CAG
(d) IABP insertion

229. All ↓ long term mortality:
(a) PTCA in CSA
(b) Stenting in RAS with HTN
(c) CRT in HF
(d) IVC filter in pulmonary embolism

230. Before elective PCI all ↓ complications *except:*
(a) Aspirin (b) Clopidogrel
(c) Eptifibatide (d) Atorvastatin

231. Prasugrel vs clopidogrel all *except:*
(a) Less nonfatal bleeding
(b) Less stent thrombosis
(c) MI
(d) Faster platelet inhibition

232. Bivalirudin vs abciximab + heparin all *except:*
(a) No HIT
(b) ↓ es stent thrombosis
(c) ↓ es 30 days mortality
(d) ↓ es bleeding

233. Match the following:
(a) Ranolazine–↑ late Ca current
(b) Tadalafil–PDE-5 inhibitor

(c) Fondaparinux–Factor Xa inhibition
(d) Bivalirudin–DTI

234. Pharmacological stress testing all *except:*
(a) More myocardial blood flow in exercise than pharmacotesting
(b) LBBB patient tolerate pharmacotesting with adenosine
(c) High dose dobutamine ↑ hypotension
(d) Less ↑ es exercise O_2 demand in pharmaco testing

235. Dor procedure is:
(a) LV aneurysm repair (b) MVR
(c) Aortic repair (d) Aortic aneurysm repair

236. Coronary angiography catheters:
(a) Sone's catheter (b) Cournard's catheter
(c) Judkin's catheter (d) Amplatzer's catheter

237. TIMI score:
(a) 6-12 (b) 7-21
(c) 10-20 (d) 21-30

238. Aspirin A/E:
(a) ↑ ses major GI and IC bleed
(b) ↑ useful than secondary prophylaxis
(c) 10-12% reduction in mortality
(d) Risk benefit ratio to be considered

239. Ranolazine mechanisms of action:
(a) Late Na^+ current (b) K^+ current
(c) Ca^+ current

240. EDHF:
(a) Arachidonic acid metabolism
(b) Acts via NO
(c) Metabolised by CYP-450, produced by cyclooxygenase
(d) Acts by hyperpolarisation vascular muscle

241. Endothelin acts via:
(a) Protein kinase C (b) Acetylcholine
(c) NO

242. Ischemic preconditioning by:
(a) GMP (b) MRK/ERK1, 2
(c) PI3k/Akt (d) RISK

243. PTE thrombolysis indicated in patient with shock in:
(a) Optimal upto 3 days but can be done upto 14 days
(b) Reteplase DOC for thrombolysis

244. Fibrinolysis C/I in A/E:
(a) Acute ischeme stroke < 3 hours
(b) Hemorrhagic stroke
(c) Aortic dissection

245. PAMI:
(a) Should be done within 24 hours
(b) Wait for 2 weeks

246. In post infarct angina to be used true:
(a) ACEI (b) Nitrates
(c) B-Blocker (d) CCB
(e) All true

247. Stent thrombosis caused by A/E:
(a) HTN
(b) Diabetes
(c) Renal failure
(d) Discontinuation of antiplatelets

248. High risk unstable angina A/E:
(a) T ↓ >0.2 mV (b) Pulmonary edema
(c) S_3 (d) Tachycardia
(e) Age

249. Pharmacoinvasive therapy:
(a) PCI preferred over thrombolysis
(b) PCI to be done only if thrombolysis not possible
(c) All patients – thrombolysis followed by PCI
(d) Facilitated PCI is preferred approach

250. Acute STEMI Management:
(a) Pharmacoinvasive is currently preferred approach
(b) Faciliated PCI
(c) Rescue PCI

251. II, III, aVF and V4R ST Elevation B.P. = 90/60, should not be done:
(a) IV fluids (b) STK
(c) NTG (d) Dopamine

252. LMCA stenosis diagnosed by:
(a) aVR ST elevation >V1
(b) aVR ST elevation <VI
(c) ST depression in II, III, aVF, I, aVL, V3,V4
(d) ST elevation in V1-V3

253. LCx CAD-ECG changes:
(a) V1- ST elevation with T inversion
(b) V1- ST elevation with T upright

(c) V1- Isoelectric with T upright
(d) V1- ST depression. T wave inversion

254. Primary angioplasty v/s thrombolysis, thrombolysis is beneficial in:
(a) Hypertensive 80 years non obese
(b) Hypertensive 80 years obese
(c) Non-hypertensive 80 years obese
(d) Non-hypertensive 80 years thin limb

255. Max risk of CAD by which ratio?
(a) TC: HDL (b) LDL: HDL
(c) Apo B 100: HDL (d) ApoB: ApoAl

256. Life saved by thrombolysis in STEMI per 100 is:
(a) 7 (b) 14
(c) 21 (d) 2

257. Most effective in decreasing cardiac mortality in MI:
(a) Beta blocker (b) Aspirin
(c) ACE1 (d) NTG

258. CAD in female true all *except*:
(a) Angina more in female
(b) CHF more in female
(c) VF and SCD less
(d) Comorbidities less

259. MI with cardiogenic shock true all *except*:
(a) Early revascularization decrease 30 days mortality in >75 years
(b) Decrease 6 months mortality
(c) No benefit with revascularization

260. On TMT more likelihood of multi-vessel and bad prognosis CAD all *except*:
(a) SBP failure to increase 120 or decrease 10
(b) ST depression (excluding aVR)
(c) Exercise <7 METs
(d) ST elevation in all leads in except aVR

261. Indication of 1ABP all *except*:
(a) AR (b) Cardiogenic shock
(c) CABG (d) PCI

262. Coronary blood flow:
(a) 8-10 ml/min (b) 7-1 ml/min
(c) 2-3 nil/min (d) 5-6 nil/min

263. Reperfusion injury involves all *except*:
(a) Accelerated necrosis
(b) Hemorrhage
(c) No reflow phenomena
(d) All true

264. Cardiogenic shock true all *except*:
(a) Systolic BP < 90 mmHg
(b) PCWP < 18 mmHg
(c) Cardiac index- 2.2
(d) Hypoperfusion

265. Clopidogrel resistance all *except*:
(a) P2 Y 12 receptor (b) Cy P polymorphism
(c) Decrease ADP (d) Alter platelet action

266. Reperfusion causes all *except*:
(a) A1VR (b) Normal BP
(c) Decrease chest pain

267. Most common cause of pulmonary edema after 1WMI:
(a) Papillary muscle dys (b) IVS rupture

268. Use of IABP T/F:
(a) Stabilization of cardiac shock patient during angioplasty
(b) AR and aortic disease
(c) Refractory HTN

269. Prinzmetal angina all *except*:
(a) 2/3 associated with stenosis
(b) RCA- normal coronary angiogram
(c) Ach - sensitive in inducing spasm
(d) ST increase in TMT

270. Fondaparinaux — all *except*:
(a) Decrease platelet function
(b) Pentasaccharide
(c) Through anti-thrombin Xa

271. Platelet deficiency presents as:
(a) Hemoarthrosis
(b) Retroperitoneal hematoma
(c) Intracranial hemorrhage
(d) Petechie and echymosis

272. t-PA deficiency present with:
(a) ↓ clot lysis (b) Abruptio placentae
(c) Abortion

273. Stress perfusion imaging versus stress echo—better stress perfusion due to:

(a) Accurate anatomical localization
(b) Accurate detection of non viable myocardium
(c) LCx visualization
(d) ↑ ed evaluation of ischemia

274. NSTEMI Marker for prognosis:
(a) CD-40 ligands
(b) BNP
(c) Myeloperoxidase

275. STEMI best marker:
(a) CPK-MB
(b) Cardiac specific troponin
(c) BNP

276. Diltiazem in ACS causes:
(a) Tachycardia
(b) Bronchodilation
(c) ↑ myocardial depression (LVF)
(d) Peripheral vasoconstriction

277. Mechanism of nitrate tolerance A/E:
(a) Plasma expansion
(b) Decreased free radicals
(c) Depletion of sulfhydryl
(d) Neurogenic

278. Linked Angina A/E:
(a) With stooping
(b) Associated with normal coronaries
(c) ↑ es with salivation
(d) ↑ with cardiac work

279. Acute MI with Angiography true:
(a) TIMI-3 and TIMI-2 patent coronary
(b) TIMI-2 has high mortality than TIMI-3
(c) TIMI-2 and TIMI-3 Similar mortality

280. Cardiac rupture true:
(a) Always fatal
(b) LV in late diastole than in early systole
(c) Atrial rupture more common
(d) Usually within 2 weeks

281. Unstable Angina, high risk A/E:
(a) Crescendo origin within 72 hrs.
(b) S_3
(c) LBBB recent origin
(d) Raised cardiac enzymes

282. High lateral wall MI with:
(a) OM of LCx (b) High OM with LCx
(c) Distal RCA (d) PDA

283. Great cardiac vein accompanies:
(a) LAD (b) LCx
(c) RCA (d) LM

284. C/I of IABP:
(a) Acute severe AR (b) Acute severe MR

285. Angiogram invented by:
(a) Grossman (b) Forssman

286. PTA not suitable in:
(a) LMCA (b) LAD
(c) TVD (d) All of above

287. Most predictive of prognosis in 1st 12 hrs of MI:
(a) Serial ECG (b) Thallium scan
(c) Persisting pain (d) LVEF

288. Result of CABG influenced by:
(a) Angina (b) Vessels
(c) Ejection fraction

289. OM is a branch of :
(a) LCx (b) LAD
(c) RCA

290. Best antihypertensive in IHD:
(a) Captopril (b) CCB
(c) α Blocker (d) Methyl dopa

291. Best patency rate seen with following:
(a) r TPA (b) STK
(c) Primary PTCA

292. In acute MI, LA pressure best correlate with:
(a) LVEDP (b) PADP
(c) Mean PAP

293. Normal LVEDP is:
(a) 2-8 mm Hg (b) 4-12 mm Hg
(c) 6-18 mm Hg

294. In STEMI all improve mortality *except:*
(a) Beta blocker (b) Nitrate

295. Primary PCI done in:
(a) Within 12 hours of STEMI
(b) NSTEMI

(c) Unstable angina
(d) MI after thrombolysis

296. Primary prevention of CAD:
(a) Aspirin (b) Statin
(c) Beta blocker

297. Which is not GP IIb IIIa inhibitor:
(a) Ximelagatran (b) Abciximab
(c) Eptifibatide (d) Tirofiban

298. Coronary artery fistula A/E:
(a) Coronary artery dissection
(b) Coronary artery thrombosis
(c) Coronary artery ectasia
(d) CAD
(e) All

299. RVMI A/E:
(a) Increased JVP (b) Increased PA

300. Pressure best in acute MI:
(a) LA pressure (b) RVEDP
(c) Mean PAP

301. Normal LVEDP:
(a) 2-8 mm Hg (b) 4-12 mm Hg
(c) 6-18 mm Hg (d) 12-18 mm Hg

302. Least likely in AWMI:
(a) ST elevation in V2-V5
(b) RBBB
(c) ST depression in II, avF
(d) Short QT interval

303. CAD least likely:
(a) Hyerlipidemia
(b) Kawasaki
(c) Supravavular AS

304. Nitrate tolerance decreased by:
(a) Eccentric dose (b) Single dose
(c) Patch

305. Earliest marker to rise in ischemia:
(a) Myoglobin (b) CK–MM
(c) CK–MB

306. ALTEPLASE true about dosage:
(a) Time dependent
(b) Vascular involvement dependent
(c) Weight dependent
(d) Fixed

307. Atherosclerosis:
(a) Autoimmune (b) Infective
(c) Inflammatory

308. Earliest after MI:
(a) Chest pain (b) ECG changes
(c) RWMA on echo (d) Myoglobin

309. ECG and chest pain after MI occur:
(a) Before relaxation abnormality
(b) Simultaneously with relaxation abnormality
(c) After relaxation abnormality
(d) No correlation

310. Coronary collateral size:
(a) 20-200 μm (b) < 100 μm
(c) 200-500 μm (d) > 500 μm

311. ESR in MI increases by:
(a) 1 to 2 days (b) 2 to 4 days
(c) 4 to 6 days (d) 1 week

312. LBBB with CAD best:
(a) Exercise stress ECG
(b) Exercise perfusion imaging
(c) Pharmacological perfusion imaging
(d) CT

313. Antiplatelet decreases mortality/MI/stroke by (risk reduction):
(a) 0.1 (b) 0.22
(c) 0.32 (d) 0.15

314. Rest ischemia when coronary stenosis of:
(a) 0.6 (b) 0.7
(c) 0.8 (d) 0.9

315. Ticagrelor A/E:
(a) PLATO – increases non CABG bleed
(b) Reversible P2 Y12 inhibitor
(c) Loading dose 150 mg
(d) Metabolized by CYP 2C9

316. Rentrop classification is for:
(a) Coronary collateral (b) Coronary stenosis

317. Lumen area on IVUS:
(a) Blood intima interface

(b) Intima media interface
(c) Media adventia interface
(d) Intima elastic lamina

318. Best view for LMCA bifurcation:
(a) LAO caudal (b) LAO cranial
(c) RAO cranial (d) RAO caudal

319. FFR significant cut off value:
(a) 0.50 (b) 0.70
(c) 0.75 (d) 1

320. MI secondary prophylaxis all *except:*
(a) Amlodipine (b) Statin
(c) B blockers (d) Aspirin

321. Plaque passivation:
(a) Statin (b) ACE- I
(c) B blockers (d) Nitrates

322. Adenosine true all *except:*
(a) Slow infusion
(b) ↑ AV block transient
(c) Useful in tachycardia
(d) Differentiates wide and narrow QRS

323. Free wall rupture:
(a) Incidence 1-3%
(b) Elderly more common
(c) Men more common
(d) Thrombolysis prevents
(e) PCI does not help

324. TIME score in USA/NSTEMI all *except:*
(a) Age > 75 years (b) Prior ASA
(c) Ischemic ST changes (d) >3 CAD risk factors
(e) Increased biomarker

325. Target organ damage subclinical:
(a) CVA (b) Microalbuminuria
(c) LVH (d) ↑ CIMT
(e) ABI < 0.9

326. Predictor of ACS all *except:*
(a) Linoleic (b) Chromogranin
(c) Platelet factor VI (d) vWF
(e) Microalbuminuria

327. Which is anticoagulant:
(a) Cangrelor (b) Tirofiban
(c) Vorapaxar (d) Ximelagatran

328. Newer antianginal:
(a) Ranolazine (b) Nitrate
(c) Fasudil (d) Ivabradine

329. Spider view is angiography:
(a) RAO cranial (b) RAO caudal
(c) LAO cranial (d) LAO caudal
(e) PA caudal

330. LBBB in MI T/F:
(a) ST ↑ 1 mm V_5-V_6
(b) ST ↑ 5 mm V_1-V_2
(c) S wave notch – mid percordial lead
(d) S wave notch I, avl, V_5,V_6
(e) qR/qS in V_1-V_2

331. Chest pain with normal angiography:
(a) Endothelial dysfunction
(b) Metabolic abnormality
(c) Sympathovagal imbalance
(d) Microvascular dysfunction
(e) All of the above

332. Metabolic modifier:
(a) Nicorandil (b) Perhexidine
(c) Fasudil (d) Regadenosan

333. Plague passivation done by:
(a) Statins (b) Beta blockers
(c) Nicorandil (d) ACE inhibitors
(e) Nitrates

334. Plague stability T/F:
(a) Smooth muscles
(b) Collagen cross struts
(c) Thick fibrous cap
(d) Significant lipid core
(e) Calcification

335. Pharmacoinvasive therapy in MI (trial):
(a) Champion (b) Everest
(c) Companion (d) Transfer AMI
(e) None

336. C/I of Prasugrel all *except:*
(a) Age > 75
(b) DM
(c) History of prior stroke/TIA
(d) Renal failure
(e) Body weight < 60 kg

337. Free wall rupture: (T/F)
(a) Incidence 1-3%
(b) Elderly more common
(c) Men more common
(d) Thrombolysis prevents it
(e) PCI does not help

338. DEB drugs eluting balloon: (T/F)
(a) Instent stenosis – side branch
(b) Side branch
(c) Small vessel
(d) Left main
(e) Bifurcation lesion
(f) Dual anticoagulant required for 6 months
(g) Less restenosis than DES
(h) Dual antiplatelet for 6 months

339. DES over BMS: (T/F)
(a) ↓ HF
(b) Very late thrombosis
(c) ↓ recurrent MI
(d) ↓ mortality

340. DES vs BMS: (T/F)
(a) Minimal 6 months of anti platelet required
(b) DES preferred in Patients on anticoagulants
(c) Left main
(d) Small vessel
(e) De novo stenosis

341. T/F:
(a) COMMIT – Clopidogrel
(b) CADILLAC – PCI with GP IIb IIIa inh.
(c) TRITON 38 – prasugrel
(d) PLATO – ticagrelor
(e) OAT no mortality benefit 3-28 days

342. Suggests RCA involvement:
(a) ST ↓ a VL > Lead I
(b) ST ↑ L II > L III
(c) ST ↓ in all precordial
(d) ST ↑ in all precordial
(e) STE is AVR

343. View for LIMA to LAD anastomosis:
(a) RAO cranial (b) LAO cranial
(c) Lt. lateral (d) LAO 30°

344. Kugel's collaterals:
(a) Px RCA to distal PDA
(b) RCA to LCX
(c) Px RCA to LAD

345. Thermodilution C.O. all *except:*
(a) Good in TR
(b) Inaccurate in low cardiac output
(c) Inaccurate in shunt
(d) Angiographic method for valves stenosis in presence of regurgitation

346. Size of guidewire in current angiographies:
(a) 0.35 (b) .50
(c) .31 (d) .18

347. Rotational atherectomy false:
(a) Diamond tip rotation at 16000 pm
(b) With GP IIb/IIIa inhibitors increases more CPKMB
(c) Perforation risk more than 10%
(d) Balloon angioplasty success rate is increased

348. Prasugrel trials all *except:*
(a) SWAP (b) PLATO
(c) Triton TIMI 38 (d) PRINCIPAL 44
(e) PRASO1 (f) Triology ACS

349. All are antiplatelet *except:*
(a) Prasugrel (b) Ticagrelor
(c) Congrelor (d) Warfarin

350. ACC/AHA recommendation for AMI:
(a) Pharmacoinvasive
(b) Thrombolysis + Rescue
(c) Thrombolysis alone
(d) Facilitated
(e) None

351. Pharmacoinvasive reperfusion:
(a) Same as facilitated
(b) Thrombolysis followed by ischemia guided PCI
(c) Recommended these days

352. MI in territory of stent irrespective of time means:
(a) Probable stent thrombosis
(b) Possible
(c) Definite
(d) Late stent thrombosis
(e) None

353. Stent thrombosis precipitated by all *except:*
(a) Diabetes (b) Renal failure
(c) Hypertensive (d) Less apposition

354. Collagen plug is used in sealing device:
(a) Angioseal (b) Noclose
(c) Çollastal

355. Plaque stabilisation by T/F:
(a) Smooth muscle (b) Thick fibrous cap
(c) Statins (d) ACE I

356. Plaque stabilisation by T/F:
(a) Amlodipine (b) Vit C and E
(c) Lipid core (d) Calcification
(e) Collagen in layers

357. IABP all *except:*
(a) AR (b) AS
(c) MS (d) VSD
(e) RV infarction

358. European guidelines 2010 for left main ostial lesion for stenting:
(a) I (b) IIa
(c) III (d) II b

359. Rotational atherectomy:
(a) FIRE II (b) EMERALD
(c) PRISM (d) REDUCE trial

360. Metabolic modulator all *except:*
(a) Fasudil (b) Perhexidine
(c) Trimetazidine (d) Etomovir
(e) Ranolazine

361. Prasugrel: (T/F)
(a) Prodrug
(b) ↓ stent thrombosis > clopidogrel
(c) No mortality benefit than clopidogrel
(d) Loading dose = 60 mg

362. Post MI angina:
(a) Nitrate (b) BB
(c) CCB (d) Ranolazine
(e) ACE I

363. T/F:
(a) Eptifibatide nonpeptide
(b) Abciximab – inhibits Vitronector receptor MAC-1
(c) Tirofiban peptide
(d) Tirofiban 6 hours = t ½
(e) PRISM trial for eptifibatide

364. Can be given in RF:
(a) Abciximab (b) Eptifibatide
(c) Tirofiban (d) Hirodin
(e) Gemilogatran

365. T/F:
(a) GEA can be used in PDA
(b) Bilateral IMA is better recommended
(c) Radial artery superior to LIMA

366. Post CABG graft stenosis: (T/F)
(a) 1 month cellular/proliferative
(b) Eccentric
(c) Venous has fibrous cap thick and eccentric
(d) Focal stenosis in venous

367. Fibrinolysis C/I in all *except:*
(a) Any haemorrhagic stroke
(b) Closed head trauma
(c) AV malformations
(d) Ischemic stroke < 3 hours

368. Viessen's collateral:
(a) RCA to LCX (b) RCA to PDA
(c) Px RCA to LAD

369. IABP C/I in:
(a) AR (b) Cardiogenic shock
(c) MR

370. Shock trial AMI with MR with shock VS AMI LVF: (T/F)
(a) More in female (b) More in anterior
(c) More in inf or post

371. CAG mortality:
(a) 1in 100 (b) 1in 1000
(c) 1in 10 thousand (d) 1 in 1000 thousand

372. IWMI with RV MI with PCWP 13 mm Hg treatment:
(a) Furosemide IV (b) IVfluids
(c) Dobutamine

373. Early accelerated atherosclerosis:
(a) Cockyane syndrome (b) Catch 22
(c) William (d) Rubinstein's

374. View for left main CA bifurcation:
(a) LAO 45 cranial 30 (b) LAO 10 cranial 60
(c) APO caudal 20 (d) PAO 20 caudal

375. ST/HR slope true is:
(a) Cornell's protocol used
(b) Bruce protocol used
(c) < 2.4 is significant
(d) Index of 1.6 is abnormal

376. Prognostic score in angina all *except*:
(a) Gregs (b) Califf
(c) Candella ricra (d) Gensini

377. FFR:
(a) Gradient between aorta and proximal to stenosis
(b) >0.75 is cut off (c) Useful for PCI
(d) Off line investigation (e) Most diagnosis test

378. Significant hemodynamic coronary artery stenosis:
(a) >50% (b) >90%
(c) 100% (d) 20-50%

379. Aspirin:
(a) T1/2- 20 min
(b) Duration of action 5 days
(c) ↓ Synthesis of thromboxane A2
(d) 30 mg daily dose ↑ max effect in 3 weeks
(e) ↑ effectiveness with ↑ dose

380. Aspirin ↓ death, MI, stroke and vascular disease:
(a) 12% (b) 22%
(c) 32% (d) 40%

381. Earliest change seen in MI:
(a) Chest pain
(b) Wall motion abnormal
(c) Trop I
(d) Myoglobin
(e) ECG

382. Coronary artery flow is mainly maintained by:
(a) NO (b) PG
(c) Adenosine (d) ATP- k channel

383. NTG:
(a) Dilates medium sized coronary arterioles
(b) ↓ preload and ↓ endocardial ischemia
(c) ↓ SVR
(d) All true

384. Coronary collaterals size:
(a) 80-20 micron (b) 20-200
(c) 200-400 (d) 400-500

385. NTG used in all *except*:
(a) CHF (b) Bradycardia < 50
(c) Severe HTN

386. All *except*:
(a) Post MI more mortality is due to ventricular arrhythmias
(b) Prehospital DC shock ↓se mortality more than thrombolytics
(c) Post MI ventricular arrhythmias have more prognosis than without it

387. AMI survival drugs all *except*:
(a) Amlodipine (b) Aspirin
(c) Ramipril (d) B blocker

388. Atherosclerotic plaque rupture true:
(a) Central area ruptures
(b) Mechanical stressed area
(c) Statins stabilize
(d) Can occur in low BP

389. Tenecteplase true is:
(a) Give I.V. over 30 min
(b) Dose 0.5 mg/kg
(c) Tims III patency approximately 60%
(d) 90 min patency 75%
(e) It has more antigenic properties

390. French guage:
(a) 0.30 (b) 0.33
(c) 0.45

391. Adenosine all true *except*:
(a) Slow IV infusion
(b) Can cause transient A-V block
(c) Used to differentiate SVT and VT
(d) Dose initially is 3 mg

392. MI in old age:
(a) May be painless
(b) Can present as fatigue/weakness
(c) Evidence based treatment is less effective
(d) More ICH with thrombolytics
(e) Less mortality benefit as compared to young

393. GP IIb/IIIa inhibitor:
(a) Abciximab (b) Tirofiban
(c) Eptifibatide (d) Gangrelor

394. Beta blocker beneficial in:
(a) STEMI
(b) Moderate-severe angina
(c) NSTEMI
(d) Post MI within 12 hours

395. After how many doses of nitro glycerine, patient is asked to come to hospital?
(a) 1 (b) 2
(c) 3 (d) 4

396. Aspirin use in secondary prevention of MI decreases mortality by:
(a) 25 (b) 30
(c) 20 (d) 15

397. All are GP IIb IIIa inhibitor, *except:*
(a) Reopro (b) Integrillin
(c) Tirofiban (d) Angiomax

398. Streptokinase is:
(a) Protein (b) Enzyme
(c) Carbohydrate

399. HERO-2 trial used:
(a) Hirulog + GP 2b 3a inhibitor
(b) Bivaluridin only

400. Exercise index:
(a) 0.4 (b) 0.8
(c) 1 (d) 4

401. Early sign of reperfusion:
(a) Early peak of CPK-MB
(b) Myoglobin ratio > 4

402. RVMI true is:
(a) RVEDP < LVEDP (b) Rise in ANP levels
(c) V_4R ST depression (d) RVEDP > LVEDP

403. Atherosclerotic aortic valve increased calcification due to:
(a) Osteopontin from macrophages
(b) Homocysteine
(c) Hypercalcemia
(d) All of the above

404. Atrial infarction true is:
(a) Occurs in 10%
(b) Mostly in right atria
(c) Causes atrial arrhythmias
(d) Associated with ↑ ed ANP

405. SVG patency rates at 10 years:
(a) 45% (b) 60%
(c) 33%

406. Rupture of heart after MI true is:
(a) 90% mortality with medical management
(b) Occurs after 2 days
(c) 50% have new murmur
(d) 50% occurs with anterior MI

407. Regarding subendocardial perfusion case is:
(a) ↑ LVEDP causes ↓ endocardial perfusion

408. Post MI prognosis true all *except:*
(a) ↑ Baroreceptor sensitivity shows poor prognosis
(b) SAECG independent marker

409. Aspirin not indicated in:
(a) Kawasaki's disease
(b) Ross shunt
(c) BT shunt
(d) Along with anticoagulation in prosthetic heart valves

410. 78 years old patient with chronic AF, no symptoms:
(a) Aspirin (b) Warfarin
(c) Amiodarone

411. Atherosclerosis epidemiology true A/E:
(a) CAD high in Japan although high fish intake
(b) Stroke in China more than India
(c) Mediterranean people less CAD than Americans

412. Theinopyrimidines MOA:
(a) P2 Y12 ADP inhibitors
(b) COX inhibitor
(c) m TOR inhibitors

413. IABP contraindicated:
(a) AR due to dissection (b) MI with VSD
(c) Post cardiogenic shock

414. In MPI, most difficult to be assessed:
(a) Anterior wall (b) Posterior wall
(c) Inferior wall (d) Lateral wall

415. All of the following statements are true about structure/origin of coronary artery *except:*

(a) Internal elastic membrane borders between intima and media
(b) Angioblasts are the precursor of endothelial cells
(c) Smooth muscle cells originate from my oblasts in blood island region
(d) Adventitia contains mostly fibroblasts and mast cells

416. A 45-year-old male has presented with chest pain of 2 hours duration with killip class II. ECG shows extensive anterior wall ST elevation MI. Since, the centre does not have PCI facility, he was thrombolysed. He is hemodynamic ally stable after treatment. Which of the following is an appropriate further management strategy?

(a) Prophylactic IABP insertion and shift to a PCI capable centre
(b) Continue medical stabilization and stress test on day 7
(c) Continue medical stabilization and shift for angiogram on day 7
(d) Early transfer to a PCI capable CENTRE

417. All of the following statements are true about coronary circulation *except:*

(a) LV Myocardium oxygen extraction is near maximal at rest (60-80%)
(b) Anaemia results in proportional reductions in oxygen delivery, while hypoxia results in relatively lesser reductions
(c) One of the major adaptations during increased demand is reduced coronary venous pressure
(d) RV oxygen extraction in lower at rest and increases substantially during exercise similar to skeletal muscle

418. All of the following situations satisfy the definition of acute myocardial infarction *except:*

(a) Stent thrombosis on angiography with c Troponin > 95% of upper reference limit (URL)
(b) Post PCI > 5 times elevation of cTroponin
(c) Post PCI > 20% elevation of cTroponin, if baseline values are elevated
(d) CABG related MI >10 times elevation of cTroponin

419. All of the following statements are true *except:*

(a) Plaque rupture is found in 75% of patients with acute STEMI
(b) Plaque erosion is more common in older women
(c) Lipid burden >70% is a risk factor for plaques that rupture
(d) Spotty calcification in a plaque also increase the chances of rupture

420. All of following are absolute contraindications for thrombolysis *except:*

(a) AV malformation in brain
(b) Concurrent ischemic stroke with a window period of 4 hours
(c) Ischemic stroke – 2 months back
(d) Intraspinal surgery 1 month back

421. All of the following statements are about mechanical complications of MI *except:*

(a) The risk of ventricular septal rupture is 1-3% without reperfusion and is 0.2-0.3% with fibrinolytic therapy
(b) The risk of ventricular free wall rupture is less with PCI
(c) Anterolateral papillary muscle rupture is more common than posteromedial papillary muscle rupture
(d) Timing of mechanical complications is different in patients undergoing reperfusion compared to those who do not get reperfusion

422. All of the following are emerging biomarkers for acute coronary syndrome *except:*

(a) SOLUBLE CD40 LIGAND
(b) Pregnancy associated plasma protein A
(c) BETA SITE APP-CLEAVING ENZYME 1 GENE (BACE 1)
(d) Growth differentiation factor 15

423. In a patient with NSTEMI, all of the following are indications for an urgent invasive (<120 min) strategy *except:*

(a) Refractory angina
(b) Heart failure
(c) LV EF <40%
(d) Ventricular tachycardia

424. 'CRUSADE-bleeding risk score' for estimating in hospital risk of major in NSTEMI include all the following parameters *except:*

(a) Baseline hematocrit
(b) Creatinine clearance
(c) Heart rate
(d) Concomitant use of proton pump inhibitor

425. Ischemic preconditioning is mediate by:

(a) Nitric oxide
(b) ADP

(c) Ryanodine receptors
(d) Adenosine

426. Which of the following is used for the diagnosis of angina pectoris in the population studies?
(a) Minnesota code (b) Borg Index
(c) Rose questionnaire (d) Framingham Score

427. Which one of the following patients with STEMI has highest mortality risk?
(a) A 58-year-old female with diabetes mellitus
(b) A 71-year-old male with an inferior MI with an S3 and basilar crackles on exam
(c) A 67-year-old male with an anterior MI and an unremarkable physical exam
(d) A 71-year-old male with prior MI with preserved ejection fraction and new inferior MI

428. Drug which acts as PART-I antagonist?
(a) Vorapaxar (b) Hirudin
(c) Bivalirudin (d) Dabigatran

429. The agent to be avoided in PCI:
(a) LMWH (b) UFH
(c) FONDAPARINUX (d) ENOXAPARIN

430. Which biomarker takes longest time to return to normal range post MI?
(a) MB-CK (b) cTn-1
(c) CTn-T (d) Myoglobin

431. Indian data on ACS comes from:
(a) Trinition TIMI 38 Trial
(b) Horizon AMI Trial
(c) Create registry
(d) Transfer AMI Trial

432. Mechanical thrombectomy is done using:
(a) Angio jet
(b) Export catheter
(c) Thrombuster catheter
(d) Basket catheter

433. Newer Marker/Markers in predicting prognosis in ACS:
(a) Thrombus precursor protein
(b) Chromogranin-A
(c) Free plasma hemocysteine
(d) All of the above

434. No benefit in Prinzmental's Angina with:
(a) ICD
(b) Aspirin
(c) Ergonorine provocation
(d) Prazosin

435. Prasugrel should be avoided in:
(a) Thin individuals
(b) Those not undergoing PCI
(c) Age more than 65 years
(d) All of the above

436. All are true for cardiogenic shock in STEMI *except:*
(a) More common in older, DM
(b) More common in prior MI
(c) C.I. < 2.4 liters/min.
(d) PCWP > 18 mm Hg.

437. All may be ECG markers of proximal LAD occlusion *except:*
(a) ST depressed in II, III aVF
(b) ST elevated in a aVR
(c) RBBB
(d) ISOLATED ST elevated in II, III, aVF

438. LCx occlusion in IWMI does not manifest as:
(a) ST elevation in lead II > III
(b) ST elevation in lead III > II
(c) ST depression in $V_1 - V_3$
(d) ST elevation in I, aVL

439. Acute Left main obstruction is diagnosed by:
(a) ST elevation in $V_2 > V_1$
(b) ST elevation in AVR > V_1
(c) ST elevation in V1 and depression in V_2
(d) ST elevation in AVR plus VI > 5 mm

440. Mark the false statement for coronary AV fistula:
(a) RCA is site of fistula in 35% of cases
(b) Most of these drain into right heart
(c) Left coronary artery is site in 35% of cases
(d) May be benign sometimes

441. Which of the following is not a feature of plaque vulnerability?
(a) Thin fibrous cap
(b) Small lipid pool
(c) Macrophage infiltrate
(d) Outward remodelling

442. Significant LMCA stenosis on IVUS:

(a) < 5 mm^2 (b) < 6 mm^2
(c) < 7 mm^2 (d) < 8 mm^2

443. CABG- 10 years patency rate:

(a) 50% (b) 35%
(c) 75% (d) 25%

444. Mach bands in angiography is for:

(a) Thrombus (b) Eccentric lesion
(c) Tortuosity (d) Guide wire

445. Persist for longer time in blood after MI:

(a) Trop-T (b) Trop- I
(c) CPK-MB (d) H-FABP

446. Drug with beta action:

(a) Procainamide (b) Flecainide
(c) Propafenone (d) Ajmaline

447. Cocaine can cause A/E:

(a) Hypotension
(b) VT
(c) MI
(d) Descending aortic aneurysm

448. Coronary artery spasm testing:

(a) α testing (b) β testing
(c) Hyperventilation (d) Valsalva maneuver

449. 30 years old female, 20 packs year smoking, past history of RF, S2 wide and fixed split:

(a) PS (b) ASD
(c) LBBB (d) RBBB

450. Which is true regarding coronary blood flow?

(a) Arterial flow is phasic while venous flow in both systole and diastole
(b) Maximum myocardial volume in diastole
(c) Subendocardial to subepicardial flow -0.6
(d) Pressure in subepicardial is more than subendocardial

451. Myocardial hibernation true A/E:

(a) Reperfusion improves it
(b) It is maladaptive phenomenon
(c) It convert metabolism from fatty acids to glucose
(d) Reduces O_2 basal requirement

452. 60 years old patient had old AWMI, q in V1-V3, undergo TMT, THR—85% of maximum, ST depression in V1- V3 at < 8 METS, true is:

(a) Proximal RCA occlusion
(b) LCx occlusion
(c) Ischemic territory cannot be localized

453. Atrial infarct A/E:

(a) Elevated Ta segment
(b) LA more common involved than RA
(c) Most common occur only with ventricle infarct
(d) Predisposes to arrhythmias/thromboembolism

454. Protamine true is:

(a) 1 mg for 1000 units of heparin
(b) Multiple infusion for subcutaneous heparin
(c) Single intravenous bolus given
(d) Pulmonary hypotension

455. Most common coronary artery in which air embolism occur?

(a) RCA (b) LAD
(c) LCA (d) Conus artery

456. Most common complication in IVUS:

(a) Coronary artery spasm
(b) Coronary artery dissection
(c) Coronary artery perforation

457. IABP true is:

(a) Position below left common carotid artery
(b) C/I in pacemaker patient
(c) Deflated in diastole
(d) Subendocardial ischemia–perfusion increases

458. ACS A/E:

(a) Complete occlusive thrombus–ST elevation
(b) Partial/non-occlusive thrombus–ST depression
(c) 75% STEMI patient have Q wave
(d) Presence of q wave reliably predict transmural ischemia

459. Myocardial bridging A/E:

(a) Most common in LAD
(b) Normal in 5-10% patients
(c) In HOCM – 40% patients
(d) Obligatory ischemia

460. LMCA stenosis by IVUS:

(a) < 5 mm^2 (b) < 6 mm^2
(c) < 7 mm^2 (d) < 8 mm^2

461. Antiplatelet shortest half life:
(a) Prasugrel (b) Ticagrelor
(c) Cangrelor (d) Clopidogrel

462. Patient with ECG showing VPC of RBBB morphology and rapidly changes to sustained VT:
(a) Ebstein anomaly (b) Uhl's anomaly
(c) Entrance to RV

463. Early post MI pericarditis true is:
(a) Steroid is DOC
(b) Aspirin provide symptomatic benefit
(c) Dose of anticoagulation need to be modified
(d) Correlates with subendocardial ischemia

464. Coronary arteriovenous fistula A/E:
(a) Cardiomegaly
(b) RCA most commonly involved
(c) Coronary steal may occur
(d) Coil embolisation may be done

465. Least useful marker in reinfarction is:
(a) Myoglobin (b) Trop T
(c) CPK (d) CPK MB

466. All of the following can be used for assessment of coronary FFR:
(a) I/V adenosine
(b) Intracoronary adenosine
(c) Intracoronary nitroprusside
(d) Intracoronary metoprolol

467. RV infarction true *except:*
(a) V1- V4 ST ↑ may occur
(b) ST ↑ in V4R disappears within 48 hours
(c) AV sequential pacing is hazardous
(d) Right atrial pulse tracing shows steep y descent

468. Patient with STEAWMI, which is suggestive of more severe CAD is:
(a) CHB within ST ↑ IN V4 – V6 leads
(b) ST ↓ in inferior leads ≥ 2 mm with ST ↑ in precordial leads
(c) ST ↑ in avR
(d) PR segment ↓

469. ACE-I in post MI settings A/E:
(a) ↓ LV remodelling's and aneurysm
(b) C/I in CRF with MI
(c) Given to all patients if tolerated and not C/I
(d) ↓ incidence of overt HF in asymptomatic patients

470. IABP C/I in:
(a) Acute AR
(b) MI in shock
(c) CABG with LV dysfunction
(d) Acute MR with MI

471. PCI versus CABG trials:
(a) SOS (b) BARI
(c) COMMIT (d) ART

472. Acute AWMI, 5 hours duration, ongoing chest pain, best treatment based on clinical trials:
(a) Primary angioplasty without stent
(b) Primary angioplasty with stent
(c) GP IIb IIIa inhibitor with half dose TNK
(d) Fibrinolysis with rt-PA

473. RV infarction with hypotension, best initial treatment:
(a) Intravenous fluids
(b) Dopamine
(c) Dobutamine

474. Cellular MOA of NTG:
(a) Phosphorylation of actin
(b) Dephosphorylation of myosin
(c) Tyrosine kinase activation
(d) Cyclic mononucleotide degradation

475. Corornary flow increased compared to resting flow by:
(a) 5 times (b) < 2 times
(c) < 3 times (d) Same as resting level

476. Cocaine overdosage A/E:
(a) Hypothermia (b) Hyperventilation
(c) Tachycardia (d) Seizures

477. A patient of stable angina on NTG, beta blocker will correct which of the side effect:
(a) Throbbing headache (b) Reflex tachycardia

478. Complications in primary PCI prevented by A/E:
(a) Thrombus aspiration (b) Filter device
(c) DES (d) BMS

479. Subclinical atherosclerosis is indicated by A/E:
(a) Flow mediated dilatation of brachial artery
(b) Carotid intimal medial thickness
(c) Aortic wall pulse wave velocity
(d) Coronary calcium score

480. Complicated plaque is characterized by A/E:
(a) Surface defect (b) Hematoma
(c) Thrombus (d) Calcification

481. Markers of vulnerable plaque A/E:
(a) Placental growth factor
(b) CD-40 ligand
(c) Fatty acid binding protein
(d) Pregnancy associated protein A

482. Antithrombotic not clinically used:
(a) Rivaroxaban (b) Cangrelor
(c) Balirudin (d) Dalteparin

483. All are oral antithrombotic A/E:
(a) Cangrelor (b) Ticagrelor
(c) Prasugrel (d) Clopidogrel

484. A patient of mechanical valve on anticoagulant, now having AWMI, PTCA with stenting done with DES (sirolimus), further management:
(a) Warfarin
(b) Warfarin + aspirin
(c) Warfarin + aspirin + clopidogrel
(d) Warfarin + aspirin + prasugrel

485. History:
(a) ASA–1988
(b) Brachytherapy–2000
(c) ICD–1980
(d) Biventricular pacing–1998
(e) Cardiac cath–1967

486. Beta blockers not used as first line anti-hypertensive now a days A/E:
(a) Increase LDL
(b) Increase weight
(c) Less decrease central aortic pressure versus peripheral pressure
(d) Increased onset of DM

487. A patient of CAD on beta blockers, CCB and nitrates. Ranolazine added because of angina, beneficial effect because of:
(a) Changes metabolism from fatty acids to glucose
(b) Decreased Na overload intracellularly
(c) Decrease myocardial oxygen demand
(d) Selective inhibition of CPT-1

488. Patient put on sirolimus stent, given LMWH, after removal of sheath found to be breathlessness, BP=90 mm Hg systolic. ECHO–shows moderate pericardial effusion with RA collapse A/E:
(a) Urgent pericardiocentesis
(b) Blood transfusion
(c) I.V. fluids and vasopressors
(d) Protamine

489. Aspirin + clopidogrel found to be useful in A/E:
(a) Stable angina (b) Acute STEMI
(c) NSTEMI (d) All of the above

490. A patient of CAD subjected to dobutamine stress echo, low dose – increase contractility and high dose – decreases contractility:
(a) Viable myocardium (b) Viable non-ischemic
(c) Scarring (d) LCx disease

491. Right gastroepiploic branch used for anastomosis with:
(a) PDA (b) LCx
(c) LAD (d) OM

492. True is:
(a) Conus artery arises from separate ostia in 10%
(b) Dominant RCA gives PDA, PLV, AV branch, SA branch
(c) Atrial branch of LCx commonly supplies SA node
(d) Left main trifurcates in LAD, LCx and intermedius in 75%

493. Osler maneuver:
(a) Pseudo HTN (b) Masked HTN
(c) White coat HTN

494. PCI to be done which anticoagulant to be used solely?
(a) Foundaparinux (b) Bavalirudin
(c) LMWH (d) UFH

495. 30 years male, midnight chest pain, took tab. sorbitrate develop shock; normal cardiac enzymes, ECG, Echo and angiography; suffering from:
(a) Erectile dysfunction (b) PVD
(c) Prinzmetal angina (d) PAH

496. Anticoagulation not to be given A/E:
(a) Moderate to severe ischemic stroke
(b) Within 24 hours of r-tPA
(c) IE + stroke
(d) None

497. Absolute C/I for fibrinolysis A/E:
(a) Ischemic stroke <3 hours
(b) Closed facial trauma <3 months
(c) Cerebral-vascular lesion
(d) All

498. Cocaine induced MI, BP= 140/90, ST↑ in II, III, aVF, V1 and ST↓ in I, AvL; best management:
(a) Catheterisation (b) Thrombolysis
(c) NTG (d) Phentolamine

499. LMCA seen best in:
(a) AP caudal (b) RAO – cranial
(c) Left lateral (d) LAO cranial

500. Cardiovascular death in India in 2000:
(a) 20% (b) 32%
(c) 44% (d) 60%

501. ↑ incidence of stent thrombosis A/E:
(a) Aspirin resistance
(b) Clopidogrel non compliance
(c) Long stent
(d) BMS

502. Exertional syncope A/E:
(a) Vasovagal (b) PAH
(c) CAD (d) None

503. Initiation of atherosclerosis A/E:
(a) Extracellular lipid deposition
(b) Intracellular lipid deposition
(c) Monocyte infiltration
(d) None of the above

504. Cardiovascular death with no vascular risk factor:
(a) 10 (b) 20
(c) 30 (d) 40

505. Coronary collaterals seen in:
(a) LVH (b) Anemia
(c) COPD (d) All

506. Prehospital fibrinolysis best:
(a) Reteplase (b) Urokinase
(c) Alteplase (d) Streptokinase

507. Free wall rupture A/E:
(a) Seen in presence of previous MI
(b) Occurs in 1 – 4 days
(c) Anticoagulation has no effect
(d) Central rupture is rare

508. Primary PTCA preferred over thrombolysis in A/E:
(a) Presentation < 3 hours
(b) Elderly patient
(c) Late presentation
(d) Post CABG

509. CABG graft true A/E:
(a) 10% at discharge had blocked venous graft
(b) 50% block at 10 years
(c) Statin ↓ graft failure
(d) Long term anticoagulant can prevent graft failure

510. Regarding primary prevention CAD in female A/E:
(a) Estrogen + progesterone combination
(b) Aspirin in high risk
(c) Hydrochlorothiazide in HTN
(d) HDL > 50 mg%

511. Direct thrombin inhibitor A/E:
(a) Danaparoid (b) Lepirudin
(c) Hirudin (d) Ximelagatran

512. Drugs for orthostatic hypotension:
(a) Fludrocortisone (b) Clonidine
(c) Esmolol (d) Phenylephrine

513. All are branches of RCA *except:*
(a) OM (b) FDA
(c) PLV

514. Decrease restenosis all *except:*
(a) Gp IIb IIIa inhibitors
(b) Everlimus eluting stent
(c) Brachytherapy
(d) Methotrexate

515. Past MI with poor prognosis:
(a) Primary VT (b) Secondary VT
(c) MR (d) Aneurysm

516. Type C lesion all *except:*
(a) Ostial (b) > 20 mm
(c) Degenerated venous graft

517. All released from endothelium *except:*
(a) Fibrinogen (b) VWF
(c) Bradykinin (d) Endothelin

518. Normal ECG in MI:
(a) 5% (b) 10%
(c) 15% (d) 20%

519. Infectious causes of atherosclerosis are all *except:*
(a) CMV (b) H. pylori
(c) Chlamydia (d) Mycoplasma

520. Which of the following is branch of left circumflex artery?
(a) Obtuse marginal (b) Acute marginal
(c) Anterior septal (d) Cornus artery

521. Restenosis rate in drug eluting stent is:
(a) 0-2% (b) 4-8%
(c) 10% (d) 12%

522. False regarding true cardiac aneurysm is:
(a) VT is seen
(b) Thromboembolism can occur
(c) Increased incidence of rupture
(d) Cardiomegaly on chest X-ray

523. Absolute contraindication for PTCA is:
(a) LAD disease
(b) Left main unprotected disease
(c) Ejection fraction <40%
(d) Double vessel disease

524. Branheim sign is seen in:
(a) Coronary AV fistula
(b) Systemic AV fistula
(c) Pulmonary AV fistula
(d) All of the above

525. Type B coronary lesion is:
(a) Irregular contour
(b) Concentric
(c) > 3 months total occlusion
(d) Friable SVG graft

526. Absolute contraindication for IABP:
(a) Acute MR (b) VSD
(c) Severe AR (d) Severe AS

527. All of the following infections are associated with coronary artery disease *except:*
(a) CMV (b) H pylori
(c) Coxsackie B virus (d) Chlamydia

528. Intracoronary thrombus can be caused by all *except:*
(a) Aspirin (b) Ticlopidine
(c) Clopidogrel (d) Abciximab

529. Catheter, which is used to hook coronary artery?
(a) Amplatz (b) NW
(c) Pig tail catheter (d) Judkins

530. All are true about nitrate *except:*
(a) Causes rebound angina on discontinuation
(b) Dilate epicardial coronary arteries
(c) Should not be given with sildenafil
(d) Reduces afterload more than preload

531. All are true about coronary arteries *except:*
(a) RCA arising from anterior coronary sinus
(b) Left dominance is less than right side dominance
(c) Sinus artery arises from left coronary artery
(d) Septal artery is the branch of anterior descending artery

532. In patients of chronic stable angina all of the following treatments are useful *except:*
(a) Aspirin (b) Beta blocker
(c) ACE-inhibitors (d) Statins

533. Which gas is used in LAB?
(a) Oxygen (b) Room air
(c) Nitrogen (d) Helium

534. Following statements are true regarding free wall rupture *except:*
(a) Incidence more in anterior wall MI
(b) Common in patients with previous MI common in old age
(c) Common in hypertensive individual

535. Most specific for MI within 48 hours is:
(a) Indium antibodies
(b) SPEC T scan
(c) TMT
(d) MRI

536. Catheter used to selectively hook the coronary artery is:
(a) Amplatz
(b) N1H
(c) PIG tail
(d) Multipurpose catheter

537. Myocardial infarction with cardiogenic shock treatment of choice is:
(a) Thrombolytic therapy
(b) CABG
(c) PTCA with IABP
(d) Heparin with aspirin

538. All of the following catheters are used in coronary angiography *except:*
(a) Judkins (b) Sones
(c) Corand's (d) Amplantz

539. Gangrene with palpable pulse is seen in:
(a) UM
(b) Lerich's syndrome
(c) Thromboembolic obstruction
(d) All of the above

540. Thrombolytic with shortest half-life is:
(a) Streptokinase (b) rTPA
(c) Reteplase (d) Tenecteplase

541. FAME trial for:
(a) FFR during PCI
(b) Rotational atherectomy in PCI
(c) IVUS for left main in PCI
(d) OCT

542. RVMI A/E:
(a) Prominent x descent (b) ↑ se RAP
(c) RAP > PCWP (d) Square root sign

543. In stent restenosis in DES, best treatment:
(a) PTCA with same DES
(b) PTCA with other DES
(c) PTCA with BMS
(d) POBA (plain old balloon angioplasty)

544. Type B lesion A/E:
(a) Concentric (b) Eccentric
(c) Moderate tortuosity (d) Tubular

545. Allen's test A/E:
(a) Done in both preterm before radial CAG
(b) +ve Allen's is C/I for radial CAG
(c) Delayed return of blush after 8-15 sec
(d) Denotes collateral in both radial and ulnar artery

546. Coronary diameter stenosis 90% correspond to area ↓ by:
(a) 90% (b) 95%
(c) 99% (d) 100%

547. Coronary vasodilator, most potent:
(a) Adenosine (b) CO_2
(c) Hypoxia (d) Hypertension

548. Atherosclerotic (native) vs Graft atherosclerosis A/E:
(a) Eccentric (b) Fibrous cap
(c) No lipid core (d) Focal

549. Atrial infarction A/E:
(a) PR elevation in inf lead
(b) PR elevation in lat lead (V_5, V_6)
(c) PR elevation in AVR with PR depression in inferolateral leads
(d) Atrial arrhythmia

550. IABP A/E:
(a) ↓ Afterload
(b) C/I in moderate severe AS

551. Type 4a MI:
(a) CABG
(b) PCI
(c) Stent thrombosis
(d) Demand supply mismatch

552. MI + MR:
(a) 5% (b) 10%
(c) 20% (d) 40%

553. Dicrotic pulse not seen in:
(a) Hyperkinetic (b) Severe HF
(c) Cardiac tamponade (d) Hypovolumic shock

554. Dicrotic notch:
(a) AV opening (b) AV closure
(c) MV opening (d) MV closure

555. MI bad prognosis rhythm A/E:
(a) A flutter (b) Sinus tachycardia
(c) Mobitz type 2 block (d) SVT

556. Heparin in PCI monitored by:
(a) aCT (b) APTT
(c) BT (d) CT

557. Shorter half life:
(a) Alteplase (b) Reteplase
(c) Tenecteplase (d) STK

558. CABG, respiratory complication:

(a) Atelectasis most common
(b) Lung plethora is increased despite normal filling pressure
(c) B1 agonist are harmful
(d) Pulmonary complication are infrequent cause of morbidity

559. True about atherosclerosis:

(a) Large plaque vulnerable to rupture
(b) Fatty streak in aorta
(c) Shear flow is related to intimal thickening
(d) Albumin is present in plaque

560. Infective cause of CAD:

(a) C. pneumonia (b) Staphylococcus
(c) Adenovirus

561. Coronary artery near mitral annulus:

(a) LCx (b) RCA
(c) LAD

562. Anterolateral papillary muscle blood supply:

(a) LCx only (b) LAD and LCx
(c) RCA only (d) PDA of RCA

563. CABG highest risk:

(a) Acute procedure (b) Women
(c) Low LVEF

564. Amylnitrate ↓ murmur of A/E:

(a) MR (b) HOCM
(c) TOF (d) AS

565. MI with cardiogenic shock appropriate treatment A/E:

(a) IABP (b) Fibrionlysis
(c) PCI (d) Vasopressors

566. Regarding use of nitrates in patients with STEMI, following is not an indication:

(a) Post MI angina
(b) Hypertension
(c) LV failure
(d) 48 hours after anterior wall MI with no angina

567. All are features of RV MI *except:*

(a) ST segment elevation in V4 R
(b) Increased LV filling pressure
(c) Increased RA pressure
(d) Steep 'Y' descent in JVP

568. Regarding allograft CAD all are true *except:*

(a) Generally diffuse and concentric
(b) Accounts for majority of late post-transplant deaths
(c) Primarily due to atherosclerosis
(d) Rarely experience angina even in advanced stages

569. The platelet bound half life is longest for:

(a) Eptifibatide (b) Abciximab
(c) Tirofiban (d) Fondaparinux

570. Resting normal coronary blood flow in ML/MIN/100 gm of myocardium:

(a) 30-60 (b) < 30
(c) 60-90 (d) 90-120

571. IABP (Intra-Aortic Balloon Counter Pulsation) is an absolute contraindication for:

(a) Aortic Dissection
(b) Postcardiotomy cardiogenic shock
(c) Post infarction angina
(d) In high risk coronary angiography

572. Restenosis with Drug-Eluting stent:

(a) 0-2% (b) 4-8%
(c) 10% (d) 12%

573. The first-line therapy for all patients with myocarditis and heart failure is:

(a) Immunosuppression therapy
(b) Hemodynamic supportive therapy
(c) Interferon therapy
(d) Immune adsorption therapy

574. TPI in AWMI is done in all *except:*

(a) RBBB with LAHB (b) Transient 2:1 block
(c) Transient CHB (d) AMI with LBBB

575. Which of the following is an independent risk factor for coronary heart disease in women but not men?

(a) Elevated total triglyceride levels
(b) Hypertension
(c) Obesity
(d) Smoking

576. Coronary restenosis will be least with:

(a) Concentric Lesion<10 mm
(b) Concentric Lesion >10 mm
(c) Promixal graft stent (SVG)
(d) Total occlusion

577. IABP (Intra-Aortic Balloon Counter Pulsation) is an absolute contraindication for:

(a) Aortic dissection
(b) Postcardiotomy cardiogenic shock
(c) Post infarction angina
(d) In high risk coronary angiography

578. Most common complication of right-heart catheterization:

(a) Non-sustained atrial and ventricular arrhythmias
(b) Pulmonary infection
(c) Pulmonary artery or right ventricular perforation
(d) Infection

579. Most common complication associated with cardiac catheterization is:

(a) Pseudoaneurysm
(b) Arterial access site bleeding
(c) Arteriovenous fistula formation
(d) Infection

580. Cardiac free wall rupture following MI, are all true *except:*

(a) More common in males
(b) Less common with multiple myocardial infarctions
(c) Occur with > 20% of myocardial involvement
(d) More common with anterior than inferior wall MI

581. What is the best view on coronary angiography to assess the left main coronary artery?

(a) RAO between 5 and 15 degrees with 25 to 35 degree caudal
(b) LAO at 45-50 degrees with 20 degree of caudal
(c) LAO at 45 degrees with 15-25 degree cranial
(d) RAO at 15 degrees with 20 degree of caudal

582. In myocardial infarction, microscopic picture of coagulation necrosis with neutrophilic infiltration is seen in:

(a) 4-12 hours (b) 12-24 hours
(c) 1-3 days (d) 3-7 days

583. The drug to be avoided in patients with known coronary artery disease when treat muscular skeletal symptoms:

(a) Acetaminophen
(b) Non-acetylated salicylates
(c) Non-Cox-2 selective non-steroidal anti-inflammatory drugs
(d) Cox-2 selective non-steroidal anti-inflammatory drug

584. The following are normally branches from the left anterior descending artery *except:*

(a) Recurrent lateral artery
(b) Posterior ascending artery
(c) Left atrial circumflex artery
(d) Septal artery

585. In setting of acute MI, severe systemic: hypoxemia due to intracardiac shunting can occur with:

(a) RV myocardial infarction
(b) Ventricular septal rupture
(c) LV papillary muscle rupture
(d) LV free wall rupture

586. Current role of GP inhibitors in acute STEMI:

(a) Immediately on arrival to all patients proceeding for primary angioplasty
(b) Half dose fibrinolytic agent with full dose GP IIb/IIIa inhibitor as reperfusion strategy
(c) GP Balla inhibitor in the cath lab, just prior to primary angioplasty
(d) GP IIb/IIIa agents as an alternative to fibrinolytic agents in all low risk STEM patients

587. Regarding Dressler's syndrome — Not true:

(a) Usually occurs 1-8 weeks after MI
(b) Leukocytosis is a feature
(c) Aspirin is the drug of choice
(d) NSAIDs and steroids are helpful in refractory cases

588. Which of the following is not associated coronary sinus?

(a) Vein of Marshall/Ligament of Marshall
(b) Thebesian valve
(c) Rahib's ASD
(d) Pectinate muscle

589. Most common mechanical complication resulting in cardiogenic shock:

(a) LV free wall rupture (b) LV septal rupture
(c) RV infarction (d) LV pump failure

590. Bivaluridin's indicators include the following, *except:*

(a) In patients with heparin induced thrombocytopenia
(b) For medical management of STEMI in place of heparin

(c) For primary PCI in STEMI
(d) For PCI in NSTEMI

591. Which statement/s is/are true for Streptokinase compared to tissue plasminogen activator?
(a) Direct plasminogen activator
(b) Longer half life
(c) Fibrin selective
(d) None true

592. The least likely finding in acute anterior MI is:
(a) Normal ECG at presentation or 3 hours later
(b) ST elevation in leads V_2-V_5
(c) New onset RBBB
(d) Hyperacute T waves in precordial leads

593. Free wall rupture following STEMI:
(a) Occurs more frequently in younger patients
(b) Appears to be more common in hypertensive patients
(c) Usually involves the inferior of posterior walls of the LV
(d) Most commonly occurs in patients with previous infarction

594. Thrombolysis for STEMI is contraindicated in all the following *except:*
(a) Systolic blood pressure greater than 180 mmHg
(b) Known structural cerebral vascular lesions
(c) Suspected aortic dissection
(d) Active menstruation

595. All the following are true regarding tPA (alteplase), *except:*
(a) It can be administered as a bolus infusion
(b) It is not antigenic
(c) Systemic fibrinogen depletion is mild
(d) Patency rate at 90 minutes approximately 75%

596. In patients who are asymptomatic following N STEMI, all the following drugs are indicated for long term therapy *except:*
(a) Aspirin (b) ACE inhibitors
(c) Statins (d) Nitrates

597. Abciximab is:
(a) A monoclonal antibody
(b) A Glycoprotein IIb/IIIa receptor blocker
(c) Useful during PTCA in patients with NSTEMI/unstable angina
(d) All of the above

598. Activated clotting time is useful in the catheterization laboratory for the monitoring of the effects of:
(a) Unfractionated Heparin
(b) Low Molecular Weight Heparin
(c) Clopidogrel
(d) Glycoprotein IIb/IIIa receptor blockers

599. Protamine is an antidote for:
(a) Unfractionated heparin
(b) Warfarin
(c) Enoxaparin
(d) Fondaparinux

600. Abciximab is a:
(a) ATP inhibitor
(b) Glycoprotein IIb/IIIa receptor antagonist
(c) Inotropic agent
(d) Anti arrhythmic agent

601. The intravenous dose of r-TPA is:
(a) 1000 mg (b) 400-500 mg
(c) 200-300 mg (d) 80- 100 mg

602. The balloon of the I ABP is inflated at the:
(a) Upstroke of the aortic pulse wave
(b) At the peak of the aortic pulse wave
(c) Immediately after the dicrotic notch of aortic pulse wave
(d) R wave of the ECG

603. Starting dose of IV nitroglycerine is:
(a) 0.5 ug/mt (b) 5 ug/mt
(c) 5 mg/mt (d) 50 mg/mt

604. Dose of IV streptokinase in the treatment of prosthetic valve malfunction due to clot is:
(a) 7.5 lakh units over ½ hour
(b) 15 lakh units over ½ hour
(c) One lakh units per hour for 24-48 hours
(d) Not indicated

605. Blood supply to AV node is predominantly by:
(a) Left circumflex artery
(b) Obtuse marginal artery
(c) Right coronary artery
(d) Left anterior descending

606. Most sensitive biochemical marker of myocardial infarction:

(a) CPK MB (b) LDH
(c) Troponin (d) Nicotinic acid

607. A 24 years old present with ST elevation least likely:
(a) Kawasaki disease
(b) Takayasu arteritis
(c) Familial hyperchylomicronemia
(d) AD homozygous familial hypercholesterolemia

608. Recommended ACT after giving heparin in CABG:
(a) > 500 (b) > 400-480
(c) 200-280 (d) 100-180

609. Absolute contraindication of STK is:
(a) Major surgery 1 week back
(b) Pregnancy
(c) Prolonged CPR > 10 min
(d) Haemorrhagic stroke > 1 year back

610. Remodelling is prevented by all *except:*
(a) ACE-I (b) ARB
(c) Digoxin (d) Spironolactone

611. A patient with H/O acute MI 7 months back on beta-blocker, aspirin, clopidogrel, ACE-I & statin came to you with no symptoms, on ECHO EF-30% so what is next recommendation?
(a) Continue same treatment
(b) Insert intra cardiac defibrillator
(c) Start amiodarone

612. Severity of angina pectoris A/E:
(a) CCS (b) SAS
(c) Califf scoring (d) Duke score

613. First coronary angiography done by:
(a) Sones (b) Forssman
(c) Seldinger

614. Rotational coronary athrectomy contraindicated:
(a) Thrombus (b) Left main disease
(c) Stent (d) Calcium

615. Vulnerable plaque A/E:
(a) Thin cap (b) Lipid rich core
(c) Increased macrophage (d) SMC rich

616. Type C lesion A/E:
(a) Bifurcation lesion
(b) > 90% angulation
(c) Degenerated friable saphenous graft
(d) CTO

617. Myocardial infarction–stent thrombosis:
(a) 4a (b) 4b
(c) 3 (d) 5

618. Stent thrombosis increased risk A/E:
(a) CRF (b) Large diameter
(c) Brachytherapy (d) Overlapping stent

619. DAPT duration in DES:
(a) 6 months (b) 12 months
(c) 24 months (d) 48 months

620. Variant angina A/E:
(a) Post menopausal female
(b) Myocardial stunning

621. Vulnerable plaque A/E:
(a) Fissured
(b) Endothelial denudation
(c) Hemorrhage
(d) 90% stenosis

622. Cocaine effect on heart:
(a) Dose has no effect
(b) Biphasic coronary spasm
(c) Intravenous-first manifestation MI

623. Stent thrombosis increased risk A/E:
(a) DM (b) CRF
(c) Omission of drugs (d) All

624. CSA A/E:
(a) 30% HF
(b) Polysomnography gold standard
(c) Insulin resistance
(d) Hypoxia lead to increased HR and BP

625. Phosphogenes is side effect of:
(a) Ivobradine (b) Ranolazine
(c) Trimetazidine (d) Pirfendione

626. Dabigatran trials A/E:
(a) Rely (b) Realign
(c) Recover

627. Ticagrelor:
(a) Dyspnoea
(b) More potent than clopidogrel
(c) High dose aspirin potentiates effect

628. Subclinical target organ damage A/E:

(a) LVH
(b) Microalbuminuria
(c) Carotid intima thickness
(d) Wide pulse pressure

629. Cardiogenic shock after acute MI:

(a) 0.03 (b) 0.06
(c) 0.09 (d) 0.12

630. Free wall rupture increased by A/E:

(a) Increased collateral (b) Female
(c) First MI (d) HTN

631. Post conditioning A/E:

(a) Initiating mechanisms same as preconditioning
(b) More clinical utility than preconditioning
(c) Reduces reperfusion injury

632. Bolus dose given in:

(a) Tenecteplase (b) Alteplase

633. Disorder with premature atherosclerosis, leathery and cobble stone appearance in axilla, angioid streak in eyes:

(a) Pseudoxanthoma elasticum
(b) Type III hypolipoproteinaemia
(c) Hemochromatosis

634. All are part of STICH trial *except:*

(a) Patient with CAD with EF < 35%
(b) Medical treatment + CABG reduces mortality due to all causes
(c) Reason for trial was that there was no previous benefit of CABG for hospitalization and all cause mortality
(d) CABG more beneficial than medical treatment

635. Serious atherosclerosis most common in:

(a) LCA (b) RCA
(c) LAD (d) LCx

636. Patient has throat discomfort since 30 min with HR– 50/min with mobitz type I second degree block, ECG likely shows:

(a) ST elevation in II, III and avF
(b) Wellen's T wave
(c) ST elevation in V_1-V_3
(d) ST elevation in I and avL

637. 45 years old patient has IWMI with HR– 130/min, BP= 90/60 mm Hg, EDM at base, pulmonary edema, what is next best plan of management?

(a) Primary PTCA
(b) Aspirin, clopidogrel, thrombolytic and inotropic
(c) Echocardiography
(d) IABP

638. 50 years old male DM, obese, wt.= 70 kg, has AWMI with killip class II, posted for PCI which is not indicated:

(a) Upstream abciximab
(b) Prasugrel 60 mg
(c) O_2, morphine and 325 mg dispersible aspirin
(d) Diuretics and NTG

639. Cystic medial necrosis seen in:

(a) Syphilitic aortitis
(b) Takayasu arteritis
(c) Congenital aortic aneurysm
(d) Ehler Danlos syndrome type IV

640. Asymptomatic patient with history of MI:

(a) Stage A HF (b) Stage B HF
(c) Stage D HF (d) Stage C HF

641. Patient undergoing PCI via transfemoral route develops increasing creatinine and bluish discoloration of distal LL are true *except*:

(a) Decreased complement level
(b) Mostly due to atheroembolism
(c) Active urinary sediment
(d) Peripheral eosinophilia

642. 70 years old male post MI with angio shows LAD lesion with plaque rupture with stenting with normal RCA and LCx before treatment. Now has asymptomatic but on echo EF= 30% anterior wall akinesia taking aspirin, ramipril, clopidogrel, B blockers, statin, furosemide, spironolactone, next line of treatment:

(a) Follow up and continue same treatment
(b) ICD
(c) Amiodarone
(d) Repeat CAG

643. Class III risk factor for intervention for CAD:

(a) HRT post menopausal
(b) Obesity
(c) Smoking
(d) Dyslipidemia

644. Blood supply of pericardium A/E:
(a) Left pulmonary Artery
(b) Intercostal Artery
(c) Epicardial coronary Artery
(d) Internal Mammary Artery

645. Sabiston firstly done:
(a) CAB through leg vein
(b) Thoracic Ao aneurysm repair
(c) First pacemaker implantation

646. Acute IWMI with BP 80/60 mm Hg with HR 40/min best initial Management:
(a) I/V dobutamine
(b) I/V fluids 300 ml over 15 min
(c) I/V atropine
(d) Temporary pacemaker

647. All are high risk for CAD *except:*
(a) Smoking (b) High vegetable diet
(c) Meat

648. Myocardial dysfunction after ischemia with normal coronary blood flow:
(a) Myocardial stunning (b) Hibernation
(c) Post ischemic conditioning

649. Resting Normal coronary flow:
(a) 40-60 ml/min/100 gm
(b) 60-89 ml/min/100 gm
(c) 100-110 ml/min/100 gm

650. True about Acute MI *except:*
(a) Max incidence between 6 am and noon
(b) Fever usually occur in most of patient at 24-48 hours
(c) Total leucocyte count may go up to 20,000/cu mm

651. Troponin T ↑ in A/E:
(a) PE (b) Pneumonia
(c) Myocarditis (d) MI

652. Kussmaul sign A/E:
(a) RVMI (b) RCM
(c) CCP (d) Cardiac tamponade

653. Coronary lesion type A:
(a) Subtotal occlusion (b) Eccentric
(c) Angulation > 90 (d) Ostial lesion

654. Direct thrombin inhibitor:
(a) Dabigatran (b) Apixaban
(c) Rivaroxaban (d) Heparin

655. Reversible P2 Y12 inhibitor:
(a) Clopidogrel (b) Prasugrel
(c) Ticlopidine (d) Ticagrelor

656. Post CABG bleeding, drugs given A/E:
(a) Aprotinin (b) Hetastarch
(c) DDAVP (d) VIIa

657. Heart rupture most common after:
(a) After 1-4 days of MI
(b) After 7 days
(c) Within 24 hours

658. Flow mediated vasodilatation due to:
(a) NO mediated shear stress
(b) G protein mediated
(c) Prostacyclin
(d) Adenosine receptor mediated

659. Adenosine super sensitivity:
(a) COPD (b) Heart transplant
(c) HOCM (d) DCM

660. DP/DV Relationship during LV filling–instantaneous DP/PV indicates:
(a) LV stiffness (b) LV compliance
(c) LV elastance (d) IVRT

661. MI least found in:
(a) HOCM (b) MS
(c) Kawasaki (d) Viral myocarditis

662. MI in < 20 years age:
(a) Left main from right coronary sinus
(b) Single coronary artery
(c) High take off coronary artery
(d) Ostial fibrotic strands in coronaries

663. Systolic murmur due to papillary muscle dysfunction:
(a) ALCAPA
(b) Fibroelastosis
(c) Glycogen storage disease
(d) Left sided Ebstein anomaly

664. Earliest histopathological change in MI:
(a) ↓ glycogen content

(b) Extracellular water
(c) Mitochondrial swelling
(d) Swelling of T-tubules

665. Ticagrelor MOA:
(a) ADP antagonist (b) Inhibit PG
(c) Gp IIb IIIa inhibitor

666. Hollenhurst plaque:
(a) Cholesterol (b) Uric acid
(c) Calcium

667. In vivo evaluation of fibrous cap:
(a) IVUS (b) OCT
(c) Multidetector CT (d) MRI

668. Tx and PTCA required in A/E:
(a) NSTEMI (b) STEMI

669. DES vs BMS:
(a) In stent restenosis (b) Acute stent thrombosis
(c) Out stent restenosis

670. O_2 therapy in MI:
(a) SaO_2 <90% (b) SaO_2 <85%
(c) Given irrespective of saturation

671. Vulnerable plaque A/E:
(a) Large plaque (b) More lipid core
(c) Angiogenesis (d) Tight stenosis on angiography

672. PTCA restenosis detected by:
(a) Contrast echo (b) Exercise ECG
(c) Exercise MPI (d) Dobutamine stress

673. Origin of smooth muscle of coronary:
(a) Proepicardial organ (b) Migratory ectoderm
(c) Regional mesoderm (d) Neuroectoderm

674. Variant angina A/E:
(a) DOC-beta blocker
(b) Associated migraine
(c) Associated Raynaud phenomenon

675. A rapid reversible, and ultra-shot acting inhibitor of platelet aggregation via competitive binding to the ADP P2Y12 platelet receptor is:
(a) Prasugrel (b) Clopidogrel
(c) Abciximab (d) Cangrelor

676. The drug that has been used to prevent vein graft failure is:
(a) Clopidogrel (b) Enoxaparin
(c) Prasugrel (d) Edifoligide

677. Which of these is least effective in reversing 'no reflow'?
(a) Verapamil (b) Nitroglycerine
(c) Nitroprusside (d) Adenosine

678. Streptokinase, when compared to tissue plasminogen activator:
(a) Is a direct plasminogen binder
(b) Has longer half life
(c) Does not cause systemic fibrinolysis
(d) Achieves higher TIME 3 flow at 90 minutes

679. A child with multiple erythematous skin lesions had 1° AV block and syncope. The most likely diagnosis is:
(a) Rheumatic carditis
(b) Kawasaki's disease
(c) Coxsackie myocarditis
(d) Lyme's disease

680. Mechanism by which transluminal angioplasty work is:
(a) Compression of plaque
(b) Dehiscence of plaque
(c) Remodelling of plaque
(d) Dissection of plaque

681. Glucose/Blood flow mismatch in PET scan of myocardium tells:
(a) Acute myocardial necrosis
(b) Old myocardial infarction
(c) Hibernating myocardium
(d) Myocardial bridging

682. IABP is absolutely contraindicated in:
(a) Aortic dissection (b) Intractable angina
(c) High risk PTCA (d) Post MI VSD

683. Reflux syncope is indicated by:
(a) Facial pallor
(b) Myoclonic jerk at onset of syncope
(c) Clonic movements at onset of syncope
(d) Alteration of smell before syncope

684. Coronary perfusion during systole instead of diastole in:
(a) ALCAPA (b) Aortic atresia
(c) RA to coronary fistula (d) Primary PAH

685. In MI true is:
(a) S4 universally present
(b) Pericardial rub most common day 1
(c) RBBB cause reverse splitting

686. GP IIb IIIa inhibitor A/E:
(a) Eptifibatide (b) Tirofiban
(c) Prasugrel (d) Abciximab

687. PDGF antagonist:
(a) Argotroban (b) Trapidil

688. Drug which needs AT III but does not affect thrombin:
(a) UFH (b) LMWH
(c) Bivalirudin (d) Fondaparinux

689. EFA A/E:
(a) Linolenic acid (b) Linoleic acid
(c) Arachidonic acid (d) Stearic acid

690. Dietary changes for CAD A/E:
(a) Fat calories 20-30%
(b) Decrease intake of complex carbohydrates
(c) Salt restricted diet <5 g/day

691. Cystic medial necrosis:
(a) Congenital aortic aneurysm
(b) Ehler Danlos syndrome IV
(c) Takayasu arteritis
(d) Syphilitic aortitis

692. Coagulation abnormality by:
(a) Gel foam (b) Dextran
(c) Hemacel (d) Albumin

693. Epicardial coronary artery maximal vasodilatation by:
(a) Serotonin (b) Adenosine
(c) Nitrates (d) Dipyramidole

694. SERM used for CAD prevention in females:
(a) Raloxifene

695. IWMI, HR=40/min, BP= 86/52, next step is:
(a) TPI
(b) Atropine 0.6 mg
(c) 300 ml NS over 15 min
(d) IABP

696. Post CABG VT treatment is:
(a) Betylium
(b) Sotalol
(c) Beta blocker + amiodarone
(d) Ignocaine

697. TACE contraindicated in:
(a) Single lesion <4 cm (b) 2 lesion of 3 cm size
(c) Patial vein invasion

698. Ticagrelor true: (T/F)
(a) PLATO (b) MATRIX
(c) BRUSIE (d) PAGASUS TIMI
(e) ARISTOTLE

699. ESC guideline 2015 NSTEMI: (T/F)
(a) Fondaparinux best side effect and mortality profile in all case of ACS
(b) Fondaparinux can be used as single agent without heparin
(c) Bivalirudin can be substituted for GPIIB/IIIA inhibitor or heparin infusion
(d) Bivalirudin dose–bolus followed by infusion over 24 hour after PCI
(e) If fondaparinux not available, LMWH or unfractionated heparin can be given

700. Preoperative revascularization more beneficial in: (T/F)
(a) LMCA > 70%
(b) TVD >70%, LAD + LCX >70%
(c) RCA – significant
(d) LCX > 50%

701. Ivabradine: (T/F)
(a) Prevent angina
(b) Never be used with β blockers
(c) Best for AF with FVR
(d) Useful with HF with tachycardia
(e) Action depend on autonomic tone

702. CAD in Indians: (T/F)
(a) Mean age 53 years
(b) ↓ incidence when migrates to west
(c) Occurs 10-15 years later than west
(d) On CAG, large coronaries
(e) Accounts for total annual death 20%

703. Ischemic VT: (T/F)
(a) 80% occur within first 48 hours
(b) 3.5 – 7% in fibrinolytic era

(c) Early and late different etiology
(d) Post MI VT not related to mortality
(e) Low EF is protective

704. Ischemic MR: (T/F)
(a) 20% incidence in fibrinolytic era
(b) MVR done in all undergoing CABG
(c) Affects mortality independent of LVEF and killip class 3
(d) Carpentier triad for classification
(e) Increased mortality only in severe MR

705. Left dominant circulation A/E: (T/F)
(a) 25% incidence
(b) LCx terminates as obtuse marginal
(c) RCA gives PDA
(d) LCx can orginate from right sinus
(e) LCx gives PDA

706. Decreased amplitude of thromboelastographic: (T/F)
(a) Low fibrinogen
(b) Low platelet
(c) Normal platelet with ↓ function
(d) Decreased factor VII
(e) Fibrinolysis

707. Troponin I mutation A/E: (T/F)
(a) RCMP (b) HCM
(c) Brugada (d) ARVD
(e) ASD

708. Shear stress: (T/F)
(a) Proportion to shear stress rate and viscosity
(b) Determined by haegen – Poiseuille equation
(c) Parallel to long axis of vessel
(d) Not proportional to blood velocity
(e) Decrease from intima towards lumen

709. Myocardial bridging: (T/F)
(a) Common in RCA
(b) More prone to atherosclerosis
(c) Decreased coronary reserve
(d) Common in HOCM
(e) SCD and arrhythmias association

710. IABP C/I: (T/F)
(a) Mild MR (b) Moderate AR
(c) PDA (d) PVD
(e) Sepsis

711. LV aneurysm: (T/F)
(a) 1-8 cm size
(b) Rarely ruptures
(c) Seen more common in AWMI
(d) Long term anticoagulation not required
(e) Seen in MVD with extensive collaterals

712. Absolute C/I for thrombolysis: (T/F)
(a) Cerebral AV malformations
(b) ICH
(c) Ischemic stroke
(d) Active peptic ulcer
(e) CPR > 10 mins

713. Primary PCI: (T/F)
(a) Within 3 hours thrombolysis preferred over PCI
(b) In elderly PCI preferred over thrombolysis
(c) Heparin preferred over enoxaparin after thrombolysis
(d) All patients to be transferred for PCI after thrombolysis
(e) Thrombosis aspiration is efficacious

714. Drug eluting balloon: (T/F)
(a) Only paxitaxel is available
(b) More effective in small vessels
(c) INDICOR trial
(d) Useful in restenosis of DES
(e) Shown to be effective over DES in acute MI

715. Dabigatran monitoring required in: (T/F)
(a) PTI
(b) PTTK
(c) Anti Xa
(d) Monitoring not required

716. In STEMI: (T/F)
(a) Patient presenting with chest pain, < 20% progress to STEMI
(b) 25% of patients presents without chest pain
(c) 50% Have ST elevation
(d) Use of biomarkers detection increases by 1/3rd
(e) Wait for biomarker to start intervention

717. End hole catheters: (T/F)
(a) Swan Ganz catheter
(b) Multipurpose catheter
(c) Berman catheter

(d) Judkin catheter

(e) AL-1

718. Type C lesion: (T/F)

(a) Ostial

(b) Moderate to heavy calcification

(c) CTO > 3 months

(d) Bifurcation lesions requiring guide wire

(e) Excessive tortuosity in proximal vessel

719. DES in: (T/F)

(a) Direct stenting – DES should be used

(b) Stent length is risk factor in restenosis rate

(c) All lesions should be tackled by primary PCI

(d) BMS is associated with more stent thrombosis

(e) DES associated with more MACE as compared to BMS

720. Stent thrombosis: (T/F)

(a) Length < 10 mm

(b) Diameter > 3 mm

(c) Underexpansion

(d) Residual dissection at margin

(e) Resistance to clopidogrel and aspirin

721. Restenosis: (T/F)

(a) In BMS > 20%

(b) Stent thrombosis most common in 1-4 days

(c) CIN defined as > 0.5% increase in creatinine

(d) CIN resolves in > 40% in 2 weeks

(e) Side branch occlusion due to slow flow phenomenon

722. VF in MI: (T/F)

(a) Lidocaine for prevention

(b) I/V Amiodarone C/I in MI

(c) Synchronized DC shock required in early VF

(d) >48 hours – large infarction and LV dysfunction

(e) Not associated with mortality

723. Fibrinolysis absolute C/I: (T/F)

(a) Active peptic ulcer

(b) Pregnancy

(c) Menses

(d) Suspected Ao dissection

(e) ICH

724. Management of STEMI: (T/F)

(a) Door to Balloon < 90 min

(b) Door to Needle < 30 min

(c) ECG should be within < 10 mm

(d) Total ischemic time should be < 120 min

(e) Within 2-3 hours PCI is equal to thrombolysis

725. IABP absolute C/I: (T/F)

(a) Severe LMCA disease

(b) Acute MI with VSD

(c) AR (severe)

(d) Refractory angina

(e) Acute MI with MR

726. Match: (T/F)

(a) Sones: 1st Angiography

(b) A. gruntzig: Angioplasty

(c) Grossman: 1st Cardiac catheterisation

(d) Heberden: 1st gave term angina

(e) Mirosky: 1st ICD

727. Antiplatelet: (T/F)

(a) Aspirin – COX-2 inhibitor only at higher dose

(b) Efficacy more at higher dose

(c) Clopidogrel and Prasugrel don't require metabolic activation

(d) Cangrelor longest acting

(e) Ticagrelor reversible

728. Fondaparinux: (T/F)

(a) Fondaparinux half life -17 hours

(b) Fondaparinux can be given for HIT

(c) LMWH bioavailability -90%

(d) Abciximab specific for GP IIb/IIIa receptors

(e) Abciximab renal excretion

729. MI localization: (T/F)

(a) RBBB indicate proximal LAD

(b) ST elevation in lead III > II indicate RCA

(c) AVR ST elevation: Left main disease

(d) ST elevation in inferior wall along with anterior wall indicate ostial LAD

(e) ST depression in V_2–V_3 in IMWI indicate LCx occlusion more than RCA

730. Radial artery versus femoral artery cath., advantage of radial artery: (T/F)

(a) Less radiation

(b) Less bleeding

(c) Large sheath can be used

(d) IABP suitable more in radial

(e) Easy assess/catheter size can be used of large size

731. Rupture free wall: (T/F)
(a) Elderly
(b) Precede by infarct expansion
(c) 1-4 day most common
(d) More in atrial due to thin wall
(e) RV > LV

732. FFR: (T/F)
(a) Absolute=maximum/Normal resting Blood flow
(b) FFR > 0.50 good prognosis
(c) Vasodilatation can increase 4-5 times of resting blood flow
(d) FFR indicate pressure distal to stenosis
(e) FFR = mean distal coronary pressure/mean aortic pressure

733. Type C lesion *except:* (T/F)
(a) Diffuse lesion > 3 cm
(b) Marked tortuosity of proximal segment
(c) Degenerated friable vein graft
(d) Inability to protect side branch
(e) Angulation > 90°

734. All true T/F:
(a) Early mortality in STEMI 6.5-7.5% with fibrinolytic
(b) Persistent ST elevation is indication for reperfusion
(c) Coronary normal in < 1%
(d) Incidence of CAD in young 10%
(e) All subjects given anticoagulation in ACS

735. All true T/F:
(a) STEMI and NSTEMI early mortality some
(b) More comorbidities with UA/NSEMI than STEMI
(c) Early mortality with STEMI 3-5%
(d) Early mortality with UA 1.5-2%
(e) Long term mortality worse with STEMI

736. 60 years, metoprolol 50 mg BD for HT after that develop syncope, rate – 40 min, 2:1 with narrow QRS, recovered after 1 day of stopping metoprolol and TPI removed advice: (T/F)
(a) Angiography must
(b) Dual chamber pacemaker
(c) Biventricular pacemaker
(d) EP study if HV interval increases – PPI
(e) After 1-3 days – Holter to rule out intermittent block

737. Prinzmetal angina: (T/F)
(a) All have normal coronary
(b) Commonly in smoker
(c) Midnight to 8 am
(d) Ach-no vasospasm
(e) ST during episode with resting chest pain

738. Free wall rupture false is: (T/F)
(a) Elderly female
(b) ↓ with fibrinolytics
(c) Common with hypertensive patient
(d) LV > RV
(e) 1-4 days after MI

739. TIMI risk score – UA: (T/F)
(a) Age > 70 years
(b) Known case of CAD
(c) ≥ 2 risk factor for CAD
(d) ≥ 2 attack of angina in last 48 hours
(e) Prior aspirin

740. Stent thrombosis: (T/F)
(a) Overlapping stent
(b) Under expansion
(c) Non polymer
(d) Bifurcating lesion

741. Troponin: (T/F)
(a) Separate gene for myocyte and skeletal muscle cell
(b) ↑ in sepsis
(c) ↑ in CRF
(d) Early ↑ FA binding protein with myocyte necrosis

742. CAD is Indians: (T/F)
(a) Younger age
(b) Diffuse disease
(c) ↑ Lp (a)
(d) ↓ Homocysteine
(e) ↓ Metabolic syndrome

743. Hypertriglyceridemia: (T/F)
(a) Tamoxifen -↑
(b) Estrogen - ↓
(c) May cause retinal vein obstruction
(d) ↑ Risk factor for CAD
(e) Niacin ↓ TG

744. DM with TVD patient do not want CABG for 3 months, drug avoided in class II angina with LV dysfunction: (T/F)
(a) Cilastazol
(b) Ivabradine
(c) Ranolazine
(d) Trimetazidine
(e) Sildenafil

745. History:
(a) DES–2001
(b) Primary PCI–1988
(c) STK–1979
(d) Angioplasty–1982

746. History:
(a) Gruentzig–1st coronary angiography
(b) Zimmerman–Retrograde left heart catheterization
(c) Sones–Radial cath
(d) Dotter–Stenting
(e) Gruentzig–PTCA

747. True regarding CSA: (T/F)
(a) Medical therapy equally effective as stenting in selected patient
(b) CAG followed by surgery in all patient
(c) Ranolazine useful
(d) Nitrates cause headache
(e) Statin is effective

748. AIVR – true: (T/F)
(a) Seen in–50% of cases with patent infarct artery
(b) Amiodarone–DOC in hemodynamically significant AIVR
(c) Most cases do not require treatment
(d) Recent studies–↑ risk of long term mortality
(e) Most common reperfusion arrhythmia

749. IVUS true: (T/F)
(a) Better for eccentric lesion than angiography
(b) Very sensitive for lipid core
(c) Useful for dissection after CAG
(d) Differentiate between thrombus and soft plaque
(e) Better for seeing vascular media in coronary artery as compared to aorta and carotid

750. Chest pain radiating to back with ST elevation in inferior leads, right brachial pulse absent, Left arm BP= 220/100, collapsed in emergency – Next line of management is: (T/F)
(a) Thrombolyse the patient
(b) Heparin
(c) Primary PCI
(d) CT for pulmonary embolism
(e) Bedside TEE to R/O dissection

751. Coronary AV fistula true is: (T/F)
(a) Causes large shunt
(b) RCA common
(c) Drain into LV
(d) Never causes I.E
(e) Present with chest pain and breathlessness in childhood

752. MET: (T/F)
(a) 1 MET = 3.5 ml/O_2
(b) 1 MET = 5 ml/O_2
(c) Prescription of exercise
(d) Exercise capacity

753. Atrial infarction: (T/F)
(a) RA> LA
(b) Lateral wall more common than appendage
(c) Reduced ANP
(d) Atrial rupture never common
(e) 15% of MI

754. Abciximab: (T/F)
(a) Monoclonal Ab
(b) Inhibit platelet aggregation
(c) Inhibit ADP induced platelet activation
(d) Used in complicated PTCA

755. Obligatory myocardial ischemia: (T/F)
(a) ALCAPA
(b) LCx from RCA
(c) Split RCA
(d) Left coronary from right sinus with inter-arterial course
(e) Myocardial bridge

756. Thrombolytic therapy C/I: (T/F)
(a) Recurrent MI in last 48 hours
(b) Non traumatic CPR
(c) Uncontrolled HTN
(d) Aortic dissection
(e) Menstruating female

757. Regarding CABG grafts: (T/F)
(a) Venous grafts better than radial artery
(b) 8-12% venous grafts blocked at hospital discharge
(c) 1 year-30% venous grafts blocked
(d) After 1 year, rate of blockage @ 5%/ 1 year
(e) LIMA–10 years patency=85%

758. Atherosclerosis in venous graft vs native CAD: (T/F)
(a) Diffuse disease

(b) Lack of fibrous cap
(c) Concentric lesion
(d) Low thrombus burden
(e) No effect of statins

759. Obligatory myocardial ischemia: (T/F)
(a) ALCAPA
(b) LCx from RCA
(c) Split RCA
(d) Left coronary from right sinus with inter-arterial course
(e) Myocardial bridge

760. AIVR: (T/F)
(a) Seen in 20% of STEMI
(b) Seen more in AWMI
(c) Highly predictive of successful perfusion
(d) Amiodarone to be given
(e) Shows worse prognosis

761. ECG – in MI: (T/F)
(a) RBBB with AWMI signifies distal LAD
(b) ST depression in avL – distal to D1
(c) AWMI ST Elevation in avR– Proximal LAD
(d) Q wave in avL – Proximal to D1
(e) ST elevation in III > II– suggestive of RCA

762. STEMI (IWMI) 3 mm ST elevation in lead II and 2 mm elevation in lead III, artery involved: (T/F)
(a) Proximal RCA (b) Distal RCA
(c) LCx (d) PDA
(e) Diagonal

763. CAD: (T/F)
(a) ↑ HDL (b) ↑ Fibrinogen
(c) ↓ Homocysteine (d) Small dense LDL
(e) ↑ D- dimer

764. Coronary AV fistula: (T/F)
(a) Large shunt
(b) Most common RCA
(c) Opening into LV
(d) Children symptomatic– Dyspnea and chest pain
(e) IE never occur

765. Coronary AV fistula: (T/F)
(a) Large AV shunt
(b) Most common RCA
(c) I.E. never occurs
(d) Drains into LV commonly
(e) Children commonly presents with chest pain and dyspnea

766. Large R wave in V1: (T/F)
(a) Apical MI (b) IWMI
(c) PWMI (d) DMD
(e) RVH

767. Atrial infarction: (T/F)
(a) Lateral wall more commonly than septum
(b) Decreased ANP
(c) RA > LA
(d) Rupture never occurs
(e) Isolated atrial infarction– 15%

768. Prazosin: (T/F)
(a) Selective $\alpha1$ antagonist
(b) Arterial and venodilator
(c) C/I in BPH
(d) Worsens lipid profile
(e) Used in HTN

769. ECG in acute pericarditis: (T/F)
(a) PR decreases
(b) LBBB
(c) RBBB
(d) ST elevation most prominent in av$\bar{R}$
(e) Prominent P waves

770. Abciximab: (T/F)
(a) Monoclonal Ab
(b) Useful in complicated PTCA
(c) Inhibits ADP mediated platelet activation
(d) Inhibits final pathway GP IIb IIIa receptors
(e) Orally effective

771. C/I STK: (T/F)
(a) Active internal bleeding
(b) Uncontrolled HTN
(c) Untraumatic CPR
(d) Reinfarction within 24 hours
(e) Suspected aortic disease

772. Cardiac enzymes: (T/F)
(a) Troponin more sensitive than CK-MB for small infarct
(b) CK-MB normalizes within 12 hours
(c) Myoglobin readily excreted in urine
(d) Specific marker is myoglobin

773. High risk factor in CAD: (T/F)
(a) Increased fibrinogen
(b) Small dense LDL
(c) Increased d dimer
(d) Increased HDL
(e) Decreased homocysteine

774. Lipid profide after AMI – correct: (T/F)
(a) TC and HDL decreases after 24-48 hours of infarction
(b) Lipid profile measured within 24-28 hours of MI
(c) Measured anytime after MI
(d) If Admitted after 48 hours measures after 5 weeks
(e) TC: HDL-C ratio proportionately after 24-28 hours and hence may be used for assessment anytime after MI

775. IABP mechanism of action: (T/F)
(a) ↑ preload (b) ↓ preload
(c) ↓ afterload (d) ↓ afterload
(e) ↑ diastolic coronary perfusion

776. ECG changes in RVMI in presence of IWMI: (T/F)
(a) 1mm ST ↑ in V_4 R to V_6 R
(b) ST ↓ I, AVL, V_4-V_6
(c) ST ↑ V_1 and ST ↓ V_2
(d) LBBB
(e) 2° AV block

777. Drugs causing coronary ischemia: (T/F)
(a) 5-FU (b) Cocaine
(c) Cisplatin (d) Verapamil
(e) Prazosin

778. Free wall rupture in MI true are: (T/F)
(a) Occus 1-4 days after
(b) Preceded by infarct expansion
(c) Common in elderly
(d) Without history of previous MI
(e) RV > LV

779. RVMI: (T/F)
(a) Shock
(b) RAP increased
(c) RV systolic pressure increased
(d) Increased PCWP

780. RA infarction: (T/F)
(a) Less than LA
(b) Decreased ANP level
(c) Isolated RA infarction in 15% of MI

781. MI: (T/F)
(a) CPK-MB excludes myocarditis
(b) Trop T better than CPK MB even in small infarction
(c) CPK MB peak at 12 hours
(d) Myoglobin leak in urine
(e) Myoglobin cardiac specific

782. CAD risk A/E: (T/F)
(a) Hypohomocyteinemia
(b) High fibrinogen
(c) Small dense LDL
(d) High HDL
(e) D-dimer

783. Discharge treatment of uncomplicated CAD: (T/F)
(a) Amiodarone (b) Amlodipine
(c) Beta blocker (d) Aspirin

784. Cells in atheroma:
(a) Platelets (b) Monocytes
(c) Histiocytes (d) Eosinophils

785. Central pain in chest OPD management:
(a) ECG (b) ECHO
(c) History (d) None

786. Nicorandil used in:
(a) HTN (b) CHF
(c) Angina (d) Intermittent claudication

787. Beta agonist causes:
(a) Increases Na ions
(b) Decreases K ions
(c) Increases c-AMP
(d) Inhibition of adenylyl cyclase

788. Post MI TMT indicated at:
(a) 2 weeks (b) 3 weeks
(c) VT (d) Persistent ST elevation
(e) Angina

789. Chronic stable angina avoid:
(a) Pushup (b) Sexual activity
(c) Jogging (d) Cycling
(e) Pushing static vehicle

790. Chronic stable angina avoid: (T/F)
(a) Push up (b) Sexual activity
(c) Jogging (d) Cycling
(e) Pushing static vehicle

791. Acute MI treatment A/E: (T/F)
(a) Intravenous metoprolol
(b) Intravenous streptokinase
(c) Oral ACE-I
(d) Oral CCB
(e) Ecoaspirin

792. Nitrates mechanisms in MI: (T/F)
(a) Antioxidant
(b) Decreases blood volume
(c) Vasodilatation
(d) Arterial dilatation
(e) Cerebral vasodilatation

793. Nitrates in MI: (T/F)
(a) CHF (b) Angina
(c) Up to 3 months (d) Upto 6 months

794. Hypotension in MI: (T/F)
(a) Sweating (b) Chest pain
(c) Tachycardia (d) Morphine
(e) Nitrates

795. Central chest pain with hemodynamic compromise: (T/F)
(a) Pulmonary embolism
(b) Oesophageal spasm
(c) Myocarditis
(d) MI

796. Drugs acting on metabolism of myocardium in angina: (T/F)
(a) Trimetazine (b) L–cartinine
(c) Nitrates (d) Beta blockers

797. Early CAG after MI: (T/F)
(a) Pericarditis (b) CHF
(c) Angina (d) Embolism
(e) PSVT

798. Maximum reperfusion after MI: (T/F)
(a) Primary PTCA (b) Streptokinase
(c) STK + aspirin (d) T-PA
(e) Urokinase

799. Volume of infarct assessed by: (T/F)
(a) ECG (b) CK-MB
(c) Echo (d) Troponin
(e) SGOT

800. Antioxidant A/E: (T/F)
(a) Pantothenic acid (b) Flavonoids
(c) α- tocopherol (d) Beta carotene
(e) Vitamin C

801. Restenosis significantly decreased by: (T/F)
(a) DCA (b) Stenting
(c) Laser (d) Aspirin + dipyridamole
(e) Anticoagulant

802. Indication of thrombolytic therapy: (T/F)
(a) Reinfarction within 1 week
(b) Only after establishing increased enzymes
(c) Hyper acute ECG changes without chest pain
(d) Typical chest pain without ECG changes
(e) Non QWMI

803. Perioperative MI most common in:
(a) With in 24 hrs of surgery
(b) With in 48 hrs of surgery
(c) With in week of surgery

804. What is to be done when guidewire in catheter in RCA cannot pass due to stenosis?
(a) Buddy wire
(b) Introduce another guide wire
(c) Guard wire

805. ASTRAL trial revealed (renal stenting vs medical therapy):
(a) Systolic BP decreased
(b) Diastolic BP reduced
(c) Better renal pressure preservation

806. Pulmonary vein wedge catheterization indicated before surgery in:
(a) Cor triatriatum with (b) HLHS with

807. Which drug not used in GUSTO-V Trial:
(a) Reteplase (b) STK
(c) Abciximab (d) TNK

808. Dabigatran dose in 60 yr old non valvular AF person with Cr Cl < 25 ml/min:
(a) 110 (b) 150
(c) 55 (d) 75

809. Which pulse can be seen in cardiogenic shock?
(a) Tardus (b) Paradoxus
(c) Corrigan (d) Alternans

810. History:
(a) William Harvey–Circulation
(b) Leannac–Stethoscope
(c) Forssman–Catheter himself
(d) Hippocrates–Auscultation
(e) Percussion–Auenbrugger

811. All have end hole *except:*
(a) NIH (b) Cunard
(c) Pigtail

812. CSA not helpful for prognosis:
(a) BNP (b) ECHO
(c) MRI (d) Calcium score

813. Mechanisms of stent restenosis:
(a) Neointimal proliferation
(b) Vascular recoil and thrombus

814. DES vs BMS, drug helps in:
(a) Prevent neointimal proliferation

815. Bioabsorbable stent used in India:
(a) Sirolimus (b) Zatarolimus
(c) Paclitaxel (d) Everolimus

816. Predictor of stent failure A/E:
(a) Present lumen diameter
(b) Post stent lumen diameter
(c) Lesion length
(d) All

817. SVG graft stenosis, PCI not done in:
(a) Chronic SVG occlusion
(b) Ostial stenosis

818. Most common complication in balloon valvotomy in COA in infants:
(a) Femoral artery infection
(b) CVA
(c) Thromboembolism
(d) Cardiac arrest

819. True statement:
(a) LCx from RCA is most common coronary anomaly

820. Least time to peak:
(a) Cangrelor (b) Ticagrelor
(c) Prasugrel (d) Clopidogrel

821. Antiplatelet to be easily reversed:
(a) Cangrelor (b) Ticagrelor
(c) Prasugrel (d) Clopidogrel

822. Course of management according to recent guidelines 60 years old hypertensive treated with streptokinase within 4 hrs of presentation:
(a) Continue with medical treatment as indicated
(b) Rescue PCI if ischemia develops
(c) Send for coronary angiography and PCI
(d) Go for stress testing 2 weeks after discharge and then decide

823. Coronary anomaly that interfere with surgery:
(a) LCA arising from RCA
(b) LCx arising anomalously

824. GP IIb IIIa inhibitor according to new rule:
(a) Useful for reducing ischemia in primary PCI
(b) Useful for reducing ischemia in rescue PCI
(c) GP IIb IIIa inhibitor causes less bleeding than when used in rescue PCI
(d) Abciximab class I indication and tirofiban class IIa indication for PCI

825. LCx best view:
(a) RAO cranial (b) RAO caudal
(c) LAO cranial (d) LAO caudal

826. Surgical mortality highest with:
(a) AVR with CABG (b) MVR with CABG
(c) DVR with CABG (d) MVR with TV repair

827. Normal M1-T1 interval:
(a) 20 msec (b) 30 msec
(c) 52 msec (d) 60 msec

828. IVS rupture in acute MI true A/E:
(a) Incidence with thrombolysis 0.2%
(b) HTN and advanced age high risk factor
(c) After thrombolysis risk ↓
(d) Posterior wall involvement – worst prognosis

829. All are end hole catheter *except:*
(a) Berman catheter
(b) Cournard catheter
(c) Angled pigtail catheter
(d) Goodale lubin

830. All are end hole *except:*
(a) Berman catheter (b) Goodale lubin
(c) Cournard catheter (d) Multipurpose catheter

831. Catheter used in selective angiography used A/E:
(a) Judkin catheter
(b) Amplatz catheter
(c) Goodhale catheter
(d) Multipurpose catheter

832. Carvedilol vs metoprolol trial:
(a) Comet (b) Capricorn
(c) CIBIS (d) Copernicus

833. High risk in MPI A/E:
(a) Multiple defects in > 1 territory
(b) Large fixed defect
(c) Transient LV dilatation
(d) ↑ lung uptake with Tl^{201}

834. High risk in USA/NSTEMI A/E:
(a) ST deviation ≥ 0.05 (b) T inversion ≥ 0.3
(c) AV block (d) LBBB

835. Basal septum supply:
(a) RCA (b) LAD
(c) LCx (d) LAD + D1

836. Left atrial blood supply:
(a) LMCA (b) LCx
(c) RCA (d) LAD

837. Least common branch of RCA:
(a) Conus (b) SA nodal
(c) Acute marginal (d) PDA

838. Restenosis risk A/E:
(a) Proximal LAD (b) Tortuosity
(c) Complete obstruction (d) SVG

839. Least specific in CSA:
(a) Exercise ECG (b) Exercise SPECT
(c) Dobutamine ECHO (d) Exercise ECHO

840. Coronary constriction A/E:
(a) Cholinergic stimulus (b) Exposure to cold
(c) Cocaine (d) Mental stress

841. Macrovascular complication A/E:
(a) Nephropathy (b) CAD
(c) PVD (d) Cerebrovascular disease

842. Heparin not true:
(a) Direct Xa inhibitor
(b) Unfractionated equal Xa and IIa
(c) ↓ ed efficacy in presence of NTG
(d) Max. benefit at ACT = 300 – 350

843. PCI vs CABG trial A/E:
(a) CASS (b) GABI
(c) ERACI (d) BARI

844. Fibrinolytic – fibrin specific max:
(a) TNK (b) Recombinant
(c) rtPA (d) Streptokinase

845. Side hole catheter A/E:
(a) Berman catheter (b) Counard catheter
(c) Swan Ganz catheter (d) Pigtail catheter

846. ST elevation may occurs in all of the following condition *except:*
(a) Hypothermia (b) Hypokalemia
(c) Pulmonary embolism (d) Hypercalcemia

847. Intravascular ultrasound (IVUS) is better than optical coherence tomography (OCT) in which of the following condition?
(a) Detection of stent malapposition
(b) Plaque morphology characterization
(c) Thrombus detection
(d) Evaluation of Ostial left main lesion

848. Cardiovascular disorders often present acutely, as a previously asymptomatic person whose first clinical manifestation is syncope or even sudden death is not seen in following condition:
(a) Acute myocardial infarction
(b) Hypertrophic QT syndrome
(c) Prolonged QT syndrome
(d) Pulmonary stenosis

849. All of the following are cardinal manifestations of cardiac disease *except:*
(a) Fatigue (b) Edema
(c) Chest discomfort (d) Syncope

850. The following statement is false regarding the first clinical manifestation of coronary artery disease in previously asymptomatic person:
(a) May present as sudden cardiac death
(b) May present as acute myocardial infarction
(c) May present as stoke
(d) May present as seizure

851. Under resting conditions, maximum pressure drop in coronary circulation occurs in:

(a) Epicardial coronaries (b) Resistance vessels

(c) Capillaries (d) Venules

852. Absolute flow reserve can be calculated by:

(a) Optical Coherence Tomography

(b) Adenosine induced vasodilation followed by thallium SPECT scanning

(c) PET perfusion scan

(d) Quantitative coronary angiography

853. Regarding fibrinolytic agents which is true?

(a) Tenectaplase dose is weight independent

(b) Alteplase is given as a double blous

(c) Tenectaplase causes maximum fibrinogen depletion

(d) Tenectaplase is the most fibrin specific

854. Among antithrombotic agents all is true *except:*

(a) LMWH have bioavailability and high factor anti-Xa to anti-IIa activity ratio producing effective blockade in coagulation cascade

(b) Unfractionated heparin is given by intravenous route

(c) Factor Xa specific antagonists were studied in OASIS 6 trial

(d) Fondaparinux was inferior in PCI patients due to higher risk of stent thrombosis

855. For acute coronary syndrome (ACS) compare the trial with the antiplatelet agent studied and identify the wrong combination:

(a) CREDO–Ticlopidine

(b) CLARITY–TIMI 28–Clopidogrel

(c) Trition–TIMI 38–Prasugrel

(d) PLATO–Ticagrelor

856. Regarding mechanical complications of Acute MI which statement is true?

(a) Fibrinolysis decreases the risk of septal and free wall rupture

(b) Mitral regurgitation produces a pansystolic murmer

(c) Ventricular septal rupture produces pan-systolic murmer

(d) Mechanical complications are commonly seen on day 2 post MI

857. IABP is not indicated in following condition:

(a) Refractory cardiogenic shock

(b) Acute MR

(c) Acute AR

(d) Acute ventricular septal rupture

858. Post myocardial Infarction pericarditis all are true *except:*

(a) Acute pericarditis occurs early within first 3 days

(b) Occurs due to antibodies to cardiac tissue casing fibrinous inflammation

(c) High does aspirin relieves the chest pain

(d) Anticoagulation is not contraindicated

859. Regarding non-invasive testing in NSTE-ACS patients which is not true:

(a) Safe after 24 hours of stabilization and pain relief

(b) Symptom limited TMT is recommended for patients with baseline ECG ST-segment abnormalities

(c) Stress Echocardiography and stress MPI have higher sensitivity than TMT

(d) CT coronary Angiography can also be used to establish diagnosis of unstable plaque

860. Regarding GP IIb IIIa inhibitors in NSTE-ACS all are true *except:*

(a) Abciximab has earliest onset action

(b) Tirofiban and ebtifibatide have longer half-lives than abciximab

(c) Current available evidence does not support the routine use in patients on DAPT

(d) They can cause severe thrombocytopenia in some patients

861. Most sensitive and specific modality of stress testing is:

(a) Exercise ECG (b) Exercise SPECT

(c) Dobutamine ECHO (d) Adenosine SPECT

862. High Risk (> 3% Annual Risk for Death or Myocardial Infarction) on noninvasive testing includes:

(a) CAC score > 1000 Agatston units

(b) Severe stress – induced LV dysfunction (Peak exercise LVEF < 45% or drop in LVEF with stress ≥ 10%

(c) ≥ 1-mm ST-segment depression occurring with exertional symptoms

(d) 1-vessel CDA with ≥ 70% stenosis or moderate CDA stenosis (50-69% stenosis) in ≥ 2 arteries o CCTA

863. Which of the following facts are true about Ivabradine *except*?

(a) Act by reducing the heart rate via specific inhibition of the funny channel (If) at SA node

(b) Indicated for the symptomatic treatment of chronic stable angina

(c) A common side effect is luminous phenomenon

(d) In beautiful study for coronary artery disease left ventricle dysfunction (ejection fraction < 40%) ivabradine showed a significant reduction in the mortality

864. Regarding management of chronic stable angina which of the following statements is true?

(a) In single vessel disease with proximal LAD involvement only PCI is recommended

(b) In two vessel disease with proximal LDA involvement surgery or PCI can be done

(c) In three vessel disease with syntax score of 40 PCI should be done

(d) In left main disease with syntax score 23-32 PCI cannot be done

865. Regarding ticagrelor with of the statement is true:

(a) Irreversible allosteric antagonist

(b) Interacts with CYP3A4 inhibitors

(c) Interacts with CYP2C9

(d) Aspirin doses less than 100 mg/day decreases its effectiveness

866. Regarding bivalirudin which of the statement is true?

(a) Irreversible direct thrombin inhibitor (DTI)

(b) It inhibits both circulating and clot-bound thrombin, while also inhibiting thrombin-mediated platelet activation and aggregation

(c) Since it is cleared from plasma by a combination of non-renal mechanisms and proteolytic cleavage clearance unrelated to renal dysfunction

(d) In HEAT-PPCI trial bivalirudin reduced the incidence of major adverse ischemic events in the setting of Primary PCI

867. Coronary perfusion: (T/F)

(a) Blood flow subendocardium during diastole and limited after CPPP < 40 mm Hg

(b) Adenosine affect arteriole < 100 μm

(c) Subepicardial blood flow mainly in systole and decreases with CPP < 50 mm Hg

(d) Compressive forces affect subepicardial blood flow

(e) With decrease in CPP subendocardium vessel dilates after subepicardial vessel

868. GRACE registry: (T/F)

(a) Serum creatinine

(b) Killip class

(c) History of cardial arrest

(d) Increase cardiac marker

(e) ECG changes

869. Does not decrease CAD: (T/F)

(a) Tocopherol

(b) Chelation

(c) HRT

(d) Folate supplementation

(e) Betacarotene

870. DES: (T/F)

(a) Drug stored between balloon and stent

(b) Monitoring not required for antimitotic drug affects

(c) Decrease stent thrombosis

(d) Requires special techniques and catheter for deployment

(e) Biodegradable DES under clinical evaluation

871. Percutaneous intervention successful: (T/F)

(a) Non rheumatic MR

(b) Calcified AS

(c) Degenerative prosthetic valve

(d) Supramitral ring

(e) Subaortic membrane

872. Anticoagulant: (T/F)

(a) Dabigatran is oral factor X inhibitor

(b) ROCKET AF – rivaroxaban single dose vs warfarin in AF

(c) Dabigatran FDA approved in rheumatic AF

(d) Vit K antidote for all three

(e) Apixaban is a prodrug, rivaroxaban is not

873. DES: (T/F)

(a) DES has no polymer

(b) DES require more inflation than BMS

(c) DES – drug between balloon and stent

(d) DES has less radial force after drug depletion

874. FFR: (T/F)

(a) Cath. in coronary distal to stenosis and in coronary sinus

(b) Can be measured instantaneous in cath lab

(c) < 0.9 = significant

(d) Adenosine can be used for post stent correct placement
(e) Cannot be done in highly tortuous

875. Coronary blood flow:
(a) Subendocardial < subepicardial in systole
(b) FFR< 0.9 is associated with other evidence of ischemia
(c) Pressure at zero flow in coronary artery is 60 to 70 mm Hg
(d) Epicardial coronary stenosis causes ↓ blood flow to endocardium
(e) Subendocardium wall stress > subepicardium

876. ↓ Periprocedural MI by: (T/F)
(a) Prasugrel ↓ incidence in elective PCI
(b) Verapamil ↓ incidence in sephanous vein graft
(c) Intra coronary urokinase
(d) Statin
(e) PTFE coated stent

877. PES: (T/F)
(a) Significantly ↓ instent thrombosis
(b) Drug between balloon and stent
(c) Regular monitoring not required for S/E of antimitotic drugs
(d) Biodegradable stent in development
(e) Special balloon/cath and techniques required

878. Absolue C/I of thrombolysis: (T/F)
(a) ICH any time
(b) Ischemic stroke >24 years
(c) History of peptic ulcer
(d) CPR > 10 min
(e) BP180/110

879. II/III generation thrombolytics: (T/F)
(a) STR less fibrin specific
(b) STK shortest half life
(c) STK early heparin started
(d) TNK better TIMI3 than STK
(e) STK indirect act on plasminogen

880. PCI done in: (T/F)
(a) Extensive AWMI
(b) IWMI + RVMI
(c) Cardiogenic shock
(d) Door to balloon time = 90 min
(e) Presenting in 1 hour of chest pain

881. Blood supply to: (T/F)
(a) RCA – AV node
(b) Conus branch – RVOT
(c) PM papillary muscle – dual blood supply
(d) Interventricular septum – RCA + LAD
(e) Acute marginal for LCx

882. Exercise: (T/F)
(a) Exercise in supine position↑ CO by ↑ HR and ↑ SV
(b) HR (max)= 220–age under estimates female
(c) Parasympathetic reactivation is main mechanism of recovery of heart rate
(d) In bicycle ergometry I W = 6 kpm (pond)

883. Myoglobin: (T/F)
(a) Released within 30 min
(b) Specific and sensitive for MI
(c) Levels correlates with CPK-MB
(d) Cocaine can increase it
(e) Myoglobin assessment not routinely recommended

884. T/F:
(a) Ticagrelor is P2 Y12 competitive antagonist
(b) Prasugrel is competitive antagonist
(c) Prasugrel has less bleeding
(d) Ticagrelor has short t½ than clopidogrel

885. TIMI in acute MI: (T/F)
(a) Killip class
(b) Body weight
(c) Age > 50
(d) Serum creatinine

886. DES: (T/F)
(a) Polymer–gives radial strength to DES
(b) Drug is put between polymer and stent
(c) Instent restenosis–drug eluting balloon used
(d) Antiplatelet not mandatory in DES
(e) In DES polymer sheath not required

887. T/F:
(a) Bivalirudin–ACT is used
(b) Bivalirudin–bleeding loss the LMWH
(c) Protamine–useful in fondaparinux
(d) Bivalirudin–in PCI catheter thrombosis is not a concern
(e) Bivalirudin–Acts on clot bound thrombin

888. T/F:
(a) Heparin activity ↓ ses in AT III def
(b) Bivalirudin–Acts in clot bound thrombin
(c) Bivalirudin–high dose–antiplatelet activity
(d) Fondaparinux DTI
(e) Idraparinux–longer acting than fondaparinux

889. CRP: (T/F)

(a) Done in high risk patient only
(b) Useful in chronic stable angina
(c) If > 6 mg/dl repeat after at least after 6 weeks
(d) Hs CRP levels to be repeated after 2 weeks
(e) CRP mainly formed in liver

890. CRP: (T/F)

(a) Normalizes after 1 week of acute infection
(b) Aspirin ↓ses hs CRP
(c) HRT ↑ses hs CRP
(d) Thiazolidiones ↓se CRP
(e) Fasting state not a requirement for CRP measurement

891. GRACE scoring includes: (T/F)

(a) History of syncope (b) Biomarker
(c) ECG changes (d) Body weight
(e) Sr. creatinine

892. In acute MI: (T/F)

(a) IV beta blocker is DOC for control of AF
(b) Primary VF does not worsen future mofosis
(c) ACE I should be started in convalescence phase
(d) ISIS-4, intravenous Mg^{2+} found to be beneficial
(e) Antioxidants have no role in prevention of recurrence

893. Vulnerable plaque suggested by: (T/F)

(a) Thin fibrous cap – < 60 μ
(b) Absent SMC
(c) Decreased macrophages
(d) Presence of necrotic core is must
(e) Type I collagen

894. True or False:

(a) Fibrinogen produced by adipose tissue
(b) Hs CRP mainly produced by liver
(c) S. amyloid – A produced in heart

895. Regarding cardiac biomarkers: (T/F)

(a) Trop T starts ↑ after 3 hours
(b) Myoglobin in most useful in ruling out MI
(c) Reinfarction – CKMB better than troponin
(d) CKMB mass better than activity
(e) Muscle disease – CKMB has plateau pattern for many days as compared to early rise and fall in MI

896. T/F:

(a) TNK – Fibrin specific
(b) Used in some specific cases of NSTEMI – TNK
(c) Used in pulmonary embolism (in most cases)– TNK
(d) Ischemic stroke of 1 hour – C/I for thrombolysis
(e) GP IIb/IIIa is useful with thrombolytic therapy

897. T/F:

(a) Electrical activation consumes 10% of total hearts energy
(b) Subepicardial perfusion continuous at low pressure
(c) Resistance occurs at 3 levels
(d) Max resistance at precapillary arteriolar level
(e) Coronary blood flow can se upto 10 times

898. T/F:

(a) Coronary O_2 extraction upto 90%
(b) Normal coronary Flow= 60-80 ml/100g/min
(c) Exercise cause more ST depression than adenosine
(d) Atropine after dobutamine stress increases diagnostic power
(e) Adenosine more sensitive than dobutamine for moderate stenosis
(f) ST depression common in exercise versus dobutamine stress

899. 1 week post MI: (T/F)

(a) Reinfarction diagnosed by CPK MB
(b) LDL is ↑ sed
(c) Trop T continued to se after 1week
(d) Clopidogrel should be given to all
(e) Angiography should be done in all at high risk

900. CABG versus stent in multivessel disease: (T/F)

(a) At 5 years ↓ revascularisation only differential
(b) DM – CABG better
(c) DES is not better than BMS
(d) Repeat revascularisation poor result
(e) CABG benefit depend on SV patency

901. TIMI risk score in UA/NSTEMI: (T/F)

(a) > 3 risk factors
(b) Aspirin within 7 days
(c) Prior PCI/CABG
(d) > 3 episodes in last 24 hours
(e) Age > 75 years

902. DES: (T/F)

(a) Radial strength more than BMS
(b) More balloon inflation time than BMS
(c) Antineoplastic used
(d) Very late stent thrombosis peculiar complication
(e) Dual antiplatelet not used

903. Thrombolysis in which condition: (T/F)

(a) Post SCD resuscitation nonspecific ST-T changes
(b) 7 months pregnancy with acute anterior STEMI
(c) 70 years female with dyspnea for 15 days with LBBB on ECG
(d) 64 years old male with chest pain with ST depression
(e) Diabetic female with having mensus and STEMI

904. Atherosclerotic plaquing: (T/F)

(a) Diffuse disease with focal luminal narrowing
(b) Type 2 DM and smoking increases negative remodelling
(c) Glasgov phenomenon is positive remodelling
(d) Macrophages secrete MMP
(e) Vulnerable plaque more at ostia and branching points

905. Coronary atherosclerosis: (T/F)

(a) Five types– I to V
(b) Type IV – fibrocalcific
(c) Can progress or regress upto stage II
(d) Proatheroma is type III
(e) Type IV/V are raised lesions

906. Trop T: (T/F)

(a) > 99th percentile in population diagnostic
(b) Changes with population under study
(c) > 30% of UA are CPK-MB negative with raised Trop T
(d) More sensitive and specific than QCPK- MB

907. Gp IIb IIIa inhibitors: (T/F)

(a) >80% receptor occupancy required for efficacy
(b) Tirofiban is non peptide mimetic inhibitor
(c) Abciximab is used in UA if PCI is to be done
(d) Epifibatide receptor occupancy for > 2 weeks
(e) Increased platelet activity lead to increased binding to fibrinogen

908. Successful thrombolysis denotes resolution of: (T/F)

(a) Chest pain
(b) Dyspnoea
(c) Incomplete ST resolution
(d) AIVR at 90/min
(e) Non sustained VT

909. New classification of MI: (T/F)

(a) MI after PCI is a new entity
(b) MI with atypical symptoms has worst prognosis
(c) CPK MB > 5 times after CABG is diagnosed as MI
(d) Rise and fall of cardiac marker very important
(e) Early thrombolysis lead to no rise of markers

910. Acute MI identified by: (T/F)

(a) PET
(b) 64 slice CT
(c) CAG
(d) Technitium pyrophosphate scan
(e) ECHO

911. Acute MI – ACE-I: (T/F)

(a) Intravenous enalapril should be given
(b) ACE-I has more mortality benefit than ASA
(c) Should be given for atleast 6 weeks
(d) Renal function should be assessed before starting ACE-I
(e) Can be started after 48 hours

912. Post MI VSD: (T/F)

(a) More in transmural MI
(b) CAG should be done before surgery
(c) IABP should be liberally used
(d) Surgery should be done even if patient haemodynamically stable
(e) Early thrombolysis increases risk

913. Vulnerable plaque: (T/F)

(a) Thin fibrous cap
(b) Increased temperature
(c) Ruptures at margin of high hemodynamic stress
(d) Coronary angiography can diagnose it
(e) Increased SMC

914. False positive trop T: (T/F)

(a) Post RFA
(b) Acute infective endocarditis
(c) Takotsubo CMP
(d) Pericarditis
(e) 20% burn

915. Cardiac surgery: (T/F)
(a) PA banding open heart surgery
(b) Pericardiectomy closed surgery procedure
(c) Increased adiponectin increases mortality
(d) Obesity increases adiponectin

916. RHD: (T/F)
(a) Development of RHD does not depend on genetic composition
(b) M protein has 20 serotypes
(c) WHO criteria has made less rigorous for recurrent RF
(d) CHF with carditis has normal LV function
(e) Echo can be diagnostic in ARF

917. IWMI and RVMI: (T/F)
(a) Surgery is indicated
(b) NTG causes HTN
(c) PCWP > 3 times JVP
(d) Hypotension and increased JVP
(e) RCA stenosis dangerous than LMCA stenosis

918. Ischemia: (T/F)
(a) Coronary blood flow decreases–diastolic dysfunction precede systolic dysfunction
(b) ECG changes first to come and disappear

919. DES: (T/F)
(a) Polymer coating can be toxic
(b) Radial force ↓ after drug depletion
(c) Paclitaxel polymerize tubules
(d) Sirolimus act on regulator genes in cells cycle
(e) Allergic reaction unknown

920. Polymer coating in DES: (T/F)
(a) Potentially toxic
(b) Act as reservoir
(c) Serolimus act later than paclitaxel on cell cycle
(d) Unavoidable for drug delivery
(e) Extracellular matrix deposition blocked

921. GP IIb IIIa: (T/F)
(a) Tirofibanmostcommoncauseofthrombocytopenia
(b) Tirofiban can be used in associated RF
(c) Tirofiban toxicity treatment by platelet transfusion
(d) Abciximab longest t ½
(e) Abciximab treatment is by cyroppt

922. Abciximab: (T/F)
(a) Ab is used for medical treatment in ACS
(b) > 90 years – of patients with ACS should not be used
(c) Cardiogenic shock with PCI – can be used
(d) LMCA stenting can be used
(e) Recent stroke – shouldn't used

923. HIT: (T/F)
(a) <50% ↓ in platelet from baseline
(b) < 1.5 lakh/cumm for diagnosis
(c) LMWH can be used
(d) After heparin use of > 4 days
(e) All of the above

924. LMWH: (T/F)
(a) Anti Xa/IIa activity correlation with efficacy
(b) Deltaparin = max IIa/Xa ratio
(c) Lepirudin= reversible DTI
(d) Dose is ↓ed in RF

925. Ant. Wall MI: (T/F)
(a) q RBBB complete is sensitive marker of proximal LAD before 1st septal
(b) ST ↑ AVR is specific for proximal LAD
(c) V5-V6 ST ↓ is indicative of distal LAD
(d) In proximal LAD – sup axis vector
(e) ST ↑ in inf. leads is indicative of distal LAD

926. IWMI: (T/F)
(a) T ↓ in v4R – is indicative of distal RCA
(b) Vector directed to lead III – LCx
(c) Ta segment in inf. lead – LCx
(d) ST Normal with T ↑ in V4R – LCx

927. IABP with cardiogenic shock all drugs can be beneficial drug given is: (T/F)
(a) Dopamine (b) Dobutamine
(c) NE (d) NTG
(e) Levosimendon

928. CABG: (T/F)
(a) 7% renal dysfunction
(b) 30% AF
(c) 1st month = 10% SVG block
(d) Bilateral IMA= sternal dehiscence
(e) 2 months-1 year : block of SVG due to atherosclerosis

929. CABG: (T/F)
(a) LIMA can be closed or left open
(b) Minimal invasive CABG always off pump surgery

(c) Thickening of aorta – off pump required
(d) In patients with LV dysfunction preoperative b blocker should be stopped
(e) Use of glucose reduction is beneficial beyond only reduction in acute infection

930. Abciximab: (T/F)
(a) Shortest acting GP IIa/IIIb
(b) Can persist upto 2 weeks in body
(c) Causes severe thrombocytopenia
(d) Monoclonal chimeric antibody
(e) Used in conservative management in UA/ NSTEMI

931. Microvascular hemolytic anemia: (T/F)
(a) CABG
(b) Prosthetic valve regurgitation
(c) Free AR
(d) Post aneurysmal repair
(e) RSOV

932. PTCA: (T/F)
(a) Prevents acute MI
(b) Prevents CHF
(c) Relieves severe angina
(d) Always reduces mortality

933. Indication of surgery in I.E.: (T/F)
(a) Culture negative fever for 10 days after optimal therapy
(b) Staph. Aureus responding to treatment
(c) Increasing HF
(d) Paravalvular abscess
(e) Recurrent PVE after optimal therapy

934. APSAC: (T/F)
(a) Antigenic
(b) Has hypotensive effect
(c) Highest mol. Wt
(d) Fibrin specific
(e) Can be given as bolus

935. LMWH: (T/F)
(a) Mol. Wt. 12000 – 15000
(b) Minimal platelet inhibition
(c) UFH excreted by renal mainly
(d) Minimal protein binding
(e) Minimal IIa activity

936. Nitrates in MI: (T/F)
(a) Completely degraded in liver
(b) Effect reversed by selective beta blocker
(c) Nitroglycerine patch best at thorax
(d) Oral better than sublingual
(e) Isosorbide dinitrate max. dose 15 mg 4 hourly

937. Post MI papillary muscle rupture: (T/F)
(a) More common with anterior than inferior wall MI
(b) Small MI more risk
(c) MR usually severe
(d) Prominent v wave in PCWP tracing diagnostic
(e) Rupture distal more than proximal
(f) Pulmonary edema common

938. MI characteristic: (T/F)
(a) RVMI in > 50% of IWMI
(b) Isolated RVMI never seen
(c) PR deviation seen in 10% of AWMI
(d) Atrial infarction LA more than RA
(e) Collateral less in RV than LV

939. Drug eluting stent: (T/F)
(a) Decreases restenosis to 0% in some trials upto 10 years
(b) Rapamycin and paclitaxel are only used
(c) Biodegradable
(d) Consists of plateform matrix and drug
(e) Inhibits all phases of cell cycle

940. IMA graft: (T/F)
(a) 90% patency after 10 years
(b) Earlier thrombus more common than SVG
(c) Early spasm
(d) Occlusion related to size of recipient artery
(e) Occlusion related to blood flow

941. True about unstable angina: (T/F)
(a) Post MI Angina < 30 days
(b) New onset angina of at least class III severity within 1 month
(c) Resting angina is angina at rest lasting at least 20 min
(d) One feature of angina suggestive of atypical angina

942. DM cardiomyopathy: (T/F)
(a) Associated mostly with type 2 DM
(b) Can be seen without CAD changes

(c) Intramyocardial microangiopathy
(d) Increased fibrosis

943. MI after 7 days: (T/F)
(a) Total cholesterol increases
(b) Antioxidant are of no value
(c) Amiodarone should be given to all patients with LV dysfunction
(d) CKMB more sensitive than troponin
(e) CKMB assay more accurate than standard CKMB within 4 hours of onset of MI

944. Coronary calcification: (T/F)
(a) Calcium score predict obstructive CAD
(b) Accurate for lumen diameter

945. Post revascularization perfusion defect: (T/F)
(a) Periprocedural MI
(b) Side branch occlusion
(c) Ulcerated plaque stenting
(d) Coronary sinus retroperfusion
(e) Post cardiotomy syndrome

946. Cardiac troponin: (T/F)
(a) Cardiac specific troponin not seen in other tissues
(b) Troponin T is less specific than Troponin I
(c) Starts to increase 3-6 hours to peak 24-72 hours
(d) Not increased in myocarditis
(e) For better than LDH of late diagnosis of MI

947. IABP: (T/F)
(a) Augmented CO and increased DBP
(b) Increased afterload
(c) Not contraindicated in aortic dissection
(d) Refractory myocardial ischemia
(e) Useful in mechanical complication

948. Exercise in CAD: (T/F)
(a) Vasoconstriction in stenotic epicardial artery is associated with decreased blood flow
(b) Related with myocardial oxygen demand and not with subepicardial– endocardial gradient

949. T/F:
(a) > 75% silent ischemia in CSA
(b) Circadian variation present and peaks in evening
(c) Basal NO is decreased in vasospastic vessels in Prinzmetal's angina
(d) Angina is caused by sensory afferent of sympathetic and vagal fibres
(e) Ischemia causes decreased RMP and increased APD

950. T/F:
(a) GISSI I – intravenous STK better at 21 days
(b) GISSI II–t-PA better than STK, no significant difference
(c) GISSI III–perindopril in post MI LVF
(d) ISIS-4 –heparin, nitrate, Mg useful in MI
(e) ISIS-3 – APSAC better than STK

951. VF in acute MI: (T/F)
(a) Intravenous amiodarone is DOC
(b) Can occur without cardiogenic shock (CHF)
(c) Suppression of VPC can prevent VF
(d) Lignocaine decreases threshold for developing VF

952. Toxins: (T/F)
(a) Cocaine cause MI
(b) Cobalt – transient biventricular dysfunction
(c) Cobalt – restrictive CMP
(d) Phenothiazine – SCD
(e) Methylsergide – right sided valvular lesion

953. Nitrate tolerance: (T/F)
(a) S-nitroso captopril decrease nitrate tolerance
(b) ACE-I decreases nitrate tolerance
(c) Develops within 48 hours of intravenous infusion
(d) Fluid retention counteracts tolerance
(e) When develops it has to be stopped

954. True or False:
(a) Intimal tear in atherosclerotic plaque due to haemorrhage in medial vessels
(b) Always leads to occlusion of artery
(c) Can lead to plaque progression
(d) Can be clinically asymptomatic
(e) Leads to thrombus formation

955. IVUS – strong indication A/E:
(a) LMCA
(b) Instant stenosis
(c) Post transplant vasculopathy
(d) All true

956. Acute marginal artery is a branch of:
(a) RCA (b) LCx
(c) CAD (d) LMCA

957. **Post MI lipids A/E:**
(a) Can be measured in 24-48 hours
(b) Total cholesterol increases
(c) HDL decreases
(d) Total cholesterol/HDL ratio unreliable

958. **IABP A/E:**
(a) Post MI
(b) AR
(c) Decrease afterload
(d) Post MI–LMCA involved

959. **False statement:**
(a) 95% plaque rupture clinically silent
(b) Class II angina non invasive test normal does not need CAG

960. **Chronic stable angina BP target:**
(a) 120/80 (b) 130/80
(c) 130/85 (d) 140/90

961. **IVUS frequency:**
(a) 10 (b) 20
(c) 20-40 (d) 40-60

962. **RVMI A/E:**
(a) Aggressive intravenous fluid
(b) Intravenous NTG
(c) Sequential AV pacing
(d) Angioplasty

963. **Adenosine causes A/E:**
(a) Pulmonary vasodilation
(b) Coronary spasm
(c) Chest pain
(d) Bronchospasm

964. **Dabigatran dose as anticoagulant:**
(a) 150 mg BD (b) 50 mg BD
(c) 75 mg BD (d) 40 mg BD

965. **After Primary PCI of AMI, primary VF treatment, normal LV function, treatment not on discharge:**
(a) Amiodarone (b) Metoprolol
(c) Statin (d) Aspirin

966. **LV free wall rupture A/E:**
(a) Transplantation ↓ risk
(b) Primary PCI ↓ risk
(c) Bimodal peak – < 24 hours and 3-5 days
(d) More common in first MI

967. **Dressler syndrome:**
(a) After 1-8 weeks
(b) Steroid used preferably within 4 weeks (DOC)
(c) ESR ↑ characteristically
(d) Leukocytosis

968. **IVUS frequency used:**
(a) <10 Hz (b) 10-15 Hz
(c) 15-20 Hz (d) >20 Hz

969. **Rate pressure produced during TMT:**
(a) Mean BP × target HR (b) Mean BP × peak HR
(c) SBP × THR (d) SBP × Peak HR

970. **Vessel used for CABG A/E:**
(a) Right IMA
(b) Left radial
(c) Inferior epigastric artery
(d) Superior mesenteric artery

971. **FFR above which it is not significant:**
(a) > 0.75 (b) > 0.8
(c) > 0.65 (d) > 0.7

972. **Dressler syndrome A/E:**
(a) 1-8 weeks
(b) NSAIDS + steroids useful in refractory cases
(c) Aspirin TOC
(d) Leukocytosis is commonly seen

973. **TNK dose is:**
(a) 10 unit double bolus
(b) 1.5 MU over 1 hour
(c) 30-50 mg according to body weight
(d) 100 mg over 90 min

974. **Trop I A/E:**
(a) Not seen in extensive skeletal muscle injury
(b) Present only in myocardial tissue
(c) Heterophile antibodies can lead to false positive
(d) Present in fetal skeletal muscle

975. **NO mediated vasodilatation by:**
(a) Carvedilol (b) Atenolol
(c) Nebivolol (d) Bisoprolol

976. **Ranolazine A/E:**
(a) Blocks late Na current (b) Prolongs APD
(c) Prolongs QT (d) Approved for CSA

977. After 72 hours of acute MI, patient is admitted, best time to do lipid profile:

(a) On admission (b) 8 weeks
(c) 2 weeks (d) 16 weeks

978. Counselling in CHD A/E:

(a) 4-10% chance of recurrence
(b) Increased chance of recurrence if first degree relative affected
(c) Fetal echo advised at first trimester
(d) CHD may be similar to parents

979. DM is concerned as CAD risk equivalent because:

(a) According to modified natural history of T2 DM with treatment macrovascular complication are responsible for most mortality than acute mortality
(b) Natural history – mortality after 7 years of DM is severe as ACS instant DM
(c) All diabetics develops ACS

980. Ivabradine A/E:

(a) Inhibits if current
(b) Decrease sinus rate
(c) Negative inotropic effect as a side effect
(d) Time to angina delayed

981. CAG contraindication:

(a) In a patient with low probability to establish diagnosis
(b) Repeatedly admitted for chest pain
(c) Morbid obesity with suspected CAD
(d) Patient with stable angina who survived SCD

982. ECG show ST ↑in lead III > Lead II and ↑ST in V_1 probable lesion in:

(a) Dominant LCX (b) Proximal to mid RCA
(c) PDA (d) Distal RCA

983. Intramural CAD seen in:

(a) RA (b) AS
(c) Scleroderma (d) MCTD

984. LMWH—which is true?

(a) More protein bound than UFH
(b) ↑ Vascular permeability
(c) ↑ Platelet inhibition
(d) Reversal with protamine easier with LMWH
(e) None

985. Accelerated atherosclerosis:

(a) Pentoxyphylline (b) Ritonavir
(c) Pentamidine (d) Cyclosporine

986. Prinzmetal angina diagnostic test for vasospasm:

(a) Ach (b) Hyperventilation
(c) Cold pressor test (d) Methylergometrine

987. Frequency of IVUS in coronaries:

(a) 2-3 MHz (b) 6-10 MHZ
(c) 20-30 MHz (d) 40-100 MHz

988. Premature CAD in female first degree relative or sibling:

(a) Age ≥ 50 (b) Age ≥ 55
(c) Age > 45 (d) Age > 65

989. Middle cardiac vein accompanies:

(a) LAD (b) PDA
(c) Diagonal (d) Acute marginal artery
(e) LCx

990. Not given in RVMI:

(a) IV NTG (b) AV sequential pacing
(c) IV fluids (d) Thrombolytics

991. Successful thrombolysis indicated by A/E:

(a) Settling of pain (b) Settling of ST segment
(c) AIVR (d) All true

992. IABP A/E:

(a) LVF with MI (b) LVF with AR
(c) Decrease afterload (d) LVF with VSD

993. Patient of stable angina with BP= 220/110, treatment A/E:

(a) Sublingual nifedipine
(b) Sublingual NTG
(c) Intravenous NTG
(d) Intravenous metoprolol
(e) Oral captopril

994. Dose of adenosine to treat PSVT to be increased if patient is taking:

(a) Theophylline (b) Dipyridamole
(c) Has CAD (d) Diabetes

995. True statement about lidocaine is:

(a) Lidocaine not used for prophylaxis of VT/VF in MI
(b) Decreased mortality by 13%
(c) Used in EF< 35%

996. New murmur in AWMI A/E:

(a) Dynamic LVOT obstruction

(b) Dynamic RVOT obstruction
(c) MR
(d) VSD

997. Patient presents with acute chest pain 2 hours with ST depression in inferior leads, intravenous NTG started, BP falls to 80/60 mm Hg and pain decreases, all possible *except:*

(a) Dissection (b) Esophageal spasm
(c) RVMI

998. True A/E:

(a) Dabigatran – DTI
(b) Rivaroxaban – Anti Xa inhibitor
(c) Fondaparinux – Anti Xa inhibitor
(d) Cangrelor – P2 Y12 inhibitor
(e) All true

999. All control CAD *except:*

(a) BP control (b) Smoking cessation
(c) Vitamin C therapy (d) Physical activity

1000. FREEDOM trial A/E:

(a) Included only diabetic
(b) Included multivessel disease
(c) Surgery beneficial in severe CAD
(d) Bare metal stent used for percutaneous revascularisation

1001. Score system for angioplasty success:

(a) Syntax (b) Euro
(c) GRACE (d) TIMI

1002. ST elevation in V3 – V6, II and avF suggest:

(a) Proximal LAD occlusion
(b) Distal LAD occlusion
(c) LMCA occlusion
(d) Simultaneous LAD and RCA occlusion

1003. RVMI present with all *except:*

(a) PCWP > 18 (b) SBP < 90
(c) RVEDP > 8 (d) CI < 2.2 $l/min/m^2$

1004. Post MI VSR after thrombolysis most common occurs:

(a) Within 48 hours (b) After 3-5 days
(c) After 5-7 days (d) After 7-14 days

1005. Ranolazine level increased A/E:

(a) Hepatic dysfunction (b) Renal dysfunction
(c) Ketaconazole (d) Digoxin

1006. IVUS suggestive ↑ future events:

(a) Lumen area < 4 mm^2 (b) Thin fibrous cap
(c) > 70% plaque burden (d) 10% necrotic area

1007. A male patient with acute onset of breathlessness with weakness lasting for 20 min, 2 hour back with no chest pain. ECG shows non specific ST/T changes. Which of the following group justify presence of silent MI?

(a) Elderly DM
(b) Premenopausal female
(c) Unstable angina on treatment
(d) Inferior wall MI

1008. Intervention is done when fractional flow reserve is:

(a) 50 (b) 75
(c) 90 (d) 30

1009. Which drug has shown benefit over clopidogrel in patient undergoing PCI and already on aspirin in mortality?

(a) Prasugrel (b) Cangrelor
(c) Ticagrelor (d) Sulfinpyrazone

1010. A 75 years old male come with typical chest pain so what will be probability of CAD?

(a) 30% (b) 70%
(c) 90% (d) 30%

1011. SA node is located in:

(a) Near right side of interatrial septum
(b) Junction of RA/SVC

1012. Duration of sublingual nitrates:

(a) 30–300 minutes (b) 10– 30 minutes
(c) 2–6 hours (d) 12–24 hours

1013. In post MI patients, predictor of mortality and SCD is by:

(a) EF (b) HR variability
(c) T – alternans (d) QT alternans

1014. In acute myocardial infarction, all of the following decreases mortality *except:*

(a) Amiodarone (b) B blockers
(c) ACE-I (d) Epelerenone

1015. Patient is currently on aspirin and clopidogrel. He has to undergo an elective major surgery. How many days before surgery should the drugs be stopped?

(a) 1 day (b) 2 days
(c) 5 days (d) 7 days

1016. Which is true?

(a) In LMCA stenosis, PCI is better
(b) In TVD, PCI is better
(c) In CAD + LV dysfunction, PCI is better than surgery
(d) Randomized trial has shown that PCI may be used as a therapy in STEMI

1017. Anterior wall STEMI which of the following is least commonly seen in ECG?

(a) Short QT
(b) ST depression in inferior lead
(c) ST elevation in avR
(d) RBBB

1018. Poly pill contains A/E:

(a) Beta blocker (b) Folic acid
(c) Thiazide diuretics (d) CCB

1019. Emergency CABG A/E:

(a) USA
(b) MI with cardiogenic shock
(c) Left main stenosis of 40%
(d) Post MI VSD

1020. DTI is:

(a) Apixaban (b) Rivaroxaban
(c) Dabigatran (d) Fondaparinux

1021. Prasugrel C/I A/E:

(a) Weight < 60
(b) Age > 60
(c) History of stroke in 6 months
(d) Thrombolytic treatment in 1 week

1022. Reversible inhibitor of P2 Y12 is:

(a) Clopidogrel (b) Prasugrel
(c) Ticagrelor (d) Ticlopidine

1023. Coronary blood supply A/E:

(a) SA node supplied by RCA in 90%
(b) PPA from LCx in 20%
(c) Both LA and LV supplied by LAD
(d) LCx descends in ant. IV groove and supplies the apex

1024. Neonate with ↓ed femoral pulsations on day 1. On day 7, develops cyanosis of lower abdomen and lower limbs appropriate treatment:

(a) PGE 1 infusion (b) Ibuprofen
(c) Balloon atrial septotomy

1025. PCI to left main ostial stenosis according to ACC:

(a) I (b) IIa
(c) IIb (d) III

1026. All true *except:*

(a) Asprin causes mortality reduction by 30%
(b) Thrombolysis causes mortality reduction by 25-50%
(c) BB are more beneficial with heart failure
(d) I/V metoprolol routinely given in AC MI

1027. On label use of DES A/E:

(a) Bifurcating lesion
(b) Stenosis—50-99%
(c) Vessel diameter 2.5-3.5 mm
(d) Length < 30 mm

1028. IVUS use most common:

(a) Vulnerability of plaque
(b) Stent apposition
(c) Bifurcation tracking
(d) Chronic total occlusion

1029. Highest mortality in MI:

(a) PCWP< 18, Cardiac Index < 2.2
(b) >18, > 2.2
(c) < 18, > 2.2
(d) >18, < 2.2

1030. Ant WMI, EF < 25%, LBBB class II at discharge:

(a) Drugs only (b) Bivent pacing + drug
(c) Drugs + AICD (d) Dual chamber + drug

1031. Use of NAC in CAG:

(a) Prophylaxis of CIN
(b) Treatment of CIN
(c) All patients of CRF
(d) High dose contrast with CHF

1032. T wave in ECG +ve deflection above isoelectric line:

(a) Change of repolarization from depolarization of ventricles
(b) Repolarization of purkinze
(c) Depolarization of his bundle

1033. RCA culprit vessel indicated by:

(a) ST ↓ in I, avl (b) Tall r in V1
(c) ST ↓ V1V2V3 (d) T inv V4R

1034. ICH with thrombolysis risk factors:
(a) High age, low BW (b) Low age, low BW
(c) Low age, high BW (d) High age, high BW

1035. On the basis of EBM true:
(a) High dose statin in all ACS
(b) 1° PCI in all STEMI TOC
(c) ICD in all stemi with low EF at discharge
(d) None

1036. Post MI on amiodarone 200 mg/d develop peripheral neuropathy next:
(a) Continue 200 + add pyridoxine
(b) Stop for 4 weeks start 100 mg
(c) Switch to flecainide
(d) Immediately ↓ dose to 100

1037. Most common coronary artery in atherosclerosis:
(a) RCA (b) LAD
(c) Left Cx (d) PDA

1038. False about dominance of coronaries:
(a) RCA 75% (b) LCA 75%
(c) 15% co-dominant (d) 10% LCA

1039. Coronary art surgery true:
(a) Claude beck – did 1st anastomosis
(b) Winberg 1st carotid endarterectomy
(c) P. Sen – direct IMA to coronary anastomosis
(d) Cervical and up dorsal sympathectomy for angina

1040. IVUS most commonly used in:
(a) Stent implantation (b) Vulnerable plaque
(c) To open CTO (d) Bifurcation lesion

1041. According to EBM true is:
(a) High dose statin in all ACS
(b) Primary PCI in all STEMI
(c) ICD at discharge in all with low EF
(d) (a) and (b) true
(e) All true

1042. Descending Ao proximal ductus in foetus:
(a) Isthmus (b) Knuckle
(c) Spiral

1043. Blood supply of heart A/E:
(a) LCx in anterior interventricular groove
(b) SA node mostly by RCA
(c) Ac. marginal branch of RCA

1044. Blood supply of bundle of HIS:
(a) Interventricular branch of RCA
(b) Interventricular branch of LCA
(c) Marginals
(d) Nodal

1045. No. of lives saved in Patient of IWMI in 12 hours of presentation with thrombolysis:
(a) 8 (b) 15
(c) 25 (d) 50

1046. Acute MI within 19 hours of presentation, best long term survival:
(a) B blockers (b) Aspirin
(c) Thrombolysis (d) PCI + Stenting

1047. Patient undergoing CAG suddenly develop blue toes azotaemia:
(a) Multiple cholesterol emboli
(b) A dissection
(c) Athero emboli
(d) Acute coronary syndrome

1048. Probability of developing HTN in life time of 45 years old till 90 years of life:
(a) 30% (b) 90%
(c) 50% (d) 10%

1049. Child with anterolateral MI with LVH, diagnosis:
(a) HOCM
(b) ALCAPA
(c) Endomyocardial fibroelastosis
(d) LV non compaction

1050. Arterial disease caused by:
(a) Intimal damage caused by shear stress
(b) Smooth muscle damage
(c) Pericytes injury
(d) Bone marrow response

1051. Thrombolysis Absolute C/I A/E:
(a) Severe dementia
(b) Embolic CVA— 6 months back
(c) GI bleed 4 weeks back
(d) Unruptured aneurysm

1052. Type B lesion A/E:
(a) Tubular lesion
(b) No ostial lesion
(c) Partial thrombotic occlusion
(d) Complete occlusion

1053. Subclinical atherosclerosis by:

(a) ABI (b) EBCT
(c) MDCT (d) All of the above

1054. GP IIb/IIIa inhibitor True:

(a) Tirofiban preferred in renal failure
(b) Tirofiban produces more thrombocytopenia compared to other GP IIb/IIIa
(c) Cryoprecipitate for abciximab toxicity
(d) Abciximab has long biological t ½

1055. Abciximab A/E:

(a) Noncompetitive inhibition
(b) Plasma t½ < 26 min
(c) Biological t ½ upto platelet life i.e. up to 7 days
(d) Persists for > 14 days after stopping infusion

1056. Infarct expansion best suggested by:

(a) Ventricular arrhythmia
(b) Systolic dysfunction with S3 with pulmonary congestion
(c) Aneurysm
(d) Pulmonary edema

1057. Venous graft vs native atherosclerosis True is:

(a) Less thrombus burden
(b) No fibrous cap
(c) Focal lesion
(d) Statin not effective

1058. True A/E:

(a) Anterolateral papillary muscle is single
(b) Most common supplied by RCA
(c) LCx close to mitral valvular apparatus
(d) Middle scallop of post MV is most common to prolapsed

1059. Epidemiology about CAD in India all *except:*

(a) Stroke 3 times more common than CAD
(b) CAD accounts of 75% of CV death
(c) CA disease accounts for 24% of total death
(d) Fat intake in Indian diet is more

1060. MI — 4 days — autopsy shows:

(a) Granulomatous inflammation
(b) Neutrophils + muscle necrosis
(c) Macrophages + collagen deposition
(d) Granulation tissue

1061. Absolute C/I of fibrinolysis:

(a) Embolic CVA 6 months back
(b) Severe dementia
(c) Duodenal ulcer with bleed × 4 weeks back
(d) Incidentally detected remote cerebral aneurysm (unruptured)

1062. Catheters in coronary angio all *except:*

(a) Ludkins (b) Amplatz
(c) Sones (d) Coumard

1063. Functional assessment of intermediate coronary lesion all *except:*

(a) FFR
(b) Coronary flow reserve
(c) Quantitative coronary angiography
(d) IVUS

1064. Most important coronary heart disease risk factor:

(a) Smoking (b) Advanced age
(c) DM

1065. Hs-CRP ↓ all *except:*

(a) Aspirin (b) Niacin
(c) Fibrate (d) Pioglitazone

1066. Interventricular septum best visualized by which view?

(a) RAO without tilt (b) RAO with caudal tilt
(c) LAO with cranial tilt (d) LAO with caudal tilt

1067. Pericarditis ST elevation seen in all *except:*

(a) avL (b) avR
(c) I (d) II

1068. About MI true:

(a) RBBB with AWMI indicate distal LAD
(b) ST ↑ II > III indicate RCA
(c) aVR ST ↑ in AWMI ind. Proximal to 1st septal perforator
(d) Q wave

1069. % of blood in venoms circulation:

(a) 45 (b) 55
(c) 65 (d) 75

1070. Most important prognostic marker after MI:

(a) Angina at end of exercise
(b) ST depression at end of exercise
(c) Inability to exercise
(d) Reversible perfusion defect

1071. Most common reperfusion arrhythmias in IWMI:

(a) Sinus bradycardia (b) CHB
(c) AIVR (d) PJRT

1072. Anterolateral papillary muscle infarction involves:

(a) LAD with LCX (b) LAD
(c) RCA

1073. Absolute contraindication of catheterization:

(a) Severe anaphylaxis
(b) Renal function deranged
(c) LVF
(d) None

1074. CAD seen with A/E:

(a) RA (b) Amyloidosis
(c) Homocystinuria (d) Hurler

1075. True in Gp IIb IIIa inhibitor A/E:

(a) Abciximab is highly specific for Gp IIb IIIa
(b) Tirofiban T ½ is 2 hours
(c) Eptifibatide is cyclic heptapeptide
(d) Gp IIb IIIa should be given with heparin

1076. UFH vs LMWH true is:

(a) LMWH cause less HIT
(b) LMWH have increase serum protein binding
(c) LMWH more renal clearance than heparin
(d) More decrease in platelet action by LMWH

1077. In acute MI, PCI by experienced operator true is A/E:

(a) Decrease stroke by PCI as compared to thrombolysis
(b) PCI has less mortality
(c) PCI with stent has less mortality and reinfection than angioplasty
(d) Post PCI flow is more than thrombolysis

1078. 30 RAO 40 Cranial is useful for:

(a) Posterior IVS (b) RVOT
(c) All 4 chamber (d) Anterior 2/3rd of IVS

1079. Most common coronary perfusion defect:

(a) Coronary AV fistula
(b) ALCAPA
(c) RCA from left cusp
(d) LAD from right cusp with path through aorta and RVOT

1080. Free wall rupture all true *except:*

(a) Common in prior MI
(b) Common in first MI
(c) In elderly
(d) Early thrombolysis decreases incidence

1081. Incidence of CAD all true *except:*

(a) CAD counts for > 50% CVS deaths
(b) Stroke/MI– 3:1
(c) Heart disease – 24% of deaths
(d) Proportion of calorie derived from fats more in India than other countries

1082. ST elevation in non Q wave lead:

(a) Specific coronary artery involvement
(b) Exercise ST elevation with Q wave – marker of CAD

1083. Endeavour stent:

(a) BMS (b) DES
(c) ASD device closure (d) VSD device closure

1084. Rupture in MI common in A/E:

(a) Previous MI (b) Old age

1085. Pericarditis A/E:

(a) Amiodarone (b) Emetine

1086. Factor predisposing the coronary artery to rupture causing acute coronary syndrome is:

(a) Distal coronary artery lesion
(b) Coronary bifurcation lesion
(c) Small lipid core in the plaque
(d) Large amount of smooth muscles with in the plaque shoulder

1087. Superficial plaque erosion (as compared to plaque rupture) is commonly associated with:

(a) Diabetes
(b) Male patients
(c) Coronary vasospasm
(d) Elderly patients

1088. Which of the following is true regarding ADP receptor antagonists?

(a) Thienopyridines predominantly act through P2Y1 receptors
(b) Prasugrel use is safe in elderly patients
(c) Ticagrelor is directly acting, oral thienopyridine agent
(d) Cangrelor is a reversible platelet inhibitor

1089. Which of the following statements is true regarding acute mitral regurgitation following acute myocardial infarction (MI)?

(a) Occurs more commonly due to anterolateral papillary muscle
(b) Can occur with both large or focal area of MI
(c) Occurs more commonly with anterior wall MI than inferior wall MI
(d) Usually occurs within 24 hours of MI

1090. The most common benign congenital coronary anomaly is:

(a) Left circumflex (LCx) coronary artery arising from right aortic sinus
(b) Left main coronary artery (LMCA) arising from right aortic sinus
(c) Single coronary artery
(d) Right Coronary Artery (RCA) arising from left aortic sinus

1091. All of the following are features of cholesterol embolization following cardiac catheterization *except:*

(a) Eosinophilia
(b) Renal dysfunction
(c) Livedo reticular is of lower limb
(d) Absent popliteal artery pulsation

1092. All of the following are true for assessment of the coronary artery using Fractional flow reserve (FFR) *except:*

(a) Intravenous nitro glycerine infusion may be used for inducing hyperaemia in place of adenosine in patients with lung disease
(b) Is affected by the amount of viable myocardium supplied by the artery
(c) Is influenced by collateral flow to the artery
(d) Is useful for physiologic assessment of side branch ostial disease in bifurcation angioplasty

1093. Absolute contraindication to thrombolytic therapy for acute myocardial infarction include(s):

(a) Prolonged CPR for more than 10 minutes
(b) Ischemic stroke of 1 hour duration
(c) Intracranial haemorrhage 3 months back
(d) All of the above

1094. Which of the following statements is true for Reteplase (Recombinant plasminogen activator, r-PA)?

(a) It is given as a single bolus dose
(b) It is less fibrin selective than alteplase (t-PA)
(c) It is given as weight adjusted doses
(d) It has a short half-life than alteplase (t-PA)

1095. In the setting of primary percutaneous coronary intervention (Primary PCI), the benefit of drug eluting stent (DES) over bare metal stent (BMS) is:

(a) Reduced stroke
(b) Reduced death
(c) Reduced target vessel revascularization
(d) Reduced stent thrombosis

1096. The most appropriate step for a patient of acute coronary syndrome who developed heparin induced thrombocytopenia (HIT) on unfractionated heparin (UFH) should be:

(a) Switch UFH to low molecular weight heparin (LMWH)
(b) Reduced the dose of UFH to half
(c) Switch to bivalirudin
(d) Switch to warfarin

1097. Which of the following patients with STEMI will have worst prognosis?

(a) 40-year male diabetic with inferior wall MI, clear chest, no LVS3
(b) 70-year-old patient with inferior wall MI and basal crepts and LVS3
(c) 60-year male with anterior wall MI and clear chest, no LVS3
(d) 75-year male with old anterior wall MI, acute IWMI, LVEF 45%, clear chest

1098. Patency rate of left internal mammary artery for LAD artery at 10 years is approximately:

(a) 75% (b) 80%
(c) 90% (d) 99%

1099. A 30-year-old patient has undergone percutaneous transvenous mitral commissurotomy (PTMC). He developed cardiac tamponade during the procedure. A total of 5,000 units of unfractionated heparin (UFH) was given during the procedure. All of the following statements are true for administration of protamine sulphate to neutralize UFH *except:*

(a) Each mg of protamine neutralizes 100 units of active heparin
(b) It should be given as fast bolus for immediate action
(c) It can cause pulmonary hypertension
(d) Maximal dose which can be given is usually 50 mg

1100. A 55-year-old man presents to emergency with acute inferior wall myocardial infarction. The blood pressure is 78/60 mm Hg. Heart rate is 50 beats/minute. Jugular venous pressure is elevated. He is still complaining of ongoing chest pain. Immediate steps should include all of the following *except:*

(a) Give aspirin (325 mg)
(b) Get right-sided precordial leads
(c) Give injection morphine for pain relief
(d) Take the patient for primary PCI

1101. A 65-year-old female suffered inferior wall myocardial infarction. The left ventricular ejection fraction is 55% with mild regional wall motion abnormality in inferior wall on echocardiography. She underwent coronary angioplasty with placement of drug-eluting stent in right coronary artery. Which of the following treatments is most likely to result in mortality benefit on follow-up:

(a) Metoprolol (50 mg/daily)
(b) Aldactone (25 mg/daily)
(c) Atorvastatin (80 mg/daily)
(d) Ramipril (5 mg/daily)

1102. A 75 years hypertensive male patient presents with severe chest pain of 2 hours duration. Blood pressure in right upper limb is 160/100 and left upper limb is 100/70. Heart rate is 110 beats/minute. There is 2 mm ST segment elevation in inferior leads. Echo reveals large pericardial effusion. The immediate management should include:

(a) Urgent pericardiocentesis
(b) Urgent coronary angiography and PCI of culprit vessel
(c) Urgent transesophageal echocardiography
(d) Urgent contrast-enhanced CT of chest and abdomen

1103. A 45-year-old patient gives history of severe contrast-induced allergy one year back. Now he presents to the emergency with extensive acute anterior wall myocardial infarction. The correct treatment strategy should be:

(a) Prefer thrombolytic agent over primary PCI
(b) Give methylprednisolone, diphenhydramine and ranitidine as early as possible and take the patient for primary PCI
(c) Give methylprednisolone, diphenhydramine and ranitidine as early as possible and wait for 2-3 hours for primary PCI
(d) Give methylprednisolone and ranitidine as early as possible and send the patient for bypass surgery after coronary angiography

1104. A 60-year-old male presented to emergency department with sudden onset chest pain and hypotension. He gives history of air travel for 12 hours, two days prior to presentation. The best diagnostic test should be:

(a) D-dimer
(b) Transesophageal echocardiography (TEE)
(c) Invasive coronary angiography
(d) Multi-slice CT angiography

1105. A 19-year-old male with mild infundibular pulmonary stenosis was found to have double aortic arch on CT angiography. On retrospective questioning, he reported dysphagia. Recommended treatment:

(a) Reassurance and no therapy
(b) Division of non-dominant arch
(c) Surgery is indicated only when life-threatening symptoms are present in view of the high risk of surgery
(d) Prokinetics like itopride

1106. All of the following constrict atherosclerotic coronaries *except:*

(a) Serotonin (b) Thromboxane
(c) Endothelin (d) Papaverine

1107. All of the following drugs are useful in coronary 'no flow' phenomenon *except:*

(a) Nitroglycerine (b) Adenosine
(c) Nicorandil (d) Sodium nitroprusside

1108. The statement regarding ventricular free wall rupture complicating myocardial infarction (MI) include all of the following *except:*

(a) It is more likely to occur in patients with a history of prior MI
(b) It typically occurs within the first 4 days after infarction
(c) It is more common in elderly patients and in women
(d) A history of hypertension is a risk factor for free wall rupture

1109. One of the following is a vasoconstrictor:

(a) Adenosine (b) Thromboxane
(c) Dipyridamole (d) Papavarine

1110. Which of the following is not a feature of right ventricular infarction?

(a) Square root sign
(b) Kussmaul sign

(c) Acute pulmonary edema
(d) Pulsus paradoxus

1111. One of the following is a mechanical complication after acute MI:
(a) Ventricular fibrillation
(b) Ventricular septal rupture
(c) Ventricular aneurysm
(d) Pericardial effusion

1112. Dressler syndrome occurs after:
(a) Acute myocardial infarction
(b) Acute rheumatic fever
(c) Infective endocarditis
(d) Congestive heart failure

1113. ST segment elevation is seen in:
(a) Acute myocardial infarction
(b) Prinzmetal angina
(c) Acute pericarditis
(d) All of the above

1114. Contraindications to beta blockers:
(a) Severe depression
(b) Raynaud phenomenon
(c) Peripheral vascular disease
(d) All of the above

1115. Ankle-Brachial index in critical limb ischemia:
(a) <0.5 (b) <0.8
(c) <0.9 (d) <1.0

1116. Euro score–the risk is high if score is:
(a) ≥ 6 (b) ≥ 4
(c) ≥ 10 (d) ≥ 15

1117. Prothrombinase contains:
(a) Va (b) Xa
(c) Both of the above (d) None of the above

1118. All of the following conditions produce hyper-coagulable state *except:*
(a) Protein C deficiency
(b) Antithrombin excess
(c) Factor V leiden mutation
(d) Prothrombin gene mutation

1119. One of the following drug has long platelet bound half life:
(a) Abciximab (b) Eptifibatide
(c) Tirofiban (d) All of the above

1120. One among the following drug has 100% bio-availability:
(a) Heparin (b) Enaxaparin
(c) Fandaparinux (d) Rivaroxaban

1121. Type C coronary lesion:
(a) Eccentric
(b) Total occlusion > 3 months
(c) Bifurcation lesion
(d) Ostial lesion

1122. Post PCI – with of the following is useful *except*:
(a) CT angio most useful after acute MI
(b) OCT – can't recognise necrotic tissue
(c) MUGA – Can differentiate between dead and hibernating myocardium
(d) ECHO

1123. Hibernating myocardium:
(a) Decrease perfusion normal function
(b) Decrease perfusion impaired function
(c) Normal perfusion decreased function
(d) Normal perfusion normal function

1124. After 15 minutes occlusion, staining is seen for:
(a) 1 hour (b) 6 hours
(c) 2 hours (d) 4 hours

1125. Absol. C/I for thrombolysis:
(a) Prolonged CPR
(b) Previous ICH
(c) BP – 180/110
(d) Active peptic ulcer

1126. Stable CAD – high risk:
(a) Stress induced LV dilation
(b) Wall motion abnormality at heart rate
(c) CAC
(d) Myo. perfusion defect > 10% @ Rest

1127. Ac. MI – Mortality benefit:
(a) β-blocker + ACEi + Aspirin
(b) β-blocker + ACEi + Nicorandil
(c) Nitrate + β-blocker + Aspirin
(d) Diuretic + CCB

1128. TRITON time 38 tiral for:
(a) Clopidogrel (b) Prasugrel
(c) Ticagrelor (d) Ticlopidine

1129. All are thienopyridines *except*:

(a) Ticagrelor (b) Ticlopidine
(c) Clopidogrel (d) Prasugrel

1130. FFR signifying non-significant stenosis:

(a) > 0.8 (b) 0.75 – 0.9
(c) < 0.75 (d) > 0.9

1131. PCI vs fibrinolysis, 300 death in 2300 patients in fibrinolysis, 200 death in 1300 in PCI, odds ratio:

(a) 0.065 (b) 0.65
(c) 0.1% (d) 9.1%

1132. Which is incorrect?

(a) $R_2 > R_3 > R_1$
(b) Without stenosis, epicardial resistance (R1) is least
(c) R_2 is resistance of arterioles and resistance vessel, which is more in subepicardial than subendocardial region
(d) R_3 is dynamic resistance, related to cardiac contraction

1133. Discrete and ostial stenosis mean:

(a) <5 mm and within 2 mm of ostium
(b) <10 mm and within 3 mm of ostium
(c) <10 mm and within 2 mm of ostium
(d) 10-20 mm and within 3 mm of ostium

1134. False statement:

(a) Collaterals can provide up to 50% of antegrade flow
(b) Chronic total occlusion with collateralizations can never cause myocardial necrosis
(c) Kugel branch between RCA proximal with PDA
(d) Vienuens collaterals between LAD and RCA

1135. All showed no benefit of thrombus aspiration in primary PCI, *except*:

(a) TAPAS (b) AIMR
(c) Expert (d) TOTAL

1136. All true about aspirin *except*:

(a) NSAID reduce antiplatelet action
(b) Irreversible Cox-1 inhibitor
(c) With chewable route, antiplatelet action can be achieved in 15 minutes
(d) Action duration 7-10 days

1137. Indication for dual antiplatelets, in patients managed with fibrinolytic therapy:

(a) 1 year (b) 6 months
(c) 3 months (d) Lifelong

1138. Failed thrombolytics, next step:

(a) PCl (b) Observe
(c) Re-fibrinolysis (d) CABG

1139. Not a class I indication for PCI:

(a) Symptom < 12 hours
(b) Cardiogenic shock, irrespective of symptom duration
(c) Symptom 12-24 hours

1140. 2 hours of MI, LVEF-20%, next management:

(a) Immediately ICD
(b) Wait till 40 days, repeat echo, in lung < 35% —ICD-
(c) ICD if EPS +ve

1141. 60 years old patient on blockers, for TMT, expected heart rate:

(a) 160 (b) 122

1142. In FFR, true statement:

(a) Significant is < 0.90
(b) NTG high dose is given in respiratory patient where adenosine cannot be given
(c) Depends on SBP and heart rate
(d) Depends on amount of infarcted myocardium

1143. Agent not causing ACS:

(a) Cisplatin (b) 5-Fluorouracil
(c) Imatinib (d) Interferon alpha

1144. ↑ sed cardiovascular mortality in CAD with diabetes:

(a) Saroglitazar (b) Empagliflozin
(c) Sitagliptin (d) Adenaxamet

1145. In diabetic patient planned for CAG, which day should be stopped prophylactically?

(a) Ramipril (b) Chlorthalidone
(c) Insulin (d) Metformin

1146. Exercise text, all have poor prognosis *except*:

(a) Early HR acceleration in 1st minute
(b) Abnormal heart rate recovery
(c) ↑ BP from baseline
(d) Low peak SBP

1147. In 2 vessel disease, NYHA-II, angina on exertion, PCI to be done for:

(a) Symptomatic relief
(b) SCD prevention
(c) Prevention of MI
(d) Prevention of asymptomatic ischemia

1148. Rotational atherectomy not done:

(a) SVG
(b) Ostial lesion
(c) 1,1,1 medina bifurcation lesion

1149. Patient with chest pain, CAG revealed 60% stenosis, next best investigation to determine functional significance of lesion:

(a) FFR (b) IVUS
(c) OCT (d) NIRS

1150. ECG:

(a) LMCA (b) Proximal LAD
(c) LCX

1151. Troponin level does not increase in following condition:

(a) STEMI (b) Myocarditis
(c) Renal disease (d) Liver disease

1152. Plaque fissuring/disruption is less common in:

(a) Lipid burden in atheroma .70%
(b) Thin cap atheroma
(c) Thick cap atheroma
(d) Luminal area of stenotic area, 4.0 mm square

1153. Following is true for atrial infarction incidence in patients with stemi:

(a) 10% (b) 5%
(c) 15% (d) 25%

1154. Infarct expansion is less in following condition:

(a) Diabetes mellitus
(b) Hypertrophied myocardium
(c) Multivessel disease
(d) Gout

1155. Following criteria favours myocardial infarction in presence of LBBB *except:*

(a) ST segment elevation greater than 1 mm and concordant with QRS complex
(b) ST segment depression greater than 1 mm in v1, v2, v3
(c) ST segment depression greater than 1 mm in II, III, AVF
(d) ST segment elevation greater than 5 mm and discordant with QRS complex

1156. Which one of the following is not true for MRI in acute myocardial infarction?

(a) It assesses perfusion in infarcted and non infarcted myocardium
(b) Repurfused myocardium
(c) Assess coronary anatomy precisely
(d) Identify myocardial fibrosis, wall thinning

1157. Which one of the following thrombolytic agent is more fibrin specific?

(a) Streptokinase (b) Tenectaplase
(c) Alteplase (d) Reteplase

1158. Which one of the following is not true in classification of TIMI flow grade?

(a) TIMI grade 1 (b) TIMI grade 2
(c) TIMI grade 3 (d) TIMI grade 4

1159. What minimum level of damage to left ventricular myocardium is required in patients with STEMI for cardiogenic shock?

(a) 50% (b) 60%
(c) 70% (d) 80%

1160. Which one of the following is not true for right ventricular infarction?

(a) Hypotension (b) Kussmaul sign
(c) Elevated JVP (d) Basal crepitations in lungs

1161. Which one of the following is not true for pseudoaneurysm of LV after infarction?

(a) It lacks any elements of myocardial wall
(b) It is made up of organized thrombus and pericardium
(c) It communicates with LV cavity through a narrow neck
(d) It communicates with LV cavity through a wide neck

1162. Which one of the following is not true for Ranolazine?

(a) It inhibits late inward sodium current
(b) It is used in angina
(c) It prolongs QT interval
(d) It decreases heart rate

1163. Which one of the following drug is not used for provocative testing for vasospastic angina?

(a) Hyperventilation
(b) Intracoronary acetylcholine
(c) Intracoronary ergonovine
(d) Intracoronary phenylepinephrine

1164. Coronary calcification on computerised tomography is helpful in predicting obstructive CAD. Which one of the following is true?

(a) Sensitivity 90% (b) Sensitivity 50%
(c) Sensitivity 60% (d) Sensitivity 80%

1165. Which one of the following has no survival benefit in coronary artery disease?
(a) Aspirin (b) Beta blockers
(c) Ace inhibitors (d) Antioxidants

1166. Which one of the following is not true for Nicorandil?
(a) It is potassium channel activator
(b) It can produce ulcerations in gastrointestinal tract
(c) It has negative chronotropic effect
(d) It is venodilator and coronary dilator

1167. Which one of the following drug is not used in drug eluting stent?
(a) Zotarolimus (b) Cyclosporine
(c) Sirolimus (d) Paclitaxel

1168. Incidence of acute MI due to aortic dissection is:
(a) 5% to 10% (b) 1% to 2%
(c) 20% to 30% (d) 40% to 50%

1169. In TRITONTIMI 38 trial clopidogrel was compared with:
(a) Cangrelor (b) Prasugrel
(c) Ticagrelor (d) Vorapaxar

1170. How much fold risk of infarction increases with use of cocaine (in first 60 minutes after cocaine use)?
(a) 2 fold (b) 5 fold
(c) 10 fold (d) 24 fold

1171. POBA:
(a) Plain old balloon angioplasty
(b) Patient oriented balloon angioplasty
(c) Post operative balloon angioplasty
(d) Post operative balloon procedure

1172. Not antiplatelet:
(a) Abciximab (b) Eptifibatide
(c) Ticagrelor (d) Dronedarone

1173. DEFER trial:
(a) Randomization done before angio and FFR
(b) Randomization done after angio and FFR
(c) Randomization done after angio and before FFR
(d) Randomization done after FFR and before angio

1174. FAME trial:
(a) FFR 0.75 (b) Done in difficult lesion
(c) FFR 0.8 (d) All of the above

1175. Atherothrombotic stroke prevention drugs–all *except*:
(a) Aspirin (b) Clopidogrel
(c) Statins (d) Warfarin

1176. Lesion predisposed to rupture:
(a) Thick cap
(b) High temperature in the superficial area
(c) Foci of calcified region > 4 mm

1177. Localisation of MI on ECG – A/E:
(a) Lead II > II – lf. circumflex
(b) q RBBB – distal to first diagonal
(c) ST depression in ant. leads rule out RWMI in patient of IWMI
(d) ST elevation in ant. and inf. leads – Mid LAD

1178. 2 times increase capillary density increase myocardial perfusion by:
(a) 10% (b) 20%
(c) 30% (d) 50%

1179. Resting Myocardial Oxygen Extraction:
(a) 20–30% (b) 80–90%
(c) 100% (d) Minimal

1180. OCT – Full form:
(a) Optical Coherence Tomography

1181. Lotus root sign:
(a) Coronary dissection in Angiography
(b) Coronary dissection in IVUS
(c) OCT post recanalization of thrombus
(d) Highly mobile mass with peduncle in ECHO

1182. Coronary Catheters – True:
(a) Pigtail – Endhole
(b) Berman – Left heart cath
(c) Swan Ganz – End + Side hole
(d) Brockenbrough needle for transseptal BMV

1183. Non-ischemic ST elevation can occur in all of the following conditions *except*:
(a) Hypothermia (b) Hypokalemia
(c) Pulmonary embolism (d) Hypercalcemia

1184. Under resting condition, maximum pressure drop in coronary circulation occurs in:
(a) Epicardial coronaries (b) Resistance vessels
(c) Capillaries (d) Venules

1185. Absolute flow reserve can be calculated best by:

(a) Using a pressure wire during coronary angiography
(b) Adenosine thallium SPECT scanning
(c) PET perfusion scan
(d) Quantitative coronary angiography

1186. Which of the following is correct statement regarding fibrinolytic agent?

(a) Tenectaplase dose is weight independent
(b) Alteplase is given as double bolus
(c) Tenectaplase causes maximum fibrinogen depletion
(d) Tenectaplase is the most fibrin specific

1187. Among antithrombotic agents, all are correct *except*:

(a) LMWH have higher bioavailability and high factor anti-Xa to anti-IIa activity ratio producing effecting blockade in coagulation cascade
(b) Unfractionated heparin is given by intravenous route
(c) Factor Xa specific antagonists were studied in OASIS 6 trial
(d) Fondaparinux was inferior in PCI patients due to higher risk of stent thrombosis

1188. Intra aortic balloon pump is indicated in all *except*:

(a) Refractory cardiogenic shock
(b) Acute mitral regurgitation
(c) Acute aortic regurgitation
(d) Acute ventricular septal rupture

1189. Which of the following is false statement regarding post myocardial infarction pericarditis?

(a) Acute pericarditis occurs early within first 3 days
(b) Anticoagulation is indicated
(c) High dose aspirin relieves the chest pain
(d) Rarely steroids may be required

1190. Regarding non-invasive testing in NSTE-ACS patients, which is false statement?

(a) Safe after 24 hours of stabilization and pain free period
(b) Recommended for patients with baseline ECG with ST/T segment changes
(c) Stress echocardiography and stress MPI have higher sensitivity than TMT
(d) CT coronary angiography can also be used to establish diagnosis of unstable plaque

1191. Most sensitive and specific modality of stress testing is:

(a) Exercise ECG (b) Exercise SPECT
(c) Dobutamine ECHO (d) Adenosine SPECT

1192. Regarding management of chronic stable angina which of the following statement is true?

(a) In single vessel disease with proximal LAD involvement only PCI is recommended
(b) In two vessel disease with proximal LAD involvement surgery or PCI can be done
(c) In three vessel disease with syntax score of 40 PCI should be done
(d) In left main disease with syntax score 23–32 PCI cannot be done

1193. All of the following statements are true regarding spontaneous coronary artery dissections *except*:

(a) Female preponderance
(b) Female post menopausal state is a risk factor
(c) Can present with chronic stable angina, acute coronary syndrome or even sudden cardiac death
(d) Smoking is a risk factor

1194. Which is true regarding ticagrelor?

(a) Irreversible allosteric antagonist
(b) Interacts with CYP3A4 inhibitors
(c) Interacts with CYP2C9
(d) Aspirin dose less than 100 mg per day decreases its effectiveness

1195. Following statements are true about surgical ventricular reconstruction *except*:

(a) Endoventricular patch plasty is also known as Dor procedure
(b) A purse-string suture is placed between the infarcted and normal myocardium. Endoventricular Dacron patch is used to exclude the infarcted segment
(c) RV Dysfunction is a contraindication to Dor procedure
(d) Ideally, the operation was designed to reduce end systolic volume by at least 50% irrespective of LV size

1196. All are true about cardiac allograft vasculopathy *except*:

(a) Annual incidence of 5–10%
(b) It results from neo intimal proliferation of vascular smooth muscle cells and majority of patients do not experience anginal pain
(c) CMV infection is one of the precipitating factors
(d) IVUS is the most specific and DSE is the most sensitive technique to detect it

1197. Anatomic variables associated with stent thrombosis are all *except*:

(a) Long lesions (b) Multivessel disease
(c) Left main disease (d) Bifurcation lesion

1198. Laboratory findings consistent with atheroembolism include all *except*:

(a) Elevated ESR (b) Eosinophiluria
(c) Polycythemia (d) Azotemia

1199. All are true about plaque characteristics on IVUS and OCT *except*:

(a) Both are good at identifying calcium in plaque, and less so at identifying fibrous and lipid tissue
(b) In IVUS images, calcium appears as a bright echogenic signal with a corresponding shadow on the far side of the calcium
(c) In OCT images, calcium appears as an area of increased signal intensity with well demarcated border
(d) Fibrous tissue appears as an area of heterogeous signal intensity beneath the media on both IVUS and OCT images

1200. All are seen best in the views *except*:

(a) LMCA – AP caudal view
(b) ORIGIN OF PDA – RAO view
(c) MID LAD – LAO cranial view
(d) OSTIUM OF RCA – LAO Caudal view

1201. Atrial infarction is characterized by all *except*:

(a) It occurs in up to 10% patients with STEMI if PR-segment displacement is used as criteria
(b) It occurs more commonly in right atrium
(c) It occurs more frequently in atrial appendage
(d) It has been linked to elevated atrial natriuretic peptide levels

1202. 54 years old female presents with chronic stable angina, normal ECG, type 2 diabetes mellitus and critical lower limb ischemia due to peripheral arterial disease of right common iliac artery. False statement regarding management of this patient is:

(a) Should undergo pharmacologic stress testing/imaging for risk stratification
(b) Aspirin and ACEI: both decrease MI and death
(c) CAG should be done to plan revascularization, if stress test shows inducible multiple perfusion defects of small size
(d) If CAG reveals significant stenosis in >1 coronary artery, CABG or PCI have similar recommendation to improve unacceptable angina despite maximum medical therapy

1203. Which among the following is most suitable for pre discharge risk stratification by exercise stress testing in STEM1?

(a) A 75 years old male who received fibrinolysis 48 hours ago is now chest pain free without ST elevation on his ECG
(b) A 65 years old female who received a PCI to her LAD artery 4 days ago and had no other stenosis > 50% on coronary angiogram
(c) A 52 years old male who received fibrinolysis 6 days ago and has pulmonary roles and a third heart sound on physical examination
(d) A 68 years old female who received thrombolysis for an inferior STEM1 4 days ago and has had intermittent atrial fibrillation

1204. A 40 years male presented in emergency with NSTEM1, on examination BP is 90/70, basal crepts+, what is the status for use of beta blocker?

(a) Beta blockers are contraindicated
(b) Only bisoprolol can be used
(c) Reassess need for beta blocker after 24 hours
(d) Metoprolol tartrate is better than metoprolol succinate in this situation

1205. Which is not true about prinz metal variant angina?

(a) Patients with associated severe fixed obstruction tend paradoxically to have a more benign course
(b) Approximately one third of patient's exhibit severe fixed coronary obstruction
(c) Elevated serum has CRP support contribution of inflammation to the condition
(d) Polymorphism of a2 presynaptic and b2 post synaptic receptors may be associated

1206. Which of the following is not a feature of atherosclerosis in diabetics?

(a) Increased apoptosis of smooth muscle cells
(b) Vascular cell adhesion molecule (VCAM) expression is increased
(c) Increased expression of matrix metalloproteinase (MMPs) 1, 2 and 9
(d) Increased adipokines

1207. A 50 years old male with a history of hypertension, diabeties and persistent atrial fibrillation for which he was receiving warfarin underwent stenting to proximal LAD using drug eluting stent. Patient comes under low haemorrhagic risk. The best combination of drugs following his interventions will be:

(a) Aspirin, clopidogrel and warfarin for 1 month, then warf and clopidogrel for 12 months followed by warf alone

(b) Aspirin, clopidogrel and warfarin for 6 months, then warf and clopidogrel for 6 months followed by warf alone

(c) Aspirin, clopidogrel and warfarin for 12 months followed by warf alone

(d) Aspirin and warfarin for 12 months followed by clopidogrel alone

1208. Which of the following statement is true regarding non-ST elevation acute coronary syndromes (NSTE–ACS) compared with ST elevation myocardial infarctions (STEMI)?

(a) Initial mortality of NSTE–ACS is higher

(b) Six-month mortality of STEMI is higher

(c) Long term mortality of NSTE–ACS is equal to or higher than STEMI

(d) STEMI patients are older with more comorbity

1209. Ticagrelor acts through:

(a) ADP receptor (b) Thromboxane

(c) GpIIb IIIa (d) Thrombin

1210. Ranolazine mechanism of action:

(a) ↓ Na late channel, ↓ Ca overload and ↑ end diastolic function and ↑ coronary blood flow

(b) ↓ coronary blood flow

(c) ↑ vasoconstriction

(d) ↑ coronary blood flow with ↑ HR and contractility

1211. Patient present with retrosternal chest pain and back with radiating to left aim, ST elevation II/III/avF, diagnosis:

(a) Post wall MI (b) RVMI

(c) Ant. wall MI (d) Inf. wall MI

1212. Patient with STEMI in II/III/avF and symptom for last 1 hour with bradycardia and hypotension, next management:

(a) V3-V4 lead to be seen if STE in V3-V4_fluid IV

(b) V3-V4 leads can be +ve of STEMI __ PCl

(c) V3-V4 __ STEMI then consider thrombolysis

(d) V3-V4 __ STEMI not seen then TPI

1213. Patient with anteroseptal wall MI with grade III/IV holosystolic murmur with PA Sat-84% and V wave in PCWP but patient in PA:

(a) VSR

(b) Acute MR

(c) Free wall rupture

(d) Aneurysmal ventricular

1214. Ranolazine mechanism of action:

(a) Inhibits late Na channels

(b) Inhibits K channel

(c) Opens Ca channels

(d) ATPase inhibitor

1215. Antianginal that has no effect on HR/CO:

(a) Nicorandil (b) CCB

(c) Ranolazine (d) Beta blockers

1216. Young boy with sudden onset breathlessness with chest pain and sweating: (See Figure 1)

(a) Acute MI

(b) Acute Pulmonary embolism

(c) Acute pericarditis

(d) Temponade

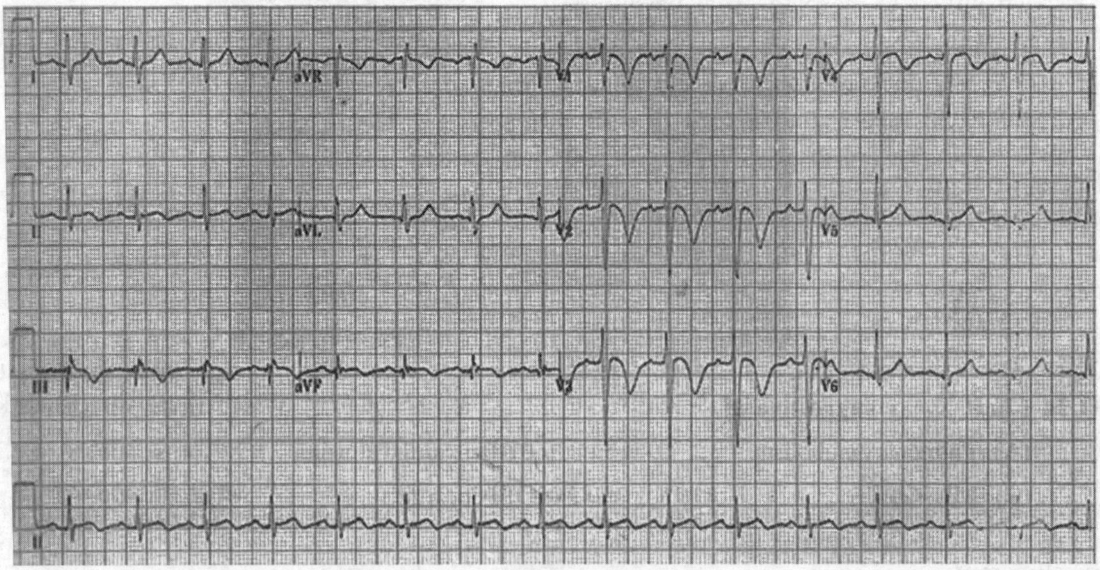

Figure 1

1217. Chest X-ray suggestive of:
(a) Pulmonary embolism
(b) Pericardial effusion
(c) MI
(d) Pericarditis

1218. IWMI, 2/6 systolic murmur best heard at apex, raised JVP:
(a) VSR (b) MR
(c) Free wall rupture (d) CHB

1219. Reversible ADP inhibitor:
(a) Ticagrelor (b) Clopidogrel
(c) Aspirin (d) Vorapaxor

1220. Atherosclerotic lesion in myocardial bridging present:
(a) Distal to bridge (b) Proximal to bridge
(c) Along with bridge (d) None

1221. Dipyridamole reversal:
(a) Aminophylline (b) Adenosine
(c) Beta blockers (d) All

1222. Systemic anticoagulation in MI:
(a) AF (b) LV clot
(c) DVT (d) All

1223. Episodic ischemia:
(a) Normal coronaries (b) Spasm of coronaries
(c) Prinzmetal (d) All

1224. Prinzmetal angina–not used is:
(a) CCB (b) Nitrates
(c) Beta blockers (d) Angiogram

1225. Newer antiplatelets–all are T/E:
(a) Cangrelor is given in infusion
(b) Prasugrel binds irreversibly
(c) Ticagrelor has antidote
(d) Clopidogrel is a prodrug

1226. Incidence of isolated RVMI:
(a) 3% (b) 10%
(c) 20% (d) 25%

1227. All are true about statin benefit groups *except*:
(a) Patient with post PCI status
(b) LDL–C more than 190 mg/dl
(c) 80 years male with LDL-C 180 mg/dl
(d) 50 years male with DM with LDL-C 100 mg/dl

1228. First coronary stent implantation was done by:
(a) Block (b) Cribier
(c) Puel (d) Simpson

1229. Inflation and deflation occurs in:

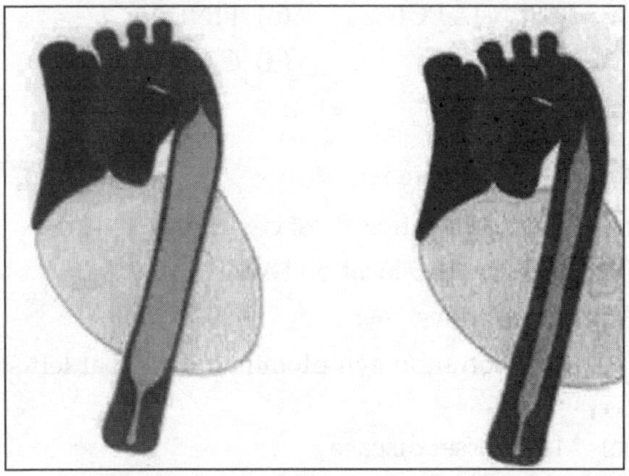

(a) Deflates in systole and inflates in diastole
(b) Inflates in systole, deflates in diastole
(c) Inflates in systole and diastole
(d) Deflates in systole and diastole

1230. First coronary angiogram was done by:
(a) Frossman (b) Sones
(c) Walter (d) Gruentzing

1231. B-blockers were discovered by:
(a) James Black (b) Smith
(c) Both (d) None

1232. Which of the following is not used in vasoreactive testing?
(a) Adenosine (b) Oxygen
(c) Bosentan (d) NO

1233. MI after non cardiac surgery most common is:
(a) <4 hours (b) 24 - 48 hours
(c) Fourth post op (d) Within 7 days

1234. MI A/E:
(a) Pseudoaneurysm has better prognosis than true aneurysm
(b) Right sided PMD rarely causes TR
(c) Inferior septal rupture associated with IWMI has poor prognosis compared to apical septal rupture associated with AWMI
(d) Posteromedial papillary muscle rupture is most common than anteromedial papillary muscle rupture

1235. MI in diabetic patients:
(a) CABG causes less stroke
(b) PCI leads to higher mortality
(c) PCI leads to higher rate of MI
(d) CABG has lesser revascularization rate

1236. Facilitated PCI trials
(a) ASSENT4 PCI (b) FINESSE
(c) WEST (d) CAPITAL AMI
(e) FREEDOM

1237. Post MI VSR true is:
(a) Anterior location most common
(b) Posterior IVS location IWMI
(c) After14 days
(d) Most common symptom is murmur at left sterna border
(e) Multivessel disease

1238. Which markers come to normal within 2 days of MI?
(a) LDH (b) Myoglobin
(c) CKMB (d) Trap I
(e) Trop T

1239. Correct about blood supply of conduction system:
(a) SAN supplied by RCA
(b) SAN can be supplied by LCX
(c) Majority of conduction system is supplied by LAD
(d) AVN is supplied by LAD
(e) AVN is mostly supplied by descending artery

1240. Prasugrel–true is:
(a) Reversible (b) More rapid inhibition
(c) Prodrug (d) Given once daily
(e) Can be given in all ACS patients

1241. Trials on PCI:
(a) ORBITA
(b) CULPRIT SHOCK
(c) EARLY–MYO
(d) ABSORB–III
(e) CRUSH

1242. Late stent thrombosis–true is:
(a) After 1 year
(b) Malapposition increases chances of late stent thrombosis
(c) Treatment needs another stenting
(d) DES is associated with delayed endothelialization
(e) More common in BMS

1243. Dabigatran–not true is:
(a) In India it's available
(b) Is easily affordable
(c) Used in ESRD
(d) Used in rheumatic MS with AF
(e) No monitoring needed

1244. ACS in women:
(a) Low exposure to emergency/medical treatment
(b) Presents in less than 45 years of age
(c) Atypical presentation
(d) Increased mortality after hospitalization
(e) Not associated with HTN/Dyslipedemia

1245. True are:
(a) Abciximab causes thrombocytopenia
(b) Cilastazole is PDE-5 Inhibitor
(c) Ambrisentan is oral selective ET-A receptor antagonist
(d) Tadalafil is PDE-5 inhibitor
(e) Selexipag is selective agonist of prostacyclin IP receptor

1246. True are:
(a) LCX–45% dominant
(b) AP view with slight caudal angulation for LM
(c) Ramus intermedius is branched from LM present in 1/3rd of cases
(d) Coronary fistula is most common coronary anomaly

1247. EXCEL trial:
(a) Paclitaxel stent vs CABG
(b) Noninferior trial
(c) 3 years follow up for primary end point
(d) CABG was associated with increased stroke
(e) PCI better than CABG in all SYNTAX score

1248. DAPT score consists of:
(a) Diabetes
(b) Everolimus stent
(c) PCI to LIMA
(d) Stent diameter <2.5 mm
(e) Acute MI

1249. OCT vs IVUS:
(a) OCT has more resolution
(b) IVUS requires bloodless field
(c) Thin fibrous cap < 65 um
(d) Thin fibrous cap less vulnerable
(e) IVUS requires contrast use

1250. AMI with fibrinolysis:
(a) 15-20% mortality reduction at the end of 1 month
(b) LBBB has lower mortality than STEMI
(c) Mortality is more in men than women
(d) Mortality of female > male
(e) Fibrinolysis in IWMI has less mortality reduction than anterior

1251. DES vs BMS restenosis rate:
(a) Venous graft stenosis 15-30% at the end of 1 year
(b) BMS restenosis 8-10% at 1 year
(c) BMS restenosis 20-30% at 1 year
(d) DES restenosis 8-10% at 1 year
(e) DES restenosis 20-30% at 1 year

1252. Septal rupture true:
(a) Fibrinolysis does not decrease risk of septal rupture
(b) Anterior is worse than inferior
(c) Percutaneous device closure is helpful
(d) Prior MI with chronic stable angina lowers risk

1253. Most important risk for CAD:
(a) HTN (b) Smoking disease
(c) Hyperlipidemia (d) Type I DM
(e) Type II DM

1254. RVMI true A/E:
(a) JVP is raised
(b) JVP is normal
(c) ST elevation most sensitive is more than 0.1 mV in V4R
(d) ST elevation most sensitive is more than 0.5 mV in V4R
(e) If associated with IWMI associated with block

1255. LV aneurysm:
(a) More in LAD disease/occlusive thrombus than multivessel disease
(b) Pseudoaneurysm rupture more common than true aneurysm
(c) More common location is apex
(d) Mortality same with or without aneurysm in MI
(e) SCD risk is very high

1256. Everolimus stent:
(a) Best among all present
(b) Inferior to BVS in acute MI
(c) 3rd generation
(d) Stent thrombosis is risk of concern
(e) Incidence of ISR same as paclitaxel

1257. Test to check for re MI after 3 days of MI:
(a) Trop I (b) Trop T
(c) CKMB (d) All

1258. Septal rupture–true is:
(a) Apical is worse
(b) Basal associated with AWMI
(c) Usually presents after 14 days
(d) Maximum mortality at 5 days

1259. Coronary artery diameter:
(a) 1-2 mm (b) 2-3 mm
(c) 3.5-4.5 mm (d) 4.5-5.5 mm

1260. Dignosis of angina by A/E:
(a) Chest pain on exertion
(b) Relieved by rest
(c) Relieved by nitrates
(d) Pricking type of pain associated with sweating

1261. Which one of the following has no survival benefit in coronary artery disease?
(a) Aspirin (b) Beta blockers
(c) Ace inhibitors (d) Antioxidants

1262. Female with CAD:
(a) Normal CAG with AMI more common than males
(b) In hospital mortality is equal to males
(c) LDL and cholesterol weak risk factor
(d) TG independent risk factor in elderly females
(e) DM2 equal risk factor as in males

1263. ARB trial:
(a) Life (b) Resolved
(c) Cibs (d) Elite
(e) Sprint

1264. Primary prevention trials for SCD:
(a) MADIT (b) CAST
(c) MUSTT (d) CIDS
(e) CASH

ANSWERS KEY

1. (a)	2. (d)	3. (b)	4. (d)	5. (d)	6. (a)	7. (b)	8. (a)
9. (b)	10. (b)	11. (b)	12. (a)	13. (a)	14. (c)	15. (a)	16. (b)
17. (a)	18. (d)	19. (d)	20. (d)	21. (b)	22. (a)	23. (a)	24. (a)
25. (a)	26. (d)	27. (d)	28. (c)	29. (b)	30. (c)	31. (a)	32. (c)
33. (c)	34. (b)	35. T	36. F	37. F	38. F	39. (a)	40. (a)
41. (c)	42. (a)	43. (a)	44. (c)	45. (b)	46. (b)	47. (a)	48. (a)
49. (?)	50. (b)	51. (c)	52. (a)	53. (d)	54. (c)	55. (b)	56. (a)
57. (d)	58. (b)	59. (b)	60. (b, d)	61. (a)	62. (a)	63. (b)	64. (a)
65. (a)	66. (a)	67. (c)	68. (a)	69. (d)	70. (d)	71. (a)	72. FFFTT
73. (a)	74. FFFTT	75. TFFFF	76. TFFTT	77. FTTTT	78. (c)	79. (d)	80. (c)
81. (a)	82. (b)	83. (c)	84. (c)	85. (b)	86. (d)	87. (d)	88. (d)
89. (d)	90. (d)	91. (b)	92. (d)	93. (a)	94. (c)	95. (b)	96. (b)
97. (b)	98. (d)	99. (b)	100. (c)	101. (b)	102. (b)	103. (b)	104. (c)
105. (b,c)	106. (a)	107. (c)	108. (a)	109. (d)	110. (a)	111. (a)	112. (d)
113. (a)	114. (c)	115. (c)	116. (a)	117. (b)	118. (b)	119. (e)	120. (a)
121. (b)	122. (a)	123. (a)	124. (b)	125. (c)	126. (c)	127. (c)	128. (a)
129. (b)	130. (d)	131. (c)	132. (d)	133. (b)	134. (c)	135. (c)	136. (b)
137. (d)	138. (d)	139. (c)	140. (d)	141. (d)	142. (c)	143. (a)	144. (a, b)
145. (c)	146. (d)	147. (b)	148. (b)	149. (a)	150. (c)	151. (c)	152. (a)
153. (a)	154. (d)	155. (a)	156. (c)	157. (b)	158. (a)	159. (c)	160. (b)
161. (a)	162. (b)	163. (a)	164. (b)	165. (d)	166. (a)	167. (c)	168. (a)
169. (a)	170. (c)	171. (c)	172. (a)	173. (a)	174. (d)	175. (a)	176. (c)
177. (a)	178. (a)	179. (b)	180. (d)	181. (b)	182. (b)	183. (b)	184. (b)
185. (a)	186. (a)	187. (d)	188. (b)	189. (c)	190. (d)	191. (d)	192. (a)
193. (a)	194. (c)	195. (c)	196. (a)	197. (b)	198. (c)	199. (c)	200. (a)
201. (a)	202. (c)	203. (a)	204. (c)	205. (a)	206. (d)	207. (b)	208. (b)
209. (b)	210. (a)	211. (b)	212. (a)	213. (c)	214. (c)	215. (d)	216. (c)
217. (a)	218. (d)	219. (a)	220. (a)	221. (b)	222. (b)	223. (b)	224. (a)
225. (a)	226. (b)	227. (b)	228. (b)	229. (c)	230. (c)	231. (a)	232. (b)
233. (a)	234. (a)	235. (a)	236. (b)	237. (b)	238. (b)	239. (a)	240. (b)
241. (a)	242. (a)	243. (a)	244. (a)	245. (a)	246. (e)	247. (a)	248. (d)
249. (c)	250. (a)	251. (c)	252. (a)	253. (d)	254. (b)	255. (a)	256. (d)
257. (b)	258. (d)	259. (b)	260. (c)	261. (a)	262. (a)	263. (d)	264. (b)
265. (c)	266. (b)	267. (a)	268. (b)	269. (d)	270. (a)	271. (d)	272. (a)
273. (c)	274. (a)	275. (b)	276. (c)	277. (d)	278. (d)	279. (b)	280. (b)
281. (a)	282. (b)	283. (a)	284. (a)	285. (b)	286. (c)	287. (d)	288. (c)
289. (a)	290. (a)	291. (c)	292. (a)	293. (b)	294. (b)	295. (a)	296. (a)
297. (a)	298. (e)	299. (b)	300. (a)	301. (b)	302. (d)	303. (b)	304. (a)
305. (a)	306. (c)	307. (c)	308. (c)	309. (c)	310. (a)	311. (b)	312. (c)
313. (b)	314. (c)	315. (c)	316. (a)	317. (a)	318. (a)	319. (c)	320. (a)
321. (a)	322. (a)	323. (c)	324. (a)	325. (a,c,d)	326. (a)	327. (d)	328. (a)
329. (d)	330. TTTFF	331. (e)	332. (b)	333. (a)	334. TTTFT	335. (d)	336. (b)
337. TTTFT	330. TTTFTFTF	339. FFTT	340. FTTTT	341. FTTTT	342. (a)	343. (c)	344. (a)
345. (c)	346. (a)	347. (c)	348. (b)	349. (d)	350. (a)	351. (b)	352. (e)

353. (c)	354. (a)	355. TTTT	356. TFTTT	357. (b, c)	358. (d)	359. (a)	360. (a)
361. TTFT	362. (b)	363. FTFFT	364. (a)	365. (b)	366. TFFF	367. (d)	368. (c)
369. (a)	370. FFT	371. (b)	372. (b)	373. (a)	374. (c)	375. (a)	376. (a)
377. (b)	378. (a)	379. (a, b, c)	380. (b)	381. (b)	382. (d)	383. (d)	384. (b)
385. (b)	386. (b)	387. (a)	388. (c)	389. (b, c, d)	390. (b)	391. (a)	392. (a, b, d)
393. (a, b, c)	394. (a,b,c,d)	395. (c)	396. (a)	397. (d)	398. (a)	399. (a)	400. (b)
401. (a)	402. (b)	403. (a)	404. (b)	405. (a)	406. (a)	407. (a)	408. (a)
409. (d)	410. (b)	411. (a)	412. (a)	413. (a)	414. (c)	415. (a)	416. (d)
417. (c)	418. (a)	419. (b)	420. (b)	421. (c)	422. (c)	423. (c)	424. (d)
425. (d)	426. (c)	427. (b)	428. (a)	429. (c)	430. (a)	431. (c)	432. (a)
433. (d)	434. (b)	435. (d)	436. (c)	437. (d)	438. (b)	439. (b)	440. (a)
441. (b)	442. (b)	443. (a)	444. (c)	445. (a)	446. (c)	447. (a)	448. (c)
449. (b)	450. (b)	451. (b)	452. (c)	453. (b)	454. (b)	455. (a)	456. (a)
457. (d)	458. (d)	459. (d)	460. (b)	461. (c)	462. (a)	463. (b)	464. (a)
465. (b)	466. (d)	467. (c)	468. (a)	469. (b)	470. (a)	471. (a)	472. (b)
473. (a)	474. (b)	475. (a)	476. (a)	477. (b)	478. (b)	479. (b)	480. (c)
481. (a)	482. (d)	483. (c)	484. (c)	485. TTTTF	486. (c)	487. (c)	488. (d)
489. (a)	490. (d)	491. (a)	492. (c)	493. (b)	494. (d)	495. (a)	496. (d)
497. (a)	498. (c)	499. (a)	500. (b)	501. (d)	502. (a)	503. (d)	504. (b)
505. (d)	506. (a)	507. (a)	508. (a)	509. (d)	510. (a)	511. (a)	512. (a)
513. (a)	514. (a)	515. (b)	516. (a)	517. (a)	518. (a)	519. (c)	520. (b)
521. (b)	522. (c)	523. (b)	524. (b)	525. (b)	526. (c)	527. (c)	528. (b)
529. (d)	530. (d)	531. (c)	532. (d)	533. (d)	534. (b)	535. (a)	536. (a)
537. (c)	538. (c)	539. (c)	540. (b)	541. (a)	542. (a)	543. (b)	544. (a)
545. (b)	546. (c)	547. (a)	548. (c)	549. (c)	550. (b)	551. (b)	552. (d)
553. (a)	554. (b)	555. (b)	556. (a)	557. (a)	558. (b)	559. (b)	560. (a)
561. (a)	562. (b)	563. (a)	564. (b)	565. (d)	566. (d)	567. (b)	568. (c)
569. (b)	570. (c)	571. (a)	572. (b)	573. (b)	574. (d)	575. (a)	576. (a)
577. (a)	578. (a)	579. (b)	580. (a)	581. (d)	582. (a)	583. (d)	584. (c)
585. (a)	586. (c)	587. (d)	588. (d)	589. (d)	590. (b)	591. (b)	592. (a)
593. (b)	594. (d)	595. (c)	596. (d)	597. (d)	598. (a)	599. (a)	600. (b)
601. (d)	602. (c)	603. (b)	604. (c)	605. (c)	606. (c)	607. (b)	608. (a)
609. (d)	610. (c)	611. (a)	612. (d)	613. (a)	614. (a)	615. (d)	616. (a)
617. (b)	618. (b)	619. (c)	620. (a)	621. (d)	622. (c)	623. (d)	624. (a)
625. (a)	626. (b)	627. (c)	628. (c)	629. (?)	630. (a)	631. (b)	632. (a)
633. (a)	634. (d)	635. (a)	636. (c)	637. (c)	638. (b)	639. (d)	640. (b)
641. (c)	642. (d)	643. (a)	644. (d)	645. (a)	646. (b)	647. (b)	648. (a)
649. (b)	650. (b)	651. (b)	652. (d)	653. (a)	654. (a)	655. (d)	656. (b)
657. (a)	658. (a)	659. (b)	660. (a)	661. (d)	662. (a)	663. (a)	664. (a)
665. (a)	666. (a)	667. (b)	668. (a)	669. (a)	670. (a)	671. (d)	672. (c)
673. (a)	674. (a)	675. (d)	676. (d)	677. (b)	678. (b)	679. (d)	680. (d)
681. (c)	682. (a)	683. (a)	684. (a)	685. (a)	686. (c)	687. (b)	688. (d)
689. (d)	690. (b)	691. (a)	692. (b)	693. (c)	694. (a)	695. (b)	696. (c)
697. (c)	698. TFFTF	699. TFTTT	700. TTFF	701. TFFFF	702. FFFFT	703. TFTTF	704. TTTTT
705. FFTFT	706. TFFFT	707. TTFFF	708. TTFTT	709. TTFTT	710. FTTTT	711. TTTFF	712. TTFFF
713. FTFFT	714. TFTTF	715. FFFT	716. FFFTF	717. TTFTF	718. FFTFT	719. FFFTF	720. FFTTT
721. FFTTT	722. FFFTF	723. FFTT	724. TTTTT	725. FFTFF	726. TTTTT	727. TFFFT	728. TTTFF
729. TTTFT	730. FTFFF	731. TTTFF	732. TFTTT	733. TTTT	734. FFTTF	735. TTTTF	736. FFFFT
737. FTTFT	738. TFTTT	739. FTFFT	740. TTFT	741. FTTF	742. TTTTF	743. FFTTT	744. TFFFT

745.	TFTF	746.	TTTFT	747.	TTFTT	748.	FTTFT	749.	TTTTT	750.	FFFFT	751.	FTFFF	752.	TFFT
753.	TFTFF	754.	TTFT	755.	TFFFF	756.	TFTTF	757.	FTFFT	758.	FTFFF	759.	TFFFF	760.	TFTFF
761.	FFTTT	762.	FFTFF	763.	FTFTT	764.	FTFFF	765.	FTFFF	766.	FFTTT	767.	FTTFF	768.	TTFFT
769.	TFFFF	770.	TTFTF	771.	TTFFT	772.	TFTFF	773.	TTTFF	774.	TTFTF	775.	FFTTT	776.	TFFTF
777.	TTTFF	778.	TTTTF	779.	TTFF	780.	TFF	781.	FTFTF	782.	TFFTT	783.	TFFT	784.	(b)
785.	(a)	786.	(c)	787.	(b)	788.	(a)	789.	(a)	790.	TFFFT	791.	FFFTF	792.	FFTTF
793.	TTFF	794.	TTTTT	795.	TFTT	796.	TFFT	797.	FTTFF	798.	TFFFF	799.	TTTTF	800.	TFFFF
801.	TTFTF	802.	TFTFF	803.	(b)	804.	(c)	805.	(b)	806.	(a)	807.	(d)	808.	(d)
809.	(d)	810.	TTTTF	811.	(a)	812.	(a)	813.	(a)	814.	(a)	815.	(d)	816.	(a)
817.	(a)	818.	(a)	819.	(a)	820.	(a)	821.	(a)	822.	(d)	823.	(a)	824.	(a)
825.	(d)	826.	(c)	827.	(b)	828.	(a)	829.	(a)	830.	(a)	831.	(d)	832.	(a)
833.	(b)	834.	(c)	835.	(a)	836.	(b)	837.	(b)	838.	(a)	839.	(b)	840.	(a)
841.	(a)	842.	(a)	843.	(a)	844.	(a)	845.	(c)	846.	(b)	847.	(d)	848.	(d)
849.	(a)	850.	(d)	851.	(b)	852.	(c)	853.	(d)	854.	(d)	855.	(a)	856.	(c)
857.	(c)	858.	(b)	859.	(b)	860.	(b)	861.	(d)	862.	(d)	863.	(d)	864.	(b)
865.	(b)	866.	(b)	867.	TTFFF	868.	TTTTT	869.	TTTTT	870.	FTTTT	871.	TTFFF	872.	FTFFF
873.	FTTF	874.	TTFTF	875.	TFFTT	876.	TTFTT	877.	FFTTF	878.	TFFFF	879.	TFFTT	880.	TTTTF
881.	TTFTF	882.	FFTT	883.	TFFTT	884.	TTFT	885.	TTFF	886.	FFTFF	887.	TTFTT	888.	TTFFT
889.	FTFTT	890.	FFTTT	891.	FTTFT	892.	FFFFT	893.	TTFTF	894.	FTF	895.	TFTTT	896.	TFFFT
897.	FTTTT	898.	FTTTTT	899.	TFTTT	900.	TTFTT	901.	TTTTT	902.	FTTTF	903.	FFFFT	904.	TTTTT
905.	FFTTF	906.	TFTT	907.	TTTFT	908.	TTFTF	909.	TTTTF	910.	FFTTT	911.	FFTTF	912.	TTTTF
913.	TTTFF	914.	TFTTF	915.	TFFF	916.	FFTTF	917.	FFFTF	918.	TF	919.	TFTTF	920.	TTFFT
921.	FTFTF	922.	FTTTT	923.	TFFTF	924.	TFFT	925.	FTFTT	926.	FFTF	927.	TTTFF	928.	TFTTT
929.	FFTFF	930.	FTTTT	931.	FTFFF	932.	FTTF	933.	TFTTT	934.	TTTFT	935.	FTFTT	936.	FTTFF
937.	FTTTTT	938.	TFTFF	939.	FTTTF	940.	TFTTT	941.	FFTT	942.	TTTT	943.	TTFFT	944.	TF
945.	TTFFF	946.	TFTFT	947.	TFFTT	948.	TF	949.	TFTTF	950.	TFFFF	951.	FTFF	952.	TTFTT
953.	TTTFF	954.	FFTTT	955.	(d)	956.	(a)	957.	(b)	958.	(b)	959.	(a)	960.	(b)
961.	(d)	962.	(b)	963.	(b)	964.	(a)	965.	(a)	966.	(a)	967.	(b)	968.	(d)
969.	(d)	970.	(d)	971.	(a)	972.	(d)	973.	(c)	974.	(b)	975.	(c)	976.	(b)
977.	(c)	978.	(c)	979.	(b)	980.	(c)	981.	(a)	982.	(b)	983.	(c)	984.	(e)
985.	(d)	986.	(a)	987.	(c)	988.	(d)	989.	(b)	990.	(a)	991.	(d)	992.	(b)
993.	(a)	994.	(b)	995.	(a)	996.	(b)	997.	(a)	998.	(e)	999.	(c)	1000.	(d)
1001.	(a)	1002.	(b)	1003.	(a)	1004.	(a)	1005.	(d)	1006.	(d)	1007.	(a)	1008.	(b)
1009.	(c)	1010.	(c)	1011.	(b)	1012.	(b)	1013.	(a)	1014.	(a)	1015.	(c)	1016.	(d)
1017.	(a)	1018.	(d)	1019.	(c)	1020.	(c)	1021.	(b)	1022.	(c)	1023.	(a)	1024.	(c)
1025.	(b)	1026.	(d)	1027.	(a)	1028.	(b)	1029.	(d)	1030.	(a)	1031.	(a)	1032.	(a)
1033.	(a)	1034.	(a)	1035.	(b)	1036.	(b)	1037.	(b)	1038.	(b)	1039.	(d)	1040.	(a)
1041.	(a)	1042.	(a)	1043.	(a)	1044.	(a)	1045.	(a)	1046.	(d)	1047.	(a)	1048.	(c)
1049.	(b)	1050.	(a)	1051.	(a)	1052.	(d)	1053.	(d)	1054.	(a)	1055.	(a)	1056.	(c)
1057.	(d)	1058.	(c)	1059.	(a)	1060.	(b)	1061.	(d)	1062.	(d)	1063.	(d)	1064.	(b)
1065.	(a)	1066.	(b)	1067.	(b)	1068.	(c)	1069.	(c)	1070.	(c)	1071.	(a)	1072.	(a)
1073.	(d)	1074.	(b)	1075.	(a)	1076.	(a)	1077.	(c)	1078.	(a)	1079.	(a)	1080.	(a)
1081.	(b)	1082.	(a)	1083.	(b)	1084.	(a)	1085.	(a)	1086.	(b)	1087.	(c)	1088.	(d)
1089.	(b)	1090.	(a)	1091.	(d)	1092.	(a)	1093.	(c)	1094.	(b)	1095.	(c)	1096.	(c)
1097.	(b)	1098.	(c)	1099.	(b)	1100.	(c)	1101.	(c)	1102.	(d)	1103.	(b)	1104.	(d)
1105.	(b)	1106.	(d)	1107.	(a)	1108.	(a)	1109.	(b)	1110.	(c)	1111.	(b)	1112.	(a)
1113.	(d)	1114.	(d)	1115.	(a)	1116.	(a)	1117.	(c)	1118.	(b)	1119.	(a)	1120.	(c)
1121.	(b)	1122.	(c)	1123.	(b)	1124.	(a)	1125.	(b)	1126.	(a)	1127.	(a)	1128.	(b)
1129.	(b)	1130.	(c)	1131.	(c)	1132.	(c)	1133.	(b)	1134.	(a)	1135.	(a)	1136.	(a)

1137. (a)	1138. (a)	1139. (c)	1140. (b)	1141. (b)	1142. (b)	1143. (c)	1144. (a)
1145. (d)	1146. (a)	1147. (a)	1148. (a)	1149. (?)	1150. (a)	1151. (d)	1152. (c)
1153. (a)	1154. (b)	1155. (c)	1156. (c)	1157. (b)	1158. (d)	1159. (d)	1160. (d)
1161. (d)	1162. (d)	1163. (d)	1164. (a)	1165. (d)	1166. (c)	1167. (b)	1168. (b)
1169. (b)	1170. (d)	1171. (a)	1172. (d)	1173. (d)	1174. (c)	1175. (d)	1176. (b)
1177. (d)	1178. (a)	1179. (b)	1180. (a)	1181. (b)	1182. (d)	1183. (b)	1184. (b)
1185. (c)	1186. (d)	1187. (d)	1188. (c)	1189. (b)	1190. (b)	1191. (b)	1192. (c)
1193. (b)	1194. (b)	1195. (d)	1196. (d)	1197. (c)	1198. (c)	1199. (d)	1200. (b)
1201. (d)	1202. (c)	1203. (d)	1204. (c)	1205. (a)	1206. (a)	1207. (b)	1208. (c)
1209. (a)	1210. (a)	1211. (d)	1212. (b)	1213. (b)	1214. (a)	1215. (c)	1216. (b)
1217. (b)	1218. (b)	1219. (a)	1220. (b)	1221. (a)	1222. (d)	1223. (d)	1224. (c)
1225. (c)	1226. (a)	1227. (c)	1228. (c)	1229. (a)	1230. (b)	1231. (a)	1232. (c)
1233. (b)	1234. (a)	1235. (d)	1236. (a, b)	1237. (a, e)	1238. (b)	1239. (a,b)	1240. (b, d)
1241. (a,b,c,d,e)	1242. (b, d)	1243. (b, c, d)	1244. (a, c, d)	1245. (a,c,d,e)	1246. (b, c, d)	1247. (b, c, d)	1248. (a, e)
1249. (a,c)	1250. (a,d)	1251. (a,c,d)	1252. (d)	1253. (b)	1254. (b, d, e)	1255. (a,b,c,e)	1256. (a)
1257. (c)	1258. (d)	1259. (c)	1260. (d)	1261. (d)	1262. TFTTF	1263. TTFFT	1264. TTFTF

CHAPTER TWO

HEART FAILURE

1. **ACE 1 in cirrhosis:**
(a) Lisinopril (b) Enalapril
(c) Rampiril (d) Delapril

2. 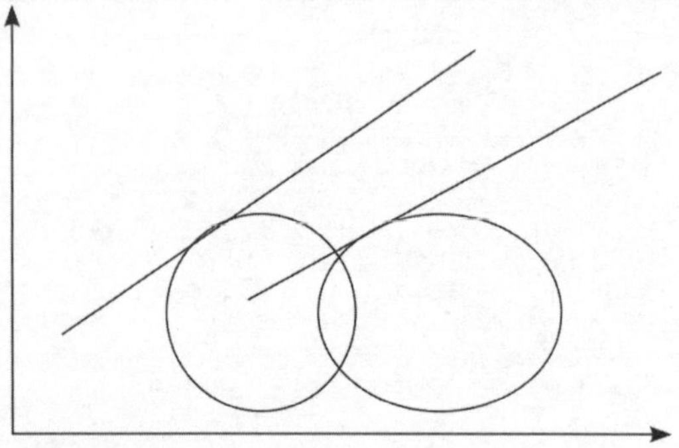

Shows:
(a) Increased afterload
(b) Loss of preload
(c) Acute loss of ionotropic
(d) MS

3. **CCP:**
(a) Equalization of diastolic pressures
(b) SAI < 1.1
(c) RV pressure > 35 mm Hg
(d) x = v

4. **Athlete heart and HOCM, not used as a differential marker:**
(a) Bizarre ECG (b) Septum 20 mm
(c) LV cavity <45 mm (d) LGE

5. **Resistance exercise not true:**
(a) Increases CO
(b) Increases DBP
(c) Increases sympathetic outflow
(d) Increased SVR

6. **Heart failure management – not true:**
(a) B blockers significantly increase exercise tolerance
(b) Digoxin mildly improves exercise tolerance
(c) Aldosterone antagonist–30% decrease in mortality
(d) ACE inhibitors – 20% decrease in mortality

7. **All of the following act through GPCR *except:***
(a) PDGF (b) Epinephrine
(c) Prostaglandins (d) Endothelin

8. **Which combination indicates beri beri?**
(a) Ao Sat 98%, SVC 85%, BP 110/40 mm Hg
(b) Ao Sat 90%, SVC 65%, BP 120/70 mm Hg
(c) Ao Sat 90%, SVC 55%, BP 110/20 mm Hg
(d) Ao Sat 85%, SVC 85%, BP 160/60 mm Hg

9. **Constrictive pericarditis–not true:**
(a) RAP 20 mm Hg; PCWP 22 mm Hg
(b) SVR 20 units; PVR 15 units
(c) LVEDP 24 mm Hg; RVEDP 28 mm Hg
(d) Mitral E>> A; tricuspid E>>A

10. **Takotsubo cardiomyopathy – all *except:***
(a) Reversible myocardial dysfunction (self limiting)
(b) LV dysfunction mechanism–due to Ca^{++} overload
(c) LVOTO not uncommon
(d) Amiodarone is useful in malignant VT

11. **ACE1 that can be used in liver failure:**
(a) Fosinopril (b) Lisinopril
(c) Ramipril (d) Captopril

12. **Diastolic heart failure causes all *except:***
(a) Left atrial enlargement
(b) Eccentric hypertrophy
(c) LVH
(d) Near normal LVEF

13. **True are all *except:***
(a) Treppe–Increase in contractility with increase in frequency
(b) Anrep–Immediate increase in force due to increase in afterload
(c) Afterload–Sum of aortic compliance and wall stress
(d) Laplace law–PR/2t

14. IE due to streptococcus–all *except:*

(a) *S. pyogenes* (b) *S. agalactiae*
(c) *E. faecalis* (d) *S. bovis*

15. Paradigm–HF:

(a) ARB (b) ARNI
(c) CCB (d) Beta blockers

16. An 18-year-old with syncope. Deep T wave inversion:

(a) Apical HCM (b) Long QT syndrome
(c) DCM (d) RCM

17. Muscle fibre, space between two z lines is:

(a) A band (b) 1 band
(c) M band (d) Sarcomere

18. Most common cause of pericarditis, 60 years worldwide:

(a) AMI (b) Viral
(c) Tubercular (d) Uremic

19. Cephalzation–A/E:

(a) ASD
(b) Moderate MS with ball valve thrombus
(c) MR with LVD
(d) Left atrial myxoma

20. B blockers CI in pregnancy:

(a) Metaprolol (b) Carvedialol
(c) Propranolol (d) Atenolol

21. Pulmonary vasoreactivity A/E:

(a) Oxygen (b) NO
(c) Adenosine (d) Isoproterolol

22. All T/E:

(a) Acetylcholine requires endothelium for vasoconstriction
(b) Hypercapnea–cerebral vasodilation
(c) Hypoxia, acidosis–pulmonary vasoconstriction
(d) Adenosine endothelium independent vasodilation

23. Adenosine T/E:

(a) Causes vasodilation
(b) Negative dromotropic effect
(c) Coronary vasodilation
(d) Bronchoconstriction

24. Mitochondrial inheritance A/E:

(a) Higher incidence and severity in females
(b) Males doesn't pass to offspring
(c) Offsprings of affected female–all affected
(d) Mosaicism common

25. A/E:

(a) ↑ Contractility ↓ rate
(b) Heart failure preload dependent
(c) Normal heart, stroke volume free of afterload
(d) Normal heart, LVEDP <20-Frank Starling has peak effect

26. Blunted y in both right and left ventricle:

(a) MS + TS
(b) Ischemic heart
(c) AF with CHB
(d) Rapidly increasing pericardial infection

27. Physiological parameter A/E:

(a) LVEDP – 18 mg (b) CO – 4.7 C/M in female
(c) PCWP – 12 mg (d) MPAP – 15 mm Hg

28. JVP–8 cm above sterna angle with PR–3 m/s calculate RVEDP:

(a) 24 (b) 27
(c) 46 (d) 60

29. Furosemide A/E:

(a) ↑ Chlorine excretions
(b) In normal person – ↑ RAAS
(c) Can be used in refractory pulmonary edema
(d) In sulfonamide allergy–furosemide replaced by torsemide

30. Class II HF and class IV HF to be taken for ICD:

(a) Class II–more HF death ratio
(b) Class II–more SCD death ratio
(c) Class IV–more chances of death by SCD
(d) Class IV–more chances of death by HF

31. Patient–HF REF resting HR 65/min, BP-90/60 mm Hg on carvidilol with postural giddiness K-4.5, gynecomastia (+) – Next drug:

(a) Aldactone
(b) Digoxin for resting HR
(c) Ivabradine
(d) Losartan if already on ACE inhibitors

32. Post menopausal with NYHA II dyspnea with DM:

(a) ACE inhibitor–start (b) Start high dose vit E
(c) HRT start (d) Do CAG→Revasc.

33. **LV dysfunction caused by A/E:**
(a) Cisplatin (b) Ifosfamide
(c) Cyclophosphamide (d) Doxorubicin

34. **HF with preserved EF, A/E:**
(a) Elderly male (b) HTN and DM
(c) Diastolic dysfunction

35. **HCM–high risk A/E:**
(a) Rest gradient > 30 mm Hg
(b) Syncope
(c) LVH > 30 mm
(d) Non sustained/multiple/VT on Holt

36. **The V wave in JVP represents:**
(a) RA compliance (b) RV compliance
(c) LA compliance (d) LV compliance

37. **Which of the findings is considered among the minor criteria for diagnosing CCF?**
(a) Neck vein distention (b) Rales
(c) S3 gallop (d) Extremity edema

DM with progressive dyspnea, 47-year-old male, pedal edema, ↑ JVP, ascites, faint MR murmur with prominent P_2 Echo–preserved EF (38–40)

38. **Diagnosis:**
(a) Bivent dysfunction (b) HF with normal EF
(c) HCM (d) RV cardiomyopathy

39. **Echo:**
(a) E/A = 1, é –N (b) E/A > 2, é ↓
(c) E/A < 0.5, é – ↓ (d) E/A > 2, é –Normal

40. **MRI finding:**
(a) Subepicardial enhancement
(b) Subendocardial enhancement
(c) CP septal bounce
(d) Midmyocardial enhancement

41. **Torsemide acts on:**
(a) Ascending limb of loop of Henle
(b) PCT
(c) DCT
(d) Descending loop of Henle

42. **Infiltrative cardiomyopathy:**
(a) Hemochromatosis
(b) Glycogen storage diseases
(c) Gaucher

43. **Karely A lines are present in MS severity:**
(a) Minimal (b) Mild
(c) Mod (d) Severe

44. **Which is seen in CCP?**
(a) Rapid y descent (b) Absent y descent
(c) PAP > 60

45. **HOCM murmur increases in A/E:**
(a) Upright (b) Squatting
(c) Valsalva (d) PVC

46. **Alcohol ablation A/E:**
(a) LVOT reduction in minority
(b) 1-4 ml used
(c) Coronary ischemia

47. **Screening for HCM after 21 years:**
(a) Every 1 year (b) Every 5 years
(c) Not required (d) Every 6 months

48. **Athlete's heart Vs HOCM:**
(a) Symmetric hypertrophy
(b) Small LV cavity
(c) Thickness < 17 mm
(d) TDI/strain normal

49. **BNP ↑ in all *except:***
(a) Obesity (b) Renal failure
(c) Cirrhosis (d) Heart failure

50. **CPR–chest rate:**
(a) 100/min (b) 200/min
(c) 50/min (d) 70/min

51. **CPR–layman:**
(a) No spontaneous respiration not responding, not breathing
(b) No pulse
(c) Not responding, breathing

52. **Nesiritide:**
(a) Bolus and IV
(b) Improves infertility and renal function
(c) Oral formation available
(d) Non expensive can be used liberally

53. **Riociguat:**
(a) Guanylate cyclase stimulator
(b) – Camp (c) G protein I

54. **Athlete's heart which is not differentiating:**
(a) Small LV cavity
(b) Symmetric hypertrophy
(c) Wall thickness < 17 mm
(d) Normal diastolic function

55. **Global diffuse subendocardial LGE seen in:**
(a) Post transplant (b) Sarcoidosis
(c) Myocarditis (d) Fabry's disease

56. **Not useful in diagnosing myocarditis:**
(a) Chest pain due to endocardial involvement in PV B19
(b) Arrhythmias and AV block suggest GCM
(c) Bilateral lobar lymph nodes S/O sarcoidosis
(d) Normal MRI

57. **All of the following are associated with calcium uptake by SERCA *except:***
(a) Calmodullin
(b) Calreticulin
(c) Phospholamban
(d) Calsequestrin

58. **All of the biomarkers indicate myocyte injury *except:***
(a) Cardiac troponins
(b) Heart type fatty acid protein
(c) Myosin light chain kinase 1
(d) Myeloperoxidase

59. **Following drug has shown to reduce mortality in heart failure with reduced EF:**
(a) Bucindolol (b) Metoprolol tartrate
(c) Nebivolol (d) Bisoprolol

60. **Regarding loop diuretics – all are true *except:***
(a) They act on $NA^+ Cl^-$ symporter of renal nephrones
(b) They increase sodium excretion by up to 20-25%
(c) Furosemide acts is venodilator and reduces right aerial and pulmonary capillary wedge pressure
(d) Bioavailability of oral torsemide is better than furosemide

61. **A 65-year-old obese female with hypertension and diabetes mellitus presents with symptoms and signs of heart failure. Identify the most appropriate statement in her:**
(a) Her 5 years survival is > 80%
(b) Her EF is likely to be < 40%
(c) β-blockers and aldosterone antagonists are likely to reduce her mortality
(d) ACEI/ARBs are important in the management of her HTN

62. **Therapy with β blockers causes significant increase in:**
(a) LDL cholesterol (b) Total cholesterol
(c) HDL cholesterol (d) Plasma triglycerides

63. **Most common morbidity 5 years after heart transplantation:**
(a) Hypertension
(b) Diabetes
(c) Renal dysfunction
(d) Cardiac allograft vasculopathy

64. **Mechanism of action of anakinra:**
(a) Anti-TNF inhibitor
(b) CD 20 inhibitor
(c) IL: 1 receptor antagonist
(d) IL: 6 receptor antagonist

65. **All true about heart failure: (T/F)**
(a) Stage C–no structural heart disease but symptoms
(b) HR > 120–minor criteria
(c) Hepatojugular reflux–major criteria
(d) Tolvaptan–non selective $V_{1a} + V_2$
(e) Salt intake < 2 in all patient with HF

66. **JVP: (T/F)**
(a) Cannon wave–regular and junctional rhythm
(b) Rapid y descent–early in TR severe
(c) Rapid y descent with deep trough in CCP
(d) Measured in mm Hg
(e) Kussmaul sign in LVMI

67. **Mechanical device: (T/F)**
(a) Jervic–pulsatile
(b) Cardiowest–not FDA approved
(c) S. creat > 5–C/I
(d) BSA > 1.7–required for all heart
(e) Tandom heart–Short acting

68. **Regarding HOCM: (T/F)**
(a) Screening to be started @ 21 years
(b) SAM is due to drag effect
(c) Atherosclerotic CAD in 50% of cases
(d) Heavy meals and exercise decrease the gradient
(e) Autosomal dominant inheritance

69. Regarding JVP waves: (T/F)
(a) a wave occurs after S_1
(b) v wave occurs after S_2
(c) Soft S_1 indicates raised LVEDP
(d) Cannon a wave occurs with A-V dissociation
(e) In tricuspid regurgitation (TR), the v wave is accentuated

70. Gradient between PCWP and LVEDP: (T/F)
(a) Parachute mitral valve
(b) Supramitral ring
(c) Submitral aneurysm
(d) Cor triatriatum
(e) Sub aortic membrane with AR and raised LVEDP

71. Regarding catheterization: (T/F)
(a) Right atrium has higher 'a' wave
(b) Left atrium has higher 'V' wave because of –RV compliance
(c) RA has steep y descent
(d) LA saturation is always 100%
(e) *a* wave is absent with AF

72. Myocarditis: (T/F)
(a) Giant cell myocarditis age 21 years
(b) Early immunosuppression improves survival
(c) Arrhythmias like heart block, VT and SVT can occur
(d) MRI is useful modality
(e) Viral infection the most common cause for myocarditis

73. Mycotic aneurysm: (T/F)
(a) Because of septic embolic due to fungal infections
(b) Infection of the arterial wall
(c) The most common organisms are *Staphylococcus aureus* and *Salmonella species*
(d) Mycotic aneurysms carry a low mortality
(e) Coined by Osler

74. Heart failure: (T/F)
(a) $\geq$ 50% cases have normal EF
(b) Heart failure increasing prevalence with age
(c) ACE inhibitors prolong life
(d) NYHA class 4–1 year mortality 30-70%
(e) CRT prolongs life

75. Carcinoid heart disease: (T/F)
(a) Present in all cases of carcinoid tumor
(b) Left sided disease–only with bronchial carcinoid
(c) Right sided disease–only with liver carcinoid
(d) TR/PS are common features
(e) Endocardial thickening is not seen

76. Tifin: (T/F)
(a) Largest protein discovered yet
(b) Connects actin filaments to M line
(c) Short and thick tifin → increased strength
(d) Transduces mechanical signals to growth signal
(e) It gives elasticity

77. True or False:
(a) Treppe effect – force of contraxn with sudden increase in afterload
(b) Anrep effect – force of contraxn with – HR (step wise – HR)
(c) Bowditch effect – force of contraxn with sudden – HR
(d) Afterload is the wall stress during LV ejection
(e) End-systolic pressure-volume relationship is considered to represent a reliable load-independent index of the contractile performance of the heart

78. Which one of the following is not true for Milrinone?
(a) It is a phosphodiesterase inhibitor
(b) It is beta receptor stimulant
(c) It has inotropic effect
(d) It has vasodilator effect

79. Which beta blocker from the following is excreted through kidney?
(a) Propranolol (b) Atenolol
(c) Carvedilol (d) Metoprolol

80. In patients with HOCM, echo screening of their son/daughter should be started at age of:
(a) 5 years (b) 9 years
(c) 12 years (d) 23 years

81. What is the incidence of dilated cardiomyopathy in Duchenne muscular dystrophy, after age of 18 years?
(a) Up to 20% (b) Up to 50%
(c) Up to 70% (d) Up to 90%

82. Following cardiomyopathy is common in Friedreich's ataxia:
(a) Asymmetrical septal hypertrophy
(b) Concentric hypertrophic cardiomyopathy
(c) Dilated cardiomyopathy
(d) Restrictive cardiomyopathy

83. **Which one of the following is not true for Takotsubo cardiomyopathy?**
(a) It is irreversible
(b) It is known as apical ballooning syndrome also
(c) ECG may mimic acute myocardial infarction
(d) Most common in postmenopausal women

84. **Which one of the following is true for development of alcoholic cardiomyopathy?**
(a) Consumption of more than 80 gm of ethanol per day for at least 10 years
(b) Consumption of more than 80 gm of ethanol per day for at least 5 years
(c) Consumption of more than 40 gm of ethanol per day for at least 5 years
(d) Consumption of more than 40 gm of ethanol per day for at least 10 years

85. **Cardiorenal syndrome (CRS) includes acute and chronic conditions where the heart or the kidney serves as the primary failing organ with resulting dysfunction in both organs. Select the statement that is false.**
(a) CRS is classified from Type I to Type V, where Type V signifies secondary CRS referring to systemic conditions like DM and sepsis causing cardiac and renal dysfunction
(b) Concomitant liver dysfunction may also play a prominent role because dysregulation of the hepatorenal reflex
(c) Baseline renal insufficiency is not an independent risk factor for the development of worsening renal function in systolic and diastolic HF
(d) Use of mineralocorticoid antagonists in the selling of CRS is offset by the risk of hyperkalemia and should be avoided when eGFR falls below 30 mL/min/1.73 m^2

86. **Following a post-premature beat the left ventricular outflow gradient is increased with a reduction in the pulse pressure of the aortic contour. In this regard, identify the false statement.**
(a) This maneuver is called as Brockenbrough maneuver
(b) A premature ventricular beat may also accentuate the spike-and-dome configuration of the aortic pressure waveform
(c) This is classically associated with restrictive cardiomyopathy
(d) The paradoxical hemodynamic response to post extra systolic potentiation is explained by dynamic narrowing of the LVOT

87. **The patho-physiology and etiologies for heart failure in children are very different from those in adults. Select the false statement in this context.**
(a) HF presenting on the first day of life are commonly due to VSD or PDA
(b) About 90% of all cases of heart failure in children occur before the end of first year of life and reflect the preponderance of congenital heart disease as a cause of HF
(c) Isolated ASD are mostly asymptomatic in children and if an infant is diagnosed to have ASD and is in failure, the likely diagnosis is TAPVC
(d) Raised jugular venous pressure, peripheral edema, effusions and chest crepitations are not seen in neonates and are unlikely in young children as a sign of HF

88. **Which of the following descriptions for assessment of cardiovascular disability is wrong?**
(a) NYHA III–Less than ordinary physical activity causes fatigue, palpitation, dyspnea or anginal pain
(b) CCS III–Marked limitation of ordinary physical activity. Walking one to two blocks on the level and climbing more than one flight in normal conditions
(c) Specific activity scale I–Patients can perform activity requiring > 5 METS
(d) Specific activity scale III–Patients can perform activity requiring > METS

89. **Which of the following is an incorrect description for dynamic auscultation?**
(a) Systolic murmur of HOCM becomes louder with Valsalva
(b) Murmur of AR decreases with handgrip exercise
(c) With squatting, murmur of MVP softens
(d) Left sided murmurs are louder during expiration

90. **Pulmonary capillary wedge mean pressure is not equal to left ventricular end diastolic pressure in:**
(a) Mitral stenosis
(b) Placement of catheter in non-dependent zone of the lung
(c) Decreased ventricular compliance
(d) All of the above

91. **Which of the following phases of cardiac cycle belongs to physiological diastole but cardiological systole?**
(a) Reduced ejection

(b) Isovolumic relaxation
(c) Maximal ejection
(d) None of the above

92. What is true about Bowditch effect?
(a) Also called as treppe phenomenon or force frequency relationship
(b) This phenomenon is muted in heart failure
(c) This phenomenon occurs only upto an optimal heart rate (usually upto 150-180/min)
(d) All of the above

93. Decreased BNP concentrations may be found in:
(a) Older individuals (b) Females
(c) Obesity (d) Cirrhosis

94. Not a major criterion in Framingham's criteria for heart failure is:
(a) PND (b) Rales
(c) Hepatomegaly (d) Hepatojugular reflux

95. Pericarditis is seen with:
(a) Lithium (b) Procainamide
(c) Methysergide (d) Indomethacin

96. Independent factor for myocardial performance A/E:
(a) Ionotropic state (b) Preload
(c) Afterload (d) Dromotropic state

97. Patient with ascites, pedal edema, early S3 ↑ JVP I inspiration, X-ray–normal heart:
(a) Constrictive pericarditis
(b) Cardiac tamponade
(c) RVMI
(d) Pulmonary embolism

98. Cardiac tamponade–All T/E:
(a) ↓ TV flow in inspiration
(b) Pulsus paradoxus
(c) Early RV diastolic collapse
(d) RA diastolic collapse

99. Decompression sickness seen in:
(a) PFO (b) HTN
(c) CCF (d) MI

100. In HF ↓ A/E:
(a) Compliance (b) Residual volume
(c) Vital capacity (d) Co-diffusion capacity

101. I.MET:
(a) 2.5 (b) 1.5
(c) 3.5 (d) 4.5

102. Inotropics shift Frank Starling curve:
(a) Lower + RT (b) Lower only
(c) Upwards + LT (d) Upwards only

103. Independent factor for cardiac performance A/E:
(a) Inotrophic state (b) Afterload
(c) Preload (d) Dromotrophic state

104. HOCM–true is:
(a) Ion channel defect
(b) Myosin heavy chain gene defect
(c) SCD not seen

105. PPH gene involved:
(a) BMPP-II (b) Endothelin
(c) PGF (d) None

106. PPH-PASP:
(a) 20 (b) 25
(c) 30 (d) 40

107. Best predictor of SCD in HOCM:
(a) AF
(b) LVH < 15 m
(c) Stress test with significant ↓ BP
(d) Gradient > 30 m

108. Dobutamine effect ↓ by:
(a) ↓ Absorption
(b) ↑ Clearance
(c) Downregulation of receptor
(d) ↑ Metabolism

109. Pulmonary HTN caused by:
(a) Schistosomiasis (b) Trypanosomiasis
(c) Amebiasis (d) Teniasis

110. All are useful in diagnosis of HFpEF *except:*
(a) BNP level of 100 pg/ral and NT-pro BNP level of 800 pg/ml supports its diagnosis
(b) LVEF-50%
(c) BNP levels are higher in obese patients and lower in women, older persons, patients with pulmonary disease and renal dysfunction
(d) PCWP > 12 mm Hg, LVEDP > 16 mm Hg, t > 48 msec, p > 0.27, E/è > 15, LAVI > 40 ml/M², LVM > 122/149 g/M²

111. All are true about cardiac allograft vasculopathy *except:*

(a) Annual incidence of 5-10%

(b) It results from neo intimal proliferation of vascular smooth muscle cells and majority of patients do not experience angina pain

(c) CMV infection is one of the precipitating factors

(d) IVUS is the most specific and DSE is the most sensitive technique to detect it

112. Which of the following is decreased in a failing myocyte:

(A) L-type calcium channel

(B) Alpha-I adrenergic receptor

(C) Troponin C

(D) Calreticulin

113. NHANES criteria to diagnose heart failure include all *except:*

(a) History

(b) Heart rate 91-110 beats/minute

(c) Abnormalities on echocardiography

(d) Abnormalities on chest X-ray

114. Which of the following statements is false?

(a) Physiologic systole lasts from the start of isovolumic contraction to the peak of the ejection phase

(b) Cardiologic systole is demarcated by the interval between the first and second heart sounds and lasts from M_1 to A_2

(c) Physiologic diastole commences as Ca^{2+} is taken back into the SR, so myocyte relaxation occurs and LV pressure starts falling

(d) Protodiastole is the early phase of atrial contraction, the time when S4 can be heard

115. The P-glycoprotein (P-gp) transporter is found in the luminal membrane of the small intestine and blood-brain barrier and in the apical membranes of excretory cells such as hepatocytes and kidney proximal tubule epithelial cells. Digoxin, is a substrate of both intestinal and renal P-glycoprotein transporter. Which of the following statements is not correct?

(a) Induction of intestinal P-gp by rifampin is shown to decrease the bioavailability of orally administered digoxin, thereby reducing plasma digoxin levels

(b) Quinidine increases plasma digoxin concentration by reducing P-gp-mediated efflux of digoxin into the gut and kidneys

(c) Amiodarone, a potent inhibitor of P-gp, increases mean serum digoxin levels

(d) Dronedarone does not interact with P-gp, and oral digoxin dose needs no adjustment when co-administered with dronedarone

116. All are true for tubercular pericarditis *except:*

(a) Pericardial involvement develops in approximately 2% of patients with pulmonary tuberculosis

(b) Late constrictive pericarditis may develop despite antitubercular treatment

(c) PCR to detect M tuberculosis can be performed with minute amounts of pericardial fluid with sensitivity of more than 70%

(d) It there is no particular contraindication, corticosteroids may be given even though they do not prevent constriction

117. Abdominojugular reflux is characterized by all, *except:*

(a) It requires firm pressure over upper abdomen preferably right u quadrant for 10 seconds

(b) A sustained rise of > 3 cm in venous pressure during continued compress

(c) Patient should avoid holding of breath

(d) It can predict heart failure and pulmonary artery wedge pressure higher than 25 mm Hg

118. Which of the following statements regarding monitoring and characterizing circulatory status in critically ill patients in ICU is not correct?

(a) Routine pulmonary artery catheterization is not indicated

(b) Static measurements of circulatory parameters (e.g., CVP, PCWP) provide reliable information on the circulatory status of critically ill patients

(c) A decrease in CVP of > 1 mm Hg during inspiration in a spontaneously breathing patient may predict an increase in cardiac output after IV fluid administration

(d) A changing pulse pressure during mechanical ventilation has been shown to predict an increase in cardiac output after IV fluid administration in patients with septic shock

119. Most common finding in myxoma is:

(a) Loud P_2 (b) Diastolic murmur

(c) Systolic murmur (d) Tumor polyp

120. True statement regarding appropriate screening protocol for family members of patients with HCM:

(a) Serial ECG and echocardiogram every 5 years for a 14-year-old child of an HCM patient

(b) Serial ECG and echocardiogram on a first degree adult relative every 10 years of an HCM patient
(c) Serial ECG and echocardiogram on a gene-negative first-degree relative of a patient who is gene positive for beta-myosin heavy-chain mutation every 5 years
(d) Serial ECG and echocardiogram every 18 months for a 17-year-old child of an HCM patient

121. The most accepted recent hypothesis for anthracycline induced cardiotoxicity is:
(a) Magnesium mediated generation of excess reactive oxygen species
(b) Formation of complexes with calcium that undergo redox cycling and generate oxygen radicals
(c) Inhibition of topoisomerase 2β
(d) Deactivation of p53 and the apoptotic pathway

122. All are true about Valsalva maneuver, *except:*
(a) Pulse amplitude ratio is a ratio of the maximal pulse pressure at the end of the strain phase to the minimum pulse pressure at initiation of the strain phase
(b) Pulse amplitude ratio has been shown to correlate very closely with ventricular filling pressures
(c) In patients with severe heart failure, Korotkoff sound appreciated during phase 2 but not phase 4
(d) In patients with mild heart failure, Korotkoff sounds are absent during both phases 2 and 4

123. Which of the following statements regarding the cardiac fibrosis is not true?
(a) Myofibroblasts are derived from cardiac fibroblasts
(b) Myofibroblasts have 2-fold higher capacity to synthesize collagen
(c) TGFP stimulates transformations of myofibroblasts to fibroblasts
(d) Among the numerous regulatory factors, angiotensin II and growth factor beta-1 are the most potent stimulators of collagen synthesis by cardiac fibroblasts

124. Which of the following statements is not true?
(a) Arterial baroreceptors (high-pressure receptors) are located in the carotid sinus and the aortic arch
(b) Cardiopulmonary baroreceptors (volume receptors) are located in the great veins and the cardiac chambers
(c) Cardiopulmonary baroreceptors (volume receptors) detect changes in the filling of the central venous circulation and are essential for short term orthostatic cardiovascular homeostasis
(d) Veno-arteriolar axon reflex, results in constriction of arterial flow to the muscles, skin and adipose tissue, leading to the increase in vascular resistance in the limbs upon standing

125. Apical HCM A/E:
(a) 7% of Japanese
(b) Ace of spade
(c) T ↓ in mid and lateral precordial leads
(d) Benign course than usual HCM

126. Tako-Tsubo cm A/E:
(a) Young Asian women
(b) ST ↑ like MI
(c) Recovers in 2 months

127. CCP A/E:
(a) Kussmaul sign
(b) Septal bounce
(c) Diff. in intrathoracic and intra pericardial pressures
(d) Square root sign in RV not LV

128. Pulsus electrical alternans in:
(a) Cardiac tamponade (b) CP
(c) RCM

129. LV = 120/120, PCWP = 19, RV = 40/20:
(a) CCP (b) RCM
(c) DCM

130. Diagnostic of HOCM:
(a) SAM
(b) Brokenbrough Braunwald
(c) LVOT gradient > 20 mm Hg
(d) LV thickness > 17 mm

131. Structural heart disease without symptoms:
(a) A (b) B
(c) C (d) D

132. MVO_2:
(a) $\frac{Q}{(A_0 - CS)}$ (b) $Q \times (A_0 - C_S)$
(c) $\frac{A_0 - C_S}{Q}$

133. Sacubitril is used for t/f:
(a) HF
(b) Myocarditis
(c) Pulmonary hypertension
(d) Angina

134. Pulmonary hypertension caused by:
(a) Schistosomiasis (b) Acyclostoma
(c) Filaria

135. Total pulmonary resistance:
(a) 100-300 (b) 300-500
(c) 700-1000

136. HCM murmur ↑ by:
(a) Amyl nitrate (b) Squatting
(c) β-blocker (d) Handgrip

137. FVR in MS predisposes most commonly to:
(a) Atrial thrombosis (b) Cardioembolic Stroke
(c) SCD (d) LV dysfunction

138. False about HOCM:
(a) Multiple gene mutation leads to severe form of phenotype
(b) Screening of all family member misprinting of result of propend
(c) Most patents have no mutation
(d) $LAMP_2$ Mutation associated with worse prognosis

139. ARVD poor prognosis A/E:
(a) THAM gene (b) Proteinuria
(c) Young age

140. Myocardial regeneration true:
(a) Systolic and diastolic heart evaluation
(b) Right and left ventricular function assessed
(c) LV relaxation time + IVCT/LVCT
(d) Reduced in LV systolic dysfunction

141. After load depends on:
(a) Viscosity of blood
(b) Myocardial wall tension
(c) Vascular distensibilty
(d) Vascular resistance

142. Takatsubo cardiomyopathy A/E:
(a) Not commonly associated with catecholamine levels
(b) RWMA extends beyond single epicardial coronary territory
(c) ST elevation is essential for diagnosis
(d) Late enhancement in MRI not seen generally

143. DP/DT all *except:*
(a) = 32 mm Hg/sec
(b) Signifies shear stress of aortic valve
(c) Accessed by eccentric MR jet
(d) Decreased by enalapril

144. Catherisation:
(a) LV pressure > RV pressure
(b) Systolic diastolic
(c) Cyanosis irrespective of pulmonary obstruction
(d) Pan systolic murmur

145. Effective pulmonary blood flow:
(a) VO2/PA-PV

146. All are pathognomic of digoxin toxicity *except:*
(a) Parasystole
(b) Bidirectional VT
(c) PAT with variable block
(d) Regularization of AF

147. Myocardial performance index:
(a) IVCT + IVRT/ET
(b) Used for systole and diastole
(c) Used for both LV and RV
(d) Decreased in LV systolic dysfunction

148. LV afterload determined by:
(a) Vascular distensibility
(b) Ventricular wall tension
(c) Vascular resistance

149. Diuretic resistance all *except:*
(a) Indomethacin (b) Dehydration
(c) Hypokalemia (d) Enalapril

150. True all *except:*
(a) Barth–tafazzin
(b) Danon disease–LAMP 2
(c) Carvajal–desmoplakin
(d) Fabry–XL GLA

151. Pseudoxanthoma elasticum:
(a) Can cause CAD (b) Angiod streaks
(c) Massive GI bleed (d) ABCC6 gene

152. Ischemic mitral involvement with SAM all *except:*
(a) β blockers (b) ACE inhibitors
(c) IV fluids (d) α agonists

153. Myocardial performance index all *except:*
(a) Indicates both LV and RV function
(b) IVCT + IVRT/ LV ejection time
(c) Both systolic and diastolic function

154. Takotsubo CMP all *except:*
(a) Variable catecholamines levels
(b) ECG changes ST ↑ must
(c) LGE seen on MRI
(d) RWMA outside vascular territory

155. Diuretic resistance all *except:*
(a) Low mean RA pressure
(b) Concomitant use of ARB
(c) NSAIDs
(d) Severe hyperkalemia

156. Nitric oxide true *except:*
(a) Selectively decreases pulmonary vascular resistance
(b) Metabolized in liver
(c) Sudden withdrawal leads to rebound increases PA pressure
(d) Prolonged usage leads to methemoglobinemia

157. In diastolic HF, findings in echo all *except:*
(a) Normal LV size (b) Increased LA size
(c) Near normal LVEF (d) Eccentric LVH

158. Potential of producing whole organisms autonomously:
(a) Pleuripotent (b) Totipotent
(c) Unipotent (d) Multipotent

159. LV afterload increased in all *except:*
(a) Systolic HTN (b) Aortic stiffness
(c) Moderate AS (d) VSD

160. Doppler echocardiography true *except:*
(a) PAEDP = 4 × (pulmonary. end regurgitation velocity)^2 + RAP
(b) LAP= 4 × (Peak mitral regurgitant velocity)^2 – aortic systolic pressure
(c) LVEDP = aortic EDP- gradient across PDA
(d) LVEDP = aortic EDP-gradient across valve in AR

161. Ambrisentan VS Bosentan all *except:*
(a) Selective ETa antagonist
(b) Common pedal edema
(c) Common LFT abnormal
(d) Similar efficacy

162. True *except:*
(a) Anrep effect- ↑ afterload
(b) Treppe- ↑ HR → ↑ ed contractility
(c) Lusitropic-↑ed cytosolic Ca+→ cause ↑ed relaxation
(d) Frank Starling- ↑ed SV→↑ed contractility
(e) All are true

163. Exercise testing in CVS disease:
(a) Isotonic exercise ↓es PVR
(b) Isotonic exercise more O_2 consumption than isometric and resistance
(c) Isometric-↑ ed SV
(d) Resistance exercise-↑ ed BP

164. All have excitable gap *except:*
(a) Ectopic AT
(b) Scar VT
(c) Bundle branch reentry tachycardia
(d) WPW

165. Worst prognosis in CHF:
(a) Warm dry (b) Warm wet
(c) Cold wet (d) Cold dry

166. Diameter of vessel if ↓ by 50%, gradient ↑ by:
(a) 2X (b) 8X
(c) 4X (d) 16X

167. Levosimenden is ADHF all *except:*
(a) ↓ 30 days mortality VS dobutamine
(b) Hypotension with I/V loading dose
(c) ↑ AF
(d) BNP markedly ↓

168. Alcohol septal ablation CI in:
(a) LBBB (b) LVOT> 80
(c) Syncope (d) SAM with MR

169. Chronic constrictive pericarditis most common cause:
(a) Viral (b) Pyogenic
(c) Tubercular (d) Recurrent idiopathic pericarditis

170. ↑ diuretic resistance all *except:*
(a) ↓ RA pr (b) ↓ K^+
(c) Associated ACE-I use (d) NSAIDs use

171. Diuretic effective in low GFR:
(a) Metalazone (b) Indapamide
(c) Chlorthalidone (d) Hydrochlor thiazide

172. Amyloidosis with multiple myeloma all *except:*
(a) Macroglossia
(b) Limp lead LVH
(c) Speckled appearance on echo
(d) Postural hypotension

173. All seen in acutely with exercise *except:*
(a) ↑ EF
(b) ↑ CVP
(c) ↓ Renal blood flow
(d) ↓ Splanchnic circulation

174. Cardiac conditioning all *except:*
(a) ↓ HR
(b) ↓ BP
(c) ↑ Parasympathetic activity
(d) ↑ Circulating volume

175. RA = 5 mm Hg, PR 3 cm/s on CW Doppler, what is PADP?
(a) 31 (b) 36
(c) 45 (d) 50

176. HOCM Brockenbrough phenomenon:
(a) ↑ LV systolic pressure
(b) ↓ Gradient
(c) ↑ Aortic pressure
(d) Interventricular dependence

177. CCP all *except:*
(a) ↑ Late diastolic filling
(b) Thoracic pressure changes not transmitted to heart
(c) Equalisation of pressure of ventricle and pulmonary arteries
(d) ↓ in flow in inspiration in left side

178. Dobutamine in cardiac failure:
(a) Weekly pulse ↓ mortality
(b) May ↑ O_2 demand
(c) In AF ↓ AV condition
(d) B_2 receptor agonist predominantly act on B_2 receptor

179. History 1st least Transplantation:
(a) Rose (b) Bernaud
(c) Wakerkey (d) Carpenter

180. B Blockers in CHF false:
(a) B blocker treatment ↓es mortality by 10-20%
(b) BEST trial-carvedilol
(c) ↓ es mortality by ↓ both SCD and non SCD
(d) RR ↓ 30%

181. Trop T/trop 1 all *except:*
(a) Only source is cardiac
(b) False Positive in CRF
(c) True Positive in pulmonary embolism
(d) False Positive in CTDs

182. ↓ CVP, ↓ PCWP, ↓CO, ↑SVR diagnosis:
(a) Cardiac tamponade
(b) Hypovolemic shock
(c) Massive MI
(d) Massive pulmonary embolism

183. CCP vs RCMP in favour of CCP all *except:*
(a) PAP > 60 mm Hg
(b) Ventricular interdependence
(c) ↑ Mitral filling velocity

184. Diuretic resistance causes all *except:*
(a) ↑ ed salt intake
(b) ↑ Vasodilation → hypotension
(c) Infusion compared to bolus dose
(d) ↓ Cardiac output

185. Tau:
(a) IV relaxation constant (b) IVCT
(c) dP/dt (d) cAMP

186. Sudden ↑ ses in aortic pressure after 1-2 min lead to ↑ inotropic effect:
(a) Anrep effect (b) Brody effect
(c) Coanda effect

187. RCMP + Constrictive pericarditis–both caused by:
(a) Radiation (b) Post cardiotomy
(c) Doxorubicin (d) Amyloidosis

188. In trials with HF, most common etiology is:
(a) HTN (b) Ischemic CMP
(c) Valvular (d) DM

189. Isovolumic contraction not seen in:
(a) AR (b) MR
(c) AS (d) MS

190. Takotsubo CMP also known as A/E:
(a) Tachycardiomyopathy
(b) Stress CMP

(c) Broken-heart syndrome
(d) Apical ballooning syndrome

191. Pulmonary circulation can ↑ without ↑ right heart pressure:
(a) Three (b) Four
(c) Six (d) Eight

192. B_2 receptors in heart:
(a) 50% (b) 20%
(c) 0% (d) 40%

193. HOCM murmur:
(a) ↑ on squatting
(b) ↑ on standing
(c) Valsalva ↓ murmur

194. Rupture of chamber during catheterization:
(a) Sign and murmur seen
(b) Nothing seen

195. HOCM septal ablation (alcohol) A/E:
(a) 1-4 ml of alcohol injected
(b) Only 10% show immediate ↓ gradient
(c) Artery visualized by contrast echo
(d) LBBB

196. Athlete's heart vs HOCM favouring athletes A/E:
(a) Ventricular cavity size ↓ ed
(b) Normal diastolic function
(c) Wall thickness < 17 mm

197. Myocardial cell specific gravity:
(a) 1.02 (b) 1.04
(c) 1.06 (d) 1.08

198. Pulmonary ↑ ITN is defined by pulmonary artery pressure:
(a) 25 (b) 30
(c) 20 (d) 40

199. True about by congenital absence of pericardium is all *except*:
(a) Left side more common
(b) Pericardiectomy TOC
(c) LBBB seen

200. In HOCM, LV pressure volume shift:
(a) Leftwards up (b) Rightwards up
(c) Upwards left (d) Downward right

201. True about angiosarcoma is all *except*:
(a) Cardio transplantation–TOC
(b) RA is most common site
(c) Cardiac sarcoma in adults is most common primary tumor
(d) Familial occurrence rare

202. Cyclophosphamide true is:
(a) 500 mg monthly for 6 months
(b) 500 mg monthly × 6 weeks
(c) 1000 mg daily for 6 weeks
(d) 500 mg daily for 6 months

203. PPH all *except*:
(a) Prostaglandin 12 (b) Indomethacin
(c) Sildenafil

204. Worst prognosis in pulmonary artery HTN:
(a) Idiopathic
(b) Eisenmenger's
(c) Anorexdyenic
(d) With connective tissue disorder

205. Which diuretic decrease mortality in STEM?
(a) Furosemide (b) Spironolactone
(c) Indapamide

206. ECG in CCP all *except*:
(a) Low voltage common
(b) AF 5-10% T
(c) ST/7′ changes are seen most common I>
(d) 50% ECG normal

207. Investigation of choice for acute viral pericarditis:
(a) ECG (b) ECHO
(c) CT (d) MRI

208. In CHF all decrease long term mortality *except*:
(a) Digoxin (b) ACE-I
(c) Hydralazine + nitrate (d) Beta blocker

209. In CCP LV pressure volume curve:
(a) Rightward (b) Leftward
(c) Upward (d) Downward

210. Which not lead to RCMP?
(a) Gaucher's
(b) Fabry
(c) Hemochromatosis disorder
(d) Glycogen storage

211. **Fabry's disease true all *except*:**
(a) Cerebroside accumulation
(b) Minimal symptomatic
(c) Normal epicardial coronaries
(d) MI can occur

212. **All increase murmur in HCM *except*:**
(a) Standing (b) Amyl nitrate
(c) Hand grip

213. **Chronic anemia all *except*:**
(a) O_2 dissociation curve shift to left
(b) Decrease after load

214. **Isovolumic phase include all *except*:**
(a) Vmax (b) Vpm
(c) Max Dp/Dt (d) Mean Vcf

215. **Pulmonary oedema all *except*:**
(a) Increase PAP
(b) Increase oncotic pressure
(c) Pulmonary venous pressure increase

216. **Cardiac tamponade all *except*:**
(a) Intrapericardial and RV diastolic pressure equal
(b) Severe tamponade leads to bradycardia
(c) Initial increase stroke volume due to equal diastolic pressure
(d) Hypovolemia difficult to diagnose

217. **CHF:**
(a) α 2 receptor normal, α 1 increase
(b) α 2 decrease, α 1 decrease
(c) G protein α 1 decrease, α 2 decrease

218. **CHF – valsalva:**
(a) Phase 1 and 4 blunt (b) Phase 2 and 4 blunt
(c) Phase 1 and 3 blunt

219. **Myocardial contractility best by:**
(a) LV end systolic pulmonary volume in Dp/dt
(b) Circumferential myocardial shortening

220. **Acute pulmonary thromboembolism, sensitive marker of screening:**
(a) D-dimer (b) FDP
(c) Oxygen saturation (d) Troponin

221. **Polycythemia Vera -EPO level:**
(a) Low (b) Normal
(c) Increases (d) Undetectable

222. **Smoker's polycythemia associated:**
(a) ↑ EPO (b) ↑ O_2 affinity to Hb
(c) Relative erythrocytosis

223. **HOCM due to:**
(a) Deficiency of tropomyosin-C
(b) Mutation of myosin binding protein
(c) Deficiency of cardiac actinin

224. **Pulsus tardus:**
(a) AS (b) PS
(c) MS (d) TS

225. **Pulsus bigeminy:**
(a) LV dysfunction (b) Digitoxicity
(c) MS with AR

226. **Rapid x-y descent:**
(a) CCP (b) Cardiac tamponade
(c) DCM (d) HOCM

227. **BNP associated with:**
(a) CHF (b) Frank-starling law
(c) PTE (d) MI

228. **OSA associated with:**
(a) AV block (b) CAD
(c) Seizure

229. **Cannon 'a' wave:**
(a) Junctional Rhythm (b) MR
(c) MS

230. **Reverse Pulsus Paradoxus in:**
(a) HOCM (b) Pulmonary Embolism
(c) Obesity (d) CCP

231. **Characteristic of RCMP:**
(a) Bilateral atrial enlargement
(b) Pulsus paradoxus
(c) Square root sign in cath study
(d) Septal bounce

232. **Which require intact endothelium for vasodilation?**
(a) Ach (b) Nitroglycerin
(c) Adenosine (d) Prostaglandins

233. **DCMP with EF <20% A/E:**
(a) Apoptosis
(b) Myocardial Slippage

(c) Perimyocardial fibrosis
(d) Myocyte Hypertrophy

234. EMF A/E:

(a) AR (b) MR
(c) TR (d) Mural thrombus

235. Predominant Venodilation:

(a) Sodium nitroprusside (b) Hydralazine
(c) NTG (d) Phentolamine

236. Least common in pulmonary hypertension:

(a) TR (b) RVS3
(c) RVH (d) Graham Steel murmur

237. Stag's antler sign:

(a) Pulmonary Arterial Hypertension
(b) Pulmonary venous hypertension
(c) Systolic HTN
(d) Renovascular Hypertension

238. Paradoxical septal movement in ASD in which Qp/Qs ratio is?

(a) 1.5 (b) 2
(c) 3 (d) 0.5

239. Reverse S2 in A/E:

(a) Pulmonary HTN (b) WPW type B
(c) HOCM (d) AS

240. Asymptomatic LV dysfunction, drug used is:

(a) ACE -I
(b) Digoxin
(c) Hydralazine + nitrates
(d) ICD

241. HOCM gene A/E:

(a) Troponin T (b) Tropomyosin
(c) β-MHC (d) X chromosome

242. Framingham major criteria for CHF A/E:

(a) Dyspnoea on exertion
(b) ↑ JVP
(c) PND
(d) Acute pulmonary Edema

243. Threshold potential of most cardiac cell:

(a) – 80 to – 90 (b) + 20 to + 40
(c) 10

244. Most important ion for RMP:

(a) Na (b) K
(c) Mg (d) Ca

245. Consensus trial benefit seen:

(a) Mild CMP
(b) Severe CMP
(c) Asymptomatic LV dysfunction

246. Which of the following is not CHF with high output:

(a) Pregnancy (b) Beri beri
(c) Paget's disease (d) Hypothyroidism

247. JVP is not raised in:

(a) Low pressure tamponade
(b) Purulent PE with tamponade

248. LV preload is increased in:

(a) MR (b) Pericardial effusion
(c) Sepsis (d) Pulmonary embolism

249. Prostaglandin treatment required in A/E:

(a) Pulmonary atresia (b) TAPVC
(c) COA

250. Austin flint murmur all *except:*

(a) MDM (b) Presystolic murmur
(c) Loud S1

251. Most specific for myocardial disease:

(a) Akinesia (b) Dyskinesia
(c) Absence of systolic thickening

252. Kerley B lines are:

(a) Short straight horizontal
(b) Curved perihilar

253. Pulmonary venous HTN seen A/E:

(a) Cortriatriatum (b) PR

254. Normal PCWP with pulmonary edema:

(a) HAPE (b) Preeclampsia

255. Mixed venous saturation:

(a) Pulmonary artery (b) SVC
(c) IVC (d) Coronary sinus

256. R → L shunt at atrial level is seen in A/E:

(a) PDA (b) ASD
(c) TAPVC

257. RCMP versus CCP best diagnosed by:

(a) Variation in inflow velocity of MV and TV
(b) PASP increased

(c) Equalization of pressure
(d) Square root sign

258. SVR decreases in A/E:
(a) Pregnancy (b) Thyrotoxicosis
(c) Standing (d) Fever

259. Pulmonary embolism-RVSP measured by:
(a) TR jet (b) PR jet

260. CO depends on:
(a) Preload (b) Afterload
(c) LV contractility (d) HR
(e) Oxygen carrying capacity

261. Myocardial oxygen consumption depends on A/E:
(a) Wall tension (b) Hemoglobin
(c) HR (d) LV volume

262. MET is:
(a) Oxygen consumption/body weight

263. Peripartum CMP:
(a) First 6 months of pregnancy
(b) Autoimmune
(c) Recurs in subsequent pregnancy

264. CCP is characterized by A/E:
(a) Kussmaul sign
(b) Equalization of systolic pressure
(c) Equalization of diastolic pressure

265. Drug used in all stages of HF:
(a) ACE-I (b) Diuretic
(c) B Blocker

266. Pericardial window used in:
(a) Amyloidosis (b) Malignancy
(c) TB

267. Pulmonary HTN drug used *except:*
(a) CCB (b) B blocker
(c) Prostanoid (d) PDE-I

268. Eplerenone:
(a) Aldoterone receptor inhibitor

269. ACE-I causes increase in creatinine A/E:
(a) Hypotension (b) HTN
(c) CCF (d) NIDDM

270. Cor pulmonale most useful in:
(a) Oxygen (b) Digoxin

271. Contractile protein *except:*
(a) Actin (b) Myosin
(c) Tropomyosin (d) None

272. Thiazide A/E:
(a) Hypouricemia (b) Hypercalcemia

273. Physiological systole consists of:
(a) Isovolumic contraction, maximal ejection and reduced ejection
(b) Isovolumic contraction and maximal ejection
(c) From M1 to A2
(d) From A2 to M1

274. Cardiological systole consists of:
(a) Isovolumic contraction, maximal ejection and reduced ejection
(b) Isovolumic contraction and maximal ejection
(c) From M1 to A2
(d) From A2 to M1

275. JVP:
(a) Variable in normal population
(b) Normal value—8 to 10 cm H_2O
(c) Prominent wave is 'c' wave

276. Levosimendan A/E:
(a) SURVIVE–it reduces AF compared to dobutamine
(b) REVIVE II–done in AHFS
(c) Increases VT incidence
(d) ATP dependent K^+ opener

277. Broadbent sign in:
(a) Constrictive pericarditis
(b) Restrictive pericarditis
(c) Tamponade
(d) MI

278. Minor criteria in Framingham criteria:
(a) PND (b) Cardiomegaly
(c) Neck vein distension (d) Pedal edema

279. EDRF is:
(a) NO (b) Adenosine
(c) Prostacycline (d) Endothelin

280. Maximum coronary flow maintained by:
(a) Adenosine (b) NO
(c) EDHF (d) Prostacycline

281. Specific activity scale III, all cannot be performed *except:*

(a) Sexual activity (b) Dancing
(c) Gardening (d) Walk 2.5 mph

282. Mebifradil is inhibitor of:

(a) L- Ca channel
(b) A1 adenosine receptor blocker
(c) T-Ca channel blocker
(d) A2 adenosine receptor blocker

283. Normal PADP:

(a) 0-4 mm Hg (b) 4-12 mm Hg
(c) 12-20 mm Hg (d) 20-24 mm Hg

284. Normal PVR:

(a) 10-50 mm Hg (b) 20-130 mm Hg
(c) 700-900 mm Hg (d) 100-200 mm Hg

285. Mortality/year of moderate HF:

(a) 0% (b) < 5%
(c) 20-30% (d) 80-90%

286. Normal upper limit of pericardial thickness in MRI:

(a) 1 mm (b) 2 mm
(c) 3 mm (d) 4 mm

287. LVEDP-RVEDP > 5 mmHg, diagnosis:

(a) CCP (b) RCM
(c) HOCM (d) MI

288. CCP A/E:

(a) LVEDP – RVEDP = 5 mmHg
(b) RVEDP > 1/3rd RVSP
(c) > 25% respiratory variation of mitral annular velocity
(d) Decreased diastolic flow reversal in hepatic vein on expiration

289. Inflammatory myocarditis true:

(a) Dallas criteria (b) Framingham criteria
(c) Jones criteria

290. Circulation first described by:

(a) William Harvey (b) Leonardo de Vinci

291. JVP true:

(a) Usually due to RV failure
(b) Increased in pericarditis
(c) Increases with inspiration
(d) Not raised in LV dysfunction

292. Extended matching—PAH drugs:

(a) Diltiazem (b) Sildenafil
(c) Bosentan (d) Iloprost
(e) Epoprostenol (f) Ambrisentan

(1) Drug without recommendation and needs high dose for full activity
(2) Increased c GMP and 25 mg TDS
(3) Inhalational prostacyclin (approved)
(4) Non selective ET receptor blocker 125 mg BD
(5) Used as continuous infusion

293. Peripheral cyanosis seen in:

(a) PVD
(b) TOF
(c) VSD with Eisenmenger
(d) ILD

294. First virus to be used in gene transfer:

(a) Adenovirus (b) Cox sackie virus
(c) Retro virus (d) Lentivirus

295. Atrial waves: (T/F)

(a) V decreased in LA in TAPVC
(b) LA mean = 3-4 mm Hg
(c) RA = a > v
(d) RA pressure increases on inspiration

296. Anthracycline toxicity: (T/F)

(a) Can be reduced by regulated doses
(b) Dextrazoxone is used for treatment
(c) CO Q is used for treatment

297. Athelete heart: (T/F)

(a) Size of LV wall < 17 mm
(b) Asymmetric hypertrophy
(c) ↓ LV dimension
(d) Tissue strain normal
(e) Ea < 7 cm/s

298. All are markers of HF, *except:*

(a) ADH (b) GDF-15
(c) ST-2 (d) Galectin
(e) BNP

299. Vasopressin differs from epinephrine on:

(a) Increases renal blood flow
(b) Decreases pulmonary blood flow
(c) Uniform action
(d) No effect HR
(e) More inotropic

300. Which drug increases cyclic GMP?
(a) Inhaled NO (b) Sildenafil
(c) Epoprostenol (d) Bosentan
(e) CCB

301. Hakki formula:
(a) Directly proportional to cardiac output
(b) Inversely proportional to square root of peak to peak gradient
(c) Simplification of Gorlin formula
(d) Directly proportional to square root of peak to peak gradient
(e) Inversely proportional to CO

302. Diastolic HF:
(a) More common in elderely
(b) HTN is a risk factor
(c) More common in female
(d) ACE I decrease mortality markedly
(e) ARB decrease mortality

303. Mitra clip–not true:
(a) Useful in primary MR
(b) Useful in secondary MR
(c) Safe for MRI
(d) Useful in rheumatic MR
(e) Based on surgical Alfieri technique

304. Grade II LV diastolic dysfunction vs normal LV function supporting prior:
(a) E/e' more than 10
(b) Deceleration less than 140 ms
(c) E/A less than 0.5 on Valsalva
(d) S wave blunting in pulmonary venous Doppler
(e) LA enlarged

305. Peripartum cardiomyopathy–not true is:
(a) Rare in less than 36 weeks
(b) Common in Caucasians
(c) Mechanism of action is unknown
(d) Partial/complete recovery is common
(e) Recurrence is common in next pregnancy if incomplete recovery

306. Central fibrous trigone true:
(a) Ligament infundibulum connects Pulmonary valve to Aortic valve
(b) Non coronary cusp of aorta is continuous with fibrous band
(c) AV node pierces central fibrous body
(d) Tendon of todaro extends from right end of fibrous body to Eustachian valve
(e) Left fibrous body is also called central fibrous body

307. Grey effect:
(a) Results from starling law
(b) Increase in coronary blood flow increases cardiac relaxation
(c) Increase in coronary blood flow increases contractility

308. NYHA class III:
(a) Asymptomatic at rest
(b) Symptomatic at less than ordinary activity
(c) Cannot do any activity without breathlessness
(d) Symptomatic at rest
(e) No symptoms

309. Changes in HF:
(a) Increased TNF
(b) Decreased aldosterone
(c) Decreased betal receptor density
(d) Decreased NE
(e) Increased BNP

310. AF with failure drug used is:
(a) Flecainide (b) Propafenone
(c) Amiodarone (d) Sotalol

311. Which beta blocker from following in excreted through kidney?
(a) Propranolol (b) Atenolol
(c) Carvedilol (d) Metoprolol

312. Normal QRS. X descent true:
(a) Occurs after S_2 (b) Occurs before S2
(c) Occurs after H (d) Not related to H

313. PVR index:
(a) 27 (b) 37
(c) 47

314. Transpulmonary gradient is:
(a) 54 (b) 60
(c) 64

315. Paradoxical split S2 all *except:*
(a) RBBB (b) RV apical pacing
(c) Severe AS (d) HOCM
(e) Ischemia

316. HOCM all *except:*
(a) Prevalence 2%
(b) Also known as Teare syndrome
(c) LVOT in 30%
(d) Block described in 1958
(e) Most common cause of SCD in young athelete

317. Treppe phenomenon:
(a) Increased HR–Increased contractility
(b) Increased preload–Increased contractility
(c) Increased afterload–Increased contractility
(d) None

318. Cardiac myocyte RMP is:
(a) -80 to -90 mV (b) -50 to -60 mV
(c) +80 to +90 mV (d) +50 to +60 mV

319. Load independent measure of LV systolic function:
(a) Isovolumic acceleration
(b) Myocardial perfusion index
(c) Fractional length shortening
(d) 3D ECHO volumetric EF

320. All are used to assess diastolic dysfunction in reduced LVEF, *except*:
(a) Left atrial size
(b) E/A
(c) Lateral and medial mitral annulus e'
(d) E/e'
(e) TR velocity

321. Sacubitril valsartan trials:
(a) DANISH
(b) ODYSSEY OUTCOMES
(c) PARAMOUNT
(d) PARADIGM-HF
(e) PARADISE-MI

322. CCP: (T/F)
(a) Pericardial knock occur after low pitch
(b) y descent slow and blunted
(c) In inspiration flow on right side ↑, on left side ↓
(d) Dip and plateau
(e) Systolic function is never impaired

323. Acute pericarditis all *except:*
(a) STE in all 12 leads
(b) Pain on inspiration and movement
(c) High pitch scratching sound
(d) ↑ Enzyme suggestive of myocardial involvement

324. Pulmonary edema least effective:
(a) CPAP 5-10 mm Hg (b) Nitrates
(c) Digoxin IV (d) Morphine

325. Normal collapsing pulse:
(a) Severe MR (b) VSD and PAH
(c) VSD without PAH (d) A and C

326. Cardiac tamponade all *except:*
(a) Hypotension (b) Bradycardia
(c) ↑ JVP (d) Pulsus paradoxus

327. CCP all *except:*
(a) Slow y descent (b) Cardiomegaly on CXR
(c) AF is common

328. Pericarditis all *except:*
(a) ST ↑ coved upward resemble transmural MI
(b) ST ↑ in all 12 leads
(c) Chest pain ↑ with deep breath
(d) Subclinical myocarditis can occur and diagnosed by enzymes
(e) Superficial high pitched scratchy rub

329. PHT caused by all *except:*
(a) Fenfluramine
(b) Chronic thromboembolism
(c) Chronic liver disease
(d) AIDS
(e) Air embolism while blood sampling

330. Normal volume collapsing pulse:
(a) Severe MR (b) VSD with PHT
(c) VSD without PHT (d) A+B
(e) All of the above

331. Continuous murmur D/D:
(a) VSD with AR
(b) AS with AR
(c) Lutembacher
(d) Bland-White Garten syndrome

332. ANTLER sign:
(a) Cephalization (b) Lateralization
(c) Equalization (d) Localization
(e) Collateralization

333. Innervation of heart all *except:*
(a) B_1 Chronotropic
(b) B_2 receptor–vascular SMC
(c) Resting rate is slow due to ↓ adrenergic drive
(d) Cholinergic SAN + AVN Muscarinic receptor
(e) Diabetic neuropathy–less variability

334. Acute pulmonary edema all *except:*
(a) CPAP 5-10 mmHg
(b) I/V digoxin
(c) I/V nitrate
(d) Standing causes relief
(e) Morphine

335. Loud S_1 all *except:*
(a) LA myxoma (b) Short PR
(c) WPW (d) MS
(e) Tachycardia

336. Athlete heart vs HCM: (T/F)
(a) Symmetric hypertrophy
(b) LVH rarely > 17mm
(c) LV dimension increased > in HCM
(d) Ea ≤ 7 cm/sec
(e) Regression of LVH after stop exercise

337. Platypnea orthodeoxia all *except:*
(a) COPD
(b) VSD
(c) ASD
(d) Hepato pulmonary syndrome
(e) PFO

338. Constrictive pericarditis: (T/F)
(a) 1/3 have pulsus paradoxus
(b) Systolic function never impaired
(c) Pericardial knock early systolic
(d) Kussmaul sign always present
(e) Calcification if present over posterior apical region of LV suggest constrictive pericarditis

339. Newer drugs in HF: (T/F)
(a) Levosimendan causes less AF/hypotension than dobutamine
(b) Cinnagulat c-GMP activator
(c) Isotroxime
(d) Omecamtiv

340. Least lipid soluble beta blocker:
(a) Atenolol (b) Carvedilol
(c) Metoprolol (d) Pindolol
(e) Propranolol

341. CCP versus restriction: (T/F)
(a) Systolic pressure time curve ↑ in CCP
(b) No equalisation occurs in CCP
(c) Pulmonary HTN more common with CCP
(d) Mitral inflow velocity >25% in CCP versus < 10% in RCMP
(e) E′ >7 in RCMP

342. Drugs induced pericarditis:
(a) Deflocort (b) Emetine
(c) Methylsergide (d) Mycophenolate

343. Infiltrative RCMP by: (T/F)
(a) Scleroderma
(b) Fabry
(c) Gaucher
(d) Glycogen storage disease
(e) Hemochromatosis

344. Kerley A lines is MS indicates:
(a) Mild (b) Mod
(c) Severe (d) Minimal
(e) MS with MR

345. HCM murmur true:
(a) ↑ on squatting (b) ↑ after PVC
(c) ↓ on standing (d) ↓ on Valsalva
(e) Leg raising

346. Alcoholic CMP, what is most specific and sensitivity for alcohol abuse?
(a) γ GGT
(b) MCV
(c) Carbohydrate related transferrin
(d) High BNP
(e) Glutaraldehyde

347. HOCM-ICD indication: (T/F)
(a) Thickness of septal > 32 mm
(b) Apical aneurysm
(c) 1st degree relative
(d) Hypotension with exercise
(e) Cardiac arrest outside hospital

348. BNP all *except:*
(a) Obesity (b) MI
(c) PE (d) CKD
(e) High output

349. Digoxin toxicity causes:
(a) Hyperkalemia (b) Anorexia
(c) N/V (d) Block
(e) Visual disturbances (f) All true

350. Furosemide:
(a) Asc. loop (b) Desc. loop

351. Athlete heart:
(a) Symmetric
(b) Echo/Doppler normal
(c) ↓ LV dimension

352. Alcohol ablation:
(a) 2-4 ml absolute alcohol
(b) Very few show immediate improved gradient
(c) C. dissection complication
(d) Perfusion to find not site of injection

353. Collapsing pulse all *except*: (T/F)
(a) Truncus arteriosus
(b) PDA reversal of shunt
(c) TOF bronchopulmonary collateral
(d) Pulmonary atresia
(e) Ebstein – low volume pulse

354. Athlete heart: (T/F)
(a) Size of LV wall < 17 mm
(b) Asymmetric hypertrophy
(c) ↓ LV dimension
(d) Tissue strain normal
(e) Ea < 7 cm/s

355. DCMP: (T/F)
(a) Associated with LV wall thickness
(b) All normal epicardial coronaries
(c) All chamber involved
(d) Valves normal annulus

356. Stress induced CMP: (T/F)
(a) Premenopausal women common
(b) ST elevation present
(c) Only apical dilation
(d) Abnormal coronaries
(e) Prognosis good

357. Opening snap: (T/F)
(a) Early diastolic event
(b) A_2OS indicate severe MS
(c) Can coexist with S_3
(d) A_2OS varies with cycle length
(e) Severe MR may rarely associated with opening snap

358. Myocarditis > 80% specific are: (T/F)
(a) Indium labelled Ab
(b) High sensitive trop I > 0.1
(c) ECG
(d) MRI
(e) Dallas criteria

359. O_2 consumption index (ml/min/m²):
(a) 50-70 (b) 70-120
(c) 120-160 (d) 170-200
(e) 200-500

360. Pulmonary artery EDP:
(a) 0-4 (b) 4-12
(c) 12-18 (d) 18-25

361. Normal pulmonary vascular resistance:
(a) 20-130 (b) 10-20
(c) 20-60 (d) 700-1600

362. LVEDP >5 mm Hg RVEDP:
(a) CCP (b) Restrictive CMP
(c) LV dysfunction (d) Ischemic CMP

363. Mortality in moderate HF person:
(a) <5% (b) 10%
(c) 10-30% (d) >30%

364. Emergency diagnosis of HF by:
(a) NT pro BNP (b) Pre pro BNP
(c) TNP (d) C-CNP

365. Indication of changing IV to oral vasodilator
(a) PCWP 18 to 22 (b) RA pressure 5-8
(c) SVR 700-1200 (d) CI > 1.5 l/min/m²

366. Pulsus alternans:
(a) Can be seen in mild HF
(b) Ppted by PVC
(c) Can only be measured by BP instrument
(d) Irregular rhythm seen

367. Electrical total alternans:
(a) PQRS-T alternans nonspecific of cardiac tamponade
(b) Freq. of swinging of heart is half the heart rate
(c) ST-T alternans S/O electrical stability

368. Major criteria of Framingham criteria:
(a) Edema feet (b) PND
(c) Cardiomegaly (d) JVP

369. HF: (T/F)
(a) Patient sleeps on left side
(b) Treponema seen in HF
(c) HF cause is PE more commonly

370. Potency of diuretic judged by:
(a) Fractional Na extraction
(b) Functional K^+ excretion
(c) Daily weight
(d) 24 hours urine output

371. Recurrent pericarditis true:
(a) 8 weeks ibuprufen
(b) Colchicine is equally effective as steroid
(c) Steroid for 1 years
(d) NSAID for 5 days

372. S_3 false:
(a) Its presence always abnormal
(b) Inspiration-loud RVS_3
(c) Always present in rapid filling phase
(d) Low pitch of LVS_3

373. ↓ murmur by amyl nitrate false:
(a) MR (b) AR
(c) VSD (d) AS

374. Dobutamine ↓ PVR by:
(a) B_2 agonist (b) α 1 agonist
(c) ↑ CO

375. LA-LV gradient affected by:
(a) HR (b) MVA
(c) CO (d) EF
(e) LVEDP

376. Paradoxical split S_2 in all *except:*
(a) RV paced
(b) LBBB peripheral
(c) LBBB proximal
(d) VSD with pulmonary HTN
(e) AS

377. Ratio of B_1B_2 in heart:
(a) 80:20 (b) 60:40
(c) 50: 50

378. Sarcomere max strength at:
(a) 2.2 μm (b) 1.6

379. A-II vasoconstriction acts through which receptor subtypes?
(a) Endothelin-A (b) A-I
(c) A-II (d) Aldosterone

380. Flamin equation:
(a) Mixed venous oxygen (b) MVA
(c) CO

381. Hyponatremia in HF treatment:
(a) Tolvaptan (b) Nestiride
(c) Omipatrilat (d) Milrionone

382. Early systolic murmur T/F:
(a) TR
(b) MR
(c) Small VSD
(d) Large VSD with Eisenmenger
(e) All true

383. Both phase IV and V BP should be mentioned when difference is:
(a) 10 (b) 20
(c) 30 (d) 40
(e) 5

384. T/F, false is:
(a) BP routinely measured in sitting position
(b) Bladder should cover 2/3 of arm
(c) Sphygmomanometer should be at level of heart
(d) 2 mm Hg/sec reduction
(e) Absence of sound used as measure of DBP

385. RCMP > CCP:
(a) PAP<50
(b) Diastolic P < 1/3 presystolic
(c) LVP > RVP by 5 mm Hg
(d) Dip and plateau

386. Cardiac syncope–characteristic:
(a) Premonitory symptoms absent
(b) 5-10 mn LOC
(c) Urine incontinence
(d) Rapid recovery

387. Factors investigation in CVP:
(a) Pulmonary artery pressure
(b) Intravascular volume

(c) Intrathoracic pressure
(d) Venous tone
(e) All

388. HCM T/F:
(a) SCD due to VF–vigorous exercise
(b) SAM of ant mitral leaflet–ASH/Mitral regurgitation
(c) Basal infarction of septum–alcohol ablation
(d) Stiff ventricle–heart failure
(e) Deep T wave inversion–apical hypertrophy
(f) All true

389. Alcohol and CVD T/F:
(a) Alcohol is a common cause of AF in < 60 years
(b) 1-2 peg/ day ↓ CVD
(c) Moderate alcohol ↓ LDL
(d) Severe alcohol intake–diastolic HF

390. Features of CCP T/F:
(a) Slow y descent
(b) LV pr ↓ on inspiration
(c) Pericardial knock has lower frequency and after S_3
(d) ↓ JVP on inspiration
(e) Dip and plateau

391. Pulmonary interstitial edema occurs at what PCWP?
(a) 20 (b) 25
(c) 18 (d) 10

392. Bowditch phenomenon also known as:
(a) Treppe phenomenon (b) Anrep effect

393. Large effusion in uremic pericarditis:
(a) Intensify dialysis (b) Pericardiocentesis

394. Still's murmur true:
(a) Early systolic murmur
(b) High frequency pulmonary fluttering
(c) Low pitched
(d) All of the above

395. DCM – mortality benefit all *except:*
(a) Digoxin (b) Aspirin
(c) Ramipril

396. Muller maneuvre:
(a) Forced inspiration (b) Open nose
(c) Open mouth (d) None

397. Angiotensin-II vasoconstriction:
(a) AT-I receptors (b) AT-II
(c) ET-A

398. S_4 all *except:*
(a) Normal in young people
(b) Absent in AF
(c) Low pitch
(d) HOCM

399. MVP all *except:*
(a) Mid systolic click (b) Benign arrhythmias
(c) Pansystolic murmur (d) Atypical chest pain
(e) Continuous after 50-60 years

400. Beta blocker in CHF:
(a) Mortality not ↓ed
(b) ↑ es EF it started slowly
(c) Decompression in patients with acute on chronic HF, its therapeutic dose given at start
(d) Antagonises harmful effects of sympathetic overactivity

401. PAWP all *except:*
(a) Correlated with mean LV pressure
(b) If balloon deflated PA pressure can be measured
(c) Correlated with CVP
(d) Correlates with LA pressure
(e) Can be calculated at midaxillary line in supine

402. Cardiac tamponade all *except:*
(a) Kussmaul sign (b) Bradycardia
(c) Y descent absent (d) Hypotension
(e) Pulsus paradoxus

403. CCP – all *except:*
(a) JVP decreases with inspiration
(b) Myocardial dysfunction can be seen in chronic cases
(c) Systolic dysfunction

404. Low cardiac output and low ejection fraction with AS true:
(a) ↑ se in CO without ↑ se in gradient–good prognosis
(b) ↑ se in CO with ↑ se in gradient–good prognosis
(c) Nitroprusside should not be given
(d) Development of AF relieves HF

405. Baroreceptors true is:

(a) Acts true NTS if MAP> 70 mm Hg

(b) Silent when MAP < 70 mm Hg

(c) MAP of 70 mm Hg set point

(d) They are mechanoreceptors

406. To demonstrate pitting edema press for:

(a) 5 to 10 sec (b) 10-20 sec

(c) 20-30 sec (d) 30-40 sec

407. All drug decrease mortality in CHF *except:*

(a) Digoxin (b) Spironolactone

(c) ACE I (d) Beta blockers

408. ITT trialist demonstrated decreased mortality incidence of:

(a) 18 (b) 24

(c) 32 (d) 36

409. Reversed splitting is caused by all:

(a) Complete LBBB (b) PDA

(c) VSD (d) RV ectopics

410. HOCM gene with most prognosis on which chromosome?

(a) 1 (b) 11

(c) 14 (d) 15

411. Sacromere length at diastasis?

(a) 2.2 µm (b) 1.8

(c) 2.4 (d) 3.2

412. Interstitial edema occurs with PCWP of:

(a) 15 (b) 18

(c) 20 (d) 25

413. Treatment of HF with hyponatremia:

(a) Tolvaptan (b) Enoximone

(c) Nesiritide (d) Dobutamine

414. DC shock can be given to all *except:*

(a) Pregnancy (b) Digitalis

(c) LA size > 40 mm

415. Snap term was given by:

(a) Thayer (b) Claude

416. Murmur word originated from:

(a) English (b) Sanskrit

(c) Latin (d) Greek

417. Fractional shortening–20%, Ef-40%, DV-125 ml, R-R interval-800 ms, cardiac output is:

(a) 3L (b) 3.75L

(c) 2.5L (d) 4.0L

418. Mechanical valve preferred over bioprosthetic valve in:

(a) Patient not on anticoagulant

(b) Pregnancy

(c) Elderly

(d) Patient on hemodialysis

419. Bowditch phenomenon is other name for:

(a) Treppe (b) Anerp

(c) Franck (d) Starling

420. ↑ systolic blood pressure causes increased contractility:

(a) Anrep effect (b) Treppe

(c) Bowditch

421. Adenosine effect on sacromere:

(a) Myocardial necrosis

(b) Prolongs QT

(c) Action reverses in 6 sec

(d) All

422. Still's murmur:

(a) High frequency murmur

(b) Medium frequency with mid systolic murmur

(c) Originates from pulmonary valve

(d) All of the above

423. Cardiorespiratory murmur:

(a) Left infrascapular murmur

(b) Right clavicle

(c) Left axilla

(d) All

424. Rytain's murmur:

(a) Early diastolic (b) Mid systolic

(c) Late systolic (d) Mid diastolic

425. Goldman specific activity scale stage–I:

(a) > 7 mets (b) > 5 mets

(c) >2 mets (d) > 10 mets

426. Korotkoff sounds phase 4 and 5 have difference of:

(a) 5 mm Hg (b) 10 mm Hg

(c) 30 mm Hg (d) 40 mm Hg

427. $B_1 : B_2$ ratio in normal heart:

(a) 80:20 (b) 60:40
(c) 50:50 (d) 75:25

428. Among following CHF mediators, which is vasodilatory?

(a) Cytokines (b) Adrenomedullin
(c) Endothelin (d) Vasopressin

429. Infiltrative pericarditis true is:

(a) Pericardiocentesis is done
(b) Frequent dialysis
(c) Balloon pericardiotomy
(d) After surgical drainage steroids given intrapericardially

430. Early changes in pericarditis, true is:

(a) ST ↑ in all leads except V_1 and AVR
(b) Mechanism of ST elevation is flow of current from epicardium to thorax

431. DCMP used is:

(a) Dor procedure (b) Maze procedure
(c) Ross procedure (d) Batista procedure

432. In CCP, pulmonary venous congestion is seen in:

(a) 10% (b) 15%
(c) 25% (d) 100%

433. Y wave occurs after:

(a) S_1 (b) S_2
(c) A_2 (d) P_2

434. Reverse pulsus paradoxus:

(a) HOCM (b) Pulmonary embolism
(c) CCP (d) RVM

435. Ventricular interdependence seen in:

(a) Constrictive pericarditis
(b) Corrected TGA
(c) HOCM

436. CHF precipitated by A/E:

(a) NSAID (b) Aspirin
(c) Trastuzumab (d) Thiazolidiones

437. Child while catching had stuck it on his chest and collapse:

(a) Cardiac thump immediately
(b) CPR within 10 minutes
(c) ACE-I within 10 minutes

438. BNP levels increased in all *except:*

(a) Obesity (b) Pulmonary disease
(c) Cirrhosis (d) Renal failure

439. IPF investigation of choice:

(a) HRCT (b) PFT
(c) Biopsy

440. ACE-I, hyperkalemia caused by mild renal disease along with:

(a) NSAID (b) Digoxin

441. HOCM:

(a) Troponin mutation causes no or minimal obstruction
(b) AD
(c) Multiple mutations in single gene
(d) 3 group mutations with different phenotype

442. Pan systolic murmur A/E:

(a) VSD with Eisenmenger syndrome

443. Cardiomyopathy due to hemochromatosis investigation of choice:

(a) MRI (b) Multislice CT
(c) 3D-echo

444. Kussmaul's sign not seen in:

(a) Constrictive pericarditis (b) RVMI
(c) Severe CHF (d) HOCM

445. In a patient with suspected heart failure which one of the following findings on Valsalva manuvre indicates elevated filling pressures?

(a) Square wave response
(b) Absence of phase IV overshoot
(c) Disappearance of S_3
(d) Disappearance of Korotkoff sound in Phase 1

446. A patient with respiratory failure has the following arterial blood gases on breathing room air – pH:7.19, PCO_2:72 mm Hg, PO_2: 64 mm Hg, SaO_2: 84% Which of the following condition is least likely?

(a) Congestive heart failure
(b) Flail chest
(c) Narcotic overdose
(d) Myasthenia gravis

447. Pulsus paradoxus may occur in all of the following conditions *except:*

(a) Pulmonary embolism

(b) Effusive – constrictive pericarditis
(c) Hypertrophic non obstructive cardiomyopathy
(d) Extreme obesity

448. All of the following statements about pulmonary artery hypertension in CRF are true *except:*
(a) Prevalence of PAH higher in PD patients as compared to HD PATIENTS
(b) Left ventricular changes are a major contributing factor to PAH in CRF
(c) AV Fistula flow and duration are related independently to the severity PAH
(d) PAH is an independent predictor for all-cause mortality in CRF

449. Which one of the following is a marker of pulmonary edema on lung ultrasound:
(a) A Profit (b) Tissue sign
(c) Shred sign (d) B line score

450. All of the following are hemodynamic hallmarks of CCP *except:*
(a) Dip and plateau in RV pressure
(b) RVEDP is > ½ of peak systolic pressure
(c) Ventricular discordance
(d) Expiratory increase in early diastolic pressure gradient between PCWP and LV

451. Which one of the following organelle constitutes the majority of the cell volume?
(a) Myofibrill (b) Mitochondria
(c) Sarcoplasmic reticulum (d) T tubule system

452. In ventricular myocytes, the L type calcium channels are located in:
(a) Mitochondria (b) T tubules
(c) Cell membrane (d) Nuclear membrane

453. Which one of the following is a load independent measure of cardiac contractility?
(a) dP/dt max (b) dP/dt min
(c) Slope of ESPVR (d) Tau

454. All of the following are true about nesiritide *except:*
(a) It is a recombinant human B-type natriuretic peptide
(b) Potent veno – and arterial dilator
(c) Has no major hemodynamic effects
(d) Vasodilatation is mediated by cGMP

455. Ototoxicity is most commonly associated with:
(a) Ethacrynic acid (b) Frusemide
(c) Torsemide (d) Indapamide

456. Paroxysmal nocturnal dyspnoea is unlikely in:
(a) Left atrial myxoma
(b) Aortic regurgitation
(c) Constrictive pericarditis
(d) Hypertensive heart failure

457. A 12-year-old boy with the Following X-ray is likely to have all of the following *except:*
(a) Minimal cyanosis
(b) Abnormalities of cartilage
(c) Systolic-diastolic murmur
(d) Pulmonary embolism on CT

458. Identify the correct statement regarding the trace given below:
(a) Shows successful procedure
(b) Balloon dilatation that resulted in regurgitation
(c) Shows artifact
(d) Trace is following alcohol septal ablation

459. An asymptomatic 22 year old male patient with nonobstructive HCM and a maximal LV wall thickness of 33 mm, three EPISODES of nonsustained VT on ambulatory 24 hour Holter, no history of syncope or family history of sudden death, and normal blood pressure response to exercise should be considered for which of the following?
(a) Surgical myectomy
(b) Electrophysiology (EP) study
(c) ICD
(d) Antiarrhythmic drug therapy

460. All the following may cause a hyperkinetic pulse *except:*
(a) Complete heart block (b) Tettralogy of Fallot
(c) Mitral stenosis (d) Cirrhosis of the liver

461. An ejection sound may be due to:
(a) Pulmonic stenosis
(b) Idiopathic dilatation of the pulmonary artery
(c) Ascending aortic aneurysm
(d) All of the above

462. Following true about Tako – tsubo cardiomyopathy *except:*
(a) Usually involves, younger woman
(b) Presentation may mimic acute myocardial infarction
(c) Sudden intense emotional or physical stress is precipitating factor
(d) LV dysfunction extends beyond a specific coronary artery territory

463. A 62 years old woman with left sided heat failure & Pulmonary Hypertension presents for a follow up. In which of the following latest WHO Pulmonary Hypertension Classification groups would her disease be categorized?

(a) Group 1 (b) Group 2
(c) Group 3 (d) Group 4

464. What is true about Riociguat?

(a) Inhibitor of soluble guanylate cyclase
(b) Anti-obesity drug
(c) New drug useful in pulmonary ARTERIAL hypertension
(d) None of the above

465. About anthracyclines, what is true:

(a) Troponin T may be used for early detection of those at High Risk
(b) Cardiac Toxicity limiting CUMULATIVE dose is < 550 mg/m²
(c) Liposomal Analogues of Anthracyclines are less Cardiotoxic
(d) All of the above

466. All of following present with circulatory collapse or CHF *except:*

(a) Aortic atresia
(b) Mitral atresia
(c) Pulmonary atresia
(d) Hypoplastic Left Heart Syndrome

467. Characteristic ECG change in pericarditis is:

(a) Generalized ST elevation with convexity upwards
(b) QT prolongation
(c) PR Depression
(d) ST elevation in V_1 more than in V_2

468. Diagnostic test for pulmonary vein stenosis is:

(a) LV Angiography (b) 2D-Echocardiography
(c) LA Angio (d) MRI

469. Endocardial fibroelastosis is not associated with:

(a) AS
(b) ALCAPA
(c) Long and thin chordate
(d) CoA

470. All are common features of fetal heart failure *except:*

(a) Scalp edema (b) Increased JVP
(c) Ascites (d) Pericardial effusion

471. Vascular resistance is expressed in:

(a) Dynes/m² (b) Dynes/kg/m²
(c) Dynes/wood units (d) Dynes.s/cm5

472. The normal pericardium:

(a) Contains 80-100 ml of fluid
(b) Is attached to the sternum
(c) Does not cover the MPA
(d) All of the above

473. Pulsus alternans:

(a) Is usually associated with an S_3
(b) Is commonly due to atrial premature beats
(c) Occurs in 2nd degree AV block
(d) Is a form of bisferien pulse

474. In LV dysfunction:

(a) Tachycardia indicates LV enlargement
(b) S_3 indicates dyskinesia
(c) S_4 indicates high LV diastolic pressure
(d) Wide split S2 indicates prolonged ejection time

475. Non ejection clicks:

(a) May be mid systolic
(b) May be multiple
(c) May be heard in the neck
(d) All of the above

476. Cannon A waves in the JVP:

(a) Are often confused with v waves
(b) Occur during ventricular systole
(c) Are a clue to AV dissociation
(d) All of the above

477. The third heart sound:

(a) Occurs just prior to opening snap
(b) Corresponds to Y descent of JVP
(c) Is common in elderly
(d) None of the above

478. Rapid Y-descent is seen in all *except:*

(a) Cardiac tamponade (b) TR
(c) CCP (d) CCF

479. Prolonging survival in CHF:

(a) Bisoprolol (b) Chlorthalidone
(c) Nifedipine

480. Levosimendon A/E:

(a) ATP dependent K^+ channel opener
(b) Inotropic and vasoconstrictor
(c) Decreases BNP
(d) Causes AF

481. **Amyloidosis true:**
(a) Thickening of interatrial septum is specific
(b) CCB are DOC
(c) Hypertension
(d) LV dilatation

482. **All are markers of CHF *except:***
(a) CRP (b) Trop-I
(c) Renin (d) Trop-C

483. **Lung disease causing PHTN:**
(a) Hypoxia (b) Hypercapnia
(c) Intracardiac shunt

484. **Patient with hypotension, bibasilar rales:**
(a) PCWP > 20 mm Hg, cardiac index < 2.2
(b) PCWP > 20 mm Hg, cardiac index > 2.2
(c) PCWP < 20 mm Hg, cardiac index < 2.2

485. **On catheterization to calculate MVA A/E:**
(a) CO (b) Systolic ejection period
(c) Gradient (d) HR

486. **PHTN of least affects:**
(a) AR (b) MR
(c) Post BMV (d) Mitral prosthetic valve

487. **All are used in cardiogenic shock *except:***
(a) Phenylephrine (b) Dopamine
(c) Dobutamine (d) Milrinone

488. **HOCM–increased risk of SCD A/E:**
(a) LVH > 30 mm
(b) Multiple VPC on Holter
(c) Family history
(d) Syncope

489. **Pulsus paradoxus seen in:**
(a) Obesity
(b) Hypovolumic shock
(c) Pulmonary embolism
(d) All of the above

490. **Pulsus paradoxus A/E:**
(a) Tension pneumothorax
(b) RVMI
(c) Pulmonary embolism
(d) CCP

491. **True:**
(a) Pulsus alternans seen in severe LV dysfunction
(b) Pulsus paradoxus – bradycardia on inspiration

492. **If radius is doubled, than blood flow will be doubled by:**
(a) 8 (b) 16
(c) 32 (d) 64

493. **Dip and plateau seen in A/E:**
(a) RVMI (b) RCMP
(c) CP (d) Cardiogenic shock

494. **S1 not loud in:**
(a) Acute AR (b) Severe MS
(c) MVP (d) Short PR

495. **Cardiac CATH study – initially the maximum pressure in chamber – 27 mm Hg. Later when catheter advanced pressure – maximum – 26, minimum -10 mm Hg, catheter was in which site during initial reading:**
(a) RA (b) RV
(c) PA (d) LV

496. **All are true about HOCM *except:***
(a) Autosomal dominant
(b) Disopyramide should not be used in obstructive HOCM
(c) Troponin carrier are not associated with LVH
(d) 2/3rd have structural abnormality of mitral valve

497. **PSM not heard in:**
(a) Roger defect
(b) MVP severe MR
(c) Hypertensive TR
(d) VSD with Eisenmenger

498. **Continuous murmur in APW is not seen in:**
(a) Pulmonary hypertension
(b) Systemic HTN
(c) PS
(d) ↑ aortic flow

499. **True statement about pulmonary ejection click (PEC):**
(a) Inspiration increase intensity of PEC
(b) No respiratory variation in mild to moderate PS
(c) PEC intensity decreases with inspiration in mild to moderate PS
(d) Timing of PEC no correlation with severity of PS

500. **Dopamine C/I in:**
(a) Septic shock
(b) Cardiac tamponade
(c) Carcinoid syndrome
(d) Pulmonary thromboembolism

501. Strongest cardiac support is:
(a) Intervalvular fibrous trigone
(b) Right fibrous trigone
(c) Left fibrous trigone
(d) Membranous septum

502. Diastolic heart failure A/E:
(a) BNP not increased
(b) Diuretics DOC
(c) Most common in elderly
(d) Echo criteria not definitive

503. M1 T1 A/E:
(a) M1 after 30 sec of LA to LV crossover
(b) Sustained handgrip ↓ M1 T1 interval
(c) T1 coincides with downslope of 'a' wave of RA
(d) ↓ PR— loud S1

504. True about pericardium A/E:
(a) Right and left pulmonary arteries are extra-pericardial
(b) Pulmonary venous confluence in TAPVC is intrapericardial
(c) Ductus arteriosus is an intrapericardial structure
(d) Pericardium is a collagenous structure with few elastic fibres

505. Cardiac output calculation: CVP–10 mm Hg, HR–70 bpm, O_2 consumption–500 ml/min, PVO_2 – 0.24 ml/min and PAO_2–0.16 ml/min, CO=:
(a) 4.55 l/min (b) 6.25 l/min
(c) 8.0 l/min (d) 5.0 l/min

506. GFR < 20 ml/min, which drug to be used?
(a) Indapamide (b) Metalazone
(c) Chlorthiazide (d) Chlorthalidone

507. Reverse splitting of S2 A/E:
(a) PDA (b) LBBB
(c) Paced rhythm (d) Left accessory pathway

508. Myocarditis caused by A/E:
(a) Diphtheria (b) Cox-sackie
(c) Chagas (d) Syphilis

509. Female with normal LVEDP and LVESP, increased PCWP (18 mmHg) cause:
(a) MS (b) AS
(c) DCMP (d) RCMP

510. Ventricular interdependence seen in:
(a) CCP (b) RCMP
(c) ASD with TR

511. Pansystolic murmur A/E:
(a) Hypertensive TR (b) VSD with Eisenmenger
(c) Roger defect

512. Exercise exacerbates A/E:
(a) Brugada syndrome
(b) CPVT
(c) NSVT with CAD
(d) Increased intensity of HOCM murmur

513. CVP in TR:
(a) Large 'v' wave
(b) 'x' and 'y' descent never seen together
(c) Prominent 'x' descent
(d) Early 'v' wave

514. HOCM A/E:
(a) Post VPC wide pulse pressure
(b) MV apparatus abnormality in 2/3rd
(c) Spike and dome pattern in arterial pulse

515. Post systolic shortening is characteristically seen in:
(a) Ischemia (b) HOCM
(c) Subaortic stenosis (d) Amyloidosis

516. A 45 years old male presents with exertional angina. Echo shows concentric LVH with characteristic binary appearance:
(a) Fabry's disease
(b) Hemochromatosis
(c) Type 2 glycogen storage disease
(d) Amyloidosis

517. LV remodelling by A/E:
(a) DOR (b) ACORN cap
(c) CRT (d) All of the above

518. A patient of RCMP with IVC diameter 20 mm with < 50% inspiratory collapse. What would be the RA pressure?
(a) 10-15 mm Hg (b) 5-10 mm Hg
(c) 15-20 mm Hg (d) > 20 mm Hg

519. DCMP with LVEF < 30% with NYHA class III/IV despite optimal medical therapy. CRT to be most suitable in:
(a) QRS > 120 msec without evaluation for dyssynchrony
(b) QRS < 120 msec with dyssynchrony on TDI
(c) QRS < 120 msec with dyssynchrony on 3D- ECHO
(d) QRS < 120 msec with dyssynchrony on M-mode

520. Niacin induced flushing prevented by:
(a) Lipropropant (b) Paracetamol
(c) Etomoxir

521. L-wave seen in:
(a) Early diastole (b) Mid-diastole
(c) Systole (d) Late diastole

522. Increase QT with pericardial effusion and myocarditis seen in:
(a) Arsenic (b) Cobalt
(c) Lead (d) Mercury

523. Atrial myxoma, systemic symptoms due to:
(a) IL-6 (b) TNF
(c) Histamine (d) Serotonin

524. 32 years old male presented with LBBB type VT with wide QRS tachycardia. Echo – mild RV dilatation, next investigation of choice:
(a) MRI (b) Cardiac cath
(c) EPS

525. Preoperative cataract in 55 years old male without HTN and DM, can walk upto 2 flights of stairs without symptoms:
(a) ECHO
(b) TMT
(c) No preoperative investigation
(d) Cardiac monitoring

526. Diuretics additive antihypertensive effect in A/E:
(a) Beta blockers (b) ARB
(c) ACE-I (d) CCB

527. A diabetes mellitus patient with BUN -40, S. creat.—1mg%, coronary angiography to be done. Dose of contrast to be safe in:
(a) 150 (b) 200
(c) 250 (d) 300

528. ACE-I indication:
(a) Symptomatic chronic severe MR not eligible for surgery
(b) Asymptomatic chronic severe MR
(c) Asymptomatic chronic severe AR
(d) All of the above

529. Diastolic HF with EF – 60%, likely finding A/E:
(a) DT – 200 msec (b) E/E′ > 17
(c) E< A (d) BNP = 500 pg/ml

530. Diastolic heart failure in 60 years female with EF = 55-60% with normal mitral inflow velocity A/E:
(a) Cath study (b) None of the above
(c) TDI (d) BNP

531. Inheritance of PAH:
(a) AD (b) AR
(c) X-linked

532. 42 years male, III/VI mid systolic murmur at base with early systolic sound, normal carotid pulse, prominent apical impulse, no change in respiration, decreases with valsalva, normalizes with seven beats, increases with PVC, no change with hand grip:
(a) Bicuspid aortic valve (b) MVP
(c) HOCM (d) Congenital PS

533. ↓ ed BNP level:
(a) Acute MR
(b) Cirrhosis
(c) Septic shock
(d) Acute pulmonary embolism

534. Normal EF with HF–A/E:
(a) ↑ in female
(b) 50-55% of total HF patients
(c) BNP usually normal
(d) LVH frequently absent

535. Least common cause of LV Dysfunction in takayasu arteritis:
(a) Myocarditis (b) HTN
(c) AR (d) Coronary vasculitis

536. Difference between athlete heart and HOCM A/E:
(a) Normal tissue doppler
(b) Normal LV dimension
(c) Normal diastolic function
(d) Septum < 17 mm

537. Most common cause of reversible constrictive pericarditis:
(a) TB (b) Radiation
(c) Postsurgical (d) Auto immune

538. AT_2 receptor:
(a) Myocyte growth
(b) Myocyte apoptosis
(c) Norepinephrine release
(d) Aldosterone

539. COPD + TR murmur + pitting edema + hepatomegaly + c-v wave in JVP:
(a) BNP > 600 suggestive of LV dysfunction
(b) NT-pro-BNP better
(c) Cor pulmonale BNP may ↑
(d) BNP ↑ es with low cardiac output

540. Which is not used in right heart catheterization?
(a) Pigtail
(b) NIH
(c) Goodale Lubin catheter
(d) Berman

541. Large v wave in PCWP not seen in:
(a) MS (b) MR
(c) VSD (d) AS

542. Echo findings in tamponade A/E:
(a) Increases mitral valve flow with respiratory variation
(b) RV systolic collapse
(c) RA late diastolic collapse
(d) Reversal of flow in tricuspid in respiration

543. Dobutamine—long use ↓ response due to:
(a) ↓ Regulation of beta receptor
(b) Saturation of hepatic enzyme
(c) Increase in NOS
(d) Renal clearance

544. Common in HCM + DCM mutation A/E:
(a) Titin (b) Troponin-T
(c) Tropomyosin-α (d) Phospholamban

545. PCWP not correlate with LVEDP:
(a) Operated LA myxoma
(b) Acute MR
(c) Catheter in dependent lung zones
(d) ↓ Compliance of ventricle

546. ↑ HR →↑ contractility:
(a) Bowditch's phenomenon
(b) Anrep's effect
(c) Laplace's law
(d) Frank-Starling's law

547. DV/DP:
(a) Elasticity (b) Compliance
(c) Elastance (d) Wall stress

548. HF with protein ↓ es:
(a) B_1 receptor (b) B_2 receptor
(c) α_1 receptor (d) Na^+-Ca^+ exchanger

549. Transient LV dysfunction + Pulmonary edema with previously normal heart A/E:
(a) Exercise
(b) Cerebral injection
(c) Emotional
(d) Post abdominal surgery

550. Cardiac transplant, indication A/E:
(a) HLHS
(b) Eisenmenger syndrome
(c) Refractory angina not responding to revascularization
(d) HCM class III/IV

551. Ventricular assist device A/E:
(a) Novacor (b) Biomed
(c) Paracor (d) Heartmate

552. Cell-based myocardial repair, true:
(a) Bone marrow delivered cells cause arrhythmia
(b) CD-34 (+ve) cells cause stenosis
(c) G-CSF cause angina in chronic ischemic cardiomyopathy
(d) G-CSF ↑ es LV function whether it is given by peripheral or intracoronary

553. HOCM gradient ↑ es with:
(a) Alcohol (b) Heavy meal
(c) VPC (d) All

554. Beta blockers not used as 1st line because:
(a) Depression
(b) Insulin sensitivity
(c) Central aortic pressure not decreased
(d) Increases MI

555. Which risk factor intervention proven to shown to ↓ cardiomortality?
(a) DM (b) LVH
(c) Obesity (d) HDL

556. Aerobic exercise main advantage by:
(a) ↑ MVO_2 - max
(b) ↑ Ventilation threshold
(c) ↑ Stroke volume
(d) ↑ Arterio venous O_2 gradient

557. Myocarditis caused by:
(a) Hepatitis A (b) Hepatitis B
(c) Hepatitis C (d) All

558. Endothelial dependent vasodilator A/E:
(a) Serotonin (b) Adenosine
(c) Endothelin (d) Histamine

559. Myocardial preconditioning A/E:
(a) ↓ regulation of adenosine
(b) ↑ NOS
(c) ↑ COX-2
(d) Mitochondrial K^+ channel opening

560. CHF class III/IV, OHA to be given:
(a) Glyburide (b) Pioglitazone
(c) Rosiglitazone (d) Metformin

561. HF in newborn A/E:
(a) Tachyarrhythmia
(b) Truncus arteriosus
(c) Pulmonary AV fistula
(d) Coarctation of aorta

562. MV repair not useful in:
(a) Chordal rupture
(b) Annular dilatation
(c) Perforation
(d) Associated with rheumatic MR

563. Graham Steel murmur seen in:
(a) PDA with Eisenmenger
(b) Rheumatic carditis
(c) Carcinoid syndrome
(d) All

564. Restrictive cardiomyopathy caused by A/E:
(a) DM (b) Adriamycin
(c) Radiation (d) None

565. Gene in PPH:
(a) ALK-1 (b) Serotonin transporter
(c) $BMPR_2$ (d) All

566. RCM cause all *except:*
(a) Hemochromatosis
(b) Fabry's disease
(c) Glyogen storage disease
(d) Gaucher's disease

567. Pulsus paradoxus all *except:*
(a) Pericardial effusion (b) Cardiac tamponade
(c) CCP (d) Pulmonary embolism

568. Compensatory short term mechanism of LV dysfunctions are all *except:*
(a) Increase preload
(b) Increase HR and ejection period
(c) Blood flow redistribution to vital organs
(d) Increase cardiac energy expenses

569. HCM true *except:*
(a) Digoxin increase gradient and murmur
(b) Isoproterenol and squatting have same effect
(c) Valsalva decrease murmur
(d) Post extrasytole increase gradient

570. Vasodilator BB are all *except:*
(a) Carvedilol (b) Labetalol
(c) Bucindolol (d) Bisoprolol

571. H wave in:
(a) RCM (b) RVM1
(c) CCP (d) All

572. Carney complex clinical criteria all *except:*
(a) Cardiac myxoma
(b) Cutaneous + myocardial
(c) Typical distribution of skin pigmentation
(d) 1st degree relative

573. LVEF 30%, poorest diagnosis:
(a) AS (b) AS + MS
(c) AR (d) Chronic MR

574. Total pulmonary resistance is:
(a) 20 to 130 (b) 100 to 300
(c) 700 to 1400 (d) 10 to 20

575. All are true about cardiac tamponade *except:*
(a) Pulsus paradoxus seen
(b) Kussmaul's sign is seen
(c) Muffled heart sounds
(d) RA collapse on echo

576. Which is the wrong combination?
(a) Merit HF trial–metoprolol
(b) CIBIS–bisoprolol
(c) ESSENCE–enalapril
(d) EPHESUS–epelerenone

577. In pulmonary artery hypertension all are decreased *except:*
(a) Prostacyclin (b) Endothelin
(c) NO (d) C-AMP

578. Potassium sparing diuretic is:
(a) Furosemide (b) Indapamide
(c) Triamterene (d) Hydrochlorothiazide

579. False regarding ANP is:
(a) A and B are clearance receptor
(b) C is clearance receptor
(c) ANP is vasodilator
(d) Increased concentration is seen in patients of heart failure

580. Bisferien's pulses seen in all *except:*
(a) Dilated cardiomyopathy
(b) AR
(c) AS+ AR
(d) HOCM

581. Decreases afterload provides the compensatory mechanism in:
(a) Mitral stenosis (b) Mitral regurgitation
(c) Aortic stenosis (d) Aortic regurgitation

582. Most common heart disease is:
(a) Coronary artery disease
(b) Sudden cardiac death
(c) Rheumatic heart disease
(d) Hypertension

583. Beck triad is:
(a) Muffled heart sound + Hypertension + distended neck veins
(b) Muffled heart sound + Hypotension + distended neck veins
(c) Muffled heart sound + Decreased JVP + hypotension
(d) Loud S I+ distended neck veins with hypertension

584. Pulmonary vascular resistance is:
(a) 5-150 (b) 20-130
(c) 10-300 (d) 750-2000

585. All are causes of early systolic murmur:
(a) Small muscule VSD
(b) Chordal rupture
(c) TR with MS
(d) VSD with pulmonary arterial HT

586. Dichrotic pulse is seen in all *except:*
(a) Septic shock (b) Hypovolemic shock
(c) CHF (d) Elderly hypertensive

587. Pericarditis is caused by all of the following *except:*
(a) Doxorubicin (b) Emetine
(c) Medrysergide (d) None of the above

588. Which of the following is phosphodiesterase inhibitor with carcinoma sensitization property?
(a) Levosimenden (b) Milrinone
(c) Amrinone (d) Cilostazol

589. All are gene polymorphism in metabolic syndrome *except:*
(a) BAR2 (b) LDL
(c) INS VNRT (d) K121 q

590. All are class side effects of ACE inhibitors *except:*
(a) Renal failure (b) Angioneurotic edema
(c) Dysguisca (d) Proteinuria

591. In all of the following conditions dicrotic pulse is seen *except:*
(a) Accelerated hypertension
(b) Hypertensive individual with low peripheral vascular resistance
(c) Hypovolemic shock
(d) Septic shock

592. All are true about treatment of HOCM *except:*
(a) Beta blockers are the drugs of choice
(b) Alcohol septal ablation decreases the gradient
(c) MVR suffice in patient having septal hypertrophy >16 mm
(d) Septal myomectomy done if alcohol septal ablation fails

593. Assymmetrical septal hypertrophy seen in the following conditions *except:*
(a) Inferior wall MI (b) Anteroseptal MI
(c) HOCM (d) Posterior wall MI

594. R wave in JVP corresponds to:
(a) Isovolumic contraction

(b) Isovolumic relaxation
(c) Ejection phase
(d) Diastasis

595. All of the following leads to square root response on valsalva maneuver *except:*
(a) ASD (b) MS
(c) CHF (d) PVA

596. All of the following are phosphodiesterase inhibitor *except:*
(a) Milrinone (b) Amrinone
(c) Epinephrine (d) Cilostazole

597. Presence of PND indicates:
(a) Alveolar edema (b) Interstitial edema
(c) Pedal edema (d) All of the above

598. All of the following are causes of pulmonary edema due to starling force *except:*
(a) CHF
(b) Overperfusion pulmonary edema
(c) Mitral stenosis
(d) Radiation pulmonary edema

599. All of the following are causes of pulmonary hypertension *except:*
(a) HIV (b) Portal hypertension
(c) Hypothyroidism (d) Anorectic drugs
(e) All true

600. Longest contractile protein is:
(a) Actin (b) Tam
(c) Myosin (d) Collagen

601. TNF alpha antagonist is:
(a) Etanercept (b) Interferon alpha
(c) Cyclosporin (d) SN 560

602. Thermodilution technique uses:
(a) Simpson's formula
(b) Steward Hamilton formula
(c) Laplace principle
(d) Bernoulli's principle

603. Continuous murmur is seen in:
(a) Cerebral AV malformation
(b) VSD with MS
(c) Pulmonary artery stenosis
(d) ALCAPA

604. All are beta-blockers with vasodilatory properties *except:*
(a) Carvidilol (b) Labetalol
(c) Bucindolol (d) Bisoprolol

605. JVP in cardiac tamponade:
(a) Absenty (b) Prominenty
(c) Prominent a (d) Absent a

606. End of isovolumetric relaxation indicated by:
(a) C wave
(b) AV valve opening
(c) Closer of semilunar valves
(d) Peak of T wave

607. Reverse split S1 in:
(a) TS (b) RBBB
(c) LA myxoma (d) AR

608. Rytand's murmur:
(a) CHB (b) Atrial myxoma
(c) AR (d) Chronic MR

609. HCM murmur ↑ by A/E:
(a) Amyl nitrite (b) Phenylephrine
(c) Extrasystole (d) Valsalva strain

610. Athlete's heart vs HCM A/E:
(a) Wall thickness < 17 mm
(b) LV carity ↓ ed
(c) Symmetric hypertrophy
(d) Normal strain value on doppler

611. Athlete's syndrome which is seen:
(a) Early repolarization (b) ↑ QRS amplitude

612. Changes with exercise A/E:
(a) ↑ P wave
(b) ↑ ed R wave
(c) Shortening of QT interval
(d) ↑ ed amplitude of T wave

613. Drug causing pericarditis:
(a) Hydralazine (b) NSAIDs
(c) Amiodarone

614. CCP vs RCMP favoring CCP:
(a) Equalization of diastolic pressure in all chambers
(b) RA dilatation
(c) Mild pericardial effusion

615. PO_2 ↓ ed in:
(a) Hypoventilation (b) Carboxyhemoglobin
(c) Anemia (d) Methemoglobinemia

616. Framingham major criteria A/E:
(a) PND (b) Neck vein distension
(c) Cardiomegaly (d) Hepatomegaly

617. S3 is not seen in:
(a) HCM (b) CCP
(c) MS (d) Ventricular aneurysm

618. Single S2 in:
(a) CC-TGA (b) Pulmonary atresia
(c) Pulmonary stenosis

619. PCWP > LVEDP in:
(a) LA myxoma
(b) Pulmonary thromboembolic disease
(c) PS

620. Hepatojugular reflux A/E:
(a) Indicates PCWP of 4-12 months
(b) +ve H-J reflux indicates ↓ ed compliance of venous system
(c) H-J reflex +ve it persists for > sec after resumption of normal respiration
(d) Valsalva during H-J reflux cause ↑ ed venous pressure

621. ↑ ed ACE level with A/E:
(a) Berylliosis (b) Sarcoidosis
(c) Silicosis (d) Bronchogenic CA

622. Specific activity scale (SAS) patient grade 3 cum performance:
(a) > 9 METS (b) >7
(c) >5 (d) >2

623. True about murmur A/E:
(a) HCM murmur ↑ se on standing
(b) MS and PS ↑ se with isometric handgrip
(c) Pulmonary ejection click ↑ se with inspiration and ↓ se with expiration

624. Isometric exercise ↑ se murmur of A/E:
(a) MVP (b) HCM
(c) MR (d) AS

625. Bisferiens pulse best seen in:
(a) Carotid (b) Brachial
(c) Radial (d) Femoral

626. Adhesion molecules A/E:
(a) Integrin (b) Metalloproteinases
(c) Selectin (d) VCAM

627. ↑ CO in post transplant (cardiac) due to:
(a) Intrisic mechanism
(b) Frank Starling law
(c) Vagal reinnervation
(d) Epinephrine from adrenal gland

628. Pericarditis ECG changes A/E:
(a) Global ST elevation occur
(b) T wave inversion occurs before ST returns to baseline
(c) PR depression in most of the cases

629. 50% ↓ diameter, ↑ area by:
(a) 50% (b) 75%
(c) 90% (d) 99%

630. Square wave response on valsalva manoeuvre:
(a) HF
(b) VSD
(c) CCP

631. Reverse pulsus paradoxus seen in:
(a) HOCM (b) RCM
(c) DCM

632. Brockenborough phenomenon:
(a) ↓ pulse pressure post VPC
(b) ↓ systolic pressure
(c) ↓ diastolic pressure
(d) ↓ aortic systolic pressure

633. Cannon A wave seen in:
(a) Bernheim syndrome (b) TS
(c) Prolonged PR (d) PHT

634. Endocardial involvement with restrictive physiology:
(a) Carcinoid (b) Amyloid
(c) Gaucher (d) Hemochromatosis

635. Reverse split S_2 A/E:
(a) LBBB (b) Severe calcific AS
(c) RV apical pacing (d) HOCM
(e) None

636. Innocent murmur:
(a) Early systolic (b) Presystolic
(c) Mid systolic (d) Diastolic

637. Valsalva phases, false is:
(a) Phase I – rise in stroke volume

(b) Phase II – tachycardia
(c) Phase III – CO increases
(d) Phase IV – tachycardia

638. 'x' wave is due to:
(a) Atrial relaxation (b) Ventricular relaxation
(c) TV closure

639. Cardiac tamponade which wave not seen?
(a) x descent (b) y descent
(c) v wave

640. ↑ vascular stiffness is indicated by A/E:
(a) Positive osler maneuver
(b) Orthostatic hypotension
(c) Wide pulse pressure
(d) Radial artery tonometry

641. Carcinoid with metastasis valve involved:
(a) TV and PV (b) MV
(c) AV (d) AV and TV

642. Excessive production of the following substance by the endothelial cells can inactivate Nitric oxide:
(a) Hydrogen peroxide
(b) Endothelium derived hyperpolarizing factor
(c) Endothelin
(d) Superoxide anion (O_2)

643. Contribution of cardiac myocytes to the ventricular mass is about:
(a) 90% (b) 50%
(c) 75% (d) 60%

644. All are true regarding conduction system of the heart *except:*
(a) SA nodal artery arises from RCA in 55-60% of persons
(b) His bundle and bundle branches have a single blood supply from 1st septal perforator of Left anterior descending artery
(c) Both SA and AV nodes are richly innervated by sympathetic and parasympathetic fibers
(d) SA node is situated on the epicardial surface of the heart

645. Bifid pulse is not seen in:
(a) Chronic severe AR
(b) HOCM
(c) IABP (intra aortic balloon pump)
(d) Severe MR

646. In JVP Kussmaul's sign may be a feature in:
(a) Mitral stenosis
(b) Right ventricular MI
(c) Severe LV failure
(d) HOCM

647. All are true regarding auscultatory gap, *except:*
(a) More likely to occur in older hypertensives with target end organ damage
(b) It may over estimate systolic pressure
(c) It may over estimate diastolic pressure
(d) It should be distinguished from pulsus paradoxus

648. S_1 (First heart sound) is likely to be loud in:
(a) PR interval of 100 msec
(b) LV EF of 30%
(c) Calcified mitral stenosis
(d) Patients on B-blockers

649. Reverse splitting of 2nd HS is not a feature in:
(a) LBBB
(b) Severe aortic stenosis
(c) Left ventricular pacing
(d) Acute myocardial ischemia

650. Ejection click may be heard in all *except:*
(a) Valvar pulmonary stenosis
(b) Dilated pulmonary artery in PH
(c) Aortic root dilatation
(d) Supravalvar aortic stenosis

651. Intensity of HOCM murmur decreases during:
(a) Valsalva strain phase (b) Standing
(c) Squatting (d) Exercise

652. Which of the following is not a non-sarcomeric protein mutation causing hypertrophic cardiomyopathy?
(a) Danon [LAMP2] disease
(b) Fabry's disease
(c) PRKAG 2 cardiac syndrome
(d) Beta Myosin Heavy chain gene mutation

653. Regarding diuretics all are true *except:*
(a) Spironolactone acts at the level of the collecting duct
(b) Loop diuretics inhibit reabsorption of NA^+, K^+ and Chloride in the descending limb of loop of Henle
(c) Thiazides lose their effectiveness when serum creatinine is >2.5 mg/dl

(d) Chronic daily use of metalazone should be avoided if possible

654. Identify the wrong statement in the management of acute heart failure:

(a) Nitroprusside can cause cyanide toxicity
(b) Infusion of dobutamine for > 72 hours can develop techyphylaxis
(c) Milrinone is a more effective vasodilator than dobutamine
(d) Levosimendon acts on B_1 and B_2 receptors

655. Systemic vascular resistance (SVR) is equal to {MAP, mean arterial pressure; RAP, right atrial pressure; PAP, pulmonary artery pressure—mean; PCWP, pulmonary capillary wedge pressure:

(a) [(MAP-PCWP)/CO] × 80
(b) [(MAP-RAP)/CO] × 80
(c) [(MAP-PAPm)/CO] × 80
(d) None of the above

656. Brockenbrough Braunwald phenomenon on aortic pulse pressure:

(a) Decreases in pulse pressure
(b) Increase in pulse pressure
(c) Wide pulse pressure
(d) None of the above

657. The prevalence of HOCM in general population:

(a) 1 : 2000 (b) 1: 500
(c) 1: 5000 (d) 1:10,000

658. The Y descent in JVP is absent in:

(a) Cardiac tamponade
(b) Constrictive percarditis
(c) Eftusive constrictive pearditiric
(d) Restrictive cardiomyopathy

659. All of the following are true about pulsus parvus *except:*

(a) Seen in aortic stenosis
(b) Decreased left ventricular output
(c) Decreased peripheral resistance
(d) Decreased pulse pressure

660. Hamilton Stewart equation is used for calculation of:

(a) Cardiac output (b) Blood volume
(c) Chamber pressure (d) Valveria

661. Features of pericardial effusion included all *except:*

(a) It is usually circumferential
(b) In the parasternal long axis view pericardial effusion is located anterior to the descending thoracic aorta
(c) Is located posterior to the aorta
(d) Detected as echo free space

662. What is the normal LV end–systolic volume index on left ventriculography?

(a) 50-90 mm/m² (b) 35-55 mm/m²
(c) 15-35 mm/m² (d) < 15 mm/m²

663. Most common complicated of right-heart catheterization:

(a) Non-sustained atrial and ventricular arrhythmias
(b) Pulmonary infarction
(c) Pulmonary artery of right ventricular perforation
(d) Infection

664. Which of the following infectious agents have been associated with development of inflamma-tory myocarditis?

(a) Coxsakie virus (b) Diphtheria
(c) Trypanosome cruzi (d) All the of above

665. Major criteria of Framingham of congestive heart failure are all *except:*

(a) Rales
(b) Positive hepatojugular reflex
(c) Cardiomegaly
(d) Pleural effusion

666. Most common cause of low output heart failure in the world is:

(a) Anaemia (b) Beriberi
(c) Thyrotoxicosis (d) Chagas' disease

667. Pulsus paradoxus can be seen in the following clinical statements *except:*

(a) Pericardial tamponade
(b) Acute severe asthma
(c) Acute myocardial infarction
(d) Massive pulmonary embolism

668. Which one of the following is the correct statement regarding findings in JVP?

(a) Cannon wave: complete heart block
(b) Slow 'y' descent: Tricuspid regurgitation
(c) Giant 'c' wave: Tricuspid stenosis
(d) Increased JVP with prominent pulsations: SVC obstruction

669. Jarvik-7 is a/an:
(a) Aortal Artifical Heart
(b) Axial flow pump
(c) Univentricular assist device
(d) Extra corporeal centrifugal pumps

670. Athletes heart differs from hypertrophic cardiomyopathy:
(a) Symmetrical hypertrophy
(b) Diastolic function is abnormal
(c) Asymmetrical septal hypertrophy
(d) LV cavity dimension is decreased

671. Pulsus paradoxus can be seen in the following clinical states *except:*
(a) Pericardial tamponade
(b) Acute severe asthma
(c) Acute myocardial infarction
(d) Massive pulmonary embolism

672. Which one of the following is the correct statement regarding findings in JVP?
(a) Cannon wave : Complete heart block
(b) Slow 'y' descent : Tricuspid regurgitation
(c) Giant 'c' wave : Tricuspid stenosis
(d) Increased JVP with prominent pulsations: SVC obstruction

673. All of the following are true about pulsus parvus *except:*
(a) Seen in aortic stenosis
(b) Decreased left Ventricular output
(c) Decreased peripheral resistance
(d) Decreased pulse pressure

674. Features of pericardial effusion include all *except:*
(a) It is usually circumferential
(b) In the parasternal long axis view pericardial effusion is located anterior to the descending thoracic aorta
(c) Is located posterior to the aorta
(d) Detected as echo free space

675. Orthostatic hypotension is:
(a) 20 mm Hg drop in systolic blood pressure within 3 minutes of standing
(b) 10 mm Hg rise in diastolic blood pressure within 3 minutes of standing
(c) Due to increase in venous return to heart
(d) 30 mm Hg drop in both systolic and diastolic blood pressure within 3 minutes of standing

676. True about carotid sinus massage:
(a) Important to perform in carotid sinus massage in both supine and upright position
(b) Pressure should be applied for 5-10 minutes
(c) Can be performed in TIA patient
(d) A normal response to carotid sinus massage is increased in atrioventricular conduction

677. What is normal LV end-systolic volume index on left ventriculography?
(a) 50-90 mm/m^2
(b) 35-55 mm/m^2
(c) 15-35 mm/m^2
(d) Less than 15 mm/m^2

678. Which of the following has proven effective and reliable in patients with hypertrophic cardiomyopathy (HCM) in prevention of sudden death?
(a) Amiodarone
(b) Beta blockers
(c) Verapamil
(d) Implantable cardioverter-defibrillator

679. The first-line therapy for all patients with myocarditis and heart failure is:
(a) Immunosuppression
(b) Hemodynamic supportive therapy
(c) Interferon therapy
(d) Immune adsorption therapy

680. Major criteria of Framingham for congestive heart failure are all *except:*
(a) Rales
(b) Positive hepatojugular reflex
(c) Cardiomegaly
(d) Pleural effusion

681. Cardiomyopathy is NOT a feature of:
(a) Duchenne's Muscular Dystrophy
(b) Friedreich's ataxia
(c) Pompe disease
(d) Lowe's syndrome

682. The systolic ejection murmur in hypertrophic obstructive cardiomyopathy is diminished when a patient:
(a) Performs the Valsalva maneuver
(b) Lies down
(c) Inhales amy nitrite
(d) Stands up

683. In the mechanism of heart failure which one is incorrect?

(a) The Frank Starling mechanism operates through an increase in after load

(b) Compensatory hypertrophy of ventricle occurs in hemodynamic overload

(c) There are changes in the size, mass and configuration of the ventricle in ventricular remodeling

(d) There is redistribution of subnormal cardiac output away from the skin, skeletal muscle and kidneys

684. Square root sign is characteristic of:

(a) Dilated cardiomyopathy

(b) Restrictive cardiomyopathy

(c) Constrictive pericarditis

(d) Cardiac tamponade

685. Rapid 'Y' descend in JVP excludes the diagnosis of:

(a) Cardiac tamponade

(b) RV myocardial infarction

(c) Restrictive cardiomyopathy

(d) Constrictive pericarditis

686. Regular pulse with changing pulse volume:

(a) Complete heart block

(b) Atrial based pacemaker (AM) for severe sinus bradycardia

(c) CHB with atrial fibrillation

(d) 2 : 1 AV block

687. Identify the condition with the highest cardiac output and the widest difference in arteriovenous oxygen content:

(a) Systemic arterior venous fistula

(b) High altitude dwellers severe anaemia

(c) Maximal exercise

688. Described as a crescendo-decrescendo murmur:

(a) Graham Steel murmur

(b) Murmur of acute AR

(c) Murmur of AR due to evened aortic cusps

(d) Pulmonary regurgitation due to absent pulmonary valve

689. Which of the following events occurs farthest from aortic component of second heart sound?

(a) Physiological third heart sound

(b) Third heart sound of LV systolic dysfunction

(c) Tumor plop of LA myxoma

(d) Pericardial knock of constrictive pericarditis

690. If systolic time interval is defined as the ratio of LV ejection time to pre ejection time, then systolic time interval is likely to be the least in:

(a) Severe systemic hypertension

(b) Aortic stenosis with preserved LV function

(c) Dilated cardiomyopathy

(d) Low gradient AS with LV dysfunction

691. The last to activate is:

(a) The anterior paraseptal wall of LV

(b) Posterior paraseptal wall of LV

(c) Left side of the septum

(d) Posterobasal area of LV

692. Turbulence of flow of fluid in duct/pipe is inversely related to:

(a) Velocity of flow

(b) Diameter of the pipe

(c) Viscosity of the fluid

(d) Density of the fluid

693. The standard background therapy for patients with heart failure is:

(a) Angiotensin converting-enzyme (ACE) inhibitors + Beta blockers

(b) ACE inhibitors + Calcium channel blockers

(c) Beta blockers + Digoxin

(d) Beta blockers + Spironolactone

694. Innocent murmurs are usually:

(a) Early systolic (b) Presystolic

(c) Mid systolic (d) Holosystolic

695. Electrical alternans is feature of:

(a) Severe left ventricular dysfunction

(b) Large pericardial effusions

(c) Ventricular bigeminal rhythm

(d) Assisted ventilation

696. Continuous murmur may be heard in all except:

(a) Coronary artery fistula

(b) BT shunt

(c) PDA with systemic pulmonary artery pressures

(d) Peripheral pulmonary artery stenosis

697. **How much myocardium is lost before LV failure occurs after a myocardial infarction?**
(a) 10% (b) 25%
(c) 40% (d) 50%

698. **All are true for Framingham major criteria for CHF, *except:***
(a) PND
(b) S3
(c) Bilateral ankle edema
(d) Circulation time -25 seconds

699. **All of the following prolong survival in CHF, *except:***
(a) Angiotension receptor blockers
(b) Thiazides
(c) ACE inhibitors
(d) Beta Blockers

700. **In CHF, all are elevated *except:***
(a) ANP
(b) BNP
(c) Effective arterial volume
(d) Endothelin

701. **Kussmaul's sign in all of the following *except:***
(a) Constrictive Pericarditis
(b) Acute pulmonary thromboembolism
(c) Right ventricular infarction
(d) Cardiac Tamponade

702. **A symptomatic subject at risk of heart failure with no structural heart disease or symptoms fall into:**
(a) Stage A (b) Stage B
(c) Stage C (d) None

703. **Heart failure with preserved systolic function:**
(a) More common in women
(b) More common in older individuals
(c) Has LVEF> 40%
(d) Has all of the following features

704. **A drug that may find its use in all stages of heart failure:**
(a) Diuretics (b) Digoxin
(c) Spironolactone (d) ACE inhibitors

705. **Eplerenone is:**
(a) An endothelin antagonist
(b) A newer ACE inhibitor
(c) An Angiotensin receptor blocker
(d) An aldosterone antagonist

706. **Brockenbrough Braunwald sign in seen in:**
(a) Restrictive Cardiomyopathy
(b) Dilated Cardiomyopathy
(c) Arrhythmogenic RV cardiomyopathy
(d) Hypertrophic obstructive cardiomyopathy

707. **Paradoxical pulse is a finding in:**
(a) Cardiac tamponade
(b) Dilated cardiomyopathy
(c) Hypertrophic cardiomyopathy
(d) Hypertension

708. **The following is a feature of constrictive pericarditis:**
(a) Prominent Y descent in venous pressure
(b) Absent X descent
(c) Pericardial rub
(d) All of the above

709. **Which of the following statement regarding pericardium is true?**
(a) The parietal pericardium is highly cellular
(b) The pericardial space contains upto 50 ml of serous fluid
(c) The left atrium is largely extrapericardial
(d) Absent pericardium is incompatible with life

710. **Regular common waves in JVP are present in:**
(a) First degree AV block
(b) Complete AV block
(c) Nodal rhythm
(d) Ventricular tachycardia

711. **Each of the following is a potential cause of constrictive pericarditis *except:***
(a) Myxedema (b) Tuberculosis
(c) Rheumatoid arthritis (d) Mediastinal irradiation

712. **The highest concentration of digoxin in a patient on digoxin therapy is present in:**
(a) Skeletal muscle (b) Myocardium
(c) Kidney (d) Brain

713. **In acute severe heart failure vasodilators should generally be used only in patients with:**
(a) Slow heart rate
(b) Systolic blood pressure of less than 90 mmHg
(c) Pulmonary capillary wedge pressure greater than 15 mmHg
(d) Patient with normal cardiac output

714. Normal pulmonary capillary pressure is:

(a) 2-6 mm Hg (b) 7-10 mm Hg
(c) 11-15 mm Hg (d) 16-20 mm Hg

715. Venus hum is a prototype of a continuous murmur that tend to peak in intensity:

(a) In systole (b) At the II heart sound
(c) In diastole (d) At the first heart sound

716. Maximum cardiac transplantation have been done at:

(a) New York (b) Chicago
(c) Cleveland (d) Stanford

717. First artificial heart was placed in the chest of a 61 years old man suffering from end stage cardiomyopathy in Salt Lake City Utah on December 1st, 1928:

(a) 1972 (b) 1976
(c) 1982 (d) 1988

718. Systolic anterior motion of the anterior mitral leaflet is a echo feature of:

(a) Dilated cardiomyopathy
(b) Hypertrophic cardiomyopathy
(c) Restrictive cardiomyopathy
(d) Endomyocardial fibrosis

719. Traube's sign is positive in:

(a) Coarctation of aorta (b) Aortoarteritis
(c) Aortic regurgitation (d) Aortic stenosis

720. Spike and dome pulse is characteristic of:

(a) Hypertension
(b) HQCM
(c) Severe mitral regurgitation
(d) Severe aortic regurgitation

721. Raised JVP from sternum manubrium:

(a) 2 (b) 3
(c) 5 (d) 7

722. BNP is elevated in all *except:*

(a) Renal failure
(b) Obesity
(c) Pulmonary embolism
(d) Congestive heart failure

723. Most sensitive finding of CHF:

(a) Hepatojugular reflex (b) S3
(c) Hepatomegaly (d) Pedal oedema

724. Which is not a sensitive marker of CHF?

(a) Pedal oedema (b) HR > 60 mm
(c) Displaced apex (d) Dyspnoea

725. Patient having dyspnoea on less than ordinary activity belong to which NYHA:

(a) I (b) II
(c) III (d) IV

726. Cystic medial necrosis is absent in:

(a) Syphilis aortitis
(b) Ehlers Danlos syndrome
(c) Takayasu arteritis
(d) Annuloaortic ectasia

727. A patient of compensated heart was given a new drug along with her old medication. One week later he comes with decompensated heart failure so which drug is not responsible?

(a) Thiazolidione (b) Metformin
(c) NSAID (d) Beta blocker

728. Furosemide resistance (Breaking phenomenon) the drug given:

(a) Torsemide (b) Metalazone
(c) Amiloride (d) Triamtrine

729. The treatment given for metabolic alkalosis due to loop diuretic is:

(a) Give oral potassium (b) Start acetazolamide
(c) Start spironolactone (d) Start amiloride

730. On inspiration which right sided sound not increase in intensity?

(a) Pulmonary ejection click
(b) TR murmur

731. HOCM ICD is indicated in all *except:*

(a) LV thickness > .30 mm
(b) Presyncope
(c) NSVT
(d) LV OT gradient

732. Post catheterisation patient develop atheroembolism with blue toe, with rise in S. creatinine, which is not true?

(a) Decrease in serum complement
(b) Presence of urine active sediment and cast
(c) Mild peripheral eosinophilia

733. Pulmonary artery catheter is used in all *except:*
(a) Cardiac output measurement
(b) Mixed venous oxygen saturation measurement
(c) Left ventricle systolic pressure
(d) Pulmonary artery occlusion pressure

734. Which is not be benign cardiac finding?
(a) Systolic murmurs (b) Diastolic murmurs

735. Loud S1 found in all *except:*
(a) LV dysfunction
(b) Short PR interval
(c) Hyperkinetic circulation

736. Regarding Bain bridge reflex which is trice?
(a) Increase in RA stretching during exercise causes tachycardia
(b) Increase in LV stretching during exercise causes tachycardia

737. Which is true regarding Frank Starling law?
(a) Stroke volume = LV end diastolic fiber length

738. Regarding heart rate variability which is not true?
(a) Respiratory sinus arrhythmia is a type of HRV
(b) Physiological ageing causes increase in HRV
(c) It indicate autonomic control of heart

739. Constrictive pericarditis A/E:
(a) Uremia (b) Irradiation
(c) Sarcoidosis (d) Acute rheumatic fever

740. Myocardial stunning A/E:
(a) Completely reversible
(b) Dobutamine–no response in initial part
(c) Variant angina
(d) Preconditioning is useful in recovery

741. Systolic myocardial bridging:
(a) HCM
(b) AV groove constriction portion
(c) Calcified LV aneurysm
(d) Taka subo CMP

742. HCM A/E:
(a) Male female equal frequency
(b) Phenotype same worldwide
(c) Male increased risk of SCD
(d) Cardiac MRI

743. Pulse wave move to periphery:
(a) Incisura less prominent
(b) Loss of dicrotic notch
(c) Amplitude reduced
(d) Initial part become steeper

744. Peripartum cardiomyopathy risk factor A/E:
(a) Africo-Caribbean race
(b) Malnutrition
(c) Previous heart disease
(d) Cocaine abuse

745. Restrictive CMP:
(a) Friedreich ataxia (b) Fabry disease

746. DCM A/E:
(a) Poor R wave progression
(b) q wave
(c) p wave abnormality
(d) RBBB

747. Na K ATPase true A/E:
(a) Increased Na intracellular
(b) 2 ATP
(c) Increased K extracellular
(d) Electrogenic

748. CINACIGUAT:
(a) Guanyl cyclase inhibitor
(b) Adenosine antagonist

749. B Blockers no mortality benefit in heart failure:
(a) Bisoprolol (b) Atenolol
(c) Metoprolol (d) Carvedilol

750. BP cuff circumference:
(a) 0.8 (b) 0.6
(c) 1.2 (d) 0.7

751. Which is true?
(a) Pulmonary ejection click increases with inspiration
(b) HCM murmur soft on valsalva
(c) MVP murmur soft on standing
(d) MVP soft on long cycle of AF

752. Myocarditis A/E:
(a) Bimodal distribution
(b) Cardiac MRI 65% sensitivity
(c) Dallas low sensitivity
(d) Fulminant myocarditis treated with IVIG

753. Constrictive pericarditis true:
(a) Square root sign
(b) X descent prominent
(c) Septal bounce absent
(d) Pulsus paradoxus in 2/3rd

754. Framingham criteria:
(a) PND (b) Rales
(c) JVP (d) Dyspnea

755. Cause of death in HF N EF:
(a) CAD (b) Non coronary cause
(c) Non CVS

756. Athlete's heart vs HOCM:
(a) Dilated LV cavity
(b) Abnormal LV filling
(c) Left atrial enlargement
(d) Symmetric hypertrophy

757. All are component of LV remodeling *except:*
(a) Beta receptor desensitization
(b) Myocardial disarray
(c) Autophagy
(d) Sphericity

758. HFnEF A/E:
(a) HTN more than normotensive
(b) Male > female
(c) Elderly > young
(d) Obese > normal BMI

759. Normal PVR in dyne.s/cm^{-5}:
(a) 20-40 (b) 40-120
(c) 220-240 (d) 1200-1400

760. True vascular ring is:
(a) Pulmonary sling
(b) Double aortic arch
(c) Aberrant right SCA with ligamentum arteiosum

761. Trials for mineralocorticoid receptor antagonist A/E:
(a) EPHESUS (b) RALES
(c) EMPHASIS (d) ASCENT–HF

762. "Second heart field" is:
(a) Reentrant circuit for VT
(b) LVH in HTN and AS
(c) Field for progenitor cells in RV
(d) Diastolic dysfunction

763. Drugs causing pulmonary arterial HTN A/E:
(a) Fenfluramine (b) Amphetamine
(c) Cocaine (d) OCP

764. Wide S1 seen in:
(a) Severe calcified MS (b) LBBB
(c) LA myxoma (d) Ebstein anomaly

765. Patient of leukemia treated with doxorubicin has dyspnea and extremity edema, best treatment:
(a) Beta 2 agonist with steroid inhalation
(b) Oxygen, digoxin
(c) Nocturnal CPAP with oxygen
(d) Diuretics with ACE-I

766. HOCM treatment A/E:
(a) Verapamil and propranolol
(b) Dual chamber sequential pacing
(c) Septal myomectomy with mitral placation
(d) Aortic valve replacement

767. PCWP > 15 mmHg clinically by:
(a) Positive abdominojugular reflux
(b) Pulmonary rales > 1/3rd of pulmonary area
(c) LV S3

768. Framingham major criteria A/E:
(a) Extremity edema (b) Pulmonary edema
(c) S3 (d) Cardiomegaly

769. Maximum loading dose of furosemide to prevent ototoxicity:
(a) 120 mg (b) 240 mg
(c) 300 mg (d) 180 mg

770. Breaking effect of furosemide drug given:
(a) Metolazone (b) Bumetamide
(c) Torsemide (d) Triamterene

771. Syncope least common with:
(a) MS (b) MR
(c) AS (d) AR

772. Systemic arterial saturation – 100% then what is coronary sinus saturation?
(a) 35% (b) 50%
(c) 60% (d) 75%

773. Most common mutation in HCM:
(a) Beta myosin heavy chain
(b) Alpha tropomyosin
(c) Titin
(d) Troponin T

774. Decreased myocardial contractility causing increased afterload limiting CO:
(a) Anrep effect (b) Bowditch effect
(c) Marie effect (d) Laplace effect

775. The neurotransmitter responsible for vascular tone in petidergic neuron:
(a) Acetylcholine (b) Substance P
(c) NO (d) Norepinephrine

776. Carotid dysphagia can be seen in:
(a) Aortic arch syndrome (b) Scleroderma
(c) Large LA (d) All of the above

777. Most common cause of heart failure:
(a) HTN (b) CAD
(c) DM (d) Valvular heart disease

778. All are true *except:*
(a) Capillaries are tubes with continuous endothelium with discontinuous pericytes
(b) Veins have small media and adventitia
(c) Small muscular arteries have prominent media
(d) Large muscular arteries have prominent media and adventitia

779. BNP not elevated in:
(a) Renal dysfunction
(b) Acute heart failure < 1 hour
(c) MS with PHT with TR
(d) MI

780. Positive hepatojugular reflux seen in A/E:
(a) LVF (b) RVMI
(c) CCP (d) Cardiac tamponade

781. Soft S1 A/E:
(a) Cardiac tamponade (b) Acute severe AR
(c) DCM (d) MVP

782. LV remodeling A/E:
(a) ↓ oxidative stress
(b) Fetal gene progressive
(c) Negative inotropic effect
(d) Apoptosis

783. Cardiomyopathies A/E:
(a) They are monogene disorder (ICM, HOCM, RCM)
(b) Familial CMP are AD
(c) Low penetrance
(d) Clinical severity variable

784. Which catheter is used in C.O. measurement by thermodilution method?
(a) Swan Ganz catheter (b) Pig tail catheter
(c) Judkin (d) Amplatzer

785. Prominent y descent in PCWP A/E:
(a) MR (b) RCM
(c) CCP (d) Myocardial ischemia

786. PCWP not equals to LVEDP A/E:
(a) Cortriatriatum
(b) Pericardial effusion
(c) Pleural pressure
(d) Pulmonary Catheter in nondependent zone

787. During demonstration of JVP a,c,v waves was named by:
(a) Potaine (b) Mackenzie
(c) Laennec

788. Beta blockers are preferred A/E:
(a) Post MI (b) High risk CAD
(c) HF (d) Renal insufficiency

789. Dobutamine S/E:
(a) Eosinophilic myocarditis
(b) DCM
(c) EMF

790. Oral β blocker, long acting used in arrhythmia:
(a) Propranolol (b) Esmolol
(c) Nadolol (d) Atenolol

791. Mechanical circulatory support in Patient in whom transplantation recovery is not feasible:
(a) Bridge to destination (b) Bridge to candidacy
(c) Bridge to recovery (d) Bridge to decision

792. OSA lead to A/E:
(a) ↑ Catecholamine (b) Renal dysfunction
(c) CAD (d) Hypoxia

793. Fabry's disease A/E:
(a) Angiokeratomas (b) CAD
(c) HOCM (d) ↑ arrhythmia

794. Heart rate turbulence A/E:
(a) Reflect reflex vagal control of heart
(b) It is benign condition
(c) Improved with beta blocker
(d) Improved with statins

795. HOCM murmer by ↑ A/E:
(a) Standing (b) Amyl nitrate
(c) Valsalva (d) Isometric handgrip

796. True A/E:
(a) Phenothiazine ↓ QRS and QT
(b) Class Ia ↑ QRS

797. All structure are present in RA *except:*
(a) Thebesian valve (b) Chiari network
(c) Coronary sinus (d) Muscle of lencini

798. Calcium ATPase is important in:
(a) Muscle contraction (b) Muscle relaxation
(c) Muscle excitation (d) All

799. Athlete's heart A/E:
(a) LVH < 13 mm
(b) Cavity dimension ↓
(c) Symmetric septal hypertrophy
(d) Family history present

800. Which is almost never occur after 8 years?
(a) Kawasaki's disease (b) Lyme disease
(c) Takayasu arteritis (d) Giant cell arteritis

801. Exercise effect A/E:
(a) Normal response exercise index >0.8
(b) Normal response exercise index <0.8
(c) Exercise factor > 60
(d) None of above

802. Atrial compliance in JVP:
(a) C wave (b) V wave
(c) A wave (d) Y wave

803. TAFAZZIN mutation associated with:
(a) Barth syndrome (b) LAMP syndrome
(c) Anderson syndrome

804. Friedreich ataxia:
(a) Fratraxin (b) Myosin
(c) MHCY7

805. Cardiogenic shock associated with A/E:
(a) ↑ ANP
(b) Renal cortical necrosis
(c) ↑ angiotensin II from liver
(d) ↑ vagal response

806. Reperfusion injury associated with typically:
(a) Diastolic dysfunction
(b) Systolic dysfunction
(c) RCMP
(d) Arrhythmia induced cardiomyopathy

807. Prognostic factor on Acute Heart Failure A/E:
(a) ↑ systolic HTN (b) Troponin T
(c) NT pro BNP (d) Sr. Creatinine/GFR

808. Nitrates MOA in Acute MI:
(a) Endothelial dependent vasodilatation
(b) ↑ perfusion in infarct area
(c) ↓ preload
(d) Venodilatation

809. Total PVR:
(a) Aorta mean – RA mean/Qs
(b) Aorta mean/Qs
(c) PA mean – LA mean/Qs

810. Afterload mismatch:
(a) Preserved contractility with systolic dysfunction due to ↑ afterload
(b) Systolic dysfunction due to ↑ afterload
(c) Diastolic dysfunction
(d) Systolic dysfunction due to ↓ preload for a given afterload

811. Acute LV dilatation:
(a) Anrep effect (b) Bowditch
(c) Bezold zarisch (d) Mary's law

812. RYR2 receptors function:
(a) Ca release from SR
(b) Ca release from SR with scaffolding protein
(c) Ca uptake
(d) SERCA (Ca release associated with Ca ATPase)

813. Pulsus paradoxus A/E:
(a) Severe Asthma (b) LV failure
(c) Myocardial disease (d) CCP

814. 7 years old, central cyanosis, Down syndrome, epigastric scar, mid systolic murmur at apex true is:

(a) HCT < 30%
(b) Hirschsprung disease in childhood
(c) CO_2 retention
(d) Dental extraction–SBE prophylaxis

815. Vanishing tumour:

(a) CCF
(b) Pneumothorax
(c) Klebsiella pneumonia

816. Reference point for CVP best:

(a) Sternal angle + 5 cm
(b) Caval sterna angle
(c) Right supraclavicular fossa
(d) 5 cm below 4th ICS left side

817. Positive hepatojugular reflex corresponds to PCWP of:

(a) < 10 (b) > 20
(c) > 15 (d) Cannot be measured

818. Giant 'a' wave:

(a) PPH (b) PDA
(c) ASD

819. ANP function A/E:

(a) ↑ RBF (b) ↑ GFR
(c) Natriuresis (d) ↓ vascular resistance

820. Continuous murmur in all *except:*

(a) Coronary artery stenosis
(b) Venous hum
(c) COA
(d) Peripheral pulmonary Artery stenosis

821. LA function A/E:

(a) ↑ BNP (b) Reservoir
(c) Boosting effect (d) Bain-bridge reflex

822. Myocardial hypertrophy with conduction defects due to deposition of:

(a) Adiponectin (b) Amylopectin
(c) Laminin A/C (d) Keratin

823. Lymphatic drainage of heart:

(a) Paratracheal left hilum
(b) Paratracheal right hilum
(c) Pretracheal below arch
(d) Mediastinum

824. DCM and conduction defects:

(a) Laminin A/C (b) JUP
(c) NOTCH 1 (d) NKX 2.5

825. Primordial prevention:

(a) Prevention of development of RF
(b) Treatment of complication

826. Cuff inflation in Lower Limb synchronised with cardiac cycle:

(a) External enhanced counterpulsation
(b) Abiomed
(c) Heartmate

827. Use of Marburg and yohimbine in:

(a) PPH
(b) Autonomic failure
(c) Primary HTN
(d) Renovascular HTN

828. The wave that occurs in the JVP with A-V dissociation and right atrial contraction against a closed tricuspid values is:

(a) Giant 'a' wave
(b) Cannon 'a' wave
(c) The 'c' wave
(d) The 'c v' wave

829. Cardiac Resynchronization Therapy has a positive inotropic effect largely due to significant increase in the level of:

(a) Apelin (b) Bradykinin
(c) Adrenomedullin (d) Nitric oxide

830. The Cardiac Danon Disease which is caused by a mutation is the X-linked lysosome-associated membrane protein (LAMP2) is characterized by:

(a) Dilated Cardiomyopathy
(b) Restrictive Cardiomyopathy
(c) Concentric hypertrophy with ventricular pre-excitation
(d) Chronic constrictive pericarditis

831. The "Thrifty Gene" hypothesis is used to explain:

(a) Predilection of salt resistant individuals to develop hypertension
(b) Relationship between low birth weight and development of hypertension
(c) Predilection for Asian Indians to develop obesity and Glucose intolerance on a Western Diet
(d) Development of hypertension and hypertrophy

832. The disorder with all features of the metabolic syndrome and associated with limb girdle fat atrophy is called:

(a) Dunnigan lipodystrophy (b) Syndrome-X
(c) Broad beta disease (d) Tangier disease

833. The mechanism of Total Electrical Alternans in cardiac tamponade is:

(a) "Bouncing Motion" of the Inter-ventricular septum
(b) "Swinging Heart Motion" as seen on echocardiography
(c) Similar to Pulsus alternans seen in heart failure
(d) Similar to Pulsus paradoxus

834. One of the following is not an action of the Atrial Natriuretic Peptide (ANP):

(a) ANP increases glomerular filtration rate
(b) ANP inhibits renal tubular sodium reabsorption
(c) ANP decreases aldosterone release from the adrenals on glomerulosa cells
(d) ANP increases renal blood flow

835. The most common innocent systolic murmur of childhood is:

(a) Venous hum
(b) Pulmonary flow murmur of childhood
(c) Pulmonary flow murmur of infancy
(d) Still's murmur

836. The width of the cuff used for measuring blood pressure in children should be:

(a) 40% of arm circumference
(b) 60% of arm length
(c) 40% of arm Diameter
(d) 60% of arm diameter

837. Beck's triad for cardiac tamponade include the following *except:*

(a) Pulsus paradoxus
(b) Hypotension
(c) Distended jugular venous pressures
(d) Muffled heart sound

838. Which one of the following is not an indicator of pericardial tamponade on a child?

(a) Collapse of Rt atrial free wall in late diastole
(b) Right ventricular free wall collapse in diastole
(c) Marked respiratory flow variation across tricuspid valve
(d) Diminished diastolic velocities in SVC

839. The drug which has no survival benefit in patients with LV dysfunction:

(a) Dobutamine (b) Eplerenone
(c) Enalapril (d) Carvedilol

840. Diastolic first heart sound occurs in:

(a) Mitral stenosis (b) Tricuspid stenosis
(c) Pulmonary stenosis (d) Aortic stenosis

841. Which one of the following causes decrease in MAP?

(a) High output with high viscosity
(b) High output with low viscosity
(c) High viscosity with low length
(d) Low tone with low viscosity

842. Which one of the following is NOT caused by Athlete's heart?

(a) RBBB
(b) QS in V_1 to V_3
(c) T inversion in V_1 to V_6
(d) Persistent Juvenile "T"

843. All are true regarding "TAKO-TSUBO" cardiomyopathy *except:*

(a) ST segment elevation
(b) Deep "T" wave inversion
(c) Obstruction of coronaries
(d) Akinesia of Distal LV

844. AC current causes:

(a) AF (b) Atrial standstill
(c) ST elevation mimicking MI

845. All drugs causes decrease mortality in CHF *except:*

(a) Digoxin (b) Metoprolol
(c) Aldactone

846. HOCM cause A/E:

(a) Systolic dysfunction
(b) 2/3rd cases structural abnormality in mitral valve
(c) Intramyocardial coronary abnormality

847. JVP true *except:*

(a) 2 trough, 2 peaks seen
(b) a > v
(c) y descent blunt in CCP
(d) Most prominent x wave on normal JVP

848. JVP A/E:

(a) IJV is preferred to EJV

(b) Inspiration increases the height of column with decrease in prominence of descents
(c) IJV is not palpable

849. Valve opened for most long time in cardiac cycle:
(a) TV (b) PV
(c) AV (d) MV

850. Trop T increases in A/E:
(a) Severe CHF (b) MI
(c) Myocarditis (d) Pneumonia

851. BNP increases in A/E:
(a) Acute MR
(b) Massive pulmonary embolism
(c) Septicemia
(d) Renal dysfunction

852. SVC PO_2:
(a) 8-10 (b) 10-12
(c) 12-14 (d) 14-16

853. PSM A/E:
(a) VSD (b) MR
(c) TR (d) ASD

854. Slope of HR related to BP is:
(a) Mary's law
(b) Sinus node dysfunction
(c) Baroreceptor sensitivity
(d) BP

855. Slope of pressure with relation of volume:
(a) Pressure volume loop (b) Elastance
(c) Compliance (d) Stiffness

856. Ventricular vascular coupling:
(a) LVEDP and SVR
(b) CI and SVR
(c) Preload and afterload
(d) End systolic elastance to vascular elastance

857. Sinus tachycardia causes:
(a) Physiological (b) Hypothyroidism
(c) Anxiety (d) None of the above

858. Cottage chesse/scrambled egg pericarditis seen in:
(a) Neisseria (b) H. influenza
(c) S. aureus (d) Salmonella

859. S4 due to:
(a) Atrial contraction
(b) Rapid ventricular filling

860. Diuretic with vasodilator with reduced renin:
(a) BNP (b) Thiazide
(c) Loop diuretics

861. Apoptosis is increased by A/E:
(a) Beta blocker (b) Angiotensin II
(c) NO (d) Superoxide

862. Neuroendocrine mediator in shock A/E:
(a) Glucagon (b) Cortisol
(c) Beta endorphin (d) Superoxide ions

863. True is:
(a) LVEDP = mean pulmonary venous wedge pressure
(b) RVEDP = PADP
(c) PADP= Mean LA pressure
(d) LAP = RAP

864. Opening snap true is:
(a) Low frequency
(b) Heard in systole
(c) More closure to S2 as severity increases

865. PAH pressure is:
(a) 18 (b) 22
(c) 15 (d) 25

866. Constrictive pericarditis/ RCMP favouring CCP: (T/F)
(a) Septal bounce (b) LVH
(c) PAH > 60 (d) RVSP > mmhg
(e) Interventricular dependence

867. LCZ-9 true: (T/F)
(a) Nephrilysin inhibitor only
(b) Nephrilysin inhibitor + ARB
(c) No added benefit with valsartan
(d) PARADIGM trial
(e) Prematurely stopped trial

868. BNP true: (T/F)
(a) Increases obesity
(b) Increases RHF
(c) Increases HFpEF
(d) Increases massive PTE

869. Diastolic HF not favouring: (T/F)
(a) Male (b) Obesity
(c) CAD (d) AF
(e) Age

870. Drugs reduces mortality in HF: (T/F)
(a) Bisoprolol (b) Carvedilol
(c) Eplerenone (d) Candesartan
(e) Digoxin F

871. Paradoxical split seen in:
(a) HOCM (b) MR
(c) AS (d) RV pacing
(e) LBBB

872. Levosimendan: (T/F)
(a) Acts on K- ATP channel , causes vasodilatation
(b) Acts on Ca channel causes vasodilatation
(c) Cardioprotective because of K- ATP
(d) Cardioprotective because of Ca channel sensitization on ventricular myocyte

873. Treprostinil true: (T/F)
(a) Can be given S/C, I/V or inhaled
(b) More stable at room temp.
(c) Eposterol has longer half life
(d) 6 minutes walk distance does not depend on dose
(e) Treprostinil causes more gram negative sepsis

874. Still murmur: (T/F)
(a) Bell of stethoscope
(b) 2nd right ICS
(c) ↑ after exercise
(d) Better in 2nd phase of systole
(e) Seldom in infants

875. Constriction of PDA: (T/F)
(a) PGE_2 (b) PGI_2
(c) NO (d) O_2
(e) Ibuprofen

876. β-MHC not associated with: (T/F)
(a) HCM (b) ARVD
(c) DCMP (d) RCMP
(e) Brugada

877. Loop diuretics: (T/F)
(a) Oral absorption of predictable torsemide better than frusemide
(b) Furosemide t1/2 -12 hrs
(c) ↑ absorption with food
(d) Hyperkalemia common
(e) Highly protein bound

878. Levosimenden: (T/F)
(a) Ca sensitizer at myofibre
(b) Blocks K^+ at sacrolemmal membrane
(c) Hyperkalemia
(d) Hypokalemia
(e) Post infusion 24 hours last for 7-9 days

879. Spironolactone: (T/F)
(a) Competitive antagonist of aldosterone
(b) Eplerenone more affinity for androgen receptors
(c) Dose related hyperkalemia
(d) Retains efficacy in renal failure
(e) ↓ mortality in systolic HF

880. Diastolic HF A/E: (T/F)
(a) Most common in elderly
(b) Most common in females
(c) HTN is risk factor
(d) ↓ mortality by ARB
(e) ↓ mortality by ACE–I

881. PAH in left heart disease: (T/F)
(a) Transpulmonary gradient ↑ early in this group
(b) To start with normal (< 10 mm Hg)
(c) Aortic > mitral disease
(d) Depends mainly on increased LAP
(e) Phasic variation in RCA

882. CVP recording in cardiac tamponade: (T/F)
(a) Prominent x (b) Prominent y
(c) Absent a (d) Absent v
(e) Higher than normal filling pressure seen

883. Septal ablation in HCM: (T/F)
(a) RBBB
(b) Septal branch of RCA
(c) Preferred in young
(d) Eliminates risk of SCD
(e) ↓ Gradient more with myomectomy

884. BB in HF: (T/F)
(a) Less effective in female
(b) Less effective in DM
(c) Not to be used in NYHA III/IV
(d) Decreased SCD in HF

885. BNP: (T/F)
(a) Increase in obesity
(b) Treatment of HF decrease level

(c) Increase in isolated RHF
(d) More in diastolic HF than systolic
(e) Does not indicate prognosis in pt. on B Blocker for HF

886. RCMP vs CCP, favouring RCMP: (T/F)
(a) Septal bounce
(b) Biatrial enlargement
(c) Increased PAP
(d) Exaggerated respiratory variation
(e) Equalization of diastolic pressure

887. Amyloid heart disease A/E: (T/F)
(a) Biatrial enlargement
(b) Most common AL type
(c) Thickness of all 4 chambers
(d) Sustained VT on Holter

888. Pulmonary arterial HTN on TEE: (T/F)
(a) TR jet velocity > 3 cm/sec
(b) Pulmonary flow acceleration > 120 msec
(c) Shift of interatrial septum to left
(d) RV enlargement
(e) Prolonged EF slope on M mode of pulm. Valve

889. Increased preload: (T/F)
(a) ESV (b) EDV
(c) SV (d) CO
(e) EF

890. S3: (T/F)
(a) Common in elderly
(b) Marker of systolic function > diastolic function
(c) Predicts increased BNP
(d) Prognostic in AMI
(e) Poor prognosis in CHF

891. Peripartum cardiomyopathy (PPCM): (T/F)
(a) Most common in last month of pregnancy
(b) Incidence-1 in 200 live pregnancy
(c) Diuretic useful in pulmonary congestion
(d) ACE-I to be continued in future pregnancy if prior PPCM
(e) More worsening of LV dysfunction if prior LV dysfunction

892. Takotsubo CMP A/E: (T/F)
(a) Due to critical stenosis of RCA
(b) Most common in adolescence
(c) Commonly involves apex
(d) Associated with AR
(e) ECG is always normal

893. Tachycardia induced cardiomyopathy A/E: (T/F)
(a) More common in frequent VPC
(b) Most common in 100-200 VPC/hour
(c) Irreversible after one month
(d) Treatment with I/V adrenaline
(e) Most patients with frequent VPC develop CMP

894. Constrictive pericarditis: (T/F)
(a) Increased pericardial thickness in all
(b) 75% develop constriction post tuberculosis
(c) < 1% viral
(d) MRI–increased gadolinium enhancement
(e) After pericardiectomy has better prognosis than post radiation

895. Cardiogenic shock: (T/F)
(a) 6-8% in NSTEMI
(b) > 10% have mechanical causes
(c) LVAD no better than IABP at 30 days
(d) Tilargine at short term mortality
(e) Multivessel intervention better than culprit vessel intervention

896. Alcohol septal ablation: (T/F)
(a) CHB in 25-30%
(b) RBBB common
(c) Contraindicated in > 15 mm septal thickness
(d) RCA septal branch
(e) Eliminates SCD risk

897. Myocarditis: (T/F)
(a) IVIg increases proinflammatory marker
(b) Cardiac transplant in acute myocarditis in survival
(c) Myocarditis common in ARF
(d) Troponin increases more than increase in CK-MB
(e) LV dysfunction with dilatation most common

898. Pericardial effusion: (T/F)
(a) Earliest seen in oblique sinus
(b) Compensation not seen in SSS
(c) Increased parasympathetic and sympathetic activity
(d) Cause identified in 90% in moderate to large effusion

899. Pulmonary diastolic pressure is less than LA pressure: (T/F)

(a) Pulmonary stenosis (b) PR

(c) RBBB (d) LBBB

(e) Increased PVR

900. Stem cell transplant: (T/F)

(a) BM derived mononuclear cell are firstly studied

(b) BM derived mononuclear cell are most commonly used

(c) Skeletal myoblasts are predisposed to arrhythmias

(d) Embryonic stem cell predisposed to teratoma formation

(e) BMC's directly differentiate into cardiomyocytes

901. Bosentan: (T/F)

(a) C/I in pregnancy

(b) Hepatoxicity

(c) Anemia is a common side effect

(d) Flushing

(e) Metabolised by cytochrome oxidase system

902. CCP versus RCMP, favouring CCP: (T/F)

(a) PAH

(b) Biatrial enlargement

(c) Square root sign

(d) Prominent y descent

(e) Pericardial knock

903. Cardiac amyloidosis: (T/F)

(a) LV wall thickness rule out amyloidosis

(b) SAM is present

(c) Systolic dysfunction is uncommon

(d) Intracavitary obstruction

(e) Intracardiac thrombus

904. HCM: (T/F)

(a) > 80% penetrance lifelong

(b) Myosin Binding protein C associated with delayed LVH

(c) MLCK associated with midcavitary obstruction

(d) Trop T with restrictive physiology

(e) Uncommon in head and hinge, common in rods

905. Valsalva maneuver: (T/F)

(a) Phase I – decrease SBP

(b) Phase II – decrease SV and pulse pressure

(c) Phase II – increases SVR

(d) Phase III – decrease intrathoracic pressure

(e) Phase IV – increases venous return

906. Cardiac physiology A/E: (T/F)

(a) Phase 0 – increased Na conductance

(b) Phase II – 1 msec

(c) RMP of SA node= -50 to -60 mV

(d) Propagation velocity of Purkinje fibres more than ventricular myocardium

(e) RMP of ventricular muscle = -80 to -90 mV

907. Verapamil: (T/F)

(a) DOC in AVNRT (adult)

(b) PSVT in neonate

(c) MS with AF

(d) Idiopathic LV VT

(e) Used in VF

908. Wide split S1: (T/F)

(a) Ebstein anomaly (b) RV pacing

(c) RBBB (d) HOCM

(e) Idiopathic LV rhythm

909. Pulsus alternans: (T/F)

(a) Severe AS with moderate AR

(b) Severe AR with moderate AS

(c) Cardiac tamponade

(d) Severe LV dysfunction

(e) VSD

910. JVP: (T/F)

(a) Prominent a wave wide QRS S/O VT

(b) v wave indicates ventricular filling

(c) Absent x wave in cardiac tamponade

(d) IJV not used due to presence of valves

(e) Left side EJV prominent S/O persistent LSVC

911. Exercise physiology: (T/F)

(a) CO more in supine than standing position

(b) Supine to standing causes decrease venous return

(c) Supine – increase CO mostly due to increased HR with little augmentation of SV

(d) EF increases more in standing than supine

(e) Old age associated with decreased peak HR

912. Digoxin in HF: (T/F)

(a) Decreases mortality

(b) Decreases hospitalisation

(c) IV calcium gluconate given for toxicity
(d) Causes increased intracellular Ca^{++}
(e) Hypokalemia precipitates toxicity

913. Murmur of PR: (T/F)
(a) PR in absence of PHT–diamond shape
(b) PR in absence of PHT gap between P_2 – onset murmur
(c) PR in absence of PHT high pitched
(d) Decreases with valsalva if PR with PHT
(e) Increases with inspiration

914. Reverse splitting of S_2: (T/F)
(a) RV pacing
(b) RBBB
(c) Severe AS
(d) Myocardial ischemia
(e) PHT

915. S_3: (T/F)
(a) Indicate systolic performance > diastolic
(b) Common in children
(c) Predicts increase in BNP
(d) Prognostic significance in CHF
(e) Worse prognosis is MI

916. Prominent y descent A/E: (T/F)
(a) RA myxoma (b) CCP
(c) RVMI (d) TR
(e) RCMP

917. CCP vs RCMP, CCP favouring (T/F):
(a) Prominent y descent
(b) Pericardial knock
(c) Bilateral enlargement
(d) Square wave response
(e) PAH

918. HOCM high risk: (T/F)
(a) Family history
(b) HT response on exercise
(c) > 20 VPC in 48 hours Holter monitoring
(d) > 35 mm thickness
(e) Unexplained syncope in young

919. Marfan–major criteria: (T/F)
(a) Ectopic lentis (b) Myopia
(c) MVP (d) Aortic dissection
(e) Lumbosacral erosion due to dural ectasia

920. Myoxamatous degeneration of all valve: (T/F)
(a) FMNA T (b) JAG-1
(c) FBN-1 (d) NOTCH-1
(e) ABCC-1

921. Physiology: (T/F)
(a) RA systole starts early than left atrial
(b) RV contraction earlier than LV
(c) RV ejection prolong than LV
(d) Ventricular contraction start near end of R wave
(e) Pulmonary artery Impedence is low

922. BNP: (T/F)
(a) Increases in obesity
(b) Increases in renal failure
(c) Increases with age
(d) May increase in PE
(e) HF with reduced EF more than HFn EF

923. HOCM true: (T/F)
(a) Trop T–restrictive cardiomyopathy
(b) Trop I–SCD
(c) Thick fibre of sarcomere involved more than thin fibre
(d) β-MHC rod region missense mutation
(e) AR inheritance

924. Wide splitting S_2 is seen in: (T/F)
(a) ASD (b) MS
(c) VSD (d) MR
(e) LBBB

925. Reverse spilit S_2: (T/F)
(a) RBBB (b) RV pacing
(c) LBBB (d) HT
(e) MS

926. Venous hum true: (T/F)
(a) Elderly more
(b) Anemia does not worsen
(c) Pregnancy does not worsen
(d) Rough and noisy
(e) More prominent in diastole

927. Valsalva maneuvre: (T/F)
(a) Phase I-↓ SV, ↓ PP
(b) Phase II- ↓SV, ↓PP
(c) Phase III- ↑ BP
(d) Phase IV- ↑ SBP with reflex bradycardia
(e) Phase IV- ↑ VR with ↑ SVR

928. Pulse: (T/F)
(a) Pulsus Alternan – severe LV dysfunction
(b) Pulsus paradoxus – tamponade > CCP
(c) Pulsus Bisferiens – HOCM
(d) Brachial pulse earlier than femoral
(e) Aortic valve closure coincides with incisura

929. Hemodynamic: (T/F)
(a) Mean RA – 6 mm Hg
(b) Mean LA – 2 mm Hg
(c) Mean PA – 8 mm Hg
(d) Normal PCWP – 4-12 mm Hg
(e) ↓ PVR – 70

930. LVDEP-PCWP discordance: (T/F)
(a) MS
(b) LA myxoma
(c) PV stenosis
(d) Placement of cath in dependent zone
(e) ↓ pleural pressure

931. JVP: (T/F)
(a) Absent y – TS
(b) Prominent y – CCP
(c) Prominent x – Tamponade
(d) Cannon 'a' wave – CHB
(e) Prominent 'a' – AF

932. S_2: (T/F)
(a) Aortic hangout interval 50 – 80 msec
(b) Expiration A2-P2 < 30 msec
(c) Pulmonary hangout interval > Aortic hangout interval
(d) P2 softer than A2
(e) P2 hangout increases with inspiration

933. HF with impaired systolic function–drug ↓ mortality rate: (T/F)
(a) Nebivolol (b) Spironolactone
(c) Valsartan (d) Digoxin
(e) Furosemide

934. HOCM drugs: (T/F)
(a) Disopyramide (b) Nifedipine
(c) Quinidine (d) Metoprolol
(e) Digoxin

935. Takotsubo CMP: (T/F)
(a) Apex involved
(b) EKG usually Normal
(c) More common in males
(d) Emotional stress
(e) TVD

936. B blocker in HF: (T/F)
(a) Metoprolol better than carvedilol in DCM
(b) Carvedilol effective in ischemic CMP
(c) C/I if ramipril given
(d) Increase survival in NYHA II
(e) Improve survival is diastolic HF

937. Wide S_2 causes: (T/F)
(a) RBBB (b) LAH
(c) LPH (d) Ebstein's anomaly
(e) PDA Eisenmenger

938. HOCM: (T/F)
(a) 30 mm of LVH (b) Trop T – LVH
(c) Trop I – restrictive (d) BP response flat
(e) Dilated type – good prognosis

939. RV dilatation A/E: (T/F)
(a) Acute pulmonary embolism
(b) ARVD
(c) TS
(d) Severe PR
(e) ASD

940. Restrictive physiology A/E: (T/F)
(a) Biatrial enlargement
(b) ↑ LVEDP
(c) ↓ RVEDP
(d) ↑ Mean RA pressure
(e) Dip and plateau in Right ventricle

941. Pulmonary paradoxus: (T/F)
(a) Acute bronchial asthma
(b) Severe LV dysfunction
(c) Effusive constructive pericarditis
(d) Acute tamponade
(e) RVMI with IWMI

942. Kussmaul's sign most common: (T/F)
(a) RV failure of any cause
(b) TAPVC (c) PAPVC
(d) ASD (e) CCP

943. Continuous murmur: (T/F)
(a) PDA with Eisenmenger

(b) RSOV to RA
(c) Coronary AV fistula
(d) AP window - 1 day age
(e) Inlet VSD

944. HOCM risk factors: (T/F)
(a) 20 mm septal thickness
(b) NSVT on Holter monitoring
(c) Family history SCD
(d) LVOT Obstruction
(e) Hypertensive response on TMT

945. Reversibility of pulmonary HTN checked by: (T/F)
(a) 40-80 NO
(b) 40-80 N_2O
(c) Prostacyclin infusion
(d) 100% O_2
(e) 50% O_2

946. LVEDP not increased: (T/F)
(a) Pulmonary vein obstruction
(b) Acute MR
(c) MS
(d) Tamponade
(e) Restrictive CMP

947. Dip and plateau in RV pressure tracing all *except:* (T/F)
(a) HOCM (b) Restrictive CMP
(c) RVMI with IWMI (d) Chronic TR
(e) CCP

948. LVS_3 – incorrect: (T/F)
(a) ↑ es on inspiration
(b) Can be heard in MR even without LV dysfunction
(c) Acute AR
(d) Heard with bell of stethoscope
(e) Normal in pregnancy

949. Alcohol septal ablation in HOCM: (T/F)
(a) RBBB seen
(b) PPI indicated is almost all patients who developed CHB
(c) 10% have MR (severe)
(d) More effective than septal myectomy
(e) Abolishes risk of SCD

950. Loeys Dietz syndrome – incorrect: (T/F)
(a) Autosomal recessive
(b) ↑ risk of aortic dissection
(c) ↑ arterial tortuosity
(d) Hypertelorism may be seen
(e) Cleft palate seen

951. HF: (T/F)
(a) Digoxin less mortality benefit
(b) Diuretics have mortality benefit
(c) CAD most common cause of HF
(d) 40% have Normal EF

952. Improved survival of ischemic CMP *except:* (T/F)
(a) Spironolactone (b) ICD
(c) Long acting b-blocker (d) ACE-I
(e) Digoxin

953. HOCM: (T/F)
(a) SCD can be presenting feature
(b) Nitrates are DOC
(c) B-blockers useful
(d) All patient require septal ablation
(e) Diabetic mother can have HOCM baby

954. Marfan–major criteria A/E: (T/F)
(a) Myopic (b) MVP
(c) Ectopic lentis (d) Aortic dissection
(e) Eorsion of L/S vertebrae by dural ectasia

955. Regarding myxoma true are: (T/F)
(a) Carney complex is AD
(b) Familial seen in 1/3 cases
(c) RA most common site
(d) Recurrence is less within familial after surgery
(e) Myxoma is most common primary tumour of heart

956. Amyloidosis in heart – false (T/F):
(a) Cardiac involvement more common in primary than secondary
(b) Primary has better prognosis than secondary
(c) Thickened IAS
(d) Marked RV dilatation is common
(e) High voltage complexes common

957. High BNP: (T/F)
(a) Severe PTE (b) RCMP
(c) CCP (d) MS
(e) Acute LVF

958. ↑ PCWP seen in: (T/F)
(a) Cortriatriatum-dexter
(b) Pulmonary vein stenosis
(c) Mitral stenosis
(d) Diastolic LV failure
(e) PPH

959. Venous hum true: (T/F)
(a) Present in elderly
(b) Less common in anemia
(c) Less common in pregnancy
(d) Murmur prominent in diastole
(e) May present as harsh and noisy

960. Isometric exercise: (T/F)
(a) S_3 reduced
(b) AS murmur increased
(c) HOCM murmur diminishes
(d) MR murmur decreases
(e) AR murmur decreases

961. Pericarditis: (T/F)
(a) LBBB
(b) RBBB
(c) ST elevation in avR
(d) P wave tall
(e) PR depression

962. Phosphodiestrase inhibitor: (T/F)
(a) Sildenafil (b) Theophylline
(c) Carvedilol (d) Losartan
(e) Cilastazol

963. Kussmaul's sign *except:* (T/F)
(a) MR (b) VSD
(c) TS (d) CCP
(e) RHF

964. Pericarditis ECG changes: (T/F)
(a) ST elevation (b) PR depression
(c) ST depression (d) RBBB

965. Paradoxical split S_2: (T/F)
(a) RV pacing (b) RBBB
(c) WPW type B (d) LVOT obstruction
(e) AR

966. Wide split S_2: (T/F)
(a) PDA
(b) MR
(c) AR
(d) Acute Pulmonary embolism
(e) Hypovolumic shock

967. Pulsus paradoxsus: (T/F)
(a) Acute massive PTE
(b) Severe COAD
(c) Tension pheumothorax
(d) Cardiac tamponade
(e) Hypovolumic shock

968. Loud S_1: (T/F)
(a) Anemia (b) Exercise
(c) Catecholamine (d) B Blocker therapy
(e) AV fistula

969. CCP vs RCMP favouring CCP: (T/F)
(a) Pulmonary Artery pressure–high
(b) Equal LV and RV end diastolic pressure
(c) Cardiomegaly on X-ray
(d) LVH

970. LVS_3: (T/F)
(a) Can be present in old age
(b) MR with Normal LV function
(c) Acute AR
(d) Better audible with bell

971. HOCM: (T/F)
(a) >30 mm thickness mortality
(b) BB improves survival
(c) Verapamil should be given in HOCM with severe pulmonary HTN
(d) Disopyramide is DOC in nonobstructive HCM
(e) Pregnancy is well tolerated

972. ↓ Mortality in CHF: (T/F)
(a) Bisoprolol (b) Candesartan
(c) Spironolactone (d) Digoxin
(e) Furosemide

973. Papillary muscle of mitral valve: (T/F)
(a) Anterolateral is single muscle usually
(b) Anterolateral supplied by RCA
(c) LCx is closest of mitral annulus
(d) Posteromedial attached to IVS
(e) AML > PML prolapsed

974. Alcohol septal ablation: (T/F)
(a) RBBB common sequelae
(b) Requires PPI in > 50% patients

(c) Dual chamber pacing is better
(d) Septal branch of RCA
(e) AR common

975. DCMP, LVIDD-65 mm, LVEF-22%, LBBB, QRS-180 ms on maximal medical treatment, NYHA class III, treatment advice: (T/F)

(a) Beta blocker (b) ACE-I
(c) CRT-P/D (d) Artificial heart
(e) Heart transplant

976. Reduced mortality in HF A/E: (T/F)

(a) Digoxin (b) Torsemide
(c) Candesartan (d) Bisoprolol
(e) Spironolactone

977. Biventricular pacing trials with favourable result: (T/F)

(a) MADIT (b) MUST
(c) DINAMIT (d) CARE-HF
(e) COMPANION

978. HCM gene A/E: (T/F)

(a) Tropomysin (b) Troponin–I
(c) Desmoplakin (d) Plakoglobin
(e) Desmin

979. S_2: (T/F)

(a) Aortic hangout interval 50-80 msecs
(b) P2 is softer than A2
(c) Pulmonary is more common than aortic hangout interval
(d) Expiration – A2 P2 interval decreases to <30 msecs
(e) A2 coincides with incisura of aortic pressure curve

980. Pulse true: (T/F)

(a) Alternans in severe LV systolic dysfunction
(b) Bisferiens pulse in HOCM often seen
(c) Brachial impulse is felt earlier than femoral
(d) Systolic BP decreases with expiration normally
(e) Pulsus paradoxus more common in tamponade than CCP

981. Valsalva manoeuvre incorrect: (T/F)

(a) Failure to overshoot seen in systolic dysfunction
(b) Square wave means low filling pressure
(c) Square wave response depends on E
(d) Systolic murmur increases
(e) Most of the murmur decreases

982. Right sided HF is seen in: (T/F)

(a) PPH (b) AR
(c) AS (d) Acute MI

983. CHB in HCM with mutation: (T/F)

(a) Trop T (b) Trop I
(c) Tropomyosin (d) PRKAG2
(e) LAMP2

984. Kussmaul A/E: (T/F)

(a) CCP (b) TS
(c) VSD (d) CHF
(e) MR

985. S_2 wide split: (T/F)

(a) MR (b) VSD
(c) LBBB (d) MS
(e) ASD

986. S_2 reverse split: (T/F)

(a) LBBB
(b) RV paced
(c) Hypertensive heart disease
(d) PDA
(e) Angina pectoris

987. Continuous murmur: (T/F)

(a) PDA (b) ALCAPA
(c) PPS (d) RSOV
(e) VSD

988. Pan systolic murmur A/E: (T/F)

(a) MR (b) TR
(c) VSD (d) AS
(e) Supravalvular AS

989. Venous hum: (T/F)

(a) Elderly (b) ↓ Pregnancy
(c) More in diastole (d) Harsh and noisy
(e) Anemia ↓

990. HCM: (T/F)

(a) Sudden death without previous symptoms
(b) Trop T mutation – severe LVH
(c) Trop I – restrictive
(d) ↓ BP on exercise – good prognosis
(e) Digoxin – DOC

991. Biomarkers: (T/F)
(a) Troponin more sensitive than CK – MB in small infarction
(b) Myoglobin : Cardiac specific
(c) Myoglobin readily excretion in urine
(d) CK-MB Normal in 12 hours
(e) CKMB ↑ rule out myocarditis

992. NYHA A/E: (T/F)
(a) Cyanosis (b) Syncope
(c) Dyspnea (d) Palpitation
(e) Fatigue

993. Peripartum CMP: (T/F)
(a) Most common in twin pregnancy
(b) Most common in 2nd trimester
(c) Most common in 3rd and 4th pregnancy
(d) Tocolytic association
(e) Age < 25 years

994. Anthracycline: (T/F)
(a) 60% have myocardial dysfunction
(b) Children at risk
(c) HF after several years usually
(d) Peak dose is important
(e) Total dose important

995. RCM vs CCP– favours RCM: (T/F)
(a) PAH (b) Square root sign
(c) ↑ JVP (d) Paradoxsus
(e) Septal bounce

996. Valsalva: (T/F)
(a) Phase I – BP ↓
(b) Phase II – Bradycardia
(c) Phase III – Right murmur ↓
(d) Square wave – CHF
(e) Square wave – MS

997. Isometric exercise: (T/F)
(a) MR murmur ↓ (b) AS ↑
(c) HCM ↓ (d) LVS3 ↓
(e) AR ↓

998. Improves survival in DCM A/E: (T/F)
(a) Digoxin (b) Carvedilol
(c) Furosemide (d) Ramipril
(e) Spironolactone

999. Cannon a wave: (T/F)
(a) TS (b) CHB
(c) VVI pacing (d) AF
(e) TR

1000. Loud S_1: (T/F)
(a) AS (b) Pliable valve
(c) Calcific MS (d) Tachycardia
(e) MR

1001. Pulsus paradoxus: (T/F)
(a) Cardiac tamponade (b) Obesity
(c) VSD (d) MR
(e) Pregnancy

1002. Kussmaul's sign A/E: (T/F)
(a) CCP (b) TS
(c) CHF (d) VSD
(e) MR

1003. NYHA A/E: (T/F)
(a) Cyanosis (b) Syncope
(c) Palpitation (d) Dyspnea
(e) Fatigue

1004. Marfan's syndrome: (T/F)
(a) Aortic dissection (b) AS
(c) MVP (d) Myopia
(e) Splenomegaly

1005. Isometric exercise: (T/F)
(a) Increased LVS3
(b) Increase AS murmur
(c) Decrease EDM of AR
(d) Decrease systolic murmur of MR
(e) Decrease HOCM murmur

1006. PDE-Inhibitor: (T/F)
(a) Amrinone (b) Theophylline
(c) Sildenafil (d) Carvedilol
(e) ARB

1007. RCMP versus CCP, favoured by RCMP are: (T/F)
(a) Increased PA pressure
(b) Square root sign
(c) Increased JVP
(d) Septal bounce
(e) Pulsus paradoxus

1008. Valsalva: (T/F)
(a) Bradycardia in phase II

(b) Hypotension in phase I
(c) Right sided murmur decreases in phase III
(d) Square wave in CHF
(e) Square wave in MS

1009. MET: (T/F)
(a) 70 kg man, 40 years age at rest
(b) 3.5 ml O_2/kg/min
(c) 5 ml O_2/kg/min
(d) Useful in exercise prescription
(e) Workloads is measured in multiples of MET

1010. Continuous murmur seen in: (T/F)
(a) RSOV (b) PDA
(c) VSD (d) ALCAPA
(e) Peripheral PS

1011. Continuous murmur noted in: (T/F)
(a) RSOV (b) PDA
(c) MR (d) VSD
(e) ASD

1012. Wide sputting of S_2 seen in: (T/F)
(a) RBBB (b) ASD
(c) VSD (d) MR
(e) MS

1013. Paradoxical splitting of S_2 seen in: (T/F)
(a) LBBB
(b) VSD
(c) RV pacing
(d) Hypertensive heart disease
(e) MS

1014. Pansystolic murmur seen in: (T/F)
(a) VSD (b) MR
(c) TR (d) Valvular AS
(e) Supravalvular AS

1015. Cervical venous hum: (T/F)
(a) Seen in elderly
(b) Rough and noisy
(c) Decrease in anemia
(d) Decrease in pregnancy
(e) Louder in diastole

1016. Pulmonary vasodilators include: (T/F)
(a) Inhaled NO (b) Milrinone
(c) Mephentine (d) NTG
(e) Dopamine

1017. C/F of CCP commonly: (T/F)
(a) Hepatomegaly (b) Increased JVP
(c) Pulsus paradoxsus (d) TR murmur
(e) Pulmonary click

1018. Dicrotic pulse seen in: (T/F)
(a) Rare in healthy adults
(b) Seen in febrile states
(c) HOCM
(d) 2nd peak in systole
(e) 2nd peak in diastole

1019. Common 'a' waves seen in: (T/F)
(a) AF (b) CHB
(c) VVI (d) TS
(e) MS

1020. Acute pericarditis: (T/F)
(a) PR depression
(b) ST elevation maximum in avR with tall T wave
(c) LBBB
(d) RBBB

1021. NYHA includes: (T/F)
(a) Chest pain (b) Dyspnea
(c) Palpitation (d) Cyanosis
(e) Clubbing

1022. HOCM: (T/F)
(a) Prognosis is bad if outflow tract obstruction present
(b) Can cause sudden death in asymptomatic
(c) Trop T mutation prognosis bad
(d) Trop I mutation restrictive physiology

1023. HCM: (T/F)
(a) DCM occur in 40%
(b) Prognosis is bad in apical HCM

1024. RCM versus CCP: (T/F)
(a) Septal bounce
(b) High PA pressure
(c) Pulsus paradoxus

1025. Pulsus paradoxus seen in: (T/F)
(a) Morbid obesity (b) Pregnancy
(c) MR (d) AR
(e) VSD

1026. Kussmaul sign A/E: (T/F)
(a) VSD (b) MR
(c) CHF (d) RCM
(e) TS

1027. Valsalva response: (T/F)
(a) Phase I – transient hypotension
(b) Phase II – reflex bradycardia
(c) Square wave response in CHF
(d) Square wave response in MS

1028. First line management in patient in patient with HF:
(a) Digoxin (b) Diuretics
(c) ACE-I (d) Beta blockers

1029. Precipitating factor of CHF in DCMP:
(a) Anemia (b) Chest infection
(c) Myxedema (d) AV dyssynergy

1030. Cause of HF in COPD:
(a) Pulmonary HTN
(b) TR
(c) Increase work of breathing
(d) Hypercapnia

1031. Wide splitting of S_2: (T/F)
(a) RBBB (b) PS
(c) Cardiac tamponade (d) VSD
(e) PHT

1032. Soft S_1:
(a) 1st degree heart block (b) Acute AR
(c) AS (d) Rheumatic MR
(e) PPH

1033. Wide splitting of S_2: (T/F)
(a) RBBB (b) PS
(c) Cardiac tamponade (d) VSD
(e) PHT

1034. Soft S_1: (T/F)
(a) 1st degree heart block
(b) Acute AR
(c) AS
(d) Rheumatic MR
(e) PPH

1035. HOCM murmur ↑: (T/F)
(a) Post VPC (b) Valsalva phase IV
(c) Inotropes (d) Leg raising
(e) Standing

1036. HAPE A/E: (T/F)
(a) Increased PCWP
(b) Increased PA pressure
(c) Hypoxia
(d) Decreased diffusion capacity
(e) Tachycardia

1037. CHF with NSR, drug to be avoided for long term use: (T/F)
(a) Digoxin (b) Aminophylline
(c) Salbutamol (d) Beta blocker
(e) Lithium

1038. Mechanisms of peripheral edema in CHF: (T/F)
(a) Increased catecholamines
(b) Venoconstriction
(c) Increased hydrostatic pressure
(d) Increased ANP

1039. CHF A/E: (T/F)
(a) Decrease pulse pressure
(b) Decrease AV O_2 difference
(c) Decreased CO
(d) Increased filling pressure

1040. Mechanisms of fatigue in CHF: (T/F)
(a) Activation of J receptor in muscle
(b) Decreased CO
(c) Decreased PaO_2
(d) Decreased metabolism in skeletal muscle
(e) Anemia

1041. Beta blocker with ISA: (T/F)
(a) Pindolol (b) Acebutalol
(c) Sotalol (d) Atenolol
(e) Propranolol

1042. Omecamtiv MOA:
(a) Myosin activator

1043. Takatsubo cardiomyopathy A/E:
(a) Due to stress
(b) In premenopausal women
(c) Mimics acute MI
(d) Benign

1044. Bosentan adverse effect A/E:
(a) Increased liver enzymes
(b) Renal dysfunction
(c) Nasopharyngitis

1045. Anthracycline cardiac toxicity risk predictor A/E:
(a) HTN (b) Male gender
(c) Age (d) Prior radiation therapy

1046. True *except:*
(a) A2-S3: 0.14-0.16 secs
(b) A2- OS : 0.04-0.12 secs
(c) A2- pericardial knock: 0.10-0.12 secs, high pitched
(d) S4 is presystolic and high pitched

1047. Pericarditis A/E:
(a) Methyldopa
(b) Emetine
(c) Methysergide

1048. S_4 A/E:
(a) No change in intensity with respiration

1049. Phasic ejection click:
(a) PS (b) TOF

1050. CCP A/E:
(a) Respiratory variation
(b) Square root sign
(c) PASP > 60 mm Hg

1051. Device which reduces afterload and increase coronary perfusion to max:
(a) IABP (b) ECMO
(c) Tandem heart (d) Impella device

1052. Pulsus paradoxus not lost in:
(a) ASD (b) AR
(c) LV dysfunction (d) All

1053. Pulsus paradoxus not lost in tamponade:
(a) Hypovolemia (b) LV dysfunction
(c) AR (d) Obesity

1054. PHT defined as pressure more than:
(a) 20 (b) 25
(c) 30 (d) 35

1055. EMF true:
(a) Common in south America and mediterranean
(b) Biopsy show eosinophilia
(c) Removal of fibrous wall and replacement of valves is standard treatment

1056. Lower right 10 intercostal vein drain into:
(a) Azygous (b) Hemizygous

1057. Orthodeoxia platypnea syndrome A/W A/E:
(a) PFO (b) Cirrhosis of liver
(c) Pulmonary AV fistula (d) LA myxoma

1058. All cause cardiomyopathy *except:*
(a) Lithium (b) Emetine
(c) Sulfonamide (d) Quinidine

1059. Vasopressin antagonist used in CHF:
(a) Tolvaptan (b) Omapralitat
(c) Moxonidine (d) Xenasentan

1060. Which is not true?
(a) PROMISE – milrinone ↑ mortality
(b) ATTACH – Vesarinone
(c) EARTH – darusentan
(d) EVEREST – tolvaptan

1061. Nesiritide A/E in CHF:
(a) More renal failure – more mortality
(b) VPC more than dobutamine
(c) More mortality compared to others
(d) ↓ PCWP more than NTG

1062. Maternal mortality 25-50% A/E:
(a) PPH
(b) MS with NYHA III
(c) Complicated CoA
(d) Marfan with aortic involvement

1063. NYHA II can do A/E:
(a) Roller skate (b) Sex without stopping
(c) Golf (d) Walking 5 mile/hr

1064. Mortality benefit proven:
(a) CRT with LVEF < 35%, class III NYHA
(b) Amiodarone with LVEF < 35%
(c) Angiography in CSA
(d) DDD in HOCM

1065. RVEF best by:
(a) First pass radionuclide angiography
(b) Equilibrium ventriculography

(c) Thermodilution
(d) Equilibrium radionuclide angiography

1066. All are mechanical valve A/E:
(a) Omniscience (b) Carpentier Edwards
(c) St. Jude (d) Medtronic valve

1067. MDM rumble in A/E:
(a) VSD without PAH
(b) ASD without PAH
(c) Moderate MR (III)
(d) Moderate PDA without PAH

1068. Long RP—short PR A/E:
(a) SNRT (b) PJRT
(c) Atrial tachycardia (d) AVNRT

1069. a = v in PCWP A/E:
(a) Constrictive pericarditis
(b) Cardiac tamponade
(c) MVP with MR
(d) Hypervolumia

1070. Prominent y descent seen A/E:
(a) Tamponade (b) CCP
(c) Restrictive CMP (d) TR

1071. Mean pulmonary diastolic pressure > PCWP A/E:
(a) Pulmonary disease
(b) PVOD – pulmonary venoocclusive disease
(c) Pulmonary embolism
(d) Tachycardia

1072. Post capillary pulmonary hypertension A/E:
(a) Truncus Arteriosus without stenosis or regurgitation
(b) TAPVC – infracardiac with obstruction
(c) Supravalvular AS in child
(d) Acute MR

1073. Heart failure minor criteria A/E:
(a) Cardiomegaly (b) Pleural effusion
(c) Hepatomegaly (d) HR > 120

1074. Amyl nitrite *except:*
(a) Intensity of OS ↓ es (b) A2- OS ↓ es
(c) S1 augmentation (d) A2 diminished

1075. Athlete's heart A/E:
(a) Symmetric hypertrophy
(b) Normal tissue Doppler velocity
(c) ↑ ed LV dimensions
(d) Grade I diastolic dysfunction

1076. Pulsus bisferiens:
(a) AS with LV dysfunction
(b) AR
(c) AS with AR
(d) Hyperkinetic circulatory state

1077. Murmur of HOCM ↑ ed by A/E:
(a) Squatting (b) Valsalva III
(c) Amyl nitrate (d) Isoproterenol

1078. S1 soft by A/E:
(a) Acute AR (b) RBBB
(c) PR > 120 msec (d) Severe MR

1079. PR > 0.2 secs, character of S_1:
(a) Soft S_1 (b) Loud S_1
(c) Normal split (d) Normal S_1

1080. All true *except:*
(a) A_2 – OS = 0.04 – 0.12
(b) Pericardial knock high pitched duration = 0.10 – 0.12 msec
(c) S4 high pitched seen in presystolic phase during ventricular filling
(d) S3 occurs in 0.12 – 0.16 msec after A2

1081. NYHA A/E:
(a) Dyspnea (b) Restlessness
(c) Angina (d) Palpitation

1082. Dip and plateau diastolic waveform occur in all the following condition *except:*
(a) Constrictive cardiomyopathy
(b) Restrictive cardiomyopathy
(c) RV ischemia
(d) Cardiac tamponade

1083. The following statement of less than ordinary activity causes symptoms in New York Heat Association Functional Classification falls into which class?
(a) NYHA 1 (b) NYHA 2
(c) NYHA 3 (d) NYHA 4

1084. Which of the following murmur is likely to be benign?
(a) Midsystolic (b) Loud systolic
(c) Holosystolic (d) Late systolic

1085. The abdominojugular reflex is used in predicting a pulmonary artery wedge pressure in excess of .... mm Hg in patients with heart failure.

(a) 5 mm Hg (b) 10 mm Hg
(c) 15 mm Hg (d) 20 mm Hg

1086. Statements are true regarding A wave in JVP:

(a) Cannon a wave occurs with atrioventricular dissociation
(b) Cannon wave during tachycardia identifies the rhythm as PSVT
(c) A wave is present with atrial fibrillation
(d) Cannon a wave occurs with sinus tachycardia

1087. Reversed or paradoxical splitting does not occurs in:

(a) Sever Aortic stenosis
(b) Right ventricular pacing
(c) Left bundle branch block
(d) Right bundle branch block

1088. Intensity of the following murmur decreases with hand grip exercise:

(a) Mitral regurgitation
(b) Ventricular septal defect
(c) Aortic regurgitation
(d) None of the above

1089. Following statement is false regarding Brockenbrough Braunwald sign:

(a) Seen in hypertrophic obstructive cardiomyopathy
(b) Seen in aortic stenosis
(c) Following a premature ventricular contraction, there is an increase in the left ventricular-aorta pressure gradient with simultaneous decrease in the aortic pulse pressure
(d) This phenomenon is elicited by delivering premature ventricular contraction beat in left ventricle

1090. Which of the following statement is true regarding chronic constrictive pericaditis?

(a) Marked increase in right ventricular systolic pressures usually more than 60 mm Hg
(b) A separation of the left and right ventricular diastolic filling pressures by > 5 mm Hg
(c) Concordant changes in left and right ventricular diastolic filling pressures with inspiration (Both increase)
(d) Discordant pressure changes in the right and left ventricles with inspiration (right ventricular systolic pressure increases while left ventricular systolic pressure decreases

1091. Which of the following finding has the highest positive predictive value in diagnosis of elevated filling pressure in patients with heart failure?

(a) Rales over more than 1/3 lung field
(b) Third heat sound
(c) Orthopnea
(d) Ascites (moderate to massive)

1092. Which of the following ionotropic agent does not have ionotropic effect?

(a) Milrinone (b) Enoximone
(c) Levosimendan (d) Nesiritide

1093. Which is not a Major Criteria in Framingham criteria for diagnosis of heart failure?

(a) PND (b) Hepatomegaly
(c) Cardiomegaly (d) Hepatojugular reflux

1094. The appropriately arranged timing sequence is:

1. Pericardial knock, 2. Tumor plop, 3. Opening snap, 4. Physiological S3, 5. Pathological S3

(a) 1,2,3,4,5 (b) 1,3,2,5,4
(c) 3,1,2,5,4 (d) 3,1,2,4,5

1095. Prominent X decent in JVP is not seen in following condition:

(a) Constrictive pericarditis
(b) Cardiac tamponade
(c) ASD
(d) TR

1096. "Square wave" arterial pressure response to vaisalva maneuvers is seen in all *except:*

(a) ASD (b) VSD
(c) MS (d) Heart failure

1097. All are true about Hangout interval *except:*

(a) Decreased by increased capacitance and decreased impedence
(b) Ventricular mechanical systole is the sum of isovolumic contraction plus the ejection period minus the hangout interval
(c) Increased hangout interval is directly proportional to the S_2 spilt duration
(d) It is about 15 ms for systemic circulation and 43-86 ms for pulmonary circulation

1098. All are true about S_2 split *except:*

(a) Type I and II S2 split can be identified bedside
(b) Paradoxical split seen in severe AS with LV dysfunction
(c) Cased due to early pulmonic valve closure or delayed aortic valve closure
(d) Valsalva maneuver in reversed 52 split patients, results in widening of 52 split in strain phase

1099. Characteristics of S3 are all *except:*

(a) Non location
(b) Low frequency
(c) Heard best with the bell of the stethoscope
(d) Augmented by maneuvers which increase blood flow into the ventricle

1100. Transient occlusion of both brachial arteries augments the murmurs of all *except:*

(a) MR (b) VSD
(c) PR (d) AR

1101. HCM: (T/F)

(a) AD
(b) 50% associated with atherosclerosis
(c) Brocken Borough phenomenon in ECHO
(d) Increases SCD

1102. HCM: (T/F)

(a) With alcohol/large meal– decreases gradient
(b) Dual chamber pacing effective in those not taking β blockers
(c) BB improves symptoms
(d) Family screening after age of 21

1103. Cardiac tumour in children: (T/F)

(a) Myxoma (b) Teratoma
(c) Fibroma (d) Rhabdomyoma

1104. Cardiac cells: (T/F)

(a) Purkinje cells are shortest
(b) T tubules max in Purkinje fibres
(c) Atrial myocyte conduct end to end
(d) Collagen max in atrial myocyte
(e) Mitochondria/sarcomere are max in Purkinje fibres

1105. Stem cell: (T/F)

(a) Hemopoietic stem cell causes thalassemia
(b) MSC causes immunosuppression
(c) Hemopoietic stem cell– pluripotent cell
(d) MSC – improves function in heart failure
(e) MSC has HLA barrier

1106. Heart transplant: (T/F)

(a) Cadaveric better than live
(b) CMV infection in < 1 month

1107. PPH: (T/F)

(a) < 50% has RVH
(b) WHO classification for functional assessment
(c) 6 min walk test has prognostic significance
(d) Max medical management with syncope– improvement with atrial septotomy
(e) Mean PAP > 50 mm Hg at rest, > 60 mm Hg with exercise

1108. Elderly: (T/F)

(a) Parasympathetic increases heart rate
(b) Dcreases collagen ratio III/I
(c) Decreases pulse wave velocity
(d) Aortic augmentation index decreases despite increases in pulse pressure

1109. Catheterization: (T/F)

(a) Pig tail catheter— both side and end hole
(b) Angio by Bermen used for RVOT obstruction
(c) Limb ischemic is limitation for transradial approach

1110. Lung zone: (T/F)

(a) Alveolar pressure > PAP in apex
(b) Pulmonary venous pressure > PAP at base
(c) PVP > PAP in mid zone
(d) Alveolar pressure < venous pressure at base

1111. S2 Split: (T/F)

(a) Wide/variable in WPW B
(b) Wide variable in VVIR
(c) Large PDA > 2:1, reverse splitting
(d) Chronic severe AR– reverse splitting
(e) Eisenmenger–single S2 due to simultaneous A2 and P2

1112. Conduction system: (T/F)

(a) Posteroinferior border of Koch triangle formed by septal tricuspid annulus
(b) Atrial myocytes shorter and broad
(c) Purkinje–shortest

1113. Cardiac tamponade: (T/F)

(a) Low pressure tamponade-hypotension

(b) RA collapse most sensitive, RV collapse specific

(c) Electrical alternans more sensitive but less specific

(d) Square root sign present

1114. JVP: (T/F)

(a) Pulsus paradoxus > 10 mm Hg decrease SBP

(b) A wave after S1

(c) V wave after S2

(d) BP cuff width > 60% of arm

1115. Acid base balance: (T/F)

(a) Decrease HCO_3 leads to decrease pH

(b) Decrease pH compensation by kidneys by retaining HCO_3

(c) Muscle spasm and tetany due to resp. acidosis

(d) Respiratory compensation starts within 1-3 hours

(e) Excess heparin decreases HCO_3 and $paCO_2$ during sample collection

1116. Receptors in HF: (T/F)

(a) b1/b2 decreases

(b) b1 decreases and b2 same

(c) Protein G decreases, b1 decrease, b2 decrease

(d) NE increases in myocardium

(e) NE increase in peripestroy

1117. Isovolumic phase related to: (T/F)

(a) DP/DT (b) V max

(c) IVRT (d) VCF

(e) VPM

1118. HOCM: (T/F)

(a) Autosomal dominant

(b) Most common mutation – trop t

(c) LVOT obst. Related to SCD

(d) LV mass is invariably increased

(e) Microvascular abnormality more common at autopsy

1119. Titin: (T/F)

(a) Attaches actin to M line

(b) Thick and short provide strength

(c) Largest protein discovery

(d) Provide elasticity

(e) Transmits mechanical signal to growth stimuli

1120. LA function: (T/F)

(a) As a reservoir

(b) Contractile chamber

(c) As a conduit

(d) Part of bainbridge reflex

(e) Volume sensor

1121. Discrepancy between PCWP and LVEDP: (T/F)

(a) Pulm. venous stenosis

(b) Submitral aneurysm

(c) Cortriatriatum

(d) Parachute mitral valve

(e) PAH

1122. PPCM: (T/F)

(a) Chimerism is a mechanisms

(b) 3 months before delivery and 12 months after delivery

(c) Beta blocker should not be used

(d) Multiparity is not a risk factor

(e) Delayed enhancement in MRI is a reliable diagnostic feature

1123. True or false:

(a) LV rapid filling period –60%

(b) Diastasis < 5%

(c) Isovolumic relaxation–mitral valve opening

(d) Isovolumic relaxation–mitral valve closure and Aortic valve opening

(e) Increase phosphocreatine/ATP ratio in HF

1124. True or false:

(a) Spironolactone increase fibrosis

(b) Carvedilol – vasodilator

1125. HF: (T/F)

(a) Increased sympathetic activity without decrease in parasympathetic activity

(b) Decreased AT-1

(c) Increased AT-1/AT-2 ratio

(d) AT-II increases aldosterone

(e) AT-II causes vasoconstriction

1126. True or false:

(a) Anrep effect–increase HR causes increased contractility

(b) Branham effect–slowing of pulse rate on compression of AV fistula

(c) Brockenbrough–loss of pulse in AV fistula

(d) Aortic recoil–wind kessel effect

(e) Impedence–pressure/flow

1127. HF: (T/F)

(a) Troponin T and I act independent of Ca for interaction of actin and myosin
(b) Inhibition of NE reuptake
(c) NE depleted in advanced HF
(d) Symptoms occur early
(e) RAS activation occur late

1128. True or false:

(a) HOCM – beta myosin mutation
(b) DCMP– AD
(c) LAMB – danon

1129. BP: (T/F)

(a) Cuff width 40% of arm circumference (b) Phase IV korotokoff sounds in AR taken as DBP
(c) Grading of pulsus alternans by sphygmanometer

1130. DCMP: (T/F)

(a) Male poor prognosis
(b) First and degree AV block poor prognosis
(c) EF inversely related to SCD
(d) Pulmonary artery DBP is atleast 1/3rd of PA SBP

1131. Pulsus paradoxus: (T/F)

(a) Severe pulmonary embolism
(b) LVF (c) RCMP
(d) CCP (e) Anemia

1132. Seen in heart failure patient A/E:

(a) Decreased ryanodine
(b) Increased SERCA
(c) Decreased Beta1 receptor
(d) Decreased cardiac capillary

1133. True/false:

(a) Hepatojugular reflux–major criteria
(b) HR > 120/min minor criteria
(c) JVP < 3 cm in Normal person
(d) Remain elevated for < 15 sec in RVF
(e) Rapid y descent is seen myocardial involvement of all cases

1134. PCWP mismatch with LVEDP: (T/F)

(a) Pulmonary vein stenosis
(b) Cortriatriatum
(c) Parachute mitral valve
(d) PAH
(e) Submitral aneurysm

1135. Endothelium: (T/F)

(a) Endothelin potent vasodilator
(b) No endothelium dependent
(c) Adenosine – NO independent
(d) Nitrate – can dilate damaged vessel
(e) Healthy endothelium required for NO for vasodilation

1136. Intensity S1 ↓ in: (T/F)

(a) Short PR
(b) Premature closure
(c) ↓ Mobility of valve
(d) ↑ Flow through MV
(e) ↑ dp/dt

1137. HOCM: (T/F)

(a) LV wall thickness – SCD
(b) Moderate to severe MR suggest other pathology (other than SAM)
(c) LV involvement in > 80% cases
(d) Fabry's X linked recessive

1138. T/F:

(a) Anrep effect— ↑ contractility with ↑ HR
(b) Treppe phenomenon– ↓ inotropic with ↑ Aortic impedence
(c) AO impedence = pressure/flow

1139. PVR: (T/F)

(a) SVR/PVR ratio of 2
(b) ↑ with hypoxia
(c) Represents drop of pressure across pulmonary arteriolar and capillary
(d) Total PVR = 80 – mean Ao
(e) Assessed by pulmonary pressure/flow

1140. Clinical examination: (T/F)

(a) Carotid pulse synchronise with apex beat
(b) Common cause of supraclavicular pulsation is kinking and tortuosity of Right carotid artery
(c) Double apex due to a wave
(d) Hyperkinetic apex due to reduced LV fraction
(e) Absence of pericardium or abnormal bony cavity – shift apex to left

1141. Pulmonary valvuloplasty: (T/F)

(a) Restenosis following it is unknown
(b) Should be done in asymptomatic patient with gradient > 40 mmHg
(c) Isolated PS in Noonan's syndrome it should not be done

(d) Gradient ↑ after valvuloplasty
(e) Contraindicated if severe cyanosis at rest

1142. T/F:

(a) Laplace law-stress directly proportional to thickness
(b) Inversely proportional to radius

1143. Acute HF: (T/F)

(a) Severe hyponatremia occurs in 25-30%
(b) ↑ BUN is poor prognostic
(c) Target PCWP < 16

1144. All are vasodilators: (T/F)

(a) Renin (b) ADH
(c) PGE2 (d) Endothelin
(e) Natriuretic peptide

1145. Cardiorenal syndrome: (T/F)

(a) Medical treatment may worsen renal function
(b) Renovascular abnormality is a common cause
(c) GFR < 60 ml/min – worse prognosis
(d) Vasopressin antagonist useful
(e) Ultra filtration useful in beneficial without neuro-hormonal effect

1146. BNP: (T/F)

(a) ↑ se in obese (b) ↓ se in female

1147. HF n EF: (T/F)

(a) Criteria > 40 EF
(b) BNP > 100 is cutoff
(c) BNP guided therapy – ↓ses mortality

1148. PPH: (T/F)

(a) CCB-DOC
(b) Endothelin antagonist – useful
(c) Prostaglandin – useful for grade IV
(d) Sildenafil – ↑ 6 min walk test
(e) Balloon atrial septostomy ↑ ses saturation

1149. NYHA class: (T/F)

(a) Less than ordinary – class II
(b) CCS more specific than NYHA
(c) Goldmann scale includes ECG
(d) Specific Activity > 2 MET is class II
(e) Califf angina scoring include tempo of angina and CCF

1150. T/F:

(a) VCAM, ICAM secreted by vessel wall
(b) HDL inhibits LDL oxidation
(c) Interleukins are secreted by a number of sources
(d) LDL oxidation occurs in vessel wall

1151. HF n/EF: (T/F)

(a) Irbesartan has mortality benefit
(b) BNP is raised both in systolic and diastolic HF
(c) Less mortality in HR normal EF
(d) More in young female

1152. Acute HF: (T/F)

(a) Sudden ↑ se in afterload does not ↓ se EF in Normal person
(b) LVEF <45% is indicator of LV dysfunction independent of loading condition
(c) ESV not dependent on preload condition
(d) VCF independent of afterload
(e) ESPVR is most reliable indicator of contractility

1153. NT Pro BNP: (T/F)

(a) Renal clearance
(b) T1/2 less than BNP
(c) BNP secreted from myocardium
(d) Pleotrophic effect
(e) Causes natriuresis, decreases renin and aldosterone

1154. Oximetry run: (T/F)

(a) > 8% step up in RA should be investigated
(b) Indocyanine dye more sensitive than oximetry
(c) Variation less in RA than any other chamber
(d) If Qp/Qs < 1.5, oximetry not beneficial
(e) In TOF negative Qp/Qs ratio

1155. Constrictive pericarditis: (T/F)

(a) X is more prominent than y wave
(b) Tricuspid valve respiratory flow changes is diagnostic
(c) Pericardiectomy is a closed procedure
(d) Filling unimpeded in late diastole
(e) Pulmonary artery banding is an open procedure

1156. Anemia with HF: (T/F)

(a) Anemia increases mortality and morbidity of CHF
(b) Cause diastolic dysfunction
(c) Prosthetic valve can cause anemia

1157. Exercise during rehabilitation: (T/F)
(a) Decreases EF
(b) Increased peak O_2
(c) Increased epinephrine levels
(d) Increased end diastolic volume

1158. T/F:
(a) Preserved flow – stunning
(b) ↑ lactate in hibernation
(c) Inotropes temporary ↑ ed contraction in hibernation
(d) Stunning may take 10 days to weeks to recover
(e) Myocardial stunning Normal lactate

1159. CHF: (T/F)
(a) ↓ B1 and B2 Receptors both primarily
(b) Spironolactone is class I indication in CHF
(c) In neonates profuse diaphoresis is S/O CHF
(d) Digitalis ↓ es mortality in CHF
(e) Cheyne-Stokes breathings is due to prolonged circulation

1160. T/F:
(a) 50% diameter stenosis – 70% ↓ in stenotic area
(b) EDV Normal is 150 ml/m²
(c) LV output > RV output
(d) SV is 75% of EDV
(e) LAO cranial view visualization of cardiac chambers without superimposition

1161. Endothelial dependent vasodilatation: (T/F)
(a) NO (b) NTG
(c) Verapamil (d) Adenosine
(e) Serotonin

1162. Vasopressin V/S dopamine in cardiac arrest – vasopressin is superior because of: (T/F)
(a) Vasopressin induced bradycardia causes reflex vasoconstriction
(b) Cerebral blood flow pressured
(c) Dopamine is less chromotropic and inotropic
(d) Cerebral V2 receptor causes vasodilation
(e) Vasopressin causes vasoconstriction and dopamine vasodilation

1163. Cardiac tamponade with absent paradoxical pulse: (T/F)
(a) Rh spondylitis (b) AR
(c) Large PDA (d) CCP
(e) OS-ASD

1164. CCP V/S RCMP favoring CCP: (T/F)
(a) Prominent y descent
(b) PASP > 50 mm Hg
(c) Intervent interdependence
(d) EDP equal RV/LV
(e) Pulsus paradoxus

1165. True or false:
(a) ↑ LV dimension ↑ es afterload
(b) EDP is directly assessed by end diastolic fiber length
(c) In isolated PS – RV curve is trapezoid

1166. Reverse split of S1: (T/F)
(a) LV pacing (b) Severe MS
(c) LBBB (d) LA myxoma
(e) Ebstein's anomaly

1167. A2 – OS gap: (T/F)
(a) Increase in bradycardia
(b) Increase in LV dysfunction
(c) Increase in AR
(d) Systemic HTN
(e) Calcified MV

1168. Loud S1: (T/F)
(a) Atrial myxoma (b) WPW
(c) Ebstein's anomaly (d) Long PR interval

1169. S3 haemodynamically influenced by: (T/F)
(a) Atrial compliance
(b) Ventricular relaxation
(c) End systolic ventricular volume
(d) Thoracic architecture
(e) Rate of ventricular contraction

1170. Paradoxical movement of septum: (T/F)
(a) RBBB
(b) TR
(c) Congenital absence of pericardium
(d) PR
(e) Post CABG

1171. First heart sound: (T/F)
(a) Muffled in AR
(b) Muffled in Ebstein's anomaly
(c) Gastric distension and pneumothorax decreases S1
(d) S1 split best heard at apex

1172. Pulsus paradoxus commonly seen in: (T/F)
(a) Tamponade (b) Hypovolemia
(c) CCP (d) RCMP
(e) RVMI

1173. Pulmonary AV fistula: (T/F)
(a) Affects lower lobe
(b) Cyanosis with mild dyspnea
(c) Will not be pick up by contrast echo
(d) Decreased by Muller's maneuver

1174. AT-II: (T/F)
(a) Vasoconstrictor
(b) Increased renin
(c) Increased aldosterone
(d) Decreased K excretion
(e) Increase Na loss

1175. Endothelial dysfunction: (T/F)
(a) ET vasoconstriction
(b) Ach vasoconstriction
(c) NO increased activity
(d) Atherosclerosis
(e) Acute coronary event

1176. ANP: (T/F)
(a) ANP and CNP released from atrium normally
(b) ANP increases renin level
(c) Increased contractility causes increased ANP
(d) Ventricular hypertrophy and dysfunction release ANP and BNP
(e) ANP release in response to hypotension

1177. ANP: (T/F)
(a) ANP antimitotic and vasodilatory
(b) Inhibit vasopressin
(c) Inhibit aldosterone
(d) In severe LV dysfunction can be released from atria and ventricles

1178. HOCM: (T/F)
(a) Post extrasystolic beat decreases pulse pressure
(b) Post extrasystolic beat decreases LV systolic pressure
(c) Squatting decreases gradient
(d) Gradient maximum in late systole
(e) Spike and dome appearance in aortic pressure waveform

1179. Squatting: (T/F)
(a) Increases venous return
(b) Causes reflex bradycardia
(c) Decreases arterial pressure
(d) Increases stroke volume
(e) Decreases peripheral resistance

1180. ACE-I and Beta blocker in HF: (T/F)
(a) Both decreases mortality even without decreasing symptoms
(b) Both synergistic
(c) ACE–I is better than ARB
(d) ACE–I does not have effect on ventricular arrhythmias
(e) ACE-I have proved antiarrhythmic effect

1181. Events in cardiac cycle: (T/F)
(a) AV open before PV
(b) TV opens before MV
(c) AV closes before PV
(d) TV closes before MV
(e) S1 just after palpable carotid upstroke

1182. Cath data: RA = 12 mm Hg, RV = 102/12 mm Hg, PA mean = 60 mm Hg (90/48), PCWP= 14 mm Hg, CI = 2 l/m²/min: (T/F)
(a) Patient in CHF
(b) Suggestive of PPH
(c) Significant pulmonary congestion
(d) Transpulmonary gradient = 12
(e) PVR > 18 wood units

1183. Measurement of CO: (T/F)
(a) LV angiography
(b) Thermodilution
(c) MUGA
(d) Thallium scintigraphy

1184. JVP: (T/F)
(a) A wave negative in atrial flutter
(b) X descent absent in tamponade
(c) PCWP is not equal to LVEDP in pulmonary venous congestion

1185. Oxygen consumption: (T/F)
(a) Resting O_2 consumption = 20 ml/ 100 gm/min
(b) Wall tension is major determinant
(c) Electrical activity consumes < 1%
(d) At maximum exercise, 30% increase in O_2 extraction only
(e) Minimal O_2 consumption before onset of contraction and relaxation

1186. Endothelium: (T/F)

(a) EDRF production (b) VWF
(c) Plasminogen (d) Prostacyclin
(e) Endothelin production

1187. Pulmonary HTN in left to right shunt: (T/F)

(a) Decreases vasodilators production
(b) 25% pulmonary bed obstruction required for Pulmonary HTN
(c) Alveolar hypoventilation without parenchymal disease causes PAH
(d) Increased CO_2 in alveoli decreases it
(e) Hypoxemia increases it

1188. Precordial examination: (T/F)

(a) Double impulse is almost always due to outward systolic and palpable movement
(b) Right supraclavicular is most common due to kinked and tortuous right carotid artery
(c) Apical impulse and carotid pulse are asynchronous
(d) Hyperkinetic impulse is associated with LVF
(e) Lateral to MCL palpable in absent pericardium and thoracic deformity

1189. Increase in murmur in HOCM: (T/F)

(a) Increases with preload
(b) Increase in contraction
(c) Decrease in LV volume
(d) Increase in HR
(e) Increase in afterload

1190. HOCM cath: (T/F)

(a) Apical pressure increases and normal outflow and inflow gradient
(b) Apical and inflow increases and outflow decreases
(c) Entrapment increases apical pressure
(d) Apical HOCM may be associated normal gradient

1191. In HF: T/F

(a) Decrease sympathetic activity
(b) Decrease adrenal medulla activity
(c) Down regulation of beat receptors
(d) Serum NE level and correlates with hemodynamic
(e) Increased central sympathetic flow

1192. T/F:

(a) Bernheim effect in HOCM
(b) Friedreich's sign in CCP
(c) Prominent y in Tamponade
(d) Persistent HJR indicates RV non compliance

1193. Angiotensin II causes: (T/F)

(a) Increased monocyte
(b) LVH
(c) Vasodilatation
(d) TNF– α increases
(e) Decreased sympathetic activity

1194. JVP: (T/F)

(a) A wave just after S1
(b) X wave between S3 and S4
(c) V wave after S2
(d) Y wave in late systole
(e) HJR persist increased shows decreased LV Compliance

1195. Pulmonary HTN: (T/F)

(a) Obliterates bronchiolitis is most common in post lung transplantation

1196. True or false:

(a) DBP increases upto 50 years then decreases
(b) Pulse pressure not important for prognosis in elderly
(c) SBP > 60 years in more than 60%
(d) Combination therapy is given if > 20/10 above normal
(e) SBP is more important than DBP

1197. Bisferien's pulse: (T/F)

(a) Double peak within systole with mid systolic dip
(b) Not seen in hyperkinetic state
(c) Dicrotic pulse–one peak in systole and 2nd in diastole with diastolic peak not seen when SBP > 130
(d) Pulsus athernans ↓ by NTG and head tilt
(e) Pulsus paradoxus because of ↑ LV stroke volume

1198. Squatting: (T/F)

(a) ↑ MR by ↑ SVR
(b) Lateral recumbency ↑ RVS3 and RVS4
(c) Amylnitrate ↑ A2 and ↓ P2
(d) Isometric handgrip ↑ es SVR and HR
(e) Isometric handgrip ↓ LVS3 and LVS4

1199. Flosequinan:

(a) Positive chronotrope
(b) Positive Ionotrope
(c) Vasoconstrictor
(d) Proved beneficial in HF
(e) First trial

1200. True or false:

(a) Effective pulmonary blood flow – adequate flow across pulmonary capillaries

(b) Thermodilution calculates cardiac output in Right sided regurgitation lesion

(c) Fick's method calculates cardiac output in rapid changes in blood flow

(d) Thermodilution Method overestimates cardiac output in low CO state

1201. Tachycardia and hypotension with NTG because of: (T/F)

(a) Direct CNS effect

(b) Effect on atrial myocyte cell

(c) Baroreceptor reflex

(d) Effect on sinoatrial node

(e) Direct chronotropic

1202. AT-I and AT-II receptor: (T/F)

(a) AT- I causes vasodilatation

(b) AT- II ↑ smooth muscle

(c) AT-I decreases Na Reabsorption

(d) In stress injury AT-II ↑ ed

(e) AT-II antigrowth

(f) AT-I endothelial dysfunction

1203. Acquired coronary AV fistula: (T/F)

(a) Kawasaki's disease

(b) Mycotic aneurysm

(c) Ablation of accessory pathway

(d) Mural thrombus

(e) Restrictive CMP

1204. Echo features of CCP: (T/F)

(a) Septal bounce

(b) Diastolic septal shudder

(c) ↑ PV flow in diastole

(d) MV respiratory variation (> 25%)

(e) Hepatic vein flow diastolic > systolic

1205. Cardiac tamponade echo: (T/F)

(a) Early RV diastolic collapse more specific

(b) IVC diameter > 2.2 cm

(c) Forward pulmonary vein flow increased

(d) LV free wall paradoxical motion

(e) LV stroke volume increases on inspiration

1206. Endothelin: (T/F)

(a) 3 types of ET- 1,2 and 3

(b) Most potent vasoconstrictor

(c) ET coverting enzyme converts ET-1 to ET-3

(d) ET causes Na and water retention

(e) ET causes VT more frequently

1207. ET antagonist: (T/F)

(a) Bosentan, darusentan, erbesentan

(b) Act on ETA and ETB receptor

(c) Helpful in CCF

(d) Reduces mortality in CHF

(e) Increased survival HF

(f) Improves hemodynamics

1208. BNP: (T/F)

(a) Marker of CHF

(b) Associated with ↑ ed mortality

(c) ↑ es urine output

(d) ↓ es Na reabsorption

(e) Reduces aldosterone antagonism

1209. Beta Receptor: (T/F)

(a) B2 Receptor – 20% in LV

(b) B1 receptor – 20% in LV

(c) B1 > B2 (isoprenaline > NE > Epinephrine)

(d) B2 > B1 in HF

(e) B2 = Epinephrine > NE > Isoprenaline

1210. LV valves: (T/F)

(a) LVEDV – 85 ml/m²

(b) LV mass – 175 mg/m²

(c) dp/dt – 1650 mmHg/sec

(d) Angiographic SV = 3.3 × EDV/S

(e) LV stroke work = 50

(f) 1 mg of Hb = 1.36 ml of O_2

1211. Valsalva: (T/F)

(a) Normal arterial waveform is sinusoidal

(b) CHF – Square response

(c) Overshoot not in CHF

(d) Overshoot causes augmentation of left sided murmur

(e) Intrathoracic pressure and venous pressure ↓ es phase 2

1212. T/F:

(a) AC wave interval ↓ es in first degree AV block

(b) Kussmaul's sign indicates increase pressure in JVP during inspiration

(c) X descent > y in CCP
(d) Large positive systolic venous pulsation in severe CCF
(e) Regular cannon wave in junctional rhythm
(f) Squatting causes reflex tachycardia and increased SVR
(g) Amyl nitrate increases A2 and decreases S2 sound

1213. Athlete's heart: (T/F)
(a) Morphological P wave changes
(b) Sinus pauses
(c) Mobity type 1 seen
(d) T wave change
(e) Prominent Q wave in anterior leads

1214. Reversible CMP: (T/F)
(a) Early alcoholic CMP
(b) Lymphocytic myocarditis
(c) Sarcoidosis
(d) Tachycardia
(e) EMF

1215. Free radical scavengers: (T/F)
(a) Repairs endothelium
(b) Prevents incorporation of oxidized LDL into atheromatous plaque
(c) Platelets adhesion
(d) Prevents progression of atherosclerosis
(e) Increases availability of adenosine

1216. Endomyocardial biopsy: (T/F)
(a) Hyperchromatic irregular nuclei in HOCM
(b) Large mitochondria with myelin body with vacuolated cytoplasm in doxorubicin toxicity
(c) Contraction band in ischemic CMP
(d) Z-band in HOCM
(d) Chronic myocardial damage with bizarre shaped nuclei in chronic myocarditis
(e) Cellular disarray–DCMP

1217. Continuous murmur: (T/F)
(a) In truncus, continuous murmur is almost always due to pulmonary stenosis
(b) In pulmonary artery branch stenosis, continuous murmur is uncommon
(c) In ALCAPA, continuous murmur due to left heart to pulmonary artery
(d) In lutembacher syndrome, continous murmur due to continuous gradient across ASD through out cardiac cycle
(e) In RSOV, continuous murmur more in systole as compared to that in PDA

1218. Cyanosis associated with: (T/F)
(a) LSVC to coronary sinus
(b) Raglib syndrome
(c) Large Eustachian valve
(d) Multiple ASD at different location
(e) PAPVC

1219. ANP: (T/F)
(a) Released in hypotension
(b) In pathological state, release from both atria and ventricle
(c) Increased renin
(d) Increased vasopressin
(e) Decreased aldosterone

1220. True of false:
(a) α-1 receptor in presynaptic position
(b) α-2 receptor in peripheral nerve and brain
(c) β1 in bronchioles
(d) β1 stimulation decreases AV conduction
(e) Norepinephrine 2-4 times more in atria than ventricles
(f) D1 dopamine receptor in splanchic is vasodilator

1221. VEGF: (T/F)
(a) Has no role in PAD
(b) Has role in vascular graft patency
(c) Arteriogenesis is budding of new vessels from persisting capillaries
(d) Angiogenesis is formation of new vessel as in embryonic development

1222. A_2 – OS gap: (T/F)
(a) Increase in AR
(b) Increase in high systolic BP
(c) Decrease in calcific MS
(d) Increases in bradycardia
(e) Decreases in LV dysfunction

1223. RCMP: (T/F)
(a) Endomyocardial biopsy is specific for amyloidosis
(b) Commonly associated with systolic dysfunction and maximum filling in late diastole
(c) Dip and plateau in atrial pressure tracing
(d) Pulmonary artery pressure > 55 mm Hg

1224. Apoptosis: (T/F)
(a) Can cause cell swelling

(b) Does not need energy
(c) Occur in terminal cases of chronic HF
(d) Nuclear fragmentation occur
(e) Is programmed cell death

1225. True or false: (T/F)

(a) Calcium binds with troponin C
(b) Raymond's model, action occurs at base of head
(c) Neck is made up of 4 light chains

1226. Paradoxical septal motion: (T/F)

(a) RBBB (b) Severe TR
(c) Severe PR (d) Post CABG
(e) Congenital absence of pericardium

1227. True or false:

(a) Post extrasystolic potentiation is bowditch effect
(b) Increase in aortic pressure cause late rise in contractility is Anrep effect
(c) Increase force increases HR
(d) Increased EDV, increased contractility– Laplace's law
(e) Preload afterload mismatch common in CHF

1228. HRV: (T/F)

(a) Time and frequency domain analysis done
(b) Decreased HRV, 2-3 weeks after acute MI is common
(c) Decreased HRV, increased chance of SCD
(d) Decreased HRV predicts recurrent ischemia
(e) Does not enhance predictive accuracy of SCD

1229. Cardiac cycle: (T/F)

(a) Protodiastolic starts with incisura
(b) Rapid filling phase with AV opening
(c) Isovolumetric contraction after MV closure
(d) Isovolumic relaxation starts after AV closure

1230. Spironolactone: (T/F)

(a) Decreases fibrosis
(b) Aspirin antagonies diuretic effect of spironolactone
(c) Along with NSAID precipitate renal failure

1231. Exercise A/E:

(a) PR decreases (b) QRS decreases
(c) QT decreases (d) PR decreases

1232. Least beneficial in CHF:

(a) Bisoprolol (b) Carvedilol
(c) Metoprolol succinate (d) Nebivolol

1233. NSAID blunt minimally of which anti-hypertensive agent?

(a) Beta blocker (b) Diuretics
(c) CCB (d) α blocker

1234. Not in Framingham risk score:

(a) Family history (b) Age
(c) Smoking (d) Diabetic state

1235. Reserved oxygen extraction ratio is:

(a) 3 (b) 6
(c) 12 (d) 18

1236. CCP A/E:

(a) Mitral valve Ea > 7 m/s
(b) Increased hepatic vein diastolic flow reversal in inspiration
(c) Normal strain imaging of interventricular septum
(d) Respiratory variation in SVC < 20 cm/sec

1237. Short duration of LV compared to RV:

(a) Ejection time (b) IVCT
(c) IVRT (d) Systole

1238. Aorta= 116/80, velocity = 4 m/s, LV systolic pressure:

(a) 180 mm Hg (b) 186 mm Hg
(c) 190 mm Hg (d) 196 mm Hg

1239. Isovolumic relaxation of ventricle not seen in:

(a) LV to aorta tunnel
(b) PA to LA fistula
(c) Aortopulmonary window
(d) Mitral prosthetic valve dehiscence with perivalvular leak

1240. Myocardial O_2 demand not depend on:

(a) Inotropic state
(b) HR
(c) Myocardial wall tension
(d) Arterial O_2 tension

1241. I.V. furosemide not given > 40 mg/min to avoid:

(a) Precipitous hypotension
(b) Hypokalemia
(c) Ototoxicity
(d) Renal shutdown

1242. Primary pulmonary hypertension–WHO grading:

(a) Angina (b) Syncope
(c) Palpitation (d) Fatigue

1243. HOCM – Mutation in which LVH can occur after 50 years age?

(a) Beta-MHC (b) α-tropomyosin
(c) Cardiac α- actin (d) Cardiac troponin I
(e) Myosin binding protein C

1244. Early systolic murmur in A/E:

(a) Acute MR
(b) VSD with pulmonary HTN
(c) Normal pressure TR
(d) Small VSD (muscular)
(e) Subvalvular AS

1245. y descent absent in:

(a) Cardiac tamponade (b) CCP
(c) RCM (d) TR

1246. Best measure of LA compliance:

(a) PCWP mean (b) A wave
(c) V wave (d) LVEDP

1247. Adequacy of systemic oxygenation on cath. accurately accessed by:

(a) Systemic venous O_2 saturation
(b) Ao O_2 saturation
(c) Hb concentration
(d) Pulmonary vien O_2 saturation

1248. Biologically inactive:

(a) Angiotensin I (b) Angiotensin II
(c) Angiotensin IV (d) Renin

1249. Stem cell transplantation:

(a) Myoblast
(b) Peripheral blood derived endothelial stem cells
(c) Embryonic stem cells
(d) Bone marrow derived mononuclear cell

1250. Selective receptor antagonist act on CT leading to diuresis:

(a) Tolvalptan (b) Conivalptan
(c) Aliskerin (d) Nesiritide

1251. Cardiomyopathy:

(a) Trastuzumab (b) Daclizumab
(c) Baciliximab (d) Rituximab

1252. Low pressure Tamponade common cause:

(a) ASD (b) Effusive pericarditis
(c) Hemodialysis (d) Cardiac perforation

1253. Constant S1 intensity seen in:

(a) Isorrhythmic AV dissociation
(b) Type II mobitz second degree AV block
(c) First degree AV block
(d) Infrahisian CHB

1254. Hemocromatosis investigation of choice:

(a) MRI
(b) Multislice CT
(c) Radionuclide angiography
(d) 3D echo

1255. Dyssynchrony can be diagnosed by A/E:

(a) Colour Doppler (b) Pulse Doppler
(c) TDI (d) M mode echo

1256. Most common with PCWP is indicated by:

(a) Loud S1 (b) Loud OS
(c) Short A2 – OS (d) Mild MDM

1257. True about HF with normal EF:

(a) Prevalence increase with age
(b) HTN seen in 20-30%
(c) Males > females
(d) Mortality is more than LV dysfunction with reduced EF

1258. Bernoulli's equation Pressure–velocity relationship:

(a) P-4 times, V-2 times (b) P-6 times, V-2 times
(c) P-2 times, V-2 times (d) P-8 times, V-2 times

1259. Calcium handling kinetics–true is:

(a) ↑ cytosolic Ca phosphorylates phospholambna and inhibits SERCA leading to ↓ Ca uptake
(b) ↑ cytosolic Ca phosphorylates phospholamban an inhibits SERCA →↓ Ca
(c) Ryanodine receptor configuration change leads to ↑ Ca uptake
(d) L-type calcium current leads to a ryanodine receptor change

1260. Aortic $SO_{2\text{-}90\%}$, PA $SO_{2\text{-}58\%}$, CO-6 l/min, 70 kg-man, O_2 consumption-250 ml/min signifies:

(a) Normal (b) Moderate exercise
(c) Anemia (d) Systemic AV fistula

1261. Walking @ 2.6 kmph-O_2 consumption:

(a) 3-5 ml/kg/min (b) 10-15 ml/kg/min
(c) 15-20 ml/kg/min (d) 20-25 ml/kg/min

1262. Which is true? (T/F)

(a) Mitral inflow during IVRT is 7 cm/sec.

(b) Mitral inflow (early) DT is 50 mm/sec.
(c) Early mitral flow blood is 300 ml/sec.
(d) Isovolumetric relaxation period < 20 msec.
(e) All of the above

1263. ↑ v wave in PCWP seen in:
(a) MS (b) MR
(c) VSD (d) All of the above

1264. True is:
(a) a > v wave is LA pressure curve
(b) a = v wave is LA pressure curve
(c) v > a wave in RA pressure curve
(d) None of the above

1265. Pulsus alternans seen in:
(a) PTE
(b) Cardiac tamponade
(c) Dual AV node physiology
(d) TdP

1266. Harmonic imaging is:
(a) Transmitted frequency = Received frequency
(b) Transmitted frequency < Received frequency
(c) Transmitted frequency > Received frequency
(d) None

1267. Loud S_1 A/E:
(a) Long PR interval (b) LA myxoma
(c) MS (d) Holodiastolic MVP

1268. DP/DT of LV measured in:
(a) Isovolumic contraction
(b) Isovolumic relaxation
(c) Diastasis
(d) Systolic ejection phase

1269. Myocardial stunning true is A/E:
(a) Recovers spontaneously mostly
(b) Persists for hour to days
(c) ↓ energy metabolism with ↓ blood flow
(d) May be due to cytosolic Ca overload

1270. Peripartum CMP true is A/E:
(a) 1 month prepartum to 3 months postpartum
(b) Spontaneous recovery in 50-60% cases
(c) Recurrence may occur in future pregnancy
(d) Classically indistinguishable from DCM

1271. True in HOCM is A/E:
(a) Trop T mutation– being prognosis
(b) ↓ Systolic thickening of septum
(c) ↑ SAM → ↑LVOT obstruction
(d) Dyspnea most common symptom

1272. Brodie's effect:
(a) ↑ QRS amplitude (b) Change in QRS axis
(c) Reciprocal changes (d) Repolarization

1273. CCP–A/E:
(a) Square root sign in ventricular tracing
(b) Prominent y descent
(c) Exaggerated respiratory variation in mitral inflow
(d) PASP > 60 mm Hg

1274. CCP vs RCM:
(a) RVSP is higher commonly in RCM
(b) Absolute ventricular diastolic pressure > 25 mm Hg commonly in RCM
(c) Inspiratory reversal in CCP and expiratory reversal in RCM hepatic venous flow patterns
(d) Increased transmitral flow > 25% with respiration in CCP

1275. Dip and plateau A/E:
(a) RCMP (b) TR
(c) CCP (d) RVMI

1276. Indicator of adequate tissue perfusion:
(a) S. lactate level (b) Blood pressure
(c) Blood O_2 saturation (d) CO
(e) Interarterial monitoring

1277. Stage II CHF on digoxin, diuretic, ACE-I presents with edema, next treatment to be started:
(a) Spironolactone 25 mg OD
(b) Carvedilol 3.125 mg BD
(c) Metoprolol 50 mg BD
(d) Losartan 50 mg OD

1278. Stage II CHF on digoxin, ACE-I, diuretics, carvedilol presents with BP = 90/60 mm Hg, inotropes to be started:
(a) Intravenous dopamine
(b) Intravenous dobutamine
(c) Intravenous amrinone
(d) Intravenous epinephrine

1279. NCPF A/E:
(a) Liver nodule, fibrosis and span decreases
(b) Biopsy shows portal fibrosis
(c) Portal HTN
(d) Arsenic and vinyl chloride causes it

1280. Subaortic AS A/E:
(a) Ejection click
(b) AR
(c) Delayed carotid upstroke
(d) Paradoxical split S2

1281. Patient with BP–220/110 mm Hg with TIA with ST elevation V1–V4, treatment:
(a) Start NTG, control BP and reassess
(b) Start NTG + GP IIb, IIIa inhibitor
(c) Start NTG + thrombolytic
(d) Start NTG, control BP and PTCA

1282. WHO has classified pulmonary hypertension into how many groups?
(a) 2 (b) 3
(c) 4 (d) 5

1283. For measurement of PAWP where (west's zone) should be tip of catheter:
(a) Zone 1 (b) Zone 2
(c) Zone 3 (d) zone 4

1284. LV afterload is decreased in:
(a) VSD with high flow (b) Aortic stiffness
(c) Moderate AS (d) Systolic HTN

1285. Pulsus alternans best felt in:
(a) Carotid (b) Brachial
(c) Femoral (d) Radial

1286. Hyperkinetic pulse seen in A/E:
(a) Hypovolemia
(b) ↑ SVR
(c) Wide pulse pressure
(d) Increased left ventricular stroke volume

1287. Valsalva increases murmur of:
(a) HOCM (b) MS
(c) VSD (d) AS

1288. Tachycardia potential side effect with:
(a) β2 – agonists
(b) Antimuscarinics
(c) Steroids
(d) Leucotriene receptor antagonist

1289. At resting fasting state, fuel for heart:
(a) FFA (b) Glucose
(c) Ketone (d) Protein

1290. HCM most common gene mutation:
(a) β-MHC
(b) Troponin-I
(c) Alpha tropomyosin
(d) Essential myosin light chain

1291. Retrograde left heart catheterization was first done by:
(a) Mason Sones (b) Wermer Forsmann
(c) Henry Ziemmerman (d) Sven Seldinger

1292. All are characteristics of CCP *except:*
(a) Septal bounce
(b) Atrial enlargement
(c) Exaggerated respiratory variation in mitral flow
(d) ↓ tissue velocity

1293. Hemorrhagic myocarditis:
(a) Cisplatin (b) Busulfan
(c) Cyclophosphamide (d) Daunorubicin

1294. 1st day heart failure A/E:
(a) Muscular VSD (b) Myocarditis
(c) Congenital CHB (d) CoA

1295. 1st day HF A/E:
(a) Coarctation of aorta (b) CHB
(c) AV fistula (d) Muscular VSD

1296. Alcohol septal ablation C/I:
(a) LBBB (b) Syncope
(c) LVOT Gradient > 80 (d) SAM

1297. Diuretic resistance A/E:
(a) ↓ RA pressure
(b) NSAID
(c) Concomitant ACE inhibitors
(d) Severe hypokalemia

1298. Pulmonary artery hypertension is defined as when mean pulmonary artery presume is more than:

(a) 15 mm Hg (b) 20 mm Hg
(c) 25 mm Hg (d) 30 mm Hg

1299. A 26 years old male patient present with compliant of acute onset of pain in right lower limb 15 days back (pain of 2 hr duration). On physical examination all peripheral pulses are normal except Right Dorsal Pedis Artery. His BP – 110/70, pulse – 100/min, regular. So What will be the next management?

(a) I/V thrombolysis
(b) Intraarterial thrombolysis
(c) Anticoagulation
(d) Embolectomy

1300. Regarding peripartum CMP, which is true:

(a) Can occur years after delivery
(b) Half of the patient recover
(c) It is a idiosyncratic and occur with the same frequency as it in general population

1301. Pulsus paradoxus is found in:

(a) Cardiac tamponade (b) Restrictive CMP

1302. Regarding NYHA III which is true?

(a) No limitation of activity
(b) Mild limitation of activity
(c) Severe limitation of activity but not at rest
(d) Severe limitation of activity at rest

1303. NYHA-II definition:

(a) Depend on I (b) Depend on II
(c) Depend on III (d) Depend on IV

1304. Regarding cardiac tamponade which is not true?

(a) Bradycardia (b) Kussmaul sign
(c) Hypotension (d) Presence of early S3

1305. The pulmonary artery pressure is 90/40 mm Hg, so pulmonary HTN is:

(a) Mild PAH (b) Moderate PAH
(c) Severe PAH (d) Normal PAP

1306. The pulmonary capillary wedge pressure is normally equal to A/E:

(a) Mean LA pressure
(b) LVEDP
(c) Pulmonary diastolic pressure
(d) Intrapulmonary pressure

1307. Pulmonary venous hypertension is seen in A/E:

(a) Mitral stenosis (b) LVF
(c) Pulmonary embolism (d) DCM

1308. Regarding pulse which is true:

(a) Pulsus bigeminus is seen in HF
(b) Diastolic time indicates myocardial oxygen consumption
(c) Pulsus bisferiens is a benign condition
(d) Area under the pulse pressure curve denotes stroke volume

1309. Normal stroke volume is:

(a) 60-120 ml/beat (b) 120-180
(c) 180-220 (d) >220

1310. Normal RVSP is:

(a) 25-50 (b) 50-70
(c) 70-90 (d) 90-110

1311. Increased myocardial length causes increased contractility across in Frank starling law, the contractility is maximally depends on:

(a) End diastolic LV size

1312. Pulsus paradoxus indicates:

(a) Decrease in pulse volume with inspiration
(b) Decrease in CVP with inspiration
(c) Tachycardia with inspiration

1313. Brockenbrough sign seen in:

(a) HOCM (b) AS
(c) MS (d) MR

1314. Not used in persistent pulmonary hypertension of neoborn:

(a) Inhaled NO (b) ECMO
(c) Surfactant (d) Indomethacin

1315. Brockenbrough Braunwald phenomenon in HOCM classically indicated by:

(a) ↓ aortic systolic pr.
(b) ↓ aortic diastolic pr.
(c) ↓ aortic pulse pr.
(d) ↑ trans valvular gradients

1316. JVP A/E:

(a) Sharp x, prominent y–CCP
(b) Sharp x, blunted y–tamponade
(c) Regular cannon A S/o complete AV block

1317. Cause of pulsatile elevated JVP:
(a) Mediastinal irradiation
(b) RVMI
(c) Atrialized RV
(d) Liver cirrhosis

1318. In large scale trials, mortality benefit in CCF A/E:
(a) Atenolol
(b) Metoprolol
(c) Carvedilol
(d) Spironolactone

1319. Portion of descending aorta prox to ductus in fetus is known as:
(a) Aortic isthmus (b) Aorticsinus
(c) Aortic spindle (d) Stenosis

1320. HF with normal EF A/E:
(a) Almost 50% of all HF cases
(b) Mortality similar as HF with EF
(c) Vasodilation primary treatment and ↓ mortality
(d) Both systolic and diastolic stiffness

1321. HF treatment A/E:
(a) ↓ Afterload (b) ↑ Preload
(c) ↑ Contractility (d) ↓ Rate

1322. Fixed split S2 A/E:
(a) ASD (b) LBBB
(c) Severe PS (d) PTE

1323. Eye opening to painful stimuli, withdraws to pain, in comprehensive speech GCS:
(a) 5 (b) 8
(c) 7 (d) 6

1324. Brockenbrough Braunwald phenomenon in PVC characterised by:
(a) ↑ LVOT gradient
(b) ↓ Systolic BP in aorta
(c) ↓ Diastolic BP in aorta
(d) ↓ Pulse pressure in aorta

1325. Elderly pulse A/E:
(a) Reflected wave comes back late
(b) Velocity: 4–5 m/s
(c) Old age–20 m/s
(d) Central aorta pressure is more than peripheral pressure

1326. Eplerenone in DM, HTN albuminuria:
(a) Hyperkalemia
(b) Acute renal shutdown
(c) Poor glycemic control

1327. Cardiac cath: a=29, V = 27, mean 20 , RV = 54/21, PA 50/22 mean 30, PCWP 22, LV 110/21:
(a) CCP (b) Severe MS
(c) Severe PPH (d) Large ASD

1328. JVP 5 cm above angle of louis:
(a) 8 mm Hg (b) 6.8
(c) 13.6 (d) 15

1329. Cuff size BP width:
(a) 40% of arm circumference
(b) 80% of arm diameter
(c) 2/3 of arm length
(d) 1/3 of arm diameter

1330. CCP, pulmonary vein flow:
(a) Atrial reversal in insp
(b) Atrial reversal in exp
(c) Atrial reversal
(d) No atrial reversal

1331. Poop prog R wave A/E:
(a) NSTEMI (b) Sp. Pneumothorax
(c) CCP (d) Vertical heart

1332. Max filling in cardiac tamponade:
(a) Early diastole (b) Late diastole
(c) Systole (d) Sys + diast

1333. Not a diagnostic criteria of Marfan syndrome:
(a) Aortic dilatation
(b) PA dilatation
(c) MV calcification > 40 years age
(d) MVP

1334. Treatment not beneficial in survival in LV dysfunction:
(a) Nitrates + hydralazine
(b) Digoxin
(c) ACEI
(d) Spironolactone

1335. S_2 in RA pressure:
(a) Peak of V
(b) Just before peak of V
(c) C wave

1336. A/E about cardiac muscle cells:
(a) Present in A and V
(b) Present in epicardium
(c) SR in < skeletal muscle
(d) Gap junction is important for conduction

1337. Major Framingham criteria A/E:
(a) HJ reflux (b) Cardiomegaly
(c) Extremity edema (d) S3
(e) PND

1338. In MS cephalization is S/O:
(a) 12-15 (b) 15-18
(c) 18-20 (d) 20-24
(e) 28-32

1339. Most common testicular tumour in infants:
(a) Teratoma (b) Seminoma
(c) Embryonal cell (d) Yolk sac
(e) Mesothelial

1340. C wave coincides with:
(a) Atrial contraction (b) Buldge of TV in RA
(c) Systolic flow in IVC (d) Atrial relaxation
(e) Opening of TV

1341. Secondary prophylaxis for RF with carditis:
(a) 5 years or 18 years (b) 10 years or 21 years
(c) Life long (d) Till 40 years
(e) Not required

1342. Rosvastatin trial in normal lipids patients:
(a) Jupiter (b) Beautiful
(c) Accord (d) Hopkin
(e) FINNESE

1343. JVP 5 cm above angle of Louis, pressure in RA is:
(a) 6.8 mm Hg (b) 8.0
(c) 13.6 (d) 16.6
(e) 18.6

1344. In RA tracing, 2nd heart sound coincides with:
(a) Tip of v wave (b) Just before v wave
(c) Just before a wave (d) Coincides with c wave
(e) Dip of y wave

1345. Typewriter cadevance seen in:
(a) DCMP
(b) Multi valvular heart disease
(c) LBBB
(d) AV canal defect

1346. Good prognosis in ischemic cardiomyopathy suggested by DST:
(a) Effective at low dose and high dose
(b) Effective at low dose and deteriorate at high dose
(c) Not effective at low dose but effective at high dose
(d) Effective at low and more effective at high dose
(e) No effect

1347. Non ejection click with murmur true is:
(a) Click earlier on standing
(b) Click earlier on lying down
(c) Click late on standing

1348. Central aortic pressure:
(a) More than brachial
(b) Indicates arterial stiffness
(c) Cannot be predicted by brachial pressure
(d) All
(e) None

1349. Cardiac tamponade clinical findings A/E:
(a) HTN (b) Raised JVP
(c) Pulses alternans (d) ↓ cardiac dullness
(e) Syncope

1350. Cardiomyopathy can present A/E:
(a) Isolated LA enlargement with MR
(b) Asymptomatic – cardiomegaly in CXR
(c) Asymptomatic – ECG change
(d) Simultaneous RV + LV failure

1351. CHF, which ↓:
(a) Na^+ (b) Bilirubrin
(c) BUN (d) Glucose

1352. True–pulmonary ejection sound:
(a) Insp ↑ intensity
(b) Insp ↓ intensity
(c) Non-phasic
(d) Insp ↑ duration between P2 – click

1353. ↑ BNP will seen in A/E:
(a) VHD (b) Cor. pulmonale
(c) PPH (d) LVH

1354. CCP cath finding:
(a) Prominent a wave
(b) Prominent v wave
(c) Equalization of pressure in all chamber
(d) Equalization of saturation in all chamber

1355. Which abnormality of myofibrils is associated with atrial arrhythmias and conduction defect?

(a) Desmin
(b) Emerin and laminin
(c) Actin, myosin and troponin
(d) Dystrophin

1356. RCMP versus CCP favouring RCMP A/E:

(a) Well defined apical impulse
(b) Gallop sound with LVH
(c) Decrease flow of pulmonary vein and across mitral valve on inspiration
(d) Q wave with BBB

1357. 'a' wave in JVP false is:

(a) Occur during atrial contraction
(b) Proceed S_1
(c) Simultaneous with p wave on ECG
(d) Increases with ↓ RV compliance

1358. K^+ ATP channel opener causes intracellular Ca accumulation:

(a) Ivabradine (b) Nicorandil
(c) Ranolazine

1359. DCM ↑ed arrival A/E:

(a) Spironolactone (b) B-block
(c) Torsemide (d) Candesartan

1360. HF mortality benefit A/E:

(a) Glycoside
(b) ACE- I
(c) Aldosterone antagonist
(d) B-blocker

1361. Bernoulli principle:

(a) $4v^2$ (b) $2v^2$
(c) $4v^4$ (d) $2v^4$

1362. Single S_2:

(a) Pulmonary atresia
(b) ASD with Eisenmenger
(c) VSD
(d) MR

1363. S_2 A/E:

(a) Pulm hangout interval > Aortic hangout interval
(b) P2 is softer than A2
(c) Expiration A2-P2 split > 30 msec
(d) A2 corresponds to incisura on aortic pressure tracing

1364. PCWP highest in:

(a) Pseudonormalisation (b) Impaired relaxation
(c) Restrictive pattern (d) None

1365. CCP vs RCM favour CCP:

(a) Equalisation of diastotic pressure
(b) PASP
(c) Cardiomegaly
(d) Thickened IV

1366. Fabry's disease true:

(a) α galactoside A deficiency
(b) AR inheritance
(c) More in females
(d) LV thinning

1367. BNP true:

(a) Indicates LV Volume pressure load
(b) ↑ ed in all heart failure cases
(c) ↑ ed only in systolic HF
(d) Renal function has no effect

1368. MVP in A/E:

(a) OI
(b) Marfan's syndrome
(c) ED Syndrome
(d) Carcinoid syndrome

1369. Rapid 'Y' descent is not seen in:

(a) TR
(b) CCP
(c) Endomyocardial fibrosis
(d) RA myxoma

1370. Beta blocker with additional vasodilatation due to calcium channel blocking at high dose:

(a) Carvedilol (b) Esmolol
(c) Propranolol (d) Nadolol

1371. BNP — True:

(a) Represents volume and/wall stretch
(b) Independent of renal function
(c) Always elevated in FIF
(d) Elevated in systolic but not in diastolic HF

1372. Variable SI seen in all *except*:

(a) AF (b) VT
(c) 2 : 1 AV block (d) CHB

1373. Cardiogenic shock all *except:*

(a) CI < 1.0 (b) BP < 80

(c) PCWP >18 (d) CVP <3

1374. At high dose Beta blocker having CCB effect causing vasodilatation:

(a) Nadolol (b) Carvidilol

(c) Propranolol (d) Esmolol

1375. B Blocker with additional alpha blocking action all *except:*

(a) Bisoprolol (b) Bucindolol

(c) Labetalol (d) Carvedilol

1376. PCWP not raised in:

(a) MS

(b) Pulmonary vein stenosis

(c) Cortriatrium

(d) PPH

1377. Dicrotic pulse absent in:

(a) Cardiac tamponade

(b) Severe cardiac failure

(c) Hypovolemia

(d) Nonobstructive HOCM

1378. Apical HOCM associated with all *except:*

(a) T wave inversion

(b) Spade appearance on angiography

(c) Severe MR common

(d) No intraventricular gradient

1379. Free wall rupture AMI all *except:*

(a) Elderly (b) HTN

(c) Previous MI (d) LV more common

1380. Hibernating myocardium:

(a) Parallel reduction in blood flow and metabolism

(b) Prolonged decreased perfusion at rest

(c) Transient decrease

(d) Reperfusion therapy

1381. Dobutamine stress echo in hibernating myocardium gives:

(a) Biphasic response

(b) Continuous increase

(c) Interrupted response

1382. S_2 splitting:

(a) Increase venous return right side

(b) Decrease VR left side

(c) Increase pulmonary valve hang out interval

(d) AI

1383. Worst prognosis CMP:

(a) HIV associated CMP

(b) Ischemic CMP

(c) Amyloidosis induced RCM

(d) Doxorubicin CMP

1384. HOCM gene not involved:

(a) Troponin T (b) Troponin I

(c) Tropomyosin (d) Desmin

1385. Constrictive pericarditis causes all *except:*

(a) Viral pericarditis (b) RA

(c) Myxedema (d) Radiation

1386. Single S2 seen in:

(a) Pulmonary atresia

(b) ASD with Eisenmenger

(c) MR

(d) VSD

1387. ↑ LV preload seen is:

(a) MR (b) Sepsis

(c) Pulmonary embolism (d) Dehydration

1388. Valsalva maneuvre all *except:*

(a) MVP Murmur ↑

(b) Most Murmur ↓

(c) Absent overshoot– systolic dysfunction

(d) Square wave response– ↓ filling pressure

1389. Mortality improved in corpulmonale in COPD:

(a) O_2 (b) Theophylline

(c) Digoxin

1390. Drugs which ↓ mortality in DCM A/E:

(a) Torsemide (b) Candesartan

(c) Spironolactone (d) ACE-I

1391. Pulsus paradoxus least common in:

(a) Cardiac tamponade

(b) CCP

(c) Massive pulmonary embolism

(d) Severe COPD

1392. Wide split S2 seen in:

(a) Severe MR (b) PHT

(c) AS (d) MS

1393. Innocent Murmur are mostly:
(a) Early systolic (b) Holo systolic
(c) Mid systolic (d) Early diastolic

1394. Mammary soufflé of pregnancy:
(a) Continuous (b) Pan systolic
(c) ESM

1395. Heart failure cells:
(a) Hemosiderin (b) Lipofuschin
(c) Ferritin

1396. All true about CCP *except:*
(a) Kussmaul sign specfic
(b) Cardiopulmonary dissociation specific
(c) Ventricular interdependence can be diagnosed by catheterization
(d) Early diastolic rapid filling

1397. Square wave response on valsalva:
(a) MS (b) VSD
(c) PAH (d) None

1398. S1 intensity true is:
(a) Loud in LBBB
(b) Soft S1 in MVP
(c) LGL syndrome– loud S1
(d) Paradoxical split S1 in RBBB

1399. Delta wave absent on exercise means for accessory pathway:
(a) Prolongs anterograde ERP
(b) Prolongs retrograde ERP
(c) Shortens anterograde ERP
(d) Shortens retrograde ERP

1400. 20 years old female with syncope on exertion:
(a) MS (b) AS
(c) PPH (d) Cardiac tamponade

1401. Difference between reversible and irreversible cardiac damage most important is:
(a) Abnormal wall motion
(b) Reduced myocardial flow
(c) Absence of metabolism
(d) ECG changes

1402. Reduced y wave in A/E:
(a) Cardiac tamponade (b) RVMI
(c) TS (d) RCMP

1403. Maximum length stress at (dp/dt):
(a) 2.2 μm (b) 2.0 μm
(c) 3 μm (d) 3.5 μm

1404. Familial HCM true is:
(a) Mainly affect sacromere
(b) Most common gene involved is tropomyosin
(c) Elderly worse prognosis
(d) X-linked

1405. Brockenbrough phenomenon:
(a) Post PVC decreases pulse pressure
(b) Post PVC increase gradient

1406. Post extrasystolic not increased in:
(a) HCM (b) Rheumatic MR
(c) Valvular PS

1407. Variable S1 A/E:
(a) VT (b) CHB
(c) AF (d) 2:1 block

1408. Prominent y descent in:
(a) Cardiac tamponade
(b) Tricuspid atresia with restrictive VSD
(c) DORV
(d) RVMI

1409. Innocent murmur is:
(a) Mid systolic murmur
(b) Mid diastolic murmur

1410. Earliest detection of systolic dysfunction:
(a) DP/DT (b) Strain imaging
(c) EF (d) LVESD

1411. Increased LAP:
(a) Rheumatic MS (b) ECD

1412. Hibernating myocarditis on stress echo-response:
(a) Increased (b) Decreased
(c) Biphasic response (d) Increase than decrease

1413. Definition of hibernating myocardium:
(a) Parallel decrease in matched flow
(b) Chronic hypoperfusion at rest

1414. P wave alternans:
(a) Pulmonary embolism

1415. WHO criteria for PAH A/E:

(a) Fatigue (b) Chest pain
(c) Palpitation (d) Syncope

1416. Syncope A/E:

(a) AS (b) Severe MS
(c) PPH

1417. Dicrotic pulse A/E:

(a) Tamponade (b) DCMP

1418. Cardiogenic shock A/E:

(a) CVP < 3 min (b) CI < 1.9
(c) PCWP > 18 (d) BP < 80 mm Hg

1419. H wave seen in A/E:

(a) RCMP (b) RVMI
(c) CCP

1420. Mitral annular calcification A/E:

(a) Most common in males
(b) Associated MR
(c) Increased in Marfan syndrome
(d) More commonly seen in AS

1421. Isometric exercise A/E:

(a) SVR (b) CO
(c) HR (d) Mean BP

1422. In Fick method, mixed venous blood derived from:

(a) SVC (b) RV
(c) PA (d) LA

1423. The longest phase of the cardiac action potential is:

(a) Phase 0 (b) Phase 1
(c) Phase 2 (d) Phase 3

1424. All of the following are physiological responses during the Phase 2 (Maintenance Phase) of valsalva maneuver in a normal person *except:*

(a) Decrease in pulse rate
(b) Decrease in aortic systolic pressure
(c) Decrease in pulse pressure
(d) Decrease in left ventricular filling

1425. Hibernating myocardium on PET testing is demonstrated by:

(a) Preserved perfusion and preserved glucose metabolism
(b) Reduced perfusion and reduced glucose metabolism
(c) Reduced perfusion and preserved glucose metabolism
(d) Preserved perfusion and reduced glucose metabolism

1426. Mortality benefit of beta blocker in congestive heart failure is seen with all of the following *except:*

(a) Bucindolol (b) Carvedilol
(c) Bisoprolol (d) Metoprolol

1427. In a patient with chronic left ventricular disease, the patient having predominant S4 gallop (as compared to having S3 gallop) will have:

(a) Higher mean left atrial pressure
(b) Higher left ventricular filling pressure in early diastole
(c) Higher atrial contractile function
(d) Higher atrial volume

1428. Which of the following is true regarding the 'v wave' in the right atrial pressure trace?

(a) It occurs just after the tricuspid valve opening
(b) It is due to filling of right atrium by blood returning from vena cava and coronary sinus
(c) It occurs during the period of ventricular diastole
(d) It is of higher amplitude than left atrial v wave

1429. Higher amplitude of 'v wave' in pulmonary capillary wedge pressure in a patient of mitral regurgitation (MR) is seen with:

(a) Marked left atrial enlargement
(b) Presence of sinus rhythm than in atrial fibrillation
(c) Chronic MR than with acute MR
(d) None of the above

1430. Drugs which have been investigated for pharmacological treatment of neurocardiogenic syncope include all of the following *except:*

(a) Midodrine (b) Pyridostigmine
(c) Diltiazem (d) Theophylline

1431. The most effective treatment which improves survival for a comatosed patient who has been resuscitated from out-of-hospital cardiac arrest is:

(a) Therapeutic hypothermia
(b) Hyperventilation using mechanical ventilation
(c) Immediate coronary angiography and PCI
(d) Dobutamine infusion

1432. Normal physiological changes during exercise in a normal adult includes:

(a) Decrease in partial pressure of oxygen in arterial blood (PaO_2)

(b) Decrease in partial pressure oxygen in mixed venous blood (PaO_2)

(c) Leftward shift of the oxy-hemoglobin dissociation curve

(d) Decrease in mean systemic blood pressure

1433. A 56-year-old male patient has Type-2 DM with micro-albuminuria, hypertension and serum creatinine of 1.5 mg%. He was started on olmesartan at the recommended doses. After 2 months, the creatinine has increased to 1.9 mg%, the blood pressure is well controlled. The appropriate step in this patient will be:

(a) Continue same treatment and monitor renal function

(b) Switch olmesartan to amlodipine

(c) Initiate dialysis

(d) Decrease the dose of olmesartan to half and reassess renal function

1434. A 40-year-old female patient is a case of idiopathic pulmonary artery hypertension (IPAH). She is hospitalized with class IV symptoms. The treatment strongly recommended to relieve her symptoms and improve survival is:

(a) Bosentan

(b) Intravenous epoprostenol

(c) Long-acting nifedipine

(d) Sildenafil

1435. A 38-year-old female is a known case of chronic thromboembolic pulmonary artery hypertension (CTEPH). She is symptomatic despite adequate treatment with warfarin and diuretics. CT angiography reveals presence of non-occluding chronic thrombus in right and left proximal pulmonary artery. The treatment of choice should be:

(a) IV prostacyclin

(b) Switch to acenocoumarol in place of warfarin

(c) Thrombolytic therapy using tenecteplase

(d) Surgical pulmonary thrombo-endarterectomy

1436. A 60-year-old chronic smoker is diagnosed to have chronic obstructive pulmonary disease. The echocardiography reveals right atrial and right ventricular enlargement with moderate PAH. The likely cause of this finding is:

(a) Pulmonary artery in-situ thrombosis

(b) Hypercapnia

(c) Alveolar hypoxia

(d) Pulmonary A-V fistula

1437. A 70-year-old feamle patient is a case of breast cancer. She is receiving active chemotherapy. She has presented to the emergency with cold extremities. The blood pressure is 100/70, heart rate 100 beats/minute, SaO_2 98%. JVP raised with blunted Y descent. The likely diagnosis is:

(a) Constrictive pericarditis

(b) Cardiac tamponade

(c) Left ventricular systolic dysfunction

(d) Acute pulmonary embolism

1438. Bezold Jarisch reflex is produced by:

(a) Atrial distension

(b) Ventricular distension

(c) Carotid sinus stimulation

(d) Carotid body stimulation

1439. Which of the following is not a major Framingham criteria for diagnosis of heart failure?

(a) Paroxysmal nocturnal dyspnea

(b) Hepatojugular reflux

(c) Hepatomegaly

(d) Response to diuretics

1440. All are established risk factors for sudden cardiac death in patients with hypertrophic cardiomyopathy *except:*

(a) Severe cardiac hypertrophy

(b) Left ventricular outflow tract gradient

(c) Causal mutations

(d) Modifier genes

1441. Which of the following drug is known to improve morbidity or mortality?

(a) Tazosentan for heart failure

(b) Ivabradine for heart failure

(c) Dalcetrapib for lipid modification

(d) Glimeperide in macrovascular disease

1442. All are risk factors for peripartum cardiomyo-pathy *except:*

(a) Primipara

(b) Older maternal age

(c) Preeclampsia

(d) Twin pregnancy

1443. Following statements are true about early repolarization pattern *except:*

(a) Prevalence of 1-13% in general population

(b) Phase 2 re-entry can be initiated with trigger VT

(c) Characterized by J point elevation with or without ST elevation in inferior limb and lateral precordial leads

(d) Early repolarization with ascending ST segment is predictor of sudden cardiac death

1444. All of the following are beneficial effects of regular exercise *except:*

(a) Favorable changes in fibrinolytic

(b) Decreased heart rate variability

(c) Increased of expression of nitric oxide synthetase

(d) Decreased systolic and diastolic blood pressure

1445. All of the following are absolute contra indications for exercise testing *except:*

(a) Acute MI (< 2 days)

(b) Acute systemic infection accompanied by fever

(c) High grade AV block

(d) Acute myocarditis

1446. A 60-year-old diabetic patient on insulin with normal renal function and BP of 160/90 is prescribed triamterene. After 2 weeks his serum K+ is 6.5 mmol/liter with no change in urea or creatinine. Most likely cause is:

(a) Recent UTI

(b) Hyporeninemic hypoaldosteronism

(c) Cushing's syndrome

(d) Primary hyperaldosteronism

1447. Each of the following statements regarding pulsus alternans in patients with marked LV dysfunction is true *except:*

(a) It is usually associated with electrical alternans of the QRS complex

(b) It is more readily detected in the femoral as compared with radial arteries

(c) It can be detected by sphygmomanometry

(d) It can be elicited by the assumption of erect posture

1448. One of the following does not belong to natriuretic peptide family:

(a) ANP (b) BNP

(c) Urodilantin (d) Urotensin

1449. Which of the following pathways contribute to cardiac dysfunction in heart failure?

(a) Necrosis (b) Apoptosis

(c) Autophagy (d) All of the above

1450. Major criteria for the diagnosis of heart failure with normal ejection fraction (EF):

(a) Ankle edema (b) Hepatojugular reflex

(c) Hepatomegaly (d) Nocturnal cough

1451. The following are therapeutic targets for gene therapy in heart failure:

(a) Adenyl cyclase (b) Phospholamban

(c) Both of the above (d) None of the above

1452. Which of the following is a marker of oxidative stress in heart failure?

(a) Myeloperoxidase

(b) Tumor necrosis factor

(c) Brain natriuretic peptide

(d) Matrix metallo proteinases

1453. Uncommon feature of acute myocardial infarction:

(a) S3

(b) S4

(c) Loud S1

(d) Paradoxical splitting of S2

1454. Killips class-III is:

(a) Shock

(b) S3 gallop

(c) Elevated JVP

(d) Frank pulmonary edema

1455. Takotsubo cardiomyopathy is related to:

(a) Peripartum (b) Stress

(c) Inflammation (d) Tachycardia

1456. Pulmonary hypertension is absent in:

(a) RV endomyocardial fibrosis

(b) LV endomyocardial fibrosis

(c) Biventricular endomyocardial fibrosis

(d) All of the above

1457. Cardiac resynchronization therapy is indicated in:

(a) HOCM (b) RCMP

(c) DCMP (d) CHB

1458. Black triad is seen in:

(a) Pericardial effusion
(b) Acute pericarditis
(c) Cardiac tamponade
(d) Constrictive pericarditis

1459. One of the following drug is not useful in primary pulmonary hypertension:

(a) Bosentan (b) Sildenafil
(c) Telmisartan (d) Iloprost

1460. The following chemotherapeutic drug produces left ventricular dysfunction:

(a) Cisplatin (b) Thalidomide
(c) Erlotinib (d) Cyclophosphamide

1461. Mechanism of contrast induced acute kidney injury:

(a) Direct toxicity
(b) Atheroembolism
(c) Intra renal vasoconstriction
(d) All of the above

1462. One of the following test is useful to assess cardiac autonomic function:

(a) Valsalva maneuver (b) Hand grip
(c) Squatting (d) Sitting

1463. Cardiovascular disability can be assessed by:

(a) Goldman specific activity scale
(b) CCS functional classification
(c) NYHA functional classification
(d) All of the above

1464. "Ventricularization" of jugular venous waveform is seen in:

(a) Severe tricuspid regurgitation
(b) Severe pulmonary stenosis
(c) Severe mitral regurgitation
(d) Severe aortic stenosis

1465. Square-wave response in sValsalva maneuver indicates:

(a) LV systolic dysfunction
(b) Elevated filling pressures
(c) Normal LV systolic function
(d) Normal LV diastolic function

1466. Gorlin formula for calculation of stenotic mitral valve area in cm²:

(a) $\{[\text{COP (liters/min)} \times 1000]/(44.3)(\text{HR})(\text{SEP})\sqrt{\text{meangradiant}}\}$
(b) $\{[\text{COP (liters/min)} \times 1000]/(37.7)(\text{HR})(\text{DFP})\sqrt{\text{meangradiant}}\}$
(c) $\{[\text{COP (liters/min)} \times 1000]/(44.3)(\text{HR})(\text{DFP})\sqrt{\text{meangradiant}}\}$
(d) $\{[\text{COP (liters/min)} \times 1000]/(37.7)(\text{HR})(\text{SEP})\sqrt{\text{meangradiant}}\}$

1467. Sellers grading is for:

(a) Mitral regurgitation (b) Aortic regurgitation
(c) Both of the above (d) None of the above

1468. Pathological 'q' waves – seen in V1–V3:

(a) Amyloidosis (b) LBBB
(c) WDW syndrome (d) All of the above

1469. Dobutamine – True:

(a) $b1 > b2 + a$
(b) $b2 > b1$
(c) Increase C.O. + increase peri. resistance
(d) Decrease HR

1470. Vasodilator:

(a) Natriuretic peptide (b) Carvedilol
(c) Endothelin

1471. Nitric oxide – MOA:

(a) Increase Na+ channel conductance
(b) Decrease Ca intracellular
(c) Increase K+ channel opening
(d) Non-ionic mech.

1472. All true about CCP *except*:

(a) Dip and plateau configuration in RV, not in LV
(b) ↑ventricular dependence
(c) Kussmaul sign
(d) No association between intrathoracic and intrapericardial

1473. Total electrical alternans specific for:

(a) Tamponade (b) DCMP

1474. Myocardial oxygen consumption feomull:

(a) $\dfrac{Q}{CAO_2 - \text{coronary sinus } O_2}$

(b) $Cl \times (CAO_2 - \text{coronary sinus } O_2)$

(c) $\dfrac{CAO_2 - \text{coronary sinus } O_2}{Cl}$

(d) Cannot be calculated

1475. Pulmonary vascular resistance:

(a) 100-300 (b) 300-500

1476. Maximum reduction in LV afterload and increase in coronary flow:

(a) IABP (b) Impella
(c) Tandem heart (d) ECMO

1477. Cardiac catheterization, BP 120/80, POWF 19 mm Hg RV pressure 40/20 diagnosis:

(a) RCMP (b) CCP
(c) Tamponade (d) RVMI

1478. Requires >10 mets:

(a) Swimming (b) 4 miles/hour
(c) Swipping floor (d) Tennis

1479. Favour CCP, all *except*:

(a) RVSP > 35
(b) SAR < 1.1
(c) Equal diastolic pressure
(d) Ventricular interdependence

1480. Prominent X and absent Y descent in:

(a) Cardiac Tamponade (b) HOCM
(c) TR (d) CCP

1481. Isometric (Resistance) exercise all *except*:

(a) ↑ DBP (b) ↑ sympathetic tone
(c) ↑ venous return (d) ↑ peripheral resistance

1482. ENGAGE heart failure trial for:

(a) Edoxaban (b) Rivaroxaban
(c) Dabigatran (d) Apixaban

1483. M mode echo of cardiac tampanode, all can be seen up:

(a) Pulsus paradoxus
(b) Friedreich's sign
(c) Preserved x and y descent

1484. Which one of the following pressure half time of AR Doppler signal is suggestive of severe AR?

(a) >800 ms (b) 400 to 800 ms
(c) 251 to 399 ms (d) < 250 ms

1485. Inverted Mercedes Benz sign on echocardiography is used for following valve:

(a) Tricuspid (b) Aortic
(c) Pulmonary (d) Mitral

1486. How many fold coronary flow can increase due to vasodilation?

(a) 23 times (b) 12 times
(c) 45 times (d) 67 times

1487. Which one of the following is not true for Milrinone?

(a) It is a phosphodiesterase inhibitor
(b) It is beta receptor stimulant
(c) It has inotropic effect
(d) It has vasodilator effect

1488. To define severe AR, vene contracta on echo should be more than:

(a) 0.5 cm (b) 0.4 cm
(c) 0.6 cm (d) 0.7 cm

1489. In patients with HOCM, echo screening of their son/daughter should be started at age of:

(a) 5 years (b) 9 years
(c) 12 years (d) 23 years

1490. What is the incidence of dilated cardiomyopathy in Duchenne muscular dystrophy, after age of 18 years?

(a) Up to 20% (b) Up to 50%
(c) Up to 70% (d) Up to 90%

1491. Following cardiomyopathy is common in Friedreich ataxia:

(a) Asymmetrical septal hypertrophy
(b) Concentric hypertrophic cardiomyopathy
(c) Dilated cardiomyopathy
(d) Restrictive cardiomyopathy

1492. Which one of the following is not true for Takotsubo cardiomyopathy?

(a) It is irreversible
(b) It is known as apical ballooning syndrome also
(c) ECG may mimic acute myocardial infarction
(d) Most common in postmenopausal woman

1493. Which one of the following is true for development of alcoholic cardiomyopathy?

(a) Consumption of more than 80 gm of ethanol per day for at least 10 years
(b) Consumption of more than 80 gm of ethanol per day for at least 5 years
(c) Consumption of more than 40 gm of ethanol per day for at least 5 years
(d) Consumption of more than 40 gm of ethanol per day for at least 10 years

1494. Which one of the following is true for electrical alternans in ECG?

(a) It is common in patients with cardiac tamponade
(b) It is ventricular bigeminy pattern
(c) It is atrial bigeminy pattern
(d) It is common in patients with rheumatic heart disease

1495. TAPSE (tricuspid annular plane systolic excursion) is determined by:

(a) M mode echo (b) 2 dimension echo
(c) 3 dimension echo (d) Doppler

1496. If inferior vena cava diameter is <2.1 cm and show >50% collapse with inspiration, than estimated RA pressure is:

(a) 5 mm of Hg (b) 10 mm of Hg
(c) 15 mm of Hg (d) 20 mm of Hg

1497. MDM all *except*:

(a) PR (b) VSD
(c) MVP (d) AR

1498. Not a fact of disorders:

(a) Tissue flap (b) Ejection click
(c) Pericardial knock (d) OS

1499. Not a fact of cardiac disorders:

(a) Isovolumic relaxation
(b) Diastasis
(c) Atrial relaxation
(d) Early filling

1500. Functional Class II true:

(a) NYHA III - Less than ordinary activity
(b) CLS II - Ordinary activity causes symptom
(c) NYHA later than CCS and specific activity side
(d) Specific Activity ——

1501. CCP – all *except*:

(a) Kussmaul sign specific
(b) Cardiopulmonary dissociation
(c) Interventricular interdependence
(d) Rapid early diastolic filling

1502. Pulsus paradoxus uncommon seen:

(a) Cardiac tamponade
(b) CCP
(c) COPD
(d) Massive pulmonary Embolism

1503. CO is not measured by:

(a) Thermodilution (b) Intracardiac ECHO
(c) Doppler (d) Ventriculography

1504. Pericardial knock:

(a) Between OS and S3 (b) Alongwith S3
(c) After S3 (d) With OS

1505. Angiotensin II – True:

(a) Decrease Aldosterene–Increase K+
(b) Increase fluid retention–by increasing vasopressin
(c) Spironolactone prolong use causes myocardial fibrosis

1506. Carvedilol:

(a) Cardioselective – with antioxidant
(b) Cardioselective – without antioxidant
(c) Non-cardioselective – without antioxidant
(d) Non-cardioselective – with antioxidant

1507. Absence of late potentials are prognostic indicator in:

(a) MCM (b) DCM
(c) AWMI (d) IWMI

1508. Increase HR increase contratility:

(a) Bowditch (b) ANREP

1509. Force Tension Relationship:

(a) Increase volume shift curve to Up and Left
(b) Increase volume shift curve Rt and UP
(c) Increase contraction shift curve to Up and Left
(d) Increase contraction shift curve Rt and Down

1510. Right ventricular systolic dysfunction on Echo is suggested when TAPSE is:

(a) < 12 mm (b) < 14 mm
(c) < 16 mm (d) < 18 mm

1511. Which of the following perfusion tracer is used for "ischemic memory"?

(a) C-palmitate (b) 1-BMIPP
(c) 2-FDG (d) C-acetate

1512. Dip and plateau diastolic waveform does not occur in:

(a) Constructive pericarditis
(b) Restrictive cardiomyopathy
(c) Right ventricular ischemia
(d) Cardiac tamponade

1513. Which of the following statement regarding NATRIURETIC PEPTIDE is false?

(a) Both ANP and BNP are only secreted in response to increasing cardiac wall tension
(b) ANP has short half life of 3 min while BNP has a half life of 20 min
(c) ANP and BNP are cleaved proteolytically by corin and furin respectively
(d) ANP and BNP bind to NPR-A while CNP binds to NPR-B

1514. Which changes does not occur in humans in heart failure?

(a) Decreased L type calcium channels
(b) Decreased beta 2 adrenergic receptor
(c) Isoform switch of titin
(d) SERCA2A levels are decreased

1515. Which of the following finding has the highest positive predictive value in diagnosis of elevated filling pressure in patients with heart failure?

(a) Rates over more than 1/3rd of lung field
(b) Presence of third heart sound
(c) Orthopnea
(d) Moderate to massive ascites

1516. Which of the following is not a major criteria in Framingham criteria for diagnosis of heart failure?

(a) PND (b) Hepatomegaly
(c) Cardiomegaly (d) Hepatojugular reflex

1517. Which of the following device does not have a pulsatile pump mechanism?

(a) Thoratec PVAD (b) Thoratec IVAD
(c) HAVD (d) Cardiowest TAH-T

1518. All are useful in diagnosis of HFpLF *except*:

(a) BNP level of 100 pg ml and NT-pro BNP level of 800 pg ml supports its diagnosis
(b) LVEF-50%
(c) BNP levels are higher in obese patients and lower in women, older persons, patients with pulmonary disease and renal dysfunction
(d) PCWP >12 mm Hg, LVEDP > 16 mm Hg, t > 48 msec, ? >0.27, E/e >15, LAVI >40 ml/M², LVM >122/149 g/M²

1519. All are true about heart rate turbulence (HRT) *except*:

(a) HRT is an index of changes in the sinus discharge rate after a PVC that is followed by a compensatory pause
(b) HRT is a measure of reflex vagal control of the heart whereas heart rate variability is more indicative of overall vagal tone
(c) Beta blocker is an absolute contraindication in patients with HRT
(d) Abnormal HRT is a strong independent predictor of mortality in patients with CAD and DCMP

1520. Which of the following is decreased in a failing myocyte?

(a) L-type calcium channel
(b) Alpha-1 adrenergic receptor
(c) Troponin C
(d) Calreticulin

1521. Which of the following statements is false?

(a) Physiologic systole lasts from the start of isovolumic contraction to the peak of the ejection phase
(b) Cardiologic systole is demarcated by the interval between the first and second heart sounds and lasts from M_1 to A_2
(c) Physiologic diastole commences as Ca^{2+} is taken back into the SR, so myocyte relaxation occurs and LV pressure starts falling
(d) Protodiastole is the early phase of atrial contraction, the time when S4 can be heard

1522. Biphasis response on dobutamine indicates all *except*:

(a) Low dose dobutamine infusion – wall thickening
High dose dobutamine infusion – wall thickening
(b) Low dose dobutamine infusion – wall thickening
High dose dobutamine infusion – wall thickening
(c) Most specific sign of myocardial viability
(d) Any improvement in RWMA by at least one grade in two or more segments during stress signify viability

1523. Which of the following is a correct statement?

(a) Arteriogenesis is the process by which new capillaries develop from the pre existing vasculature
(b) Angiogenesis is the process of collateral vessel enlargement, caused by remodeling or growth of pre existing arteriolar collateral connections
(c) Vasculogenesis, is defined as the de novo formation of a primitive vascular network from differentiating precursor mesodermal cells, such as endothelial progenitor cells, in the absence of pre existing vasculature
(d) Bevacizumab causes angiogenesis through VEGF

1524. The P-glycoprotein (P-gp) transporter is found in the luminal membrane of the small intestine and blood brain barrier and in the apical membranes of excretory cells such as hepatocytes and kidney proximal tubule epithelial cells. Digoxin is a substrate of both intestinal and renal P-glycoprotein transporter. Which of the following statements is not correct?

(a) Induction of intestinal P-gp by rifampin is shown to decrease the bioavailability of orally administered digoxin, thereby reducing plasma digoxin levels

(b) Quinidine increases plasma digoxin concentration by reducing P-gp-mediated efflux of digoxin into the gut and kidneys

(c) Amiodarone, a potent inhibitor of P-gp, increases mean serum digoxin levels

(d) Dronedarone does not interact with P-gp, and oral digoxin dose needs no adjustment when co-administered with droneadaerone

1525. All are points of ABCD SCORE, *except*:

(a) Age >65 years

(b) Unilateral weakness

(c) Blood pressure > 140/90 mm Hg

(d) Diabetes

1526. All are true about adenosine *except*:

(a) Adenosine dilates coronary arteries through activation of A2 receptors

(b) Adenosine mediated vasodilation is enhanced by lowering LDL levels

(c) It has a differential sensitivity for the micro-circulation

(d) None of the above

1527. Which of the following statements regarding monitoring and characterizing circulatory status in critically ill patients in ICU is not correct?

(a) Routine pulmonary artery catheterization is not indicated

(b) Static measurements of circulatory parameters (e.g., CVP, PCWP) provide reliable information on the circulatory status of critically ill patients

(c) A decrease in CVP of >1 mm Hg during inspiration in a spontaneously breathing patient may predict an increase in cardiac output after IV fluid administration

(d) A changing pulse pressure during mechanical ventilation has been shown to predict an increase in cardiac output after IV fluid administration in patients with septic shock

1528. A 40 years old female has VSD with L-R shunt and a dilated RV with severe systolic dysfunction on echocardiography, Catheterization study reveals arterial oxygen saturation 95% SVC oxygen saturation 48%, IVC oxygen saturation 52%, RA oxygen saturation 61%, RV oxygen saturation 78%, PA oxygen saturation 77%, RA 12 mm Hg, RV 62/12 mm Hg, PA 63/39(47) mm Hg, PCWP 14 mm Hg, Pulmonary to systemic shunt fraction is:

(a) 1.8 (b) 2.2

(c) 2.6 (d) 3.0

1529. Catheterization study in a patient of pulmonary hypertension reveals following findings: RA–8 mm Hg, RV–68/8 mm Hg, PA–68/32/43 mm Hg, PCWP–25 mm Hg, CO–3 L/min, Cl–1:5 L/min/m. The pulmonary vascular resistance (PVR) expressed in wood units (WU) is:

(a) 18 WU (b) 24 WU

(c) 12 WU (d) 6 WU

1530. True statement regarding appropriate screening protocol for family members of patients with HCM:

(a) Serial ECG and echocardiogram every 5 years for a 14 years old child of an HCM patient

(b) Serial ECG and echocardiogram on a first degree adult relative every 10 years of an HCM patient

(c) Serial ECG and echocardiogram on a gene-negative first-degree relative of a patient who is gene positive for beta-myosin heavy-chain mutation every 5 years

(d) Serial ECG and echocardiogram every 18 months for a 17 years old child of an HCM patient

1531. The most accepted recent hypothesis for anthracycline induced cardiotoxicity is:

(a) Magnesium mediated generation of excess reactive oxygen species

(b) Formation of complexes with calcium that undergo redox cycling and generate oxygen radicals

(c) Inhibition of Topoisomerase 2β

(d) Deactivation of p^{53} and the apoptotic pathway

1532. All are true about Valsalva maneuver, *except*:

(a) Pulse amplitude ratio is a ratio of the maximal pulse pressure at the end of the strain phase to the minimum pulse pressure at initiation of the strain phase

(b) Pulse amplitude ratio has been shown to correlate very closely with ventricular filling pressures

(c) In patients with severe heart failure, Korotkoff sounds are appreciated during phase 2 but not phase 4

(d) In patients with mild heart failure, Korotkoff sounds are absent during both phases 2 and 4

1533. Regarding cardiac amyloidosis, all statements are true *except*:

(a) Two types of amyloid commonly infiltrate the heart: AL or primary systemic and Transthyretin (TTR) amyloid
(b) Transthyretin (TTR) related amyloid cardiomyopathy is slowly progressive and clinically well tolerated
(c) ^{123}I-SAP (Serum amyloid P) can assess the amyloid burden affecting the heart, permitting its use for diagnosis or serial quantification of cardiac amyloidosis
(d) Tafamidis is a TTR stabilizing drug

1534. Early repolarization is present if all of the following criteria are met *except*:

(a) There is an end-QRS notch or slur on the down slope of a prominent R-wave
(b) If there is a notch, it should lie entirely above the baseline. The onset of a slur must also be above the baseline
(c) J peak is ≥ 0.1 mV in 2 or more contiguous leads of the 12-lead ECG, excluding leads V1 to V3
(d) QRS duration is > 120 ms

1535. Which of the following statements regarding the Transcranial Doppler is not true?

(a) It is useful for diagnosis of acute occlusion of middle cerebral artery
(b) Valsalva manoeuvre helps in detection of patent foramen ovale on transcranial Doppler
(c) Transcranial Doppler studies can differentiate between a shunt at atrial, ventricular and pulmonary level
(d) Transcranial Doppler with contrast has a greater sensitivity than transthoracic echocardiography with contrast at identifying PFO

1536. Most potent endogenous cardio stimulatory peptide is:

(a) Asopressin (b) Endothelin
(c) Urotensin (d) Apelin

1537. Most potent cardiostimulatory peptide:

(a) Endothelin (b) Urotensin II
(c) Angiotensin (d) Neuropeptide γ

1538. Riociguat mechanism of action is:

(a) Soluble cGmp stimulation
(b) Phosphodiesterase
(c) Endothelin receptor antagonist
(d) Prostaglandin analogues

1539. ANP – mechanism true:

(a) Cause ↑ GFR and smooth mg relaxation
(b) ↑ ca and mg retention
(c) ↑ Na and water retention
(d) Vasoconstriction ↑ aldosterone

1540. JVP–true:

(a) Kussmaul sign pathognomonic of constrictive pericarditis
(b) X and Y are more prominent seen than a, c and v
(c) Tamponade X is less prominent than y prominent
(d) C wave is different ventricular diastole and ↑ only in ventricular diastole

1541. Apical thrombotic obliteration difference with inflow/outflow tract:

(a) EMF
(b) Hypereosinophilic syndrome
(c) Amyloid
(d) Saicoid

1542. True of false: (T/F)

(a) Bisoprolol – non cardioselective vasoconstrictor
(b) Carvedilol – non cardioselective vasoconstrictor
(c) Nebivolol – non cardioselective vasoconstrictor
(d) In moderate HF, beta blocker decreases mortality more than ACE-I

1543. c wave of JVP correlates with:

(a) Isovolumetric relaxation
(b) Isovolumetric contraction
(c) Diastole
(d) Atrial systole

1544. Mean pulmonary artery pressure:

(a) 25 mm Hg (b) 15
(c) 30 (d) 20

1545. Myocyte changes during remodeling in HFREF:

(a) Apoptosis
(b) Autophagy
(c) Beta adrenergic desensitization
(d) Hypertrophy

1546. In HF myocyte changes all seen *except*:

(a) Necrosis (b) Apoptosis
(c) Autophagy (d) Atrophy

1547. Parasite causing myocarditis:

(a) Coxsackie (b) Tenia
(c) Trypanosoma (d) Borrelia

1548. All are risk factors for peripartum cardiomyopathy *except*:
(a) Increased maternal age
(b) Preeclampsia
(c) Twin pregnancy
(d) Obesity

1549. All are true about Takotsubo cardiomyopathy *except*:
(a) Ventricle shows segmental wall motion abnormality
(b) Stress induced
(c) Typically in older woman
(d) CAG is advised

1550. PASP is more than 50 mm Hg in:
(a) Constrictive pericarditis
(b) Restrictive cardiomyopathy
(c) Cardiac temponade
(d) IWMI

1551. Broadbent sign is seen in:
(a) Constrictive pericarditis
(b) Restrictive cardiomyopathy
(c) Cardiac temponade
(d) IWMI

1552. Pleural effusions are common in:
(a) Left ventricular failure
(b) Right ventricular failure
(c) Biventricular failure
(d) Cor pulmonale

1553. Omecamtiv mecarbil is:
(a) Selective myosin activator
(b) Nonselective myosin activator
(c) Selective actin activator
(d) Nonselective actin activator

1554. Cause of unilateral pulmonary edema:
(a) Acute AR (b) Acute MR
(c) Acute TR (d) Acute VSR

1555. Isovolumetric relaxation phase ends with:
(a) AV valve opening (b) T wave beginning
(c) C wave of JVP (d) None

1556. Acute onset heart failure with preserved ejection fraction. Treatment of choice:
(a) ACEI (b) Beta blockers
(c) ARB (d) CCB

1557. CCB used in CHF:
(a) Verapamil (b) Amlodipine
(c) Diltiazem (d) None

1558. Sacubitril/valsartan mechanism of action:
(a) Decrease BNP (b) Increase BNP
(c) Decrease ANP (d) None

1559. HFPEF promising drug:
(a) Sacubitril (b) ACEI
(c) ARB (d) BB

1560. LVAD indication:
(a) <14 mlO_2 (b) <10 ml
(c) <18 ml (d) <12 ml

1561. Tissue harmonic imaging:
(a) B mode (b) A mode
(c) M mode (d) None

1562. Causes of RCM A/E:
(a) Amyloid (b) Sarcoid
(c) Hemochromatosis (d) Alcohol

1563. PDE 5–inhibitor:
(a) Riociguat (b) Vardenafil
(c) Macitentan (d) Iloprost

1564. What is more important in heart transplantation?
(a) ABO-compatibility (b) Uncontrolled DM
(c) Obesity (d) CKD

1565. 2 years boy with ht–81 cm, weight–8.5 kg, BMI–12.95 kg/m², Hb–10 gm/dl, O_2 conc–175 ml/min/mt², BSA–0.48 m². Cath data–saturation %–RV–67.5/PA–83.4/FA–94.9/PV–98. Qp/Qs is:
(a) 0.9 (b) 1.2
(c) 1.8 (d) 2.0

1566. In a person with 70 kg and Hb of 13 mg/dl, arterial saturation of 95% and pulmonary artery saturation of 65%. Cardiac output is:
(a) 2 L/min (b) 4 L/min
(c) 5 L/min (d) 6 L/min

1567. PND is least likely with:
(a) LA myxoma (b) CCP
(c) AR (d) MI

1568. Diuretic resistance is seen due to A/E:
(a) NSAID
(b) ARB use
(c) Decreased RA pressure
(d) Severe hypokalemia

ANSWERS KEY

1. (a)	2. (b)	3. (a)	4. (b)	5. (d)	6. (b, d)	7. (a)	8. (a)
9. (b)	10. (d)	11. (b)	12. (b)	13. (c)	14. (a)	15. (b)	16. (a)
17. (a)	18. (b)	19. (a)	20. (d)	21. (d)	22. (a)	23. (a)	24. (a)
25. (a)	26. (b)	27. (a)	28. (c)	29. (d)	30. (b)	31. (b)	32. (a)
33. (a)	34. (?)	35. (a)	36. (a)	37. (d)	38. (d)	39. (b)	40. (b)
41. (a)	42. (a)	43. (d)	44. (a)	45. (d)	46. (a)	47. (a)	48. (b)
49. (a)	50. (a)	51. (a)	52. (a)	53. (a)	54. (a)	55. (a)	56. (d)
57. (a)	58. (c)	59. (d)	60. (a)	61. (d)	62. (d)	63. (a)	64. (c)
65. FTTFT	66. TTTFF	67. FFFFT	68. FTFFT	69. FTTTT	70. FTTTF	71. TFTTT	72. FTTTT
73. FTTFT	74. TTTTT	75. FFFTF	76. TFFTT	77. FFFTT	78. (b)	79. (b)	80. (c)
81. (d)	82. (b)	83. (a)	84. (b)	85. (c)	86. (c)	87. (a)	88. (c)
89. (b)	90. (d)	91. (a)	92. (d)	93. (c)	94. (c)	95. (c)	96. (d)
97. (a)	98. (a)	99. (a)	100. (a)	101. (c)	102. (c)	103. (d)	104. (b)
105. (a)	106. (b)	107. (c)	108. (c)	109. (a)	110. (c)	111. (d)	112. (a)
113. (c)	114. (d)	115. (d)	116. (c)	117. (d)	118. (b)	119. (c)	120. (d)
121. (c)	122. (a)	123. (c)	124. (d)	125. (a)	126. (a)	127. (d)	128. (a)
129. (a)	130. (b)	131. (b)	132. (b)	133. (a)	134. (a)	135. (b)	136. (a)
137. (d)	138. (b)	139. (a)	140. (c)	141. (d)	142. (a)	143. (c)	144. (d)
145. (a)	146. (a)	147. (d)	148. (c)	149. (d)	150. (c)	151. (c)	152. (b)
153. (a)	154. (c)	155. (b)	156. (c)	157. (d)	158. (b)	159. (d)	160. (a)
161. (c)	162. (e)	163. (c)	164. (a)	165. (c)	166. (d)	167. (a)	168. (a)
169. (c)	170. (c)	171. (a)	172. (b)	173. (b)	174. (d)	175. (b)	176. (a)
177. (a)	178. (b)	179. (b)	180. (b)	181. (a)	182. (b)	183. (a)	184. (c)
185. (a)	186. (a)	187. (a)	188. (a)	189. (b)	190. (a)	191. (a)	192. (b)
193. (b)	194. (?)	195. (d)	196. (a)	197. (c)	198. (a)	199. (c)	200. (a)
201. (a)	202. (a)	203. (b)	204. (b)	205. (b)	206. (d)	207. (d)	208. (a)
209. (b)	210. (a)	211. (a)	212. (c)	213. (a)	214. (a)	215. (a)	216. (a)
217. (c)	218. (a)	219. (b)	220. (a)	221. (a)	222. (b)	223. (b)	224. (a)
225. (a)	226. (a)	227. (a)	228. (a,b)	229. (a)	230. (a)	231. (a)	232. (a)
233. (b)	234. (a)	235. (c)	236. (d)	237. (b)	238. (a)	239. (a)	240. (a)
241. (d)	242. (a)	243. (a)	244. (a)	245. (b)	246. (d)	247. (a)	248. (a)
249. (b)	250. (c)	251. (c)	252. (a)	253. (b)	254. (a)	255. (a)	256. (a)
257. (b)	258. (d)	259. (a)	260. (e)	261. (b)	262. (a)	263. (a)	264. (b)
265. (a)	266. (b)	267. (b)	268. (a)	269. (b)	270. (a)	271. (d)	272. (a)
273. (b)	274. (a,c)	275. (a)	276. (a)	277. (a)	278. (a, d)	279. (a)	280. (b)
281. (d)	282. (c)	283. (b)	284. (b)	285. (c)	286. (c)	287. (b)	288. (d)
289. (a)	290. (a)	291. (a)	292. (a,b,d,c,e)	293. (a)	294. (c)	295. FTTF	296. TFF
297. FFFFF	298. (a)	299. (a,b,d)	300. (a,b)	301. (a,b,c)	302. (a,b,c)	303. (a,c,e)	304. (a,d,e)
305. (b)	306. (a,b,d)	307. (b)	308. (a,b)	309. (a,c,e)	310. (c)	311. (b)	312. (a)
313. (a)	314. (a)	315. (a)	316. (a)	317. (a)	318. (a)	319. (a)	320. (a)
321. (c,d,e)	322. FFTTT	323. (a)	324. (c)	325. (d)	326. (b)	327. (b)	328. (b)
329. (e)	330. (c)	331. (a)	332. (a)	333. (c)	334. (d)	335. (b, c)	336. TTTFT
337. (b)	338. TFFTT	339. TTFT	340. (a)	341. TTFTT	342. (c)	343. FFTFF	344. (c)
345. (b)	346. (c)	347. TFFTT	348. (a)	349. (f)	350. (a)	351. (c)	352. (a)

353.	FTTTF	354.	FFFFF	355.	FTTT	356.	FTFFT	357.	TFFFT	358.	FTFTT	359.	(c)	360.	(b)
361.	(a)	362.	(b)	363.	(c)	364.	(a)	365.	(a)	366.	(c)	367.	(b)	368.	(a)
369.	FTF	370.	(c)	371.	(b)	372.	(a)	373.	(d)	374.	(b)	375.	(b)	376.	(d)
377.	(a)	378.	(a)	379.	(b)	380.	(a)	381.	(a)	382.	(e)	383.	(a)	384.	TFFTT
385.	(c)	386.	(d)	387.	(e)	388.	(f)	389.	(c)	390.	(e)	391.	(c)	392.	(a)
393.	(a)	394.	(c)	395.	(a)	396.	(a)	397.	(a)	398.	(a)	399.	(c)	400.	(a)
401.	(c, e)	402.	(a)	403.	(a)	404.	(b)	405.	(a,b,c,d)	406.	(b)	407.	(a)	408.	(a)
409.	(c)	410.	(b)	411.	(a)	412.	(c)	413.	(a)	414.	(b)	415.	(a)	416.	(d)
417.	(b)	418.	(d)	419.	(a)	420.	(c)	421.	(c)	422.	(d)	423.	(a)	424.	(d)
425.	(a)	426.	(b)	427.	(a)	428.	(a)	429.	(b)	430.	(a)	431.	(d)	432.	(c)
433.	(d)	434.	(a)	435.	(a)	436.	(b)	437.	(a)	438.	(a)	439.	(a)	440.	(a)
441.	(d)	442.	(a)	443.	(a)	444.	(d)	445.	(a)	446.	(a)	447.	(c)	448.	(a)
449.	(d)	450.	(b)	451.	(a)	452.	(b)	453.	(c)	454.	(c)	455.	(a)	456.	(c)
457.	(d)	458.	(b)	459.	(c)	460.	(c)	461.	(d)	462.	(a)	463.	(b)	464.	(c)
465.	(d)	466.	(c)	467.	(c)	468.	(d)	469.	(c)	470.	(b)	471.	(d)	472.	(b)
473.	(a)	474.	(c)	475.	(d)	476.	(d)	477.	(b)	478.	(a)	479.	(a)	480.	(b)
481.	(a)	482.	(c)	483.	(a)	484.	(a)	485.	(b)	486.	(b)	487.	(a)	488.	(b)
489.	(d)	490.	(b)	491.	(a)	492.	(b)	493.	(d)	494.	(a)	495.	(b)	496.	(d)
497.	(d)	498.	(a)	499.	(b)	500.	(c)	501.	(b)	502.	(b)	503.	(c)	504.	(c)
505.	(b)	506.	(a)	507.	(a)	508.	(d)	509.	(a)	510.	(a)	511.	(b)	512.	(a)
513.	(a)	514.	(a)	515.	(a)	516.	(a)	517.	(d)	518.	(a)	519.	(d)	520.	(b)
521.	(a)	522.	(d)	523.	(a)	524.	(b)	525.	(a)	526.	(c)	527.	(a)	528.	(d)
529.	(a)	530.	(d)	531.	(c)	532.	(a)	533.	(a)	534.	(c)	535.	(d)	536.	(b)
537.	(c)	538.	(b)	539.	(c)	540.	(b)	541.	(a)	542.	(b)	543.	(a)	544.	(d)
545.	(a)	546.	(a)	547.	(b)	548.	(a)	549.	(a)	550.	(b)	551.	(c)	552.	(c)
553.	(d)	554.	(c)	555.	(b)	556.	(a)	557.	(c)	558.	(b)	559.	(a)	560.	(a)
561.	(b)	562.	(d)	563.	(a)	564.	(d)	565.	(c)	566.	(d)	567.	(a)	568.	(d)
569.	(c)	570.	(b)	571.	(d)	572.	(d)	573.	(d)	574.	(b)	575.	(b)	576.	(c)
577.	(b)	578.	(c)	579.	(a)	580.	(a)	581.	(b)	582.	(d)	583.	(b)	584.	(b)
585.	(c)	586.	(d)	587.	(a)	588.	(a)	589.	(b)	590.	(c)	591.	(a)	592.	(c)
593.	(a)	594.	(d)	595.	(d)	596.	(c)	597.	(b)	598.	(b,d)	599.	(e)	600.	(b)
601.	(a)	602.	(b)	603.	(c)	604.	(d)	605.	(a)	606.	(b)	607.	(c)	608.	(a)
609.	(b)	610.	(b)	611.	(b)	612.	(b)	613.	(a)	614.	(a)	615.	(a)	616.	(d)
617.	(c)	618.	(b)	619.	(a)	620.	(a)	621.	(d)	622.	(d)	623.	(c)	624.	(b)
625.	(c)	626.	(b)	627.	(b)	628.	(b)	629.	(b)	630.	(a)	631.	(a)	632.	(a)
633.	(c)	634.	(a)	635.	(d)	636.	(a)	637.	(d)	638.	(a)	639.	(b)	640.	(b)
641.	(a)	642.	(d)	643.	(c)	644.	(b)	645.	(d)	646.	(b)	647.	(b)	648.	(a)
649.	(c)	650.	(d)	651.	(c)	652.	(d)	653.	(b)	654.	(d)	655.	(b)	656.	(a)
657.	(b)	658.	(a)	659.	(c)	660.	(a)	661.	(c)	662.	(c)	663.	(a)	664.	(d)
665.	(d)	666.	(d)	667.	(c)	668.	(a)	669.	(a)	670.	(a)	671.	(c)	672.	(a)
673.	(c)	674.	(c)	675.	(a)	676.	(a)	677.	(c)	678.	(d)	679.	(b)	680.	(d)
681.	(d)	682.	(b)	683.	(a)	684.	(c)	685.	(a)	686.	(d)	687.	(a)	688.	(d)
689.	(a)	690.	(a)	691.	(d)	692.	(b)	693.	(a)	694.	(c)	695.	(b)	696.	(c)
697.	(b)	698.	(c)	699.	(b)	700.	(c)	701.	(d)	702.	(a)	703.	(d)	704.	(d)
705.	(d)	706.	(d)	707.	(a)	708.	(a)	709.	(b, c)	710.	(c)	711.	(a)	712.	(a)
713.	(c)	714.	(b)	715.	(c)	716.	(d)	717.	(c)	718.	(b)	719.	(c)	720.	(b)
721.	(c)	722.	(b)	723.	(a)	724.	(b)	725.	(c)	726.	(c)	727.	(d)	728.	(b)
729.	(c)	730.	(a)	731.	(b)	732.	(b)	733.	(c)	734.	(b)	735.	(a)	736.	(a)
737.	(a)	738.	(b)	739.	(d)	740.	(c)	741.	(a)	742.	(b)	743.	(a)	744.	(b)
745.	(b)	746.	(c)	747.	(a,c)	748.	(a)	749.	(b)	750.	(a)	751.	(a)	752.	(b)

753. (a)	754. (d)	755. (a)	756. (a)	757. (b)	758. (b)	759. (b)	760. (b)
761. (d)	762. (c)	763. (d)	764. (d)	765. (b)	766. (d)	767. (a)	768. (a)
769. (b)	770. (a)	771. (b)	772. (a)	773. (a)	774. (a)	775. (b)	776. (b)
777. (b)	778. (c)	779. (b)	780. (a)	781. (d)	782. (a)	783. (c)	784. (a)
785. (d)	786. (b)	787. (b)	788. (d)	789. (a)	790. (c)	791. (a)	792. (b)
793. (b)	794. (b)	795. (d)	796. (a)	797. (d)	798. (d)	799. (a, d)	800. (a)
801. (a)	802. (b)	803. (a)	804. (a)	805. (c)	806. (b)	807. (a)	808. (a)
809. (b)	810. (d)	811. (a)	812. (b)	813. (b)	814. (b)	815. (a)	816. (d)
817. (c)	818. (a)	819. (a)	820. (a)	821. (a)	822. (b)	823. (c)	824. (a)
825. (a)	826. (a)	827. (b)	828. (a)	829. (a)	830. (c)	831. (c)	832. (a)
833. (b)	834. (d)	835. (d)	836. (a)	837. (a)	838. (d)	839. (a)	840. (a)
841. (d)	842. (d)	843. (c)	844. (c)	845. (a)	846. (a)	847. (c)	848. (b)
849. (a)	850. (d)	851. (a)	852. (d)	853. (d)	854. (c)	855. (b)	856. (d)
857. (b)	858. (?)	859. (a)	860. (a)	861. (a)	862. (d)	863. (c)	864. (d)
865. (d)	866. TFFFT	867. FTFTT	868. FTTT	869. TFFFF	870. TTTTF	871. (a,c,d,e)	872. TFTT
873. TTFFT	874. TFTFF	875. FFFTT	876. TFTFF	877. TFFFT	878. TFFTT	879. TFTTT	880. TTTFF
881. FTFFF	882. TFFFT	883. TFFFT	884. FFTT	885. FTTFF	886. FTTFF	887. TTFF	888. TFTTF
889. FTTTF	890. FFTTT	891. FFTFT	892. TTFFT	893. FTTTT	894. FFFTT	895. FTTFT	896. FTFFF
897. FFFTT	898. FTFTF	899. FTFFF	900. FFTTT	901. TTTFT	902. FFTTT	903. FTTFT	904. TTTTF
905. FTTTT	906. TTTTT	907. FTFTF	908. TFTFT	909. FFFTF	910. TFTFT	911. TTTFT	912. FTFTT
913. TTFTT	914. TFTTF	915. FTFTT	916. FTFTT	917. TTFTF	918. TFFTT	919. TFFTT	920. TFFFF
921. FFTFT	922. FTTTT	923. FFTFF	924. TFTTF	925. FTTTF	926. FFTTT	927. FTFTF	928. TTTTT
929. FFFTT	930. TTTFF	931. TTTTF	932. FTTTT	933. FTTFF	934. TFFTF	935. TFFTF	936. FTFTF
937. TFFTF	938. TTFTT	939. TTFTT	940. TTFTT	941. TFTTT	942. TFFFT	943. FTFFF	944. FTTFF
945. TFFTF	946. TFTFF	947. FTTFT	948. FFTTT	949. TFFFF	950. TFFFF	951. TTFT	952. FFFFT
953. TFTFT	954. FFFFF	955. TFFFT	956. TTFTT	957. TTTTT	958. TTTTF	959. FFFTT	960. FFTFF
961. FFFFT	962. TTFFT	963. TTFFF)	964. TTFF	965. TFFTF	966. FTTFF	967. TTTTT	968. TTTFF
969. FTFF	970. FFFT	971. FTFFT	972. TTTFF	973. TFTFF	974. FFTFF	975. FFTFT	976. TTFFF
977. FFFTT	978. FFTTT	979. FTTTT	980. TTTFT	981. FTTTF	982. TFFT	983. TFFTF	984. FFTFT
985. TTFFT	986. TTTTT	987. TTTTF	988. FFFTT	989. FFTTF	990. TFTFF	991. TFTFF	992. TTFFF
993. TFTTF	994. FTTTT	995. FFFTF	996. FFFTT	997. FFTFF	998. TFFFF	999. FTTFF	1000. FTFTF
1001. TTFF	1002. FFFTT	1003. TTFFF	1004. TFTTF	1005. TFFFT	1006. TTTFF	1007. TFFFF	1008. FFFTT
1009. FTFTT	1010. TTFTT	1011. TTFFF	1012. TTTTF	1013. TFTTF	1014. TTTFF	1015. FTFFT	1016. TTFFF
1017. TTTTF	1018. TTFFT	1019. TTTFF	1020. TTTF	1021. TTTFF	1022. TFTT	1023. FF	1024. TTF
1025. TTFFF	1026. FTFTT	1027. FFTT	1028. (b)	1029. (a,b)	1030. (a)	1031. (a,b,d)	1032. (d)
1033. TTFTF	1034. TTFTF	1035. TFTFT	1036. TFFFF	1037. TTTFT	1038. TFTF	1039. FTFF	1040. FTTTT
1041. TTFFF	1042. (a)	1043. (b)	1044. (b)	1045. (b)	1046. (d)	1047. (a)	1048. (a)
1049. (a)	1050. (c)	1051. (a)	1052. (d)	1053. (d)	1054. (b)	1055. (b)	1056. (a)
1057. (a)	1058. (d)	1059. (a)	1060. (b)	1061. (d)	1062. (b)	1063. (d)	1064. (a)
1065. (a)	1066. (b)	1067. (c)	1068. (d)	1069. (c)	1070. (a)	1071. (b)	1072. (b)
1073. (a)	1074. (a)	1075. (d)	1076. (a)	1077. (a)	1078. (c)	1079. (a)	1080. (c)
1081. (b)	1082. (d)	1083. (c)	1084. (a)	1085. (c)	1086. (a)	1087. (d)	1088. (d)
1089. (b)	1090. (d)	1091. (d)	1092. (d)	1093. (b)	1094. (c)	1095. (c)	1096. (b)
1097. (a)	1098. (a)	1099. (a)	1100. (c)	1101. TFFT	1102. FTTF	1103. TTTT	1104. TTFFT
1105. FFTTT	1106. TF	1107. FFTTF	1108. FTFT	1109. FTF	1110. TFFT	1111. FFTTT	1112. TTF
1113. TTFF	1114. TFFF	1115. TFFTF	1116. FTFTT	1117. TTTFF	1118. TTTTT	1119. FTTTT	1120. TTTTT
1121. TTTTF	1122. TFFFF	1123. FTFTT	1124. FT	1125. TTTFT	1126. TTFTT	1127. FTFTT	1128. TTT
1129. TTT	1130. FTTF	1131. TFTTF	1132. (b)	1133. TTTFF	1134. TTTFT	1135. FFTTF	1136. FFTFT
1137. TTTT	1138. FFT	1139. FTTFT	1140. TTTFT	1141. TTFFF	1142. FF	1143. FTF	1144. FFTFT
1145. TFTTT	1146. TT	1147. FTF	1148. TTTTF	1149. FTFFT	1150. TTTT	1151. FTTF	1152. TFFFT
1153. TFTTT	1154. TTTTT	1155. FTFFT	1156. TFT	1157. FTFT	1158. TFTTT	1159. FTTFT	1160. FFTTT

1161. FFFFT	1162. TTFFF	1163. FFFTF	1164. TFTTT	1165. TFT	1166. FTTFT	1167. TTTTF	1168. TTTF
1169. TTTTF	1170. TTTTT	1171. FFTF	1172. TTTFF	1173. TTFF	1174. TFTFF	1175. TTFTT	1176. FFFTF
1177. TTTT	1178. TFTTT	1179. TTFTF	1180. TTTFT	1181. FFTFF	1182. FTFFF	1183. TTTT	1184. TFT
1185. FTFFT	1186. TTFTT	1187. TTTFT	1188. FTTFT	1189. FTTTF	1190. FFTT	1191. FFTTT	1192. TTFT
1193. FTTTF	1194. FFTFT	1195. T	1196. TFTTT	1197. TFTTF	1198. FFFTF	1199. (d)	1200. TFFT
1201. FFTFF	1202. FFFTTT	1203. FFTTF	1204. TTTTF	1205. TTTTF	1206. TTFTT	1207. TTTFFT	1208. TTTTF
1209. TFFTF	1210. TFTFTF	1211. TTTTT	1212. FTFTTFF	1213. TTTTF	1214. TTFTF	1215. TTTTF	1216. TTFFF
1217. FFFTF	1218. FTTFF	1219. FTFFT	1220. FTFFTT	1221. FFFF	1222. TTFTF	1223. TFTT	1224. FFTTT
1225. TTF	1226. TTTTT	1227. FTTFT	1228. TTTFF	1229. TFTT	1230. TTT	1231. (a)	1232. (d)
1233. (b)	1234. (a)	1235. (b)	1236. (b)	1237. (c)	1238. (a)	1239. (a)	1240. (a)
1241. (d)	1242. (d)	1243. (e)	1244. (e)	1245. (a)	1246. (c)	1247. (d)	1248. (a)
1249. (d)	1250. (a)	1251. (a)	1252. (c)	1253. (c)	1254. (a)	1255. (a)	1256. (a)
1257. (a)	1258. (a)	1259. (b)	1260. (a)	1261. (b)	1262. TT?F	1263. (b,c)	1264. (d)
1265. (b)	1266. (a)	1267. (a)	1268. (a)	1269. (c)	1270. (a)	1271. (a)	1272. (a)
1273. (d)	1274. (b)	1275. (c)	1276. (a)	1277. (b)	1278. (b)	1279. (a,c)	1280. (a)
1281. (a)	1282. (d)	1283. (b)	1284. (a)	1285. (d)	1286. (b)	1287. (a)	1288. (a)
1289. (a)	1290. (a)	1291. (c)	1292. (d)	1293. (c)	1294. (a)	1295. (d)	1296. (a)
1297. (c)	1298. (c)	1299. (c)	1300. (b)	1301. (a)	1302. (c)	1303. (a)	1304. (d)
1305. (c)	1306. (d)	1307. (c)	1308. (d)	1309. (a)	1310. (a)	1311. (a)	1312. (a)
1313. (a)	1314. (d)	1315. (c)	1316. (c)	1317. (b)	1318. (a)	1319. (a)	1320. (c)
1321. (b)	1322. (b)	1323. (b)	1324. (a)	1325. (d)	1326. (a)	1327. (a)	1328. (a)
1329. (a)	1330. (a)	1331. (c)	1332. (c)	1333. (c)	1334. (b)	1335. (b)	1336. (b)
1337. (c)	1338. (b)	1339. (e)	1340. (b)	1341. (b)	1342. (a)	1343. (b)	1344. (b)
1345. (b)	1346. (b)	1347. (a)	1348. (b)	1349. (a)	1350. (a)	1351. (a)	1352. (b)
1353. (a)	1354. (c)	1355. (a)	1356. (c)	1357. (c)	1358. (b)	1359. (c)	1360. (a)
1361. (a)	1362. (a)	1363. (b)	1364. (b)	1365. (a)	1366. (a)	1367. (b)	1368. (d)
1369. (d)	1370. (a)	1371. (a)	1372. (c)	1373. (d)	1374. (b)	1375. (a)	1376. (d)
1377. (d)	1378. (c)	1379. (c)	1380. (a)	1381. (a)	1382. (d)	1383. (a)	1384. (d)
1385. (c)	1386. (a)	1387. (a)	1388. (d)	1389. (a)	1390. (a)	1391. (b)	1392. (a)
1393. (a)	1394. (a)	1395. (a)	1396. (a)	1397. (a)	1398. (a)	1399. (a)	1400. (c)
1401. (c)	1402. (d)	1403. (a)	1404. (a)	1405. (a)	1406. (c)	1407. (d)	1408. (d)
1409. (a)	1410. (b)	1411. (a)	1412. (c)	1413. (b)	1414. (a)	1415. (c)	1416. (b)
1417. (a)	1418. (a)	1419. (?)	1420. (a)	1421. (a)	1422. (c)	1423. (c)	1424. (a)
1425. (c)	1426. (a)	1427. (c)	1428. (b)	1429. (b)	1430. (c)	1431. (a)	1432. (b)
1433. (a)	1434. (b)	1435. (d)	1436. (c)	1437. (b)	1438. (b)	1439. (c)	1440. (b)
1441. (b)	1442. (a)	1443. (d)	1444. (b)	1445. (c)	1446. (b)	1447. (a)	1448. (d)
1449. (d)	1450. (b)	1451. (c)	1452. (a)	1453. (c)	1454. (d)	1455. (b)	1456. (b)
1457. (c)	1458. (c)	1459. (c)	1460. (d)	1461. (d)	1462. (a)	1463. (d)	1464. (a)
1465. (b)	1466. (b)	1467. (c)	1468. (d)	1469. (b)	1470. (a)	1471. (c)	1472. (a)
1473. (a)	1474. (a)	1475. (a)	1476. (d)	1477. (b)	1478. (d)	1479. (b)	1480. (a)
1481. (b)	1482. (a)	1483. (a)	1484. (d)	1485. (b)	1486. (c)	1487. (b)	1488. (c)
1489. (c)	1490. (d)	1491. (b)	1492. (a)	1493. (b)	1494. (a)	1495. (a)	1496. (a)
1497. (c)	1498. (a)	1499. (d)	1500. (b)	1501. (d)	1502. (d)	1503. (b)	1504. (a)
1505. (b)	1506. (d)	1507. (b)	1508. (a)	1509. (b)	1510. (c)	1511. (b)	1512. (d)
1513. (c)	1514. (b)	1515. (b)	1516. (b)	1517. (c)	1518. (c)	1519. (c)	1520. (a)
1521. (d)	1522. (b)	1523. (c)	1524. (d)	1525. (a)	1526. (d)	1527. (b)	1528. (c)
1529. (d)	1530. (d)	1531. (c)	1532. (a)	1533. (c)	1534. (d)	1535. (c)	1536. (c)
1537. (a)	1538. (a)	1539. (a)	1540. (a)	1541. (a)	1542. FFFT	1543. (a)	1544. (b)
1545. (c)	1546. (d)	1547. (c)	1548. (d)	1549. (a)	1550. (b)	1551. (a)	1552. (c)
1553. (a)	1554. (b)	1555. (a)	1556. (c)	1557. (b)	1558. (b)	1559. (a)	1560. (a)
1561. (b)	1562. (d)	1563. (b)	1564. (a)	1565. (c)	1566. (b)	1567. (b)	1568. (b)

CHAPTER THREE

VALVULAR HEART DISEASE

1.

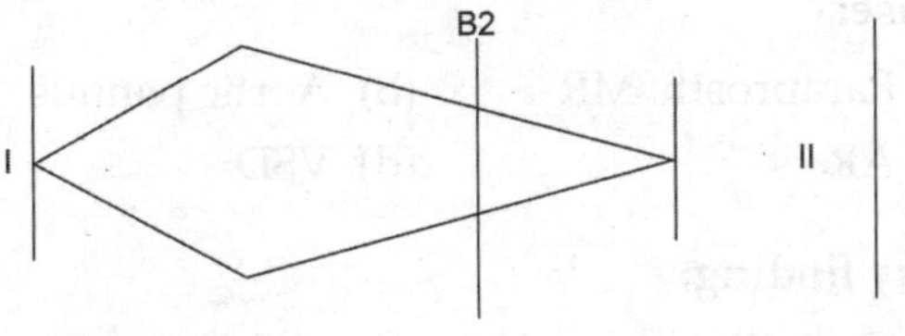

12-year-old with:
(a) TOF (b) AS
(c) PS (d) Supracristal VSD

2.

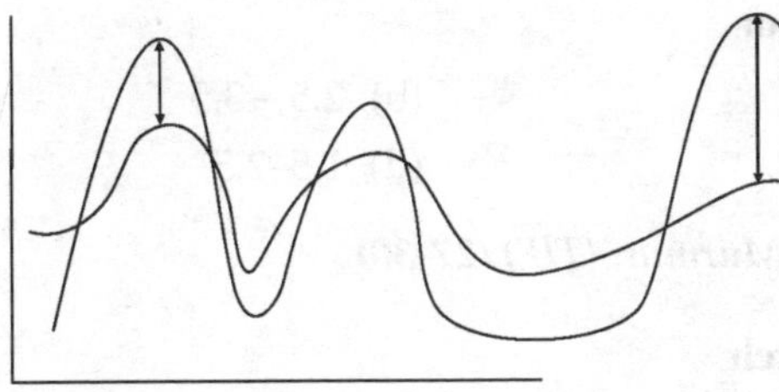

Clinically seen:
(a) Bisferiens pulse
(b) Ejection click
(c) Family history of cardiac disease
(d) Murmur–on standing

3. **Y descent not seen in:**
(a) Tamponade (b) CP
(c) RCM

4. **Chronic AR severity marker:**
(a) Graham Steel murmur
(b) ESM
(c) Reverse S_2 split
(d) Loud diastolic murmur

5. **Endocarditis by listeria is seen in patients with:**
(a) Burn (b) Ureteric stent
(c) Tooth extraction (d) IV drug user

6. **Severe MS with left atrial enlargement, not associated with:**
(a) HTN (b) PAPVC
(c) Severe anemia (d) MI

7. **2nd IC space thrill in ASD A/E:**
(a) Lutembacher (b) Eisenmenger
(c) MR (d) Pulmonary murmur

8. **Elderly patient on examination not seen:**
(a) LVS_4
(b) Orthostatic hypotension is not normal
(c) Wide PP
(d) Wide pulse pressure

9. **Major criteria for rheumatic fever in Indian scenario:**
(a) Polyarthralgia
(b) Fever-
(c) –ESR
(d) 1st degree HB

10. **Aortic valve gradient A/E:**
(a) Peak instantaneous > peak to peak gradient
(b) Low gradient may be seen severe AS
(c) Peak instantaneous measured by Doppler
(d) Catheter pullback from LV to aorta decrease pressure

11. **Which is least common in streptococcal sore throat?**
(a) Fever
(b) Cough
(c) Tender lymphadenopathy
(d) Painful deglutition

12. **IE least common in:**
(a) Small PDA
(b) Small VSD
(c) TOF
(d) Obstructive TAPVC

13. **Elevated LAP in MS is caused by all *except*:**
(a) SV-ASD
(b) Anemia

(c) Systemic hypertension
(d) LV dysfunction

14. Acute rheumatic – all T/E:
(a) RHD–1/3rd have infection history
(b) In epidermic 3%
(c) In endemic 1/10th of epidemic
(d) Erythromycin is better in epidermic areas

15. Criteria for acute rheumatic (recurrent) fever:
(a) 2 major or 1 major + 2 minor or 3 minor
(b) 1 major
(c) 1 major + 2 minor
(d) 1 major + 2 minor

16. Updated ARF epidemiology low endemic risk defined as:
(a) < 1/100000 school age
(b) < 2
(c) < 3
(d) < 4

17. Updated ARF – low endemic risk area, minor criteria:
(a) > 38.0 (b) > 38.5
(c) > 37.5 (d) 39.5

18. Minor criteria in modified Duke *except*:
(a) Predisposing heart disease
(b) IV drug abuse
(c) Fever
(d) New cardiac murmur

19. AS patient asymptomatic, could walk for 4 miles/hr but wife tells the patient was breathless, management is:
(a) Echo to measure gradient and monitor
(b) Treadmill test
(c) Wait and watch for symptoms
(d) CAG

20. Coel-Cecil murmur:
(a) AR (b) MR
(c) TR (d) PR

21. Diastolic murmur seen in:
(a) CHB (b) PDA with PAH
(c) Small PDA (d) CoA

22. C/I of BMV – A/E:
(a) Moderate AR
(b) Large clot
(c) MR severe
(d) Commissural calcification

23. High risk peg A/E:
(a) MR (b) 1 PHTN
(c) Cyanotic heart lesion (d) Prosthetic heart valve

Young patient with History of – DVR→fever, taken medication from local practitioner, fever resolved. After some time patient has murmur at apex→radiation to parasternal, with mild basal crepts/normal JVP (24–26)

24. Cause:
(a) Paraprosth. MR (b) Aortic pannus
(c) AR (d) VSD

25. X-ray finding:
(a) Cephalization only→upper lob diversion
(b) ↑ PBF
(c) Normal CXR
(d) Kerley B line

26. INR ratio:
(a) 2.3 (b) 2.5 – 3.5
(c) 3–4 (d) 1.5–2.5

Graham Steel Murmur: (T/F) (27-30)

27. High pitch

28. Positive in absent PV

29. Decresendo

30. Hyperkinetic PHTN

31. Thrombosis in prosthetic valve A/E:
(a) Tilting disc in aortic position is low risk
(b) Mitral 1.5 times the risk compared to low risk patients
(c) 9% annual risk of thrombosis due to discontinuation of warfarin in aortic prostheses

32. Paradoxical pulse absent in A/E:
(a) ASD
(b) AR
(c) LV dysfunction
(d) Malignant etiology

33. The most prevalent anatomy for a bicuspid valve:
(a) Fusion of the right and left coronary cusps

(b) Fusion of the left and non coronary cusps
(c) Fusion of the right and non coronary cusps
(d) None

34. All are causes of late systolic murmur *except:*

(a) Acute myocardial ischemia
(b) Mitral valve prolapse
(c) Normotensive TR
(d) Tricuspid valve prolapse

35. Identify the wrong statement in infective endocarditis:

(a) Fever may be absent in 20% of patients
(b) Risk of IE in patients with bicuspid aortic valve is high, about 10%
(c) Bicuspid aortic valve is a strong independent predictor of periannular complications
(d) Preexisting valvular regurgitant lesions are fax more prone to infection than stenotic lesions

36. Following organism is likely to cause acute presentation during infective endocarditis:

(a) Streptococcus sanguis
(b) Staphylococcus epidermidis
(c) Staphylococcus aureus
(d) Enterococcus fecalis

37. Which of the following is not true about HACEK organisms?

(a) Slow growing
(b) Require carbon dioxide
(c) Normally reside in oral cavity
(d) Gram positive bacteria

38. On cultures Brucella species may be misidentified as:

(a) Agro bacterium (b) Ochrobacterium
(c) Both A and B (d) A only

39. Antibiotic prophylaxis to a child with rheumatic heart disease should be given minimum till:

(a) At least 5 years after onset
(b) Lifelong
(c) Till 17 years
(d) Till 21 years

40. 1st heart sound: (T/F)

(a) Due to high frequency comp. of closure of mitral and tricuspid valve
(b) Can be loud in wpw
(c) Can be loud in AS
(d) Auscultatory alternans in severe card. tamponade
(e) S1 coincides/just after carotid downstroke

41. ARF: (T/F)

(a) Muddy brown granular cast–acute glomerulonephritis
(b) Flank pain – S/O – acute pyelonephritis
(c) Pre. Renal ARF fr Na > 1
(d) Hyperphosphatemia – S/O–tumor lysis syndrome
(e) Cosinophiluria in interstitial nephritis

42. Regarding prosthetic heart valves: (T/F)

(a) Tilting disc valves have superior hemodynamic compared to bileaflat and caged ball valves
(b) Dabigatran is superior to warfarin for thromboprophylaxis in mechanical heart valves
(c) Tilting disc and bileaflet valves have mild (5-10 ml) regurgitation
(d) Short diastolic murmur is normal finding in tilting disc valve in aortic position
(e) Structural deterioration is lesser in elderly > 65 years compared to young patients

43. Auscultatory findings of 'Squatting': (T/F)

(a) Augmentation of LVS$_3$ and LVS$_4$
(b) Muffling of RV S$_3$ and S$_4$
(c) Diastolic murmur of MS becomes louder
(d) Systolic murmur of MR decreases
(e) Murmur of HCM soften

44. Regarding 'acute MR': (T/F)

(a) Soft low pitched, early systolic decrescendo murmur
(b) Heard in apex and radiates to axilla
(c) IABP has no benefit
(d) 50% cases of moderate to severe MR have minimal auscultatory findings
(e) Nitroprusside decreases regurgitation by decreasing SVR

45. Aortic regurgitation: (T/F)

(a) de Musset sign positive in mild AR
(b) Becker's sign–alternate constriction and dilation of retinal artery and pupils
(c) Murmur intensity may be decreased in severe LV dysfunction
(d) Muller sign present
(e) Soft S1

46. PAH in MS: (T/F)

(a) It completely resolves after balloon mitral valvotomy

(b) Dyspnea improves with the onset of obliterative vascular changes
(c) It has fibrinoid necrosis and plexiform lesion
(d) Fick's method of CO is unreliable
(e) In suprasystemic RV pressure–BMV CI

47. Regarding acute rheumatic fever: (T/F)
(a) History of pharyngitis in 2/3rd of cases
(b) Elevated levels of serum mannose binding protein
(c) Chorea has long latent period
(d) M protein reacts with myosin
(E) Oligoarthritis is most common

48. Regarding acute rheumatic fever: (T/F)
(a) Carditis in 50% of cases
(b) Polyarthritis is present in 60-75%
(c) Erythema marginatum 10%
(d) Subcutaneous nodules 4%
(e) Prevalence of chorea 50%

49. Wilkin score is used for:
(a) Mitral stenosis (b) Pulmonary stenosis
(c) Aortic stenosis (d) Tricuspid stenosis

50. Rupture of chordae tendinae to posterior mitral leaflet produces prominent murmur over following area:
(a) Apex (b) Axilla
(c) Base of heart (d) Left scapular

51. Which one of the following is not used for the surgical treatment of tricuspid regurgitation?
(a) Metalic valve (b) Bioprosthesis
(c) Suture annuloplasty (d) Ring annuloplasty

52. Which one of the following is not true for mechanical prosthetic valve?
(a) Bileaflet valve (b) Trileaflet valve
(c) Ball and cage valve (d) Tilting disc valve

53. Which one of the following is true for oral anti-coagulation after bioprosthetic mitral valve surgery?
(a) It is not required
(b) It is required for the first 1 year
(c) It is required for the first 3 months
(d) It is required lifelong

54. Which one of the following is recommended after mechanical valve replacement?
(a) Only vitamin K antagonist anticoagulant
(b) Aspirin + Clopidogrel
(c) Vitamin K antagonist anticoagulant + aspirin
(d) Vitamin K antagonist anticoagulant + Dipyridamole

55. Which one of the following organisms is associated with culture negative endocarditis?
(a) Salmonella (b) Coxiella burnetii
(c) Pseudomonas species (d) Enterococcus faecalis

56. Streptococcus gallolyticus endocarditis is commonly associated with:
(a) Cirrhosis of liver (b) Gastrointestinal lesion
(c) Skin lesions (d) Uremia

57. Following is not true for Janeway lesions:
(a) It is painless hemorrhagic macules
(b) Common over soles and palms
(c) Commonly associated with staphylococcal endocarditis
(d) It results from immune complex deposition and focal vasculitis

58. According to modified Duke's criteria, following is not true for diagnosis of infective endocarditis:
(a) 2 major criteria
(b) 5 minor criteria
(c) 1 major and 2 minor criteria
(d) 1 major and 3 minor criteria

59. Which one of the following is not an indication for surgery in patients with infective endocarditis?
(a) Persistence of vegetation after antimicrobial therapy
(b) Highly mobile vegetation of > 10 mm size over anterior mitral leaflet
(c) Embolic episodes during first 2 weeks of therapy
(d) Valve perforation

60. In AIDS patients with infective endocarditis following organism is uncommon as a causative organism for endocarditis:
(a) Salmonella species
(b) Streptococcus pneumoniae
(c) Streptococcus aureus
(d) Clostridium septicum

61. Which one of the following is not true for Jaccoud arthritis?
(a) It occurs after repeated attacks of rheumatic fever

(b) It is painless without signs of inflammation
(c) Ulnar deviation of 4th and 5th fingers are common
(d) Hyperextension of metacarpophalangeal joints are common

62. **Which one of the following is not true for Sydenham chorea in rheumatic fever?**
(a) It may persist for 2 years
(b) It is never unilateral (hemichorea)
(c) It does not occur simultaneously with arthritis
(d) Emotional lability is common

63. **Which one of the following is not true for subcutaneous nodules in rheumatic fever?**
(a) Usually firm and painful
(b) Freely movable over the subcutaneous tissue
(c) Usual size is 0.5 cm to 2 cm
(d) Occurs in crops

64. **Which one of the following is not true for erythema marginatum in rheumatic fever?**
(a) The rash is evanescent, pink and non pruritic
(b) It has irregular serpingious border
(c) It becomes less prominent after taking hot bath
(d) It extends centrifugally, whereas skin at centre returns to normal

65. **Regarding native valve endocarditis (NVE), which of the following statements is true?**
(a) Modified Duke's criteria emphasize on persistently positive blood cultures, except for Cardiobacterium species where single positive blood culture is sufficient
(b) Hacek NVE has been associated with large vegetations and a high incidence of systemic emboli
(c) Mobile vegetations > 10 mm is a Class I indication of surgery for NVE
(d) Ceftriaxone 2 gm once daily for 4 weeks plus gentamycin 3 mg/kg/day IM for 2 weeks may be the standard therapy for enterococcal endocarditis

66. **Prophylaxis of infective endocarditis in highest risk patients is indicated for which of the following procedures?**
(a) Bronchoscopy or laryngoscopy
(b) Placement or adjustment of removable prosthodontic or orthodontic appliances or braces
(c) Colonoscopy or transesophageal echocardiography
(d) None of the above

67. **Absolute contraindications for transcatheter aortic valve implantation include all *except:***
(a) Estimated life expectancy > 1 year
(b) Annulus size < 18 mm
(c) Annulus size > 29 mm
(d) Thrombus in the left ventricle

68. **Contraindications to percutaneous mitral commissurotomy includes:**
(a) Mild mitral regurgitation
(b) Unicommissural calcification
(c) Left atrial thrombus
(d) Moderate tricuspid regurgitation

69. **Which of the following factors does not favor choosing mechanical prosthesis over bioprosthesis?**
(a) Patients at risk of accelerated structural valve deterioration
(b) Age > 65 years
(c) For whom future redo valve surgery would be at high risk
(d) Patients already on anticoagulation as a result of having a mechanical prosthesis in another valve position

70. **Which of the following is not an auscultatory finding of severe mitral stenosis?**
(a) Loud S1 (b) Opening snap
(c) Loud P2 (d) LV S3

71. **Normotensive TR occurs in all *except:***
(a) Ebstein's anomaly (b) Right sided EMF
(c) Pulmonary embolism (d) Trauma

72. **Paradoxically split S2 is heard in:**
(a) VSD (b) MR
(c) Severe AS (d) All of the above

73. **Prominent X descent is seen in:**
(a) Tricuspid stenosis (b) Cardiac tamponade
(c) Both of the above (d) None of the above

74. **Hemodynamic improvement not seen only with rate control and rhythm control–necessary in:**
(a) MS (b) AR
(c) MR (d) HOCM

75. Rheumatic fever without carditis–prophylaxis for:
(a) 10 years or 21 years (b) 40 years
(c) 5 years or 21 years (d) Lifelong

76. Amyl nitrate–murmur increased is:
(a) MR/ (b) AR/
(c) TR/ (d) Austin Flint murmur

77. Inflammation in severe AS–reflected by:
(a) CRP (b) Trop T
(c) CPK (d) BNP

78. Severe AS–24 weeks pregnancy, best approach:
(a) Aortic balloon valvotomy
(b) AVR
(c) Medical therapy
(d) Termination

79. Most common cause of IE post prosthetic valve replacement:
(a) S. aureus
(b) Coagulase negative staph
(c) Streptococcus
(d) Pneumococcus

80. IE major criteria is:
(a) New valve regurgitation
(b) Fever
(c) ICH
(d) Roth spots

81. Loeffler's carditis A/E:
(a) CCF
(b) Eosinophilia
(c) Asthma and nasal polyps
(d) Thromboembolism

82. Most common cause of early prosthetic valve IE:
(a) Staph. epidermidis (b) Staph. aureus
(c) Streptococcus (d) E. coli

83. Split SI common in A/E:
(a) MS (b) TS
(c) RBBB (d) Ebstein

84. Severe AR A/E:
(a) Diastolic MR
(b) Jet occupying most of LV
(c) Diastolic flow reversal in aorta
(d) PHT > 500

85. Severe patient-prosthetic mismatch for aortic prosthesis is indexed orifice area less than:
(a) 0.55 cm^2/m^2 (b) 0.65 cm^2/m^2
(c) 0.75 cm Vm^2 (d) 0.85 cm^2/m^2

86. All are true about transcatheter aortic valve implantation *except:*
(a) Catheter implantation of aortic valve was first accomplished in 2002
(b) SAPIEN valve incorporates a balloon-expandable stainless steel stent frame
(c) Transvalvular regurgitation is rare, but paravalvular regurgitation is common
(d) Cardiac arrhythmias are a major cause of mortality and morbidity complicating TAVI

87. A 32-year-old premenopausal married female presented with rheumatic heart disease and severe aortic stenosis (LVEF 40%) with 2 early abortions due to APLA syndrome. True statement is:
(a) AVR: only if symptoms present
(b) Must undergo CAG followed by AVR with metallic valve ± CABG
(c) CAdG not required before AVR
(d) AVR with bioprosthetic valve preferred over metallic valve

88. According to revised Jones criteria 2015, 'low risk' population is defined as incidence of ARF in:
(a) <4/100000 school aged children
(b) <3/100000 school aged children
(c) <2/100000 school aged children
(d) <1/100000 school aged children

89. Juvenile mitral stenosis is defined as predominant or pure mitral stenosis in age:
(a) < 20 years (b) < 18 years
(c) < 15 years (d) < 12 years

90. Strongest association of clinical risk factor in epidemiological studies and calcific aortic valve disease is found in:
(a) Age (b) Male sex
(c) Body mass index (d) Dyslipidemia

91. Type IIIA mitral regurgitation in caused by:
(a) Ischemic cardiomyopathy
(b) Marfan syndrome
(c) Barlow syndrome
(d) Radiation

92. Findings in congenital mitral stenosis includes all *except:*
(a) Loud S_1

(b) MDM with presystolic accentuation
(c) No opening snap
(d) AF is rare in children

93. A homograft is the preferred valve choice in the following scenario:
(a) A 45-year-old man with aortic valve endocarditis and aortic root abscess in the presence of a bicuspid aortic valve
(b) A 30-year-old man with a non-repairable aortic bicuspid valve in the setting of severe symptomatic aortic insufficiency
(c) A 68-year-old woman with chronic lymphocytic leukemia, who has rheumatic mitral stenosis that is not amenable to valvuloplasty
(d) A 70-year-old woman with a non-repairable aortic bicuspid valve in the setting of severe symptomatic aortic insufficiency

94. All are true regarding primary prevention of rheumatic fever *except:*
(a) Involves antibiotic treatment of presumed/proven GAS pharyngitis
(b) Simpler than primordial prevention
(c) Oral penicillin preferred over benzathine penicillin in young children
(d) There is one fewer case of rheumatic fever for every 50-60 patients of GAS pharyngitis treated with antibiotics

95. All are criteria for pathological MR in rheumatic valvulitis *except:*
(a) Seen in atleast 2 views
(b) Jel length > 2 cm in at least 1 view
(c) Peak velocity > 2 m/s
(d) Pansystolic jet in at least one envelope

96. According to revised Jones criteria 2015, in high risk population for ARF, all are true *except:*
(a) Subclinical carditis is a major criterion
(b) Mono arthritis is a major criterion
(c) ESR > 60/hour is a minor criterion
(d) Fever > 38°C is a minor criterion

97. In chronic MR or AR, LVEDP doesn't increase due to:
(a) Right shift of PV curve
(b) Left shift of PV curve
(c) ↑ contractility of LV

98. Paradoxical split A/E:
(a) AS (b) PDA
(c) VSD (d) DCM

99. Acute AR A/E:
(a) Hypotension
(b) S_3 and S_4
(c) Absent Austin Flint

100. RHD patient anticoagulant alternate to warfarin:
(a) Dabigatran (b) Rivaroxaban
(c) Apixaban (d) None

101. PARTNER trial:
(a) Aortic valve (TAVI) (b) AVR
(c) Perulaneous MVR (d) MS

102. IE prophylaxis for:
(a) PFO closure of 3 months
(b) PDA closed 1 year back
(c) BAV

103. Surgery for IE done for A/E:
(a) Mobile veg > 10 min
(b) Not responding to antibiotics after 2 weeks
(c) New heart failure
(d) New heart block

104. AS patient with syncope, survival:
(a) 5 years (b) 3 years
(c) 2 years (d) 1 year

105. 12 years + mild AS + ESM radiating to carotid S/O:
(a) BAV fusion Rt and Lt cusp
(b) BAV fusion Rt and NC cusp
(c) Unicuspid
(d) Quadricuspid

106. Pul ejection click A/E:
(a) ↑ with inspiration (b) ↓ with inspiration
(c) Variable effect (d) No effect

107. 72/male insulin require DM, create—2.1 mg%, post CABG for TVD. AS Gradient–104 mm Hg, NYHA II dyspnoea, management should be:
(a) Medical (b) Bioprosthetic valve
(c) Mechanical (d) TAVI

108. Severity of MS does not depend on:
(a) Intensity of murmur
(b) Duration of murmur
(c) A2- OS gap
(d) Severity of pulmonary HTN

109. Highest risk for I.E.:

(a) Large VSD (b) Severe AR
(c) Severe MS (d) TAPVC

110. True regarding infective endocarditis A/E:

(a) Cerebral angiography should be done in children with streptococcal infection
(b) Salmonella typhi is uncommon organisms for IE
(c) Methicillin should not be prescribed for staph epidermidis
(d) Colonoscopy should be done in elderly with streptococcal bovis infection

111. Acute streptococcal pharyngitis in children. Not seen:

(a) Fever
(b) Tonsil enlargement
(c) Coryza
(d) Tender cervical lymphadenopathy

112. Recurrent rheumatic fever–WHO criteria:

(a) Any 1 major
(b) Minor + H/O strepicoccoal infection RHD patient
(c) Scarlet Fever history not included
(d) Evidence of recent streptococcal infection recurrence

113. Most severe IE infections:

(a) Fungal (b) Staph aureus
(c) Enterococci (d) Streptococcus viridans

114. I.E. prophylaxis A/E:

(a) Prosthetic valve
(b) Ischemic MR
(c) Post transplant vasculopathy
(d) Prior I.E.

115. AS A/E:

(a) RHD most common cause in < 10 years
(b) Annuloaortic ectasia in 12-20 % of RHD
(c) Surgical valvotomy is TOC in children

116. RHD echo A/E:

(a) School health programme include echo
(b) Suspected RHD do not need penicillin prophylaxis
(c) Echo criteria increases prevalence than present criteria
(d) World federation criteria

117. Pansystolic murmur all *except:*

(a) MVP (b) Ebstein anomaly
(c) PAH (d) Ischemic VSD

118. Diagnostic criteria for recurrent RF true:

(a) Gp A streptococci evidence must
(b) 1 major criteria with RHD
(c) 1 minor criteria
(d) Scarlet fever not included in strep. infection evidence

119. Recurrent IE common with:

(a) Fungal (b) Staph. aureus
(c) Viridans streptococci (d) Enterobacter

120. Not a sign of streptococcal pharyngitis:

(a) Coryza (b) Cervical LAP
(c) Fever (d) Tonsillar swelling

121. I.E. in aortic valve all *except:*

(a) Subaortic membrane high risk factor for I.E.
(b) Risk of I.E. in AS is directly proportional to degree of severity of AS
(c) Chances of I.E. in AR is > 50% than AS
(d) I.E. in aortic valve rarer than mitral valve

122. Relapse of I.E. is most common in:

(a) Candida albicans
(b) Strept. Viridans
(c) Enterobacteriace family
(d) Staph. aureus

123. Pansystolic murmur all *except:*

(a) Traumatic TR (b) Post MI VSD
(c) MVP (d) Pulmonary HTN

124. Latent tricuspid stenosis detected by all *except:*

(a) IV atropine (b) Isometric exercise
(c) Passive leg raising (d) Slow IV fluid infusion

125. Primigravida variable S1, mild MS, MVA-1.6, PASP= 30 mm Hg HR-140, BP-90/50. Best management would be:

(a) Rate control by digoxin and diltiazem
(b) Cardioversion
(c) Emergency BMV
(d) Amiodarone

126. IE in elderly true:

(a) Majority from GI/GU source

(b) More in women
(c) Good prognosis because effects degenerated valve
(d) Peripheral signs are common

127. TS all *except:*
(a) PND (b) EF slope ↓ed
(c) Fatigue (d) Atrial arrhythmia

128. Gorlin formula for MV include all *except:*
(a) HR
(b) Mean gradient
(c) Systolic ejection period
(d) CO

129. BAV with gradient > 45 mm Hg with aortic root dilatation of 46 mm with class II angina treatment:
(a) Medical management (b) Bioprosthetic valve
(c) Mech valve (d) Bental procedure

130. Syncope in AS:
(a) Cardio inhibitory
(b) Does not affect prognosis
(c) Varodepressor
(d) Pacemaker required

131. 15/F presented with HF with significant radio-femoral delay:
(a) Takayasu arteritis (b) SLE
(c) COA (d) Neurofibromatosis

132. Rh fever cause of abdominal pain:
(a) Peritoneal inflammation
(b) Gastritis
(c) Splanchnic Vc
(d) Pyuria

133. IE highest risk:
(a) RHD (b) Prosthetic valve
(c) I/V drug user (d) MVP with MR

134. IE all *except:*
(a) Mycotic aneurysm common in splenic and splanchnic
(b) Gram +ve organisms
(c) Embolism in vasovasorum
(d) Routine screening not recommended

135. May recurrence of following treatment in RF:
(a) I/V Benztheine penicillin < 3 weeks
(b) I/V benztheine penicillin 4 weekly
(c) Sulfonamide
(d) Oral penicillin

136. Most common site of Aschoff nodule in RF:
(a) Atrial surface of MV
(b) Ventricular surface of AV
(c) Ventricular surface of MV
(d) Subendothelium of atria and ventricule

137. All can be seen in acute RF *except:*
(a) Isolated pericarditis (b) Pancarditis
(c) Isolated myocarditis (d) Isolated valvulitis

138. M1 T1 all *except:*
(a) M1 after 30 msec of LA to LV pr. crossover
(b) Sustained hand grip ↓ M1 T1 interval
(c) T1 concides with down slope of 'a' wave of RA
(d) ↓ PR loud S1

139. False statement:
(a) Most common community acquired staph MRSA
(b) I/E ↑ with age
(c) Rifampicin 6 weeks for PVE staph
(d) Strept. viridans–vancomycin better than penicillin

140. False statement:
(a) Endocarditis in MVP female common
(b) Chance of IE, MS < MR
(c) Staph bacteremia is major duke criteria
(d) Prophylaxis for GI is not recommended

141. Acute RF 1944 not in a criteria:
(a) Erythema nodosum
(b) Subcutaneous nodules
(c) Carditis
(d) Chorea

142. Cor bovinum:
(a) AR (b) MR
(c) TR (d) PR

143. Anasarca, ascites in a case of MS:
(a) PA pressure
(b) TR
(c) Decrease lymphatic drainage

144. Double valve replacement done, new onset AR A/E:
(a) Murmur seen (b) Peripheral sign seen
(c) S_1 soft (d) S_3 present

145. Severe AS suggested by gradient:
(a) 70 (b) 50
(c) 25 (d) > 100

146. Kerley 'A' line in MS indicate:
(a) Mild MS (b) Moderate MS
(c) Severe MS (d) Associated MR

147. Maximum effective orifice area in which condition of mitral valve?
(a) Bileaflet (b) Heterograft
(c) Ball cage valve

148. Which is not a vascular phenomenon?
(a) Roth spot
(b) Janeway lesion
(c) Mycotic aneurysm
(d) Septic pulmonary infarct

149. Mitral annular calcification seen in all *except*:
(a) HOCM (b) Juvenile MS
(c) Hyperparathyroidism

150. Severe MR true are all *except*:
(a) Axillary radiation of murmur
(b) Flow murmur of mitral valve
(c) Loudness (intensity IV or more)
(d) Cardiomegaly

151. Mitral valve used with pressure half time 540 ms:
(a) 0.6 (b) 0.7
(c) 0.8 (d) 0.9

152. Migratory arthritis in rheumatic fever all *except*:
(a) Mostly involve small joints
(b) HIP rarely involvement
(c) NSAIDs and salicylates after confirmation
(d) Last for few weeks

153. Valvular AS is diagnosed by:
(a) Clinical examination (b) ECG
(c) History

154. AF with highest risk of embolism with previous 1E:
(a) AF with previous history of previous embolism
(b) AF with DVT month
(c) AF with prosthetic valve 1 month
(d) AF recent onset

155. Indication of surgery in PVE:
(a) Fungal infection (b) HF
(c) Large Vegetation (d) Conduction block
(e) All

156. Indication of AVR in AS:
(a) Mean gradient >50 mm Hg
(b) Peak to peak gradient >50 mm Hg
(c) Area — 0.7-0.9 cm/BSA

157. IE–most common renal manifestation is:
(a) Interstitial GN (b) Crescentric GN
(c) Membranous GN (d) FSGS

158. S3 associated with:
(a) Rapid filling phase (b) Protodiastolic filling
(c) Atrial contraction

159. Reverse splitting:
(a) LBBB (b) RBBB
(c) MR

160. Tricuspid aortic stenosis calcification risk factor A/E:
(a) Age (b) ↑ LDL
(c) Unequal cusps (d) HTN

161. Mitral stenosis with absent OS:
(a) Mild AS
(b) Severe AR
(c) Thickened mitral leaflet
(d) CAD

162. Original Jones criteria in:
(a) 1940 (b) 1942
(c) 1944

163. A2—Mitral valve opening interval is:
(a) IVRT (b) DT
(c) IVCT

164. Subaortic stenosis, best view:
(a) 60° LAO with 25° cranial
(b) RAO
(c) AP
(d) 30° LAO

165. Rheumatic nodule A/E:
(a) In severe carditis
(b) Tender
(c) On extensor surfaces
(d) Peanut size

166. Severity of AR is indicated by:
(a) HILL sign
(b) Width of regurgitant jet
(c) Fluttering of AML
(d) All

167. Continuous murmur seen in A/E:
(a) ASD + MS (b) PA + VSD
(c) Peripheral PS (d) Coronary AV fistula

168. Diastolic murmur seen in A/E:
(a) Subaortic AS (b) Supraaortic AS
(c) Dysplastic PV

169. Best valve for unmarried women with MR with EF =50%:
(a) Star Edwards (b) MV Repair
(c) Bjork Shaily (d) Medronic Hall

170. Following is a minor criteria of rheumatic fever in India:
(a) Prolonged PR interval
(b) Polyarthralgia
(c) Raised ESR
(d) Recurrent rheumatic fever

171. All cause increase in intensity of S1 *except:*
(a) LA myxoma (b) Decreased dp/dt
(c) Shunt lesion (d) Short PR interval

172. Paradoxical split of both S1 and S2 seen:
(a) LBBB (b) HOCM
(c) Severe AS (d) All of the above

173. MVP best view is:
(a) PLAX (b) 4 chamber view

174. MR seen in A/E:
(a) SLE
(b) Pseudoxanthoma elasticum
(c) Carcinoid
(d) Methylsergide

175. Loeffler's endocarditis A/E:
(a) Eosinophilia
(b) Biventricular failure
(c) Normal LV systolic function
(d) Asthma

176. Hangout interval crossover seen is:
(a) Ao and PA (b) RV and PA
(c) LV and RV (d) LV and LA

177. TR true:
(a) Carvallo sign absent in CHF
(b) TR murmur decreases in expiration
(c) Holosystolic murmur
(d) All

178. LVS$_4$ A/E:
(a) HTN (b) HOCM
(c) AS (d) Acute MR

179. MS + AS–pressure gradient of AS:
(a) Overestimate severity of AS
(b) Underestimate severity of AS

180. All following occur after S2 *except:*
(a) Ejection click (b) Tumour plop
(c) OS

181. All following increases with inspiration *except:*
(a) Ejection sound

182. Loud S1 A/E:
(a) RA myoxoma (b) Decreased dp/dt
(c) Short PR (d) Shunt lesion

183. Jones criteria used in:
(a) Acute rheumatic fever
(b) Chronic rheumatic fever
(c) Sydenham chorea
(d) Recurrence of RF

184. Most common cause of I.E. in young:
(a) Streptococci viridans (b) Staphylococci

185. Reverse split S2 A/E:
(a) RBBB (b) RV pacing

186. Continuous murmur:
(a) From start of S1 to end of S2
(b) Late systolic overlapping S2 and continues in diastole
(c) Mid of systole to early part of diastole

187. Infective endocarditis not caused by:
(a) Pneumococci (b) HACEK
(c) Pseudomonas (d) Enterococci

188. A2 to P2 ans A2 to OS behave in opposite direction on:
(a) Inspiration (b) Expiration
(c) Standing (d) Squatting

189. Difference between AS and MR:

(a) Squatting (b) Standing
(c) Inspiration (d) Expiration
(e) None

190. Hangout interval false statement:

(a) Pulmonary hangout interval is 60-80 ms
(b) Aortic hang out interval is 20 ms
(c) Second heart sound is widely split because the pulmonary hangout interval is wide
(d) Pulmonary hangout interval less than systemic hangout interval

191. S4 A/E:

(a) Severe MR (b) HTN in elderly
(c) AS (d) Acute MI

192. JVP—'y' descent present:

(a) CCP (b) Cardiac tamponade
(c) TR

193. Hepatojugular reflex false statement:

(a) Sustained rise in the JVP of at least 4 cm or more–positive
(b) Abdomen is compressed for 10 to 30 seconds
(c) Sensitivity of 80%

194. Splitting of S_2:

(a) Inspiration–50 msec (b) Expiration–30 msec
(c) Inspiration–30 msec (d) Expiration–50 msec

195. Severe TR A/E:

(a) Late systolic concavity on continous Doppler wave signal
(b) > 7 mm vena contracta
(c) ERO > 0.3 cm^2
(d) Volume > 45 ml

196. Congenital MS A/E:

(a) Less calcification (b) AF common
(c) Male > female (d) Parachute valve

197. ESR in I.E. returns to normal in:

(a) < 2 weeks (b) 2-4 weeks
(c) 4-6 weeks (d) 6-8 weeks

198. Most common cause of early PVE < 2 months:

(a) S. aureus (b) Enterococci
(c) Staph. Epidermidis (d) Fungi

199. Most common cause of NVE:

(a) S. aureus (b) Klebsiella
(c) Candida (d) S. viridans

200. Prussian helmet sign:

(a) AS (b) MR
(c) AR (d) MS

201. Extended matching:

(a) Muller's sign (b) Carvallo's sign
(c) Demusset's sign (d) Light house sign
(e) Abrahim Lincoln sign (f) Lancini's sign
(g) Seller's sign:
(1) Parasternal PSM increases on inspiration
(2) Large v wave with parasternal PSM
(3) Head nodding with valvular lesion
(4) Alternate flushing and blanching on forehead
(5) Pulsating uvula

202. Well's index: (T/F)

(a) Based on interval on echo in AS
(b) Used in MS
(c) Used in AS and AR
(d) Used in AR and MS

203. Least chance of I.E.:

(a) ASD (b) VSD
(c) MR (d) PDA

204. All seen with aortic regurgitation all *except:*

(a) Ao aneurysm (b) Ao dissection
(c) Truncus arteriosus (d) Austin flint murmur
(e) Gram Steel murmur

205. Cole Cecil murmur:

(a) AS (b) AR
(c) MR (d) TS
(e) MS

206. Mimic MS: (T/F)

(a) Ball valve thrombi
(b) Parachute MV
(c) Large mitral valve vegetation
(d) Tumour of MV
(e) Myxoma

207. IE prophylaxis given in: (T/F)

(a) AS
(b) MVP
(c) Unrepaired congenital HD
(d) Post transplant valvuloplasty
(e) Prosthetic valve

208. Blood sample in IE:
(a) Better result if taken at the time of fever
(b) >3 samples
(c) Better results with arterial and I/D catheter
(d) Aseptic techniques to be used
(e) All of the above

209. Congenital MR all *except:*
(a) COA (b) Sub Ao stenosis
(c) Cortriatum (d) Ostium 1° ASD
(e) VSD with prolapsed of AML

210. Prosthetic valve embolism:
(a) 1.5 times in MV than low risk
(b) Tilting disc in Ao less risk
(c) 9%/year patient not anticoagulated
(d) Max in 1st year

211. IE minor immunological all *except:*
(a) Osler (b) R. factor
(c) Janway (d) GN
(e) Roth spot

212. IE prophylaxis new indication:
(a) MVP without MR for tooth extraction
(b) ASD post 2 months
(c) AS with appendicectomy

213. Acute severe AR: (T/F)
(a) IE T
(b) ALCAPA
(c) MR
(d) Unicuspid valve
(e) Ac rheumatic fever

214. Chronic compensated AR: (T/F)
(a) ↑CO (b) ↑EF
(c) ↑LVESV (d) ↑Filling pressure
(e) Eccentric hypertrophy

215. AS with velocity 4 m/s then gradent is:
(a) 64 (b) 74
(c) 84

216. IE least:
(a) ASD (b) VSD
(c) MR (d) PDA

217. Infective endocarditis: (T/F)
(a) Yield is higher if sample taken during fever
(b) Same venepuncture can be used if not infected for multiple samples
(c) Arterial blood has better results
(d) If culture is to come +ve occurs in 1st 2 samples in 95% cases (12 hours apart) in absence of antibiotics
(e) 5 ml blood is taken in each of anerobic and anaerobic media

218. Natural history of AS:
(a) Mortality risk of 5 years after syncope
(b) Latency period, high starts after 60 years
(c) In 50% cases CAD is cause of angina
(d) Syncope more common on exertion

219. Correct matching:
(a) Genitourinary and intestinal infection–enterococcus fecalis
(b) Immunosuppressed–candida
(c) Blood culture + in prolonged duration–bartonella
(d) Post surgical infection–staph epidermidis
(e) With brushing–viridans streptococci
(f) All true

220. I.E.: (T/F)
(a) Aqueous penicillin G. 12-18 million unit/24 hours in 6 doses with gentamicin 3 mg/kg in 3 doses for 2 weeks
(b) Ceftriaxone IV 2 gm/d × 2 weeks
(c) Vancomycin 30 mg/kg in 2 divided doses × 2 weeks
(d) Ceftriaxone (2 gm)/d I/M × 4 weeks
(e) Aqueous penicillin G for 2 weeks

221. Severe MS–ECG true:
(a) AS severity ↑ ses S_1 comes close to QRS
(b) Middiastolic Murmur ↑ ses
(c) A_2 OS gap ↓ ses
(d) On inspiration 3 sounds heard in order of A_2-OS P_2

222. Fever in IE false:
(a) In most cases–fever occur after bacteremia
(b) Fever may not be present in elderly patient
(c) Fever usually occurs in most patients
(d) Fever may not be seen in staph epidermidis
(e) None

223. LA dilation seen after how much period of mitral regurgitation?
(a) 1 month (b) 3 months
(c) 6 months (d) 12 months

224. St. Jude valve, true is:

(a) 3 discs

(b) 4 truts

(c) Titinium

(d) Useful especially in children

225. Lutembacher syndrome–true all *except:*

(a) Increased pulmonary vascular congestion

(b) Clinical features of MS obscured

(c) More in females

226. Early systolic murmur is heart in all *except:*

(a) Acute MR (b) Normotensive TR

(c) Small VSD (d) MVP

227. In infective endocarditis, 6 weeks course is given in:

(a) PVE (b) NVE

(c) Libmann sack

228. All are time in low gradient AS with LV dysfunction *except:*

(a) Na nitroprusside used

(b) Dobutamine used

(c) ↑ Cardiac output is good prognosis

(d) ↑ Gradient good prognosis

229. I.E. by streptococcus viridans A/E:

(a) Backache

(b) ASO titre

(c) Progressive GN

(d) Positive RA factor

230. All are true about Mitral valve *except:*

(a) The annulus is saddle shaped

(b) Posterior mitral leaflet prolapsed is more common than that of anterior

(c) Posterior mitral leaflet is broader than the anterior mitral leaflet

(d) Attachment of posterior mitral leaflet is longer than the anterior mitral leaflet

231. All of the following are ABSOLUTE contraindications for mitral balloon valvuloplasty *except:*

(a) Clot limited to LA appendage – persisting despite 3 months of anticoagulation

(b) More than moderate mitral regurgitation

(c) Mitral bicommissural calcification

(d) Ball valve thrombosis

232. Echocardiographic diagnosis of rheumatic heart disease may be made using:

(a) Australian RF/RHD guidelines

(b) World health organization (WHO) criteria

(c) Modified Jones criteria 2014

(d) World heart federation (WHF) criteria

233. Which among the following condition is at the highest risk of endocarditis:

(a) Patent ductus arteriosus in a 5 years child

(b) TOF with central shunt in a 13 years old girl

(c) Mitral valve prolapse with regurgitation in an elderly

(d) Ebstein's anomaly in a pregnant patient

234. A 65-year-old male who underwent colestomy for carcinomas of the colon 2 months back is being evaluated for prolonged fever. Echo reveals small sized vegetations on the mitral valve and severe mitral regurgitations. The most likely organism is:

(a) Streptococcus sanguis

(b) Streptococcus mutans

(c) Streptococcus GALLOLYTICUS

(d) Enterococcus

235. Which of the following statements is correct when severe tricuspid stenosis is diagnosed?

(a) Pulmonary capillary wedge > 18 mm Hg and right atrial pressure> 10 mm

(b) A men diastolic tricuspid gradient of greater than equal to 7 mm Hg is present and the valve area is less than equal to 1 centimeter square.

(c) A Wilkins score of > 8 is observed in the echocardiogram

(d) The right atrial pressure is increased, but the RV systolic pressure is normal

236. Following are true about Infective Endocarditis in I.V. drug abusers *except:*

(a) Most commonly involves normal valves

(b) S. aureus is most common causative agent

(c) Most commonly Tricuspid valve involved

(d) Risk in lower than that of prosthetic valves endocarditic

237. True about aortic stenosis, all *except:*

(a) Exercise testing should be avoided in symptomatic patients

(b) Normal splitting of second heart sound less likely in severe aortic srenosis

(c) Severity of aortic stenosis is inversely related in symptomatic patients

(d) Paradoxical splitting of second heart sound may be associated with dysfunction

238. Mayen sign is positive in:
(a) MVP
(b) Aortic regurgitation
(c) Hypertrophic cardiomyopathy
(d) Dissection of Aorta

239. The following is true for aortic regurgitation in rheumatic fever:
(a) It always occurs with MR
(b) Isolated AR occurs in less than 10% cases
(c) Results from valve perforation
(d) Murmer is longer and louder than IN chronic AR

240. Acute rheumatic activity is established RHD is diagnosed by:
(a) Regurgitant murmurs
(b) Increasing heart failure
(c) Two minor criteria and evidence of preceding streptococcal infection
(d) One major criterion and raised ASO titre

241. The following is true for syndenham chorea:
(a) It is characterized by the "supinator sign"
(b) It is common in males after puberty
(c) Occurs equally in males and females in younger age
(d) It is indicative of severe cardiac involvement

242. Duration of prophylaxis in rheumatic carditis without residual valvular disease:
(a) 10 years or till age 40 years whichever is longer
(b) 5 years or till age 21 years whichever is longer
(c) 10 years or age 21 years whichever is longer
(d) Till age 40 years in endemic areas

243. Formula for balloon sizing in BMV (Balloon Mitral Valvotomy):
(a) Height in cm/10+10 mm
(b) Height in cm/10+5 mm
(c) Height in cm/10 mm
(d) Height in inches/10

244. Melody valve is:
(a) Aortic valve (b) Pulmonary valve
(c) Tricuspid valve (d) Mitral valve

245. True:
(a) AR – quincke sign
(b) AS – Hill's sign

246. Carey comb valvulitis A/E:
(a) Mitral valvulitis
(b) Disappear with time
(c) Begin with S3
(d) It indicate obstruction during activity

247. Vena contracta in AR A/E:
(a) Best visualized in apical 4 chamber view
(b) Specific finding of AR > 6 mm
(c) Seen near constriction of flow

248. Low flow low gradient AS, dobutamine infusion → valve replacement done in:
(a) Increase in gradient with same valve area
(b) Increase in gradient with decrease in valve area
(c) Increase in gradient only

249. 20 years old female with chest pain, breath-lessness, mid systolic click at apex:
(a) MVP (b) BAV
(c) MS

250. Prosthetic valve endocarditis least:
(a) Streptococcus (b) Staphylococcus
(c) Co NS (d) Gram negative bacilli

251. Native valve endocarditis *except:*
(a) Enterococci (b) Staphylococci
(c) Streptococci (d) Co NS

252. I.E. in intravenous drug abuser true is:
(a) Most common in HIV
(b) Spares left sided valves
(c) Involves native valves
(d) Usually culture negative

253. Infective endocarditis most common in:
(a) VSD (b) PS
(c) PDA (d) ASD

254. Acute MR A/E:
(a) Ejection systolic murmur
(b) Increased PVR
(c) Displaced/hyperdynamic impulse

255. Modified Duke criteria (minor) A/E:
(a) Fever
(b) Immunological phenomenon
(c) Predisposing heart condition
(d) IE on echo

256. Patient of severe AR, which would be the best hemodynamic scenario immediately post AVR?

(a) ↓ in EDV, ↓ ESV with ↓ in EF
(b) ↓ in EDV, ↓ ESV with ↑ in EF
(c) ↓ in EDV, ↓ ESV with ↑ in forward SV with initial ↓ in EF
(d) ↓ in EDV, ↓ ESV with ↑ in forward SV with initial ↑ in EF

257. Patient of acute MR, put on I.V. diuretics, I.V. nitroprusside, I.V. nitroglycerine. On day 4 develop cyanosis, SOB, ABG–pH– 7.2, PO_2 – 90 mm Hg, PCO_2– 33 mm Hg, HCO_3– 12. treatment of choice:

(a) I.V. methylene blue (b) MVR
(c) O_2 therapy (b) $NaHCO_3$

258. Severity of TR on ECHO:

(a) Annular dilatation > 4 cm
(b) Late systolic flow reversal in hepatic veins
(c) TR velocity > 4 cm/sec
(d) Jet regurgitant area > 8 cm^2

259. AR true A/E:

(a) Hill's sign is an artifact in BP measurement
(b) Cooing dove murmur occurs in everted prolapsed of aortic valve
(c) In HF, DBP may rise
(d) Chronic AR, EF is maintained till late due to dilatation and hypertrophy

260. All are indications for AVR *except:*

(a) Asymptomatic severe AR, LVIDd= 60-65 mm, EF> 50%
(b) Asymptomatic severe AR, LVIDs > 55 mm , EF< 50%
(c) Symptomatic severe AR
(d) Asymptomatic severe AR, LVIDd < 55 mm, EF < 50%

261. Lowest risk of I.E. in:

(a) HCM
(b) VSD
(c) MVP with severe MR

262. Early prosthetic valve I.E. most common:

(a) S. epidermidis
(b) Streptococcus
(c) HACEK
(d) Coagulase negative staph.

263. HACEK- DOC:

(a) Ceftriaxone (b) Ampicillin + salbactum
(c) Vancomycin (d) Imepenem

264. Recurrence of rheumatic fever in a child suffered from acute RF 2 years back who had stopped penicillin prophylaxis:

(a) 50% (b) 75%
(c) 3 % (d) 25%

265. 55 years old male CAD (chronic stable angina) risk of acute MI over next 1 year:

(a) 3-4 % (b) < 1 %
(c) 5-6 % (d) 10 %

266. Jai Vigyan mission project true:

(a) Carried out in rheumatic fever patients
(b) Under AIIMS and CMC Vellore
(c) Significantly differentiates between nephrogenic and rheumatogenic strain
(d) All of the above

267. A 5 years old child with BAV with severe AS. Balloon angioplasty done – gradient abolished with mild AR, but symptoms class III/IV persists. What would be the next management?

(a) Dobutamine infusion
(b) Intravenous nitroprusside as child not tolerating mild AR
(c) Intravenous diuretics
(d) BNP

268. All are true about PPH *except:*

(a) Bosentan decreases sildenafil effect
(b) Silfenadil decreases bosentan effect
(c) Post marketing surveillance–more hepatotoxicity is found as compared to trials (bosentan)
(d) All of the above

269. Prosthesis valve preferred at tricuspid position:

(a) Bioprosthesis (b) Tilting disc
(c) Bileaflet

270. A patient admitted for aortic valve endocarditis with severe AR, during hospitalization have dense embolic stroke. True is:

(a) Immediate AVR (b) AVR within 2 weeks
(c) AVR after 3 weeks (d) Warfarin

271. End of diastole indicated by:
(a) Peak of R wave (b) End of T wave

272. C/I of coronary angiography A/E:
(a) Digitoxicity (b) Hypokalemia
(c) VT (d) Decompensated HF

273. Most common cause of renal failure in I.E.:
(a) Drugs
(b) Immune mediated GN
(c) Embolic
(d) Focal glomerulonephritis

274. Intravenous drug abuser–TR with pneumonia treated with 3 weeks of piperacillin + tazobactum, no response and positive blood culture with pseudomonas, next strategy:
(a) Tricuspid valvectomy without prosthesis + antibiotic
(b) Tricuspid valvectomy with prosthesis
(c) Change antibiotic to ceftazidine + tobramycin
(d) Continue same treatment for 4 weeks

275. Dallas criteria—used in:
(a) Endomyocardial biopsy
(b) IE
(c) Diastolic heart failure

276. AS with GI bleeding:
(a) Associated with severity
(b) Because of ↑ flow + ↓ platelet aggregability
(c) ↑ vWF
(d) All of the above

277. Progression of rheumatic disease arrested by (in study):
(a) Steroid (b) IVIG
(c) Aspirin (d) None of the above

278. Asymptomatic MR, surgery indicated in:
(a) LVESD > 40 mm (b) New onset AF
(c) PAH (d) All

279. Rheumatic fever increase manifestation in elderly:
(a) Arthritis (b) Carditis
(c) Chorea (d) Subcutaneous nodules

280. MV calcification all *except:*
(a) Males common
(b) Stroke
(c) LV inlet obstruction

281. Severity of MS in presence of AR:
(a) Overestimated (b) Underestimated
(c) Depends on heart rate

282. Not seen in IE:
(a) MCD (b) MPGN
(c) FSG (d) RPGN

283. IE absolute indication for surgery are all *except:*
(a) Unstable prosthesis (b) Perivalvular leak
(c) CHF

284. Absolute indication of surgery in IF are all *except:*
(a) Large hypermobile vegetation > 10 mm
(b) Relapse of PVE
(c) Fistula to pericardiac sac

285. Seven AS asymptomatic N LV function treatment by:
(a) AVR (b) Ross
(c) Echo follow up (d) Valvotomy

286. Late manifestation of RF:
(a) EM (b) Arthritis
(c) Carditis (d) Subcutaneous nodule

287. All are causes of acute infective endocarditis *except:*
(a) S aureus
(b) Beta hemolytic streptococcus
(c) HACEK
(d) Pneumococcus

288. In MVP infective endocarditis prophylaxis is indicated in all *except:*
(a) Severe MR on auscultation
(b) Valve thickness >5 mm
(c) Only click no MR
(d) Severe MR on echocardiography

289. Severity of MS is proportional to:
(a) Intensity of the murmur
(b) Loud S2
(c) Length of the murmur
(d) Presence of opening snap

290. Drug of choice for HACEK organism infective endocarditis is:
(a) Vancomycin (b) Ceftraxone
(c) Ampicillin (d) Rifampicin

291. Skin manifestation of infective endocarditis is:
(a) Erythema marginatum
(b) Erythema nodosum
(c) Janeway lesions
(d) Tendon xanthomas

292. Infective endocarditis prophylaxis is indicated in:
(a) Flexible branchoscopy
(b) Sclerotherapy of esophageal varices
(c) Cesarean section
(d) Upper GI endoscopy

293. Acute AR not useful in:
(a) NTG (b) Nitroprusside
(c) Surgery (d) Labetalol

294. Carey Coombs' murmur A/E:
(a) Like diastolic
(b) Low pitched
(c) Associated with AR
(d) Associated with Ac Rh fever

295. LA compliance does not ↓ se in:
(a) Chronic MR (b) SLE
(c) Cardiac surgery (d) Rheumatic fever

296. Rheumatic fever true is:
(a) Coexist with arthritis and chorea
(b) ↑ ses in severity in pregnancy (chorea)
(c) Erythema multiforme seen
(d) Tender subcutaneous nodule

297. Vegetations on undersurface of A-V values:
(a) NBTE
(b) Libman sacks endocarditis
(c) Rheumatic
(d) Infective

298. Mortality in chronic severe AR (NYHA III/IV) after 4 years without surgery:
(a) 10% (b) 20%
(c) 30% (d) 40%

299. Falsely high cardiac output in:
(a) AS (b) MS
(c) AR (d) MR

300. Least common organism in IE:
(a) S typhi (b) P aeruginosa
(c) Staph albus (d) Strepto faecalis

301. Severity of MR by:
(a) Wide split S2
(b) Low volume, early peaking pulse

302. Osler's node more common with:
(a) Staph aureus (b) Streptococcus
(c) Candida

303. Primary pulmonary HTN gene:
(a) BMPR II (b) Homeobox
(c) TBX

304. Pure rheumatic MR without MS:
(a) 5 % (b) 10%
(c) 15% (d) 20%

305. Severe AR seen by:
(a) PHT <200
(b) AML flutter
(c) LVEDD > 55
(d) Annular diameter > 50%

306. Severe AR (NYHA Class III/IV) survival without surgery–4 years:
(a) 10% (b) 20%
(c) 30% (d) 40%

307. Functional OS:
(a) TS (b) VSD
(c) Vascular aneurysm (d) Tricuspid atresia

308. Acute IE A/E:
(a) Beta hemolytic streptococcus
(b) HACEK
(c) Staph. aureus
(d) Pneumococcus

309. Late prosthetic valve endocarditis A/E:
(a) Streptococcus (b) Enterococcus
(c) Staph. epidermidis (d) HACEK

310. Patient of AS with angina – life expectancy:
(a) 1 year (b) 2 years
(c) 3 years (d) 5 years

311. Risk of anaphylaxis with benzathine penicillin is:
(a) 2% (b) 3.2%
(c) 5% (d) 0.2%

312. Risk of recurrence of rheumatic fever after group A beta hemolytic streptococcal pharyngitis in those with prior rheumatic fever is about:

(a) 0.3% (b) 3%
(c) 30% (d) 50%

313. Evidence of preceding group A streptococcal infection is not essential in the diagnosis of acute rheumatic fever in patients with:

(a) Previous rheumatic fever
(b) Subcutaneous nodules
(c) Low grade carditis
(d) Established rheumatic heart disease

314. All are causes of early systolic murmur *except:*

(a) Acute MR
(b) Infundibular pulmonary stenosis
(c) Acute TR with normal PA pressure
(d) Muscular VSD

315. All are true about Tricuspid Stenosis *except:*

(a) Almost always rheumatic in origin
(b) A mean diastolic gradient of 2 mm Hg is sufficient to establish the diagnosis
(c) Generally accompanies mitral valve disease
(d) In severe TS, dyspnea, orthopnea and PND are common symptoms due to associated mitral stenosis

316. Following is not a cause of organic Tricuspid Regurgitation (primary TR):

(a) Carcinoid syndrome
(b) Right ventricular MI
(c) Endomyocardial fibrosis
(d) Infective endocarditis in IV drug users

317. Identify the wrong statement about mechanical prosthetic valves:

(a) All mechanical valves have an excellent record of durability upto 40 years for the STARR- EDWARD valve and over 25 years for St. JUDE valve
(b) Thromboembolic risk is greatest in the first post operative year
(c) Aspirin–75 to 100 mgs should be given to all patients with MV prosthesis only
(d) Target INR is 2.5- 3.5 for post AVR patients with associated atrial fibrillation

318. Bioprosthetic valve is most preferred in the following patient:

(a) 40 years old female with severe calcified MS
(b) 60 years old male with severe MS and long standing AF
(c) 30 years old male with severe MS and hemophilia
(d) 18 years old male with severe AR

319. In the management of MVP with MR all true *except:*

(a) B-Blockers are recommended for all patients
(b) MV repair is possible in > 90% of patients
(c) Repair of anterior leaflet prolapse is more challenging
(d) Aspirin should be given to patients with MVP who had documented focal neurologic event and in whom no other cause is apparent

320. All are causes of acute MR *except:*

(a) Spontaneous chordal rupture
(b) Cleft mitral valve
(c) Infective endocarditis with leaflet perforation
(d) AML tear following balloon mitral valvotomy

321. In the management of MR, systemic vasodilator therapy is recommended in all *except:*

(a) Acute severe MR
(b) Asymptomatic severe MR with preserved LV function
(c) Chronic severe MR with LV dysfunction
(d) Symptomatic severe MR who is not a candidate for surgery

322. Following is not a cause of AR due to aortic root dilatation:

(a) Ankylosing spondylitis
(b) Systemic hypertension
(c) Sub pulmonic VSD with AR
(d) Osteogenesis imperfecta

323. All are features of low flow, low gradient Aortic Stenosis *except:*

(a) Aortic valve area < 1 cm^2
(b) LV EF < 40%
(c) AV mean gradient < 30-40 mm Hg
(d) LV EF <50%

324. Antibiotic Prophylaxis to a child with Rheumatic Heart Disease should be given minimum till:

(a) At least 5 years after onset
(b) Lifelong
(c) Till 17 years
(d) Till 21 years

325. Drug of choice for HACEK is:

(a) Rifampicin (b) Ceftriaxone
(c) Gentamicin (d) Imipenem

326. What is the murmur of Rheumatic Mitral Regurgitation?

(a) A low-pitched diastolic ruble with an opening snap, best heard at the apex

(b) A decrescendo, high-pitched diastolic murmur heard best at the lower self sternal border, starting almost with the second heard sound
(c) A holosytolic, high pitched murmur that starts with the first heard sound and continues through the second heard sound, best heard at the apex and radiated either to the axilla or lower left sternal border
(d) A mid-systolic high-pitched murmur best heard at the apex and left sternal border, accompanied by one or more systolic clicks in half the cases

327. In a patient with bacterial endocarditis, which of the following echocardiographic lesions is most likely lead to embolization?
(a) 5 mm mitral valve vegetation
(b) 5 mm tricuspid valve vegetation
(c) 11 mm aortic valve vegetation
(d) 11 mm mitral valve vegetation

328. Mitral stenosis is frequently, complicated by hypertension. Which of the following is a cause of pulmonary hypertension in mitral stenosis?
(a) Passive transmission of elevated left atrial pressure
(b) Obliterative changes in the pulmonary vascular bed
(c) Pulmonary arteriolar constriction
(d) All of the above

329. Which of the following physical examination findings suggests severe aortic regurgitation?
(a) Corrgan's pulse (b) Pulses alternans
(c) Pulses bigeminus (d) Pulses paradoxus

330. Most common cause of Aortic stenosis in India is:
(a) Degenerative valvular calcification
(b) Rheumatic disease
(c) Medication toxicity
(d) Hypereosinophilia

331. Cardiovascular diagnostic criteria phenotypic manifestations include MVP endocarditis, dysrhythmia, dilated mitral annulus, MR, TVP, AR, aortic dissection and dilatation of the aortic root. The syndrome is:
(a) Marfan syndrome
(b) Ehlers-Danlos syndrome
(c) Down syndrome
(d) Turner syndrome

332. Most common cause of Aortic stenosis in India is:
(a) Degenerative valvular calcification
(b) Rheumatic disease
(c) Medication toxicity
(d) Hypereosinophilia/Radiation

333. The following are true in third degree heart block, *except:*
(a) No atrial impulse propagates to the ventricles
(b) A.V. Nodal Block is probably when the ventricular rate is around 50/minute
(c) The QRS complex is always wide
(d) Pacemaker syndrome may develop if a simple ventricular pentricular pacemaker is used

334. Drug of choice for HACEK is:
(a) Rifampicin (b) Ceftriaxone
(c) Gentamicin (d) Imipenem

335. Causative organism of Early Prosthetic Valve Endocarditis is:
(a) Coagulase negative Staphylococci-Staphylococcus epidermidis
(b) Staphylococcus aureus
(c) Enterococci
(d) Streptococci

336. A 25 years old lady presents with arrythmias, palpitations, substernal chest pain poorly related to exertion and finds mid systolic clicks on auscultation. What is the investigation to be done?
(a) Arteriography
(b) Echocardiography
(c) Chest X-ray
(d) Electrophysiological test

337. The most common presenting symptom of mitral stenosis is:
(a) Chest pain
(b) Hemoptysis
(c) Palpitations
(d) Fatigue and decreased exercise tolerance

338. Mitral valve vegetations do not usually embolise to:
(a) Lung (b) Liver
(c) Spleen (d) Brain

339. In mitral regurgitation Jet spectral envelop, if the time taken for the MR jet velocity to attain velocity 3 m/s from velocity 1 m/s is 30 milliseconds, then DP/DT is:
(a) 1200 mm Hg/sec (b) 1066 mm Hg/sec
(c) 920 mm Hg/sec (d) 1080 mm Hg/sec

340. Least common organism isolated in early prosthetic valve endocarditis from the following:

(a) Staph aureus (b) Gram negative bacilli
(c) Streptococci (d) Fungi

341. Each of the following heart sound may occur after S2 *except*:

(a) Opening snap (b) S3
(c) Ejection click (d) Pericardial knock

342. Rheumatic Fever:

(a) Follows Group A streptococcal sore throat
(b) Follows Group B streptococcal infection
(c) May be a complication of streptococcal skin infection
(d) In an infection affecting the large joints

343. The following are major Jones criteria for diagnosis of Rheumatic Fever, *except:*

(a) Carditis (b) Polyarthritis
(c) Chorea (d) Raised ASO titre

344. In Rheumatic heart disease, pure mitral stenosis is seen in approximately:

(a) 50% of all patients (b) 40% of all patients
(c) 25% of all patients (d) 10% of all patients

345. The following finding indicates severe mitral stenosis:

(a) A soft first heart sound
(b) A third heart sound (LV S3)
(c) A short A2-OS interval
(d) Absent opening snap

346. "Osborne wave" is an ECG finding present in:

(a) Hypovolaemia (b) Hypervolaemia
(c) Hyperthermia (d) Hypothermia

347. The percentage of culture negative infective endocarditis in India is:

(a) >25% (b) 20%
(c) 10% (d) 5%

348. Aortic balloon valvoplasty is safer as compared to surgery in:

(a) Children
(b) Elderly people
(c) Patients with LV dysfunction
(d) All of the above

349. The least common among Jones Criteria:

(a) Polyarthritis
(b) Erythema marginatum
(c) Subcutaneous modules
(d) Carditis

350. In pulmonary ballon valvoplasty the balloon size should be:

(a) Equal to annular diameter
(b) 50-79 mm Hg
(c) More than 80 mm Hg
(d) More than 150 mm Hg

351. Severity of AS in 60 years old male:

(a) Delayed carotid upstroke
(b) Presence of click
(c) Severity of murmur
(d) Duration of murmur

352. Severity of MR is suggested by all *except:*

(a) AF (b) Presence of S3
(c) Presence of S4 (d) Displaced apex

353. Worst prognosis in. Aortic stenosis:

(a) CHF (b) Syncope
(c) Angina (d) Palpitation

354. A young male with mitral valve replacement came with low grade fever for 1 month with normal ECHO, with normal CT abdomen/chest, so which organisms will grow in the culture?

(a) Staph epidermidis (b) Staph aureus
(c) H. influenza (d) Pseudomonas

355. Regarding RHD secondary prophylaxis which is true?

(a) In benzathine (Regular) is better than oral penicillin
(b) Oral penicillin is given
(c) Sulphonamide is not given because it is bacteriostatic
(d) PSRA not require secondary prophylaxis

356. Preceding streptococcal (Essential) criteria is not required for diagnosing Rheumatic fever:

(a) Recurrent rheumatic fever
(b) Primary rheumatic fever
(c) Establised RHD
(d) Low grade chronic carditis

357. On rapid standing what happen to MVP:
(a) Murmur and click move closer to S1
(b) Murmur and click move closer to S2
(c) Murmur and click move closer to S1
(d) Murmur and click away from S2

358. Wide pulse pressure A/E:
(a) AR (b) Severe MR
(c) HOCM (d) Thyrotoxicosis

359. Bisferiens pulse with slow rise:
(a) Severe AS (b) Severe AR
(c) AS + AR (d) HOCM

360. Propagation velocity highest in:
(a) Purkinje fibre (b) Bundle of his
(c) AV node

361. Enterococcal endocarditis treatment:
(a) Penicillin + gentamicin
(b) Ceftriaxone + gentamicin
(c) Vancomycin
(d) Ampicillin

362. Staphylococcus endocarditis A/E:
(a) Large vegetation (b) Purulent meningitis
(c) Large abscess (d) IV drug abuse

363. Severe AS:
(a) < 0.6 cm^2 (b) < 1 cm^2
(c) < 2 cm^2 (d) < 1.2 cm^2

364. Syncope in AS survival rate:
(a) 1 year (b) 10 years
(c) 3 years

365. Wilkin score—severe MS:
(a) Diastolic dooming
(b) Valve thickness > 9 mm
(c) Distal

366. I.E. prophylaxis mostly indicated in following:
(a) Ligated PDA
(b) Repaired OS-ASD
(c) Repaired COA
(d) Repaired subaortic VSD

367. Patient with MVR after 1 month has low grade fever. Normal echo with no vegetation, normal CT abdomen, thorax and chest. Which organisms probably be grown in culture?
(a) Pseudomonas aeruginosa
(b) Staph. Aureus
(c) Hemophilus sp.
(d) S. epidermidis

368. Primary cause of TR A/E:
(a) Subendocardial fibroelastosis
(b) Radiation
(c) Ebstein's anomaly
(d) Carcinoid syndrome

369. 45 years old female with NYHA–III, easy fatiguability since 1 year with PSM at apex, Carvallo's sign on cardiac cath., diagnosis:
(a) Severe AS (b) Severe MR
(c) HOCM (d) Severe LV dysfunction

370. "Cabot locke" murmur:
(a) Severe anemia (b) LAD stenosis
(c) Severe AR (d) HOCM

371. Patient with rheumatic fever with carditis– bacterial prophylaxis:
(a) Daily penicillin V
(b) PnG with procaine I.M. every 3 weeks
(c) Amoxy– clav daily
(d) Azithromycin daily

372. Echo criteria for severe AR A/E:
(a) PHT – 150
(b) ER volume – 50 ml
(c) ER fraction – 55%
(d) Jet area / LVOT area – > 65%

373. Post VPC, PSM of MR decreases in:
(a) MR with HOCM
(b) Chronic rheumatic MR
(c) Papillary Muscle rupture– MR
(d) MR with VSD

374. Feature of chronic severe MR A/E:
(a) Wide splitting of S2
(b) Soft S1
(c) S4
(d) Left parasternal impulse

375. Medical valvotomy:
(a) IE in severe PS
(b) PPI lead in severe TS
(c) Non penetrating trauma in severe MS

376. **'O' Brien valve:**
(a) Bioprosthetic MV (b) Mechanical MV
(c) Bioprosthetic AoV (d) Mechanical AoV

377. **Complication specific for severe bicuspid AoV stenosis A/E:**
(a) Congenital CHB (b) Hyede syndrome
(c) Ao dissection (d) IE

378. **Calcific severe Aortic Stenosis:**
(a) Subvalvular
(b) Valvular and severe
(c) Associated with atherosclerosis

379. **Severe Aortic Stenosis A/E:**
(a) Subvalvular in William syndrome
(b) Calcific AS
(c) Atherosclerotic

380. **Hyede syndrome treatment:**
(a) vwF (b) VIIa
(c) AoVR

381. **About prosthetic valve A/E:**
(a) Bioprosthetic preferred in young
(b) Bioprosthetic preferred in young lady expected with pregnancy
(c) Thrombosis is more of mitral than aortic valve
(d) Durability of bioprosthetic is less than mechanical

382. **Erythematic, nontender lesion at palm and sole in IE:**
(a) Janeway lesion (b) Osler node
(c) Roth spot

383. **Gallavardin phenomenon dissociation with:**
(a) Fibrocalcific AS
(b) Valvular AS
(c) BAV

384. **Fall of sound in gallaverdin is due to:**
(a) S4 fused with S1 (b) Multiple S4
(c) Multiple S3 (d) S3 and S4 summation

385. **Heyde syndrome:**
(a) Valvular AS
(b) Sub valvular AS
(c) Supravalvular AS

386. **ARF, 2004 modification:**
(a) Issue of recurrent RF
(b) Erythema marginatum incorporated
(c) Group A strept. Essential criteria

387. **6 years old with fever, what add to diagnosis of RHD?**
(a) ↑ PR on ECG
(b) Target lesion on hand
(c) Tendon nodule on finger pulp
(d) + ve Romberg sign

388. **NBTE most common involved is:**
(a) Aortic Valve (b) Mitral Valve
(c) Tricuspid Valve (d) Pulmonary Valve

389. **Mild to moderate AS per year progression (mean gradient):**
(a) 4-7 mm Hg (b) 15-20 mm Hg
(c) > 50 mm Hg

390. **Aortic valve commissure:**
(a) Right and posterior valve commissure– over membranous septum
(b) Right and Left valve–pulm. valve
(c) Left and Posterior–mitral valve
(d) Roof of RA–Right sinus

391. **MS, IE prophylaxis not needed in:**
(a) Dental scaling (b) Cystoscopy
(c) Bronchoscopy (d) Cardiac catheterization

392. **Least common thromboembolism:**
(a) Bioprosthetic valve (b) Tilting disc valve
(c) Saint Jude valve (d) Ball and cage valve

393. **Which of the following cardiac lesion require infective endocarditis prophylaxis?**
(a) Hypertrophic cardiomyopathy
(b) Previous coronary artery bypass surgery
(c) Cardiac pacemakers and implanted defibrillators
(d) Previous rheumatic fever without valvular dysfunction

394. **In severe mitral incompetence the tall 'V' waves in LA pressure wave from tracing will decrease in the following sitting *except:***
(a) Phenylephrine infusion
(b) Intra aortic balloon pump
(c) I/V nitroprusside
(d) I/V Amyl nitrite

395. **Identify the wrong statement in Rheumatic carditis:**
(a) Rheumatic cardities is a pancarditis
(b) New onset cardiomegaly is suggestive of myocarditis

(c) MV disease is seen in 70-75% of patients
(d) Carditis episodes are common in order patients

396. All are true regarding congenital bicuspid aortic valve *except:*
(a) All are inherently stenotic
(b) Frequency is as high as 2% of all live birth
(c) Male preponderance of 4:1
(d) It is an important risk factor for aortic dissection

397. Identify the correct statement regarding of prosthetic valves:
(a) Bioprosthetic valves have a longer durability than mechanical prosthetic valves
(b) All patients with bioprosthetic valves require lifelong anticoagulation
(c) Risk of valve thrombosis is highest for aortic valve prosthesis
(d) Starr-Edward caged ball valve is inherently stenotic

398. Qualification of mitral stenosis is done by measuring:
(a) Peak systolic gradient
(b) Mean diastolic gradient
(c) Pressure half time
(d) Pulmonary vein velocity

399. Regarding percutaneous balloon mitral vavotomy, all are true *except:*
(a) It is recommended in symptomatic moderate to severe mitral stenosis irrespective of age of the patient
(b) It is recommended in symptomatic mitral stenosis with resting pulmonary systolic pressure of more than 50 mm of Hg.
(c) It is contraindicated in patients with mitral stenosis and presence or evidence of left atrial thrombus
(d) It is contraindicated in patients with moderate mitral stenosis and recent onset atrial fibrillation

400. S1 is modified A/E:
(a) Atrial contraction
(b) Forced ventricular contraction
(c) Vagal stimulation
(d) PR interval

401. In acute rheumatic fever least consequence is:
(a) Apical diastolic murmur
(b) Apical systolic murmur
(c) EDM in left sternal border
(d) MSM in aortic area

402. RHD least tolerated:
(a) MS (b) MR
(c) AS (d) AR

403. Acute MR causes A/E:
(a) I.E. (b) RHD
(c) MI (d) Trauma

404. Penicillin prophylaxis in RHD is:
(a) Primordial prevention
(b) Primary prevention
(c) Secondary prevention
(d) Tertiary prevention

405. Austin flint murmur:
(a) High flow through stenotic AV valves
(b) High flow through normal AV valves
(c) High flow through partial closed AV valves

406. Tuft of red finger:
(a) I.E. (b) R to L shunt
(c) Scleroderma (d) Polycythemia

407. AS false A/E:
(a) RHD most common cause of AS in North America and western Europe
(b) AS more common in female
(c) Valvular gradient more in LV dysfunction
(d) Symptomatic only with 0.5 cm/m²

408. MS gradient LA-LV not increased in: (T/F)
(a) Tachycardia
(b) Hypocalcemia
(c) New onset AF
(d) Central neuaxial block
(e) RHF

409. Hemolysis in prosthetic valve true: (T/F)
(a) More in mechanical valve than bioprosthetic valve
(b) Hemolysis mainly due to paravalvular leak
(c) Pentoxiphylline decreases risk
(d) Gold standard treatment surgery

410. Prosthetic valve thrombosis A/E: (T/F)
(a) St. Jude mechanical > cage ball at mitral
(b) Mitral > tricuspid
(c) Max. within 1 year post operative
(d) Incidence 0.2%
(e) Mechanical > bioprosthetic

411. I.E. prophylaxis: (T/F)

(a) MV repair
(b) Mechanical valve
(c) Congenital repair < 12 months
(d) Palliative shunt in situ
(e) Ostium secundum ASD

412. Bioprosthetic valve A/E: (T/F)

(a) Star Edwards (b) Edwards HIRA
(c) Hancock II (d) Paramount – Magna
(e) On – X prosthetic valve

413. Acute MR versus chronic MR: (T/F)

(a) Cardiomegaly (b) Aneurysmal LA
(c) S4 (d) Systolic thrill at apex
(e) Increased PCWP

414. CMV not indicated: (T/F)

(a) LA clot with calcified MS
(b) Severe subclavian thickening
(c) Severe MS with mild MR
(d) Severe MS with sinus rhythm
(e) Prior CMV with pliable valve

415. RHD prophylaxis: (T/F)

(a) Oral penicillin better than benzathine penicillin
(b) Oral erythromycin better than benzathine penicillin
(c) Rheumatic fever vaccination to be used
(d) 4 weeks not better than 3 weeks
(e) No previous reaction with penicillin can present with anaphylaxis

416. True or False:

(a) S3 does not always indicate LV dysfunction
(b) Pulsus bisferiens indicate LV dysfunction
(c) Volume overload – sustained apical impulse
(d) AS – heaving apical impulse
(e) Apical impulse on left 5th ICS medial to MCL in severe MS

417. PHT not useful for MVA in: (T/F)

(a) Mild MR (b) Severe AR
(c) Raised LVEDP (d) Post BMV
(e) Post CMV

418. Percutaneous mitral valve repair A/E: (T/F)

(a) EVERSET trial
(b) Mitraclip is used
(c) Useful in rheumatic MR
(d) Not frequently done in India
(e) Commonly done through coronary sinus

419. All are mechanical valves *except*: (T/F)

(a) Carpentier Edwards (b) Hancock
(c) Carbomedics (d) Starr Edwards
(e) St. Jude valve

420. I.E. prophylaxis: (T/F)

(a) BT shunt
(b) Prior I.E
(c) ASD closure after 1 year
(d) Prosthetic cardiac valve
(e) Rheumatic MR

421. AR: (T/F)

(a) Isolated aortic valve involvement 5-8%
(b) Asymptomatic severe AR progresses to asymptomatic LV dysfunction in 6%
(c) In presence of LV dysfunction, Hill's sign false positive
(d) Asymptomatic LV dysfunction to symptomatic LV dysfunction
(e) Severe symptomatic AR mortality 20%/year

422. BMV: (T/F)

(a) Has 4 types of in one balloon
(b) Wilkin score not useful now-a-days
(c) Post BMV severe MR occur in 2=9%
(d) LAA clot is not a C/I
(e) Successful if mean gradient < 5 mm Hg

423. Rheumatic TS: (T/F)

(a) Most common in females
(b) Isolated TS never seen
(c) Calcification seen
(d) Prominent a wave
(e) Gradient > 5 mm Hg associated with systemic venous congestion

424. AS: (T/F)

(a) At 25 years isolated AS is rheumatic
(b) At 75 years isolated AS is degenerative
(c) May present with SCD
(d) Treatment at 50 years age with AS – balloon dilatation
(e) TOC in neonates – balloon dilatation

425. Acute AR versus chronic AR, favour Acute AR: (T/F)

(a) Tachycardia

(b) Loud EDM murmur
(c) Long duration EDM
(d) Absence of peripheral sign
(e) Soft S_1

426. Mitral MS, A2-OS gap increases: (T/F)
(a) HT (b) Bradycardia
(c) Old age (d) MR
(e) LV dysfunction

427. Murmur (dynamic auscultation): (T/F)
(a) Right sided murmur increases with inspiration
(b) After valsalva Right murmur return to Normal early
(c) PS murmur soft with isometric Exercise
(d) MS murmur soft with isomeric Exercise
(e) After PVC semilunar/stenotic murmur increases

428. Prosthetic valve: (T/F)
(a) Tilting disc most common used
(b) Star Edward valve not suitable for aortic valve with small aortic annulus
(c) Bioprosthetic valve require anticoagulation for 6 months
(d) Thrombosis in Aortic Valve > mitral valve
(e) Aspirin Indicated in all Prosthetic Valve

429. BMV WILKIN scoring not criteria: (T/F)
(a) Subvalvular (b) Age
(c) Mobility (d) Calcification
(e) Thickening

430. Transcatheter aortic valve replacement A/E: (T/F)
(a) Paravalvular regurgition is rare
(b) Valvular regurgitation is common
(c) AV block may occur after surgery
(d) Indicated only in high risk surgery
(e) Hemodynamic similar to surgery patient

431. Pansystolic murmur: (T/F)
(a) MR (b) TR
(c) VSD (d) Supravalvular AS
(e) Valvular AS

432. 10 years old, SM on auscultation–diagnosis - PS, peak gradient= 36 mm Hg, asymptomatic–Management: (T/F)
(a) Pulmonary balloon valvuloplasty
(b) Pulmonary valvotomy
(c) Medical follow up
(d) Diuretic
(e) Prescribe sport

433. TR-organic versus functional, in favour of organic TR: (T/F)
(a) Murmur ends well before S2
(b) Does not become louder in inspiration
(c) More louder than functional
(d) Hepatic pulsation more prominent
(e) Parasternal heave more prominent

434. Acute MR: (T/F)
(a) Murmur always pansystolic
(b) May radiate to axilla
(c) Radiate to back
(d) Associated with palpable presystolic impulse
(e) Palpable S4

435. Rheumatic MS: (T/F)
(a) OS indicates seventy
(b) Presystolic accentuation presence denotes severity
(c) MDM ↑ with ASD
(d) If AF+ then start anticoagulation
(e) Heart rate reduction can improve symptom

436. MS with LAA clot: (T/F)
(a) BMV
(b) MVR
(c) Open mitral commissurectomy
(d) Closed mitral commissurectomy
(e) Warfarin for 3 months → TEE→ dissolves→ BMV

437. IE in VSD with shunt of < 1.5 :1 false: (T/F)
(a) IE incidence 1-2:1000 patient years
(b) Life time risk of dying due to I.E. - 5-7%
(c) Depends on size of VSD
(d) Surgery closure dominates IE risk
(e) Previous endocarditis in small VSD – should be closed

438. Causes of diastolic MR: (T/F)
(a) Acute AR
(b) DCMP with first degree heart block
(c) Restrictive physiology
(d) VSD
(e) MS (Rheumatic)

439. Acute vs chronic MR – favouring acute MR *except:* (T/F)
(a) Sinus tachycardia (b) Hypotension
(c) Tachypnea (d) Rales
(e) Loud holysystolic murmur

440. BAV – true: (T/F)
(a) Associated with NOTCH-1 gene
(b) Root dilatation seen
(c) Seen in 5% of general population
(d) ↑ ed risk of aortic dissection
(e) More common in females

441. I.E. prophylaxis indicated in: (T/F)
(a) MVP with no MR (b) MR
(c) PDA (d) OP ASD > 1 year
(e) OS ASD

442. Murmur of AS ↑ ed by: (T/F)
(a) Amyl nitrate (b) Isoproterenol
(c) Handgrip (d) Exercise
(e) Leg raising

443. Murmur of MVP – length ↑ ed by: (T/F)
(a) Standing (b) Handgrip
(c) Bradycardia (d) Leg raising
(e) Exercise

444. LVOT obstruction – causes are: (T/F)
(a) Subaortic membrane (b) HOCM
(c) Shone complex (d) Bicuspid aortic valve
(e) Cortriatriatum

445. Mitral annular calcification – Risk factors are: (T/F)
(a) Hurler Syndrome (b) Marfan Syndrome
(c) Young age (d) DM
(e) HTN

446. Organic versus hypertensive TR: (T/F)
(a) Former louder
(b) Ends before S_2 in organic
(c) Hepatic pulsation more prominent
(d) Left parasternal heave more in hypertensive
(e) Organic does not increase on inspiration

447. Tricuspid opening snap: (T/F)
(a) Augmented by leg raising
(b) Radiates to a wider area than mitral OS
(c) Augmented by inspiration
(d) Usually follows mitral
(e) Augmented by Muller's monliver

448. MVP seen in: (T/F)
(a) Metabolic syndrome (b) Obesity
(c) Pectus excavatum (d) Straight back
(e) Scoliosis

449. I.E. true: (T/F)
(a) From infection to symptomatic > 2 weeks duration
(b) Splenomegaly more in acute I.E.
(c) ICH seen in 5%
(d) Emboli moore in MCA
(e) Emboli seen after 4 weeks of treatment

450. Prophylaxis for I.E.: (T/F)
(a) Tooth extraction
(b) Tonsillectomy
(c) Intubation
(d) Cardiac catheterization
(e) Cholecystectomy

451. Early PV endocarditis organisms involved: (T/F)
(a) Coagulase -ve staph (b) Staph aureus
(c) HACEK (d) Gram -ve cocci
(e) Candida

452. All true about rheumatic fever: (T/F)
(a) Arthralgia less common in Indians
(b) WBC < 5,000 in synovial fluid
(c) Arthritis and carditis often co-exist with inverse severity
(d) Sydenham's chorea never coexist with arthritis
(e) Polyarthritis migratory with each joint involvement upto 1 month

453. Mitral valve: (T/F)
(a) AML has more annular attachment
(b) PML separates LV outflow versus outflow tract
(c) PML has 3 scallops
(d) Middle scallop is involved more commonly in MVP
(e) Both leaflets have equal area

454. Rheumatic fever true is: (T/F)
(a) ASO positive for 8 months
(b) Anti DNAse B positive for 35 months
(c) ASO paired sera positive in 99.9%
(d) ASO positive, anti DNAse positive in 99.9%
(e) ASO positive in 70% patients

455. BAV: (T/F)
(a) Common in females
(b) Aortic dilatation common
(c) Aortic dissection is common
(d) NOTCH-1 gene is involved
(e) Infective endocarditis is not common

456. Acute MR murmur: (T/F)
(a) May radiate to axilla
(b) May radiate to back
(c) Palpable LVS4
(d) Palpable systolic impulse is common
(e) Always pan systolic

457. Organic versus hypertensive TR differentiated by: (T/F)
(a) Louder intensity
(b) Better hepatic pulsations
(c) Ends well before S2
(d) Para-sternal heave is more prominent
(e) Does not increase with inspiration

458. I.E.: (T/F)
(a) Bactremia within 2 weeks of infection
(b) MCA most common territory involved
(c) ICH-5%
(d) Splenomegaly in acute IE > SARE
(e) Embolic after 2 weeks of treatment

459. I.E. prophylaxis required in: (T/F)
(a) Endotracheal intubation
(b) CAG
(c) Tonsillectomy
(d) GB surgery
(e) Tooth extraction

460. Rheumatic fever: (T/F)
(a) Is a streptococcal infection
(b) Chorea
(c) Pancarditis
(d) Carey Coombs' murmur
(e) Permanent joint damage

461. Infective endocarditis: (T/F)
(a) Embolic events common in acute I.E.
(b) I.E. manifestation within 2 weeks of bacteremia
(c) Splenomegaly more common in acute I.E.
(d) ICH in 5%
(e) Most common in MCA territory

462. Major Jone's criteria include: (T/F)
(a) Chorea (b) Arthritis
(c) Carditis (d) PR interval
(e) Sore throat

463. X-ray features of LAE include: (T/F)
(a) Double density of atrial shadow
(b) Widened carinal angle
(c) Prominent aortic knuckle
(d) Anterior displacement of lower esophagus
(e) Boot shaped heart

464. C/I of CMV include: (T/F)
(a) LA clot
(b) Severe calcific MS
(c) Mild AR
(d) Pregnancy
(e) Pliable mitral valve leaflets

465. Conditions commonly causing IE: (T/F)
(a) Small VSD (b) PDA
(c) Tricuspid atresia (d) TOF
(e) Ebstein's anomaly

466. Common presenting features of AS: (T/F)
(a) Blue tues and nails (b) Angina
(c) Syncope (d) Breathlessness
(e) Pedal edema

467. I.E.: (T/F)
(a) Embolism in MCA territory most common
(b) Embolism maximum 2 weeks of antibiotics
(c) Bacteremia and fever have interval of 2 weeks
(d) Splenomegaly more in acute than subacute

468. Cause of AR:
(a) PAN (b) Paget's disease
(c) HTN (d) Mucopolysccharidosis
(e) Rheumatic MS

469. Non rheumatic MR ↑ by: (T/F)
(a) Expiration (b) Squatting
(c) Standing (d) Leg raising
(e) Hand grip

470. Severe AR A/E:
(a) Regurgitation volume > 50 ml
(b) Regurgitation fraction > 50%
(c) Aortic orifice area eH 0.3
(d) Vena contracta > 0.6

471. Severe TR A/E:

(a) Annular diameter > 4 cm
(b) Regurgitation fraction > 40% of RA
(c) Regurgitation orifice > 0.4
(d) Regurgitation volume > 45 ml

472. PARTNER TRIAL:

(a) TAVI (b) CRT-D
(c) AICD

473. Severe AS, worst predictor of bad prognosis:

(a) Gradient > 60 mm Hg
(b) Systolic BP fall during exercise
(c) Velocity > 4 cm/s
(d) Dobutamine injection increase gradient > 20%

474. True about rheumatic fever:

(a) Subcutaneous nodule more common in west
(b) Erythema marginatum more in Indians
(c) Chorea more in Indian
(d) Carditis more in west

475. In AR true:

(a) Rosenbach sign- liver palbable
(b) Ewart sign- spleen palpable

476. True is:

(a) Mitral valve open 30 sec before tricuspid valve
(b) Mitral valve open 12-15 sec before tricuspid valve
(c) Both open simultaneously in sinus rhythm

477. Parachute mitral valve A/E:

(a) Single papillary muscle may be present
(b) Presents as MS/MR
(c) Can present without symptoms
(d) Sometime corrective surgery not needed

478. Clinical severity of rheumatic MR A/E:

(a) Systolic thrill (b) S_3
(c) Length of murmur (d) MDM

479. Murmur in acute AR A/E:

(a) PSM (b) ESM
(c) EDM (d) MDM

480. Tricuspid valve A/E:

(a) Circumference 10-12 cm
(b) Anterior papillary muscle large and attached to anterior and septal leaflet
(c) Posterior papillary muscle large with posterior and septal leaflet
(d) Septal leaflet rudimentary/absent

481. Rheumatic carditis A/E:

(a) Fibrinous pericarditis
(b) Fibrinoid necrosis with neovacularisation of valve
(c) Myocyte necrosis
(d) Pin head vegetation on valve

482. Severe TS gradient:

(a) > 3.5 (b) > 7
(c) > 10 (d) > 12

483. Malar telangiectasias are seen in patients:

(a) Advanced pulmonary stenosis
(b) Advanced Aortic stenosis
(c) Advanced Tricuspid stenosis
(d) Advanced Mitral Stenosis

484. Following statement is false regarding lesion/nodule on body:

(a) Janeway lesions are nontender
(b) Janeway lesions are typically seen on palms & soles
(c) Oslers nodes are nontender
(d) Oslers nodes are typically seen on the pads of fingers or tones

485. Which of the following is the wrong statement about bioprosthetic valve?

(a) Bioprosthetic valve in mitral position is usually associated with a mid systolic murmur
(b) In normally functioning aortic prosthesis, a mild diastolic murmur can be heard
(c) Decrease in OC or CC of prosthetic valve needs further evaluation
(d) High pitched or holosystolic apical murmur signifies paravalvular or regurgitation

486. M model in MS following is true:

(a) Decreased EF slope
(b) Posterior movement of PML
(c) Paradoxical septal movement
(d) Systolic anterior motion

487. All of the following are common cause of acute AR *except:*

(a) Infective endocarditic (b) Aortic Dissection
(c) Marfan's syndrome (d) Myocardial Infarction

488. All of the following true regarding acute onset AR *except:*

(a) S4 is consistently present
(b) Absent peripheral sign
(c) Presystolic accentuation is present
(d) LV dilatation is absent

489. Which of the following is abnormal finding of aortic prosthesis?

(a) Opening click
(b) Diastolic murmur
(c) Closing click
(d) Systolic ejection murmur

490. All of the following are typical complication of standing MS *except:*

(a) Atrial fibrillation
(b) Systemic embolism
(c) Right ventricular hypertrophy
(d) Left ventricular systolic dysfunction

491. In which of the following condition presence of LV S3 is least likely?

(a) Mitral stenosis
(b) Mitral regurgitation
(c) Aortic stenosis
(d) Aortic regurgitation

492. In a patient with indication for AVR, concomitant aortic root surgery is indicated if aortic root dimension is more than:

(a) 35 mm (b) 45 mm
(c) 50 mm (d) 55 mm

493. Regarding explanation for syncope in aortic stenosis which of the following statement is false?

(a) Decrease cerebral perfusion
(b) Vasodepressor response during exercise
(c) Transient AF
(d) Malfunction of chemoreceptor

494. Rheumatic fever: (T/F)

(a) I penicillin allergic azithromyin 250 mg OD
(b) Revised JONES criteria – arthralgia – major
(c) Second RF in established RHD – one major with e/o GABHS infection
(d) IVIG delays onset of RHD when given in rheumatic carditis

495. Chorea: (T/F)

(a) Recurrence is common
(b) In 50% RF
(c) Permanent sequelae (CNS)
(d) Chorea not associated with valvular lesion

496. I.E.: (T/F)

(a) Strepto. Viridans most common
(b) Fungal – embolism more common than bacteria
(c) I.E. prophylaxis given in VSD
(d) Right side – hemoptysis/cough
(e) Libmann sach's – sterile

497. Hangout interval: (T/F)

(a) Aortic – 0.02 sec
(b) Pulmonary– 0.04-.12 sec
(c) Pulmonary hangout interval increases due to increased capacitance with decreased resistance
(d) 75% of the S2 split is due to increased hangout interval
(e) Hangout interval is proportional to impedence

498. Chorea: (T/F)

(a) More common in young
(b) Recurrence is common
(c) In 50% cases
(d) CNS sequelae is permanent

499. MS: (T/F)

(a) LV S3 in critical MS
(b) RV S3 is a measure of RV dysfunction
(c) OS heard best at apex and low pitched
(d) Decrease murmur in presence of ASD
(e) Loud S1 because of persistent LA- LV gradient in late diastole

500. Valve replacement surgery: (T/F)

(a) Lifelong anticoagulation in bioprosthesis and AF
(b) Anticoagulation for 66 months in all patients
(c) Less degeneration of bioprosthetic valve in young

501. BMV: (T/F)

(a) Long term outcome OMV > BMV
(b) Low valve score and low baseline MP are imp factor
(c) Brockenbrough needle
(d) I.E. prophylaxis not required after BMV

502. TAVI: (T/F)
(a) Edward Sapiens – self expandable
(b) BAV – relative C/I
(c) Rapid vent pacing required for Edwards
(d) Edwards can be implanted transjugular/femoral/apical
(e) Core valve balloon expandable

503. True/False:
(a) Plasma density 1.060
(b) Chylomiron/ chylomicron remnants more dense than plasma
(c) LP (a) is less dense than plasma
(d) Lp (a) levels directly correlation with kringles
(e) Classification depends on density on ultrafiltration

504. NVE: (T/F)
(a) 10 mm vegetation class 1 indication for surgery
(b) HACEK – large vegetation with systemic emboli
(c) Ceftriaxone 2 g I/V 4 weeks + gentamicin 3 mg/kg/d – 2 weeks for enterococci
(d) Revised Duke – persistent positive culture and single culture for cardiobacterium
(e) Treatment for NVE and PVE is same except staph but longer duration

505. Dynamic auscultation: (T/F)
(a) AS decreases with squatting
(b) VSD increases with hand grip
(c) MR increases with amyl nitrate
(d) MR murmur – no change with post VPC
(e) MVP– squatting, click and murmur closer to S1

506. True or False:
(a) AR murmur decreases with vasopressor
(b) AS murmur increases post VPC

507. PVE: (T/F)
(a) Duke's criteria not applied
(b) Early PVE upto 90 days
(c) Streptococci infection most common cause of late PVE
(d) Fever is less in early PVE

508. True or false:
(a) Cage ball valve – stenotic
(b) Flexible endoscopy and bronchoscopy– ampicillin and gentamicin 1 hour prior

509. BAV: (T/F)
(a) M:F= 4:1
(b) Associated with aortic dissection
(c) Inherent aortic stenosis
(d) COA in 50%
(e) Incidence 2% live birth

510. Rheumatic carditis: (T/F)
(a) Pancarditis
(b) Carditis elderly > young
(c) New onset cardiomegaly indication myocarditis
(d) Life long prophylaxis is not mandatory
(e) Mitral Valve 70-75% involvement

511. Bicuspid Aortic valve: (T/F)
(a) M:F= 4 : 1
(b) Associated with Aortic dissection
(c) Inherent Aortic stenosis
(d) COA 50%
(e) Incidence 2%/live birth

512. Percutaneous intervention is therapeutic in: (T/F)
(a) Calcified AS
(b) Calcfied MS
(c) Degenerated prosthetic valve
(d) Supramitral ring
(e) Sub Aortic membrane

513. Prosthetic valve: (T/F)
(a) Bioprosthetic valve longer duration
(b) Life long anticoagulation with bioprosthetic
(c) Once thrombosis maintain INR: 2-3
(d) Star Edward valve inherently stenotic
(e) Aortic valve–maximum thrombosis

514. I.E. in prosthetic valve: (T/F)
(a) Early < 90 days
(b) Fever less common with early PVE
(c) Dukes may not diagnostic
(d) Late mainly due to streptococci

515. Rheumatic carditis: (T/F)
(a) Pancarditis
(b) Carditis elderly > young
(c) New onset cardiomegaly indication myocarditis
(d) Life long prophylaxis is not mandatory
(e) Mitral Valve 70-75% involvement

516. Rheumatic arthritis: (T/F)
(a) Mainly monoarthritis
(b) Jaccould's arthritis – small joint
(c) Resolves in 3-4 weeks
(d) α- hemolytic streptococci

517. Cause of Chest pain MS: (T/F)
(a) Bronchitis (b) PE
(c) Coronary embolism (d) Pericarditis
(e) RV ischemia

518. BMV: (T/F)
(a) Transjugular preferred approach
(b) C/I in severe pulmonary HTN
(c) CMV long term result better than BMV
(d) IE prophylaxis not required for post BMV
(e) Main criteria for success– mild MR and less echo valve score
(f) Success is indicated by no commissural fusion after BMV

519. Murmur: (T/F)
(a) MR not affected by AF/VPC
(b) Squatting ↑ AS murmur
(c) Valsalva strain ↑ MS murmur
(d) Murmur of MS and OS–↑ with expiration/↓ with inspiration

520. Rheumatic MS: (T/F)
(a) Murmur of MS and OS– ↑ with expiration/ ↓ with inspiration
(b) RVH severe silent MS
(c) ↓ symptom with severe PAH
(d) Intensity of murmur not suggest severity
(e) Fick method murmur over estimates CO

521. AS: (T/F)
(a) Severe when jet velocity > 4 m/s
(b) Valve areas < 0.4 cm^2/m^2 BSA
(c) Moderate 1.5-2cm^2
(d) Peak gradient > 60 mm Hg with normal LVCO
(e) Low flow low gradient suggest 1.2 cm^2 valve area

522. AS severity: (T/F)
(a) High risk – >5% SCD/yr
(b) ≥ Grade III murmur required for severe AS
(c) Peak to peak gradient same on echo and cath

523. IV drug abuse: (T/F)
(a) Staph. aureus is most common
(b) TV is most commonly involved by staphylococcus
(c) TOF – bronchial biopsy requires prophylaxis
(d) Pericardial fistula is absolute Indication for Surgery
(e) Intracardiac fistula – Absolute indication for Surgery

524. BMV: (T/F)
(a) Antegrade approach is better
(b) Gives better result in metallic commisurotomy than balloon
(c) LAA thrombus absolute C/I
(d) Iatrogenic ASD can occur
(e) Double balloon most useful
(f) Retrograde less complication

525. Acute rheumatic fever: (T/F)
(a) 0.3 – 3.0% primary attack rate
(b) 60% ASO positivity in rheumatoid arthritis
(c) Jones criteria in 1994
(d) Established RHD requires atleast 2 minor criteria with GABHS
(e) Increased immune response to GABHS relates with damage

526. Acute rheumatic fever: (T/F)
(a) GABHS has 20 serotypes
(b) Genetic predisposition not seen

527. Aortic stenosis: (T/F)
(a) Pseudo AS— increase valve area after dobutamine stress
(b) Asymptomatic severe AS can be safely followed
(c) Asymptomatic severe AS – absolute C/I for TMT
(d) Increase BNP in severe AS
(e) Normal valve area 2-3 cm

528. BMV: (T/F)
(a) Successful BMV > 1.5 cm^2
(b) Dense spont echo contrast is a relative contraindication
(c) LA thrombus relative C/I
(d) Metallic commissurotomy is better than Inoue balloon
(e) Early successful BMV prevents recurrence

529. BAV: (T/F)
(a) Mild AR is usual
(b) Can be used as bridge in severe AS with CHF
(c) Curative in neonatal AS
(d) Subvalvular memb. AS-BAV is better than surgery
(e) Femoral complication can occur in 1/3rd patients of congenital AS

530. Balloon atrial septostomy: (T/F)
(a) Can be done upto 3 months of age
(b) Umbilical vein can be used in neonates
(c) 1/3 neonates develop femoral complication
(d) Can be used in ASD dependent circulation
(e) Can be used in TGA, TAPVR, MV/PV/TV atresia

531. Post streptococcal reactive arthritis: (T/F)
(a) Involves small joints of hand
(b) No response to salicylates
(c) Required sec prophylaxis for RF
(d) Lasts longer than RF
(e) Occurs early

532. Rheumatie fever: (T/F)
(a) In chorea – inf in cerebellum and basal ganglia
(b) Ashoff nodules – s/o active carditis
(c) Mucoid strain more pathogenic
(d) 25 subtypes of GABHS based on M proteins
(e) Max recurrence in previous Rheumatic fever patients

533. IE prophylaxis A/E:
(a) Ebstein's anomaly (b) Secundum ASD
(c) Cleft MV (d) Muscular VSD
(e) PDA post op > 3 months

534. Bioprosthetic valve: (T/F)
(a) Aspirin is always indicated
(b) BPV less effective in CRF patients undergoing hemodialysis
(c) MV – INR – 2.5 – 3.5
(d) AV – INR = 2.0-3.0

535. Prosthetic valve: (T/F)
(a) Starr-Edwards less suitable for small cavity
(b) Omniscience=ball caged valve
(c) Best hemodynamic = bileaflet valve
(d) Ball–caged valve = hemolysis
(e) Thromboembolism is not always due to valve

536. Bioprosthetic valve preferred: (T/F)
(a) Adolescence
(b) Elderly 70 years with severe MR with LV dysfunction
(c) Prosthetic valve leak
(d) Prosthetic valve thrombosis
(e) Hemodialysis

537. Treatment of Acute Rheumatic Fever: (T/F)
(a) Sulfadiazine 0.5 gm/d
(b) Erythromycin 0.5 gm/d in sulfadiazine allergic patients
(c) 3 weeks of benzathine penicillin does not assure protection always
(d) Recurrent episodes mimic first episode
(e) Penicillin V 250 mg BD

538. I.E.: (T/F)
(a) Janeway lesion – embolisation macule
(b) Osler node – tender immune
(c) N splinter hemorrhage – distal 1/3rd nail bed
(d) Roth spot – conjunctiva pale central spot
(e) Third generation cephalosporin DOC for HACEK group

539. AS: (T/F)
(a) HF survival 2 years
(b) Angina most common symptoms
(c) Syncope survival 8-10 years
(d) Mild AR in 10% cases
(e) Anacrotic notch appear due to AR

540. I.E. uncommon in: (T/F)
(a) Severe MS with PAH
(b) Moderate MR
(c) ASD with severe PAH
(d) Large VSD
(e) Small PDA

541. Prosthetic valve endocarditis: (T/F)
(a) Early PVE > 90 days
(b) Duke's criteria is not applicable
(c) Streptococci common in late PVE
(d) Fever is uncommon in early PVE
(e) Flexible bronchoscopy and endoscopy with I.E. prophylaxis

542. Coronary artery aneurysm: (T/F)
(a) Mucocutaneous LN syndrome

(b) Mycotic
(c) Atherosclerotic
(d) Post PCI
(e) Marfan

543. Prophylaxis I.E.: (T/F)
(a) Endoscopy (b) Tonsillectomy
(c) Cystocopy (d) LSCS
(e) Cardiac catheterization

544. Rheumatic fever prophylaxis: (T/F)
(a) Sulfadiazine dose is 500 mg OD
(b) Erythromycin dose is 500 mg OD
(c) Oral penicillin 250 mg BD
(d) Failure has been seen even with 3 weeks prophylaxis
(e) Erythromycin is indicated only in patient sensitive to sulfadiazine

545. Rheumatic fever: (T/F)
(a) IL-1, IL-2 are decreased
(b) CD-4 are increased and ratio of CD-4/CD-8 increased
(c) Aschoff nodule is not pathogonomic
(d) Can occur after 8-12 weeks of throat infection
(e) No association with HLA-2 antigen
(f) Second attack of RF does not mimic initial attack

546. Myxoma: (T/F)
(a) Chance of recurrence after excision is 10%
(b) Arises from posterior wall
(c) Can lead to mitral valve destruction
(d) Systemic effect can cause clubbing
(e) Leimyosarcoma aparts from myxoma is most common

547. HIV: (T/F)
(a) Can cause lymphoma
(b) Decreases atherosclerosis
(c) Pulmonary HTN
(d) Myopericarditis
(e) Marantic endocarditis

548. Chronic AR: (T/F)
(a) Landolfi's sign – pulsating spleen
(b) Rosenbach's sign – pulsating liver
(c) Traube's sign – nodding of head
(d) Quincke's sign – pulsating nail beds
(e) Gerhardt's sign – pulsating spleen

549. Chronic MR:
(a) Normal filling pressure in compensated
(b) Increased intraventricular contraction time
(c) Decreased intraventricular contraction time
(d) Increased filling pressure in compensated
(e) EF = 50% is considered normal

550. Severe AS symptomatic true:
(a) SCD can be seen without symptoms
(b) CXR– not diagnostic in old age without calcified valve
(c) In dissection of aorta, BP should be reduced to 130/90 in 30 mins

551. Systolic murmur after MI A/E:
(a) MR (b) VSD
(c) Dynamic LVOT (d) Dynamic RVOT

552. I.E. organisms predominant for both early and late PVE A/E:
(a) S. aureus (b) Streptococci
(c) Co NS (d) Enterococci

553. Pressure half time – 250 msec, MVA= :
(a) 0.46 cm^2 (b) 0.88 cm^2
(c) 1.26 cm^2 (d) 2.52 cm^2

554. All are features of Renal artery thrombosis *except:*
(a) Abdominal pain (b) Proteinuria
(c) C. hematuria (d) ↓ ed LDH

555. I.E. present in all *except:*
(a) Heart transplant – severe MR
(b) Biscuspid Ao valve –severe AR
(c) Normal functioning prosthetic valve
(d) Previous I.E.

556. Rheumatic fever:
(a) Incidence 3% in treated pharyngitis
(b) 50% of Rheumatic fever involves heart
(c) Vulnerable age– 50% of pharyngitis due to GBHS
(d) Recurrence in previous RF patient is 3%

557. Rheumatic fever false is:
(a) Jaccold arthritis – chronic RF-periarticular fibrosis
(b) Polyarthritis within 2-3 weeks of pharyngitis
(c) Recurrence on benzathine penicillin – 10%
(d) Subcutaneous nodule after 1 month of pharyngitis

558. BMV all contraindicated *except:*
(a) Calcified commissures
(b) LA body clot
(c) Moderate and more MR
(d) Moderate subvalvular disease

559. AVR in AR – class I indication:
(a) Symptomatic NYHA II with EF – 55%
(b) Symptomatic NYHA III with EF – 55%
(c) Asymptomatic patient with LVEDD > 55 mm
(d) EF = 22%

560. Systolic tenting of MV in MR:
(a) MVP (b) RHD
(c) Chordal rupture (d) DCMP with MR

561. BMV contraindicated in A/E:
(a) AF (b) Severe MR
(c) Calcified MV (d) LA thrombosis

562. I.E.:
(a) Erythromycin in penicillin allergy
(b) Echo is not cost effective in patients with low probability
(c) Most common precipitating factor is invasive procedure
(d) Leucocytosis is a reliable feature

563. AS all *except:*
(a) SCD only in severe AS
(b) Surgery only in symptomatic
(c) Angina can occur without CAD
(d) Measurable gradient if AVA decreases by 50%

564. HACEK I.E. DOC:
(a) Ceftriaxone
(b) Vancomycin + Rifampicin + gentamicin
(c) Crystalline Penicillin + gentamicin + rifampicin
(d) Vancomycin + gentamicin

565. Nosocomial IE—organism:
(a) Candida (b) Gram +ve cocci
(c) Staph. aureus (d) Strep viridans

566. Epsilon waves seen in:
(a) ARVD (b) Hypothermia
(c) Brugada

567. 20 years old female non-calcific MS, TOC:
(a) BMV (b) CMV
(c) OMV (d) MVR

568. Prosthetic valve patient presents with thrombosis of valve treatment:
(a) Thrombolysis (b) Urgent surgery
(c) IV heparin + warfarin

569. Patient with murmur since birth presents with palpitations, on exam. Mild cyanosis, elevated JVP, S1 loud with second component loud and delayed, PSM in LPS, mechanisms of PSVT:
(a) WPW (b) AF
(c) AVNRT (d) VT

570. Patient presents with elevated JVP with a wave, edema, loud S1, MDM at apex and LPS, chest clear, OS present diagnosis:
(a) MS (b) MS with TS
(c) MS with AR (d) MS with TR

571. Patient with loud S1, normal S2, diastolic sound 0.10 sec after S2 between apex and LPS, no murmur, diagnosis made by:
(a) Exercise (b) Handgrip
(c) Squatting (d) Valsalva

572. Soft S1 A/E:
(a) Short PR interval
(b) Severe MR
(c) MS with a rigid valve
(d) Large pericardial effusion

573. S3 true:
(a) May be heard in CCP
(b) Caused by systolic filling of the ventricles
(c) Associated with ASD
(d) Is characteristically soft in aortic stenosis

574. All of the following statements regarding opening snap in mitral stenosis are true *except:*
(a) S2 opening snap interval correlated with MS intensity
(b) Best heard with diaphragm
(c) Best heard with calcified valve
(d) ↓ with MR

575. Pulmonary edema with cardiomegaly seen in A/E:
(a) MR (b) AR
(c) Pure MS (d) ASD

576. Most common cause of aortic stenosis in an 8 years old child in India is:
(a) RHD (b) BAV
(c) Subaortic membrane (d) HOCM

577. True A/E:
(a) MR and AR decreases with isometric hand grip
(b) MVP increases with valsalva maneuver

(c) HOCM softens on squatting
(d) Murmur of PR increases in intensity on deep inspiration

578. 8 months of prosthetic valve endocarditis most common organism:
(a) HACEK group (b) S. viridans
(c) S.aureus (d) S. epidermidis

579. Fever, anemia, splenomegaly and cardiac murmur in I/V drug addicts:
(a) Vancomycin (b) Penicillin G
(c) Ceftriaxone (d) Moxifloxacin

580. Class I indication for surgery in native valve endocarditis A/E:
(a) Perivalvular abscess
(b) Fungal endocarditis
(c) Heart failure
(d) Large mobile vegetation

581. BMV C/I A/E:
(a) Left atrial clot
(b) Fixed orifice MR
(c) Calcified mitral commissure
(d) Wilkin score > 12

582. OS with MS A/E:
(a) OS and S2 interval are related to severity MS
(b) Best heard with diaphragm
(c) OS disappear in presence of MR
(d) OS classically heard with calcified and severely fibrosed valve

583. Erythema marginatum A/E:
(a) Pathognomonic of rheumatic fever
(b) Sparing of face
(c) Blanches on pressure
(d) No effect of NSAIDS

584. According to new guidelines, severe MS is defined as:
(a) < 1 cm^2 (b) < 1.5 cm^2
(c) < 0.7 cm (d) < 1.0 cm^2/m^2 BSA

585. Paradoxical splitting of S_2 occurs in:
(a) LBBB (b) RBBB
(c) RV failure (d) TAPVC

586. PHT for mitral valve area is affected by:
(a) Mitral regurgitation (b) Low cardiac output
(c) LV compliance

587. Infective endocarditis in children, which is true?
(a) Staph. Aureus is most common cause
(b) PDA is the most common lesion causing I.E.
(c) VSD is not a risk factor for I.E.
(d) 2D ECHO usually shows no vegetation in most of the cases

588. Major criteria for diagnosis of RHD includes A/E:
(a) Syndeham chorea (b) Carditis
(c) Polyarthritis (d) ASO titre

589. Echocardiographic criteria for severe MR is A/E:
(a) Regurgitant volume > 60 ml
(b) ERO > 0.4 mm
(c) Vena contracta > 0.5 mm
(d) LVESD > 45 mm

590. Regarding aortic stenosis which is true?
(a) Presence of S4 indicates impending LV dysfunction
(b) BAV causes 4 times more commonly calcific aortic stenosis than acquired causes
(c) To relieve angina, nitrates is to be used
(d) Digoxin is used for treatment of atrial fibrillation in AS

591. A patient with loud S1, MDM at apex with presystolic accentuation heard best at the left lateral position. Diagnosis is:
(a) MR (b) MS
(c) AS (d) AR

592. In aortic stenosis, gradient calculated using 4v2 is:
(a) Peak instantaneous gradient
(b) Mean gradient

593. In AR loud S3 suggests:
(a) LV dysfunction (b) LV hypertrophy
(c) Associated MR (d) Severe AR

594. High risk for IE, A/E:
(a) VSD
(b) HOCM
(c) MS
(d) MVP with severe MR on echo

595. IE A/E:
(a) Strep viridans responsible for > 50% of NVE
(b) Staph epidermidis responsible for > 50% of PVE
(c) Partial antibiotic treatment is most common reason for culture -ve IE

596. AS A/E:
(a) AVR is common modality of treatment
(b) Syncope is ominous sign
(c) Carotid shudder is common
(d) All true

597. Regarding MS, all true *except:*
(a) S3 seen in young male
(b) S2-0S interval inversely relates to severity of MS
(c) Even with severe MS, 20% patient would be in sinus rhythm

598. Cephalization in MS denotes LA pressure:
(a) 12-15 mm Hg (b) 15-18
(c) 18-24 (d) > 24

599. Rh fever age group:
(a) 5-15 (b) 5-10
(c) 5-20 (d) 12-18

600. TS severe:
(a) TVG>5 (b) >7
(c) PHT > 150 (d) TVG>5 + PHT> 150

601. 60-year-old male with CHF presyncope in ace I ↓ ed carotid pulse, TV aortic valve gradient 100 on single extrasystole, best management:
(a) AVR
(b) Balloon aortic valvoplasty
(c) BB
(d) Furosemide

602. Most common cause of AS in 10-year-old child in India:
(a) Bicuspid (b) Unicuspid
(c) Rheumatic (d) SABE AS

603. AS true is:
(a) 1st symptom is syncope
(b) Palpitations – ominous sign
(c) Angina is due to concomitant usually CAD
(d) Gradients > 25 mm Hg is indication of surgery

604. Cardiac ms A/E:
(a) Most abundant in epicardium
(b) Most abundant in atrium and ventricle
(c) T tubules are present
(d) Ionic transmission through gap junction
(e) Sacroplasmic reticulum more abundant in skeletal than myocardium

605. Subcutaneous nodules in RF true:
(a) Most specific for RF
(b) More seen in chronic cases and incidence <2%
(c) Painful 0.5-2 mm and immobile over extensor surface
(d) Present over trunk and extremities
(e) More prominent over legs

606. True for IE is:
(a) Fever and new onset murmur hallmark for IE
(b) Right sided murmur can be absent
(c) I/V drug user right sided valve commom
(d) Mortality high despite treatment
(e) All

607. Severe TS suggested by:
(a) Gradient > 3 mm Hg
(b) Gradient > 5 mm Hg
(c) Gradient > 7 mm Hg
(d) Gradient > 5 mm Hg with PHT > 150 msec
(e) PHT > 150 msec

608. Symptoms in AS true is:
(a) Presence of palpitations is S/O ominous prognosis
(b) Syncope is earliest symptoms
(c) Chest pain usually due to CAD
(d) Severe AS > 25 mm Hg – surgery

609. Severity of AR can be assessed by:
(a) Hill sign (b) Quincke
(c) Traube (d) De musset
(e) Water hammer pulse

610. True about MS:
(a) OS –p2 interval indicates severity
(b) Calcified valve – absent OS
(c) BMV is C/I in MI
(d) Presystolic accentuation present in AF
(e) Earliest sign is pedal edema

611. Prosthetic valve–what is definitely abnormal in bioprosthesis?
(a) AR murmur in AV prosthesis
(b) Grade 2-3 mid systolic murmur at left sternal border in mitral tissue prosthesis
(c) Grade 2-3 diastolic murmur in mitral position
(d) MSM at suprasternal and upper right area in aortic prosthesis

612. Major criteria of Jones:
(a) Chorea (b) Arthralgia
(c) Fever (d) PR interval

613. Bileaflet valve false:

(a) St Judes (b) Medtronic heart valve
(c) Star Edward

614. Acute MR A/E:

(a) Hypovolemia with MVP
(b) Hypertension with MVP
(c) IE
(d) Acute MI

615. Second stenosis in rheumatic MS:

(a) Development of rheumatic AS
(b) Pulmonary vasoconstriction
(c) Development of rheumatic TS
(d) Subvalvular fibrosis

616. AR is not associated with:

(a) Barlow's syndrome
(b) Subaortic stenosis
(c) Bicuspid aortic valve
(d) Ankylosing spondylitis

617. Acute MR not a feature of:

(a) HOCM (b) I.E.
(c) Trauma to chest (d) Angina pectoris

618. Severe MS A/E:

(a) A2-0S short
(b) Hepatomegaly
(c) Presystolic accentuation
(d) Loud P2

619. Tricuspid stenosis for diagnosis, mean diastolic gradient >:

(a) 2 (b) 4
(c) 5 (d) 10

620. BAV:

(a) More in female
(b) NOTCH 1 gene
(c) Associated with abdominal aortic aneurysm
(d) No high IE risk

621. Severe AR surgical indication:

(a) NYHA ≥ 3 (b) LVEDD > 65
(c) LVESD > 45 (d) EF 60%

622. Acute severe AR associated with all *except:*

(a) Loud SI (b) Austin Flint murmur
(c) S3 (d) S4

623. Native valve endocarditis + MRSA 1st line of treatment:

(a) Ceftriaxone
(b) Vancomycin
(c) Naficillin/Oxacillin + Gentamycin

624. AR common with all *except:*

(a) Subaonic VSD (b) TOP
(c) BAV (d) Truncus arteriosus

625. AR common with all *except:*

(a) Subaortic VSD (b) TOP
(c) BAV (d) Truncus arteriosus

626. 70 years female had 3 episodes of syncope in last 2 weeks. Sputum produce breathlessness × 2 days. Afebrile. Cholesterol = 170. X-ray prominent left heart border ano no, increase in any other chamber size with pulmonary edema BP = 130/90°. Most likely cause:

(a) Calcific AS (b) I.E.
(c) MS (d) MVP

627. Dynamic LVOT obst. all *except:*

(a) Amyloid
(b) Hypereosinophilic syndrome
(c) Post op AS
(d) Anteroapical MI with posterobasal hypertrophy

628. I.E. prophylaxis is to be given in:

(a) Ostium secundum ASD + Dental extraction
(b) Ligated PDA + Cystoscopy
(c) CoA +Catheterization
(d) AVR + Dental cleaning and scaling

629. NBTE most common cause:

(a) Adenocarcinoma GIT (b) GIT mucinoma
(c) GIT sarcoma (d) DVT

630. Severity of MS indicated by all *except:*

(a) A2-OS interval (b) Loud S1
(c) PND (d) Duration of murmur

631. Severity of MS indicated by all *except:*

(a) Loud P2
(b) Hepatomegaly
(c) Shot A2 OS
(d) Presystolic accentuation

632. MS seen in:

(a) S3
(b) Reversed splitting of S2

(c) Pre systolic murmur
(d) PND

633. Echo Doppler assessment of MR include all *except:*
(a) Vena contracta
(b) Intensity of regurgitant flow
(c) Holosystolic flow
(d) Regurgitant flow as % of LA

634. BAV true is:
(a) Click seen only in severe AS
(b) Click intensity prop to severity
(c) Click heard after end of Murmur
(d) In non severe AS, click widely separated by S1

635. Organic TR differ from hypertensive TR:
(a) Organic TR end before A2
(b) Organic TR are more loud
(c) Systolic hepatic pulsation more in organic TR
(d) RV heave more prominent with organic TR

636. Mitral valve false:
(a) Anterolateral papillary muscle usually single
(b) Anterolateral papillary muscle supplied by RCA commonly
(c) Middle cusp is most common prolapse in PML

637. Gradient to diagnosis TS:
(a) 2 mm Hg (b) 4 mm Hg
(c) 5 mm Hg (d) 10 mm Hg

638. Acute MR shows:
(a) Wide split S2, variable
(b) Narrow split S2
(c) Reverse split
(d) Normal

639. TR without PAH:
(a) Holosystolic (b) ESM
(c) MSM (d) MDM

640. Serology in I.E. A/E:
(a) Legionella (b) Barotenella
(c) HACEK (d) Coxiella

641. Vena contracta seen in:
(a) MR (b) MS
(c) HOCM

642. Acute severe AR – all marker indicate severity *except:*
(a) Loud S1 (b) Austin flint murmur
(c) S3 (d) S4

643. Patients with chronic aortic regurgitation are likely to have (as compared to acute aortic regurgitation):
(a) Normal pulse pressure
(b) Elevated left ventricular end-diastolic pressure
(c) Dilated left ventricle
(d) Sinus tachycardia

644. All of the following findings suggest severe tricuspid regurgitation on echocardiography *except:*
(a) Vena contracta width >7 mm
(b) Systolic flow reversals in hepatic veins
(c) Jet velocity > 4 m/s
(d) None of the above

645. Which of the following is an abnormal finding in a patient who had undergone mitral valve replacement with bileaflet valve?
(a) Opening click (b) Closing click
(c) Diastolic murmur (d) Systolic murmur

646. Which of the following is true of arthritis associated with acute rheumatic fever?
(a) Spine and axial joints are frequently affected
(b) Usually painless
(c) Resolves in most patients within 3-4 weeks
(d) Joint aspirates are usually acellular

647. A 40-year-old man is admitted with fever, dyspnea, hypotension and new murmur of aortic regurgitation. Which of the following is typical of acute aortic regurgitation?
(a) A widened systemic pulse pressure
(b) A long, decrescendo diastolic murmur
(c) Delayed closure of the mitral valve on echocardiography
(d) Diastolic mitral regurgitation on echocardiography

648. A 25-year-old woman of suspected primary pulmonary arterial hypertension undergoes right sided catheterization study. The mean pulmonary artery pressure is 44 mm Hg, and PCWP is 11 mm Hg. Infusion of epoprostenol reduces the mean PAP to 31 mm Hg with no change in systemic blood pressure or PCWP. Following statements are true *except:*
(a) Both intravenous adenosine and inhaled nitric oxide are alternative useful agents to assess vasoreactivity
(b) The observed drop in mean PAP is predictive of a favourable response to oral calcium channel blockers

(c) The failure of the systemic blood pressure to decline suggests that the vasodilator challenge was ineffective
(d) Very high doses of chronic calcium channel blocker therapy would likely be necessary for clinical benefit

649. Wilkins score is for:
(a) Mitral stenosis (b) Mitral regurgitation
(c) Aortic stenosis (d) Aortic regurgitation

650. In severe aortic regurgitation:
(a) Vena contracta width <0.3 cm
(b) Regurgitant orifice area ≥0.3 cm^2
(c) Regurgitant fraction 40%
(d) Regurgitant volume 50 ml

651. Mechanism of syncope in severe aortic stenosis:
(a) Systemic vasodilatation
(b) Abnormal baroreceptor mechanism
(c) Vasodepressor response
(d) All of the above

652. Low flow low gradient aortic stenosis:
(a) Valve area <1.0 cm
(b) LV ejection fraction <40%
(c) Mean pressure gradient <30 mm Hg
(d) All of the above

653. One of the following disease become symptomatic early in the course of disease:
(a) Mitral regurgitation
(b) Aortic stenosis
(c) Mitral stenosis
(d) Aortic regurgitation

654. False statement about mitral valve prolapse syndrome:
(a) Female (b) Click
(c) Malignant (d) Thin leaflets

655. Example for single tilting disc valve:
(a) CarboMedics valve (b) Medtronic Hall valve
(c) St. Jude valve (d) Hancock valve

656. Normal finding in Bileaflet tilting disc mitral prosthesis:
(a) Diastolic murmur
(b) Systolic murmur
(c) Both systolic and diastolic murmur
(d) No murmur

657. Most common organism in early prosthetic valve endocarditis:
(a) Streptococci
(b) Staphylococcus aureus
(c) Enterococci
(d) Staphylococcus epidermidis

658. Modified Duke criteria is for the diagnosis of:
(a) Primary pulmonary hypertension
(b) Acute rheumatic fever
(c) Chronic rheumatic heart disease
(d) Infective endocarditis

659. Drug of choice for methicillin resistant Staphylococci:
(a) Vancomycin (b) Nafcillin
(c) Oxacillin (d) Cefazolin

660. Criteria for severe mitral stenosis:
(a) MVA ≤ 1 cm^2
(b) PHT ≥ 220 m.sec
(c) Mean gradient ≥ 10 mm Hg
(d) All of the above

661. Bioprosthetic value – True A/E:
(a) Preferred in young due to more durability
(b) Mech. value not preferred in female preferring pregnancy

662. In isolated chronic MR or chronic AR, CO is maintained because of:
(a) Right shift of LV pressure volume curve
(b) Left shift of LV pressure volume curve
(c) Relaxation of LV
(d) None

663. Prophylaxis of IE to be given:
(a) Percutaneous closure of PFO for 3 months
(b) PDA occluder for > 1 year
(c) TOF with VSD patch

664. Indication for surgery all except in bacterial endocarditis:
(a) > 10 mm mobile vegetation
(b) No decrease in size of vegetation after 2 weeks of therapy
(c) New CHB
(d) Heart failure

665. Acute AR all *except*:
(a) Soft S1

(b) S3 and S4 present
(c) Austin flint murmur absent

666. Incorrect statement (about mitral regurgitation):
(a) Overestimation of severity when width of eccentric jet is used
(b) 3D echo can be used to calculate value area by planimetry
(c) Severe AR jet with > 6 mm

667. Expected survival after syncope in AS:
(a) 5 years (b) 3 years
(c) 2 years (d) 1 year

668. Infective endocarditis with Listeria Monocytogenes cause:
(a) Ureteric stent (b) Pulmonary
(c) IV drug use (d) Dental procedure

669. Not a criteria for RVH:
(a) qR in V_1
(b) RSR_1 in V_1 with R > 0.8
(c) $S_1 Q_3$
(d) $S_1 S_2 S_3$

670. Severe M.S., LA pressure increased by, all *except*:
(a) Severe anemia
(b) PAPVC
(c) M.R.
(d) Hypertensive heart disease

671. AR severity:
(a) Loudness of murmur
(b) Reverse S2 split
(c) Graham Steel murmur
(d) ESM

672. True regarding AS, all *except*:
(a) Instantaneous gradient > peak to peak gradient
(b) In some cases, low gradient can be present in severe AS
(c) Pulling of catheters from LV to aorta can decrease gradient in critical AS
(d) Instantaneous gradient is done by Doppler

673. Wilkin score is used for:
(a) Mitral stenosis (b) Pulmonary stenosis
(c) Aortic stenosis (d) Tricuspid stenosis

674. Mechanism of balloon mitral valvuloplasty is:
(a) Chordal separation
(b) Commissural separation
(c) Leaflet stretch
(d) Papillary muscle separation

675. Which one of the following echo finding is suggestive of severe MR?
(a) Effective regurgitant orifice 0.40 cm square
(b) Vene contracta 0.30 cm
(c) Central jet MR area > 50% LA area
(d) Regurgitant fraction 40%

676. Rupture of chordae tendinea to posterior mitral leaflet produces prominent murmur over following area:
(a) Apex (b) Axilla
(c) Base of heart (d) Left scapular

677. Which one of the following is not used for the surgical treatment of tricuspid regurgitation?
(a) Metalic valve (b) Bioprosthesis
(c) Suture annuloplasty (d) Ring annuloplasty

678. Which one of the following is not true for mechanical prosthetic valve?
(a) Bileaflet valve (b) Trileaflet valve
(c) Ball and cage valve (d) Tilting disc valve

679. Which one of the following is true for oral anti-coagulation after bioprosthetic mitral valve surgery?
(a) It is not required
(b) It is required for the first 1 year
(c) It is required for the first 3 months
(d) It is required lifelong

680. Which one of the following is recommended after mechanical valve replacement?
(a) Only vitamin k antagonist anticoagulant
(b) Aspirin + clopidogrel
(c) Vitamin k antagonist anticoagulant + aspirin
(d) Vitamin k antagonist anticoagulant + dipyridamole

681. Which one of the following organism is associated with culture negative endocarditis?
(a) Salmonella
(b) Coxiella burnetii
(c) Pseudomonas species
(d) Enterococcus faecalis

682. Streptococcus gallolyticus endocarditis is commonly associated with:
(a) Cirrhosis of liver
(b) Gastrointestinal lesion

(c) Skin lesions
(d) Uremia

683. Following is not true for janeway lesions:
(a) It is painless hemorrhagic macules
(b) Common over soles and palms
(c) Commonly associated with staphylococcal endocarditis
(d) It results from immune complex deposition and focal vasculitis

684. According to modified Duke's criteria, following is not true for diagnosis of infective endocarditis:
(a) 2 major criteria
(b) 5 minor criteria
(c) 1 major and 2 minor criteria
(d) 1 major and 3 minor criteria

685. Which one of the following is not an indication for surgery in patients with infective endocarditis?
(a) Persistence of vegetation after antimicrobial therapy
(b) Highly mobile vegetation of > 10 mm size over anterior mitral leaflet
(c) Embolic episodes during first 2 weeks of therapy
(d) Valve perforation

686. In aids patients with infective endocarditis following organism is uncommon as a causative organism for endocarditis:
(a) Salmonella species
(b) Streptococcus pneumoniae
(c) Streptococcus aureus
(d) Clostridium septicum

687. Which one of the following is not true for Jaccoud arthritis?
(a) It occurs after repeated attacks of rheumatic fever
(b) It is painless without signs of inflammation
(c) Ulnar deviation of 4th and 5th fingers are common
(d) Hyperextension of metacarpophalangeal joints are common

688. Which one of the following is not true for sydenham chorea in rheumatic fever?
(a) It may persist for 2 years
(b) It is never unilateral (hemichorea)
(c) It does not occur simultaneously with arthritis
(d) Emotional lability is common

689. Which one of the following is not true for subcutaneous nodules in rheumatic fever?
(a) Usually firm and painful
(b) Freely movable over the subcutaneous tissue
(c) Usual size is 0.5 cm to 2 cm
(d) Occurs in crops

690. Which one of the following is not true for erythema marginatum in rheumatic fever?
(a) The rash is evanescent, pink and non pruritic
(b) It has irregular serpingious border
(c) It becomes less prominent after taking hot bath
(d) It extends centrifugally, whereas skin at centre returns to normal

691. Which one of the following is not true for echo finding in patients with severe diastolic dysfunction?
(a) E/A >1.5
(b) Deceleration time of E wave >220 msec
(c) E/A >10
(d) E/A < 5 cm/sec

692. 3 years child post ARF incidence of PSGN:
(a) 50% (b) 30%
(c) 80% (d) 90%

693. Post streptococcal rheumatoid arthritis:
(a) 6 Record very well to NSAID
(b) In severe condition can be given for 6 months with steroid tapering
(c) After 6 months of treatment, 5% of patients have recurrence
(d) Similar to rheumatic arthritis

694. Post Streptococcal rheumatic arthritis. True:
(a) Aspirin dose – 10 mg/kg
(b) Prophylaxis for rheumatic fever should be given

695. Class I Indication of MR with good indication:
(a) Symptom with EF–25% NYHQ 3
(b) EF–30% NYHA 2 with PAH
(c) ESD > 48 with EF–50% Asymptomatic Age
(d) Asympt Age 60 EF–6%, Asymptomatic

696. Mid diastolic murmur – all *except*:
(a) PR (b) Sev. MR
(c) Sev. AR (d) Large VSD

697. I.E. – 8 months old – prosthetic value + Most common org.:
(a) Staph. aureus (b) Staph. epidermidis
(c) HACEK (d) Streptococci

698. Rheumatic fever dose of oral penicillin:

(a) 400 mg bd (b) 250 mg bd
(c) 1.2 g bd (d) As per wt

699. All occur close to S2 *except*:

(a) Physiological S3 (b) Pericardial knock
(c) Ejection click (d) Opening snap

700. Acute aortic regurgitation is not associated with:

(a) Infective endocarditis of aortic valve
(b) Aortic dissections
(c) Margan's syndrome
(d) RV myocardial infarction

701. Which of the following auscultatory finding is abnormal in prosthetic aortic valve?

(a) Opening click
(b) Diastolic murmur
(c) Short systolic ejection murmur
(d) Closing click

702. All of the following are typical complications of long standing mitral stenosis *except*:

(a) Atrial fibrillation
(b) Systemic thromboembolism
(c) Pulmonary arterial hypertension
(d) Left ventricular systolic dysfunction

703. Which of the statement is False regarding mitral valve prolapse murmur?

(a) Increases on squatting
(b) Decreases on squatting
(c) Increases on valsalva
(d) Increases on standing

704. Lyme carditis is characterized by all, *except*:

(a) It is caused by Borrelia burgdorferi
(b) It usually begins in winter month with a characteristic rash
(c) 10% of untreated patients with Lyme disease demonstrated transient cardiac disease
(d) The most common manifestation is atrioventricular block of variable degree

705. All are true about transcatheter aortic valve implantation *except*:

(a) Catheter implantation of aortic valve was first accomplished in 2002
(b) SAPIEN valve incorporates a balloon-expandale stainless steel stent frame
(c) Transvalvular regurgitation is rare, but paravalvular regurgitation is common
(d) Cardiac arrhythmias are a major cause of mortality and morbidity complicating TAVI

706. All are true for tubercular pericarditis *except*:

(a) Pericardial involvement develops in approximately 2% of patients with pulmonary tuberculosis
(b) Late constrictive pericarditis may develop despite antitubercular treatment
(c) PCR to detect M. tuberculosis can be performed with minute amounts of pericardial fluid with sensitivity of more than 70%
(d) If there is no particular contraindication, corticosteroids may be given even though they do not prevent constriction

707. According to revised JONES criteria 2015, "low risk" population is defined as incidence of ARF in:

(a) < 4/100000 school aged children
(b) <3/100000 school aged children
(c) <2/100000 school aged children
(d) <1/100000 school aged children

708. Juvenile mitral stenosis is defined as predominant or pure mitral stenosis in age group:

(a) <20 years (b) <18 years
(c) <15 years (d) <12 years

709. Type IIIA mitral regurgitation is caused by:

(a) Ischemic cardiomyopathy
(b) Marfan syndrome
(c) Barlow syndrome
(d) Radiation

710. A homograft is the preferred valve choice in the following scenario:

(a) A 45 years old man with aortic valve endocarditis and aortic root abscess in the presence of a bicuspid aortic valve
(b) A 30 years old man with a non repairable aortic bicuspid valve in the setting of severe symptomatic aortic insufficiency
(c) A 68 years old woman with chronic lymphocytic leukemia, who has rheumatic mitral stenosis that is not amenable to valvuloplasty
(d) A 70 years old woman with a non repairable aortic valve in the setting of severe symptomatic aortic insufficiency

711. All are true regarding primary prevention of rheumatic fever *except*:

(a) Involves antibiotic treatment of presumed/proven GAS pharyngitis
(b) Simpler than primordial prevention
(c) Oral penicillin preferred over benzathine penicillin in young children
(d) There is one fewer case of rheumatic fever for every 50–60 patients of GAS pharyngitis treated with antibiotics

712. All are true about rheumatic valvulitis *except*:

(a) Lasts for 2 weeks
(b) Length > 2 cm, increases embolism
(c) Usually < 2 cm
(d) Preantibiotic era, last longer

713. According to revised JONES criteria in high risk population for ARF, all are true *except*:

(a) Subclinical criteria major criteria
(b) Arthritis major criteria
(c) Raised ESR minor criteria
(d) Fever minor criteria

714. Rifampin is used in prosthetic valve endocarditis due to:

(a) Staph
(b) Streptococcus (nutritional vallent) - granulibattela
(c) Hacek
(d) Bartonella

715. Which of the following does not require urgent cardiac intervention before planned surgical procedure?

(a) Severe asymptomatic AS
(b) Severe AR
(c) Wenckebach
(d) Symptomatic severe MS

716. All are class I indication for surgery in severe AR:

(a) Symptomatic severe AR
(b) Asymptomatic severe AR posted for other cardiac surgery
(c) LVEDD more than 65 mm
(d) Severe asymptomatic AR with EF less than 50%

717. Culture negative IE are A/E:

(a) Coxiella (b) Bartonella
(c) Legionella (d) T. cruzi

718. AS severity:

(a) > 4 m/s – severe AS
(b) AVA – < 1.0 cm^2 – moderate AS
(c) Severe AS – EF <50%
(d) Edema – survival less than 5 years

719. TS A/E:

(a) Edema
(b) PND
(c) Female predominance
(d) Diastolic rumble +

720. Inappropriate sinus tachycardia:

(a) HR >100/min (b) Beta blockers
(c) Physical training (d) All

721. Exercise ECG in valvular heart disease:

(a) Confirm the absence of symptoms
(b) Assess the hemodynamic response to exercise
(c) Determine prognosis
(d) All

722. Most common valve in RHD:

(a) Tricuspid (b) Mitral
(c) Aortic (d) Pulmonary

723. Acute MR murmur:

(a) Early systolic (b) Late systolic
(c) Holosystolic (d) All

724. Chronic MR – not related to severity:

(a) LV dilated (b) S3
(c) Systolic thrill (d) Loud P2

725. In a patient with HR–74/min, CO–5 L/min, Mean gradient–40 mm Hg, SEP–0.33 sec/beat. What is the aortic valve area?

(a) 0.7 cm^2 (b) 0.9 cm^2
(c) 1.0 (d) 0.5

726. Diagnosis is:

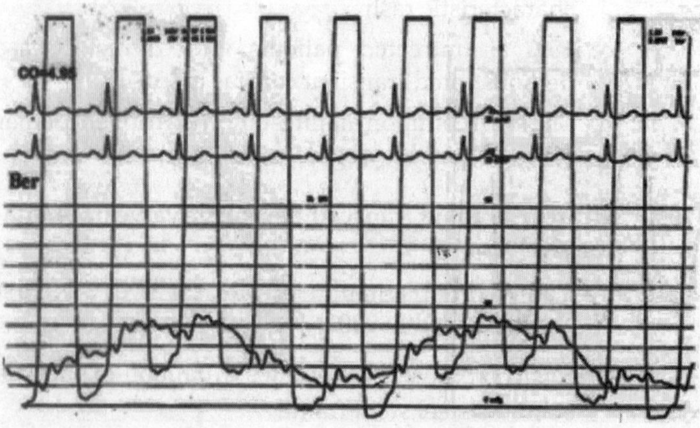

(a) AS (b) MS
(c) MR (d) PS

727. Calculate the MV area according to Gorlin formula with data below: CO–2.8 L/min, HR–75/min, MVG–16 mm Hg, Diastolic filling period–0.4 sec/beat

(a) 1 (b) 1.2
(c) 0.6 (d) 0.8

728. Recurrence of IE is most common with:

(a) Staph. aureus
(b) Candida
(c) Streptococcus viridans
(d) Enterococcus

729. Rheumatic fever A/E:

(a) Antibodies against M protein are protective
(b) Valve involvement is more important than myocardial damage
(c) Several ASLO titres are better than single titre
(d) Subclinical carditis is major manifestation

730. TAVR–true is:

(a) My valve is self expandable valve
(b) My valve is balloon expandable valve
(c) Heart team is required
(d) CT not required
(e) PARTNER trial is done with TAVR

731. Chronic AR–true is:

(a) Diastolic dysfunction
(b) Pressure volume curve shift to left
(c) Abnormal isometric relaxation
(d) Abnormal isometric contraction
(e) Normal EF

732. Severe MS:

(a) MVA less than 1 cm^2
(b) PHT more than 220
(c) Triangular MV Doppler pattern
(d) Calcified MV
(e) Commissural closure

733. Acute MR:

(a) Increased preload
(b) Decreased afterload
(c) Increased EF
(d) Increased afterload
(e) Decreased contractility

734. Low dose dobutamine test in severe AS is done if:

(a) Velocity more than 4 m/s
(b) EF less than 50%
(c) Aortic valve gradient less than 40 mm Hg
(d) Severely calcified valve
(e) Slow systolic opening of valve

735. FRC defines as:

(a) Lung volume at end of normal inspiration
(b) Lung volume at end of normal expiration

ANSWERS KEY

1.	(c)	2.	(b)	3.	(a)	4.	(a)	5.	(b)	6.	(b)	7.	(d)	8.	(b)
9.	(a)	10.	(c)	11.	(b)	12.	(d)	13.	(a)	14.	(d)	15.	(a)	16.	(b)
17.	(b)	18.	(d)	19.	(a)	20.	(a)	21.	(c)	22.	(a)	23.	(a)	24.	(a)
25.	(a)	26.	(b)	27.	T	28.	F	29.	T	30.	T	31.	(b)	32.	(d)
33.	(a)	34.	(c)	35.	(b)	36.	(c)	37.	(d)	38.	(c)	39.	(b)	40.	TTFTF
41.	FTFTT	42.	FFTFT	43.	TFTTT	44.	TFFTT	45.	FFTTT	46.	TTTFT	47.	FTTTT	48.	TTFTF
49.	(a)	50.	(c)	51.	(a)	52.	(b)	53.	(c)	54.	(c)	55.	(b)	56.	(b)
57.	(d)	58.	(c)	59.	(a)	60.	(d)	61.	(d)	62.	(b)	63.	(a)	64.	(c)
65.	(b)	66.	(a)	67.	(a)	68.	(c)	69.	(b)	70.	(d)	71.	(c)	72.	(c)
73.	(b)	74.	(d)	75.	(c)	76.	(c)	77.	(a)	78.	(a)	79.	(c)	80.	(a)
81.	(c)	82.	(a)	83.	(a)	84.	(d)	85.	(b)	86.	(d)	87.	(b)	88.	(c)
89.	(a)	90.	(a)	91.	(d)	92.	(a)	93.	(a)	94.	(c)	95.	(c)	96.	(c)
97.	(a)	98.	(c)	99.	(c)	100.	(d)	101.	(a)	102.	(a)	103.	(b)	104.	(b)
105.	(a)	106.	(a)	107.	(d)	108.	(a)	109.	(a)	110.	(a)	111.	(c)	112.	(b)
113.	(a)	114.	(b)	115.	(c)	116.	(b)	117.	(a)	118.	(a)	119.	(a)	120.	(a)
121.	(a)	122.	(a)	123.	(a)	124.	(b)	125.	(b)	126.	(a)	127.	(a)	128.	(c)
129.	(d)	130.	(c)	131.	(a)	132.	(a)	133.	(c)	134.	(a)	135.	(c)	136.	(d)
137.	(c)	138.	(c)	139.	(d)	140.	(a)	141.	(a)	142.	(a)	143.	(a)	144.	(b)
145.	(a)	146.	(c)	147.	(a)	148.	(a)	149.	(a)	150.	(c)	151.	(a)	152.	(a)
153.	(a)	154.	(a)	155.	(e)	156.	(a)	157.	(a)	158.	(a)	159.	(a)	160.	(c)
161.	(c)	162.	(c)	163.	(a)	164.	(a)	165.	(b)	166.	(d)	167.	(b)	168.	(c)
169.	(b)	170.	(b)	171.	(b)	172.	(d)	173.	(b)	174.	(d)	175.	(d)	176.	(b)
177.	(d)	178.	(d)	179.	(b)	180.	(a)	181.	(a)	182.	(c)	183.	(a)	184.	(a)
185.	(a)	186.	(d)	187.	(a)	188.	(a)	189.	(e)	190.	(d)	191.	(a)	192.	(a)
193.	(c)	194.	(a,b)	195.	(c)	196.	(b)	197.	(d)	198.	(c)	199.	(d)	200.	(a)
201.	(b,f,c,d,a)	202.	FFFF	203.	(a)	204.	(e)	205.	(b)	206.	TTTTT	207.	TTTTT	208.	(e)
209.	(a,d,e)	210.	(a)	211.	(c)	212.	(e)	213.	TFFFT	214.	TTTFT	215.	(a)	216.	(a)
217.	FFFTF	218.	(a)	219.	(f)	220.	TFFTF	221.	(b,c)	222.	(e)	223.	(c)	224.	(d)
225.	(a)	226.	(d)	227.	(a)	228.	(d)	229.	(c)	230.	(c)	231.	(a)	232.	(d)
233.	(b)	234.	(c)	235.	(b)	236.	(d)	237.	(c)	238.	(b)	239.	(b)	240.	(c)
241.	(c)	242.	(c)	243.	(a)	244.	(b)	245.	(a)	246.	(c)	247.	(a)	248.	(b)
249.	(a)	250.	(a)	251.	(d)	252.	(c)	253.	(a)	254.	(c)	255.	(d)	256.	(c)
257.	(a)	258.	(b)	259.	(c)	260.	(d)	261.	(a)	262.	(a)	263.	(a)	264.	(d)
265.	(d)	266.	(d)	267.	(a)	268.	(a)	269.	(c)	270.	(a)	271.	(a)	272.	(a)
273.	(a)	274.	(a)	275.	(a)	276.	(a)	277.	(d)	278.	(d)	279.	(a)	280.	(a)
281.	(a)	282.	(a)	283.	(b)	284.	(a)	285.	(c)	286.	(d)	287.	(c)	288.	(c)
289.	(c)	290.	(b)	291.	(c)	292.	(b)	293.	(a)	294.	(c)	295.	(a)	296.	(c)
297.	(b)	298.	(c)	299.	(d)	300.	(a)	301.	(a)	302.	(a)	303.	(a)	304.	(a)
305.	(a)	306.	(c)	307.	(c)	308.	(b)	309.	(d)	310.	(d)	311.	(d)	312.	(d)
313.	(c)	314.	(b)	315.	(d)	316.	(b)	317.	(c)	318.	(c)	319.	(a)	320.	(b)
321.	(b)	322.	(c)	323.	(d)	324.	(b)	325.	(b)	326.	(c)	327.	(d)	328.	(d)
329.	(a)	330.	(b)	331.	(a)	332.	(b)	333.	(c)	334.	(b)	335.	(a)	336.	(b)

337.	(d)	338.	(a)	339.	(b)	340.	(a)	341.	(c)	342.	(b)	343.	(d)	344.	(c)
345.	(c)	346.	(d)	347.	(a)	348.	(c)	349.	(c)	350.	(a)	351.	(a)	352.	(b)
353.	(a)	354.	(a)	355.	(d)	356.	(c)	357.	(c)	358.	(c)	359.	(c)	360.	(a)
361.	(b)	362.	(b)	363.	(a)	364.	(a)	365.	(b)	366.	(b)	367.	(b)	368.	(a)
369.	(c)	370.	(a)	371.	(b)	372.	(a)	373.	(a)	374.	(b)	375.	(a)	376.	(c)
377.	(a)	378.	(b)	379.	(a)	380.	(c)	381.	(a)	382.	(a)	383.	(a)	384.	(a)
385.	(a)	386.	(a)	387.	(d)	388.	(b)	389.	(a)	390.	(a)	391.	(b)	392.	(a)
393.	(a)	394.	(a)	395.	(d)	396.	(b)	397.	(d)	398.	(b)	399.	(d)	400.	(a)
401.	(d)	402.	(d)	403.	(b)	404.	(c)	405.	(c)	406.	(b)	407.	(d)	408.	FTFFF
409.	TTTT	410.	TF?TT	411.	FTFTF	412.	FFTTF	413.	FFTTT	414.	FFTTT	415.	FFTTT	416.	TFFFF
417.	TTTFF	418.	FFTFT	419.	TTFFF	420.	TTFTF	421.	FTFFF	422.	TFTTF	423.	TTFTT	424.	FTTFT
425.	TFFTT	426.	TTTFT	427.	TTFFT	428.	TTFFT	429.	TFTTT	430.	FFTTT	431.	TTTFF	432.	FFTFT
433.	TFFFF	434.	FFFFT	435.	FFFTT	436.	FTTFT	437.	TTFFF	438.	TTFFF	439.	TTTTF	440.	TTTTF
441.	FFFFF	442.	TTFFF	443.	TFFFF	444.	TTTFF	445.	FTFTT	446.	FTFFF	447.	TFTTF	448.	FFTTT
449.	FFTTF	450.	TFFFF	451.	TTFFT	452.	FFTFF	453.	FFTTT	454.	TFTFF	455.	FTTTF	456.	FFTFF
457.	FFTFT	458.	TTTFF	459.	FFTTT	460.	FTTTF	461.	FTFTT	462.	TTTFF	463.	TTFTT	464.	TTFFF
465.	TTTTF	466.	FTTTF	467.	TFTF	468.	(a,b,c,d)	469.	TTFTT	470.	(a)	471.	(b)	472.	(a)
473.	(b)	474.	(a)	475.	(a)	476.	(a)	477.	(b)	478.	(c)	479.	(a)	480.	(c)
481.	(b)	482.	(b)	483.	(d)	484.	(c)	485.	(b)	486.	(a)	487.	(d)	488.	(c)
489.	(b)	490.	(d)	491.	(a)	492.	(b)	493.	(d)	494.	FFTT	495.	TFFF	496.	TTTTT
497.	TTTTT	498.	TTFF	499.	FTFTT	500.	TFF	501.	TTTT	502.	FTFTF	503.	TFTTT	504.	FTFFT
505.	FTFTF	506.	FT	507.	FFTF	508.	TT	509.	TTTFT	510.	TFTTT	511.	TTTFT	512.	TFFFF
513.	FFFTF	514.	FFFT	515.	TFTTT	516.	FTTF	517.	FFTFT	518.	FFFFTF	519.	TTFT	520.	TTFTF
521.	TFFTF	522.	TTF	523.	TTTTF	524.	TFTTFF	525.	TFTTT	526.	FF	527.	TTFTT	528.	TTFFF
529.	TTTFT	530.	TTTTT	531.	TTTTT	532.	TFTFT	533.	FTTTF	534.	TTTT	535.	TFTTT	536.	FTFFF
537.	FFTFT	538.	TTFFT	539.	TFFFF	540.	FFTFF	541.	FFTFF	542.	TTTTT	543.	FTFFF	544.	TFTTF
545.	FTFFFF	546.	FFFTF	547.	TFTTT	548.	FTFTT	549.	(b,d)	550.	(a)	551.	(d)	552.	(b)
553.	(b)	554.	(d)	555.	(b)	556.	(b)	557.	(d)	558.	(d)	559.	(a)	560.	(d)
561.	(a)	562.	(b)	563.	(c)	564.	(a)	565.	(b)	566.	(a)	567.	(a)	568.	(a)
569.	(d)	570.	(b)	571.	(c)	572.	(a)	573.	(a)	574.	(c)	575.	(c)	576.	(a)
577.	(a)	578.	(d)	579.	(a)	580.	(d)	581.	(b)	582.	(d)	583.	(a)	584.	(b)
585.	(a)	586.	(c)	587.	(d)	588.	(d)	589.	(c)	590.	(b)	591.	(b)	592.	(a)
593.	(c)	594.	(c)	595.	(b)	596.	(d)	597.	(a)	598.	(b)	599.	(a)	600.	(b)
601.	(c)	602.	(b)	603.	(c)	604.	(a)	605.	(d)	606.	(e)	607.	(c)	608.	(c)
609.	(a)	610.	(b)	611.	(a)	612.	(a)	613.	(a)	614.	(b)	615.	(b)	616.	(a)
617.	(a)	618.	(c)	619.	(a)	620.	(b)	621.	(b)	622.	(a)	623.	(c)	624.	(b)
625.	(b)	626.	(a)	627.	(b)	628.	(d)	629.	(a)	630.	(b)	631.	(d)	632.	(d)
633.	(c)	634.	(d)	635.	(a)	636.	(b)	637.	(a)	638.	(d)	639.	(d)	640.	(c)
641.	(a)	642.	(a)	643.	(c)	644.	(c)	645.	(d)	646.	(c)	647.	(d)	648.	(c)
649.	(a)	650.	(b)	651.	(d)	652.	(d)	653.	(c)	654.	(c)	655.	(b)	656.	(a)
657.	(d)	658.	(d)	659.	(a)	660.	(d)	661.	(b)	662.	(b)	663.	(a)	664.	(c)
665.	(b)	666.	(a)	667.	(d)	668.	(a)	669.	(d)	670.	(b)	671.	(a)	672.	(d)
673.	(a)	674.	(b)	675.	(a)	676.	(c)	677.	(a)	678.	(b)	679.	(c)	680.	(c)
681.	(b)	682.	(b)	683.	(d)	684.	(c)	685.	(a)	686.	(d)	687.	(d)	688.	(b)
689.	(a)	690.	(c)	691.	(b)	692.	(b)	693.	(a)	694.	(b)	695.	(b)	696.	(a)
697.	(b)	698.	(b)	699.	(d)	700.	(d)	701.	(b)	702.	(d)	703.	(a)	704.	(b)

705. (d)	**706. (c)**	**707. (c)**	**708. (a)**	**709. (d)**	**710. (a)**	**711. (c)**	**712. (c)**
713. (c)	**714. (a)**	**715. (c)**	**716. (c)**	**717. (d)**	**718. (a)**	**719. (b)**	**720. (d)**
721. (d)	**722. (b)**	**723. (d)**	**724. (b)**	**725. (a)**	**726. (b)**	**727. (c)**	**728. (a)**
729. (b)	**730. (b,c,e)**	**731. (a,c,e)**	**732. (a,b,c)**	**733. (a,b)**	**734. (c,e)**	**735. (a)**	

CHAPTER FOUR

ARRHYTHMIAS

1. CPVT treatment all are true *except:*

(a) Verapamil (b) Amiodarone
(c) Flecainide (d) Carvedilol

2. Which does not affect accessory pathway conduction?

(a) IA (b) III
(c) IV (d) IC

3. Drug causing methemoglobinemia:

(a) Cocaine (b) Lidocaine
(c) Dapsone (d) Furosemide

4. CPR:

(a) 100-120 (b) 60-80
(c) 100-150 (d) 120-140

5. Ectopic atrial pacemaker with presyncope/giddiness next step:

(a) EPS (b) Pacemaker
(c) Loop recorder (d) Holter monitoring

6. ECG-SVT with aberrancy Rx:

(a) Ca gluconate (b) DC version
(c) Adenosine

7. Long RP arrhythmia:

(a) PJRT
(b) AVRT Manheim
(c) Atypical AVNRT
(d) Ectopic atrial tachycardia

8. Need not be treated:

(a) Asymptomatic hyperuricemia
(b) Asymptomatic LQTs (Romano-Ward syndrome)
(c) Subclinical hypothyroidism
(d) Asymptomatic heterozygous hypercholesterolemia

9. CPVT – Mechanism:

(a) DAD (b) EAD
(c) Reentry

10. A 35-year-old patient with LVH (> 14 mm) on ECG develops AF. Best drug for long term management is:

(a) Amiodarone (b) Sotalol
(c) Flecainide (d) Propafenone

11. Class I antiarrhythmic drugs do not cause:

(a) Propafenone – ↑ ventricular rate in AF with WPW
(b) Incessant monomorphic VT
(c) Torsade de pointes
(d) Antidromic conduction in AF

12. Epsilon waves........................ Young male with syncope. Evaluation method:

(a) Cardiac MRI (b) Body temperature
(c) Chest X-ray (d) CAG

13. Irregular rhythm, Narrow complex QRS. Negative P waves in 2.3 aVF? Positive in V_1 isoelectric segment present between P waves:

(a) Ectopic AT
(b) 2 : 1 AVNRT
(c) Atrial flutter (Counter clockwise flutter)
(d) PJRT

14. CXR–bilateral infiltration, patient on AF therapy. False is amiodarone toxicity:

(a) Alveolar, interstitial, or both alveolar and interstitial infiltrates can be seen
(b) DLCO is preserved till late in the course of disease
(c) Can occur 6 days and 60 months of treatment
(d) Corticosteroids can be tried

15. VT (monomorphic) with LBBB pattern, inferior axis. Treatment RVOT-VT:

(a) Propafenone (amiodarone)

(b) Verapamil
(c) Flecainide
(d) Sotalol

16. **Phosphene (colored version) in A/E:**
(a) Ivabridine (b) Nicorandil
(c) Sildenafil (d) Tadalafil

17. **Recurrent idiopathic VT all T/E:**
(a) Adenosine can be used
(b) Most common side – left ventricular outflow
(c) Exercise ↑ it
(d) ↑ CAMP with triggered activity with DAD

18. **VVI with following reading HR set at 60:**

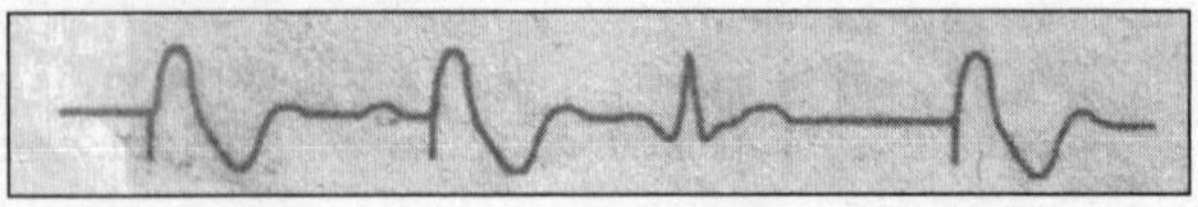

(a) Oversensing (b) Undersensing
(c) Hysteresis (d) Capture defect

19. **Epicardiac and endocardium – action potential A/E:**

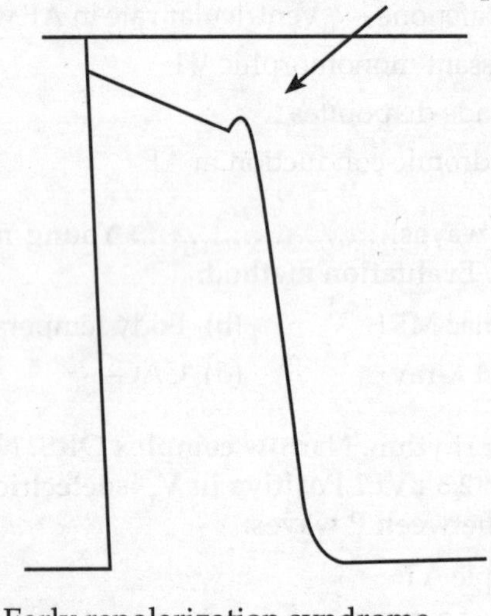

(a) Early repolarization syndrome
(b) Brugada
(c) Digitalis toxicity
(d) Flecainide

20. **SCD–true is:**
(a) Total death–7 million worldwide
(b) 25% of all deaths by CAD–SCD
(c) 25% of all presentations of CAD–SCD
(d) 25% all natural deaths–SCD

21. **ECG with AF with broad QRS axis around 90° RBBB:**
(a) AF with aberrancy
(b) AF with access pathway
(c) Pacemaker induced tachycardia

22. **CRT–changes:**
(a) QRS ↓
(b) QRS does not change, only CO ↑
(c) Only MR will decrease
(d) CO will not change, only ↑ contractility

23. **WPW patient with AF drug not used:**
(a) Digoxin (b) Ibutilide
(c) Amiodarone (d) Procainamide

24. **Indoor patient with AF, pharmacotherapy, which drug is not used?**
(a) Amiodarone (b) Ibutilide
(c) Propafenone (d) Quinidine

25. **Drug that does not cause QT prolongation (least):**
(a) Propafenone (b) Sotalol
(c) Procainamide (d) Amiodarone

26. **Pill in pocket:**
(a) Procainamide (b) Propafenone
(c) Ibutilide (d) Sotalol

27. **Prolonged QT in amiodarone due to:**
(a) ↑ ST (b) ↑ QRS
(c) ↑ Widening of QRS (d) PR prolongation

28. **Hypotension due to I/V bolus of amiodarone due to:**
(a) Class III action
(b) Beta blockers
(c) CCB action
(d) Coronary artery dilation

29. **Most common fetal arrhythmia:**
(a) APC
(b) PC
(c) Type 1, 2nd degree AV block
(d) Sinus tachycardia

30. **Atrial rate in AFI:**
(a) 200 (b) 250
(c) 300 (d) 350

31. **Feature of SVT A/E:**
(a) LAD
(b) Time to peak R < 50
(c) Vagal maneuver respond
(d) Premat. P starts

32. **Epsilon wave seen in:**
(a) ARVD (b) Brugada
(c) CPVT

33. DAD seen in:

(a) CPVT (b) LQT
(c) AIVR (d) AT

34. Concealed pathway in WPW:

(a) Less in children
(b) Mostly narrow QRS
(c) Antegrade conduction by accessory pathway
(d) Accessory pathway–hidden–no conduction

True/False (35-38)

VT

35. R in aVR diagnostics

36. Negative concordance in QRS

37. RBBB with axis + GO

38. Previous history of post MI

39. MAT:

(a) Variable P wave (b) Digoxin used for Rx
(c) PR prolonged (d) Short QT

40. Digoxin A/E:

(a) VT (b) Visual disturbance
(c) AV block (d) Hyperkalemia

41. Drugs acting on both AV node and accessory pathway:

(a) Class IC (b) IA
(c) Adenosine (d) Digoxin

42. MADIT – 1 A/E:

(a) QRS > 150 ms (b) EF < 30%
(c) Inducible VT on EPS (d) NSVT

43. CPVT all *except:*

(a) Bi-directional VT is specific
(b) B blockers useful
(c) Prolonged exercise causes sustained VT
(d) Drug of choice is dronedarone

44. SQTS true is:

(a) Syncope is common
(b) Cardiac arrest is most common presentation
(c) T wave changes are not specific

45. Digoxin is metabolized by:

(a) P-glycoprotein (b) CYP3A4
(c) CYP2C19 (d) N-acetyl transferase

46. Bidirectional VT is a characteristic feature of:

(a) Long QT syndrome (b) Short QT syndrome
(c) Brugada syndrome (d) Andersen Tawil

47. Drug very useful in children with congenital heart disease and serious ventricular arrhythmias:

(a) Amiodarone (b) Flecainide
(c) Mexiletine (d) Propafenone

48. Following may be a marker of imminent risk of "Torsade de pointes" in long QT syndrome:

(a) QRS alternans
(b) Microvolt T wave alternans
(c) T-U wave alternans
(d) Total electrical alternans

49. Factors which favor SVT in a wide QRS tachycardia–all are true *except:*

(a) "Short long" sequence preceding initiation
(b) QRS duration ≤ 0.14 sec
(c) Onset of QRS to its peak < 50 msec
(d) Slowing or termination with Valsalva maneuver

50. In AVNRT–recurrence rate after slow pathway ablation is approximately:

(a) 1% (b) 5%
(c) 10% (d) 12%

51. Drugs that slow conduction in the accessory pathway:

(a) Adenosine (b) Verapamil
(c) Bucindolol (d) Ajmaline

52. EAD/DAD: (T/F)

(a) EAD due to phase ¾
(b) Digoxin toxicity–DAD
(c) Both congenital and acquired LQT–EAD
(d) Post repolarization refractoriness–due to Tachycardia induced block
(e) Overdrive pacing in DAD – ↑ amplitude and ↑ cycle length

53. Class of drug antiarrhythmic: (T/F)

(a) Ia–↓ Vmax and ↑ APD
(b) Ia–Faster than Ib and Ic
(c) Ic–slowest
(d) Ib–↑ Vmax and ↑ APD
(e) Ic–↓ Vmax and ↑ refractoriness

54. Ca Channel: (T/F)

(a) Ca-ATPase–4 Ca^+ – inside for 1 ATP
(b) T type – atria.

(c) L type – ventricle near T tubule
(d) Conventional drug don't act on T-type
(e) In voltage gated channel during normal RMP, activation gate is open and inactivation gate is closed

55. **CRT/ICD true or false:**
(a) CRT is useful in NYHA class II, W EF < 35%
(b) Useful in all class 4 patients (NYHA)
(c) CRT for QRS ≥ 120 msec irrespective of morphology
(d) ICD is useful in NYHA class 2 class 3 with LVEF < 35%
(e) Left lead is placed via coronary sinus

56. **Which one of the following drugs is not used for pharmacological conversion of atrial fibrillation of recent onset?**
(a) Dofetilide (b) Flecainide
(c) Ismolol (d) Ibutilide

57. **Following is not true for dronedarone:**
(a) It is used to maintain sinus rhythm after conversion from AF
(b) It has structural similarities with amiodarone
(c) It can be used in patients with IVdysfunction
(d) It does not contain iodine

58. **Arrhythmogenic right ventricular dysplasia (ARVD) was coined for the first time in 1978 for "total or partial replacement of right ventricular muscle by adipose and fibrous tissue associated with arrhythmias." True regarding ARVD is:**
(a) No familial predilection of ARVD/C has been recognized
(b) The sites of involvement are found in the so-called "triangle of dysplasia", namely, the right ventricular inflow, tricuspid valve and moderator band
(c) The ECG in patients with ARVD/C usually shows sinus rhythm and a terminal deflection within or at the end of the QRS complex (called epsilon wave) in leads V5 and V6
(d) The tachyarrhythmias occurring in ARVD are characteristically monomorphic and LBBB morphology, usually with inferior QRS axis

59. **Which of the following statements is false regarding diagnosis and management of tachyarrhythmias?**
(a) CHADS2 score assesses risk of stroke in patients with non valvular AF
(b) Bundle branch re-entry (BBR) tachycardia is a type of sustained monomorphic VT, common in patients with dilated cardiomyopathy
(c) Bidirectional VT can be a manifestation of digitalis excess, typically in older patients and severe myocardial disease
(d) Belhassen's VT or idiopathic left fascicular VT is due to re-entry and is resistant to verapamil

60. **What is not correct regarding Brugada syndrome?**
(a) Male preponderance
(b) Cardiac events never occur during sleep or rest
(c) Concealed forms may be unmasked by provocative drugs like ajmaline and flecainide
(d) Quinidine may be used as an adjunct to ICD

61. **Which is not a class IA antiarrhythmic agent?**
(a) Ajmaline (b) Disopyramide
(c) Moricizine (d) Procainamide

62. **What is not true regarding amiodarone?**
(a) Prolongs APD and refractoriness of all cardiac fibres without affecting resting membrane potential
(b) Amiodarone is a peripheral and coronary vasodilator
(c) Doses need not be reduced in renal diseases
(d) With concomitant use of warfarin with amiodarone, dose of warfarin should be increased

63. **False about NASPE generic code for antibradycardia pacing is:**
(a) Position I–Chamber(s) paced
(b) Position III–Rate modulation
(c) Position II–Chamber(s) sensed
(d) Position V–Multisite pacing

64. **The management of polymorphic VT in the setting of myocardial infarction in acute phase may include all *except:***
(a) I/V Beta blockers
(b) I/V Amiodarone
(c) Urgent angiography when myocardial ischemia cannot be excluded
(d) I/V Sotalol

65. **Complications are least in radiofrequency ablation of which accessory pathway?**
(a) Left anteroseptal pathway
(b) Left posteroseptal pathway
(c) Right posteroseptal pathway
(d) Left lateral pathway

66. **Which is true regarding different parameters tested during pacemaker testing?**

(a) In case of lead dislodgement, pacing threshold will be increased
(b) In case of insulation failure, lead impedance will be increased
(c) In battery depletion, lead impedance will be decreased
(d) On loose setscrew, pacing threshold will be decreased

67. **Mechanism of counterclockwise atrial flutter is:**
(a) Automaticity in the cavotricuspid isthmus
(b) Triggered activity
(c) Reentry using cavotricuspid isthmus
(d) Any of the above

68. **Digoxin does not cause:**
(a) Ventricular extrasystoles
(b) Mobitz type 2 block
(c) Complete heart block
(d) Sinus arrest

69. **AICD–Secondary prevention trial is:**
(a) MADIT II (b) AVID
(c) CIDS (d) CASH

70. **The sinus node is predominantly characterized by depolarization in which phase of the action potential?**
(a) Phase 0 (b) Phase 1
(c) Phase 2 (d) Phase 4

71. **Long RP A/E:**
(a) Orthodromic AVRT (b) Antidromic AVRT
(c) AT (d) JPRT

72. **AF oral drug for acute termination:**
(a) Amiodarone (b) Procainamide
(c) Propaferone (d) Quinidine

73. **Ashman–phenomenon associated – A/E:**
(a) AF (b) Digoxin toxicity
(c) Long short cycle (d) ↑ refractory period

74. **Pacemaker–asymptomatic–T wave inversion in rhythm (Internal):**
(a) VT (b) Ischemia
(c) Pacemaker memory (d) LVH

75. **Managed ventricular pacemaker–true is:**
(a) ↑ battery life
(b) Right ventricular pacemaker not necessary
(c) Rate control
(d) Automatic threshold

76. **"Slew rate"–important:**
(a) Pacemaker (b) IHSS
(c) Bradyarrhythmia (d) MS

77. **Acute termination of SVT in a patient with acute asthma on theophylline:**
(a) IV verapamil (b) IV esmolol
(c) IV adenosine (d) IV digoxin

78. **Endless loop tachycardia Rx:**
(a) ↑ PVARP
(b) AV nodal delay
(c) Amiodarone
(d) ↑ effective ventricular RP

79. **↑ QRS in A/E:**
(a) Antidromic SVT (b) Orthodromic SVT
(c) SVT with aberrency (d) SVT with previous block

80. **QT prolonged by A/E:**
(a) Amiodarone (b) Procainamide
(c) Mexiletine (d) Quinidine

81. **All can be used in atrial fibrillation *except:***
(a) Amiodarone (b) Dofetilide
(c) Ranolazine (d) Mexiletine

82. **All are true about Ajmaline *except:***
(a) Inhibits platelet activity more potently than aspirin
(b) Can cause torsade de pointes
(c) Ajmaline infusion is useful in establishing diagnosis of WPW syndrome, occult Chagasic cardiomyopathy and Brugada syndrome
(d) Can cause a decrease in defibrillation threshold

83. **All are true regarding Andersen Tawil syndrome *except:***
(a) Long stature, low set ears, macrognathia and hypertelorism
(b) Weakness can be triggered by low, normal or high potassium levels
(c) Mutation of KCNJj gene are responsible for the majority of cases
(d) It has been given a long QT syndrome 7 nomenclature

84. **Bundle branch re-entry tachycardia is a feature of:**
(a) Myotonic dystrophy type 1
(b) Myotonic dystrophy type 2

(c) Emery-Dreifuss muscular dystrophy
(d) None of the above

85. A 50-year-old male patient with ICD for secondary prevention of SCD in setting of old MI with moderate LV dysfunction presented to ED with 4 ICD shocks dispersed over last 24 hours without loss of consciousness. Immediate ICD interrogation revealed all ICD shocks were appropriate for fast VT and VF events only. Which statement is true?

(a) By definition, this is not electrical/VT storm
(b) By definition, this is electrical/VT storm and ICD is to be turned off to prevent further ICD shocks
(c) Reset ICD settings to increase number of ATP therapies and increase detection rate of VF zone
(d) Catheter mediated radiofrequency ablation on an urgent basis may be an ideal modality of management (after reversible cause of VT is ruled out)

86. Following are true about CARDIOVERSION/Defibrillation shocks *except:*

(a) Monomorphic VT can often be terminated by low energy synchronized shock energy < 5 J
(b) Weak shocks risk acceleration of VT to VF
(c) High energy > 50 J shocks are generally used for VT termination
(d) Shock pain is directly proportional to shock strength

87. Short QT syndrome is characterized by all *except:*

(a) Increase risk for sudden death because of VF
(b) Persistently short QT intervals, short or absent ST segments and tall and narrow T waves in the precordial leads
(c) Hypokalemia, hypocalcemia or hypothermia can cause shortening of QT interval
(d) Quinidine has been shown to be effective in patients with a gain of function mutation in the HERG (KCNH2) gene

88. "Inverse saw-tooth" appearance on ECG is seen in which type of atrial flutter?

(a) Typical clockwise
(b) Typical counter clockwise
(c) Upper loop re-entry
(d) Septal atrial flutter

89. All are true about chaotic atrial tachycardia *except:*

(a) Atrial rates 100-130 beats per min
(b) Atleast 3 P waves contours are noted
(c) Commonly occur in older patients with COPD and CHF
(d) Digitalis is useful in treatment of this tachycardia

90. Which of the following statements is true?

(a) Maximum score of $CHADS_2$ is 10.T
(b) Score of 0 on $CHADS_2$ have stroke rate of 2% while CHA_2DS_2-VASc score of 0 indicate stroke rate of 0
(c) Dabigatran is preferred over warfarin in valvular AF
(d) None of the above

91. Conduction/Propagation velocity is slowest for:

(a) SA nodal cells
(b) AV nodal cells
(c) Purkinje fibers
(d) Atrial muscles

92. Genetic loci for ARVD-5 is:

(a) Transforming growth factor-β_3
(b) Ryanodine receptor-2
(c) Transmembrane protein-43
(d) Desmoplakin-3

93. Recommended period to avoid driving/flying after ICD implantation for secondary prevention is:

(a) 6 months
(b) 3 months
(c) 2 months
(d) Not required

94. All statements regarding autonomic innervations of atria are true, *except:*

(a) Sympathetic nerves originate inside the vertebral column and reach the stellate ganglion
(b) At the synapses within the ganglia, preganglionic neurons release acetylcholine
(c) Stimulatory beta adrenergic response is initiated via G protein subunit alpha complexes (Gα), leading to the activation of adenylcyclase
(d) Beta-1-receptors compose 20% to 30% of all beta receptors in the normal atrium

95. All statements regarding Bachmann's bundle are true, *except:*

(a) Disruption of the bundle's structure causes interatrial conduction block
(b) Based on electron microscopy, there are 5 different types of myocardial cells in Bachmann's bundle
(c) The SA nodal artery "invariably supplies Bachmann's bundle"
(d) BB action potentials are characterized by a gradual upstroke followed by a prolonged plateau phase

96. A 79-year-old retired service man with known aortic stenosis (AS) comes for his annual check-up. He remains physically active with no symptoms but his blood pressure is 180/110 mm Hg. Following echo findings were obtained:

Severe AS-peak velocity has increased from 3.8 m/sec a year ago to 4.0 m/sec at present, mean gradient 40 mm Hg, aortic valve area 1 cm², mild LVH and good overall LV systolic function.

Which one of the following statements is correct?

(a) A statin should be prescribed to reduce the rate of AS progression
(b) An antihypertensive drug should be prescribed
(c) The increase in peak velocity of > 0.2 ms/year suggests that surgery should be considered
(d) An exercise tolerance test (ETT) is unsafe in asymptomatic severe AS

97. Effect of digitalis on atrial myocyte:

(a) Effective refractory period is reduced due to direct effect
(b) Effective refractory period is reduced due to vagomimetic effect
(c) Effective refractory period is reduced due to vagolytic effect
(d) Effective refractory period is reduced due to sympathomimetic effect

98. Which of the following statements regarding the delayed after depolarizations (DADs) is not true?

(a) DADs are oscillations in membrane voltage that occur after completion of repolarization of the action potential (i.e., during phase 4)
(b) The most important influence that causes subthreshold DADs to reach threshold is a decrease in the initiating cycle length, because that increases both the amplitude and rate of the DADs
(c) Digitalis causes DAD-dependent triggered arrhythmias by inhibiting the NaVK[4] exchange pump
(d) Drugs that prolong action potential duration (e.g., class IA antiarrhythmic agents) can decrease DAD amplitude, whereas drugs that shorten action potential duration (e.g., class IB antiarrhythmic agents) can increase DAD amplitude

99. Muscle repolarization by:

(a) Inward Na
(b) Outward K
(c) Inward Ca

100. RMP in atrial and ventricular muscles by:

(a) INa (b) IK
(c) IK1 (d) If

101. Class III A/E (K blocking action):

(a) Procainamide (b) Ibutilide
(c) Bretylium (d) Sotalol

102. Class II A/E:

(a) Moricizine (b) Ibutilide
(c) Bretylium (d) Sotalol

103. TdP A/E

(a) Due to EAD (b) Short long cycle
(c) A/W ↑ QT (d) Amiodarone causes

104. ARVC A/E:

(a) Sustained monomorphic VT
(b) Genetically determined
(c) RFA relieved in 85% at 3 years
(d) Can affect both ventricles

105. Carto mapping:

(a) Alcohol ablation for HOCM
(b) RFA for VT
(c) Detection of complex long HD

106. Entrainment type of:

(a) Reentry (b) Paranystole
(c) Automaticity

107. Pill in pocket:

(a) Flecainide (b) Procainamide
(c) Dilzem

108. 16 years old boy with exercise induced syncope:

(a) HCM (b) LQTS
(c) Coronary anomaly

109. Pacemaker-III stands for:

(a) Rate response (b) Mode
(c) Senring (d) All of the above

110. Long QT in the SCN5A predisposes to SCD during:

(a) Stress (b) Auditory stimuli
(c) Sleep (d) Swimming

111. Not true about RFA in atrial fibrillation:

(a) Anticoagulation to be discontinued after RFA in patent of proxysmal AF

(b) Isolation of arrhythmic matrix in addition to pulmonary vein isolation for permanent AF
(c) Multiple sessions may be needed
(d) Ablation of ganglionated plexus

112. DOC in hyperdynamic shock with tachyarrhythmia's:
(a) Phenylephrine (b) Epinephlrine
(c) Dopamine (d) Dobutamine

113. Ventricular arrhythmias:
(a) Ectopic atrial tachycardia
(b) BB re-entrant VT
(c) Atrial flutter with variable block
(d) VT with LV aneurysm

114. Lignocaine A/E:
(a) Not used in SVT
(b) Effective in Ischemic myocardium
(c) Hypercalcemia decrease effect
(d) Not effective in NYHA-IV

115. Idiopathic LV VT:
(a) BB are DOC
(b) Precipitated by atrial pacing
(c) Commonly due to false tendon
(d) MC with inferoposterior part of septum

116. Least arrhythmogenic antidepressant:
(a) Doxepin (b) Duloxetine
(c) Imipramine (d) Amitrylline

117. ICD in HF A/E:
(a) Patient with ICD dies with progressive CHF
(b) Worse outcome in ICD and appropriate shock as compared to ICD without shock
(c) Dual chamber better than single chamber
(d) All of the above

118. ILVT A/E:
(a) Most common at inferolateral septum
(b) Precipitated by atrial pacing
(c) Beta blocker DOC
(d) Associated with false tendon

119. All true *except:*
(a) Digoxin level to be measured 6-8 hours after drug
(b) Amiodarone has distribution more than total body water
(c) Use of loading dose increases time to achieve equilibrium
(d) Digoxin is substrate for P-glycoprotein

120. RFA used in A/E:
(a) Varicose vein (b) Recurrent pericarditis
(c) CTO (d) Liver mass Ca

121. ICD all *except:*
(a) Double chamber better than single chamber
(b) EF < 30%
(c) Patient mortality in ICD is due to progressive HF
(d) Defibrillating shocks worse outcome than non-shockable

122. Drugs all *except:*
(a) Perhexiline inhibit FA oxidation
(b) Ivabridine impair night vision
(c) Ranolazine increases QT
(d) Trimetazidine increases glucose levels

123. Lignocaine all *except:*
(a) Efficacy ↓ in hypercalcemia
(b) Efficacy ↓ in class IV failure
(c) Effective in ischemic myocardium
(d) Not useful in SVT

124. ARVD poor prognosis:
(a) Young (b) TMEM43 gene
(c) LV involvement (d) Naxos disease

125. Antidepressant with higher arrhythmias:
(a) Doxepin (b) Imipramine
(c) Amitryptiline (d) Duloxetine

126. Idiopathic LV tachycardia true:
(a) B blockers used
(b) Atrial pacing ↑ arrhythmias
(c) False tendons associated with ILVT

127. Brugada syndrome true is:
(a) Female preponderance
(b) AR inheritance
(c) Exertional syncope
(d) Functional phase 2 rentry

128. TdP caused by drugs all *except:*
(a) Propafenone (b) Disopyramide
(c) Quinidine (d) Dofetilide

129. Bidirectional VT all *except:*
(a) Digoxin toxicity
(b) Anderson's syndrome
(c) CPVT
(d) Cerebrovasular accident

130. Most common cause of SCD:

(a) IHD (b) HOCM
(c) Brugada syndrome (d) ARVD

131. Digoxin toxicity all *except:*

(a) Cl ↑ ed (b) Advanced age
(c) Hypothyroidism (d) Amyloidosis

132. Dronedarone C/I all *except:*

(a) Permanent AF–PALLAS study
(b) Hepatic dysfuncton
(c) CHF
(d) Prior TIA

133. 60 years old DM-2, HTN, Normal ECG/Echo Intermittent AF with symptoms:

(a) Amiodarone with dabigatran
(b) Flecainide with warfarin
(c) Propafenone with aspirin
(d) Aspirin + clopidogrel

134. All ↑ se defibrillation threshold *except:*

(a) Dofetilide (b) Amiodarone
(c) Disopyramide (d) Flecainide

135. All have proarrhythmia effect due to ↑ed QT dispersion *except:*

(a) Amiodarone (b) Terfenadine
(c) Cisapride (d) Grepofloxacin

136. Short QT all *except:*

(a) Acidosis (b) Ischemia
(c) Hyperkalemia (d) Digoxin

137. Match all *except:*

(a) ARVD–Desmosome
(b) CPVT–Ry R2
(c) Brugada–loss of function SCN 5a
(d) I Ca Lchannel–AF

138. Genetic testing least useful:

(a) CPVT (b) Short QT syndrome
(c) Long QT syndrome (d) Brugada syndrome

139. External pacemaker:

(a) Paul Zoll (b) Burton
(c) Kriklin

140. Amiodarone pulmonary toxicity all *except:*

(a) Young age
(b) Serum level of deoxy amiodarone
(c) High daily dose
(d) ↓ baseline DLCO

141. Advanced heart block not seen in:

(a) Gout (b) Behcet
(c) Conn's syndrome (d) Fabry disease

142. Short QT syndrome all true *except:*

(a) QTc < 300 msec
(b) QTc < 88 percentile
(c) Treated with hydroquinine
(d) HERG mutation

143. Calcium channel all *except:*

(a) Membrane influx with L type channel
(b) Membrane efflux with T type channel
(c) SERCA for flux Ca into SR
(d) Ryanodine for Ca mediated Ca release

144. Osborn wave mechanism:

(a) Hyperpolarisation of cell memb
(b) ↑ Epicardial action potential
(c) Dissociation of repolarisation, depolarization
(d) Intracellular conduction defect

145. All true *except:*

(a) Vernacline is used in AF
(b) Dronedarone effective in VT
(c) Ranolazine prevents VT in NSTEMI
(d) Ivabradine in Inappropriate sinus tachycardia

146. β blocker C/I in renal failure all *except:*

(a) Atenolol (b) Carvedilol
(c) Sotalol (d) Nodalol

147. Most common cause of SCD:

(a) IHD
(b) HCM
(c) Congenital coronary anomalies
(d) ARVD

148. Reverse use dependence:

(a) III (b) II
(c) IV (d) I

149. Lignocaine all *except:*

(a) No role in SVT
(b) Hypocalcemia ↓ Effective

(c) Better than procainamide
(d) Usually has no hemodynamics SE

150. Dronedarone all *except*:
(a) Not contain iodine
(b) Has liver toxicity
(c) Better than amiodarone in AF
(d) CI in adv HF

151. Short QT syndrome:
(a) QT < 300 (b) Tall T wave
(c) AF (d) Sotalol DOC

152. ICD indicated in all *except*:
(a) ARVD (b) RVOT VT
(c) Short QT (d) Brugada

153. CPVT all *except*:
(a) ICD is treatment
(b) Mutation calsequestrin
(c) Ca mediated EAD
(d) Polymorphic bidirectional VT

154. RF ablation most effective all *except*:
(a) Counterclockwise AFL
(b) AVRT
(c) AVNRT tachycardia
(d) Paroxysmal AF

155. Syncope of quinidine:
(a) Torsades
(b) Monomorphic VT
(c) ↓ K^+
(d) Conduction disturbances

156. SCD all *except*:
(a) ALCAPA (b) LCx from RCA
(c) LAD from right sinus (d) Kawasaki

157. Match the following:
(a) AF–Reentry
(b) RVOT–Triggered activity DAD
(c) TDP–Triggered activity EAD
(d) Brugada syndrome–Triggered activity EAD

158. AF with FVR, rate can be ↓ed by all *except*:
(a) Ivabradine (b) Propranolol
(c) Verapamil (d) Carvedilol

159. Patient of AF, cardioversion unsuccessful with 360 J all *except*:
(a) Repeat 360 J→reverts
(b) Ibutilide helps in cardioversion
(c) Intracardiac version 2-15 J effective
(d) Converted to atrial flutter

160. Sick sinus syndrome:
(a) 10% dev. AF
(b) 0.6-1% develop AV block per year
(c) Atrial better than ventricular pacing
(d) Asymptomatic with 3 sec sinus pause indication of PPI

161. LQTS-7 also known as:
(a) Anderson syndrome
(b) Timothy syndrome
(c) Romano-Ward syndrome

162. Vernakalant A/E:
(a) Atrial specific
(b) Recent onset AF conversion
(c) Acts on early K^+ channel
(d) Long half life like amiodarone

163. Brugada syndrome true:
(a) ECG RBBB with ST ↑ in V1-V3
(b) K^+ channel
(c) Autosomal recessive

164. RVOT-VT: ECG:
(a) LBBB with inferior axis
(b) RBBB
(c) LBBB with superior axis
(d) LAHB

165. Belhassens tachycardia A/E:
(a) Narrow QRS
(b) RVOT
(c) Treatment with verapamil
(d) Fascicular VT

166. Amenable to radiofrequency ablation A/E:
(a) Polymorphic VT (b) AVNRT
(c) AVRT (d) Belhassen tachycardia

167. Long RP tachycardia A/E:
(a) Typical AVNRT (b) PJRT
(c) AT (d) Sinus tachycardia

168. AVNRT ablation successful rhythm:
(a) Junctional tachycardia
(b) Sinus shythm

(c) VT
(d) AF

169. Brugada gene is SCN-5A, other gene:
(a) GPDL1
(b) HCN5A
(c) SCN4B

170. Wenckebach phenomenon A/E:
(a) Incremental increments
(b) Longest RR < 2 shortest RR
(c) PR ↓ ed
(d) PR progressively ↑ ses till dropped

171. Atrial specific channel:
(a) I ks (b) I kur
(c) I kr (d) I ki

172. Digitalis side effect A/E:
(a) Vomiting (b) Anorexia
(c) Visual disturbances (d) Hyperkalemia

173. ICD indicated in A/E:
(a) LQTS with syncope of undetermined origin
(b) Resuscitated cardiac arrest
(c) EF < 50%

174. Patient inclusion criteria in MADIT- I:
(a) LVEF < 35%
(b) Inducible arrhythmia on EPS
(c) NSVT on Holter spontaneously
(d) QRS > 150 msec

175. Preoperatively in a patient with pacemaker A/E:
(a) Bipolar cautery not to be used within 15 cm
(b) VOO mode should be used
(c) Preoperative testing for impedence, battery conduction

176. Defibrillation in children:
(a) 1 J/kg (b) 2 J/kg
(c) 3 J/kg (d) 4 J/kg

177. Brugada with VT – mechanism:
(a) Phase 0 (b) Phase 1
(c) Phase 2 (d) Phase 4

178. Pacemaker in sinus node dysfunction with normal AV node:
(a) AAI (b) VVI
(c) DDD

179. WPW all *except*:
(a) Short PR interval (b) QRS -120 ms
(c) Delta + wide QRS (d) Short QT

180. Antiarrhythmic drugs all *except*:
(a) Ia decrease Vmax, increase APD
(b) Ib increase Vmax, increase APD
(c) Ic decrease Vmax, increase APD
(d) III increase repolarisation

181. AF with renal failure DOC is:
(a) Dofetilide (b) Sotalol
(c) Flecainide (d) Propafenone

182. EAD:
(a) Increase by CCB
(b) Decrease by catecholamine
(c) Increase by long cycle

183. VDD all *except*:
(a) AV syndrome
(b) Atrial pacing at slow rate
(c) Both chamber sensed

184. Class I indication for PPM — all *except*:
(a) Mobitz I AV block
(b) Neurocardiogenic + Bradycardiac response with HUTT

185. Chronic AF:
(a) Sarcoidosis
(b) Amyloidosis
(c) ↑ Thyroid

186. A. Flutter best Rx:
(a) Cardioversion-DC (b) Pacing
(c) Atropine (d) Isoproterenol

187. Isoproterenol DOC for:
(a) SVT (b) AV block
(c) VF (d) LGL syndrome

188. Deafness with fatal heart disease:
(a) Long QT syndrome
(b) Brugada syndrome
(c) CPVT

189. Best drug for ARVD:
(a) Metoprolol (b) Amiodarone
(c) Sotalol (d) Digoxin

190. Pacing on LV A/E:
(a) LBBB
(b) RBBB
(c) Wide split S2

191. CRT useful in A/E:
(a) AF (b) PR>150
(c) QRS>120 msec (d) NYHA III/IV

192. Quinidine with paradoxical tachycardia:
(a) Sick sinus (b) AF
(c) APC (d) VPC

193. Amiodarone causes A/E:
(a) ↑ PR interval
(b) Minimal effect on QRS duration
(c) ↑ QT
(d) Causes sinus tachycardia

194. Drug of choice of Broad QRS tachycardia:
(a) I/V procainamide (b) I/V digoxin
(c) I/V verapamil (d) I/V amiodarone

195. Which drug not causes TdP?
(a) Digoxin (b) Flecainide
(c) Verapamil

196. Drug of choice of SVT:
(a) Verapamil (b) Adenosine
(c) Amiodarone

197. Digoxin not useful in:
(a) MR (b) AR
(c) TOF (d) DCM

198. Increased mortality in Ia and Ic drugs demon-strated in:
(a) CASH (b) CAST
(c) CIDS (d) EMIAT

199. Least proarrhythmic drug:
(a) Flecanide (b) Encainide
(c) Amiodarone

200. Lowest energy in DC shock in:
(a) Atrial flutter
(b) Junctional tachycardia
(c) Atrial fibrillation

201. Mechanism of atrial flutter:
(a) Enhanced automaticity
(b) Increased triggered activity
(c) Reentry
(d) Unknown

202. T ½ of adenosine:
(a) 10 sec (b) 30 sec.
(c) 60 sec (d) 80 sec

203. Brugada mechanisms of arrhythmias:
(a) Reentry
(b) Triggered activity
(c) Increased automaticity

204. Plateau of action potential by:
(a) Increased Ca reflux and K efflux
(b) K and Ca influx
(c) K influx and Ca efflux
(d) K and Ca deflux

205. Calcium influx seen in:
(a) Phase I (b) Phase III
(c) Phase II

206. Normal P wave seen:
(a) AVRT (b) AVNRT
(c) VT (d) Ectopic

207. All used in SVT *except:*
(a) Digoxin (b) Beta blocker
(c) CCB (d) Adenosine

208. Atrial flutter due to:
(a) Reentry in RA (b) Reentry in LA
(c) Ectopic focus in pulmonary vein

209. AF (non valvular):
(a) Rate control better than rhythm control
(b) Rhythm better than rate control
(c) Both strategies equivalent
(d) Strategy has to be individualized

210. Accessory pathway seen in:
(a) Ebstein anomaly (b) C c-TGA
(c) HLHS (d) All

211. Ashman phenomenon seen:
(a) AF (b) Second degree CHB
(c) WPW (d) VT

212. SVT versus VT A/E:
(a) Fusion beat-VT (b) Hypotension-VT
(c) CSM-VT (d) IHD-VT

213. Last part to be excited in LV:
(a) Posterobasal (b) Anterior wall
(c) Septum

214. Percentage of energy utilized for electrical activation:
(a) 1% (b) 5%

215. Most common mode of pacing:
(a) AAI (b) VVI
(c) DDD (d) VDD

216. Sick sinus syndrome pacing indicated in:
(a) Symptomatic (b) Asymptomatic
(c) Asystole > 2 sec

217. AIVR treatment:
(a) I/V amiodarone (b) I/V lignocaine
(c) Atropine (d) No treatment

218. DDD pacemaker third 'D' stand for:
(a) Pacing (b) Sensing
(c) Response to sensing (d) Rate modulation

219. AF and AV block, best PPI:
(a) AAI (b) VVI
(c) DDDR (d) DDDI

220. Congenital CHB best management:
(a) AAI (b) VVI
(c) DDD (d) DDD + AICD

221. Recommended oral anticoagulant in AF before DC:
(a) Apixaban (b) Rivaroxaban
(c) Heparin (d) Dabigatran

222. Vernaklant A/E:
(a) Half life–2.9 to 3.3 mins
(b) Increases only atrial ERP
(c) Majority excreted by bile
(d) New drug for AF

223. ERP increaseas A/E:
(a) Ia (b) Ic
(c) II (d) III

224. VT; ECG criteria all true *except:*
(a) avR-initial r wave
(b) avR-if r absent, initial q > 20 ms
(c) avR-slurred descending limb of predominant negative qRS
(d) vi/ve ≤ 1

225. Energy used for electrical activity:
(a) 1% (b) < 5 %
(c) 10 % (d) 15 %

226. Most common cause of sudden death in young athelete:
(a) HOCM (b) Ischemia

227. Extended matching–drugs:
(a) Adenosine (b) Amiodarone
(c) IV NTG (d) Labetolol
(e) Disopyramide (f) Clopidogrel
(g) Heparin (h) Fondaparinux
(i) Bivalirudin
(1) Used in tachycardia of 220/min in 25 years age
(2) Used during CPR in cardiac arrest
(3) T inversion in right precordial leads
(4) HIT with unstable angina
(5) HTN in pregnancy

228. Which of the following drugs are not recommended for pharmacological conversion of atrial fibrillation?
(a) Amiodarone 5 mg/kg I/V over 1 hour
(b) Metoprolol 5 mg I/V over 5 minutes
(c) Ibutilide 1 mg I/V over 10 minutes
(d) Propafenone 2 mg/kg I/V over 10 min or 450-600 mg P/O

229. Electrical alternans true:
(a) Non specific sign in cardiac tamponade
(b) Due to swinging motion of heart
(c) Due to ½ the rate of HR
(d) Due to alteration in electrical activity of heart

230. Beta blockers: (T/F)
(a) Contraindicated in all COPD
(b) Can be used in CCF NYHA III

231. Amiodarone:
(a) T1/2 – 53 days
(b) Bioavailability 30 – 60%
(c) Conc. = 1-2.5 ng
(d) Continued I/V for > 3 weeks
(e) Dose < 300 mg to reduce pulmonary toxicity

232. B blockers lipid soluble no CNS effect:
(a) Carvediolol (b) Propranolol
(c) Metoprolol (d) Atenolol

233. SCD:
(a) 80% of SCD cause is CAD
(b) 30% of non MI SCD recur within a year
(c) LMCA occlusion most common in patients with SCD than general
(d) 50% of CAD have SCD as presentation

234. Worst prognosis:
(a) Pulseless electrical activity with rupture
(b) Fine VF
(c) Asystole with sudden CHB
(d) VT with LV dysfunction

235. HR-175/min, regular heart rate, every P is followed by QRS all *except:*
(a) AVRT (b) AVNRT
(c) Sinus tachycardia (d) AT
(e) A flutter

236. If RP is 60 msec (RP<PR) diagnosis:
(a) AVRT (b) AVNRT
(c) Sinus tachycardia (d) AT
(e) A flutter

237. If vagal manoeuvre fails – next management in haemodynamically stable patient:
(a) Digoxin (b) Adenosine
(c) DC shock (d) B blockers
(e) CCB

238. Amiodarone all *except:*
(a) Peripheral and coronary artery dilator
(b) More effective at slow HR
(c) Maintenance < 300 mg to reduce pulmonary toxicity

239. Short QT:
(a) <100 msec (b) <200 msec
(c) <300 msec (d) <400 msec

240. If RP is 60 msec (RP<PR) diagnosis:
(a) AVRT (b) AVNRT
(c) Sinus tachycardia (d) AT
(e) A flutter

241. Long QT syndrome True or False:
(a) QT = QTc of heart rate of 60
(b) Females has prolonged QT than males
(c) Beginning from Q to start of T wave
(d) Signifies both ventricular depolarisation and repolarisation
(e) Maximum in V_2-V_3

242. AV conduction decreased by all *except:*
(a) Lignocaine (b) Beta blocker
(c) CCB (d) Adenosine

243. ARVD: (T/F)
(a) AD
(b) LV involvement may be seen
(c) In 80%, 1st events are syncope/SCD
(d) Epsilon wave in V_1 is characteristic
(e) Malignant arrhythmia in naxo's disease

244. Management of asystole cardiac arrest:
(a) CPR immediately
(b) External trancutaneous pacing may be used
(c) Adrenaline may be given
(d) Atropine should be given
(e) Defibrillation only if shockable rhythm

245. HR-175/min, regular heart rate, every P is followed by QRS all *except:*
(a) AVRT (b) AVNRT
(c) Sinus tachycardia (d) AT
(e) A flutter

246. If vagal manoeuvre fails – next management in haemodynamically stable patient:
(a) Digoxin (b) Adenosine
(c) DC shock (d) B blockers
(e) CCB

247. DDD pacemaker:
(a) Senses both ventricle and atria
(b) Paces both atria and ventricle

(c) Senses p and initiate pacing
(d) Senses QRS and inhibit ventricle

248. Embolic protection device all *except:* (T/F)

(a) Watchman (b) Angioguard

249. Pacemaker patient for non cardiac surgery evaluation:

(a) Put on VOO mode
(b) Preoperative evaluation of impedence pulse generator and lead
(c) Bicautery avoid in 15 cm
(d) ECG can easily detect pulse changes

250. MAT: (T/F)

(a) Seen in young
(b) PP irregular
(c) P. morphology same
(d) Digoxin is treatment
(e) Class Ia is TOC

251. Both accessory and AV node:

(a) Ia (b) Ic
(c) Adenosine (d) Digoxin

252. MADIT I patient selection all *except:*

(a) QRS > 150 ms (b) NSVT
(c) EPS – inducible VT (d) CAD – sustained VT
(e) EF < 35%

253. RVOT VT: (T/F)

(a) RBBB morphology
(b) LBBB morphology
(c) Benign
(d) Associated with ARVD

254. A flutter: (T/F)

(a) P –ve in avR and +ve in I, II avF
(b) Mechanism can be reentry, triggered automaticity
(c) Macroentrant in right atrium
(d) First P wave different from remaining tachycardia

255. CPR with $NaHCO_3$: (T/F)

(a) Hypercarbic intracellular acidosis
(b) Venous acidosis in arterial alkalemia
(c) Successful CPR is best buffer
(d) Previous acidosis is an indication

256. CPR in SCD early defibrillation is preferred because: (T/F)

(a) VF progress to asystole in few min
(b) Most common is VF
(c) Early defibrillation most effective
(d) Only treatment of VF is defibrillation

257. A-V nodal dual pathways:

(a) Slow path long refractory period
(b) Fast path–short refractory period
(c) In sinus rhythm short path conduction occurs
(d) In fast path–rapid conduction and longer refractory period

258. RVOT VT mechanism:

(a) Triggered
(b) Abnormal automaticity
(c) Eeentry

259. Amiodarone:

(a) Use in LV dysfunction, diastolic dysfunction, with supraventricular and ventricular tachycardia
(b) Pulmonary toxicity in 1st week
(c) Can be used in LQTS

260. DOC for AF prevention due to HT:

(a) Dofetilide (b) Amiodarone
(c) Sotalol (d) Class IC

261. Lignocaine true:

(a) 1st drug used in VT and VF due to MI
(b) Recurent VT – bolus dose 0.1mg/kg
(c) Infusion continue in cardiac arrest resuscitation
(d) Prophylactic use ↓ mortality in MI

262. C/I of DC shock:

(a) Digitalis (b) LV dysfunction

263. CRT false is:

(a) LBBB (b) Mod sev HF
(c) LVEF=35 (d) NSR
(e) All true

264. Worst prognosis after cardiac arrest:

(a) Pulseless electrical activity with cardiac rupture
(b) Asystole with CHB
(c) VT
(d) Fine VF

265. DC shock: (T/F)

(a) Biphasic–AC current used
(b) Start from 100 J
(c) Max 150 J
(d) Adrenaline after 3 shocks
(e) None

266. Contraindication of PPI in all *except:*
(a) Suprahisian type 1, asymptomatic
(b) Awake patient > 3 sec pause, asymptomatic

267. Class III antiarrhythmic drugs:
(a) Amiodarone (b) Lignocaine

268. Amiodarone true all *except:*
(a) Dose not reduced in renal failure
(b) Coronary and peripheral vasodilation
(c) No pulmonary toxicity if <300 mg maintenance dose
(d) Corneal microdeposits in 100% after 6 months

269. Torsade (TDP) seen in all *except:*
(a) Pheochromocytoma (b) Sotalol
(c) Bradycardia (d) Ischemia
(e) None

270. Basic life support all *except:*
(a) Thump version
(b) Chest compression
(c) Mouth to mouth respiration
(d) Restoration of airway

271. AF restoration of rhythm all *except:*
(a) < 48 hours DC shock + heparin
(b) >48 hours 3 weeks prior anticoagulation of INR= 2-3
(c) Post conversion anticoagulation ideally till 6 months
(d) Flecainide to be given in cases of structural heart disease

272. Atrial flutter all *except:*
(a) Macroreentrant RA
(b) Atrial rate = 450-600
(c) AV Block present/occurs
(d) Hemodynamic collapse if 1:1 conduction

273. AF all not seen *except:*
(a) Presystolic accentuation of murmur present
(b) 'a' present
(c) S_4 present
(d) Normal QRS

274. ARVD true:
(a) Autosomal recessive
(b) Endocardium is replaced by fibrous tissue
(c) MRI used in diagnosis
(d) RV type of configuration–VT with LBBB

275. Class III antiarrhythmics:
(a) Metoprolol
(b) Procainamide
(c) Amiodarone

276. WPW syndrome true all *except:*
(a) Structurally normal heart
(b) Incidence ↑ es with increasing age

277. Risk of thromboembolism in AF ↑ all *except:*
(a) Smoking (b) History of HT
(c) Diabetes (d) RHD

278. SCD occur in A/E:
(a) RCMP
(b) Non obstructive HCM
(c) Left circumflex from RCA
(d) Tako-tsubo cardiomyopathy

279. Accessory pathway A/E:
(a) Loss of delta wave on exercise testing is suggestive of high risk
(b) Q in inferior leads
(c) Tachycardia in foetus
(d) Can present without delta wave on ECG

280. ARVD least specific ECG finding:
(a) VT with LBBB
(b) Incomplete RBBB
(c) Epsilon wave in V1-V3
(d) T wave inversion in V1-V3

281. Least dangerous VPC:
(a) VPC on descending limb of T wave
(b) Parasystole VPC
(c) Bundle branch reentry VPC
(d) VPC with QR morphology in v6

282. Paroxysmal AF with EF < 30%:
(a) Amiodarone (b) Propafenone

283. Torsade de pointes treatment not given:
(a) Intravenous amiodarone
(b) Mg
(c) Beta blockers
(d) Overdrive pacing

284. AF caused by A/E:

(a) Surgery of oesophagus
(b) Submassive PE
(c) AAI pacing
(d) Atrial infarction

285. Flecainide MOA:

(a) Na channel inhibitor

286. Exercise precipitate SCD:

(a) Can be caused by all exercise
(b) VT in HOCM
(c) NSVT in CAD
(d) RVOT VT in structural heart disease

287. Identify the WRONG match regarding the target molecule involved in the channelopathies:

(a) Arrhythmogenic RV dysplasia–Desmosome
(b) Catecholaminergic Polymorphic VT–Ryanodine receptor (RyR2)
(c) Brugada syndrome–loss of function in SCN5A
(d) Sick sinus syndrome–Voltage gated L-type cannel

288. Which one of the following is not among the major diagnostic criteria for ARVC?

(a) Epsilon wave
(b) Nonsustained or sustained VT of LBB morphology with superior axis
(c) ARVC confirmed pathologically or current task force criteria in a second degree relative
(d) Inverted T waves in right precordial lead (V_1, V_2, & V_3) or beyond in individuals> 14 years (in absence of complete RBBB QRS > 120 msec)

289. Atrioventricular node re-entry tachycardia is due to re-entry within the AV node with dual AV node physiology. Which one of the following type of re-entry is not seen in this tachycardia?

(a) Slow-fast
(b) Fast-slow
(c) Slow-slow
(d) Fast- fast

290. All of the following statements with true about sudden cardiac death *except:*

(a) Aortic rupture is an uncommon cause of sudden cardiac death
(b) History of survival after syncope is protective against sudden cardiac death
(c) Sudden cardiac death has bimodal peak
(d) One third of heart failure deaths are sudden cardiac death

291. An AICD is mandatory in symptomatic patient with ventricular tachycardia in:

(a) Right ventricular outflow tract (RVOT) VT
(b) Left ventricular outflow tract (LVOT) VT
(c) Fascicular VT
(d) Arthythmogenic right ventricular dysplasia

292. Re-entry is NOT the tachycardia mechanism in which of the following arrhythmias?

(a) AVNRT
(b) WPW syndrome
(c) EAT
(d) Atrial Flutter

293. Gene responsible for familial WPW syndrome is:

(a) KCNJ5
(b) PRKAG2
(c) HERG
(d) None of the above

294. Which of the following is not a recommended provocative test for unmasking long QT syndrome?

(a) Exercise Test
(b) Epinephrine BOLUS
(c) Epinephrine Brief Infusion
(d) Procainamide Test

295. You are evaluating a 20-year-old patient in a clinic with no previous medical history who has been having presyncope. You obtain an ECG which demonstrates a corrected QT interval of 510 ms but no other abnormalities, This patient most likely which of the following?

(a) Romano-Ward Syndrome
(b) Jervell and Lange – Nielson syndrome
(c) Brugada syndrome
(d) Timothy syndrome

296. A previously asymptomatic 17-year old female presents with a syncopal episcode occurring upon acute emotion. Her ECG shows QT prolongation with QTs ST 490 ms and low voltage/biphasic T wave in all leads. A second-degree cousim died suddenly at age 36. Which of the following is the first line of therapepils strategy?

(a) ICD and propranolol 2.5 mg/kg
(b) Nadolol 1 mg/kg
(c) ICD
(d) Nadolol and potassium supplements

297. Following criteria are useful in the diagnosis of ventricular tachycardia in a patient of wide complex tachycardia:

(a) Kindwall criteria
(b) Wellen's criteria
(c) Brugada criteria
(d) All of the above

298. A patient who has undergone AICD implantation reports to emergency room with multiple AICD shocks in last one hour. ECG done in emergency room shows AF with rapid ventricular rate. Immediate management would be:

(a) I.V. adenosine
(b) Apply magnet over AICD pulse generator
(c) I.V. verapamil
(d) I.V. amiodarone bolus followed by infusion

299. Inducible ischemia can be diagnosed by exercise testing in symptomatic patients with:

(a) Complete RBBB
(b) WPW syndrome
(c) Complete LBBB
(d) Electronically paced ventricular rhythm

300. QRS duration widening occurs due to:

(a) Sudden death is rare
(b) Mitral regurgitation can occur
(c) Can cause heart failure
(d) Surgery is curative

301. True about Catecholaminergic Polymorphic Ventricular Tachycardia

(a) Bidirectional ventricular tachycardia can occur
(b) Exercise induced AF nay occur
(c) Base line EGC may show bradycardia
(d) All of the above

302. CRT in Heart failure NYHA class 1/11 was studied in:

(a) MADIT CRT (b) Reverse Trial
(c) Both (d) None

303. Vagal manoeuvre in automatic atrial tachycardia commonly:

(a) Restore sinus rhythum
(b) Cause transient AV blocks
(c) Cause slowing of the atrial rate
(d) Can lead to atrial fibrillation

304. ICD is not a class I indication 40 days post MI in:

(a) NYHA-II, III LVEF < 35%
(b) NYHA-I, LVEF < 35%
(c) NYHA-I, LVEF < 30%
(d) NSVT-I, LVEF < 40%, provocable VT

305. All are primary prevention trials of ICD *except*:

(a) MADIT (b) MUSTT
(c) AVID (d) SCD-HeFT

306. Treatment of choice for fascicular VT:

(a) Amiodarone (b) Propafenone
(c) ICD (d) RF Ablation

307. Pill in pocket:

(a) Propafenone (b) Sotalol
(c) Amiodarone

308. All are used for new onset AF *except*:

(a) Betaxolol (b) Amiodarone
(c) Ibutalide (d) Flecainide

309. Accessory pathway most commonly associated with congenital heart disease:

(a) Tricuspid atresia
(b) Ebstein's anomaly
(c) HOCM
(d) Glycogen storage disease

310. Long RP tachycardia A/E:

(a) Atypical AVNRT
(b) SNRT
(c) AVRT with retrograde conduction through fast pathway
(d) PJRT

311. SVT versus VT, favouring SVT is:

(a) Irregularly irregular pulse
(b) North west axis
(c) QRS duration > 140 msec
(d) Ventriculo-atrial dissociation

312. All true about pacemaker syndrome A/E:

(a) Intact VA association
(b) Can be relieved by converting into VVIR mode
(c) Common in elderly population
(d) Causes presyncope and heart failure

313. Bipolar versus unipolar leads A/E:

(a) Reduction in spike artifact
(b) Increased crosstalk
(c) Decreased farfield signals
(d) Decreased myogenic stimulation

314. After Fontan surgery, most common arrhythmias

(a) Atrial flutter
(b) VT
(c) Junctional tachycardia

315. Lead impedence–100 ohm seen in:

(a) Lead fracture (b) Loose screw
(c) Depletion of battery (d) None of the above

316. LQTS-1:
(a) ECG– broadbase T waves
(b) Rest and sleep precipitate

317. EPS is least useful:
(a) Brugada syndrome (b) LQTS
(c) ARVD (d) Idiopathic VT

318. SCD due to VT (low risk):
(a) Sarcoid (b) Chagas
(c) Thyrotoxicosis (d) DCMP

319. 60 years old female presents with haemo-dynamically unstable VT, DC shock given–haemodynamically stable, but comatose, according to ACC guidelines:
(a) Hypothermia given and neurosurgery opinion
(b) Neurosurgery opinion
(c) Hypothermia and PCI
(d) Hypothermia give and observe for 6 hours

320. Amiodarone A/E:
(a) < 100 mg maintenence dose
(b) Increased QT commonly predisposes to VT
(c) Warfarin dose increases, if amiodarone is added
(d) Amiodarone to be stopped in hypothyroid

321. Digoxin induced VT- treatment:
(a) Phenytoin (b) Amiodarone
(c) Sotalol (d) Quinidine

322. Brugada syndrome true is:
(a) Quinidine is DOC
(b) Females > males
(c) Flecainide used for provocative agents

323. 1,2,3,4 points for action potentials propagation velocity in cath lab–EPS Study: 1—1.1 cm/s, 2— 0.05 cm/s, 3—2.2 cm/s, 4—0.3 cm/s
(a) Atrial – ventricular – purkinje – AV node
(b) Atrial – purkinje – ventricular – AV node
(c) Purkinje – atrial – ventricular – AV node
(d) Atria – AV node – ventricle – purkinje

324. Brugada syndrome true *except:*
(a) AD transmission
(b) More common in males
(c) PR prolongation may be less
(d) Supraventricular arrhythmia are very uncommon

325. CHB responding to antibiotic:
(a) Lyme carditis (b) Congenital syphilis
(c) Diphtheria

326. In accessory pathway all true *except:*
(a) Q in inferior leads
(b) Surface ECG may be normal
(c) Narrow complex VT most common
(d) Disappearance of delta wave suggest severe disease

327. ICD not treatment of choice in:
(a) RVOT VT (b) Brugada
(c) ARVC (d) Short QT

328. Mexilitine true A/E:
(a) t1/2 is 10-12 hours
(b) Should be avoided in seizure disorders
(c) Decreased APD
(d) May cause prolonged QRS

329. Reverse use dependence with prolongation in APD:
(a) Class I (b) II
(c) III (d) IV

330. CPVT all true *except:*
(a) Calsequetrin mutation
(b) Polymorphic and bidirectional VT
(c) Calcium induced EAD is MOA
(d) Exercise induced

331. Abdominal CPR all true *except:*
(a) Better outcome than in-hospital resuscitation
(b) Compression between xiphesternum and umbilicus
(c) Abdominal compression to be given when chest is not being compressed by second rescuer
(d) Better outcome than out-hospital resuscitation

332. Least dangerous arrhythmias:
(a) NSVT in DCM
(b) VPC with bundle branch reentry
(c) Parasystole VPC
(d) VPC on descending limb of T wave

333. 78 years old male with lone AF with HR of 70/min:
(a) Aspirin (b) Warfarin
(c) Metoprolol (d) Diltiazem

334. SA node phase IV depolarization channel:
(a) Increased Na conductance
(b) Increased K conductance
(c) Decreased Ca conductance
(d) Decreased Cl conductance

335. Initial intracellular event responsible for MOA of digoxin:

(a) Decreased efflux of Na
(b) Increased influx of K
(c) Increased influx of Ca
(d) c- AMP

336. The following ECG finding suggest AVNRT:

(a) Inverted 'p' wave
(b) 'p' wave merged with QRS
(c) Tall 'p' wave

337. Mismatch:

(a) Ranolazine–shortest QT
(b) Digoxin–xanthopsia
(c) Furosemide–metabolic alkalosis
(d) Nifedipine–gum hyperplasia

338. True statement is:

(a) Dronedarone does not contain iodine
(b) Amiodarone is more effective than beta blockers in HF
(c) Dronedarone is safely given in HF

339. Short QT A/E:

(a) Sotalol DOC
(b) AF can occur
(c) T wave abnormalities
(d) QT < 300 msec is diagnostic

340. SCD A/E:

(a) Short QT
(b) Kawasaki's disease
(c) WPW syndrome
(d) Anomalous LCx from RCA
(e) All

341. Temporary pacing indication after acute MI:

(a) Wenkebach (b) Mobitz type II block
(c) LBBB (d) Bifascicular block

342. Class I indication for permanent pacemaker implantation:

(a) Third degree AV block and high degree AV block with exercise
(b) Unexplained syncope with vasodepressor response on HUTT
(c) Alternating BBB with type II AV block in MI
(d) Symptomatic sinus node dysfunction

343. A young male run towards bus and died. Least likely diagnosis:

(a) LQT-2 (b) LQT-3
(c) HOCM (d) LQT-1

344. Patient on VVI pacemaker, there are no pacing artifact with HR 55/min, least likely:

(a) Undersensing (b) Oversensing
(c) End of life (d) Hysteriasis

345. A patient on PPI during monitoring, resistance – 50 ohm, likely cause:

(a) Lead fracture (b) Lead displacement
(c) Insulation break (d) Pocket infection

346. DOC in SVT with asthma:

(a) Adenosine (b) Verapamil
(c) Esmolol

347. VT in 13 years old treatment:

(a) Lignocaine (b) Amiodarone
(c) Verapamil

348. EP study A/E:

(a) SNRT–last paced beat to onset of spontaneous beat
(b) HV interval–from H to onset of ventricular excitation
(c) AH interval–atrial excitation to onset of his activity
(d) SACT measures conduction of atrial tissue includes SA and AV node

349. Drug used in maintaining of sinus rhythm in structurally normal heart:

(a) Dofetilide (b) Flecainide
(c) Amiodarone (d) Sotalol

350. Short QT syndrome:

(a) Na^+ channel mutation
(b) Flecainide + propafenone corrects QT
(c) Atrial + ventricular fibrillation
(d) ↑ ed ERP in atria + ventricle muscle fibre

351. CPVT A/E:

(a) Bidirectional VT
(b) Autosomal (dominant + recessive)
(c) Amiodarone corrects VT
(d) Structurally normal heart

352. VPC murmur↑ es:

(a) Rheumatic MR
(b) MVP + MR

(c) Normal semilunar valve
(d) Papillary muscle dysfunction

353. Phase-O:

(a) Na^+ entry (b) K^+- efflux
(c) K^+- influx (d) Digoxin

354. VT versus SVT – supports VT A/E:

(a) Absence of RS complex in precordial lead
(b) Long short sequence
(c) Change in R-R precede P-P sequence
(d) LAD (-90 to -180)

355. Class-I indication for pacing:

(a) Trifascicular + alternating bundle branch block
(b) Inferior wall MI + CHB
(c) HOCM
(d) Neurocardiogenic syncope

356. Cardarone + pulmonary toxicity - A/E:

(a) Hypersensitivity
(b) In 6 - 60 days
(c) Steroids can be helpful
(d) High dose (maintenance) may be a cause

357. RFA complication A/E:

(a) Stroke
(b) Pulmonary artery stenosis
(c) LA - esophageal fistula
(d) Tamponade

358. SCD in:

(a) Coronary AV fistula (b) PS
(c) ARVD (d) All

359. CHB seen in:

(a) Myotonic dystrophy
(b) Limb-girdle muscular dystrophy
(c) Becker's dystrophy
(d) All

360. VT (Monomorphic) with structurally N heart an all *except:*

(a) CPVT
(b) Propranolol sensitive idiopathic VT
(c) Idiopathic LV VT
(d) RVOT VT

361. Entrainment seen in:

(a) RV extrasystole VT
(b) RVOT VT
(c) Fascicular VT
(d) Idiopathic LVOT VT

362. Systolic HTN *except:*

(a) Alcohol withdrawal (b) Beriberi
(c) Thyrotoxicosis (d) AR

363. Least energy for cardioversion:

(a) VT (b) Sinus tachycardia
(c) AF (d) Mahaim tachycardia

364. Short RP tachycardia are all *except:*

(a) AVNRT (b) AVRT
(c) AT (d) AT with increase PR

365. Blocks accessory pathway all *except:*

(a) IA (b) IC
(c) Amiodarone (d) IV

366. Torsade de pointes is seen with all *except:*

(a) Procainamide (b) Sotalol mexilitene
(c) Disopyramide

367. All of the following are used for postoperative AF prophylaxis *except:*

(a) Over drive pacing (b) Beta blockers
(c) Amiodarone (d) Sotalol

368. Following causes QT prolongation *except:*

(a) Amiodarone (b) Sotalol
(c) Flecainide (d) Digoxin

369. Poor prognosis on non invasive testing: (T/F)

(a) ↑ lung uptake
(b) LV dilatation with exercise
(c) -10 TMT score
(d) >2 RWMA on stress echo
(e) Resting LVEF – 40%

370. All are types of long RP/short PR tachycardia *except:*

(a) SNRT (b) Atrial tachycardia
(c) ANRT (d) Atypical AVNRT

371. All are secondary trials *except:*

(a) MADIT (b) AVID
(c) CASH (d) CIDS

372. All are true about ARVD *except:*
(a) Epsilone waves are seen in ECG
(b) Autosornal recessive
(c) Male predominant
(d) Most common cause of death ventricular arrhythmia

373. Long QT by A/E:
(a) Digoxin
(b) Hypocalcaemia
(c) Hypothermia

374. WPW syndrome A/E:
(a) More common in females
(b) RV aberrancy is common
(c) Structurally normal heart
(d) Incidence ↓ es with age

375. Exercise changes in WPW syndrome A/E:
(a) δ-wave disappear in 20-50% cases
(b) Abrupt disappearance of δ-wave indicates short refractory period of accessory pathway
(c) Presence of WPW does not limit physical work capacity
(d) Presence of WPW causes difficulty in interpretation

376. Lenient rate control in AF is defined as:
(a) < 80 resting and < 110 with exercise (moderate)
(b) Resting < 70
(c) Resting <110

377. EP studies A/E:
(a) A-H jump s/o dual pathways
(b) Slow pathway ablation less successful these fast
(c) 90% of cases due to slow past pathway

378. Torsade de pointes with:
(a) Long QTc (b) Short QTc
(c) Wide QRS (d) Short QRS

379. Wide QRS tachycardia A/E:
(a) Orthodromic AVRT
(b) Antidromic AVRT
(c) SVT with previous LBBB
(d) VT

380. SCD in young athlete A/E:
(a) HCM in 36% (b) ARVD - 10%
(c) CAD - 19% (d) AS - 4%

381. Pulseless electrical activity with A/E:
(a) Massive AWMI (b) Cardiac tamponade
(c) Cardiogenic shock (d) Hypothermia

382. SIDS seen in:
(a) Brugada (b) LQTS
(c) Romanoward (d) JLN syndrome

383. DAD's cause of A/E:
(a) Digitalis (b) LQTS
(c) RVOT VT (d) AIVR

384. ICD indicated most beneficial in trial:
(a) MADIT-I (b) MADIT-II
(c) CIDS (d) AVID

385. Pacemaker needed in non cardiac surgery:
(a) Alternate BBB
(b) RBBB with ↑ PR
(c) Old MI with LBBB

386. In idiopathic outflow tract VT–All are true *except:*
(a) Typically has a LBBB pattern in V1
(b) Vagal maneuvers can terminate the VT
(c) High risk of sudden cardiac death
(d) More common in women

387. Identify the correct statement in concealed aomalous pathway:
(a) Can preseut with incessant tachycardia and tachycardia induced LV cardiomyopathy
(b) There is no retrograde conduction but antegrade conduction is preserved
(c) High risk of developing rapid ventricular response to AF
(d) Anomalous pathway is manifest in sinus rhythm

388. Bidirectional VT in digoxin toxicity is due to:
(a) Triggered activity associated with calcium overload
(b) Increased automaticity
(c) Reentry
(d) Suppression of phase–0

389. Stimuli for sudden death in Brugada syndrome is:
(a) Auditory (b) Sleep
(c) Swimming (d) Visual

390. Who discovered SA node?
(a) Shamroth (b) Fleak and Keith
(c) E Braunwald (d) Joseph Perloff

391. The following are true in third degree heart block, *except:*

(a) No atrial impulse propagates to the ventricles
(b) A.V. Nodal Block is probably when the ventricular rate is around 50/minute
(c) The QRS complex is always wide
(d) Pacemaker syndrome may develop if a simple ventricular pacemaker is used

392. Which of the following is the most common electrical mechanism to explain sudden cardiac death?

(a) Asystole
(b) Pulseless electrical activity (PEA)
(c) Pulseless ventricular tachycardia (PVT)
(d) VF

393. Adverse effects of amiodarone include all *except:*

(a) Corneal deposits (b) Thyroid dysfunction
(c) Pulmonary fibrosis (d) Hypertension

394. Most common cardiovascular cause of sudden death in young athletes includes:

(a) Coronary-artery anomalies
(b) Hypertrophic cardiomyopathy
(c) Myocarditis
(d) Aortic valve stenosis

395. Brugada syndrome include all *except:*

(a) ST elevation in right precordial leads ECG (V_1-V_3)
(b) Phase 2 reentry
(c) Mutation in SCN5A gene
(d) Triggered activity

396. VT with hemodynamic instability:

(a) Amiodarone
(b) Lidocaine
(c) DC cardioversion
(d) Calcium gluconate

397. First-line pharmacologic therapy of Wolff-Parkinson-White Syndrome includes:

(a) Propranolol (b) Verapamil
(c) Diltiazem (d) Amiodarone

398. Sinus bradycardia is associated with all *except:*

(a) May be a manifestation of heart failure
(b) Occurs more commonly during inferior than anterior myocardial infarction
(c) During reperfusion with thrombolytic agents
(d) It can be associated with syncope caused by abnormal autonomic reflex

399. Most common cardiac mechanism of cardiac arrest is:

(a) Ventricular fibrillation
(b) Rupture of ventricle
(c) Asystole
(d) Sustained VT

400. In MADIT clinical trial, following is true:

(a) ICD indicated if EF < 35%
(b) ICD indicated if EF > 35%
(c) Amiodarone better if EF > 35%
(d) Amiodarone better if EF < 35%

401. Most common cardiovascular cause of sudden death in young athletes includes:

(a) Coronary-artery anomalies
(b) Hypertrophic cardiomyopathy
(c) Myocarditis
(d) Aortic valve stenosis

402. Congenital long QT syndrome is associated with neonatal:

(a) Sinus bradycardia
(b) Sinus tachycardia
(c) Supra ventricular tachycardia
(d) Ventricular tachycardia

403. Anti-arrhythmic drug which causes QFtS widening, without significant QT lengthening:

(a) Sotalol (b) Amiodarone
(c) Quinidine (d) Flecainide

404. Proarrhythmic effect is typically occurrence of monomorphic VT rather than torsade de pointes:

(a) Flecainide (b) Sotalol
(c) Quinidine (d) Dofetilide

405. Drug with K^+ channel blocking and Ns^+ channel enhancing action:

(a) Flecainide (b) Ibutilide
(c) Dofetilide (d) Anilide

406. Brugada Syndrome, all are true *except:*

(a) Beta blockers decrease mortality
(b) Sudden cardiac death in sleep
(c) Procainamide unmasks ST elevation in VI
(d) Genetic abnormality SCN 5a

407. Permanent pacemaker implantation is NOT indicated in an asymptomatic patient with:

(a) Sinus Pause > 4 seconds
(b) Trifascicular block after MI
(c) Sick sinus syndrome
(d) Bundle branch block with Mobitz II AV block

408. Radio-frequency ablation is least effective in:

(a) AVNRT (b) Atrial Flutter
(c) Ischemic VT (d) AVRT

409. Permanent cryoablation of accessory pathway occurs at:

(a) -20 C (b) -45 C
(c) -65 C (d) -80 C

410. Permanent pacemaker implantation is required for:

(a) Symptomatic congenital complete heart block
(b) Chronic complete heart block due to Lengre's disease
(c) Persistent complete heart block after acute myocardial infarction
(d) All of the above

411. The sinus node is described by:

(a) Bachman (b) James
(c) Keith and Flack (d) His

412. In the human ventricular myocardium calcium enters the cell during __________ phase of the action potential.

(a) Phase 1 (b) Phase 2
(c) Phase 3 (d) Phase 4

413. In interpolated beat the subsequent P-R interval is:

(a) Shortened (b) Normal
(c) Increased (d) Variable

414. In alternating ventricular tachycardia:

(a) QRS alternate in polarity
(b) QRS alternate in amplitude
(c) QRS sometimes upright and sometimes inverted
(d) QRS is unpredictable

415. 0.3 mg of atropine given IV produces:

(a) Tachycardia
(b) No change
(c) Bradycardia
(d) Tachycardia following bradycardia

416. Sudden cardiac death occur during sleep in:

(a) All LQT (b) LQT1
(c) LQT2 (d) LQT3

417. A 25 years old female diagnosed with LQT2, which will precipitate TDP?

(a) Auditory stimuli (b) Sleep
(c) Exercise (d) Swimming

418. Pill in packet:

(a) Digoxin (b) Propafenone
(c) Verapamil

419. Acute termination of AF is done by which during:

(a) Propafenone (b) Doronedrone
(c) Ibutilide (d) Verapamil

420. The mechanism of arrhythmia in digoxin toxicity is:

(a) Reentry
(b) Triggered
(c) Abnormal automaticity
(d) Normal automaticity

421. Ventriculophasic arrhythmia occur in:

(a) TGA (b) CHB
(c) ASD (d) VSD

422. AVNRT is suggested by:

(a) Bounding sensation in chest
(b) Abrupt termination
(c) Termination by vomiting
(d) Gradual onset

423. Definition of SCD is:

(a) 1 hour (b) 2 hours
(c) 30 min (d) 6 hours

424. Calcium channel blocker, belong to which class in William-Vaughan classification?

(a) I (b) II
(c) III (d) IV

425. Regarding adenosine which is not true?

(a) It can be terminate some VT
(b) Its half life is few seconds
(c) Theophylline increase its systemic effect
(d) Transient AV block occur during termination of PSVT

426. All infection causes AV block *except:*

(a) Trypanosomiasis (b) Chagas diseases
(c) Diphtheria (d) Lyme disease

427. All channel $Na^+ - K^+ -Ca2^+$ are involved as funny if in which phase of action potential?

(a) I (b) II
(c) III (d) IV

428. Paroxysmal AF which is true?

(a) Both sympathetic and parasympathetic mechanism are responsible
(b) Always subside in 24 hours spontaneously
(c) No anticoagulation is needed
(d) Paroxysmal AF always terminated by beta blocker

429. Regarding ARVD which is true?

(a) Epsilon wave

430. Long RP tachycardia A/E

(a) PJRT (b) Orthodromic AVRT
(c) Atypical AVNRT (d) SANRT

431. Tall R in V_1:

(a) DMD
(b) Right sided accessory pathway
(c) Brugada syndrome
(d) Early repolarization

432. SCD risk in HCM true A/E:

(a) LVOT gradient does not have risk
(b) Abnormal ECG in 1st degree relative
(c) Amiodarone may be useful in elderly

433. Pill in pocket approach:

(a) Flecainide (b) Sotalol
(c) Amiodarone

434. All are primary prevention trials A/E:

(a) CAMIAT (b) Cascade
(c) CABG-PATCH (d) Companion

435. CPVT arrhythmias mechanisms:

(a) Automaticity (b) EAD
(c) DAD (d) Re-entry

436. Digitalis intoxication characteristic arrhythmias:

(a) Bundle branch Re-entry VT
(b) Fascicular VT
(c) Outflow VT
(d) Idiopathic VT

437. Digitalis toxicity A/E:

(a) Cholestyramine (b) Quinidine
(c) Amiodarone (d) Erythromycin

438. AF with aberrancy, fast ventricular rate which is not used:

(a) IV procainamide (b) IV digitalis
(c) RFA (d) Cardioversion

439. Bifid T wave:

(a) LQT1 (b) LQT2
(c) LQT3 (d) LQT4

440. Last ventricular activation:

(a) Posterobasal (b) Free wall
(c) Settum

441. Cannon wave in WCT:

(a) S/o VT
(b) S/o SVT with aberrancy

442. Bachmann bundle is:

(a) Interatrial (b) Anterior intermodal
(c) Posterior intermodal (d) Middle intermodal

443. Disorder with involvement of His bundle has incomplete LBBB in sinus rhythm and LBBB with superior axis left axis in VT, diagnosis:

(a) ARVD
(b) Idiopathic outflow tract VT
(c) Fascicular/left septal VT
(d) Bundle branch reentry VT

444. Most common mechanisms for pulseless activity:

(a) Acidosis
(b) Hypovolemia
(c) Cardiac tamopnade
(d) Tension pneumothorax

445. Most common cause of cardiac arrest:

(a) VF (b) Asystole
(c) PEA (d) None

446. Least useful in treatment of asystole:

(a) External pacemaker
(b) Epinephrine 1: 10000 (10 ml)
(c) Atropine 0.5 mg
(d) Ca gluconate 10%, 10 ml

447. Sinus node dysfunction caused by A/E:

(a) Lithium (b) Orciprenaline
(c) Amitryptiline (d) Cimetidine

448. Adenosine least given in:
(a) Patient with CAD with wide QRS tachycardia
(b) CAD with narrow QRS tachycardia
(c) Irregular rhythm with wide QRS
(d) Narrow QRS with preexcitation

449. HF with maximum arrhythmias risk:
(a) Pulsus alternans with T wave alternans
(b) Pulsus alternans with multiple VPC's
(c) Pulsus paradoxus
(d) Dicrotic pulse

450. Brugada syndrome A/E:
(a) 30% idiopathic VF
(b) Structurally normal heart
(c) K^+ channel defect
(d) ST elevation V1-V3

451. Concerted action of K channel, Na Ca exchanger, if current involved in:
(a) Phase 1 repolarisation (b) Phase 2
(c) Phase 3 (d) Phase 4

452. Which is not a class III antiarrhythmic drugs?
(a) Sotalol (b) Bretylium
(c) Amiodarone (d) Moricizine

453. True about antiarrhythmics regarding accessory pathway is:
(a) Class Ia prolongs refractoriness in accessory pathway only
(b) Class III prolongs refractoriness in AV node only
(c) Class II prolongs refractoriness in AV node and accessory pathway
(d) Class Ic prolongs refractoriness and conduction in AV node only

454. Most common arrhythmia in WPW:
(a) Normal QRS irregular rate 160-200
(b) Normal QRS regular rate 160-200
(c) Wide QRS irregular rate 160-200
(d) Wide QRS regular rate 160-200

455. Arrhythmia is cause of syncope in all A/E:
(a) AS (b) HOCM
(c) CAD (d) ARVD

456. CRT indication A/E:
(a) ORS > 120 msec (b) Class III or more
(c) EF < 35% (d) RBBB

457. Best treatment for TdP:
(a) $MgSO_4$ (b) B blocker
(c) Potassium infusion

458. Most common correctable cause of AF:
(a) Hyperthyroidism (b) OSA
(c) MS

459. Most common cause of pulseless electrical activity:
(a) Acidosis (b) Hypovolemia
(c) Pneumothorax (d) Tamponade

460. Amoidarone interaction A/E:
(a) Potentiate digoxin effect
(b) Decrease effect of warfarin level
(c) 30% Iodine by weight
(d) May cause hypo and hyperthyroidism

461. Ta (Atrial repolarization) in ECG is not visible because of:
(a) Occur at the time of ventricular repolarization
(b) Occur during P wave loop
(c) During ventricular depolarization

462. Which is associated aberrant conduction?
(a) Bachmann bundle (b) Kent bundle
(c) Mahaim's fibre (d) James' fibre

463. Conduction from RA to LA occur via:
(a) Bachmann bundle (b) Wenkebach bundle
(c) Thoral bundle (d) Kent bundle

464. Antiarrhythmic drug with antiplatelet action like aspirin:
(a) Ajmaline (b) Quinidine
(c) Procainamide (d) Amiodarone

465. Pacemaker of choice in CSH:
(a) AAI (b) AAIR
(c) VVI (d) DDI

466. WPW A/E:
(a) Verapamil DOC
(b) Amiodarone ↑ ERF of accessory pathway
(c) Wide QRS > narrow QRS
(d) Accessoary pathway between LA and LV

467. Macroentrant tachycardia most common:
(a) Atrial flutter
(b) Atrial fibrillation

(c) MAT
(d) Left atrial tachycardia

468. SCD least with:
(a) AS (b) PPH
(c) AVSD (d) Cardiomyopathy

469. The tract that preferentially conducts impulses from the right Atrium to the Left Atrium is:
(a) The Bachmann bundle
(b) The middle Inter Nodal Tract
(c) The posterior Inter nodal Tract
(d) The James Fibres

470. Quinidine may be appropriate for management of:
(a) Long QT syndrome
(b) Catecholaminergic polymorphic VT
(c) Brugada syndrome
(d) Arrhythmogenic RV dysplasia

471. All are cause of long QT *except:*
(a) Digoxin (b) Quinidine
(c) Liquid protein diet (d) Hypomagnesaemia

472. Type I second degree SA block is characterized by all *except:*
(a) Normal PR interval
(b) Lengthening of PR interval
(c) Shortening of RR interval
(d) Incomplete pause

473. In tachycardia the term "Wide QRS tachycardia" is used when duration of QRS Exceeds ___seconds.
(a) 0.02 (b) 0.04
(c) 0.06 (d) 0.08

474. Fibres connecting RA to LA:
(a) Bachmann bundle (b) Thorell bundle

475. VT is cause of syncope A/E:
(a) Atrial myxoma (b) Post MI
(c) HOCM (d) Valvular AS

476. RFA is used for:
(a) AVRT (b) AVNRT
(c) AF (d) Atrial flutter

477. Reversible fluctuating heart block:
(a) Lyme's disease

478. QT prolongation with TdP caused by:
(a) Mitoxantrone (b) Amsarine
(c) Herceptin (d) Cyclophophamide

479. CHB treatment of choice:
(a) Pacemaker (b) Quinidine
(c) Beta blocker (d) Digoxin

480. Adult basic life support false is:
(a) 30:2 ratio
(b) Compression for 2 inch (5 cm)
(c) Give rescue breath after every 2 secs
(d) 100 compression/minute

481. Ivabradine true: (T/F)
(a) Involves funny channel
(b) Beautiful trial reduces mortality
(c) Stable angina used
(d) Not used in CHF
(e) Causes luminous phenomenon

482. Brugada syndrome false: (T/F)
(a) SCN 5A most common
(b) During sleep
(c) Intermittent ST elevation
(d) Amiodarone reduces SCD
(e) Flecainide increases ST elevation

483. VT/SVT favouring VT: (T/F)
(a) Fusion beat
(b) Capture beat
(c) Short fixed RP interval
(d) AV dissociation
(e) RBBB morphology

484. Drugs used as antiarrhythmic in pregnancy: (T/F)
(a) Digoxin (b) Procainamide
(c) Quinidine (d) Disopyramide
(e) Flecainide

485. Drugs increases QT: (T/F)
(a) Procainamide (b) Flecainide
(c) Quinidine (d) Digoxin
(e) Lignocaine

486. Brugada criteria for VT false: (T/F)
(a) Absence of RS complexes
(b) R-S < 100 msec
(c) Vi/vt <1

(d) AV dissociation
(e) Morphology seen in V1-V6

487. Congenital CHB: (T/F)
(a) Best in 18-24 weeks
(b) Steroid only in third degree heart block to prevent complication
(c) Anti Ro + with cardiac rosary fibre (30-50%)
(d) Anti SSA + in SLE with CHB
(e) If positive in previous birth, risk in next is 70-90%

488. Structurally normal heart, risk of SCD: (T/F)
(a) LQTS (b) ARVD
(c) Commotion cordis (d) CAD
(e) Brugada

489. Polymorphic VT A/E:
(a) SQTS
(b) LQTS
(c) CPVT
(d) Left anterior fascicular
(e) Left posterior fascicular

490. Sotalol A/E:
(a) ↓ threshold of DC
(b) Mortality benefit in MI with ↓ EF
(c) Non selective
(d) Poor oral bioavailbility
(e) ↑ QT

491. CPR latest guidelines: (T/F)
(a) CAB instead of ABC
(b) Sternal compression 1 inch instead of 1.5 – 2 inch
(c) 30 : 2
(d) For layman perform both chest compression and breathing
(e) VF most common arrhythmia

492. AF: (T/F)
(a) Persistent < 7 days
(b) Males > females
(c) Rhythm control no need for anticoagulation
(d) Digoxin control heart rate during exercise
(e) PV ablation with vagal denervation newer techniques

493. Brugada A/E: (T/F)
(a) Common in females
(b) ECG may be transient
(c) Most common – SCN5A
(d) Associated with AF
(e) Procainamide decreased SCD risk

494. Polymorphic VT A/E: (T/F)
(a) RVOT VT
(b) Brugada
(c) SQTS
(d) Post MI scar ischemia
(e) LQTS

495. Prognostic marker for SCD in HCM: (T/F)
(a) Wall thickness > 34 mm
(b) Hypertensive response to exercise
(c) EPS induced VT
(d) NSVT on Holter
(e) Family history of sudden death

496. RVOT VT treatment A/E: (T/F)
(a) Adenosine (b) Verapamil
(c) Beta blocker (d) RFA
(e) Digoxin

497. AF–anticoagulation A/E: (T/F)
(a) INR= 1.5-2
(b) Dabigatran can be used
(c) PTTK monitoring of dabigatran
(d) Clopidogrel + aspirin is better than warfarin
(e) Clopidogrel to be added in all patients on warfarin

498. SQTS: (T/F)
(a) Associated with AF
(b) ICD is C/I
(c) Gain of function of K + channel
(d) SCD is common
(e) Quinidine helpful

499. Increase digoxin level: (T/F)
(a) Verapamil (b) Quinidine
(c) Amiodarone (d) Ranitidine
(e) Rifampicin

500. CRT indicated in A/E: (T/F)
(a) LVEF < 35%
(b) AF
(c) NYHA class II, III and ambulatory IV
(d) QRS > 120 msec
(e) Survival of more than 1 year

501. Coding system NASE/BGSE: (T/F)
(a) I – pacing
(b) II– multisite pacing

(c) III– rate modulation
(d) IV– response to pacing
(e) V – sensing

502. Pacemaker related infection: (T/F)
(a) Incidence 5%
(b) Erosion suggest indolent infection
(c) Irrigation of pocket with antibiotic has favourable outcome
(d) Removal of complete pacemaker system
(e) S. aureus – early infection most common

503. CPVT: (T/F)
(a) Mutation of ankyrin B protein
(b) Bidirectional VT with exercise
(c) Swimming predisposes to VT
(d) AR
(e) Structurally normal heart

504. ARVD: (T/F)
(a) Desmin (b) Plakophilin
(c) Plakoglobin (d) Troponin I
(e) Ankyrin B

505. Brugada: (T/F)
(a) ST coving up with T wave inversion in right precordial leads
(b) Death most common in sleeping
(c) Monomorphic VT
(d) Fever most common precipitant

506. WPW syndrome: (T/F)
(a) RF ablation definite treatment
(b) Disappear with age
(c) Digoxin alone worsen tachycardia
(d) Associated with cardiac arrest
(e) Associated with Ebstein anomaly

507. VF: (T/F)
(a) DC cardioversion TOC
(b) Amiodarone used for VF with increased QT
(c) Most common with CAD
(d) AICD is TOC

508. AF: (T/F)
(a) PPI is indicated
(b) Causes stroke
(c) RF ablation always successful
(d) Anticoagulation indicated
(e) LV dysfunction with fast ventricular rate

509. Long cycle in AF: (T/F)
(a) Papillary muscle dysfunction murmur decrease
(b) AS murmur increased
(c) MR murmur no change
(d) PS decreases
(e) TR decreases

510. AF: (T/F)
(a) More in elderly
(b) < 60 years age not risk factor
(c) OSA Risk factor
(d) Obesity is risk factor
(e) Presence does not increase mortality

511. CRT: (T/F)
(a) Only Indicated in EF < 35%
(b) QRS > 140 msec only
(c) NYHA III-IV with refractory to Rx
(d) Has proven better in RBBB than LBBB
(e) Prove to regress in NYHA class to I-II

512. Family history of SCD due to HCM and patient having syncope-3 episode, 2 sibling asymptomatic which are true (T/F)?
(a) Patient need ICD
(b) Start B Blocker in patient
(c) Need EP study to decide eligibility for ICD
(d) To establish diagnosis–Histology showing for disarry is must
(e) Sibling–2D echo-even asymptomatic

513. CPVT: (T/F)
(a) Exercise induced syncope with QTc < 460 is suggestive
(b) Characteristic bidirectional
(c) Swimming – precipitating factor
(d) Mutation – Ankyrin B

514. ARVD genes: (T/F)
(a) Desmin (b) Titin
(c) Plakaglobin (d) Desmoplakin
(e) Trop T

515. Brugada syndrome: (T/F)
(a) Quinidine can be given
(b) Male – ↑ risk
(c) Type I – coved ST ↑ with T ↓ in V1-V3

(d) SCN 5B
(e) Polymorphic VT

516. CPR in pregnant women: (T/F)
(a) DC cardioversion C/I
(b) Right lateral position preferred
(c) 1-2 mm larger ET tube
(d) Cricoid pressure during PPV
(e) Hysterectomy if < 20 weeks

517. ARVD true: (T/F)
(a) Titin (b) Transferrin
(c) Plakophilin (d) Desmoplakin
(e) Phakoglobin

518. ↑ QT drugs except: (T/F)
(a) Sotalol (b) Disopyramide
(c) Aniline (d) Amiodarone
(e) Digoxin

519. Cardiac K^+ channel gene: (T/F)
(a) Brugada syndrome
(b) LQT-3
(c) Andersen Tawil syndrome
(d) LQT-1
(e) SQTS

520. RVOT VT A/E: (T/F)
(a) Typically superior axis
(b) RVOT more common than LVOT
(c) ↑ Ca^{2+} overload
(d) DAD with triggered activity
(e) Ppt. by catecholamines

521. ARVD: (T/F)
(a) Treatment – EPS with RFA
(b) Treatment – ICD
(c) Quinidine prevents electrical storm

522. CHB: (T/F)
(a) c-TGA (b) d-TGA
(c) DORV (d) Maternal lupus
(e) Tricuspid atresia

523. Ventricular arrhythmia ↑ with exercise: (T/F)
(a) CPVT (b) RVOT
(c) Fasicular VT (d) Idiopathic VF
(e) ARVD

524. Disopyramide – incorrect: (T/F)
(a) Class Ic
(b) Causes urinary retention
(c) Acts on phase 3 of action potential
(d) Most effective in non obstructive HCM
(e) ↑ QT

525. LQTS: (T/F)
(a) In children manifestation more common in girls vs boys
(b) QT > 500 ↑ es risk of SCD more than short QT
(c) LQT2 associated with bifid T wave
(d) LQT2 associated with noise (SCD associated)
(e) LQT3 beta-blocker effective

526. Wide QRS VT vs SVT favoring VT: (T/F)
(a) Fusion beat (b) Capture beat
(c) HR = 140/- (d) AV dissociation
(e) Inferior axis

527. Causes of long RP tachycardia: (T/F)
(a) Atypical AVNRT
(b) AF
(c) A Flutter
(d) Ectopic atrial tachycardia
(e) Orthodromic AVRT

528. Long RP tachycardia: (T/F)
(a) Typical AVNRT
(b) Atypical AVNRT
(c) Decrementel concealed pathway
(d) Atrial tachycardia
(e) AF

529. Drug effective in AF for pharmacological conversion: (T/F)
(a) Sotolol (b) Ibutilide
(c) Dofetilide (d) Flecainide
(e) Verapamil

530. Pharmacological maintenance of NSR in AF by: (T/F)
(a) Metoprolol (b) Verapamil
(c) Sotalol (d) Amiodarone
(e) Ibutilide

531. VT with LBBB morphology: (T/F)
(a) Fascicular VT (b) BB re-entry VT
(c) RVOT VT (d) VT - ARVD
(e) Mitral annulus VT

532. Indication of EPS in asymptomatic pre-excitation syndrome: (T/F)
(a) Intermittent pre-excitation
(b) In pilots
(c) Left sided pathway
(d) Anteroseptal pathway
(e) On fast HR – pre-excitation disappears on TMT

533. PPI required in A/E: (T/F)
(a) Paroxymal AF
(b) Inter-atrial re-entrant Tachycardia
(c) AVNRT
(d) HOCM
(e) DCM with LBBB

534. Sudden cardiac death – cause: (T/F)
(a) HCM (b) LQTS
(c) SQTS (d) ARVD
(e) CAD

535. Patient on metoprolol 50mg BD developed giddiness, ECG showed 2 : 1 AV block with normal QRS duration with ventricular rate—40 min, TPI done block reverted after stopping metoprolol for 1 day further management: (T/F)
(a) Biventricular pacing
(b) Dual chamber pacing
(c) EPS done and pacing if HV interval prolonged
(d) Holter after 3-4 days for intermittent A-V block

536. AV dissociation seen: (T/F)
(a) CHB (b) Typical AVNRT
(c) Atypical AVNRT (d) VT
(e) AF

537. WPW–true are: (T/F)
(a) RFA done in asymptomatic WPW
(b) 100% success rate in AF
(c) Pregnancy improves AVRT
(d) VF can lead to SCD
(e) Recurrent AVRT indication for ablation

538. 3 episodes of syncope with family history of SCD in two younger brothers asymptomatic, septal thickness 34 mm and posterior wall 18 mm–true is: (T/F)
(a) B-blocker should be given
(b) EPS followed by ICD
(c) ICD implantation
(d) Echo for asymptomatic brothers

539. Drugs causing LQTS: (T/F)
(a) Metoprolol (b) Amiodarone
(c) Esmolol (d) Cisapride
(e) Mg

540. LQTS: (T/F)
(a) Most common involves Na channel
(b) LQT_1 cause death in sleep
(c) LQT_2 causes events in arousal
(d) Most common cause of death in athlete
(e) LQT_3 causes events in exercise

541. LQTS: (T/F)
(a) LQT_1 on exercise
(b) LQT_2 on auditory
(c) LQT_3 on sleep
(d) LQT_3 k^+ channel mutation
(e) BB therapy – effective in LQT_3

542. Paradoxical split S_2: (T/F)
(a) RV pacing
(b) RBBB
(c) WPW type B
(d) LVOT obstruction
(e) AR

543. Wide split S_2: (T/F)
(a) PDA
(b) MR
(c) AR
(d) Acute pulmonary embolism
(e) Hypovolumic shock

544. Short QT interval: (T/F)
(a) QTc < 300 mse
(b) ↑ Frequency of AF
(c) ↑ Frequency of VF
(d) ↑ SIDS
(e) RyR mutation

545. Atrial fibrillation:
(a) Absent S1 (b) Absent S2
(c) Absent S3 (d) Absent S4

546. SCN 5A gene mutation A/E: (T/F)
(a) HCN

(b) LQT_3
(c) Brugada
(d) Progressive Conduction block

547. Secondary trials of ICD A/E: (T/F)
(a) AVID (b) AIDS
(c) CASH (d) SCD-HEFT
(e) MADIT-II

548. Indications of pacing in congenital CHB A/E: (T/F)
(a) Sleeping HR=58/min
(b) Pre-syncope
(c) Frequent VPC
(d) On TMT – exercise intolerance
(e) Complex congenital heart disease

549. Amiodarone: (T/F)
(a) Prolongs AH interval
(b) Prolongs PR interval
(c) Short QT interval
(d) Short A-H with I/V administration
(e) ↑ ERP of bypass tract

550. Quinidine: (T/F)
(a) Causing α-stimulation
(b) I/V adm - T ½ = 5 min
(c) Long QT
(d) Prolonged PR
(e) QRS duration shorten

551. Long RP tachycardia: (T/F)
(a) Typical AVNRT
(b) PJRT
(c) EAT
(d) Junctional tachycardia
(e) AF

552. AV dissociation seen in: (T/F)
(a) CHB
(b) VT with no retrograde atrial capture
(c) Mahaim tachycardia
(d) AVNRT
(e) Junctional tachycardia

553. Symptomatic SSS with chronotropic incompetence with 3-5 secs sinus pauses in 58 years old man, PPI of choice: (T/F)
(a) VVI (b) VDD
(c) VVIR (d) AAIR
(e) No PPI

554. PSVT in infant – drug not used is: (T/F)
(a) Metoprolol (b) Verapamil
(c) Adenosine (d) Digoxin
(e) Amiodarone

555. Digoxin causes A/E: (T/F)
(a) Reduced peripheral tone
(b) Shortens atrial refractoriness
(c) Effectively control ventricular response in AF undergoing exercise
(d) Hypothyroidism increases sensitivity digoxin induced arrhythmias
(e) Hypomagnesemia increases toxicity of digitalis

556. ARVD genes involved: (T/F)
(a) Desmin (b) Titin
(c) Desmoplakin (d) Troponin–T
(e) Plakoglobin

557. ARVD causes: (T/F)
(a) Partial/complete replacement of RV with adipose tissue
(b) RV segmental hypokinesia with RVOT dilatation on echo
(c) SCN5A gene is involved
(d) Incomplete RBBB with broad QRS in V1> V6
(e) LBBB type VT

558. SCD in HOCM factor true are: (T/F)
(a) LV thickness is > 20 mm
(b) Family history of CSD
(c) Flat BP response on TMT
(d) History of syncope
(e) 1 episode of NSVT on Holter (6 beat at 140/min)

559. LQTS: (T/F)
(a) Ionic channelopathy
(b) LQTS1 is higher risk
(c) Amiodarone is DOC
(d) Notching of T wave may be seen
(e) Raised QTc correlates with increased SCD

560. 20 years old male with LBBB with LAD morphology, rate—200/min on ECG: (T/F)
(a) RVOT VT
(b) RV inflow VT
(c) Mahaim fibre VT
(d) ILVT
(e) Bundle branch re-entry VT

561. LQTS: (T/F)

(a) Na channel mutation most common defect
(b) LQT2 – SCD during arousal
(c) LQT1 – SCD less in exercise than rest
(d) LQT3 – SCD less in rest than exercise
(e) Most common cause of SCD in athlete

562. Open chest CPR done in: (T/F)

(a) Anterior flail chest
(b) Tension pheumothorax
(c) Pericardial tamponade
(d) AMI
(e) Dissection of aorta

563. Long QT syndrome: (T/F)

(a) Most common Na channel defect
(b) LQT1 more on arousal
(c) LQT1 more on sleeping
(d) LQT3 more on exertion
(e) Most common cause of SCD in young athlete

564. Digoxin: (T/F)

(a) Cross placenta
(b) Stimulates Na^+K^+ ATPase
(c) Decrease mortality in CHF
(d) DOC in HOCM with obstruction

565. PSVT with CHF management is:

(a) Diltiazem (b) CSM
(c) Beta blockers (d) Amiodarone

566. Features suggestive of SVT:

(a) LAD (b) RBBB
(c) Presence of P waves (d) Responds to CSM

567. PSVT over VT: (T/F)

(a) LAD (b) RBBB
(c) Visible p waves (d) Capture beat
(e) CSM

568. High incidence of SCD: (T/F)

(a) MVP
(b) Romanoward syndrome
(c) PDA
(d) Rapid weight lowering protocol
(e) HTN

569. Rapid early depolarization is:

(a) Phase 0 (b) Phase 1
(c) Phase 2 (d) Phase 4

570. 16 years old with sudden syncope, most common diagnosis is:

(a) HOCM (b) LQTS

571. Superior boundary of triangle of Koch:

(a) Tendon of tadaro
(b) Septal attachment of tricuspid valve
(c) Coronary sinus

572. Concealed pathway most common is:

(a) Right anteroseptal (b) Left anteroseptal
(c) Right posterosaptel (d) Left posteroseptal

573. BB rentry VT occur in:

(a) Type III SMA
(b) Type I muscular dystrophy
(c) Limb girdle dystrophy
(d) Friedreich's ataxia

574. Resting membrane potential A/E:

(a) SA node = 50 to -60 mV
(b) Purkinje = -90 to – 95 mV
(c) LV muscle APD 300 to 500 msec
(d) Purkinje fibres has max. conduction velocity (2-3 m/sec)

575. Not metabolized in liver:

(a) Procainamide (b) Quinidine
(c) Lidocaine (d) Phenytoin

576. Absence of p wave A/E:

(a) SA exit block
(b) Left lateral accessory pathway
(c) Hyperkalemia
(d) AF

577. Short QT A/E:

(a) Hyperkalemia (b) Acidosis
(c) Digoxin (d) Hypothermia

578. Diastolic murmur at mitral area A/E:

(a) Star Edwards (b) St. Jude
(c) Medtronic valve (d) Carpentier Edward

579. AS asymptomatic A/E:

(a) Asymptomatic after 2 years survival > 72%, Velocity. 4 m/s
(b) AVA ↓ es by 0.12 ± 1 cm^2/year
(c) Gradient – mean ↑ es by 7 ± 7
(d) Velocity ↑ es by 0.34 - 0.39

580. RVOT VT A/E:

(a) Superior axis (b) LBBB in V1
(c) Adenosine DOC (d) Precipitated by exercise

581. SCN 5A A/E:

(a) CPVT
(b) LQT 3
(c) Brugada
(d) SSS with conduction block

582. AD mutation CPVT:

(a) RyR2 (b) Calsequestrin
(c) HERG

583. Early after depolarization:

(a) TdP (b) Digoxin
(c) AIVR (d) RVOT

584. CPR A/E:

(a) Ratio compression: RR – 30: 1 single rescuer
(b) Sternum ↓ in 5 – 7 cm
(c) Palm of hand over dorsum of other hand
(d) Compression ≥ 100/min

585. QRS complex on surface ECG corresponds to which part of transmembrane action potential?

(a) Phase 0
(b) Phase 1
(c) Phase 1 and initial part of 2
(d) Phase 2 and 3

586. Which of the statement is true regarding with reference to cardiac disease?

(a) Transient atrial arrhythmia could cause stroke
(b) Transient bradycardia can cause stroke
(c) Sinus arrhythmia can cause stroke
(d) Sinus tachycardia can cause stroke

587. Which of the following statement is false regarding class 1indication for pacemaker in sick sinus syndrome:

(a) Atrial fibrillation with bradycardia and pauses > 5 s
(b) Atrial fibrillation with bradycardia and pauses > 3 s
(c) Atrial fibrillation with bradycardia and pauses > 2 s
(d) Atrial fibrillation with bradycardia and pauses > 6 s

588. Which of the following PSTV most common among PSVT referred for ablation?

(a) Atrial tachycardia
(b) AV node reentry tachycardia
(c) Concealed pathway mediated tachycardia
(d) Manifest pathway mediated tachycardia

589. Which of the following statement regarding junctional ectopic Atrial tachycardia is false?

(a) Rarely seen in children
(b) Commonly seen in post-operative period in children with congenital heart disease
(c) AV dissociation may be present
(d) May occur for short period after AVNRT ablation

590. Accessory Pathway and Wolf Parkinson White syndrome is associated with which heart disease?

(a) Restrictive cardiomyopathy
(b) Hypertrophic cardiomyopahy
(c) Dilated cardiomyopathy
(d) Uhl's anomaly

591. Adenosine is contraindicated in following situation:

(a) PSVT in children
(b) PSVT in patient with prior cardiac transplant
(c) Atrial Tachycardia
(d) Right ventricular outflow ventricular tachycardia

592. In wide complex tachycardia which of the following is not suggestive of Ventricular Tachycardia?

(a) AV dissociation
(b) A monophasic S wave in AVR lead
(c) A monophasic R wave in AVR lead
(d) A concordant R wave in V1-V6 lead

593. Sudden death during sleep is feature of which of the following condition?

(a) Arrythmogenic right ventricular dysplasia
(b) LQTS-1
(c) LQTS-2
(d) LDTS-3

594. Which of the following drug has been used to suppress frequent episode of ventricular tachycardia in Brugada syndrome?

(a) Flecainide (b) Ivabradine
(c) Amiodarone (d) Quinidine

595. Which of the following was a negative trial in primary prevention ICD trials?

(a) MADIT (b) DEFINITE
(c) CABG PATCH (d) MUSTT

596. All of the following gene mutations are seen in long QT Syndrome *except:*

(a) KCNQ1 (b) KCNH2
(c) SCN5A (d) RYR2

597. All are caused by loss function mutation in gene SCN5A *except:*

(a) LQT3
(b) CPVT
(c) Sick sinus syndrome
(d) Cardiac conduction disorder

598. The bidirectional ventricular tachycardia seen in:

(a) Brugada syndrome (b) CPVT
(c) LQTS (d) SQTS

599. Drug of choice in WPW syndrome and AF with FVR:

(a) Adenosine (b) Beta blockers
(c) Digoxin (d) Procainamide

600. All of the following are specific for ventricular tachycardia *except:*

(a) QRS duration 120 msec
(b) Fusion beat
(c) Capture
(d) AV dissociation

601. All are true about ARVD *except:*

(a) Mutation in genes encoding desmosomes
(b) Associated with sudden cardiac death
(c) Ventricular tachycardia with LBBB morphology
(d) ECG show epsilon wave

602. All are true about catecholamine sensitive polymorphic ventricular tachycardia (CPVT) *except:*

(a) Caused by mutation in ryanodine receptor
(b) Exercise associated with sudden cardiac death
(c) Bidirectional VT not seen
(d) Treatment of choice is beta blocker and ICD

603. CRT: (T/F)

(a) NYHA II < 35%
(b) Can be given with wide QRS > 120 ms with normal EF
(c) Prolongs survival
(d) Indicated in all NYHA IV
(e) ICD improves survival in EF < 30%

604. EPS: (T/F)

(a) AH interval > 110 ms
(b) Sinus to atrial conduction is not visible in ECG
(c) Type 1 mobitz more serious than mobitz 2
(d) PR prolongs with normal QRS – His Purkinje block

605. Wide QRS tachycardia: (T/F)

(a) SVT aberrancy is most common cause of WCT
(b) Orthodromic tachycardia is least common of WCT with aberrancy
(c) > 35 years is SVT with aberrancy common
(d) RS < 100 ms in VT
(e) R on T due to APC predisposition for VT

606. Wide QRS tachycardia: (T/F)

(a) Procainamide can be used irrespective of SVT or VT
(b) Adenosine DOC in irregular rhythm
(c) Verapamil in preexcitation with AF
(d) Monomorphic R in RBBB with SVT
(e) Hemodynamically unstable–treatment cardioversion

607. SQTS: (T/F)

(a) Alkalosis
(b) Hypothermia
(c) Hyperkalemia
(d) Tachycardia is the most common cause
(e) Sudden death is common

608. SQTS: (T/F)

(a) Autosomal recessive
(b) Calcium channel
(c) Paroxysmal AF is frequent
(d) Family history of SCD is common
(e) In symptomatic patient most common is cardiac arrest

609. EPS: (T/F)

(a) Atropine worsen AV nodal block
(b) Isoprotenol/exercise improves his Purkinje block
(c) Carotid massage decreases his Purkinje block
(d) Sometimes cannot differentiate between type II Mobitz and Wenkebach
(e) His bundle has two spikes

610. EPS: (T/F)

(a) HV interval < 65 msec
(b) PA = 25 msec
(c) Cycle that follows the missed beat in Wenkebach is twice the preceded beat

611. Conduction system: (T/F)
(a) AV node is subendocardial
(b) Ach is 60-80% in ventricle vs SA node
(c) Acetyl cholinestrases more in SA node
(d) Purkinje is less sensitive to ischemia
(e) Sarcomere and mitochondria more in ventricle myocytes

612. Conduction system: (T/F)
(a) T tubule more ventricle myocyte
(b) Large gap junction more in Purkinje
(c) Ach is very less in ventricle vs atria
(d) SA nodal artery from RCA 70%
(e) Tendon of tadaro absent in 2/3rd

613. Class I antiarrhythmias: (T/F)
(a) 1a- increases v max, increases APD
(b) Ib- increases v max, decreases APD
(c) Ic- slow offset and onset
(d) Ia- fastest offset and onset
(e) Ic- decrease v max, increases ERP

614. LQTS: (T/F)
(a) LQT1 – loss of K channel function
(b) LQT2 – gain of K channel function
(c) LQT3 – loss Na channel function
(d) Romanoward – autosomal recessive
(e) Jerval and Neilson – autosomal recessive

615. True or false:
(a) SA node – spindle shaped cell with fibrous tissue mixed with packed cell
(b) AV node subendocardial
(c) AV node supplied by RCA
(d) SA node supplied by RCA in 60%
(e) TOK – infero posterior septal leaflet of tricuspid valve

616. True or false:
(a) Brugada is AD
(b) Brugada syndrome mechanisms–abnormal automaticity
(c) Brugada – loss of Na channel
(d) Loss of AP duration in RV epicardium
(e) Origin is RV

617. True or false:
(a) Parasystole – interaction of 2 autonomic foci
(b) CPVT – DAD
(c) WPW reentry mechanisms is reflection
(d) Inappropriate sinus tachycardia or bradycardia – abnormal automaticity
(e) TdP– DAD

618. LQTS: (T/F)
(a) LQTS associated with deafness
(b) LQTS genetic and acquired both causes VT and same molecular mechanisms
(c) LQTS correction of hypokalemia by K decreases repolarisation
(d) LQTS – K channelopathy

619. True or false:
(a) Ia – reduces v- max and increased APD
(b) Ib – reduces v- max and increased APD
(c) Ic – reduces v- max and increased APD
(d) Ic has slow onset kinetics
(e) Class III –increased repolarisation time

620. True or false:
(a) Ach more in ventricle than atria
(b) AV node and Purkinje fibres more cholinergic and parasympathetic than ventricle

621. Long QT syndrome: (T/F)
(a) Digoxin (b) Liquid protein
(c) Hypokalemia (d) Hypomagnesia
(e) Quinidine

622. ARVD: (T/F)
(a) Acquired cardiomyopathy
(b) Fibrofatty involvement of RV
(c) MRI – gold standard
(d) ICD – treatment of choice
(e) Heart failure can occur

623. True or false:
(a) Nonstructural heart with stage C
(b) Salt restriction < 2 gm in all stages

624. Antiarrhythmic: (T/F)
(a) Ia – ↓ Vmax ↑ APD
(b) Ic – ↑ Vmax ↓ ERP
(c) Ib – ↑ V max ↓APD
(d) Ic – slowest onset of action/offset
(e) Ia – rapid onset of action/offset

625. AF with MS: (T/F)
(a) LVEDP ↑

(b) LVEDV within Normal limit
(c) Regional hypokinesia
(d) LV compliance ↓ leading to early RV rapid filling
(e) Increased LVEF

626. LQT: (T/F)
(a) Digoxin
(b) Liquid protein
(c) Hypokalemia
(d) Hypomagnesia
(e) Quinidine

627. T/F:
(a) Digitalis – DAD
(b) LQT – DAD
(c) Overpacing causes increased membrane potential and ↓ cycle length
(d) EAD-phase III/IV

628. CSM: (T/F)
(a) AVNRT – sudden stop or no response
(b) PAT– gradual slowing to terminate
(c) Atrial flutter – transient ↓ ventricular rate
(d) Sinus tachycardia – gradual ↓ rate
(e) Circus movement – stood gradually ↓ normal

629. Wide QRS tachycardia: (T/F)
(a) SVT with accessory pathway
(b) Orthodromic with aberrancy
(c) Nodoventricular pathway
(d) Antidromic
(e) AF with functional block

630. In AF – Acute: (T/F)
(a) Oral ibutilide treatment of choice for cardioversion
(b) Propafenone C/I in structural heart disease
(c) Amiodarone can be use in WPW with AF
(d) AF > 48 hours – anticoagulant required for 4 weeks after DC shock
(e) I/V digoxin has limited success is controlling rate

631. SVT/VT: (T/F)
(a) PP variation preceding RR change S/o SVT
(b) Long – short sequence suggestive of SVT
(c) Absent rS in all precordial leads – SVT
(d) Starting with premature P – SVT
(e) Concordance in precordial leads– SVT

632. EPS: (T/F)
(a) HV < 65 ms
(b) PA interval is 25 ms
(c) His bundle may have 2 deflection (spikes)
(d) Hidden A-V dissociation may not be detected by intracardiac recording
(e) Always can detect mobitz type I and II

633. T/F:
(a) SQTS – risk of AF
(b) LQTS – 2 = SCD on exercise can occur
(c) Brugada syndrome– beta blocker is DOC
(d) LQTS 3 > LQTS 2 > LQTI – risk of SCD
(e) LQTS – gene abnormality present, QT Normal – beta blocker may ↓ mortality

634. Pacemaker: (T/F)
(a) Lead Dislodgement max in 1st weak
(b) Improper placement can lead to extracardiac stimulation
(c) Oversensing may lead to pacing inhibition
(d) Runaway pacemaker is usually associated low battery
(e) Decreased impedance is S/O lead fracture

635. AF cardioversion: (T/F)
(a) AF with <12 months for cardioversion – favourable outcome
(b) Dilated CA–favourable outcome
(c) AF with Digoxin–DC shock favourable
(d) AF with AV block–favourable
(e) Post DC shock–mechanical asystole S/O better prognosis

636. AEDS: (T/F)
(a) Bipolar DC – ↓ sed energy required
(b) Monopolar – usually max is 360 J
(c) AED – can diagnose rhythm
(d) AED has ↓ mortality in out of hospital

637. Cardiopulmonary resuscitation: (T/F)
(a) Bystander – 15 : 2
(b) Mouth to mouth resp – 30 : 2
(c) EMS should DC shock the patient irrespective of tissue
(d) Extrahospital DC shock has decreased mortality by 2 times
(e) Coronary perfusion – only 10-20% by CPR

638. Brugada syndrome: (T/F)
(a) Sodium channel mutation
(b) Normally presents with VT
(c) Right precordial leads – RBBB with ST depression

(d) ECG indicates abnormality of RV
(e) Has long QT

639. Brugada syndrome: (T/F)
(a) Changes in RV always required for arrhythmias production
(b) Death occurs during sleep

640. Digoxin: (T/F)
(a) Does not shorten QT
(b) Does not action on HP bundle and ventricular fibres
(c) T ½ = 48-72 hours
(d) DC shock to be given in infranodal block
(e) ECG always diagnostic of digitoxicity

641. Digoxin: (T/F)
(a) Narrow therapeutic window
(b) Redigitalization after CABG due to absorption after CPB
(c) Ion based treatment for removal of digoxin
(d) T ½ – 12 hours
(e) Decreases hospitalization in HF

642. Pacing: (T/F)
(a) First code – sensing
(b) Second code – pacing
(c) Third code – response to sensing
(d) Fourth code – multisite pacing
(e) Fifth code – rate modulation and programming

643. Pacing threshold: (T/F)
(a) Threshold decreases within weeks after implantation
(b) Depends on circadium rhythm
(c) Depends on pulse width and pulse amplitude

644. Amiodarone: (T/F)
(a) Hypothyroidism more than hyperthyroidism
(b) Pulmonary toxicity – 25%
(c) Cardiac side effects in < 5%
(d) Decreases level of warfarin
(e) Pulmonary toxicity is most common serious non cardiac side effect

645. ARVD: (T/F)
(a) QRS > 110 msec in V4-V6
(b) Heart transplantation is definite treatment
(c) Non-familial predisposition
(d) Terminal notch in V1-V3
(e) Fibrofatty in RV myocardium

646. Anatomy of conduction system: (T/F)
(a) RBBB divides at the level of anterior papillary muscle
(b) His bundle has rich autonomic supply

647. Pacemaker: (T/F)
(a) Insulation failure ↑ impedance
(b) Set screw loose ↓ threshold
(c) Lead dislodgement ↓ threshold
(d) Battery depletion ↑ impedance
(e) Insulation failure ↓ threshold

648. ICD: (T/F)
(a)
(b) MI with EF < 30% reasonable indication
(c) May itself cause arrhythmic storm sometimes
(d) All long QT require ICD
(e) Idiopathic VT with LBBB with inf. axis is an indication

649. T/F:
(a) IA – ↓ cond. velocity
(b) Ic – ↓ cond. velocity
(c) III – ↓ velocity in AV node
(d) IB – ↑ APD
(e) IB – ↓ conduction velocity

650. Brugada: (T/F)
(a) RBBB c ST ↑
(b) K + channelopathy
(c) ICD is TOC
(d) User common in Asia
(e) SCD during exercise

651. ARVD: (T/F)
(a) Epsilon in early part of QRS
(b) LBBB + RAD–during VT
(c) RFA is good option of treatment
(d) CPVT having strong genetic basis
(e) RVOT, idiopathic VT with inf. axis with LBBB ICD is quite useful

652. T/F:
(a) PJRT – short RP
(b) VA= < 55 msec S/O AVNRT

(c) WPW with orthodromic tachycardia–IV procainamide is TOC
(d) Metoprolol metabolism is inhibited by quinidine so it is not given in patient of AF
(e) Verapamil ↓ es AV nodal ERP
(f) Postcardiac transplant heart shows super sensitivity to adenosine

653. TDP: (T/F)
(a) AF is a risk factor
(b) LQT2 is most common
(c) LQTS death – SCD is less common in children
(d) For polymorphic VT diagnosis both variation in duration and axis of QRS is required
(e) Disopyramide in high risk

654. True or false:
(a) QT dispersion < 50 ms is normal
(b) QTc – QT/√RR
(c) QRS amplitude is more in African American
(d) QRS amplitude is more in male than female
(e) QRS amplitude is more in obese person than thinner persons
(f) QRST angle < 60

655. Voughan-Williams: (T/F)
(a) CCB – class III
(b) D-sotalol – class II
(c) Quinidine – IB
(d) Morcizine – IC
(e) Dofetilide – III

656. APD: (T/F)
(a) Phase – 4 – Na+ exit
(b) Phase – 2 – slow Ca^{+2} entry
(c) Phase – 1/3 – K^+ entry
(d) SAN/AVN – AP due to slow Ca^{+2}
(e) Atrial/vent fast AP due to K^+ channel

657. Digoxin toxicity: (T/F)
(a) ST/T changes
(b) PR prolongation
(c) V wave prominent
(d) QT prolongation
(e) Mobitz type II block

658. TdP: (T/F)
(a) Due to DAD
(b) Frequently occur after short coupling after pause
(c) Precipitated by severe bradycardia
(d) Pacing prevents by decreasing c-QT interval
(e) Giant T wave inversion suggest recent syncope

659. Reentrant arrhythmias: (T/F)
(a) Atrial flutter
(b) WPW
(c) AIVR
(d) Sinus tachycardia
(e) TdP

660. Sinus arrhythmias: (T/F)
(a) Digitalis toxicity non respiratory Sinus arrhythmia
(b) Longest shortest cycle > 60 sec
(c) Ventriculophasic arrhythmia in CHB
(d) Loss of variability predicts sudden death

661. True or false:
(a) SNRT > 550 msec
(b) AH interval < 80 msec
(c) HV interval = 25 – 55 msec
(d) Sinoatrial time < 150 msec
(e) PA time < 25 msec

662. AF: (T/F)
(a) Oral ibutilide treatment of choice of cardioversion
(b) High intravenous amiodarone for conversion in WPW syndrome
(c) Dofetilide for recurrent VF and does not increase QT
(d) Propafenone contraindicated in structural heart disease
(e) Intravenous digoxin does not effectively decreases AV conduction and not good for rate control

663. Class I indication for PPI: (T/F)
(a) Asymptomatic trifascicular block
(b) Recurrent syncope with LBBB
(c) IWMI < 3 days
(d) Congenital CHB asymptomatic HR< 45/min with wide QRS
(e) Chronotropic incompetence
(f) Asymptomatic sick sinus syndrome

664. Wide QRS tachycardia: (T/F)
(a) Antidromic tachycardia
(b) Orthodromic with aberrancy pathway
(c) AT with LBBB
(d) SVT with accessory pathway
(e) Nodoventricular/fascicular with antegrade conduction

665. T/F:
(a) Diastolic depolarization less negative in ischemic cells

(b) During systolic depolarization early rise to positive
(c) ST depression is sum of TQ elevation and true ST depression
(d) RMP in diastole – 85 mV

666. **T/F:**
(a) Phase I early rapid repolarization progress to plateau
(b) Phase III is brief and few msec similar to skeletal and nerve potential
(c) Phase III related to terminal repolarization to rest potential
(d) Fast depolarization in conduction tissues
(e) Phase IV slow depolarization

667. **T/F:**
(a) Sotalol with ISA and prolonged repolarization
(b) Propafenone C/I in structural heart disease
(c) Amiodarone decreases slope of phase IV of sinus node action potential
(d) Sotalol effective in ARVD
(e) Disopyramide can be given intravenous
(f) Bertylium causes hypotension

668. **SNRT (sinus node reentrant tachycardia): (T/F)**
(a) More common in females
(b) Rate = 80-200/min
(c) Initiation by APC
(d) Termination by APC
(e) 20% of total supraventricular arrhythmias

669. **Digoxin levels increased by: (T/F)**
(a) Verapamil (b) Dilzem
(c) Nitrendipine (d) Captopril
(e) Amiodarone

670. **Antiarrhythmias drugs: (T/F)**
(a) Ia- ↑ APD and ↓ v-max
(b) Ia causes ↓ RMP
(c) Ic ↓ v max
(d) Class III ↑ repolarisation time
(e) Ic ↓ APD

671. **Long RR cycles causes changes in EAD/DAD: (T/F)**
(a) ↑ EAD (b) ↓ DAD
(c) ↓ EAD and ↓ DAD (d) ↓ EAD
(e) ↑ DAD

672. **Conduction velocity – slowest to fastest: (T/F)**
(a) SA > AVN > ventricle > Purkinje fibres
(b) SA < AVN < ventricle < Purkinje fibres
(c) SA =AVN < ventricle < Purkinje fibres
(d) SA < AVN < ventricle = Purkinje fibres
(e) None of the above

673. **ARVD: (T/F)**
(a) 55-60% LV is involved
(b) AR inheritance
(c) VPC has RBBB morphology
(d) VT induced by reentry
(e) Epsilon wave seen in 40-50%

674. **LQTS Chromosome: (T/F)**
(a) LQT3–Na channel
(b) LQT1–max mortality
(c) LQT1– K channel
(d) LQT2–arousal/emotional most common stimuli
(e) B Blocker indicated in symptomatic patients

675. **Torsade de pointes: (T/F)**
(a) Terfenadine (b) Astemizole
(c) Roxithromycin (d) Mosapride
(e) Liquid protein diet

676. **Triggered activity: (T/F)**
(a) Digoxin induced (b) TDP
(c) RVOT VT (d) Fascicular VT
(e) Atrial flutter

677. **Pacemaker: (T/F)**
(a) Short electrode – ↓ Threshold
(b) Insulation breakage – ↓ impedance
(c) Bipolar – cathode at tip and anode at proximal ring
(d) Unipolar – pulse generator inactive
(e) Steroid elution lead – ↓es acute and chronic threshold

678. **LQTS chromosome: (T/F)**
(a) Chr 7 – LQTS 1 (b) Chr 3 – LQTS 3
(c) Chr 7 – LQTS 2

679. **Drugs improve outcome in CPR: (T/F)**
(a) Epinephrine (b) Vasopressin
(c) Calcium chloride (d) Sodium bicarbonate

680. **True or false about CPR:**
(a) Epinephrine can be given by above the level of diaphragm

(b) Epinephrine converts coarse fibrillation to fine fibrillation
(c) Epinephrine and lidocaine can be given by endotracheal tube
(d) High dose epinephrine can cause LV systolic dysfunction after recovery from deleterious effect
(e) Somatosensory evoked potential can detect irreversible brain damage

681. **CPR: (T/F)**
(a) Survivors of cardiac arrest can develop psychosis
(b) After 90 sec of cardiac arrest initial chest compression better than defibrillation
(c) Intravenous epinephrine prevent carotid artery collapse
(d) Coronary perfusion is insignificantly decreased if chest compression is stopped for ventilation
(e) Active chest compression increases survival

682. **CPR: (T/F)**
(a) Abdominal compression interposed with chest compression
(b) Vest CPR inflated to 100-200 ATM pressure
(c) Patient is inflated with air in CPR
(d) Thoracic compression increase brain blood flow even without cardiac compression
(e) Cerebral blood flow depend upon gradient between jugular vein and right atrium

683. **CPR: (T/F)**
(a) Coronary perfusion depends upon pressure gradient between aorta and pulmonary artery
(b) Epinephrine increases carotid blood flow
(c) During asystole thump version restores cardiac contractility
(d) Automatic external defibrillation improves survival
(e) Defibrillation in primary VF within time improves survival

684. **CPR: (T/F)**
(a) Amiodarone can be used in recurrent VT/VF
(b) Compression more than 2 inches
(c) Rate > 100/min
(d) Abdominal binder increases cerebral blood flow with simultaneous chest compression
(e) After electrocution, there may be delayed recovery

685. **Primary prevention trials of amiodarone in SCD: (T/F)**
(a) GESICA (b) CHF-STAT
(c) CAMIAT (d) SWORD-D
(e) CIDS

686. **DAD: (T/F)**
(a) Decreased by catecholamines
(b) Decreased by CCB
(c) Decreased by long cycle
(d) Due to triggered activity
(e) Due to automaticity

687. **Doefitilide: (T/F)**
(a) It prevents atrial flutter better than AF
(b) Used in both oral and intravenous form
(c) Used for prevention of recurrent AF
(d) Can give rise of TdP
(e) Decreases QTc

688. **TdP: (T/F)**
(a) Due to DAD
(b) Class Ia don't cause
(c) Flecainide normally do not cause it
(d) Chronic bradycardia can lead to TdP
(e) Short cycle after pause can cause TdP
(f) Pacemaker prevent TdP by decreasing QT interval

689. **Lignocaine: (T/F)**
(a) Increased AV conduction
(b) Inward Na current is responsible for long QT in Romano-Ward syndrome

690. **True or false:**
(a) CSNRT < 550 msec
(b) SACT < 150 msec
(c) PA interval – 25 msec
(d) AH interval < 80 msec
(e) HV interval 25—55 msec

691. **Sinus node: (T/F)**
(a) Length = 10-20 mm
(b) Supplied by RCA in 70-80% of cases
(c) Impulse generation by T cells
(d) Posterior intermodal carries impulse from RA to LA
(e) NE ratio–4:1 in atria: ventricle

692. **Sinus arrhythmias: (T/F)**
(a) Max. – min. cycle length difference is 60 msec
(b) Digitalis can cause non respiratory sinus arrhythmias
(c) Always asymptomatic

(d) Ventriculophasic due to CHB
(e) Loss of sinus arrhythmias – poor prognosis

693. Digoxin: (T/F)
(a) Blocks Na^+K^+ pump is mechanism of action
(b) Spironolactone decreases digoxin level
(c) DOC in chronic AF without CHF
(d) Digoxin is better than diuretic in CHF in children
(e) Frequent manifestation of toxicity – bidirectional VT

694. Koch's triangle A/E:
(a) Crista terminalis (b) Tendon of tadaro
(c) Tricuspid valve (d) Coronary sinus

695. Single chamber asynchronous sensing:
(a) AAIR (b) DDDR
(c) VOOR (d) DOOR

696. Brugada syndrome–drug used for VF prevention:
(a) Quinidine (b) Amiodarone
(c) Sotalol (d) Metoprolol

697. No effect on Action potential:
(a) Class IA (b) Class IB
(c) Class IC (d) Class III

698. SCD in young athlete:
(a) HOCM (b) CAD
(c) ARVD

699. Digoxin toxicity A/E:
(a) Activated charcoal (b) Digibind
(c) Pacing (d) Hemodialysis

700. Sick sinus syndrome ME:
(a) Low unbound Sr total T3
(b) Normal 14
(c) Increased TSH
(d) Increased Reverse T3

701. Preexcitation brought out by all *except:*
(a) Verapamil (b) Atrial pacing
(c) Adenosine (d) Isoprenaline

702. Atrial specific anti-arrhythmic:
(a) Vernakalant (b) Dronedarone
(c) Ajmaline (d) Ibutilide

703. AF treatment true is:
(a) Long term antiarrhythmic treatment better than pill in pocket
(b) Long term antithrombotic irrespective frequency of sign and symptoms
(c) Rhythm control – ↓ recurrent hospitalisation
(d) Amiodarone not used for rate control

704. Short QT interval A/E:
(a) AD
(b) Loss of function mutuation in K channel
(c) AF common
(d) ICD – Treatment of Choice

705. Atrial flutter – DC shock of:
(a) 50 J (b) 150 J
(c) 250 J (d) 200 J

706. Accessory pathways:
(a) Left side less antidromic tachycardia
(b) Left side less AF
(c) Sinus tachycardia reveals preexcitation better
(d) Intermittent preexcitation– marker of SCD

707. Defibrillation A/E:
(a) Most common efficacious in automaticity
(b) No need to stop digoxin, if no toxicity
(c) Higher energy higher damage
(d) Dofetilide – facilitates

708. Short RP tachycardia A/E:
(a) Orthodromic AVRT
(b) Typical AVNRT
(c) PJRT
(d) Ectopic junctional tachycardia

709. DDD is useful in CHB and:
(a) AF (b) Sinus node dysfunction
(c) LV dysfunction (d) TR

710. Young male narrow QRS tachycardia (180/min) each QRS followed by p wave, carotid sinus massage (165/min), RBBB morphology diagnosis:
(a) Orthodromic AVRT with right sided bypass tract
(b) AVNRT
(c) VT with 1:1 VA dissociation
(d) VT + AVNRT

711. SCD in a patient with no structural heart disease A/E:
(a) PR= 0.36
(b) QTc = 254

(c) QTc = 538
(d) Epsilon wave in right precordial leads

712. Koch triangle boundary:
(a) Tendon of todaro (b) Crista terminalis
(c) Tricuspid annulus (d) Coronary sinus

713. Brugada syndrome—most dangerous:
(a) Typical ECG spontaneously
(b) Syncope + Spontaneous ECG changes
(c) Syncope + Drug induced ECG changes
(d) Asymptomatic but malignant arrhythmia on EPS

714. SCD incidence after 35 years of age:
(a) 0.1-0.2% (b) 0.01-0.02%
(c) 1-2% (d) 0.001-0.002%

715. Class I ICD indication A/E:
(a) Incessant VT/VF
(b) Symptomatic sustained VT with structural heart disease
(c) NSVT with CAD with LV dysfunction with sustained VT on EPS

716. PSVT drug of choice:
(a) Adenosine (b) Verapamil
(c) Diltiazem (d) Metoprolol

717. Long RP interval tachycardia A/E:
(a) Slow fast AVNRT (b) Atrial tachycardia
(c) PJRT (d) SANRT

718. Trough digoxin level:
(a) 0.5-1 ng/ml (b) 3-4 ng/ml
(c) 0.5-1 ng/ml (d) 1-2 mg/ml

719. CHB is typically seen in:
(a) Friedreich ataxia (b) Becker's dystrophy
(c) Myotonic dystrophy (d) All

720. RF ablation A/E:
(a) Frequency used 300-10,000 Hz
(b) Resistive heating
(c) Painless
(d) Polymorphic VT can occur

721. Patient present with narrow complex tachycardia of 180/min with p wave following every QRS. CSM cause a rate of 165/min with LBBB morphology, diagnosis:
(a) AVNRT
(b) Orthodromic AVRT with left sided tract
(c) VT with 1: 1 conduction
(d) Combined AVRT and VT

722. Patient present with BP=80/60 mm Hg, rate = 210/min with LBBB morphology, diagnosis:
(a) RVOT VT
(b) Orthodromic AVRT with left pathway
(c) AVNRT with LBBB
(d) Antidromic AVRT with right sided pathway
(e) All

723. Patient with AICD complains of repeated shocks. Clinical exam normal rhythm, has multiple shocks in spite of normal rhythm treatment:
(a) Arrange for urgent reprogramming of AICD
(b) Put a magnet on AICD
(c) Urgent EPS
(d) Intravenous amiodarone
(e) Intravenous lignocaine

724. Atrial flutter and AF, all true *except:*
(a) Pulmonary vein isolation is treatment of choice for typical atrial flutter
(b) Anticoagulation is required for atrial flutter as for AF
(c) AF is more common than a flutter
(d) Rate control may be considered as management option for Atrial Flutter

725. All of following are properties of an accessory (WPW) pathway A/E:
(a) Usually have decremental conduction properties
(b) Intermittent preexcitation means long effective refractory period
(c) May conduct both antegrade and retrograde pathway
(d) Slow conduction in antegrade pathway cause subtle ECG changes

726. Most common cause of SCD:
(a) IHD (b) HOCM
(c) Brugada (d) ARVD

727. Ryanodine receptors associated with:
(a) CPVT (b) Brugada
(c) LQTS (d) SQTS

728. Drug used in stable monomorphic VT A/E:
(a) Verapamil (b) Sotalol
(c) Lidocaine (d) Procainamide

729. Most common type of wide complex tachycardia:
(a) Monomorphic VT
(b) SVT with bundle branch block
(c) Pseudo ventricular tachycardia
(d) Antidromic tachycardia

730. Digoxin toxicity A/E:
(a) Paroxysmal atrial tachycardia
(b) Ventricular ectopy
(c) AF
(d) VT

731. Digoxin toxicity A/E:
(a) Hyperkalemia (b) Hypomagnesium
(c) Hypercalcemia (d) Renal impairment

732. PPI indication A/E:
(a) CHB
(b) Mobitz type I block
(c) Symptomatic bradycardia
(d) Alternating right and left bundle branch block

733. Flecainide C/I A/E:
(a) Patient on Beta blocker
(b) Myocarditis
(c) RBBB with LAHB
(d) Post MI patients

734. SCD most common cause:
(a) Ischemic Heart Disease
(b) HCM
(c) ARVD
(d) Congenital coronary anomalies

735. Ivabradine true:
(a) ↑ PR (b) ↑ QT
(c) ↑ QTc (d) ↑ QRS

736. Digoxin toxicity associated with A/E:
(a) AF (b) VPC
(c) PAT (d) VT

737. WPW syndrome A/E:
(a) Both retrograde and antegrade
(b) Usually have decremental response
(c) It slow conduction through antegrade pathway than there is subtle ECG manifestation
(d) Intermittent preexitation occur if there is long effective refractory period

738. Long RP interval A/E:
(a) Atypical AVNRT
(b) AT with first degree block
(c) Sinus tachycardia
(d) PJRT

739. In the intracardiac ECG, maximum contribution to AV conduction time is by:
(a) PA (b) AH
(c) HV (d) Conduction through bundle branch

740. Peak T wave with short QT occur in:
(a) Hypokalemia with hypocalcemia
(b) Hypokalemia with hypercalcemia
(c) Hyperkalemia with hypocalcemia
(d) Hyperkalemia with hypercalcemia

741. What is true about fascicular VT?
(a) No AV dissociation
(b) Indeterminate axis
(c) Concordant ST changes
(d) Relatively narrow QRS

742. Regarding MADIT trial which is true?
(a) Secondary prevention of ICD
(b) Primary prevention of ICD
(c) Secondary prevention of CRT
(d) Primary prevention of CRT

743. When you advise CRT?
(a) Class I NYHA LBBB QRS > 120 ms
(b) Class III Non LBBB QRS > 150 ms
(c) Class IV NYHA with AF
(d) Class III NYHA Non LBBB QRS > 120 ms

744. Regarding CPR, which is true regarding cardiac respiratory ratio?
(a) 20:2 (b) 30:2
(c) 40:2 (d) 60:2

745. About LQTS A/E:
(a) Autosomal dominant
(b) Mutation in chr 11
(c) Children presents with syncope
(d) CCB are DOC

746. In pulseless electrical activity according to PALS recommendation which drug is used?
(a) Adenosine
(b) Atropine
(c) Epinephrine
(d) Amiodarone

747. CRT indication A/E:

(a) RBBB (b) QRS>120
(c) Sinus rhythm (d) EF < 35%

748. Long QT caused by A/E:

(a) Hypo K^+ (b) Hypocalcemia
(c) Hypomagnesemia (d) Rheumatic carditis

749. Most common tachycardia in a structurally normal heart:

(a) RBBB with LAD (b) LBBB with LAD
(c) RBBB with RAD (d) LBDD with RAD

750. Wide QRS RVOT VT:

(a) RBBB with LAD (b) RBBB with RAD
(c) LBBB with LAD (d) LBBB with RAD

751. AS on colour dopplers $4v^2$ denotes:

(a) Peak to peak gradient
(b) Mean gradient
(c) Peak instantaneous gradient
(d) All of the above

752. Mobitz type II block:

(a) 1° AV block (b) 2° AV block Type II
(c) Wenkebach (d) Infrafasicular block

753. Conducting system of heart made by:

(a) Modified nerves
(b) Modified cardiac muscle cell
(c) Neurons
(d) Connective tissue

754. 2:1 heart block, atrial rate 80/min, N QRS duration site of block:

(a) Bundle of his (b) AV node
(c) Bundle branch (d) Can't be determined

755. Mobiz-2 block:

(a) AV-Type – 2 block (b) Wenckebach
(c) 1° AV block (d) Unifascicular

756. ARVD all are major criteria *except*:

(a) SAECG late potential
(b) Segmental RV dilatation
(c) Epsilon wave
(d) Parietal block

757. Criteria of VT A/E:

(a) V1 R > RS
(b) aVR R positive initial deflection
(c) Absent RS in primordial lead
(d) AV dissociation

758. Frontal QRS anis in CRT (BV pacing) axis:

(a) $+30^\circ$ to $+60^\circ$ (b) -90° to -120°
(c) -30° to -60° (d) $+120^\circ$ to $+180^\circ$

759. Most common VT in structurally normal heart axis:

(a) RBBB superior axis (b) LBBB superior axis
(c) RBBB inferior axis (d) LBBB inferior axis

760. Structurally normal heart RBBB with superior axis VT broad QRS. DOC to terminate VT:

(a) Amiodarone (b) Xylocaine
(c) Verapamil (d) Adenosine

761. Post SCD survival true:

(a) Amiodarone and sotalol > ICD
(b) Amiodarone DOC
(c) Amiodarone can be added adjust ICD
(d) ICD aborts ventricular arrhythmia but no effect on mortality

762. Trial of CRT mortality benefit:

(a) Miracie ICD (b) Path CHF
(c) Care HF (d) None of the above

763. AIVR is not caused by:

(a) Digoxin toxicity (b) Cocaine intoxication
(c) Rheumatic carditis (d) MI
(e) None

764. CHB not caused by:

(a) Chagas disease (b) Lyme disease
(c) Diphtheria (d) TB pneumonia

765. Phase 2 plateau correspond to:

(a) End of QRS (b) ST segment
(c) T wave inflection (d) Onset of QRS

766. Endless loop tachycardia treatment:

(a) ↑ sing PVARP (b) Switching mode
(c) Beta blocker

767. WPW syndromes A/E:

(a) Wide QRS during sinus rhythm
(b) Narrow complex SVT
(c) δ wave, in sinus rhythm
(d) ↑ ed H-V interval

768. (JUP) Plakoglobin mutation in:
(a) ARVD (b) CPVT
(c) HOCM

769. SVT vs VT favouring VT A/E:
(a) AV dissociation
(b) Fusion beats
(c) RSR in V1 during RBBB
(d) Nonconcordance in precordial leads

770. NKX 2.5 A/E:
(a) AF (b) VF
(c) Sick sinus syndrome (d) Wenckebach block

771. TDP A/E:
(a) Commonly seen on amiodarone infusion
(b) Prolonged QT
(c) Long-short cycles with bradycardia precipitate it
(d) EAD phase II and III with triggered activity

772. 30 years male, transient syncope ECG showing VT drug to be avoided:
(a) Adenosine (b) Verapamil
(c) DC shock (d) Amiodarone

773. Which component of PR internal is maximally influenced by vagal discharge:
(a) PA interval
(b) AH
(c) HV
(d) All are equally influenced

774. 30 years male presents with history of transient loss of consciousness and palpitations ECG shows VT. Drug to be avoided:
(a) Adenosine (b) Verapamil
(c) DC shock (d) Amiodarone

775. All are causes of SCD due to VF *except:*
(a) Hyperthyroidism (b) DCM
(c) Chagas (d) Sarcoidosis

776. Vagal stimulation maximum affect which part of PR interval:
(a) PA (b) AH
(c) HV (d) All are equally affected

777. Amiodarone all *except:*
(a) ↑ Conversion of T4→T3
(b) ↑ QT prolongation
(c) ↑ PR

778. Narrow QRS tachycardia with AV dissociation true is:
(a) Digoxicity
(b) AVNRT
(c) Dual AV node pathway
(d) WPW syndrome

779. Autosomal dominant associated with SCD in newborn:
(a) ALCAPA
(b) Jervell Lange syndrome
(c) Romano-Ward syndrome
(d) Brugada syndrome

780. Indication for pacing A/E:
(a) Sinus bradycardia with first degree AV block
(b) Should be done in asymptomatic CHB

781. True about ICD / EPS:
(a) EPS should be done to detect type of arrhythmias
(b) EPS done before ICD implantation for sustained VT
(c) Done in VT to detect usefulness of RFA
(d) Surgery is preferable for LV aneurysm than ICD with VT

782. Drugs causing torsade de pointes A/E:
(a) Amiodarone (b) Mexilitine
(c) Sotalol (d) Quinidine

783. DDD vs VVI choice:
(a) HOCM with 2:1 infranodal block
(b) AF with ventricular rate– 40/min
(c) 46 years old male with HR– 46/min
(d) First degree heart block

784. AF will not have variable S1 in:
(a) AF with FVR (b) AF with slow VR
(c) AF with CHB (d) None

785. Mechanisms TDP:
(a) Automaticity (b) Reentry
(c) Triggered activity

786. Brugada syndrome all true *except:*
(a) Curve differentiate it from long QT 3
(b) Pseudo bundle branch
(c) ST elevation with T inversion in V1-V3
(d) N a channel

787. WPW – B associated with cardiac lesion:

(a) Ebstein anomaly (b) cc-TGA

788. Genetic testing is most appropriate for:

(a) Long QT syndrome
(b) Dilated cardiomyopathy
(c) Coronary artery disease
(d) Atrial fibrillation

789. The most common energy source used for catheter ablation for treatment of arrhythmias is:

(a) Cryoablation
(b) Radiofrequency
(c) High frequency ultrasound
(d) Laser

790. Which of the following statements is true regarding peristent junctional reciprocating tachycardia (PJRT)?

(a) It is an antidromic variety of AVRT
(b) It has short R-P interval
(c) The tachycardia rates are usually slower than other tachyarrhythmias
(d) It is usually seen in elderly patients

791. Arrhythmias causing tachycardia-mediated cardiomyopathy include all of the following *except:*

(a) Ectopic atrial tachycardia
(b) Atrial fibrillation
(c) Persistent junctional reciprocating tachycardia (PJRT)
(d) Bidirectional ventricular tachycardia

792. Bundle branch re-entrant ventricular tachycardia (BBRVT) is usually associated with:

(a) RBBB morphology during tachycardia
(b) HV interval during VT is typically shorter than during sinus rhythm
(c) Patients with no structural heart disease
(d) Poor response to pharmacological therapy

793. All of the following drugs may be useful for treatment of catecholaminergic polymorphic ventricular tachycardia (CPVT) *except:*

(a) Quinidine (b) Nadolol
(c) Verapamil (d) Flecanide

794. Out-of-hospital self-treatment of recent-onset atrial fibrillation (Pill-in-the-Pocket approach) can be done by taking:

(a) Quinidine (b) Amiodarone
(c) Sotalol (d) Flecainide

795. All of the following are true regarding multifocal atrial tachycardia (MAT) *except:*

(a) Variable P wave morphologies
(b) Variable P-P interval
(c) Constant PR interval
(d) Variable R-R interval

796. A 15-year-old athlete is diagnosed to have Ebstein's anomaly. He has no limitation in his physical activity. There is no cardiomegaly. Recently, he had two episodes of palpitations and dizziness but no syncope. The likely arrhythmia in this patient will be:

(a) Atrial fibrillation
(b) Atrial flutter
(c) AVRT
(d) Ventricular tachycardia

797. A 45-year-old male patient is a case of CAD, post CABG, LVEF 28%. He is having class II symptoms (dyspnea) on optimal medical management. His ECG shows sinus rhythm, PR interval 220 msec and QRS duration of 112 msec. There is no history of syncope or pre-syncope or palpitations. The likely management should include:

(a) ICD implantation
(b) CRT implantation
(c) Combo (ICD and CRT implantation)
(d) No device therapy (at present)

798. Arrhythmogenic right ventricular cardiomyo-pathy is a disease of:

(a) Tropomyosin (b) Intercalated disc
(c) Myosin light chain (d) Mitochondrial DNA

799. A 50-year-old patient of VVI pacemaker for complete heart block has to undergo surgical treatment using cautery. Any of the following perioperative strategy is useful *except:*

(a) Place a magnet over the pacemaker during the procedure
(b) Program the pacemaker to VOO mode
(c) Switch off the hysteresis
(d) Use bipolar electro cautery

800. In the beat after long cycle length in atrial fibrillation, which of the following murmur increases in intensity?

(a) Pulmonary stenosis
(b) Rheumatic mitral regurgitation
(c) Mitral regurgitation due to papillary muscle dysfunction
(d) Mitral regurgitation due to mitral valve prolapse

801. Which of the following diseases has been linked to mutation in the cardiac sodium channel?

(a) Long QT syndrome (b) Brugada syndrome
(c) Sinus node disease (d) All of the above

802. Which of the following is not true about atrioventricular nodal re-entrant tachycardia?

(a) It is a cause of short RP supraventricular tachycardia
(b) Mostly manifests as incessant tachycardia leading to ventricular dysfunction
(c) May be controlled with beta blockers
(d) Is quite suitable for radiofrequency ablation

803. In patient with atrial fibrillation and fast conduction through accessory pathway, all drugs can be used *except:*

(a) Quinidine (b) Flecanide
(c) Amiodarone (d) Digoxin

804. A 70-year-old woman presents with chronic atrial fibrillation and ventricular rate of 30 per minutes. Pacemaker of choice is:

(a) DDDR (b) AAIR
(c) VVIR (d) VVI

805. One of the following is not a boundary for triangle of Koch:

(a) Tendon of Tadaro
(b) Anterior tricuspid leaflet
(c) Septal tricuspid leaflet
(d) Mouth of coronary sinus

806. False statement about parasystole:

(a) Intervals are multiples of basic interval
(b) Functions like fixed rate asynchronous pacemaker
(c) Functions like fixed rate synchronous pacemaker
(d) Can exhibit entrance block or exit block

807. Entrainment is a feature of:

(a) Reentry (b) Automaticity
(c) Triggered activity (d) All of the above

808. False statement about Brugada syndrome:

(a) Phase 4 reentry
(b) Mutations in SCN5A
(c) Ventricular fibrillation
(d) ST elevation in V1-V3

809. The following anti arrhythmic drug has no place in Vaughan Williams classification:

(a) Lignocaine (b) Adenosine
(c) Ibutilide (d) Verapamil

810. Epsilon waves are seen in:

(a) Ebstein anomaly
(b) Endomyocardial fibrosis
(c) Arrhythmogenic right ventricular dysplasia
(d) Hypertrophic cardiomyopathy

811. Capture beats are characteristic of:

(a) Ventricular tachycardia
(b) Atrial flutter
(c) PSVT
(d) Atrial fibrillation

812. In dual chamber pacemakers important feature to prevent endless loop tachycardia:

(a) AV interval (b) PVARP
(c) Hysteresis interval (d) Automatic interval

813. LQTS:

(a) Romano-Ward – no hearing loss
(b) Jarnell large – autosomal recessive
(c) Starnation prolongs QT
(d) All of the above

814. Which is not a reasonable cause of SA node dysfn?

(a) Radiation (b) Lithium toxicity
(c) Hypothyroidism (d) Hypothermia

815. Einthoven's law:

(a) II = III + I

816. Class II NYHA class of indication for non LBBB with QRS> 130 mm:

(a) I (b) IIa
(c) IIb (d) III

817. Fill in pocket:

(a) Flecainide

818. Not acting on K channels:

(a) Amiodarone (b) Sotalol
(c) Ibutilide (d) Propafenone

819. Not class III:

(a) Mexilitine (b) Bretylium
(c) Sotalol (d) Amiodarone

820. False regarding Tdp:

(a) Commonly seen with amiodarone
(b) Due to EAD in phase 2 and 3
(c) Presented by short long sequences (Bradycardia)
(d) Associated with long QT

821. Entrainment phenomenon:

(a) Reentrant tachycardia (b) Parasystole

822. CARTO for:

(a) RVOT ablation

823. What does 'R' stand in pacemaker coding?

(a) Rate response

824. True about ARVD *except*:

(a) Present with monomorphic VT
(b) Biventricular involvement in 20%
(c) RFA ablation lead to event free survived in > 85%

825. Responsible for maintaining resting membrane potential:

(a) IK (b) IK1
(c) IT (d) I Na

826. Main ion responsible for cardiac repolarisation:

(a) Ca (b) Na
(c) Cl (d) K

827. Desmosomal mutation likely diagnosis finding:

(a) Arrhythmogenic right ventricular DYSPLASIA
(b) HOCM
(c) RCMP
(d) Renovascular hypertension → may be due to obstruction at any .....

828. Drug not acting as accessory pathway:

(a) Ia (b) Ic
(c) III (d) IV

829. CPVT not used:

(a) Flecainide (b) Carvedilol
(c) Verapamil (d) Amiodarone

830. Long RP tachycardia all *except*:

(a) AVRT with mayhaim
(b) Atypical AVNRT
(c) PJRT
(d) Ectopic atrial tachycardia

831. ECG broad complex tachycardia, presented in casualty treatment:

(a) Ca gluconate (b) D.C. shock
(c) Adenosine (d) Thrombolysis

832. Which one of the following ECG pattern is not true for left anterior fascicular block?

(a) rS pattern in leads I and aVL
(b) qR pattern in lead aVL
(c) Time to peak r wave in aVL 45 msec
(d) Frontal plane mean QRS axis is 45 to 90 degrees

833. Which one of the following drug is not used for pharmacological conversion of atrial fibrillation of recent onset?

(a) Dofetilide (b) Flecainide
(c) Ismolol (d) Ibutilide

834. Following is not true for dronedarone:

(a) It is used to maintain sinus rhythm after conversion from AF
(b) It has structural similarities with amiodarone
(c) It can be used in patients with LV dysfunction
(d) It does not contain iodine

835. Which one of the following is not true for left posterior hemiblock in ECG?

(a) North west axis deviation [usually (120 degree)]
(b) Small q in 2,3 and aVF
(c) Increased QRS voltage in limb leads
(d) No evidence of right ventricular hypertrophy

836. Which one of the following is not true Osborn waves in ECG?

(a) It is seen in hypothermia
(b) It is an elevated j waves
(c) It represents distortion of the earliest stage of repolarisation
(d) QT interval shortens

837. Which one of the following is not true for sino ventricular rhythm in ECG?

(a) It is seen in hyperkalemia
(b) Absent P wave
(c) It is common after heart transplant
(d) Conduction between SA node and AV node persists

838. Which one of the following are most common accessory pathways?

(a) Right lateral (b) Left lateral
(c) Left posteroseptal (d) Right anteroseptal

839. Atrial flutter – DC shock

(a) 25 J (b) 50 J
(c) 100 J (d) 200 J

840. Atrial fibrillation drives:

(a) LA appendage (b) Pulm vein
(c) Tricuspid valve

841. In AF, embolic risk increases with all *except*:

(a) OHR (b) HT
(c) DM (d) LA > 4 cm

842. Class A recommendation for ARDS:

(a) High PEEP (b) Low tidal volume
(c) Prove position (d) In LA filling pressure

843. Class I Indication of EPS study:

(a) Nocturnal asymptomatic type 1 and 2 heart block
(b) Differential between 2° and 3° AV block
(c) Recurrent SVT requiring drug with suspicion of proarrhythmia
(d) IVCD to know site of origin

844. Na^+ channel all *except*:

(a) Selective pirmobh (b) Elect-worth exchange
(c) Neurotoxin

845. Long QT all *except*:

(a) Decrease K^+ (b) Decrease Mg
(c) Digoxin (d) Quinidine

846. Conduction system all *except*:

(a) SA node – Spindle shaped, made of dense fibrous tissue
(b) In C – TGA, Bundle branch block
(c) SA node is most commonly supplied by LCA
(d) AV node and SA node have more ——— supply compared to vent. myocardium

847. SVT vs VT – Can be diff. by (M. imp. for VT):

(a) AV dissociation (b) QRS > 120 ms

848. SVT vs VT (can be diff.):

(a) Prior history of MI (b) Carotid sinus massage
(c) Fusion beat (d) Extreme LAD

849. Persistence of AV block even after carotid sinus massage by:

(a) AVRT (b) AVNRT
(c) AT (d) All

850. Long RP:

(a) SNRT with long PR (b) SNRT
(c) AT (d) AVNRT typical

851. AICD – Indication:

(a) Fascicular VP
(b) Idiopathic RV Tachycardia
(c) VT storm
(d) CPVT

852. Lewis leads:

(a) V6 @ V1
(b) Right leg placed @ V1
(c) V1 – suprasternal
(d) Limb leads over out chest

853. Which of the following has poor prognosis?

(a) VPC at high rates
(b) NSVT in elderly male
(c) Late heart rate recovery post exercise
(d) All of the above

854. Which of the following gene mutation is not seen in long QT syndrome?

(a) KCNQ1 (b) KCNH2
(c) SCN5A (d) RYR2

855. The bidirectional ventricular tachycardia is seen in:

(a) Brugada syndrome
(b) Chanelopathies ventricular tachycardia
(c) Long QT syndrome
(d) Short QT syndrome

856. Drug of choice in WPW Syndrome presenting with atrial fibrillation with fast ventricular rate is:

(a) Adenosine (b) Metoprolol
(c) Digoxin (d) Procainamide

857. Which of the following was a negative trial in primary prevention?

(a) MADIT (b) DEFINITE
(c) CABG PATCH (d) MUSTT

858. Percentage of patients that revert to sinus rhythm from atrial fibrillation after treatment of thyroid state alone is:

(a) 20% (b) 50%
(c) 70% (d) 90%

859. All can be used in atrial fibrillation *except*:

(a) Amiodarone (b) Dofetilide
(c) Ranolazine (d) Mexiletine

860. Bundle branch re-entry Tachycardia is a feature of:

(a) Myotonic dystrophy type 1
(b) Myotonic dystrophy type 2
(c) Emery-Dreifuss muscular dystrophy
(d) None of the above

861. QT-interval response to exercise in long QT syndrome-1 is:

(a) Normal QT during exercise but with exaggeration of QT-hysteresis
(b) Attenuated QTc shortening and an exaggerated QTc prolongation during early and peak exercise
(c) Supernormal QT-shortening
(d) No change in QT interval

862. A 55 years old patient with history of M1 (LVEF 35%) on optimal medical treatment for the last 6 months, now presented with exertional dyspnea NYHA class II. Patient's survival expectancy is good. True statement regarding the management of this patient is:

(a) Should receive subcutaneous ICD to reduce all cause mortality
(b) Should receive CRT to reduce SCD only (if LBBB > 150 ms with normal sinus rhythm)
(c) Should receive CRT-D to reduce SCD only (if LBBB > 120 ms with normal sinus rhythm)
(d) Should receive ICD to reduce SCD only

863. 50 years old male patient with ICD for secondary prevention of SCD in setting of old MI with moderate LV dysfunction presented to ED with 4 ICD shocks dispersed over last 24 hours without loss of consciousness. Immediate ICD interrogation revealed all ICD shocks were appropriate for fast VT and VF events only. Which statement is true?

(a) By definition, this is not electrical/VT storm
(b) By definition, this is electrical/VT storm and ICD is to be turned off to prevent further ICD shocks
(c) Reset ICD settings to increase number of ATP therapies and increase detection rate of VF zone
(d) Catheter mediated radiofrequency ablation on an urgent basis may be an ideal modality of management (after reversible cause of VT is ruled out)

864. Following are true about CARDIOVERSION/ Defibrillation shocks *except*:

(a) Monomorphic VT can often be terminated by low energy synchronised shock energy ≤ 5 J
(b) Weak shocks risk acceleration of VT to VF
(c) High energy ≥ 50 J shocks are generally used for VT termination
(d) Shock pain is directly proportional to shock strength

865. Short QT syndrome is characterised by all *except*:

(a) Increase risk for sudden death because of VF
(b) Persistently short QT intervals, short or absent ST segments and tall and narrow T waves in the precordial leads
(c) Hypokalemia, hypocalcemia or hypothermia can cause shortening of QT interval
(d) Quinidine has been shown to be effective in patients with a gain of function mutation in the HERG (KCNH2) gene

866. "Inverse saw-tooth" appearance on ECG is seen in which type of atrial flutter?

(a) Typical clockwise
(b) Typical counter clockwise
(c) Upper loop re-entry
(d) Septal atrial flutter

867. All are true about chaotic atrial tachycardia *except*:

(a) Atrial rates 100–130 beats per min
(b) At least 3 P waves contours are noted
(c) Commonly occur in older patients with COPD and CHF
(d) Digitalis is useful in treatment of this tachycardia

868. Which of the following statements is true?

(a) Maximum score of $CHADS_2$ is 10
(b) Score of 0 on $CHADS_2$ have stroke rate of 2% while CHA_2DS_2-VAS score of 0 indicate stroke rate of 0
(c) Dabigatran is preferred over warfarin invalvular AF
(d) None of the above

869. Conduction/Propagation velocity is slowest for:

(a) SA nodal cells (b) AV nodal cells
(c) Purkinje fibers (d) Atrial muscles

870. Recommended period to avoid driving flying after ICD implantation for secondary prevention is:

(a) 6 months (b) 3 months
(c) 2 months (d) Not required

871. All statements regarding Bachmann's bundle are true, *except*:

(a) Disruption of the bundle's structure causes interatrial conduction block
(b) Based on electron microscopy, there are 5 different types of myocardial cells in Bachmann's bundle
(c) The SA nodal artery invariably supplies Bachmann's bundle
(d) BB action potentials are characterized by a gradual upstroke followed by a prolonged plateau phase

872. Effect of digitalis on atrial myocyte:

(a) Effective refractory period is reduced due to direct effect
(b) Effective refractory period is reduced due to vagomimetic effect

(c) Effective refractory period is reduced due to vagolytic effect
(d) Effective refractory period is reduced due to sympathomimetic effect

873. Which of the following statements regarding the delayed after depolarizations (DADs) is not true?
(a) DADs are oscillations in membrane voltage that occur after completion of repolarization of the action potential (i.e., during phase 4)
(b) The most important influence that causes subthreshold DADs to reach threshold is a decrease in the initiating cycle length, because that increases both the amplitude and rate of the DADs
(c) Digitalis causes DAD-dependent triggered arrhythmias by inhibiting the Na^+/K^+ exchange pump
(d) Drugs that prolong action potential duration (e.g., class IA antiarrhythmic agents) can decrease DAD amplitude, whereas drugs that shorten action potential duration (e.g., class IB antiarrhythmic agents) can increase DADs amplitude

874. EF-50%, AF with FVR, patient started on metoprolol tartarate, patient achieved good rate control. Resident asked that dofetilide a newer and better drug, so why not use dofetilide:
(a) Beta blockers and dofetilide have comparable efficacy and outcome
(b) Dofetilide useful in EF <35%
(c) Dofetilide reserved in chronic renal insufficiency
(d) Dofetilide mortality same as compared to amiodarone

875. Reverse use dependence true:
(a) Has better prevention as compared to treatment and has better proarrhythmic effect at slower heart rate
(b) Has better prevention as compared to treatment and has lesser proarrhythmic effect at slower heart rate
(c) Has lesser prevention as compared to treatment and has better proarrhythmic effect at slower heart rate
(d) Has lesser prevention as compared to treatment and has lesser proarrhythmic effect at slower heart rate

876. AVNRT drug used all *except* to prevent recurrences:
(a) Flecainide (b) Propafenone
(c) Sotalol (d) Amiodarone

877. QRS axis at 60° isoelectric waves in which lead:
(a) II (b) III
(c) aVR (d) aVL

878. Sprouting of nerve growth factor leading to VT/VF seen in:
(a) Brugada (b) Long QT
(c) Short QT (d) Post MI scarring

879. CAST-I and CAST-II trial true:
(a) Propafenone, moricizine, flecainide used
(b) Effectively suppress VPC
(c) ↑ mortality in patient without heart disease
(d) ↓ mortality IC drugs

880. ECG low voltage complex, Echo and biopsy:
(a) Sarcoid
(b) Amyloid
(c) Endomyocardial fibrosis
(d) Rheumatic valvulitis

881. Athlete with sudden fall and arrest: (See Figure 1)
(a) Brugada (b) ARVD
(c) Wellens (d) Acute PE

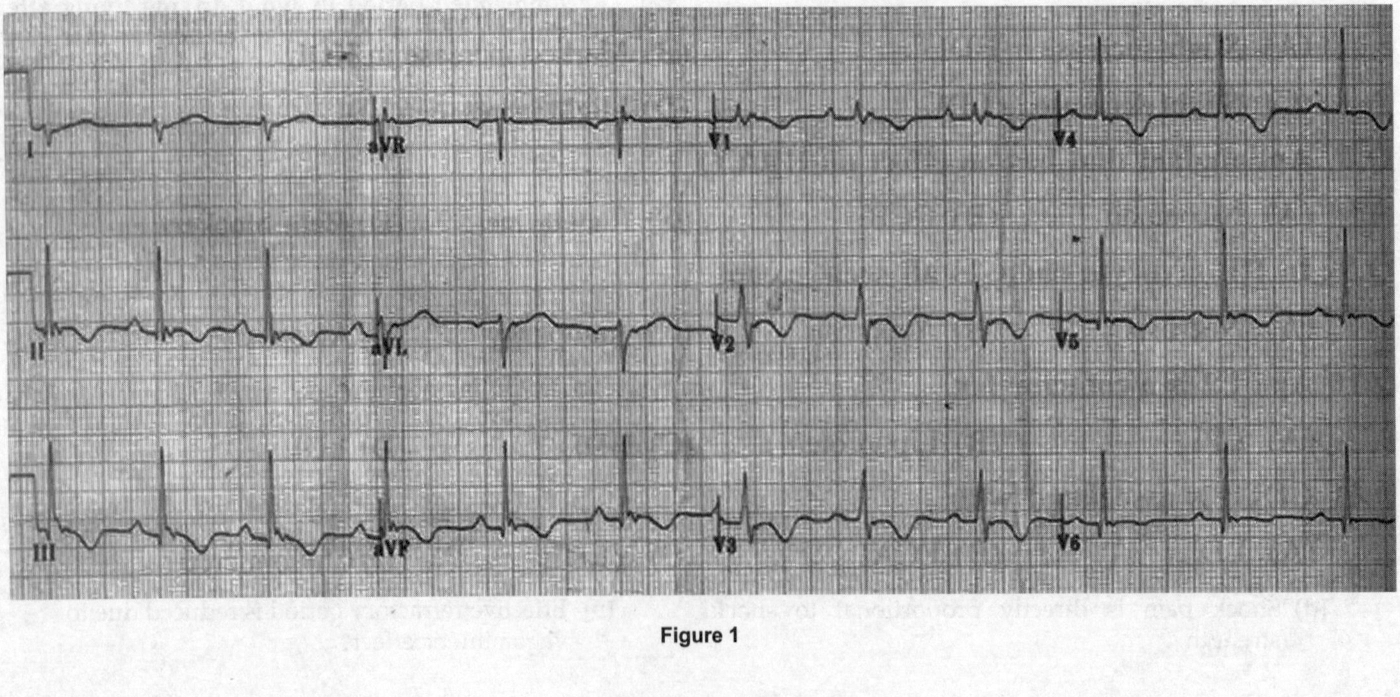

Figure 1

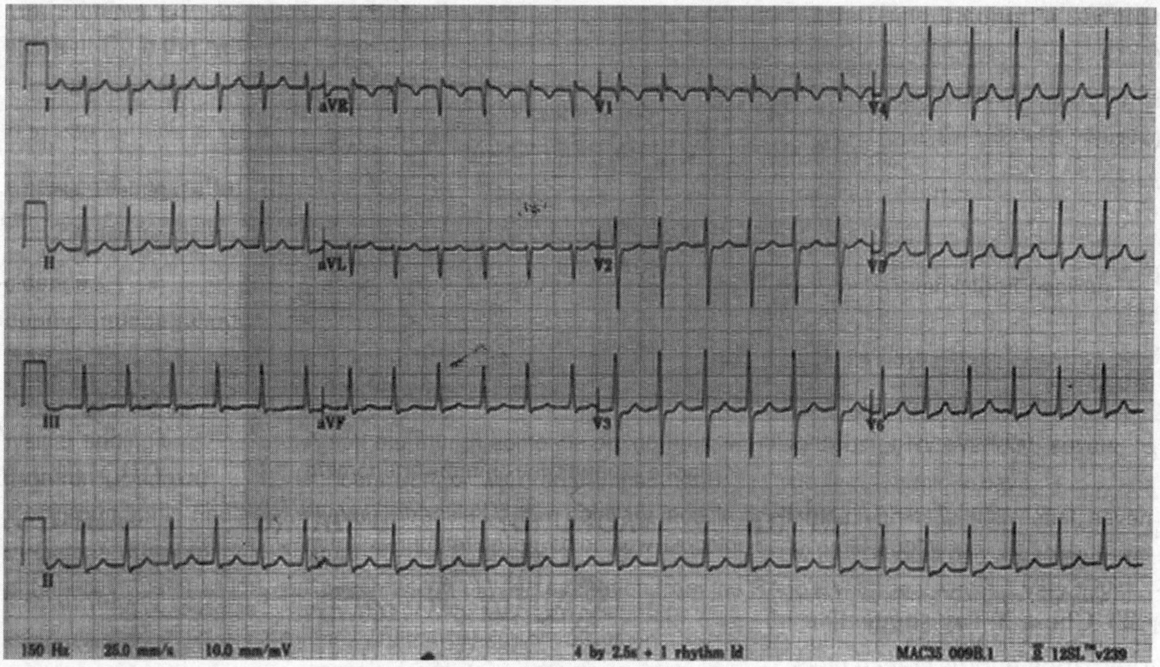

Figure 2

882. Young female with breathlessness and palpitations sudden onset: (See Figure 2)

(a) AVNRT (b) Antidromic AVRT
(c) VT (d) Sinus tachycardia

883. Atrial flutter mechanism is:

(a) Excitable gap reentry
(b) Leading circle reentry
(c) Triggered automaticity
(d) EAD

884. Causes of physiologic sinus tachycardia are A/E:

(a) Fever (b) Anemia
(c) Pheochromocytoma (d) Carcinoid

885. Inappropriate sinus tachycardia all are T/E:

(a) Sinus rate increases inappropriately out of proportion to Physiological stimulus
(b) Fatigue, dizziness may present
(c) Beta blockers/CCB is useful
(d) Ivabradine is not useful

886. POTS all true *except*:

(a) Sinus rate increases by 20 beats/min
(b) Within 10 min of standing symptoms appear
(c) Symptoms similar to inappropriate sinus tachycardia
(d) Midodrine is useful

887. ICD contraindicated in:

(a) VT with structurally normal heart
(b) VT with structurally abnormal heart
(c) LV dysfunction
(d) Incessant VT

888. WPW includes:

(a) Prolonged PR interval
(b) Short PR interval
(c) QS complex
(d) ST elevation

889. Treatment of preexcited tachycardia:

(a) Dilzem (b) Beta blockers
(c) Procainamide (d) Amiodarone

890. TDP caused by A/E:

(a) Propafenone (b) Amiodarone
(c) Disopyramide (d) Ibutalide

891. HR control in AF:

(a) 80 during rest and 110 during exertion
(b) 70,110
(c) 70,120
(d) 90,110

892. SVT first line Rx:

(a) Adenosine (b) DC shock
(c) Dilzem (d) Face in cold water

893. Epsilon waves are seen in:

(a) ARVD (b) CPVT
(c) Brugada (d) Long QT syndrome

894. SA node is the pacemaker because:

(a) Is the most rapidly discharging part
(b) Is the most richly supplied by nerve endings
(c) Located in the atrium
(d) All of the above

895. SA nodal location:

(a) Between SVC and RA
(b) Between IVC and RA
(c) Between coronary sinus and RA

896. Non-physiological tachycardia is associated with:

(a) Always underlying structural heart disease
(b) All cases need immediate intervention
(c) Most of them present with palpitations

897. Paroxysmal heart block:

(a) Intermittent III degree AV block
(b) Alternating bundle branch block
(c) II degree AV block
(d) I degree block

898. PPI is advised for:

(a) Asymptomatic I degree heart block
(b) Asymptomatic II, type I
(c) Degeneration of SA node with HR <40/min
(d) None

899. Drug for induction of brugada syndrome:

(a) Sotalol (b) Procainamide
(c) Adenosine (d) Amiodarone

900. Mutation in Brugada syndrome associated with poor prognosis is:

(a) CACNB2b gene (b) CN10A
(c) SCN5A (d) HEY2

901. Class Ic antiarrhythmic among the following:

(a) Sotalol (b) Procainamide
(c) Tocainide (d) Moricizine

902. A 50 years female with no risk factors diagnosed with AF on routine evaluation. Treatment is:

(a) Beta blockers
(b) Reassurance
(c) Oral anticoagulants
(d) Heparin + oral anticoagulants

903. AVNRT vs AVRT supporting AVNRT:

(a) Delta wave on baseline ECG
(b) Pseudo s in lead V1
(c) Short RP interval
(d) HR of 250/min

904. ECG in ARVD:

(a) The tachyarrhythmias occurring in ARVD are characteristically monomorphic and LBBB morphology, usually with inferior QRS axis
(b) The ECG in patients with ARVD/C usually shows sinus rhythm and a terminal deflection within or at the end of the QRS complex (called epsilon wave) in leads V5 and V6
(c) ST elevation in anterior leads
(d) The tachyarrhythmias occurring in ARVD are characteristically monomorphic and LBBB morphology, usually with superior QRS axis

905. ECG showing VT, next step is:

(a) Cardioversion
(b) Adenosine
(c) Amiodarone
(d) Check for hemodynamic stability

906. All are criteria for CRT *except*:

(a) LBBB
(b) QRS >150 ms
(c) RBBB
(d) Symptomatic on maximal Rx

907. Atrial flutter with negative P in II, III, aVF:

(a) Reverse typical (b) Typical
(c) Atypical (d) Clockwise

908. TdP is least with drug:

(a) Propafenone (b) Quinidine
(c) Disopyramide (d) Dofetalide

909. AF in India:

(a) Mostly still treated with aspirin
(b) Sub therapeutic INR common
(c) Mortality less due to young age
(d) RHD is most common cause
(e) Idiopathic is most common

910. Sotalol:

(a) Non selective BB
(b) Increase QT
(c) Decrease mortality
(d) Decrease defibrillation threshold
(e) Poor oral bioavailability

911. AF:

(a) More common in elderly

(b) Pulmonary vein ablation with vagal denervation is latest therapy
(c) <7 days persistent AF
(d) Rhythm control eliminates anticoagulation
(e) M > F

912. Pacemaker–true is:

(a) Position I–sensing
(b) II–pacing
(c) III–"I" means inhibits pacing after sensing activity
(d) III–"T" means activated by triggered pacing
(e) V–Multiple pacing

913. AICD–true is:

(a) AVID, CASH are secondary prevention trials
(b) MADIT is primary prevention trial
(c) No benefit of ICD in primary prevention
(d) DEFINITE is a secondary prevention trial
(e) MUSTT had EF more than 40%

914. Brugada–true is:

(a) Role of potassium channel
(b) Problem in depolarization
(c) Persistent ST-T change
(d) RBBB is incomplete
(e) Changes in anterior lead

915. Idiopathic VT–not true is:

(a) 10% of VT
(b) LVOT-VT is common
(c) RVOT-VT is LBBB with inferior axis with early transition
(d) Ablation is less useful
(e) Reentry is one of the mechanisms

916. LQTS–not true is:

(a) Beta blockers in all
(b) Mexiletine treatment in LQT3
(c) Procainamide treatment in LQT3
(d) Exercise precipitates VT in LQT 1
(e) Pacing is useful in LQT3

917. Treatment of TdP:

(a) IV Magnesium
(b) IV Amiodarone
(c) Procainamide
(d) Beta blocker
(e) Mexiletine

918. Leadless pacemaker–true is:

(a) Rule out embolus
(b) Not used in AF
(c) Comes with ICD
(d) Retrievable
(e) Most suitable for DDD

919. ARVC–true is:

(a) Epsilon wave is not specific
(b) LV involvement is seen
(c) SVT is common
(d) SCD is well known
(e) VT is not common

920. True are:

(a) RBBB with more than 150 ms QRS advised CRT–class I indication
(b) REVERSE, MADIT-CRT and RAFT are positive trials
(c) DANISH trial showed no benefit of ICD
(d) CRT helpful if EF less than 35%
(e) NYHA class II are benefited from CRT

921. Catheter ablation:

(a) In AF only refractory to medical management
(b) In AF class I AAD and rhythm control is desired
(c) First line of choice in idiopathic VT
(d) First line of choice in SVT
(e) Is helpful in atrial flutter

922. True in AF catheter ablation is:

(a) Ice and fire are used in trials
(b) Pulmonary vein isolation is done commonly
(c) Phrenic nerve inury common in cryoablation
(d) RF ablation has lower cost
(e) Cryoablation is easy to learn

923. SVT with aberrant conduction versus VT:

(a) R/S > 100 ms suggest VT
(b) Absence of RS in all precordial leads suggest VT
(c) Concordant negative suggest VT
(d) All negative QRS in II, III and aVF suggest VT
(e) All positive QRS in II, III, aVF suggest VT

924. Idiopathic fascicular left ventricular VT:

(a) 10-15% of all VT
(b) Anterior fascicle origin more common
(c) Digoxin doesn't precipitate LV VT
(d) Mechanism is macro reentry
(e) Most common of all LV VT

925. **Digoxin toxicity:**
(a) VPC is specific marker for digoxin toxicity
(b) Nonparoxysmal atrial tachycardia does not occur
(c) AV dissociation indicate toxicity
(d) Ventricular bigeminy with variable morphology
(e) Bradyarrhythmias due to vagal stimulation and tachyarrhythmias due to DAD

926. **Monogenic cardiac inheritance in which genetic analysis is done?**
(a) LQTS (b) MVP
(c) HOCM (d) Marfan
(e) RCM

927. **Atrial fibrillation:**
(a) ECG is required for documenting diagnosis
(b) Anticoagulation
(c) INR is measured weekly for 1 month then every 3 months
(d) No need for evaluation of renal function before starting NOAC
(e) Atrial flutter same anticoagulation

928. **Pacemaker:**
(a) VVI improves AV synchrony
(b) DDIR best in AF
(c) AAT/VVT increases battery depletion
(d) AAI in sick sinus with AV nodal dysfunction
(e) VVI not useful in chronotropic incompetence

929. **CPVT–all are T/E:**
(a) AR–CASQ2 (b) Bidirectional VT
(c) Stress induced VT (d) AR–RYR2

930. **Dengue with diffuse T wave inversion:**
(a) Myocarditis (b) MI
(c) DCM (d) Metabolic imbalance

931. **ECG suggests: (See Figure 3)**
(a) Sinus pauses (b) VT
(c) SVT (d) Atrial flutter

932. **ECG suggests: (See Figure 4)**
(a) MAT (b) SVT
(c) Wandering atrial pacemaker (d) APCs

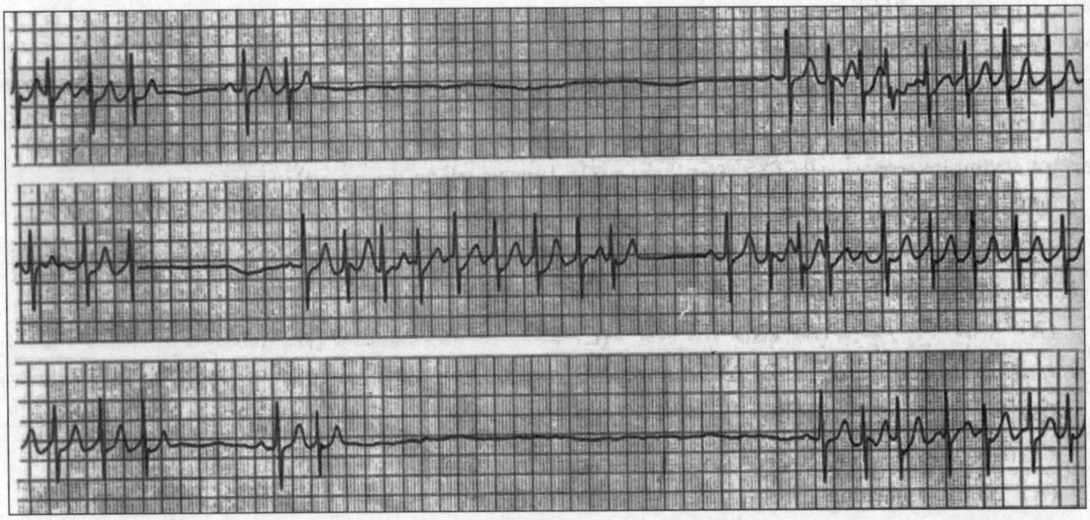

Figure 3

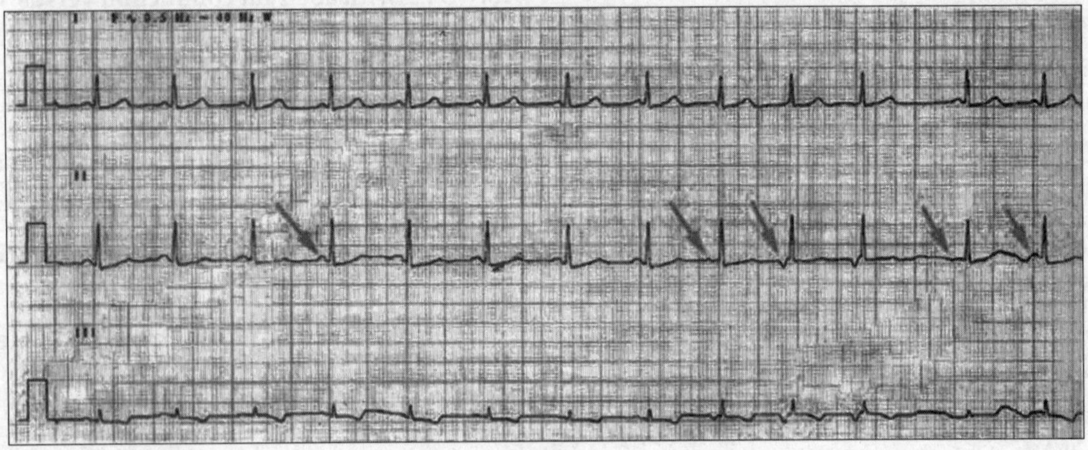

Figure 4

933. ECG suggestive of: (See Figure 5)
(a) MAT
(b) SVT
(c) Wandering atrial pacemaker
(d) APCs

934. ECG suggestive of: (See Figure 6)
(a) MAT
(b) SVT
(c) Wandering atrial pacemaker
(d) APCs

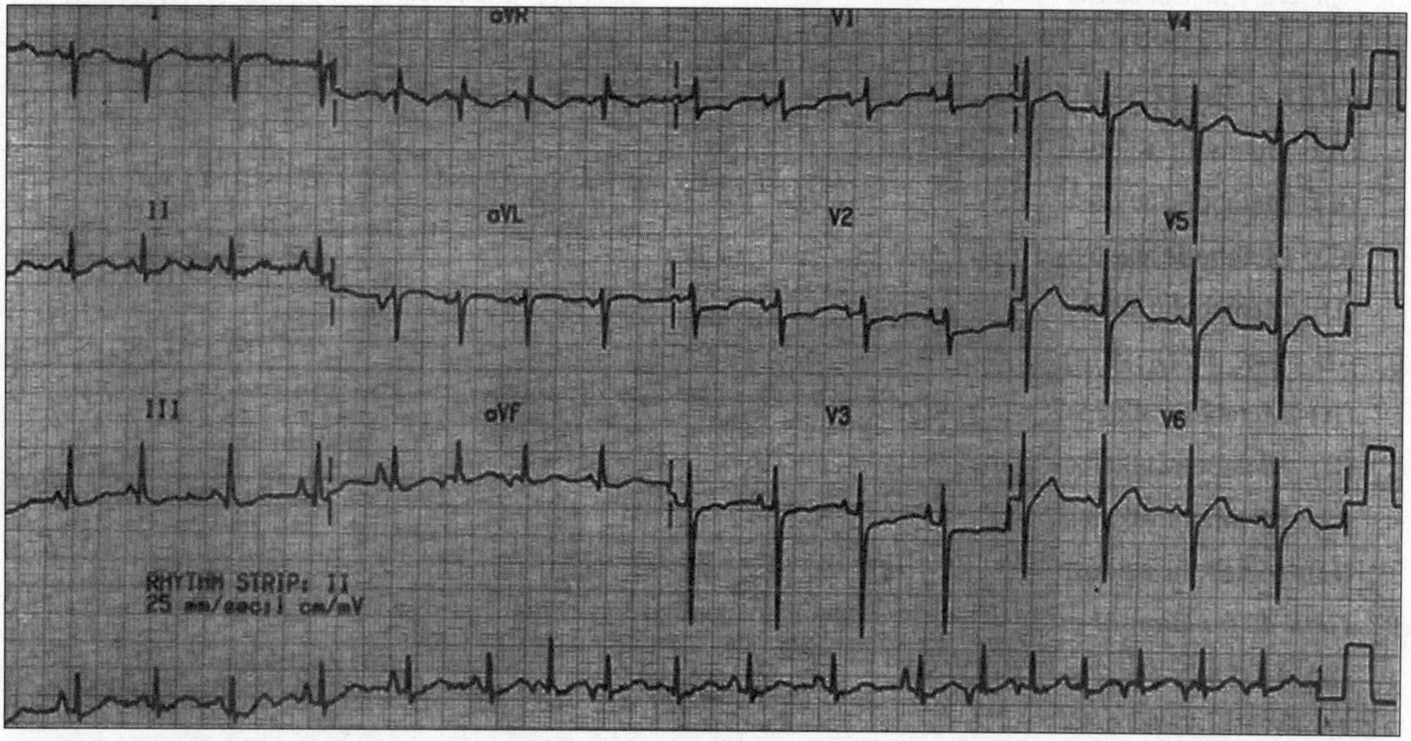

Figure 5

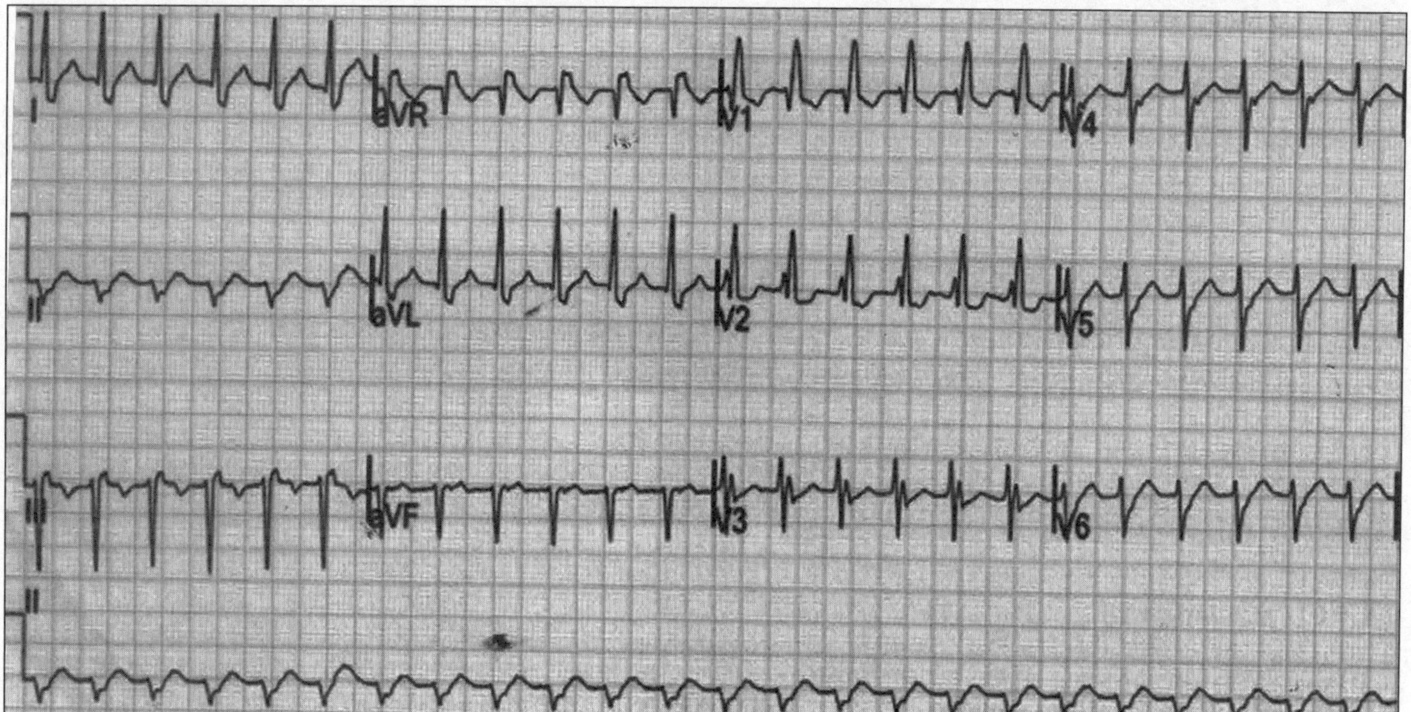

Figure 6

935. Gain of function of calcium channel is seen in:

(a) LQTS 2 (b) LQTS 4
(c) LQTS 6 (d) LQTS 8

936. Digoxin toxicity A/E:

(a) VT with exit block
(b) Monomorphic VPCs
(c) AF
(d) Bidirectional VT

937. Atriofascicular pathway is:

(a) Orthodromic
(b) Antidromic
(c) Both
(d) None

938. Electromechanical asystole all are T/E:

(a) Need continuous monitoring
(b) At least 2 ECGs should show asystole
(c) Carotid pacing
(d) DC shock

939. Normal AH interval is:

(a) 50-130 msec (b) 20-50
(c) 70-180 (d) 10-20

ANSWERS KEY

1.	(b)	2.	(c)	3.	(b, c)	4.	(a)	5.	(b)	6.	(c)	7.	(c)	8.	(a)
9.	(a)	10.	(a)	11.	(a)	12.	(a)	13.	(c)	14.	(b)	15.	(b)	16.	(d)
17.	(b)	18.	(c)	19.	(c)	20.	(c)	21.	(a)	22.	(a)	23.	(a)	24.	(d)
25.	(a)	26.	(b)	27.	(b)	28.	(b)	29.	(a)	30.	(c)	31.	(a)	32.	(a)
33.	(a)	34.	(b)	35.	T	36.	T	37.	F	38.	T	39.	(a)	40.	(d)
41.	(c)	42.	(a)	43.	(d)	44.	(b)	45.	(a)	46.	(d)	47.	(c)	48.	(c)
49.	(a)	50.	(b)	51.	(d)	52.	FTTTT	53.	TFTFT	54.	FTTTF	55.	TTFTT	56.	(c)
57.	(c)	58.	(b)	59.	(d)	60.	(b)	61.	(c)	62.	(d)	63.	(b)	64.	(d)
65.	(d)	66.	(a)	67.	(c)	68.	(b)	69.	(b,c,d)	70.	(d)	71.	(a)	72.	(c)
73.	(b)	74.	(c)	75.	(b)	76.	(c)	77.	(a)	78.	(a)	79.	(b)	80.	(c)
81.	(d)	82.	(d)	83.	(a)	84.	(a)	85.	(d)	86.	(d)	87.	(c)	88.	(a)
89.	(d)	90.	(b)	91.	(a)	92.	(c)	93.	(a)	94.	(d)	95.	(d)	96.	(b)
97.	(b)	98.	(d)	99.	(b)	100.	(c)	101.	(a)	102.	(a)	103.	(b)	104.	(c)
105.	(b)	106.	(a)	107.	(c)	108.	(a)	109.	(a)	110.	(c)	111.	(a)	112.	(a)
113.	(d)	114.	(c)	115.	(b)	116.	(b)	117.	(d)	118.	(c)	119.	(a)	120.	(b)
121.	(d)	122.	(d)	123.	(a)	124.	(c)	125.	(c)	126.	(c)	127.	(d)	128.	(a)
129.	(d)	130.	(a)	131.	(a)	132.	(d)	133.	(b)	134.	(a)	135.	(a)	136.	(b)
137.	(d)	138.	(d)	139.	(a)	140.	(a)	141.	(c)	142.	(b)	143.	(b)	144.	(b)
145.	(b)	146.	(b)	147.	(a)	148.	(a)	149.	(c)	150.	(c)	151.	(d)	152.	(b)
153.	(c)	154.	(d)	155.	(a)	156.	(b)	157.	(d)	158.	(a)	159.	(d)	160.	(d)
161.	(a)	162.	(d)	163.	(a)	164.	(a)	165.	(a)	166.	(a)	167.	(a)	168.	(a)
169.	(a)	170.	(a)	171.	(c)	172.	(d)	173.	(c)	174.	(d)	175.	(c)	176.	(b)
177.	(c)	178.	(a)	179.	(d)	180.	(b)	181.	(d)	182.	(c)	183.	(c)	184.	(a)
185.	(c)	186.	(a)	187.	(b)	188.	(a)	189.	(c)	190.	(a)	191.	(a)	192.	(d)
193.	(b)	194.	(d)	195.	(c)	196.	(b)	197.	(c)	198.	(b)	199.	(c)	200.	(a)
201.	(c)	202.	(a)	203.	(a)	204.	(a)	205.	(c)	206.	(c)	207.	(a)	208.	(a)
209.	(c)	210.	(a)	211.	(b)	212.	(b)	213.	(a)	214.	(a)	215.	(b)	216.	(a)
217.	(d)	218.	(c)	219.	(b)	220.	(c)	221.	(d)	222.	(a)	223.	(c)	224.	(b)
225.	(?)	226.	(a)	227.	(a,b,g,i,d)	228.	(b)	229.	(b)	230.	FT	231.	(d)	232.	(d)
233.	(a)	234.	(c)	235.	(e)	236.	(b)	237.	(b)	238.	(b)	239.	(c)	240.	(b)
241.	TTFTT	242.	(a)	243.	FTTTT	244.	(c)	245.	(e)	246.	(b)	247.	(a,b)	248.	TT
249.	(b)	250.	FTFFF	251.	(b)	252.	(a)	253.	FTTT	254.	FTTF	255.	TFTF	256.	FTTT
257.	(d)	258.	(a)	259.	(a)	260.	(b)	261.	(b,d)	262.	(a)	263.	(e)	264.	(b)
265.	(e)	266.	(a)	267.	(a)	268.	(c)	269.	(e)	270.	(a)	271.	(d)	272.	(b)
273.	(d)	274.	(c)	275.	(c)	276.	(a)	277.	(a)	278.	(c)	279.	(a)	280.	(d)
281.	(b)	282.	(a)	283.	(a)	284.	(c)	285.	(a)	286.	(d)	287.	(d)	288.	(c)
289.	(d)	290.	(b)	291.	(d)	292.	(c)	293.	(b)	294.	(d)	295.	(a)	296.	(b)
297.	(d)	298.	(b)	299.	(a)	300.	(b)	301.	(d)	302.	(c)	303.	(b)	304.	(b)
305.	(c)	306.	(d)	307.	(a)	308.	(a)	309.	(b)	310.	(c)	311.	(a)	312.	(b)
313.	(b)	314.	(a)	315.	(d)	316.	(a)	317.	(b)	318.	(c)	319.	(c)	320.	(b)
321.	(a)	322.	(c)	323.	(d)	324.	(d)	325.	(a)	326.	(d)	327.	(a)	328.	(c)
329.	(c)	330.	(c)	331.	(a)	332.	(c)	333.	(b)	334.	(b)	335.	(a)	336.	(b)
337.	(a)	338.	(a)	339.	(a)	340.	(e)	341.	(d)	342.	(c)	343.	(a)	344.	(b)
345.	(a)	346.	(a)	347.	(b)	348.	(d)	349.	(b)	350.	(c)	351.	(c)	352.	(c)

353. (a)	354. (b)	355. (a)	356. (c)	357. (b)	358. (d)	359. (d)	360. (a)
361. (c)	362. (b)	363. (d)	364. (c)	365. (d)	366. (c)	367. (d)	368. (d)
369. TTTTT	370. (c)	371. (a)	372. (b)	373. (a)	374. (a)	375. (b)	376. (a)
377. (b)	378. (a)	379. (a)	380. (b)	381. (d)	382. (b)	383. (b)	384. (b)
385. (a)	386. (c)	387. (a)	388. (a)	389. (b)	390. (b)	391. (d)	392. (d)
393. (d)	394. (b)	395. (?)	396. (c)	397. (d)	398. (a)	399. (a)	400. (a)
401. (b)	402. (a)	403. (d)	404. (a)	405. (b)	406. (a)	407. (c)	408. (c)
409. (d)	410. (b)	411. (c)	412. (b)	413. (c)	414. (a)	415. (a)	416. (a)
417. (a)	418. (b)	419. (c)	420. (b)	421. (b)	422. (b)	423. (a)	424. (d)
425. (c)	426. (a)	427. (d)	428. (a)	429. (a)	430. (d)	431. (a)	432. (a)
433. (a)	434. (c)	435. (c)	436. (a)	437. (d)	438. (b)	439. (b)	440. (a)
441. (a)	442. (a)	443. (d)	444. (c)	445. (a)	446. (d)	447. (b)	448. (b)
449. (a)	450. (c)	451. (b)	452. (d)	453. (a)	454. (b)	455. (a)	456. (d)
457. (a)	458. (a)	459. (b)	460. (b)	461. (b)	462. (a)	463. (a)	464. (a)
465. (d)	466. (a)	467. (a)	468. (d)	469. (a)	470. (c)	471. (a)	472. (b)
473. (a)	474. (a)	475. (a)	476. (a)	477. (a)	478. (a)	479. (a)	480. (c)
481. TFTFT	482. FFTTF	483. TTFTF	484. TTTTT	485. TFTFF	486. FFFFT	487. FFTFT	488. TFTFT
489. TTTFF	490. TTTFT	491. TFTFT	492. FFFFT	493. FTTTF	494. FTTFT	495. TFFTT	496. TTTTF
497. FTFFF	498. TFTTT	499. TTTFF	500. FFTFF	501. TFFFF	502. FTTTT	503. FTTFT	504. FTTFF
505. TTFT	506. TTTTT	507. TFTF	508. FTFTT	509. TTTFF	510. TTTTF	511. TFTFT	512. TFFFT
513. TTTT	514. FFTTF	515. TTTFT	516. FTTTT	517. FFTTT	518. FFFFT	519. TTTTT	520. FTTTT
521. FTF	522. TFFTF	523. TTFFF	524. FTFTT	525. FTTTF	526. TTFTF	527. TFFTF	528. FTFTF
529. FTFTF	530. FFTTF	531. FTTTF	532. FTTFF	533. TFTTF	534. TTTTT	535. FFFT	536. TFFTF
537. TFTTF	538. TFFT	539. FTTTF	540. FFTFF	541. TTTFF	542. TFFTF	543. FTTFF	544. TTTTF
545. (d)	546. FTTFF	547. TTTFF	548. TFFFF	549. TTFFT	550. FFTTF	551. FTTFF	552. TTFFT
553. FFFTF	554. FTFFT	555. FFTTF	556. FFTFT	557. TTFTT	558. FTTTF	559. TFFTT	560. FFTFT
561. FTFFF	562. TTFFF	563. FTFFF	564. TFFF	565. (d)	566. (d)	567. FFFFT	568. FTFFF
569. (a)	570. (a)	571. (a)	572. (c)	573. (b)	574. (c)	575. (a)	576. (b)
577. (d)	578. (a)	579. (a)	580. (a)	581. (a)	582. (a)	583. (a)	584. (a)
585. (a)	586. (a)	587. (a)	588. (b)	589. (a)	590. (b)	591. (b)	592. (b)
593. (d)	594. (d)	595. (c)	596. (d)	597. (a)	598. (b)	599. (d)	600. (a)
601. (c)	602. (d)	603. FFTTT	604. FTFF	605. FFFFT	606. FFFFT	607. FFT?T	608. FTTTF
609. FTFTT	610. FFF	611. TFTTT	612. TTTFF	613. FFTFT	614. TFFFF	615. TTTTF	616. TFTFF
617. TTFFF	618. TTTT	619. TFTTT	620. TT	621. FTTTT	622. FTTTT	623. FF	624. TFTTT
625. FTTFF	626. FTTTT	627. TFTF	628. TFTTF	629. TTTTF	630. FTTTT	631. TTFTF	632. FTTFT
633. TFFTT	634. TTTTF	635. TFFTF	636. TTTT	637. FTFTT	638. TTFTF	639. TT	640. FTFFF
641. TFTFT	642. FFTFF	643. FFT	644. TFTFT	645. FFFTT	646. FT	647. FFFFF	648. FTTFF
649. TTFFT	650. TFTTF	651. FTFTF	652. FTFTF	653. TFFFT	654. TTTTTF	655. FFFTT	656. FTFTF
657. TTTFF	658. FTTTT	659. TTFFF	660. TFTT	661. TFTTF	662. FTFTF	663. FFFTFF	664. TTTTT
665. TTFT	666. TFTTT	667. FTTFTT	668. FTTTF	669. TTFTT	670. TFFTF	671. TTFFF	672. FTFFF
673. TFFTT	674. TFTTT	675. TTTTT	676. TTTFF	677. FTTFT	678. FTT	679. TTTT	680. TFTFT
681. TFTFF	682. FFFTF	683. TTTTT	684. TFFTT	685. TTTFF	686. FTTTF	687. TFTTF	688. FFTTTT
689. FT	690. TTTFT	691. TFFFT	692. FTFTT	693. TFFFF	694. (a)	695. (a)	696. (a)
697. (b)	698. (a)	699. (d)	700. (c)	701. (a)	702. (a)	703. (c)	704. (b)
705. (a)	706. (b)	707. (a)	708. (c)	709. (a)	710. (a)	711. (a)	712. (b)
713. (b)	714. (a)	715. (c)	716. (a)	717. (a)	718. (a)	719. (c)	720. (d)
721. (d)	722. (a)	723. (b)	724. (a)	725. (a)	726. (a)	727. (a)	728. (a)
729. (a)	730. (c)	731. (a)	732. (b)	733. (a)	734. (a)	735. (c)	736. (a)
737. (b)	738. (b)	739. (b)	740. (d)	741. (d)	742. (a)	743. (b)	744. (b)

745. (d)	746. (c)	747. (d)	748. (d)	749. (d)	750. (d)	751. (c)	752. (b)
753. (b)	754. (b)	755. (a)	756. (a)	757. (a)	758. (b)	759. (d)	760. (c)
761. (c)	762. (c)	763. (e)	764. (d)	765. (b)	766. (b)	767. (b)	768. (a)
769. (d)	770. (d)	771. (a)	772. (b)	773. (b)	774. (b)	775. (a)	776. (b)
777. (a)	778. (a)	779. (c)	780. (a)	781. (c)	782. (b)	783. (a)	784. (c)
785. (c)	786. (a)	787. (a)	788. (a)	789. (b)	790. (c)	791. (d)	792. (d)
793. (a)	794. (d)	795. (c)	796. (c)	797. (a)	798. (b)	799. (c)	800. (a)
801. (d)	802. (b)	803. (d)	804. (c)	805. (b)	806. (c)	807. (a)	808. (a)
809. (b)	810. (c)	811. (a)	812. (b)	813. (d)	814. (b)	815. (a)	816. (d)
817. (a)	818. (d)	819. (a)	820. (b)	821. (a)	822. (a)	823. (a)	824. (b)
825. (a)	826. (d)	827. (a)	828. (c)	829. (d)	830. (a)	831. (b)	832. (a)
833. (c)	834. (c)	835. (a)	836. (d)	837. (c)	838. (b)	839. (a)	840. (b)
841. (a)	842. (d)	843. (c)	844. (a)	845. (d)	846. (c)	847. (a)	848. (c)
849. (d)	850. (b)	851. (c)	852. (d)	853. (c)	854. (d)	855. (b)	856. (d)
857. (c)	858. (a)	859. (d)	860. (a)	861. (b)	862. (d)	863. (d)	864. (d)
865. (c)	866. (a)	867. (d)	868. (b)	869. (a)	870. (a)	871. (d)	872. (b)
873. (d)	874. (a)	875. (c)	876. (a)	877. (a)	878. (d)	879. (c)	880. (b)
881. (b)	882. (a)	883. (a)	884. (d)	885. (d)	886. (a)	887. (d)	888. (b)
889. (c)	890. (a)	891. (a)	892. (d)	893. (a)	894. (a)	895. (a)	896. (c)
897. (a)	898. (c)	899. (b)	900. (c)	901. (d)	902. (b)	903. (c)	904. (d)
905. (d)	906. (c)	907. (b)	908. (a)	909. (a,b,c,d)	910. (a,b,d)	911. (a,b)	912. (c,d,e)
913. (a,b)	914. (e)	915. (a,e)	916. (c)	917. (a,d,e)	918. (a,d)	919. (a,b,d)	920. (b,c,d,e)
921. (b,c,d,e)	922. (b,c,d,e)	923. (a,b)	924. (a,d,e)	925. (c,d,e)	926. (a,c,d,e)	927. (a,b,e)	928. (b,c,e)
929. (d)	930. (d)	931. (a)	932. (c)	933. (a)	934. (b)	935. (d)	936. (c)
937. (b)	938. (b)	939. (a)					

CHAPTER FIVE

VASCULAR DISEASES

1. **Submassive PE, not ture:**
   (a) Involve > 1/3 lung field
   (b) BNP (N)
   (c) Thrombolysis in low bleeding risk
   (d) (N) LV function

2. **Type B dissection with uterine rupture:**
   (a) EDS (b) Marfan
   (c) LDS (d) Turner

3. **Renal artery stenosis:**
   (a) NF (b) Williams
   (c) Turner

4. **Elderly with CrCl < 25 ml/min, pulmonary embolism with breathlessness, treatment of choice:**
   (a) I.V. LMWH (b) I.V. UFH
   (c) Fondaparinux (d) Oral apixaban

5. **Aorta–tensile strength is determined by:**
   (a) Adventitial collagen (b) Medial collagen
   (c) Elastin (d) SMCs

6. **Neurogenic syncope – all *except:***
   (a) Syncope following exercise–cardiac cause
   (b) NTG–useful in provocative testing
   (c) Use of provocative tests decrease specificity
   (d) No change in vital signs–psychogenic syncope

7. **Massive PTE–all *except:***
   (a) Hemoptysis (b) Cyanosis
   (c) Rv hypokinesis (d) Syncope

8. **All are true about PTE *except:***
   (a) Mc Connell sign is highly specific
   (b) Normal troponin T rules out PTE
   (c) D-dimer-varying specificity with age
   (d) RA dilated

9. **CT angiography–showing pulmonary thromboembolism. What is not seen in the patient?**
   (a) Right arm BP >> left arm
   (b) Cardiogenic shock
   (c) Pulsus paradoxus
   (d) Irregular rhythm

10. **A-a gradient ↑ all *except:***
   (a) V-P mismatch (b) Shunt
   (c) Sedative overdose (d) Pulmonary edema

11. **Bad prognosis in pulmonary embolism A/E:**
   (a) Ventricular strain (b) Syncope
   (c) Right pulm infarct (d) Cyanosis

12. **Carotid baroreceptor activation is used in:**
   (a) HTN
   (b) NO use in cardio
   (c) AF paroxysmal
   (d) Neurocardiogenic shock

13. **Sign of severe PE–indication on echo:**
   (a) Global RV hypokinesia
   (b) RV hypokinesia with apical sparing
   (c) RV dysfunction with severe TR
   (d) Diastolic dysfunction

14. **Takayasu arteritis diagnosis A/E:**
   (a) Age > 40 (b) Carotidynia
   (c) Art. bruit (d) Pulse difference

15. **Renal artery stenosis may occur in all of the following *except:***
   (a) Atherosclerosis
   (b) Fibromuscular dysplasia
   (c) Takayasu's arteritis
   (d) Polyarteritis nodosa

16. **Ideal emergency imaging modality for unstable patient with proximal aortic dissection is:**
(a) Retrograde aortography
(b) MRI
(c) Transesophageal echocardiography
(d) Intravascular ultrasound/transthoracic echocardiography

Takayasu Arteritis (T/F) (17-20)

17. **Macaroni sign on MRI**

18. **Type IV most common in India**

19. **Coronary artery involvement absent**

20. **MR–Most common valve abnormality**

21. **Embolic protection devices for CAS A/E:**
(a) Watchman (b) Percusurge
(c) Angioguard (d) Accunet

22. **Fontain classification < 100 m:**
(a) I (b) IIa
(c) IIb (d) III

23. **Angioplasty (PTRA) non ostial disease:**
(a) FMD–good prognosis
(b) Atherosclerotic–useful
(c) Takayasu arteries–excellent results

24. **Sildenafil:**
(a) PPH (b) BPH
(c) HTN

25. **Fontaine classification of peripheral artery disease class 2b indicates:**
(a) Pain free, claudication walking more than 200 m
(b) Pain free, claudication walking less than 200 m
(c) Pain free, claudication walking more than 400 m
(d) Pain free, claudication walking less than 200 m

26. **All are features of submassive pulmonary embolism *except:***
(a) Pro BNP is elevated
(b) Clot is present bilaterally, sometimes as "saddle" embolus occupying at least half of pulmonary arterial vasculature
(c) Severe RV hypokinesia
(d) Normal systemic arterial pressure

27. **All are causes of Group I pulmonary arterial hypertension *except:***
(a) Scleroderma
(b) Portal hypertension
(c) Schistosomiasis
(d) Chronic thromboembolic pH

28. **"Painless aortic dissection is common in:**
(a) Previous aortic aneurysm
(b) Hypertension
(c) Bicuspid aortic valve
(d) Marfan's syndrome

29. **PVR: (T/F)**
(a) ↓ with nitrous inhalation
(b) ↑ with isoprenaline
(c) Chronic hypoxia–PVR
(d) PVR–1/6 of SVR
(e) Measured with flow regulated balloon catheter tip thermister

30. **Pulmonary thromboembolism: (T/F)**
(a) Majority of patients have normal echo finding
(b) D-dimer–>95% sensitivity
(c) CT chest with contrast–for stratification and diagnosis
(d) Pleuritic chest pain S/O–massive PE
(e) Post OP pulmonary embolism–6 months anticoagulation sufficient

31. **FDP–interfere with: (T/F)**
(a) S. Ca level
(b) Thrombin
(c) Intrinsic pathway
(d) Formation of fibrin cross linking

32. **SVC syndrome: (T/F)**
(a) Most common features–dry cough and arm swelling
(b) Most common neoplasm causing SVC–lymphoma
(c) 2/3rd of cases have malignant etiology
(d) Hodgkin lymphoma–though mediastinal involvement is common–SVC syndrome is rare
(e) The clinical picture is milder if the obstruction is located above the azygos vein

33. **Ross procedure is used for:**
(a) Diseased aortic valve

(b) Diseased mitral valve
(c) Diseased tricuspid valve
(d) Diseased pulmonary valve

34. Surgery is indicated in ascending aortic aneurysm if diameter of ascending aorta or aortic sinus is:

(a) 4.5 cm (b) 5.5 cm
(c) 6.5 cm (d) 7.5 cm

35. In a patient with Marfan's syndrome pregnancy is contraindicated if diameter of ascending aorta is greater than:

(a) 4 cm (b) 5 cm
(c) 6 cm (d) 3 cm

36. Which one of the following statements is not true for inferior vena cava filters?

(a) It is used in patients in whom anticoagulants are contraindicated
(b) It is used in patients with recurrent pulmonary embolism despite therapeutic levels of anticoagulation
(c) It is used in patients with massive pulmonary embolism with very poor cardiopulmonary reserve
(d) Anticoagulants are must

37. Which drug is approved by FDA for thrombolysis in massive pulmonary embolism?

(a) Streptokinase (b) Alteplase
(c) Urokinase (d) Tenectaplase

38. Bosentan belongs to one of the following groups:

(a) Endothelin receptor antagonist
(b) Phosphodiesterase inhibitors
(c) Soluble guanylate cyclase stimulators
(d) Prostanoids

39. Acute limb ischemia (ALI) is defined as a sudden decrease in limb perfusion that could threaten limb viability. In this context, state which is false?

(a) ALI may be the first manifestation of arterial disease in a previously asymptomatic patient
(b) Patients with ALI may initially present with five symptoms known as the "5 Ps": pain, pulselessness, pallor, paralysis and paraesthesia
(c) Category I of the severity of ALI refers to irreversible damage and may benefit from revascularization
(d) Myoglobinuria may occur in up to 20% of patients following revascularization and elevated urine myoglobin levels may be predictive of acute renal failure

40. Aortic dissection is an uncommon but potentially catastrophic illness. Which of the following statements is false?

(a) Stanford Type A dissections are all dissections not involving the ascending aorta
(b) In a small minority of patients with ascending aortic dissection, the proximal dissection flap may involve ostium of right coronary artery more commonly than left coronary artery
(c) Antihypertensive choice in cases of aortic dissection should include combination of both vasodilator and beta blocker
(d) In cases of aortic dissection associated with cardiac tamponade, pericardiocentesis may sometimes in fact deteriorate the hemodynamics

41. Pulmonary embolism (PE) and deep venous thrombosis (DVT) are collectively termed under VTE (venous thromboembolism). Which of the following statements is false?

(a) McConell sign is echocardiographic evidence of right ventricular hypokinesia (free wall) in cases of PE
(b) Hampton's hump is a peripheral wedge shaped opacity above the diaphragm seen in cases of PE
(c) Classic Well's criteria is used to assess clinical likelihood of death in pulmonary embolism
(d) Alteplase has been approved for massive PE in a dose of 100 mg in continuous infusion during 2 hours without concomitant heparin

42. Carotid artery stenting is not recommended in patients with the following features *except:*

(a) Heavily calcified aortic arch or protruding atheroma
(b) Internal carotid artery lumen diameter < 3 mm
(c) Post-radiation or post-surgical stenosis
(d) Contraindication to DAPT

43. Clinical situations where the diagnosis of renal artery stenosis should be considered include all *except:*

(a) Onset of hypertension before the age of 30 years
(b) Onset of hypertension after 55 years
(c) Malignant hypertension (hypertension with coexistent end-organ damage, i.e., acute renal failure, flash pulmonary edema)
(d) White coat hypertension

44. **Sitaxentan used in primary pulmonary hypertension is a:**
(a) Prostanoid
(b) Phosphodiesterase type 5 inhibitor
(c) Endothelin receptor antagonist
(d) Calcium channel blocker

45. **Branham's sign is seen in:**
(a) Pulmonary AV fistula
(b) Systemic AV fistula
(c) Pulmonary embolism
(d) Cardiac tamponade

46. **Subclavian artery stenosis A/E:**
(a) TAO (b) Takayasu arteritis
(c) Atherosclerosis (d) GCA

47. **Cause Type III aortic dissection:**
(a) Marfan (b) GCA
(c) Takayasu (d) HTN

48. **Most common risk factor for PVD:**
(a) HTN (b) Smoking
(c) ↑ CRP (d) Atherosclerosis

49. **Pulmonary embolism bad prognosis A/E:**
(a) RV dysfunction (b) ↑ troPT
(c) ↑ BNP (d) ↑ Transaminase

50. **IOC–noninvasive in suspected pulmonary embolism:**
(a) D-dimer (b) Multislice CT angio
(c) MRI (d) Catheter angiography

51. **For aortic stiffness, all statements are true, *except:***
(a) Pulse-wave velocity is the most validated method to noninvasively quantify
(b) Predictor of future changes in systolic blood pressure and future development of hypertension in healthy volunteers
(c) MRI enables detection of more subtle changes in regional stiffness
(d) An increase of aortic pulse wave velocity of 10 m/s raises CV risk by more than 10%

52. **Aortic dissection most common coronary affected:**
(a) RCA (b) LAD
(c) LCX

53. **Stenting not showing promising result in:**
(a) Carotid (b) Renal
(c) Subclavian (d) Iliac

54. **Strongest vasoconstrictor of coronary arteries:**
(a) Acetylcholine (b) Bradykinin
(c) Adenosine (d) Endothelin

55. **Sotalol not contraindicated in:**
(a) Amiodarone (b) Flecainide
(c) Dofetilide (d) Quinidine

56. **True regarding PTE A/E:**
(a) V/Q scan investigation of choice in parents having renal dysfunction
(b) Dyspnoea with normal C X R suggestive of PTE
(c) D-dimer useful screening test for ill hospitalises person
(d) Pulmonary ejection acceleration velocity > 60 indicate severe PTE

57. **Patient of PAD, having ABI - 1 undergone TMT, after TMT, At what value of ABI, PAD is diagnosed:**
(a) 0.9 (b) 1.0
(b) 0.6 (d) 0.7

58. **AAA expansion presented by all *except:***
(a) BB (b) Cholchicine
(c) Doxycydine (d) Losartan

59. **Thromboangitis obliternans (TAO) all *except:***
(a) Anti-endothelial antibodies in majority
(b) Superficial thrombophlebitis- early presentation
(c) Involvement of internal elastic lamina in thrombus formation
(d) Toe and finger gangrene most common presentation

60. **TAO all *except:***
(a) Anti endothelial cell abnormality
(b) Superficial thrombophlebitis can be an early sign
(c) Can involve all layers with necrosis
(d) Most common present as toe/digit gangrene

61. **Massive PTE all *except:***
(a) Pleuritic chest pain (b) RV dysfunction
(c) Cyanosis (d) Hypotension

62. **Hemorrhagic stroke risk factors all *except:***
(a) Hyperlipidemia (b) Cigarette smoking
(c) Alcohol (d) Hypertension

63. **Transcranial Doppler useful in:**
(a) PFO
(b) PDA

(c) Pulmonary thromboembolism
(d) VSD

64. 55 years old hypertensive presents with sudden onset of severe chest pain, right arm BP=180/90, left arm BP= 100/80 mmHg, ECG–ST elevation in inferior leads, next investigation of choice:
(a) CT angiography
(b) Cardiac cath
(c) MR angiography
(d) Upper limb USG colour Doppler

65. Massive PTE all *except:*
(a) Syncope (b) Hemoptysis
(c) RV strain (d) Cyanosis

66. AS all/*except:*
(a) MR (b) AR
(c) Sick sinus (d) CHB

67. Acute most common cause of aortic rupture seen:
(a) Marfan (b) LD syndrome
(c) Familial A. dissection (d) EDS-IV

68. Risk factor for abdominal aortic dil *except:*
(a) DM (b) Smoking
(c) HTN (d) Dyslipidemia

69. Drug used to prevent aortic root dilatation:
(a) Amlodipine (b) Losartan
(c) Eplerenone (d) Tadafil

70. Athero embolism true *except:*
(a) Eosinophiluria (b) Thrombocytosis
(c) Livedo reticularis (d) Hollenhorst plaque

71. Carotid artery stenosis all *except:*
(a) Symptomatic > 50% stenosis on angiography with < 60% mortality, CEA indicated
(b) In asymptomatic CAS better than CEA
(c) USG duplex IOC
(d) Aspirin + clopidogrel not indicated in 1st 3 months of stroke/TIA

72. Ankle 60 mm Hg, brachial 120 mm Hg all *except:*
(a) Intermittent claudication
(b) Critical limb ischemia
(c) ↓ ABI an exercise
(d) ↑ CV risk

73. May Thurner syndrome:
(a) Iliac vein compression between iliac artery and body of vertebra
(b) Uterine artery compression
(c) Femoral artery compression

74. Infrapopliteal PVD Indication to operate:
(a) Rest pain and claudication
(b) Diffuse nature of disease
(c) Active smoker

75. Claudication on walking 100 m on ground:
(a) I (b) IIa
(c) IIb (d) III

76. Carotid sinus hypersensitivity:
(a) Sinus pause > 3 sec or SBP decrease of 50 mm Hg
(b) Sinus pause > 3 sec and SBP decrease of 50 mm Hg
(c) Sinus pause > 5 sec and SBP decrease of 30 mm Hg
(d) Sinus pause > 5 sec or SBP decrease of 30 mm Hg

77. Pain in interscapular area and coldness in right hand:
(a) Type I A dissection (b) Type 2 dissection
(c) Takayasu arteritis

78. About atheroembolism all are true *except*:
(a) Catheter induced
(b) Livedo reticularis
(c) Retinal artery shows Cholestrol Crystal
(d) All

79. S1Q3T3 is seen in how many cases of pulmonary embolism?
(a) 10% (b) 30%
(c) 50% (d) 90%

80. Pulmonary opacification in aortic angiography not seen in:
(a) RSOV to RA (b) RSOV to RV
(c) RSOV to LA (d) RSOV to PA

81. In aortoarteritis coronary artery involvement seen in:
(a) 10% (b) 20%
(c) 5%

82. Coronary sinus true is:
(a) Tributary to great cardiac vein

(b) Runs in posterior AV groove
(c) 9 cm long
(d) All

83. Most common sign of pulmonary embolism:
(a) Tachycardia (b) Tachypnea

84. Mechanisms of PAH:
(a) Increased plasma oncotic pressure
(b) Increased pulmonary venous pressure

85. Treatment of aortic dissection A/E:
(a) Na nitroprusside
(b) Beta blocker
(c) Surgery for distal dissection
(d) Surgery for proximal dissection

86. RAS all *except:*
(a) > 65 years 7% incidence
(b) Resistance index ↑ worst outcome
(c) FFR is useful
(d) Captopril not good for screening

87. Aortic dissection: (T/F)
(a) Pain radiating to back in between scapula
(b) Asymmetrical pulse
(c) Most common in female
(d) 3-4th decade
(e) AR

88. Aortic aneurysm most common site:
(a) Infrarenal aorta (b) Aortic arch
(c) Descending aorta (d) Supra renal aorta
(e) Ascending aorta

89. Aortic dissection: (T/F)
(a) Associated with AR
(b) Pain radiates to back
(c) Most common in 3rd to 4th decade
(d) Females > Males
(e) Assymetrical pulses

90. Indication for tibioperoneal revascularisation all *except:*
(a) Diabetes
(b) Rest pain and ischemia
(c) Low profile stents with success available
(d) Distal runoff absent

91. CAS vs CEA: (T/F)
(a) CEA is choice but approach multidisciplinary
(b) CEA indicated for 50% stenosis with previous stroke/TIA
(c) CEA ↑ preoperative MI while CAS ↑ perioperative stroke
(d) Significant stenosis means > 50% in male, > 70% is female

92. Takayasu arteritis:
(a) Type IV more in females than males
(b) Mid SCA stenosis is major criteria
(c) Stenosis, aneurysm mix lesion
(d) Panarteritis all layers including intima

93. RAS:
(a) Stent better in FMD
(b) Surgery better in FMI
(c) Stent good result in atherosclerosis

94. Aortic dissection: (T/F)
(a) Type A medical management
(b) Type B surgical management
(c) Instead trial type B medical alone vs medical + stenting – same mortality
(d) Endovascular stenting reduces thrombosis
(e) Endovascular stenting indication in type B with branch occlusion, symptomatic

95. Chronic pulmonary thromboembolism:
(a) Non contrast CT show mosaic pattern
(b) Angiography not useful
(c) 80% APLAS
(d) RA pressure is less than primary PHT with same degree of HT
(e) It is non progressive

96. Most common cause of DVT:
(a) Protein C deficiency
(b) Protein S deficiency
(c) Protein C activated resistance
(d) AT 3 deficiency

97. X-ray sign of pulmonary embolism most common:
(a) Oligemia
(b) Elevation of hemidiaphragm

(c) Peripheral wedge shaped opacity
(d) Atelectasis

98. Drug induced PE:
(a) Dandrolene (b) Methylsergide
(c) Cyclophosphamide (d) Proctitis

99. Eosinophilic PE:
(a) Parasitic (b) Drug induced
(c) Pancreatitis (d) Trauma

100. Abdominal aortic aneurysm true:
(a) >95% occur in infrarenal aorta
(b) M:F ↑ 9:1
(c) Definition > 1.5 enlargement of diameter
(d) If diameter >7 cm chance of rupture 20%/years
(e) All of the above

101. Critical limb ischemia:
(a) Ankle BP < 50 (b) Gangrene present
(c) Resting pain (d) Duration < 2 weeks

102. Normal RV apex with free wall hypokinesia in PTE is known as:
(a) Hampton's sign (b) Mc Connell's sign
(c) Palla's sign (d) Westermark's sign

103. Aortic arch aneurysm, true is:
(a) Infrarenal aneurysm is 95% of all abdominal aneurysm
(b) Defined as more than 1.5 times diameter of corresponding segment of normal aorta
(c) Male : Female ratio 1:1
(d) All of the above

104. All of the following conditions are at higher risk for aortic dissection:
(a) Loeys-Dietz syndrome
(b) Bicuspid aortic value
(c) Turner syndrome
(d) Syphilitic aortitis

105. Type III in deBakey classification of aortic dissection tachycardia:
(a) Ascending aorta alone
(b) Descending aorta alone
(c) Both ascending and descending aorta
(d) None of the above

106. Ideal emergency imaging modality for unstable patients with proximal aortic dissection:
(a) Retrograde aortography
(b) TEE
(c) MRI
(d) TIE

107. Pulmonary embolism, diagnostic test is:
(a) Elevated FDP (b) Elevated D-dimer
(c) Oxygen saturation (d) CT angiography

108. Pulmonary embolism A/E:
(a) Westermark's sign (b) Pleural rub
(c) Hampton's hump (d) Rose's sign

109. Signs of pulmonary embolism A/E:
(a) Westermark sign (b) Hampton's hump
(c) Rose's sign (d) Pleural friction rub

110. Risk of rupture of aortic aneurysm of 6.5 cm in 55 years old male over 1 year:
(a) 6.5% (b) 0.3%
(c) 10% (d) 0.5%

111. PAD:
(a) Cilostazol in CHF increases arrhythmias
(b) Stenting disappointing results in infrapopliteal involvement
(c) Percutaneous treatment better for femoral
(d) All of the above

112. Carotid endarterectomy versus carotid stenting in A/E:
(a) Tortous arch of aorta
(b) Visible thrombus
(c) Calcification
(d) Contralateral carotid artery occlusion

113. Which is more common in distal third of Aortic dissection?
(a) HTN
(b) Aortic medial degeneration
(c) Marfan
(d) Bicuspid aortic valve

114. Aortic dissection + Pericardiac tamponade + shock, next to be done:
(a) Immediate shift to OT

(b) Pericardiocentesis
(c) Conservative as pericardiocentesis cause ↓ BP

115. Most common cause of ascending aorta aneurysm:
(a) Syphilis (b) Atherosclerosis
(c) Medial necrosis (d) Hypotension

116. Massive PTE, not done:
(a) IVC filter
(b) Thrombolysis
(c) Thrombolysis + IVC filter
(d) UFH

117. Surgery for dissection all *except:*
(a) Proximal (b) AR
(c) Isolated arch (d) Marfan's

118. Takayasu arteritis related with all *except:*
(a) Rheumatoid arthritis (b) UC
(c) PPH (d) Rheumatic fever

119. Asymptomatic carotid artery stenosis stroke rate:
(a) 2%/year (b) 7%/year
(c) 5%/year (d) 13%/year

120. Best Ix for diagnosis in PE (most definitive):
(a) D-dimer
(b) Pulmonary arteriography
(c) Perfusion scintigraphy
(d) Venogram

121. Retinal artery pulsations:
(a) Becker sign (b) Demusset's sign
(c) Duroziez's sign (d) Traube's sign

122. Takayasu arteritis most common major complication:
(a) HF (b) Stroke
(c) Aortic dissection (d) Aortic rupture

123. Beaded renal artery:
(a) COA (b) HTN
(c) Hypercholesterolemia

124. Thoracic aortic aneurysm cause:
(a) CMD (b) HTN
(c) Atherosclerosis

125. The most accurate diagnostic imaging test for pulmonary embolism is:
(a) Lung scanning
(b) Chest CT
(c) Pulmonary angiography
(d) Magnetic Resonance Imaging

126. Not a risk factor for aortic dissection:
(a) Diabetes mellitus (b) Pregnancy
(c) Coarctation of aorta (d) Bicuspid aortic valve

127. Most common splanchnic artery aneurysm:
(a) Hepatic artery
(b) Splenic artery
(c) Superior mesenteric artery
(d) Inferior mesenteric artery

128. Most common site of peripheral arterial aneurysm from the following:
(a) Iliac arteries (b) Femoral arteries
(c) Popliteal arteries (d) Posterior tibial arteries

129. Risk factors for aortic aneurysm rupture include the following *except:*
(a) Male gender
(b) Hypertension
(c) Aneurysm diameter
(d) Rate of increase in aneurysm diameter

130. The following drugs have been found to be therapeutically useful in treatment of active Takayasu's arteritis, *except:*
(a) Cyclophosphamide (b) Methotrexate
(c) Colchicine (d) Prednisolone

131. Popliteal artery entrapment syndrome is often linked to:
(a) Soleus muscle (b) Gastrocnemius muscle
(c) Quadriceps muscle (d) Sartorius muscle

132. A patient has aortic dissection from aortic valve to left brachiocephalic artery so belong to which group in. Debakey classification:
(a) I (b) II
(c) III a (d) III b

133. Most common artery involved in takayasu arteritis is:
(a) Carotid (b) Subclavian
(c) Renal

134. All are complication of aortic dissection *except:*
(a) Paraparesis
(b) Syncope
(c) Mitral regurgitation
(d) Renal failure (acute)

135. Regarding thromboangitis obliterans which is not true?

(a) Anticoagulant is the main treatment
(b) Veins and nerves are also involved
(c) Upper and lower limb small vessels are involved
(d) Segmental vasculitis with collaterals are present

136. Takayasu arteritis A/E:

(a) 50% has pulmonary artery involvement
(b) Aneurysm not feature
(c) Left subclavian involvement in 90%
(d) 2nd and 3rd decade

137. Dissection of aorta A/E:

(a) Loye Dietz syndrome (b) Nonnan syndrome
(c) TOF (d) BAV

138. Pulmonary embolism rule out test:

(a) CXR (b) D dimer
(c) Echo (d) ABG

139. RAS system inhibitor trials for HF n EF A/E:

(a) Topcat (b) Senior
(c) I–preserve (d) PEP-CHF

140. Clinical indicator of renal artery stenosis A/E:

(a) Isolated systolic HTN
(b) Flash pulmonary pulmonary edema
(c) Asymmetric kidney
(d) HTN < 30 years

141. CREST trial for treatment carotid stenosis by stenting:

(a) Symptomatic patient > 50% stenosis
(b) Asymptomatic patient > 70% stenosis
(c) Both
(d) None

142. RAS due to atherosclerosis with renal HTN (resistant) A/E:

(a) Flash pulmonary edema
(b) Active urinary sediment
(c) Abdominal bruit

143. Abdominal aortic aneurysm size above what is indication for surgery?

(a) 4.5 cm (b) 5 cm
(c) 5.5 cm (d) 6 cm

144. Incidence of asymptomatic carotid stenosis > 50% in CABG patients:

(a) 16% (b) 22%
(c) 28% (d) 32%

145. Aortic dissection A/E:

(a) Aortic angiography is gold standard
(b) CT-angiography 99% specific and 95% sensitive
(c) MRI cannot be done in 100% because of patient factor
(d) AR best detected by TEE

146. Fontain classification claudication free distance of >300, will be classified in:

(a) I (b) IIa
(c) IIb (d) III

147. Kawasaki disease coronary aneurysm with thrombi with inflammation are classified in:

(a) I (b) II
(c) III (d) IV

148. Ao aneurysm inflammation detected by:

(a) PET-FDG (b) OCT
(c) IVUS (d) MRI spectroscopy

149. Popliteal artery entrapment syndrome:

(a) Insertion of medial heart of gastrocnemius muscle compresses the popliteal A
(b) Bilateral in 1/3
(c) Young male athlete present as claudication
(d) At rest popliteal artery pulsation may be absent

150. Sequential cuff pressure difference in lower limbs S/O severe PAD:

(a) 10 mm Hg (b) 20 mm Hg
(c) 30 mm Hg (d) 40 mm Hg

151. String sign in angiography:

(a) Takayasu arteritis (b) FMD with RAS
(c) Moya moya disease

152. The typical angiographic appearance of Takayasu's non-specific aorto-arteritis is:

(a) Long areas of smooth narrowing interspersed with areas that appear normal
(b) Seccular Aneurysms
(c) "Rat tailing" of Aorta
(d) Predominant involvement of Aortoiliac bifurcation

153. PVD: (T/F)
(a) Fontaine III gangrene
(b) Fibrinolysis upto 7 days
(c) Stent in below knee vessel
(d) Cilastazol is effective
(e) Intermittent claudication < 0.4

154. Aortic dissection: (T/F)
(a) Highest most in first 24 hours
(b) Type I – Surgery acutely required
(c) Smoking is risk factor
(d) Type II – debakey proceeds to proximal aorta
(e) > 2 week – definition of chronic dissection

155. Mid aortic syndrome: (T/F)
(a) Takayasu arteritis
(b) GCA
(c) Wegener's granulomatosis
(d) SLE
(e) Behcet's syndrome

156. Visceral artery aneurysm: (T/F)
(a) Takayasu arteritis (b) Behcet's syndrome
(c) Dermatomyositis (d) PAN
(e) Polymyositis

157. Most common RAS cause in children: (T/F)
(a) FMD (b) Takayasu
(c) PAN (d) Atherosclerosis
(e) None

158. Takayasu arteritis: (T/F)
(a) Aneurysm formation may occur
(b) Adventitia commonly involved
(c) Arch involvement equal in Indians and Japanese population
(d) Acute phase intervention leads to more restenosis
(e) In children most common cause of RAS in Indians

159. Takayasu arteritis A/E: (T/F)
(a) 5 years mortality 50%
(b) Stenosis more common than aneurysm
(c) Tropomyosin
(d) Coronary ostia commonly involved
(e) Disease progression even with normal ESR

160. Thoracic aortic aneurysm: (T/F)
(a) Syphilis (b) SLE
(c) PAN (d) Cystic medial necrosis
(e) Atherosclerosis

161. Aortic root dilatation surgical operations are: (T/F)
(a) Kanno's (b) Nissen S
(c) Nick's (d) Adam's
(e) Hardy's

162. Aortoarteritis: (T/F)
(a) Most common in males
(b) Stenosis is more than aneurysm
(c) Coronary ostia involved often
(d) Normal ESR can be with active disease

163. Diagnosis in P.E.:
(a) FDP
(b) V/Q scan
(c) Peripheral venous scan
(d) ECG

164. Aortoarteritis typically involve: (T/F)
(a) Mid subclavian artery
(b) Renal artery
(c) Axillary artery
(d) Femoral artery
(e) Internal carotid artery

165. Chronic PTE treatment:
(a) Embolectomy (b) Anticoagulation

166. Sinus tachycardia with S1Q3T3 is typically seen in:
(a) Acute rheumatic fever
(b) Acute pericarditis
(c) Acute myocarditis
(d) Acute pulmonary embolism

167. Spontaneous coronary dissections following statement is false:
(a) Female preponderance
(b) Can present with chronic stable angina, coronary syndrome or even sudden cardiac death
(c) In female post menopausal state is a risk factor
(d) Smoking is a risk factor

168. Wreathlike AV anastomosis on fundus examination is seen in:
(a) Pseudoxanthoma elasticum

(b) Coarctation of aorta
(c) Takayasu arteritis
(d) Malignant hypertension

169. Pulmonary embolism: (T/F)
(a) D-dimer-sensitive not specific
(b) Dyspnea is most common symptom
(c) CT–inv of choice
(d) CT replaced V/Q scan
(e) If pain (pleuritic)–small and distal infarct

170. AAA: (T/F)
(a) Surgery in > 4.5 cm
(b) CT used for screening
(c) Diameter > 4 cm – diagnostic
(d) 5.5-6 cm 5 years rupture 30-40%
(e) After surgery screening 1 month 6 months and annual

171. Aortic dissection: (T/F)
(a) Type A does not involve whole ascending aorta
(b) CMD is a common underlying condition
(c) If coronary artery involved LCA> RCA
(d) Beta blocker + vasodilator should be included in treatment
(e) If associated tamponade cardocentesis can worsen the condition

172. Aortic dissection: (T/F)
(a) Usually present with hypotension
(b) Pulse deficit more in distal dissection
(c) Distal dissection – endovascular graft treatment of choice
(d) Surgery in proximal dissection
(e) 64 MDCT is diagnostic

173. Carotid sinus hypersensitivity: (T/F)
(a) > 2 secs pause
(b) Atropine is useful in vasopressor
(c) Aura is usually present
(d) Single chamber pacing useful than dual chamber
(e) Sensation from carotid body is carried by glossopharyngeal nerve

174. Fibromuscular dysplasia: (T/F)
(a) Common in young female
(b) Medial dysplasia most common
(c) Common in proximal 1/3rd
(d) Common in black
(e) Unilateral

175. Fibromuscular dysplasia: (T/F)
(a) String of beats sign
(b) ACE-I may precipitate ARF

176. Renal artery stenosis: (T/F)
(a) ACE-I can sometime lead to ARF
(b) DTPA diagnostic
(c) Most common etiology aortoarteritis

177. Carotid artery stenosis: (T/F)
(a) Asymptomatic, risk of stroke 3%/year
(b) Aspirin decreases event risk > 50%
(c) Cause less cerebral embolism than coronary
(d) If AF present, warfarin used

178. ABI: (T/F)
(a) ABI < I abnormal
(b) <0.2 S/O tissue loss
(c) > 0.5 rest pain
(d) Dopper probe ideal
(e) Segmental vol. plethysmography can be used for non compressible vessel

179. Carotid sinus massage: (T/F)
(a) Decreases rate of AT and terminates it same in AF
(b) AVNRT–sudden decreases in rate or no effect
(c) Sinus tachycardia–gradual transient decrease rate
(d) Circus movement–slowdowns or no effect
(e) Reentry–sudden decrease in rate or no effect
(f) PAT–decrease slowly and then stop
(g) Atrial flutter–transient slowing of ventricular rate

180. Aneurysm: (T/F)
(a) 15% Abdominal aorta have multiple aneurysm
(b) Abdominal aorta most common site infrarenal aorta
(c) AAA 10-year survival rate after surgery < 50%
(d) Thoracic aorta are almost asymptomatic

181. Annuloaortic ectasia: (T/F)
(a) More in females
(b) Progress to AR
(c) 5-10% stigmata of Marfan
(d) Cystic medial necrosis seen
(e) Aortic calcification with aortic root dilation

182. PTE: (T/F)

(a) RVH and RAD commonly seen

(b) ↑ es limb voltage < 5 mm

(c) Clockwise rotation and persistent S in V6

(d) Tachycardia only sign

(e) Atrial arrythmias commonly seen

183. True or false:

(a) In secondary pulmonary HTN, PCWP more than PA diastolic pressure

(b) In acute pulmonary embolism, 10–20% has resolution in 24 hours

(c) RV failure when total obstruction is > 60%

(d) RV enlargement is most sensitive sign for pulmonary HTN in chest X-ray

(e) Lung is largest endothelial bed

(f) Lung perfusion scan can differentiate between thrombotic and primary pulmonary HTN

(g) PE moratlity without treatment – 30%

184. Fontaine classification–patient has no rest pain and claudication at < 200 m:

(a) Class II b (b) Class II a

(c) Class III a (d) Class III b

185. PTE true:

(a) RV dysfunction with normal BP – low risk

(b) Normal ECG – 20%

(c) CXR– helpful in diagnosis

(d) Cardiac biomarker may helpful in management

186. Most common vascular ring:

(a) Double Ao arch

(b) Right Ao arch

(c) Left Ao arch

(d) Aneurysm with aberrent LSA

(e) Aneurysm with right subclavian artery

187. Dissection of aorta A/E:

(a) Bicuspid Ao valve (b) Marfan syndrome

(c) Ao valve repair (d) Bilateral RAS

188. Ao dissection A/E:

(a) Most common – ascending Ao (2/3 cases)

(b) Most common – site – just distal to left SCA

(c) Type B– medical Mx

(d) Pregnancy – Most common in 1st trimester

189. Abdominal aortic aneurysm strongest risk factor:

(a) Smoking (b) Age

(c) Gender (d) Hypertension

190. Asymptomatic most common vascular ring:

(a) Aberrant right subclavian artery

(b) Right aortic arch

(c) Double aortic

(d) Cervical arch

191. Intramural aortic hematoma A/E:

(a) Rupture of vaso vasorum

(b) Rare in elderly

(c) Contrast enhancement absent in CT

(d) Aortography may miss it

192. True about PE is A/E:

(a) D dimer is sensitive but not specific

(b) IVC filter ↓ both PE and DVT

(c) OCP ↑ both PE and DVT

(d) Low probability V/Q scan with symptoms may still have PE

193. Pulmonary embolism A/E:

(a) Hypercapnia (b) PHT

(c) RV dilatation (d) Increased Troponin T

194. Patient with severe calcific AS with CHF with global hypokinesia, EF= 35% treatment:

(a) Medical treatment (b) AVR C/I

(c) AVR absolutely C/I (d) None

195. Surgery advised in 30 years old female:

(a) Asymptomatic severe AR with EF – 65%

(b) Asymptomatic severe MR with EF – 65%

(c) Asymptomatic MS with MVA – 0.9 cm^2

(d) Asymptomatic AS with AVA –1.1 cm^2

(e) Asymptomatic PS with PV gradient 50 mm Hg

196. Patient presents with sudden onset chest pain, dyspnoea, S1 soft, S2 soft, EDM at aortic area, basal crepts, non displaced apex diagnosis is:

(a) Pulmonary embolism

(b) Chronic AR with acute insufficiency

(c) Dissection involving aortic root

(d) Myocarditis

(e) Acute MI

197. Which one of the following is not a component of the Wells criteria for pulmonary embolism?

(a) Acute dyspnea
(b) Previous DVT
(c) Heart rate > 100 bpm
(d) Presence of hemoptysis

198. RAS association:

(a) William syndrome (b) Neurofibromatosis
(c) Refsum disease (d) Turner syndrome

199. True about abdominal aortic aneurysm A/E:

(a) M:F - 10:1
(b) Infrarenal most common
(c) Duration of smoking is more important but not amount
(d) Rupture more likely in male than female

200. Which is the most common finding on chest X-ray in a patient of aortic dissection?

(a) Calcium sign
(b) Nonspecific superior mediastinal widening
(c) Widening of Aortic sillhoutte
(d) Left pleural effusion

201. Type 1 Aortic dissection Risk increased A/E:

(a) BAV (b) Marfan
(c) AR (d) HTN

202. Pulmonary embolism prognostic scoring is:

(a) Geneva score (b) PESI
(c) Well's score (d) William's score

203. In carotid artery pulse, diachrotic notch indicates:

(a) End of ventricle systole
(b) Atrial distension
(c) Early ventricle filling
(d) Rapid ventricle filling

204. RAS by A/E:

(a) Atherosclerosis (b) FMD
(c) Takayasu disease (d) PAN

205. Central aortic pressure:

(a) Is more than brachial
(b) Signifies stiffness of arteries
(c) Can't be calculated from brachial
(d) All of the above

206. Aortic root dilatation A/E:

(a) TOF
(b) COA
(c) Interrupted aortic arch
(d) BAV with AS

207. Aortic dissection with hypotension DOC:

(a) Phenylephrine (b) Dobutamine
(c) Epinephrine (d) Norepinephrine

208. C/I for TMT:

(a) Advanced CHB
(b) Pericarditis
(c) AS
(d) USA with crescendo angina

209. Which of the following is true of acute aortic intramural hematoma?

(a) It has benign self-limiting course in majority of cases
(b) TEE is better than CT angiography for early diagnosis
(c) Occurs due to bleeding from the damaged vasa vasorum
(d) Usually associated with acute aortic regurgitation

210. Which of the following peripheral revasculari-zation techniques is associated with worst patency rate at 5 years?

(a) Femoro-popliteal bypass graft using saphenous venous graft
(b) Femoro-popliteal stenting using self-expanding stents
(c) Iliac artery stenting
(d) Infra-popliteal peripheral angioplasty

211. All are true for mesenteric vein thrombosis leading to mesenteric ischemia *except:*

(a) Associated with oral contraceptives
(b) Presents with weight loss, lower GI bleeding
(c) Inferior mesenteric vein is more commonly involved than superior mesenteric vein
(d) Less common than the mesenteric arterial involvement (as a cause of mesenteric ischemia)

212. Carotid artery stenting is preferred over carotid endarterectomy in the presence of:

(a) Visible thrombus
(b) Contralateral carotid artery occlusion
(c) Platelet disorder
(d) Tortuous aortic arch

213. A 40-year-old man develops thrombocytopenia following heparin administration for acute pulmonary embolism. For further management which statement is true?

(a) Low molecular weight heparin can be safely substituted for intravenous unfractionated heparin
(b) A direct thrombin inhibitor, such as lepirudin, could be safely substituted for heparin
(c) Intravenous heparin should be continued because the low platelet count represents a laboratory artefact without clinical significance
(d) This is a transient reaction to heparin and does not preclude future heparin treatment for this patient

214. Absolute contraindication for fibrinolytic therapy:

(a) Aortic dissection
(b) Recent internal bleeding
(c) Active peptic ulcer
(d) Prolonged CPR

215. Stanford classification is for:

(a) Aortic aneurysm (b) Aortic dissection
(c) Aorto arteritis (d) All of the above

216. Fontaine classification of peripheral artery disease stage-III is:

(a) Necrosis (b) Gangrene
(c) Rest pain (d) Claudication

217. Clinical predictors of renal artery stenosis:

(a) Flash pulmonary edema
(b) Resistant hypertension
(c) Unexplained renal dysfunction
(d) All of the above

218. Well's criteria is for the diagnosis of:

(a) Acute pulmonary embolism
(b) Right ventricular infarction
(c) Primary pulmonary hypertension
(d) Cardiac tamponade

219. Window period for thrombolysis in acute pulmonary embolism:

(a) 7 days (b) 14 days
(c) 24 hours (d) 21 days

220. Most common artery to be involved in arotic dissection:

(a) RCA (b) LAD
(c) LCX

221. Patient with back pain, BP in Rt arm 180/95, new diastolic murmur, next step:

(a) CT chest (b) TF
(c) Angio

222. According to recent trials, stenting of which vessels is not beneficial?

(a) Carotid (b) Renal
(c) Illiac (d) Subclavian

223. Female 40 years with type B aortic dissections had history of uterine rupture in past, most likely diagnosis:

(a) Ehlers-Danlos syndrome
(b) Loeys-Dietz syndrome
(c) Turner's syndrome
(d) Marfan's syndrome

224. Submassive pulmonary embolism all *except*:

(a) BNP normal
(b) SBP normal
(c) > 1/2 of pulmonary vascular bed
(d) Thrombophlebitis in low bleeding risk

225. Surgery is indicated in ascending aortic aneurysm if diameter of ascending aorta or aortic sinus is:

(a) 4.5 cm (b) 5.5 cm
(c) 6.5 cm (d) 7.5 cm

226. In patient with Marfan's syndrome pregnancy is contraindicated if diameter of ascending aorta is greater than:

(a) 4 cm (b) 5 cm
(c) 6 cm (d) 3 cm

227. Which drug is approved by FDA for thrombolysis in massive pulmonary embolism?

(a) Streptokinase
(b) Alteplase
(c) Urokinase
(d) Tenectaplase

228. Bosentan belongs to one of the following group:

(a) Endothelin receptor antagonist
(b) Phosphodiesterase inhibitors
(c) Soluble guanylate cyclase stimulators
(d) Prostanoids

229. Renal artery stenosis all *except*:

(a) Atherosclerosis (b) FMD
(c) Takayasu (d) PAN

230. Odds ratio with PVD – Max. with:

(a) Diabetes (b) Smoking

(c) HT (d) Hypercholesterolemia

231. Endovascular vs surgery for Abdominal Aortic aneurysm:

(a) Dream (b) Over

(c) Ever (d) All of the above

232. For aortic stiffness, all statements are true, *except*:

(a) Pulse-wave velocity is the most validated method to non-invasively quantify arterial stiffness

(b) Predictor of future changes in systolic blood pressure and future development of hypertension in healthy volunteers

(c) MRI enables detection of more subtle changes in regional stiffness

(d) An increase of aortic pulse wave velocity of 10 m/s raises CV risk by more than 10%

233. Pulse:

(a) For assessing pulse character radial is better than carotid

(b) AS with LV dysfunction–delayed upstroke is absent, only pulsus parvus is present

(c) Brachiofemoral delay in COA, arteries are palpated simultaneously

(d) Normal aorta palpable above and below umbilicus

(e) Pulses bisferiens better in isolatedAR than AS+AR

234. PAD:

(a) ABI sensitive but less specific

(b) Toe brachial index in non compressible ankle vessel

(c) Surgery is required in critical limb without clinical feature

(d) Pulse volume recording can be used for diagnosis

(e) Post exercise ABI can unmask PAD in normal ABI

ANSWERS KEY

1. (b)	2. (a)	3. (a)	4. (b)	5. (a)	6. (a)	7. (a)	8. (b)
9. (a)	10. (c)	11. (c)	12. (a)	13. (b)	14. (b)	15. (d)	16. (c)
17. F	18. F	19. F	20. T	21. (a)	22. (c)	23. (a)	24. (a)
25. (b,d)	26. (b)	27. (d)	28. (d)	29. TFTTT	30. TTTFT	31. FTTTT	32. TFTTT
33. (a)	34. (b)	35. (a)	36. (d)	37. (b)	38. (a)	39. (c)	40. (a)
41. (c)	42. (c)	43. (d)	44. (c)	45. (b)	46. (a)	47. (d)	48. (b)
49. (d)	50. (b)	51. (d)	52. (a)	53. (b)	54. (d)	55. (b)	56. (c)
57. (d)	58. (b)	59. (c)	60. (b)	61. (a)	62. (a)	63. (a)	64. (a)
65. (d)	66. (c)	67. (d)	68. (a)	69. (b)	70. (b)	71. (b)	72. (b)
73. (a)	74. (a)	75. (c)	76. (b)	77. (a)	78. (d)	79. (a)	80. (c)
81. (c)	82. (d)	83. (b)	84. (b)	85. (c)	86. (d)	87. TTFFF	88. (a)
89. (d)	90. (a)	91. TTFT	92. (a)	93. (c)	94. FFF??	95. (a)	96. (c)
97. (d)	98. (b)	99. (b)	100. (a,b,c)	101. (a,b,c)	102. (b)	103. (d)	104. (d)
105. (b)	106. (b)	107. (d)	108. (b)	109. (d)	110. (b)	111. (a)	112. (d)
113. (a)	114. (a)	115. (c)	116. (c)	117. (c)	118. (d)	119. (a)	120. (b)
121. (a)	122. (b)	123. (b)	124. (a)	125. (c)	126. (a)	127. (b)	128. (c)
129. (a)	130. (c)	131. (b)	132. (b)	133. (b)	134. (c)	135. (a)	136. (b)
137. (c)	138. (b)	139. (b)	140. (a)	141. (c)	142. (b)	143. (c)	144. (?)
145. (a)	146. (b)	147. (b)	148. (a)	149. (d)	150. (b)	151. (d)	152. (c)
153. FTFTF	154. TTTFT	155. TTFFF	156. FTFTF	157. FTFFF	158. TTFTT	159. TFFTF	160. TFFTT
161. TFFFF	162. FTFT	163. (b)	164. FTFFF	165. (b)	166. (d)	167. (c)	168. (c)
169. TTTTT	170. FTFTF	171. FTFTT	172. FTFTT	173. FFFFT	174. TTFFF	175. TT	176. TFF
177. FTFT	178. FFFFT	179. FTTTFF	180. TTTT	181. FTFTF	182. TFTTT	183. TTTFT	184. (a)
185. (a)	186. (a)	187. (d)	188. (d)	189. (a)	190. (b)	191. (b)	192. (b)
193. (a)	194. (c)	195. (b)	196. (c)	197. (a)	198. (b)	199. (d)	200. (c)
201. (c)	202. (b)	203. (a)	204. (d)	205. (b)	206. (c)	207. (a)	208. (a)
209. (c)	210. (d)	211. (c)	212. (b)	213. (b)	214. (a)	215. (b)	216. (c)
217. (d)	218. (a)	219. (b)	220. (b)	221. (a)	222. (b)	223. (a)	224. (a)
225. (b)	226. (a)	227. (b)	228. (a)	229. (d)	230. (b)	231. (d)	232. (d)
233. (b,c,e)	234. FTFTT						

CHAPTER SIX

CONGENITAL HEART DISEASE

1. **Most common CHD at birth:**
(a) ASD (b) VSD
(c) TGA (d) PDA

2. **Straight left heart border A/E:**
(a) TA (b) EA
(c) TGA (d) Absent pericardium

3. **Tricuspid atresia obstruction to pulmonary blood flow:**
(a) Valvular
(b) Infundibular
(c) Pulmonary artery
(d) VSD

4. **Small VSD 2 m/s which is not seen?**
(a) PS
(b) PAH
(c) Gerbode
(d) Double chamber RV

5. **Atrial septostomy in infants most common for:**
(a) TA (b) TGA
(c) TOF (d) Tricuspid atresia

6. **Bicuspid aortic valve associated with A/E:**
(a) AS (b) AR
(c) Dissection (d) SAH

7. **False match is:**
(a) Adenoma sebaceum–Rhabdomyoma
(b) IIa–Tuberoeruptive xanthoma
(c) NF with RAS
(d) Marfan–Abdominal aortic aneurysm

8. **Heart development all are T/E:**
(a) PDA–6th arm
(b) LA–Pulmonary veins
(c) Left superior vena cava–duct of Cuvier
(d) RA–Right horn

9. **SaO_2–100%**
PaO_2–88%
MVO_2–64%
QP QS =
(a) 5:2 (b) 3:2
(c) 2:1 (d) 3:1

10. **Continuous murmur–all *except:***
(a) TOF with absent pulmonary valve
(b) Obstructive TAPVC
(c) MS with restrictive ASD
(d) Peripheral pulmonary stenosis

11. **Least PaO_2 is found in all *except:***
(a) Methemoglobinemia
(b) TOF
(c) TGA
(d) Pulmonary AV fistula

12. **Features of severe TS are all *except:***
(a) Fatiguability
(b) PND
(c) Systemic congestion
(d) Atrial arrhythmias

13. **Congenital complete heart block–false is:**
(a) Neonatal lupus
(b) Most mothers do not have SLE
(c) Most common site of block is infrahisian
(d) Most require pacemaker by middle age

14. **Eisenmenger's complex–what is not required for diagnosis?**
(a) Cyanosis

(b) Unrestrictive septal defect

(c) PVR increased

(d) Bidirectional shunt

15. Normal heart – true is:

(a) Aorto-tricuspid continuity is not seen

(b) Aortic valve is posterior and to the right of pulmonary valve

(c) Aortic valve is anterior and superior to pulmonary valve

16. Development mismatch:

(a) Left SVC–Duct of Cuvier

(b) PDA–6th arch

(c) Pulmonary vein–Left atrium

(d) RA–Right sinus horn

17. Not true:

(a) TGA with Pm. HTN–Reversed differential cyanosis

(b) ES with VSD–Narrow S_2 is commonly seen

(c) MVP murmur decreases in pregnancy

(d) ASD with R-L shunt–No flow murmur at pulmonary area

18. Regarding AV node–all are true *except:*

(a) Dual AV nodal physiology is seen in 1/3rd of individuals

(b) Decremental conduction

(c) Conduction velocity does not depend on refractoriness

(d) It is the only electrical connection between atria and ventricles

19. CXR – concave PA, LV apex, which is not seen?

(a) Cyanosis

(b) RAD

(c) Restrictive VSD

(d) RV hypoplasia

20. 4-day neonate, with ground glass appearance on CXR:

(a) Obstructive TAPVC

(b) Truncus arteriosus

(c) TGA

(d) ASD

21. Echocardiography of Ebstein's anomaly is shown. Not seen in Ebstein's anomaly:

(a) Cyanosis (b) Loud P_2

(c) Multiple heart sounds

22. All T/E:

(a) Fetal echo–fetal tachycardia

(b) FFR–cardiac transplantation atherosclerosis

(c) Cardiac MRI–RT ventricular function

(d) CT–cardiac calcification

23. A/E:

(a) HHT–TGF – β

(b) Carney complex–sentigess

(c) Noonan–by lymphedema

(d) LQT3–Potassium channel

24. Cyanosis present in A/E:

(a) ASD with severe PHT

(b) ASD with severe RV dysfunction

(c) ASD with PAPVC

(d) ASD with unroofed coronary sinus

25. Cardiomegaly in A/E:

(a) DCM

(b) CCF

(c) Ebstein

(d) After long space trip

26. 12 years cyanosis with X-ray–ECG shows:

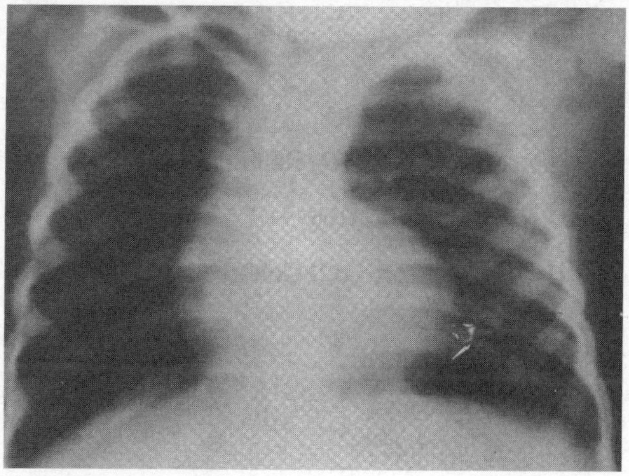

(a) LVH with LAD

(b) RVH with RAD

(c) RVH with extreme axis deviation

(d) RVH with LAD

27. RV and LV pressure trainings in corrected TOF patient:

(a) Pulmonary valve stenosis

(b) LVD

28. Cardiac pressure tracing LV with catheter withdrawn to aorta shows:

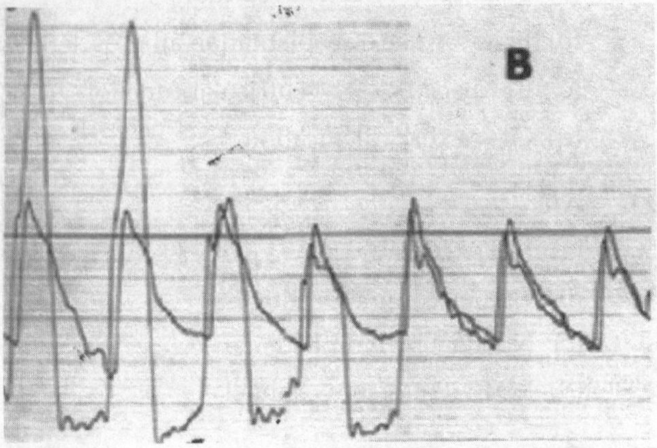

(a) Subaortic membrane (b) CoA
(c) AS (d) Williams syndrome

29. Location of vieussens valve:
(a) Junction of great cardiac vein→cavernous sinus
(b) Junction of basian vein→RA
(c) Ant/middle/post cardiac vein→coronary sinus
(d) All the ant cardinal veins→coronary sinus

30. Eisenmenger in VSD (large) at age:
(a) < 6 months (b) 2 years
(c) 10 years (d) 20 years

31. All *except* Ebstein anomaly ECG:
(a) Tall and wide P wave
(b) Deep S in V_1
(c) Prolonged q in V_1–V_4
(d) Low amplitude QRS in right precordial lead

32. Fontan done in A/E:
(a) Tricuspid atresia (b) AVSD large
(c) DORV (d) TOF

33. TOF RV pressure:
(a) > systemic pressure
(b) = systemic pressure
(c) < systemic pressure

34. Congenitally diagnosed ASD initially, was done cath study which revealed equal oxygenation in all 4 chambers:
(a) Done wrong (b) TAPVC supra cardiac
(c) Sinus venous ASD (d) Primum ASD

35. Cardiac cath – RV step up is not in:
(a) PDA with PR (b) Outlet VSD
(c) Inlet VSD (d) PAPVC

36. Cardiac situs is diagnosed by:
(a) Cardiac apex position
(b) Atria
(c) Ventricle
(d) Great vessel

37. Turner surgery, risk of AD–A/E:
(a) BAV
(b) CoA
(c) –length of transverse arch
(d) HTN

38. Uncomplicated large VSD with Eisenmenger not a feature:
(a) Cardiomegaly (b) Palpable P2
(c) Single S2 (d) No parasternal thrill

39. All true *except*:
(a) Eisenmenger–prog. now has good prog. with advanced technology
(b) PAH–poor prog. than 1° PHTN
(c) HF–Most common cause of death
(d) Eisenmenger has good prog.

40. COA in pregnancy:
(a) Eclampsia lesser in COA than non COA
(b) ICH risk high even after correction
(c) IE can be seen
(d) AD (+)

Case Scenario (41-43)

24-year-old history of childhood murmur, after lifting weight→dyspnea

41. Diagnosis:
(a) RSOV (b) BAV with AR
(c) PDA with PR (d) VSD with AR

42. Initial investigational for diagnosis:
(a) TTE (b) TEE
(c) Cath. (d) MRI

43. Type of murmur:
(a) Continuous murmur throughout cycle
(b) Continuous murmur loud around S_1
(c) Continuous murmur loud around S_2
(d) Variable intensity with multiple peak

8-week child, large VSD/tachypnea, otherwise stable (44-46)

44. Sign of CHF A/E:
(a) Sweating over forehead while feeding
(b) ↓ hunger

(c) ↑ hunger
(d) Growth lesser

45. **X-ray finding:**
(a) Right pulmonary artery dilation
(b) Prom. aortic knuckle
(c) Pulmonary artery/Bronchus ratio increased
(d) Peripheral pruning

46. **↑ shunt detected by:**
(a) Lund A_2 (b) Soft P_2
(c) Loud P_2 (d) Absent parasternal heave

Patient right retrosternal chest pain, radiating to back, BP upper limbs–equal in lower limb and ECG–IWMI (47-49)

47. **Diagnosis:**
(a) Type A AD with IWMI with AR
(b) Type B AD with IWMI with AR
(c) AR with IWMI

48. **Investigation:**
(a) TTE
(b) TEE
(c) CT angio with aortic root secondary
(d) MR angio

49. **Treatment:**
(a) Urgent surgery (b) PCI
(c) Stenting (d) Thrombolysis

CCTGA (50-53)

50. **CHB (+)**

51. **Can proceed to adult life**

52. **TR murmur–leaflet–three**

53. **Moderate band–identify RV**

Sinus Venous ASD (54-57)

54. **Association with anomalous pulmonary connection**

55. **Can present even without setup**

56. **Atrial rhythm can be non-sinus**

57. **Needn't operate/Inter vein**

58. **PDA type A:**
(a) Wide @ aortic end
(b) Wide @ pulmonary end
(c) Tabular
(d) Multiple indentation

59. **Clubbing after cyanosis:**
(a) Immediately (b) Within 2 months
(c) 3 months (d) 1 year

60. **The least prevalent anatomy for a bicuspid valve:**
(a) Fusion of the right and left coronary cusps
(b) Fusion of the left and non coronary cusps
(c) Fusion of the right and non coronary cusps
(d) None

61. **Surgery not indicated in:**
(a) Large VSD (b) VSD × AR
(c) Sub pulmonic VSD (d) Restrictive VSD

62. **TGA ECG changes:**
(a) RVH (b) LAE
(c) RAE

Case Scenario Type (63-64)

63. **Aortic stenosis, 56 years, asymptomatic, velocity > 5.5 m/sec AVR in this patient is:**
(a) Class 1 (b) Class 2a
(c) Class 2b (d) Class 3

64. **Valve for replacement:**
(a) Mechanical (b) Bioprosthetic
(c) TAVI (d) ROSS

65. **Fetal bradycardia with 2:1 AV blocks at birth is a feature of:**
(a) Timothy syndrome (b) Andersen-Tawil
(c) Brugada (d) Long QT syndrome

66. **Physiologic right to left shunt results from:**
(a) Pulmonary AV fistula
(b) LSVC draining to coronary sinus
(c) Bronchial veins draining to pulmonary veins
(d) Cardinal veins draining to pulmonary veins

67. **Identify the wrong statement in Ebstein's anomaly:**
(a) ASD is present in 90%
(b) Accessory conduction pathway is seen in 25%
(c) Typical X-ray appearance–"water bottle"
(d) "Sail sound" is a feature

68. All are cyanotic heart diseases with decreased pulmonary blood flow *except:*

(a) TOP
(b) Single ventricle with PS
(c) Trilogy of Fallot
(d) Taussig Bing anomaly

69. On chest X-ray prominent pulmonary vessels in the periphery of the lung is seen in all *except:*

(a) Sickle cell disease with severe anemia
(b) Hyperthyroidism
(c) Large VSD with right to left shunt
(d) Large PDA with L→R shunt

70. Sinus venous defect (ASD) results from:

(a) Malformation of septum primum
(b) Malformation of septum secundum
(c) Persistence of common cardinal vein
(d) Deficiency of the wall of the common pulmonary vein

71. D. George/Velocardiofacial syndrome is due to deletion of:

(a) 15 q11-q13 (b) 7 q11.23
(c) 17 p11.2 (d) 22 q11.2

72. Congenital heart–cyanotic disease: (T/F)

(a) Complete repair of TOF should be done < 1 year
(b) Chr. 22q11 most common presentation of congenital cyanotic heart
(c) TOF desaturation seen in LA
(d) More collateral seen in pink POF
(e) Rib notching seen < 6 years

73. Genetic surgery: (T/F)

(a) In AR, early death than AD
(b) Consanguineous marriage ↑ transmission in both AD and AR
(c) Mitochondrial inheritance from mother to both sons with daughter
(d) X linked disorder most common in female
(e) Thalassemic parents (AR) have 2 healthy and 1 affected, chance of transmission in next child – 25%

74. Genetics: (T/F)

(a) Penetrance is genotype manifested as phenotype
(b) Epigenetics–inheritance of genes without alteration DNA codon
(c) Real time PCR–gives degree of gene expression
(d) Next generation gene sequences for multigenic disorder line HTN

75. LTGA: (T/F)

(a) Right side looping of primitive heart
(b) Coronary artery mirror image
(c) MV anomaly–30%
(d) VSD–50% (Isolated)
(e) PS–50-60%

76. Surgical management: (T/F)

(a) Pulmonary A-banding–closed heart surgery
(b) Bentall is open heart surgery
(c) TA (tricuspid atresia) with severe cyanosis–Glenn shunt TOC
(d) Pott's shunt–central shunt
(e) Modified BT shunt–Direct connection of pulmonary artery to subclavian artery

77. Regarding shunt operations: (T/F)

(a) Modified BT shunt directly connects subclavian artery to pulmonary artery
(b) Pott's shunt connects ascending aorta to pulmonary artery
(c) Glen shunt–SVC to RPA
(d) Watersten's shunt–IVC to pulmonary artery
(e) Classic BT shunt can be done on either side of aortic arch

78. Regarding Turner syndrome: (T/F)

(a) Patient has 45 X0 karyotype
(b) PS is common manifestation
(c) Short fourth metacarpal
(d) Nondisjunction is the mechanism of monosomy
(e) Most common cause of HTN in TS is COA

79. Regarding congenital lesions: (T/F)

(a) Turner syndrome–obstructive mitral and aortic diseases
(b) Noonan syndrome has butterfly vertebrae, intrahepatic chelestanis
(c) Leopard syndrome–85-100% have cardiac lesions
(d) Holt–Oram syndrome–IX a single gene disorder
(e) DiGeorge syndrome–TBX1

80. Regarding congenital heart disease: (T/F)

(a) LAD with widely split fixed P_2 indicates AVSD
(b) TAPVC has LV hypertrophy
(c) DORV with PS has widely split S_2
(d) Characteristic triple or quadruple rhythm is audible in Ebstein's anomaly
(e) LVH with RAH in tricuspid atresia

81. CC-TGA: (T/F)

(a) 80% cases have VSD
(b) 50% cases have left AV valve regurgitation
(c) Aorta and pulmonary artery are parallel
(d) Acquired complete AV block continues to develop at a rate of 2 percent per year
(e) A single S_2 is heard

82. What is incidence of right aortic arch in tetralogy of Fallot?

(a) 5% to 10% (b) 10% to 20%
(c) 20% to 30% (d) 30% to 40%

83. Which one of the following types ASD is suitable for device closure?

(a) Ostium primum
(b) Ostium secundum
(c) Sinus venosus
(d) Unroofed coronary sinus

84. Which one of the following genetic conditions is not associated with aortic dissection?

(a) Marfan syndrome (b) Down syndrome
(c) Turner syndrome (d) Biscuspid aortic valve

85. Which one of the following is not true for corrected transposition of great arteries?

(a) Atrioventricular discordance present
(b) Ventriculo arterial discordance present
(c) Cyanosis is common
(d) It produces loud second sound at left basal area

86. What is incidence of complete heart block in patients with corrected transposition of great arteries?

(a) 10% (b) 5%
(c) 30% (d) 50%

87. Williams syndrome does not include:

(a) Supravalvular aortic stenosis
(b) Pulmonary artery stenosis
(c) Elfin faces
(d) Hyperuricemia

88. Coarctation of aorta is common in:

(a) Marfan's syndrome (b) Turner's syndrome
(c) Down's syndrome (d) All of the above

89. Which one of the following is not a part of Shone's complex?

(a) Subaortic stenosis
(b) Coarctation of aorta
(c) Parachute mitral valve
(d) Atretic aortic valve

90. First trimester maternal rubella infection makes fetus vulnerable for:

(a) Supravalvar pulmonary stenosis
(b) Pulmonary artery stenosis
(c) Infundibular pulmonary stenosis
(d) Pulmonary atresia

91. What apical displacement of septal leaflet of tricuspid valve is used as a cut off limit for diagnosing Ebstein's anomaly in adults?

(a) 25 mm (b) 10 mm
(c) 15 mm (d) 20 mm

92. Which one of the following is not common in ECG of patient with Ebstein's anomaly?

(a) Himalayan P wave
(b) Type A, WPM syndrome
(c) RBBB
(d) Prolonged PR interval

93. Which one of the following is not true for Uhl's anomaly?

(a) Aplasia or hypoplasia of RV myocardium
(b) Ventricular arrhythmias are common
(c) RV is enlarged
(d) Paradoxical movement of septum

94. Which one of the following is not true for total anomalous pulmonary venous connection?

(a) Right atrium and ventricle are significantly dilated
(b) ASD with left to right shunt
(c) Snowman appearance is common on X-ray
(d) Pulmonary hypertension is common

95. What is the incidence of congenital heart disease in Down syndrome?

(a) 20% (b) 30%
(c) 70% (d) 50%

96. Cleft mitral valve is common in:

(a) Ebstein's anomaly

(b) Cor triatriatum

(c) Atrioventricular septal defects

(d) Congenital mitral stenosis

97. Most common ventricular septal defect is:

(a) Perimembranous VSD

(b) Muscular VSD

(c) Inlet VSD

(d) Subpulmonic VSD

98. Spontaneous closure of VSD occurs up to:

(a) 1 year age (b) 4 years age

(c) 8 years age (d) 15 years age

99. Which one of the following is not a component of Taussig Bing anomaly?

(a) Double outlet right ventricle

(b) Subpulmonic VSD

(c) Pulmonary stenosis

(d) Severe PAH

100. Which one of the following are most common accessory pathways?

(a) Right lateral (b) Left lateral

(c) Left posteroseptal (d) Right anteroseptal

101. Which type of atrial septal defects are associated with partial or complete connection of pulmonary veins to right side of heart?

(a) Secundum ASD

(b) Superior sinus venosus defect

(c) Primum ASD

(d) Inferior sinus venosus defect

102. Supravalvular aortic stenosis accounts for nearly 7% of all fixed forms of LVOT obstruction. Which of the following is true regarding supravalvular AS?

(a) Its occurrence has been associated with a loss-of-function mutation of the elastin gene on chromosome 7q11.23

(b) It frequently occurs as part of the William-Beuren syndrome, and may be associated with stenosis of major branches of the aorta or pulmonary arteries

(c) Due to a preferential jet of blood flow from a Supra AS into the left brachiocephalic artery (Coanda effect), there might be marked increase in the left upper extremity systolic pressure relative to the right

(d) Since the coronary arteries are under high pressure, surgery might be considered earlier than in patients with valvular AS, particularly when no valve substitute is required

103. Ebstein's anomaly is characterized by abnormally apical displacement of tricuspid valve leaflets. Which of the following statements is true in this context?

(a) The septal leaflet is characteristically described as being sail-like

(b) The most frequently associated anomaly is pulmonary atresia

(c) Echocardiography is the key diagnostic technique with apical distal displacement of the septal or posterior leaflet of 8 cm/m° BSA

(d) ECG shows prolonged PR interval, RBBB and bizarre "second" QRS attached to preceding normal QRS

104. Regarding cyanotic congenital heart diseases select the true statement:

(a) Hyperviscosity that occurs by the virtue of erythrocytosis may be aggravated by iron deficiency

(b) The total cholesterol levels of these patients is higher than that of general population

(c) Glenn shunt is a palliative shunt connecting ascending aorta to right pulmonary artery

(d) Right aortic arch exists in more than 70% of patients with tricuspid atresia

105. Which of the following matches of genetic channelopathies with the affected gene is not correct?

(a) LQT 1–Loss of function KCNQ1

(b) LQT 3–Loss of function SCN5A

(c) CPVT 1–Gain of function RyR2 (Ryanodine receptor)

(d) Timothy syndrome–Gain of function CACNA1c

106. Incorrect regarding Noonan syndrome:

(a) Autosomal dominant

(b) Short stature

(c) Dysplastic valvular pulmonic stenosis

(d) Coarctation of aorta

107. Normal wedge mean pulmonary capillary pressure is:

(a) 2-4 mm Hg (b) 4-12 mm Hg

(c) 12-18 mm Hg (d) 18-24 mm Hg

108. Which of the following cardiac malpositions is associated with highest chances of 0012060 congenital heart disease?

(a) Dextrocardia with situssolitus
(b) Dextrocardia with situsinversus
(c) Levocardia with situssolitus
(d) Levocardia with situsinversus

109. Choussat's criteria are operability criteria for which operation?
(a) Norwood's procedure
(b) Glenn's shunt
(c) Fontan's operation
(d) BT shunt

110. Central cyanosis seen in:
(a) PAPVC (b) RSOV
(c) ASD (d) Pulmonary AV fistula

111. Central cyanosis in congenital HD influenced by A/E:
(a) O_2 desaturation (b) PCO_2
(c) Hb concentration (d) Pulmonary blood flow

112. Left atrial pressure:
(a) A>V (b) V>A
(c) V=A (d) None

113. Suprasystemic right ventricular pressure A/E:
(a) Eisenmenger VSD (b) Eisenmanger ASD
(c) PPH (d) PS without VSD

114. Pulmonary AP-140 mm Hg, aortic pressure 120 mm Hg possible in:
(a) ASD
(b) VSD
(c) PDA
(d) Aortopulmonary septal defect

115. ToF in cyanotic spell A/E:
(a) Systolic murmur heard
(b) Syncope
(c) Central cyanosis

116. ToF–CCF aggravated by A/E:
(a) Anemia (b) Syncope
(c) Volume overload (d) TR

117. ToF with right ventricular outflow–5 m/s with systemic BP-120/70 mm Hg, pulmonary artery systolic pressure is:
(a) 10 (b) 20
(c) 30 (d) 40

118. CC-TGA:
(a) Atrial inversion
(b) Ventricular inversion
(c) Pulmonary vein inversion
(d) Vena caval inversion

119. PDA must for A/E:
(a) TA (tricuspid atresia) (b) PA
(c) COA (d) Hypoplastic left heart

120. ASD must for A/E:
(a) TA (b) TGA
(c) PA (d) TAPVC

121. ↑ risk of cryptogenic embolism maximum in:
(a) PFO I septal aneurysm
(b) PFO I VSD
(c) PFO I ASD

122. RV morphology all A/E:
(a) Moderator band (b) Coarse trabeculation
(c) Triangular (d) No septal attachment

123. False is:
(a) PV superior to AV
(b) Anterior left ventricle continuous I septum
(c) TV superior to MV
(d) Posterior aortic valve continuous I mitral valve

124. Left SVC derived from:
(a) Left anterior cardinal vein
(b) Supracardiac cardinal vein
(c) RT common cardinal vein
(d) RT innominate vein

125. Late onset cyanosis in A/E:
(a) TA (b) Ebstein
(c) ASD (d) VSD

126. ASD with JVP-12 CM H_2O, what is the right ventricular filling pressure?
(a) 12 (b) 17
(c) 20 (d) 25

127. Asplenia/polysplenia–Most common with:
(a) D-TGA

(b) Mirror image dextrocardia

(c) Ambigouse

(d) TA

128. Young lady with ASD with ↑ JVP treatment is:

(a) Termination

(b) Decongestive therapy

(c) Closure (ASD)

(d) Elective closure after pregnancy

129. In congenital heart disease–I cyanosis I polycythemia ↑ risk of:

(a) Premature atherosclerosis

(b) CHB

(c) Cholelethiasis

130. O_2 Step up in right atria:

(a) VSD (b) PDA

(c) Gerbode defect (d) MR

131. Patient SPO_2 in aorta–98%, SVC–64, IVC–68. Upper RT atrium–68, middle RT atrium–88%, lower right atrium–88, pulmonary A–88% diagnosis is:

(a) VSD (b) PDA

(c) ASD (d) ASD with bidirectional shunt

132. Doppler showing flow towards right ventricle in both systole and diastole:

(a) RSOV (b) VSD

(c) TR (d) PDA

133. Digoxin toxicity:

(a) 0.5-1 ml (b) 1-15

(c) 1.5-2 (d) > 2.4 ng/all

134. Brugada syndrome–false is:

(a) Na^+ channel defect

(b) Men while sleeping (SCD)

(c) B blocker ↓ mortality

(d) Idiopathic VF

135. Congenital rubella syndrome A/E:

(a) IgG persists for 6 months after delivery

(b) IgM can be detected immediately after birth

(c) Mainly involves hearing defect and cardiac defects

(d) ↑ incidence of defects if infected > 16 weeks

136. Venous to artery shunt:

(a) Blalock-Taussig (b) Glenn

(c) Pott's (d) Waterson

137. Brokenbrough Braunwald phenomenon is:

(a) ↓/normal pulse pressure

(b) ↑ in the gradient

(c) ↓ in the gradient

(d) ↑ in Co

138. Which of the following statements regarding anatomy of tricuspid valve is not correct?

(a) The anterior tricuspid leaflet is the largest

(b) The posterior leaflet is usually the smallest

(c) The septal leaflet is the most mobile

(d) The anterior tricuspid leaflet separates the inflow and outflow tracts of the right ventricle

139. Persistent left superior vena cava results from failure of normal regression of:

(a) Left superior cardinal vein

(b) Right superior cardinal vein

(c) Left inferior cardinal vein

(d) Right inferior cardinal vein

140. Knott-Craig approach is used in the treatment of:

(a) Transposition of great arteries

(b) Ebstein anomaly

(c) Tricuspid atresia

(d) Tetralogy of Fallot

141. True about total anomalous pulmonary venous connection is:

(a) The anomalous connection is most often subdiaphragmatic

(b) ECG shows left axis deviation

(c) ECHO shows marked enlargement of right ventricle and left atrium

(d) In asymptomatic children without pulmonary hypertension, surgery can be deferred to 3-6 months of age

142. All are more common in females than males *except:*

(a) HLHS (b) TGA

(c) Pulmonary atresia (d) None of the above

143. Rashkinds procedure is done in all *except:*

(a) HLHS with restrictive ASD

(b) dTGA without ASD

(c) Tricuspid atresia

(d) ECMO with severe pulmonary edema

144. Manifestations of supra-azygos SVC-obstruction includes all *except:*

(a) Distended arm and neck veins

(b) Congested mucous membrane (mouth)

(c) Dilatation of collateral vessels on anterior and posterior abdominal wall

(d) Edema of neck, face and arms

145. All are ECG findings in Ebstein anomaly *except:*

(a) Peaked P waves in lead II and V_1 reflect RAE

(b) Low voltage is typical

(c) PR interval is generally prolonged

(d) LBBB is common in adults

146. Correct match, all *except:*

(a) PROSPECT–PFO device closure reduces risk of cryptogenic stroke significantly

(b) PROTECT AF–Watchmen device closure of LAA in AF patients is non inferior to warfarin in reducing stroke in AF

(c) EVEREST–Mitraclip reduces morbidity in degenerative mitral regurgitation

(d) PARTNER–TAVR is superior to medical management

147. Goal of phlebotomy in management of cyanosis is:

(a) Control of symptoms (b) Haematocrit <65%

(c) Hb<16 gm/dl (d) Normal MCV

148. All are true about cardiac Situs *except:*

(a) Situs solitus with dextro version is associated with congenital heart disease in more than 90% of cases

(b) Situs inversus with dextrocardia carries a high incidence of congenital heart disease

(c) Situs inversus with levocardia is associated with severe congenital disease in 100% of cases

(d) Upto 80% of patients of situs solitus with dextro version have c-TGA

149. ECG in hypoplastic left heart syndrome shows all *except:*

(a) RAD (b) RAE

(c) RV enlargement (d) Q wave in V6

150. Protein loosing enteropathy following Fontan surgery is characterized by:

(a) High αl-antitrypsin stool clearance

(b) High serum albumin and protein

(c) High plasma lymphocyte

(d) 5-year survival rate of 25-30%

151. Which of the following statements is false regarding echocardiography in post Fontan patient?

(a) Superior and inferior vena cava biphasic and pulmonary artery triphasic flow suggest unobstructed flow in the Fontan circuit

(b) Mean gradient between the Fontan circuit and the pulmonary artery should be 4 mm Hg or greater to represent significant obstruction

(c) Assessment of the pulmonary venous flow is important in detecting pulmonary venous obstruction caused by an enlarged right atrium

(d) TEE may be required if visualization of the Fontan anastomosis is inadequate

152. Which of the following statements is false regarding device closure of an ASD?

(a) Patients should undergo echocardiography every 5 years or so following device closure because of the possibility of late issues like erosion

(b) Device closure is available only for patients with a secundum ASD of stretched diameter of less than 41 mm and adequate margins

(c) Patients should take aspirin and endocarditis prophylaxis for 1 year following device closure

(d) For patients with pulmonary hypertension, closure can be recommended if there is L-R shunt of at least 1.5:1 or evidence of pulmonary artery reactivity to pulmonary vasodilator

153. A 17-year-old male is referred for evaluation of a murmur. Cardiac examination shows normal S1 and S2, no ejection sound with grade III/VI ejection systolic murmur at the right upper sternal border with radiation to the carotids. Blood pressure of the patient is 110/70, the carotid pulses are slightly delayed and the murmur softens with Valsalva. Most likely diagnosis is:

(a) Bicuspid aortic valve

(b) Subvalvular aortic stenosis

(c) Hypertrophic cardiomyopathy

(d) None of the above

154. A 40-year-old female has VSD with L-R shunt and a dilated RV with severe systolic dysfunction on echocardiography. Cauterization study reveals: arterial oxygen saturation–95%, SVC oxygen saturation–48%, JVC oxygen saturation–52%, RA oxygen saturation–61%, RV oxygen saturation–78% PA oxygen saturation–77%, RA–12 mm Hg, RV–62/12 mm HG, PA–63/39 (47) mm Hg, PCWP–14 mm Hg. Pulmonary to systemic shunt fraction is:

(a) 1.8 (b) 2.2

(c) 2.6 (d) 3.0

155. Catheterization study in a patient of pulmonary hypertension reveals following findings: RA–8 mm Hg, RV–68/8 Hg, PA–68/32/43 mm HG, PCWP–25 mm Hg, CO–3 L/min, CI–1.5 L/min/m². The pulmonary vascular resistance (PVR) expressed in wood units (WU) is:
(a) 18 WU (b) 24 WU
(c) 12 WU (d) 6 WU

156. Which of the following statements regarding RA anatomy is true?
(a) The venous component is located anteromedially and receives the systemic venous return from SVC, IVC and coronary venous return from the coronary sinus
(b) Vestibule is a coarsely trabeculated muscular wall around the tricuspid orifice and supports the leaflets of the TV
(c) The right atrial appendage lies over the antero-superior aspect of the right AV groove
(d) Right atrial appendage contains single pectinate muscle, which arise from the crista terminalis

157. Which of the following derivatives of the aortic arches is correctly matched?

ARCH	Arterial derivative
(a) 4th arch left side	Left common carotid and first part of the internal carotid arteries
(b) 4th arch, right side	Arch of the aorta from the left common carotid to the left subclavian arteries
(c) 5th arch	Right and main pulmonary artery
(d) 6th arch, left side	Left pulmonary artery and ductus arteriosus

158. Atrial septostomy done for all *except:*
(a) TOF (b) Tricupid atresia
(c) Pulmonary atresia (d) TGA

159. Down associated with all *except:*
(a) TAPVC (b) ASD
(c) VSD (d) PDA

160. Nakata index for:
(a) > 100 (b) > 200
(c) > 150 (d) > 250

161. Type IV tricuspid atresia:
(a) LTGA (b) DTGA
(c) Pulmonary atresia (d) Truncus arteriosus

162. PA oxygen saturation > mixed venous O_2 sat. S/O:
(a) L → R shunt (b) R → L shunt

163. Graph:

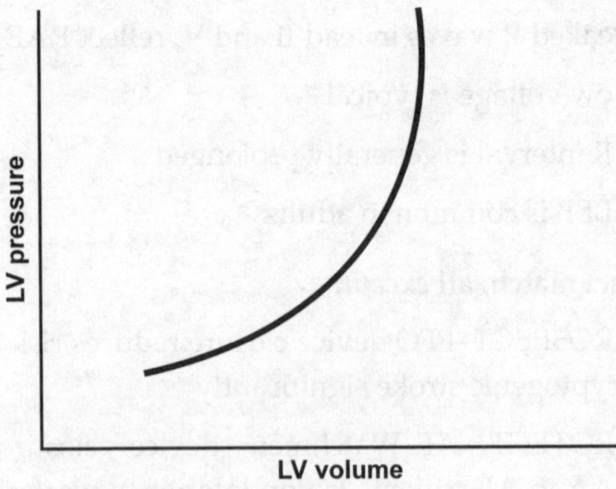

(a) ↓ compliance (b) ↓ compliance

164. Straight left heart border A/E:
(a) Ebstein
(b) Congenital absent left pericardium
(c) CCTGA
(d) None

165. False is:
(a) Situs inversus with dextrocardia has high incidence of CHD
(b) Situs solitus with dextrocardia 80% associated with CCTGA
(c) Situs solitus with dextrocardia 90% associated with CHD
(d) Situs solitus with levocardia associated with–incidence of CHD

166. LA and RA develop from:
(a) Pulmonary vein and sinus venous
(b) Sinus venous and PV
(c) Pulmonary vein and primitive atrium

167. Coronary sinus ostium associated with:
(a) Thebesian valve
(b) Eustachian valve
(c) Chiari network

168. False is:
(a) Maxillary artery develops from 2nd arch
(b) 3rd arch–CCA and ICA
(c) Right 4th–Initial most right SCA
(d) Left 4th arch–arch aorta

169. Diagram–Coronary catheter taken back from LV to aorta:

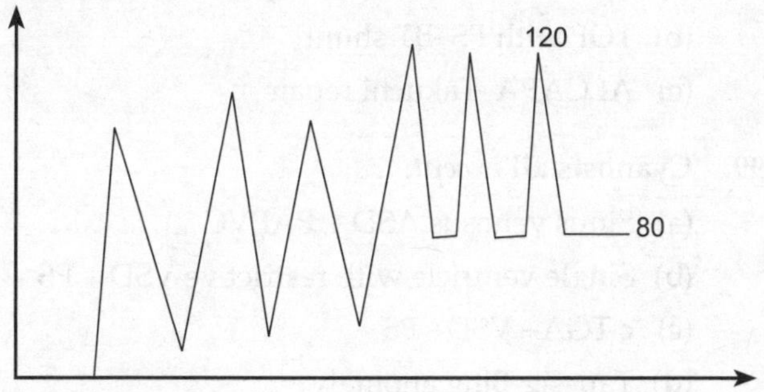

(a) Severe AS
(b) Coronary obstructing flow (LM disease)
(c) HOCM
(d) MS

170. Polydactyly 2 years old + ASD + Finger dysplasia S/O:

(a) Holt-Oram (b) Alagille
(c) Ellis-van Crevald

171. A 2 years old, 3/6 ESM no click, elfin facies + engrossed activity S/O:

(a) Chr 7 (b) Chr 8
(c) Chr 12 (d) Chr 16

172. Patient operated for PS by balloon valvotomy RV pressure becomes = systemic pressure:

(a) Infundibular spasm (b) PR
(c) Re-PS (d) Rupture

173. Crochetage S/O all *except:*

(a) Seen in secundesive ASD, sinus venous ASD and PFO
(b) Notch in R wave (inf. leads)
(c) May be suggested as PFO with aneurysm
(d) Never associated with severity of ASD

174. Wide split S_2 in ASD due to:

(a) ↑ pul. hangout (b) ↓ pul. hangout
(c) ↑ aortic hangout

175. False is:

(a) Veissuns–RAD and LAD
(b) Kugels–Pron RADS PDA of RAD
(c) Collateral never cause myocardial necrosis

176. Ross procedure:

(a) Transport of pulmonary value at aortic valve
(b) Useful in elderly
(c) Mechanical valve

177. OS ASD best view:

(a) Subcostal view (b) Suprasternal view
(c) PLAX (d) PSAX

178. Difference in BP in 2 arms in supravalvular AS is due to:

(a) Conda (b) Ohm law
(c) Bernoulli

179. BP difference in 2 arms > 10 mm Hg and murmur radiating to carotid:

(a) Supravalvular AS (b) Valvular AS
(c) HOCM

180. Single ....S2 in Eisenmenger.

(a) PDA (b) VSD
(c) ASD (d) AV canal defect

181. Ground glass appearance:

(a) Obstructed TAPVC
(b) AS with AR
(c) PAPVC
(d) Obstructed systemic venous return

182. Stenosis at pulmonary valve in TOF:

(a) Infundibular level (b) Valvular level
(c) Subpulmonary level (d) Supravalvular level

183. Most common congenital heart disease:

(a) Bicuspid aortic valve (b) VSD
(c) ASD (d) PDA

184. Noonan syndrome A/E:

(a) AS (b) Left axis deviation
(c) Lymphedema (d) Mental retardation

185. 12-year-old child of Pink TOF with 93% saturation, which is in correct:

(a) MAPCAs are uncommon
(b) PS is mild
(c) Early surgical intervention

186. True about tricuspid atresia:

(a) Current treatment are only palliative
(b) Associated with Down syndrome
(c) LAD is universal
(d) Always associated with reduced PBF

187. Full term neonate, highest oxygen saturation is:

(a) Ductus arteriosus (b) Pulmonary artery
(c) Descending aorta (d) Carotids

188. Shone's complex A/E:
(a) Supramitral rug (b) Cortriatriatum
(c) Congenital MS (d) AS

189. Cyanosis A/E:
(a) Single ventricle without PS
(b) ccTGA with VSD with PS
(c) Taussig-Bing anomaly
(d) Sinus venosus ASD with PAPVC

190. Bicuspid aortic valve–inheritance:
(a) AD (b) AR
(c) XR (d) XD

191. For PFO *except:*
(a) Special Doppler required
(b) Probe at internal carotid artery
(c) Agitated normal saline
(d) Can be used in SAH

192. Cath data—saturation MvO_2= 73%, PA= 85%, Ao = 98% true for L-R shunt:
(a) 2 : 1 (b) 3 : 1
(c) 3 : 2 (d) 5 : 3

193. Right to left shunt through atrial septum A/E:
(a) Ebstein (b) Eisenmenger
(c) RVMI (d) Coronary sinus ASD

194. All true *except:*
(a) VSD Eisenmenger can have cardiomegaly
(b) ASD Eisenmenger can have TR
(c) TR may be seen in PDA Eisenmenger
(d) No heave seen in VSD Eisenmenger

195. Part of atrial septum A/E:
(a) Limbus of fossa ovalis
(b) Torus aorticus
(c) Nodule arensis

196. Noonan syndrome A/E:
(a) AS (b) Lymphedema
(c) LAD

197. Congenital CHB A/E:
(a) QT prolongation has no role in prognosis
(b) HR > 80/min does not need PPI
(c) R-R interval varying with phasic arrhythmias

198. All true *except:*
(a) Truncus arteriosus–venopulmonary anastomoses
(b) TOF with PS–BT shunt
(c) ALCAPA–Takuchi repair

199. Cyanosis all *except:*
(a) Sinus venosus ASD + PAPVC
(b) Single ventricle with restrictive VSD + PS
(c) c TGA+ VSD+ PS
(d) Taussig-Bing anomaly

200. Bicuspid aortic valve:
(a) AD (b) AR
(c) XD (d) XR

201. Shone complex all *except:*
(a) Cortriatriatum
(b) AS
(c) Congenital MS
(d) Supravalve mitral membrane

202. Procedure all *except:*
(a) ALCAPA–Takauchi
(b) Truncus arteriosus–REV
(c) Single ventricle–Takashewa procedure
(d) TOF with VSD with PS–Blalock-Taussig shunt

203. Pulmonary blood flow by:
(a) VO_2/ pulmonary Venous O_2 saturation–pulmonary arterial O_2 saturation
(b) VO_2/pulmonary Venous O_2 saturation – IVC satuartion
(c) VO_2/ pulmonary Venous O_2 saturation – aortic saturation

204. Ross procedure indications all *except:*
(a) Young individual (b) BAV
(c) Rheumatic AS (d) C/I for anticoagulation

205. Day 1 neonate with soft systolic murmur with hepatomegaly, no cyanosis all *except:*
(a) Large VSD with PAH
(b) Ebstein's anomaly
(c) Severe AS
(d) Vein of Galen malformation

206. 25-year-old female presents with history of syncope and breathlessness on exertion, CXR–PA view and lateral view–prominent right descending PA, oligemia, diagnosis:

(a) IPAH (b) Valvular PS
(c) Scimitar syndrome (d) Sarcoidosis

207. Aorto-tricuspid continuity seen in:
(a) Holmes heart
(b) TGA (complete)
(c) DORV with transposition
(d) Normal heart

208. Which one is wrong?
(a) Holt Oram–12q 24 (b) Carney–12q
(c) William–7q 11.23 (d) Digeorge–22q 11

209. Continuous mumur all *except:*
(a) Obstructive TAPVC
(b) Peripheral PA stenosis
(c) TOF with absent PV
(d) Restrictive ASD with MS

210. All true *except:*
(a) Absent Q in V5 V6 in D–TGA
(b) LAD with LVH in SV with PS
(c) RVH with early transition in TOF
(d) Himalayan 'P' wave–Ebstein's anomaly

211. Pulmonary venoclusive disease all *except:*
(a) Resemble PPH
(b) > 2/3rd have vasodilator response
(c) PCWP ↑ed
(d) CTPE common

212. ↑ed LA pressure in MS all *except:*
(a) Ball valve thrombus
(b) ASD
(c) Acute MI
(d) LA myxoma

213. Day 1 neonate tachypnoea, S3+, JVP ↑ed, Hepatomegaly, no cyanosis with soft systolic murmur all *except:*
(a) Severe PAH with VSD
(b) Severe anemia
(c) Vein of galen malformation
(d) COA

214. Neonates 2 days cyanosis Pa O_2=80%, PFO +, R-L shunt least likely:
(a) PPH of newborn (b) TGA with IVS
(c) Severe Ebstein (d) TAPVC

215. All associated with 22q11 *except:*
(a) TOF (b) Truncus arteriosus
(c) TAA (d) ECD

216. 1 day old neonate loud precordial murmur:
(a) TGA
(b) Transient ischemia of newborn
(c) Supracristal large VSD
(d) HLHS

217. Cyanosis in 1 week child all *except:*
(a) Ebstein (b) Critical AS
(c) AP window (d) TGA

218. Ebstein anomaly indication for surgery all *except:*
(a) CT ratio > 0.65 (b) Carpenter type IV
(c) SpO_2– 65% (d) Paradoxical embolism

219. Continuous murmur all *except:*
(a) Gerbode defect
(b) Peripheral PS
(c) COA
(d) Mitral atresia with ASD

220. ECG of ASD with 'P' wave inversion in II III AVF:
(a) Sinus venosus ASD (b) ECD primary ASD
(c) TAPVC (d) Lutembacher

221. 6 years old female evaluated for congenital HD ECG showing ↓ P in I, AVL with –ve QRS:
(a) Lead reversal (b) DORV
(c) Dextrocardia

222. Gerbode defect:
(a) LV-RA shunt (b) LV-RV shunt
(c) LA-RA shunt

223. Pseudo beats of stokes:
(a) CHB with atrial contraction
(b) MVP
(c) TR

224. Taussig-Bing syndrome is a type of:
(a) DORV (b) DILV
(c) TGA

225. Infant bounding pulse with large heart and normal echo:
(a) Vein of galen malformation
(b) Infracardiac TAPVC
(c) Intracardiac TAPVC
(d) AR

226. Type B PDA:
(a) Aortic root is large
(b) Pulmonary root is larger
(c) Both same
(d) PDA with constriction

227. Eisenmenger seen in A/E:
(a) TAPVC
(b) Large VSD
(c) Large ASD in 4th decade
(d) A-P window
(e) VSD with AR

228. Loud P_2 A/E:
(a) PAH
(b) PS
(c) Eisenmenger's syndrome
(d) VSD

229. Cyanosis in a patient clubbing develops after:
(a) 3 months (b) 1 year
(c) 2 months (d) Simultaneously

230. Pulmonary stenosis true:
(a) Most adults present asymptomatic
(b) Dysplastic PV in 50% cases
(c) Surgery is TOC

231. Pregnancy C/I in:
(a) Eisenmenger syndrome
(b) CoA
(c) MR
(d) ASD

232. BAV fusion most common between:
(a) Right and non coronary cusp
(b) Left and non coronary cusp
(c) Right and left coronary cusp
(d) None

233. Most common type of ECD in Down's:
(a) Type A (b) Type B
(c) Type C (d) None

234. Highest risk of congenital malformation in baby with mother of:
(a) Madan's (b) ASD
(c) VSD (d) TOF

235. Most common coronary anomaly in TGA:
(a) Single left anterior descending
(b) Single RCA
(c) LCX from RCA

236. Inverted IVC seen in:
(a) Asplenta (b) Polysplenia
(c) Down's syndrome (d) All

237. In situs solitus with dextroversion most common:
(a) D-TGA (b) C-TGA
(c) TAPVC (d) TOF

238. Increase pulmonary blood floss in all *except*:
(a) Tr. atresia (b) HLHS
(c) TGA (d) Device malformation

239. 2 months old with ESM with cyanosis with decrease pulmonary vascularity with LAD diagnosis is:
(a) Ebstein (b) Tricuspid atresia
(c) TOF (d) WA

240. Both Stridor and Dyspnoea seen in:
(a) Double aortic arch
(b) Left aortic arch + aberrant right subclavian artery
(c) Right aortic arch + aberrant left subclavian artery
(d) Right aortic arch with mirror image

241. TOF all *except*:
(a) VSD distal to RVOT obstruction in some patients
(b) 4 criteria
(c) Pseudo TOF resembles TOF

242. Most common coronary artery anomaly:
(a) AV fistula (b) ALCAPA
(c) LCx from RCA (d) LCA from right sinus

243. Eisenmenger all *except*:
(a) Familial disposition→small size
(b) Worse prognosis with congenital than PPH
(c) All may not have cyanosis at rest
(d) All

244. Pulmonary AV fistula associated with:
(a) Osler Weber Rendu syndrome
(b) Wegener granulomatosis

245. Increase pulmonary blood flow + cyanosis:
(a) Ebstein (b) TAPVC
(c) TA

246. Congenital absence of pericardium:
(a) Heart shift to left
(b) Hypermobility on Echo and paradoxical septal movement
(c) Bradycardia
(d) Apical impulse

247. Most common coronary arterial anomaly:
(a) ALCAPA
(b) LAD from Right Anterior sinus
(c) LCX from RCA
(d) Coronary AV fistula

248. Ideal time for surgery in asymptomatic CoA:
(a) < 1 year (b) 3-5 years
(c) 5-10 years (d) 20-30 years

249. RVSP > LVSP in:
(a) Eisenmenger VSD (b) Valvular PS
(c) Eisenmenger PDA (d) TOF

250. Conotruncal anomaly beyond 1 month of age:
(a) HLHS (b) Interrupted aortic arch
(c) Severe TOF (d) TGA

251. Which of the following not diagnosed in 1 week:
(a) Large VSD (b) TOF
(c) AS (d) PS

252. Asplenia-polysplenia syndromes are associated with:
(a) Situs ambiguous
(b) Mirror image dextrocardia
(c) Single atrium

253. All are features of CHF in infants *except*:
(a) Flaring of alar nasi (b) Oedema
(c) Thready pulse

254. PCWP =30 which correspond to:
(a) PASP = 60 PADP = 30 MEAN = 40
(b) PASP = 60 PADP = 20 MEAN = 30

255. Bounding pulse in infant is seen in 1st day:
(a) PDA (b) Hypoxia
(c) Systemic AV fistula

256. Most common cause of CHF in 1st week:
(a) HLHS (b) TGA
(c) Large VSD

257. BT shunt:
(a) PA to ipsilateral SCA (b) PA to descending aorta

258. Rib notching seen in all *except*:
(a) BT shunt (b) COA
(c) Aortoarteritis (d) All

259. Treatment of TOF in less than 1 year of age:
(a) Total correction (b) BT shunt

260. ASD with systolic thrill at pulmonic area s/o:
(a) MS (b) AS
(c) Large ASD

261. Continuous murmur seen in A/E:
(a) PDA with Eisenmenger
(b) Coronary AV fistula

262. Peripheral PS all *except:*
(a) William syndrome (b) Noonan syndrome
(c) Rubella (d) Holt-Oram syndrome

263. LA dilatation seen in all *except:*
(a) Large ASD (b) Large VSD
(c) Large PDA (d) Severe MS

264. Supra systemic pressure seen in:
(a) PS with intact IVS
(b) Eisenmenger syndrome

265. Earliest sign of pulmonary venous pressure increase:
(a) Kerley B line (b) Cephalisation

266. Cannon a waves in:
(a) VT (b) Pulmonary stenosis
(c) Tricuspid stenosis

267. cc- TGA A/E:
(a) Ventricular inversion
(b) Systemic venous return to RA
(c) Die as young
(d) CHB seen

268. Egg on side appearance:
(a) d-TGA (b) Ebstein anomaly
(c) DORV

269. Maximum life expectancy:
(a) Ebstein anomaly (b) TGA

270 ASD not seen:
(a) TAPVC (b) COA
(c) Ebstein anomaly (d) TGA

271. In ECD which is not seen:
(a) Inlet VSD (b) Primum ASD
(c) Thickened AML

272. Supracristal VSD view:
(a) PLAX (b) PSAX
(c) AP-4C (d) AP- 2C

273. Pulmonary valvuloplasty not useful in:
(a) Infundibular PS (b) Pulmonary atresia
(c) PS with cyanosis (d) PS with CCF

274. CHB A/E:
(a) cc-TGA (b) Anti-Ro
(c) All true

275. **LV saturation:**
(a) 95% (b) 97%
(c) 100% (d) 85 %

276. **LAD A/E:**
(a) ECD
(b) TOF
(c) Multiple VSD
(d) Single ventricle LV type

277. **Ostium primum A/E:**
(a) Cleft MV (b) Inlet VSD
(c) RAD

278. **Pulmonary venous desaturation seen:**
(a) ARDS (b) Pulmonary AV fistula

279. **10 weeks child with MI:**
(a) ALCAPA (b) Hyper cholesterolemia

280. **Fondaparinux:**
(a) Anticoagulant (b) Antianginal agent
(c) Antiplatelet

281. **Single S2 seen in A/E:**
(a) Pulmonary atresia (b) Eisenmenger
(c) Moderate PS (d) Truncus arteriosus

282. **Fetal echocardiography best:**
(a) 16-29 weeks (b) 29-36 weeks
(c) 26-29 weeks

283. **Cyanotic spells A/E:**
(a) TOF (b) Tricuspid atresia
(c) Pulmonary atresia (d) Pulmonary stenosis

284. **Most common cause of CNS involvement in TOF:**
(a) Polycythemia (b) Brain abscess
(c) Paradoxical emboli

285. **Ebstein anomaly A/E:**
(a) Reverse split of S2 (b) Pre excitation
(c) Atrial flutter (d) ASD

286. **Cyanosis not caused by:**
(a) Hb-6 gm% with 50% saturation
(b) Hb-20 gm% with 75% saturation
(c) Hb-18 gm% with 60% saturation

287. **SVR:**
(a) 10-20 wood units (b) 20-30 wood units
(c) 50-100 wood units (d) 5-10 wood units

288. **PVR:**
(a) 30-130 dyne cm^{-5} (b) 10-20 dyne cm^{-5}
(c) 20-30 dyne cm^{-5}

289. **LVEDP normal value:**
(a) < 12 mm Hg (b) <18 mm Hg
(c) < 22 mm Hg (d) < 25 mm Hg

290. **Mean PAP:**
(a) < 19 mm Hg (b) < 25 mm Hg
(c) < 30 mm Hg (d) 35 mm Hg

291. **Cyanosis begin in TOF at:**
(a) 2–6 months (b) 1 year
(c) 2 years (d) 18 months

292. **Most common congenital abnormalities:**
(a) BAV (b) VSD
(c) ASD (d) MVP

293. **Neonate–COA, best management**
(a) Surgery with patch correction
(b) Angioplasty
(c) Stent insertion
(d) Medical treatment

294. **ASD in mother, recurrence in child:**
(a) 2% (b) 4%
(c) 6% (d) 8%

295. **Asplenia all true *except:***
(a) Eparterial bronchi
(b) More common in males
(c) Superior p axis
(d) Bilateral right atria

296. **Likely diagnosis:**
(a) ASD (b) VSD
(c) PDA (d) Veno-occlusive disease
(e) PPH

297. **TOF with pregnancy: (T/F)**
(a) Fully corrected without residual shunt tolerate well
(b) ↓ Peripheral resistance and ↑ CO, cyanosis improved
(c) BT shunt before pregnancy tolerate well because of ↑ CO

(d) In p/o PR, patient with RVD
(e) Pregnancy causes improvement in symptoms

298. Turner's syndrome:
(a) COA (b) Male sex
(c) PAPVC (d) Aortic dissection
(e) Tall stature

299. Female preponderance in CHD *except:*
(a) PDA (b) ASD
(c) Ebstein (d) TA
(e) Juxtaposition of atrial appendage

300. ASD true all *except:*
(a) MDM at apex, large L-R shunt
(b) F > M = 2:1
(c) Wide and fixed split
(d) Systolic murmur at pulmonary area

301. Eisenmenger all *except:*
(a) In VSD develops at 2-5 years
(b) Rare in VSD with AR
(c) Irreversible
(d) Differential cyanosis with PDA

302. Heart border on CXR above downward:
(a) Ao-PT-LAA-LV (b) Ao-PT-LA-LV
(c) PT-Ao-LA-LV (d) PT-Ao-LAA-LV

303. A/E:
(a) PDA runs is post IV groove
(b) Supply inferior IVS
(c) PDA supply collateral if proximal LAD block
(d) Left dominant more common than right

304. Eisenmenger: (T/F)
(a) ↑ Maternal mortality
(b) VSD with AR seldoms occur with Eisenmenger
(c) Large VSD develops 2-5 years

305. Cyanosis spell in TOF: (T/F)
(a) Ppt by crying, feeding
(b) Inaudible murmur
(c) <2 years uncommon
(d) Apnoea + loss of consciousness
(e) RVOT dynamic obstruction ↑ adr. activity

306. Most common right aortic arch anomaly:
(a) Double AO arch (b) Common type
(c) Avion (d) Gothic
(e) None

307. Device closure:
(a) Small muscular VSD
(b) PDA
(c) Coronary AV fistula
(d) Primum ASD

308. ASD all *except:*
(a) F : M – 2:1
(b) Operate if Qp/Qs=1.5:1
(c) Systolic flow murmur in pulmonary area
(d) Diastolic flow murmur at apex if large L-R shunt
(e) Wide fixed split

309. Cortriatriatum true *except:*
(a) Because defective resorption of common pulmonary vien
(b) Surgical correction is treatment of choice
(c) ↑ PVR and PCWP
(d) Presentation resembles congenital pulmonary vein stenosis

310. Reversible differential cyanosis in:
(a) TGA with PDA with COA
(b) cc-TGA with PDA with COA
(c) Taussig Bing with PDA with COA
(d) PDA with reversal

311. Female preponderance in CHD *except:*
(a) PDA (b) ASD
(c) Ebstein's anomaly (d) TA
(e) Juxtaposition of atrial appendage

312. Peripheral PS all *except:*
(a) Rubella (b) Alegille's syndrome
(c) William's syndrome (d) Down's syndrome
(e) TOF

313. 2 years child with weak distal pulses true:
(a) Immediate surgery
(b) Ribnotching in X-ray in majority of cases
(c) Most will have claudication
(d) Survival without surgery upto 30 years

314. Cyanotic with wide pulse pressure all *except:*
(a) PDA with reversal (b) TOF with collateral
(c) Pulmonary atresia (d) Ebstein

315. Pulsus paradoxus absent in all *except:*

(a) ASD (b) LV dysfunction
(c) Malignant etiology (d) IPPV

316. Epigastric pulsations: (T/F)

(a) TOF
(b) Descending aortic aneurysm
(c) RV aneurysm
(d) Left lobe liver aneurysm
(e) RVH

317. Indication of VSD surgery all *except:*

(a) Restrictive VSD
(b) All subpulmonary VSD
(c) VSD with AR
(d) Large VSD

318. 2 days old, acyanotic with murmur left sternal SM with ECG/X-ray chest normal:

(a) VSD (b) PDA
(c) TOF (d) TGA

319. Loud P_2:

(a) Ebstein (b) TOF
(c) TGA (d) Truncus arteriosus
(e) TAPVC (f) Common atrium

320. Type A PDA:

(a) Wider at pulmonary end
(b) Tubular lesion
(c) Multiple indentations
(d) Difficult to close by catheter
(e) Wider at aortic end

321. Clubbing after cyanosis:

(a) 1 month (b) 12 months
(c) 3 months (d) 1 year

322. Marfan major criteria:

(a) Ectopic lentis
(b) Ao dissection
(c) Spontaneous pneumothorax
(d) Dolicosternomelia

323. Eisenmenger syndrome not seen in:

(a) AP window (b) ASD after 40 years
(c) VSD with AR (d) TAPVC

324. Pulmonary stenosis all *except:* (T/F)

(a) Valvuloplasty is best for infant/neonate
(b) Most valvular
(c) In valvular PS/dysplastic
(d) Most adult asymptomatic
(e) Valvular replacement in dysplastic

325. 8-11 old sport grade III ejection murmur asymptomatic thumb like finger normal growth:

(a) Holt-Oram (b) Leopard
(c) Turner (d) Noonan
(e) Kartagener

326. Pregnancy C/I:

(a) Eisenmenger (b) MR
(c) HOCM (d) COA

327. Himalayan p wave seen in:

(a) Ebstein anomaly (b) Eisenmenger
(c) ASD

328. VSD: (T/F)

(a) Size of VSD directly proportional to endocarditis
(b) Doubly committed with Eisenmenger has more AR
(c) Muscular VSD may close in child and young adult
(d) May cause progressive sub aortic and sub pulmonary obstruction

329. Incomplete AV defect T/F:

(a) Cleft anterior mitral valve
(b) Down's syndrome
(c) Right axis deviation
(d) Ostium primum

330. Nonnan's all *except:*

(a) AR
(b) 80-90% cardiac involved
(c) Valvular PS most common
(d) Dysplastic pulmonary valve seen
(e) Asymmetric HCM

331. Most common in Turner's all *except:*

(a) Post ductal coarctation
(b) HLHS
(c) BAV
(d) Asc. Ao dilatation

332. Neonatal coarctation:
(a) Angioplasty (b) Angioplasty + stent
(c) PG infusion (d) Surgery with patch

333. Peripheral cyanosis seen in:
(a) TOF
(b) Peripheral vascular disease
(c) COPD
(d) VSD
(e) Pulmonary embolism

334. Treatment of congenital CHB:
(a) AAI pacemaker
(b) Dual chamber pacemaker
(c) Dual chamber ICD
(d) α-agonist

335. Down's false is:
(a) Primum ASD (b) RAD
(c) Cleft MV (d) Hyperthyroidism
(e) ↑ incidence of pulmonary HTN

336. ↑ birth weight with cyanosis is seen in:
(a) d–TGA (b) l-TGA
(c) HLHS

337. Norwood procedure is done in:
(a) HLHS (b) DORV with PS
(c) C-TGA (d) D-TGA

338. O_2 step up in PA in all *except:*
(a) AVSD (b) AP window
(c) TAPVC (d) Subpulmonic VSD

339. Precocious PAH in Down's syndrome is due to:
(a) ↑ Adenoid, tonsils
(b) Small nose, small pharynx
(c) ↓ sed/malformation by terminal alveolar units
(d) Flaccid hypopharynx
(e) All

340. Fetal circulation factors ↑ O_2 in brain all *except:*
(a) HbF
(b) Most of IVC blood shunted to LA
(c) Most SVC blood shunted to RV, PA and descending aorta
(d) Aorta isthmus stenosis

341. Down's syndrome associated with:
(a) Ostium primum ASD
(b) RAD
(c) Cleft mitral valve
(d) Hyperthyroidism
(e) Rapid progression of pulmonary vascular disease

342. Turner's syndrome false: (T/F)
(a) AO dissection can occur
(b) COA
(c) Long stature
(d) Male sex

343. Subarterial VSD:
(a) Pulmonary regurgitation occurs/associated
(b) Spontaneous closure occur
(c) Should be followed up if <5 mm and asymptomatic
(d) Should be closed even if R-L shunt occurs
(e) More in caucasians

344. Cyanotic spells:
(a) Can be absent in mild right out flow obstruction
(b) Precipitated by crying and feeding
(c) ↑ sed by adrenaline
(d) Afterload ↑ sed by squatting–cyanosis ↓ ses

345. VSD pansystolic murmur all *except:*
(a) Large VSD associated with loud murmur
(b) Eisenmenger with VSD

346. Single S_2:
(a) TOF (severe) (b) Pulmonary atresia
(c) Single ventricle (d) VSD with Eisenmenger

347. Norwood procedure true is:
(a) HLHS (b) TGA
(c) TOF (d) Tricuspid atresia

348. Which of the following is a cyanotic condition?
(a) Hemi anomalous pulmonary venous connection 36
(b) Post Hemi Fontan surgery
(c) Hernitruncus
(d) AV canal defect

349. Increased body weight at birth in:
(a) TOF (b) PS
(c) TGA (d) HLHS

350. ASD with cyanosis in all *except:*
(a) ASD with Eisenmenger
(b) ASD with TAPVC
(c) Common atrium
(d) ASD with PAPVC
(e) AVSD

351. Down's syndrome all *except:*
(a) Incidences rise exponentially with increasing maternal age
(b) 40-50% associated with congenital heart diseases
(c) ECD most common
(d) Surgery gives poor result in comparison to W/O down syndrome
(e) Increased incidence of pulmonary hypertension

352. O_2 step up at PA level:
(a) Outlet VSD
(b) Aorto pulmonary window
(c) TAPVC

353. TAPVC all *except:*
(a) Infradiaphragmatic type is non-obstructive
(b) O_2 saturation same in all 4 chambers
(c) 80% mortality in first year of life

354. Non dysplastic pulmonary valve:
(a) Usually unicuspid and a commissural
(b) Pulmonary valvulotomy useful
(c) S_1-EC duration increases with severity
(d) Post stenotic dilatation

355. Congenital AS true all *except:*
(a) Usually bicuspid
(b) Diamond shape murmur and symmetry of murmur does not change with severity
(c) Male > female

356. Clubbing occurs in cyanosis after:
(a) At appearance (b) 1-2 years
(c) 2-4 years (d) 5-6 years

357. Hypoxic spell true all *except:*
(a) Initiated by feeding
(b) Child becomes limpless
(c) Occur in pulmonary stress
(d) Related to degree of cyanosis

358. In TOF, aortic click:
(a) Varies with inspiration
(b) Varies with expiration

359. TOF after corrective surgery:
(a) SCD after 10 years–10%
(b) Normal prognosis
(c) VT never occurs

360. Ebstein's anomaly all *except:*
(a) Type A WPW (b) Type B WPW

361. Coarctation of aorta, true all *except:*
(a) Figure of E due to aorta above C_3
(b) Bilateral rib notching
(c) Occur below age 2 years
(d) CCF in infancy

362. Supravalvular AS gene:
(a) Elastin gene (b) Troponin
(c) Beta MHC

363. Prostaglandin infusion worsen:
(a) Obstructive TAPVC
(b) Hypolastic left ventricle
(c) Interrupted aortic arch
(d) Pulmonary atresia without VSD

364. Continuous murmur A/E:
(a) Peripheral PS (b) BT shunt
(c) ASD with MS (d) RSOV into LV

365. Pink TOF due to A/E:
(a) Degree of RV hypertrophy is minimal
(b) No cyanosis
(c) No significant left to right shunt
(d) All true

366. Which of the following presents with NYHA class III HF with near normal JVP?
(a) ASD with MS
(b) Ebstein's anomaly
(c) Ruptured sinus of valsalva aneurysm
(d) EMF

367. All of the following are examples of early systolic murmur *except:*
(a) Acute MR
(b) Non-restrictive VSD with pulmonary ARTERIAL hypertension
(c) TOF with absent pulmonary valve
(d) Low pressure tricuspid regurgitation

368. A balloon atrial septostomy may be beneficial in all of the following condition *except:*
(a) Mitral atresia
(b) Primary pulmonary hypertension
(c) Unbalanced AV septal defect
(d) Pulmonary atresia with intact septum

369. Indentify the wrong match:

(a) Corrected transposition–Rastelli

(b) Tricuspid atresia–Fontan

(c) Transposition physiology–Rev operation

(d) Single ventricle physiology with IVC interruption – Kawashima repair

370. All of the following indicate operability in a child with VSD with severe pulmonary ARTERIAL hypertension *except:*

(a) Q waves in lateral leads

(b) RA/RV overload in echocardiogram

(c) Absence of exercise induced ARTERIAL desaturation

(d) Cardiomegaly on X-ray

371. In which Eisenmenger syndrome, cardiomegaly is noted?

(a) ASD (b) VSD

(c) PSD (d) AP Window

372. Complication of PGE2 infusion include all of the following *except:*

(a) Apnea (b) Hypercalcemia

(c) Hypotension (d) Pyloric stenosis

373. All are true about coronary sinus *except:*

(a) It lies posterior to the tricuspid valve

(b) It lies in the right AV groove

(c) It may be absent in left isomerism

(d) It is dilated in the presence of persistent left superior vena cava

374. Right ventricle is identified by the:

(a) Absence of gross trabeculations

(b) Connection to the right atrium

(c) Connection to the pulmonary artery

(d) Septal attachment of the atrioventricular value

375. Best way to determine situs is:

(a) Assessment of the abdominal visceral situs

(b) Assessment of the relationship of abdominal aorta and IVC

(c) Assessment of the relationship of aortic and pulmonary valve

(d) Assessment of bronchial situs

376. Which of the following is not an anatomical part of the interatrial septum?

(a) Limbus fossa ovalis (b) PFO

(c) Noduli arranti (d) Torus aorticus

377. Which of the following is an accepted indication for percutaneous pulmonary valve replacement:

(a) Severe PR following TOF repair

(b) Truncus arteriosus

(c) Severe pulmonary artery bifurcation narrowing

(d) ToF with absent pulmonary valve

378. Which one of the following is FALSE about sinoatrial node location?

(a) Located in Myocardium Just Internal to Epicardium

(b) At posterolateral aspect of right atrium

(c) Right atrium SVC junction

(d) Identified as a bulge on the surface of heart

379. A 5-year-old boy with cyanosis and 2/6 ESM in pulmonary area is likely to have:

(a) DORV, large VSD with PS

(b) Valvular PS with intact septum

(c) Tricuspid atresia, VSD with PS

(d) Ebstein's anomaly

380. A 6-day-old neonate had presented to casualty with the following X-ray. The likely diagnosis is:

(a) Tetralogy of Fallot

(b) Transposition of great vessels

(c) Obstructed infra-diaphragmatic TAPVC

(d) Diaphragmatic hernia

381. Following are true about Lambl's excrescences *except:*

(a) Age related thickening along nodule of Arantis and closing edges cusps

(b) Associated with cardioembolic stroke

(c) May have appearance of a sea anemone

(d) Present on posterior wall of left atrium

382. Following are true about cardiac skeleton *except:*

(a) Right fibrous trigone forms the largest and strongest component

(b) Bundle of His passes through Right fibrous trigone

(c) It welds together all cardiac valves

(d) Fibrous trigone forms the anatomic substrate for direct mitral-aortic continuity

383. About scimitar syndrome, all are true *except:*
(a) Connection of right pulmonary veins to IVC
(b) Hypoplasia of ipsilateral lung
(c) Supply of right lung by systemic veins
(d) Left lung involvement common

384. Ebstein's anomaly commonly A/E: (T/F)
(a) PSVT–75%
(b) Accessory Pathway–25%
(c) Gross cardiomegaly can be seen
(d) Bimodel age distribution
(e) Mild cases can survive upto adult hood

385. Following are true about ruptured sinus of valsalva aneurysm *except:*
(a) M:F ratio 4:1
(b) Continuous murmur peaks around S2
(c) Mostly occurs in young <30 years age
(d) Unruptured aneurysm may cause ejection murmur

386. In choussat's criteria for Fontana operation in Tricuspid Atresia, all are true *except:*
(a) Age of operation <4 years
(b) Presence of normal right atrial volume
(c) Mean pulmonary artery pressure <15 mm Hg
(d) Pulmonary vascular resistance <4 woods unit/m^2

387. What is not true about risk of SCD in patients post-TOP repair surgery?
(a) Upto 100 times greater risk than general population
(b) Usually occurs in first 20 years after repair
(c) QRS duration > 180 msec predicts SCD
(d) Further increases 20 years after repair

388. In cor-triatriatum, all are true *except:*
(a) Loud first heart sound
(b) Physical signs are due to pulmonary hypertension
(c) Interatrial membrane is proximal to LA appendage
(d) Associated with high frequency diastolic oscillations of mitral valve

389. Anomalous origin of the left coronary artery from the pulmonary artery in adult true all *except:*
(a) Sudden death is rare
(b) Mitral regurgitation can occur
(c) Can cause heart failure
(d) Surgery is curative

390. Fetal heart failure is least likely to be caused by:
(a) Ebstein anomaly (b) Isolated large VSD
(c) Bradycardia (d) Haemoglobinopathy

391. Notch 1 mutations are identified in patients with:
(a) Long QT syndromes
(b) Transposition of Great Vessels
(c) Left sided obstructive lesions
(d) Right sided obstructive lesions

392. The arterial switch surgery requires:
(a) Reduced pulmonary blood flow
(b) Oxygen saturation of >80%
(c) Functionally competent LV
(d) Infant aged at least 6 months

393. Long term results in treatment for coarctation of aorta depends upon:
(a) Systemic arterial hypertension
(b) Age at repair
(c) Residual coarctation
(d) All of the above

394. In a new born HF is not a resenting symptom in:
(a) TOP
(b) HLHS
(c) Sustained tachycardia
(d) Myocarditis

395. Which is not a feature of Alagille syndrome?
(a) Butterfly like vertebral anomaly
(b) Autosomal recessive
(c) Peripheral PS
(d) Intrahepatic cholestasis

396. Goose neck is described for:
(a) VSD (b) TGA
(c) AVSD (d) ASD

397. Presence of a pan systolic murmur at birth means:
(a) A large VSD
(b) A PDA with increased PVR
(c) A tricuspid regurgitation
(d) An innocent murmur

398. Left to right shunt in a given size of ADS depends mainly upon:
(a) Location of defect
(b) Compliance of the ventricles
(c) Gradient between LA and RA
(d) Pulmonary blood flow

399. Left atrial isomerism is associated with all *except:*
(a) Male predominance
(b) Bilateral Bilobed Lungs
(c) Absent or atretic sinus node
(d) Polysplenia

400. Batista procedure:
(a) Endoventricular repair Dacron patch (DOR procedure)
(b) Percutaneous mitral valve repair
(c) Latissmus dorsii myoplasty
(d) LV reduction surgery–partial ventriculectomy

401. Ross procedure true is:
(a) Used in elderly population
(b) Long term anticoagulation not required
(c) Can be used in rheumatic heart disease
(d) Pulmonary and aortic homograft are used in it

402. Most common arrhythmias in children:
(a) AVRT (b) AVNRT
(c) Junctional tachycardia (d) VT

403. True is:
(a) Sones–performed first angiography
(b) Grossman–pulmonary valve implantation
(c) Kirklin–ICD

404. Venous drainage of RV through:
(a) Thebesian vein
(b) Coronary sinus
(c) Oblique vein of Marshall
(d) Anterior cardiac vein

405. True about ASD:
(a) Sinus venosus ASD–negative p wave in inferior lead
(b) ASD primum–RAD
(c) ASD secundum–LAD

406. In ASD, possible reason for cyanosis:
(a) Sinus venosus ASD
(b) Unroofed coronary sinus
(c) Persistence of Eustachian valve directing blood from IVC to LA
(d) ASD with severe PS

407. Duct dependent lesion A/E:
(a) HLHS (b) COA
(c) PA with intact IVS (d) TAPVC

408. COA true:
(a) HTN persist after surgery in elderly
(b) With repair of COA, survival is like normal person
(c) Patient is asked to do static exercise

409. DiGeorge syndrome:
(a) Abnormal genitalia (b) Cardiac defects
(c) Thymus hypoplasia (d) Cleft palate

410. Suicidal RV:
(a) RV cardiomyopathy
(b) Conal artery ablation
(c) RVOT VT
(d) Transient RVOT obstruction following BPV

411. PA with intact ventricular septum A/E:
(a) LAD stenosis/atresia
(b) Tricuspid valve abnormality
(c) R to L shunt
(d) Collateral–myocardial sinusoids

412. Supravalvular AS A/E:
(a) Above aortic valve but below origin of coronary arteries
(b) BP difference in arms
(c) Coronary ostial stenosis
(d) Aortic valve thickening

413. PAPVC most common form is:
(a) Right pulmonary vein → SVC
(b) Left pulmonary vein → coronary sinus
(c) Left pulmonary vein → innominate artery

414. Most common coronary anomaly:
(a) LCx from RCA
(b) RCA from left sinus
(c) LAD from RCA

415. Vascular ring A/E:
(a) RAA with aberrant left SCA
(b) RAA with aberrant left ligamentum arteriosum
(c) Left aortic arch with common brachiocephalic trunk
(d) Double aortic arch

416. ↑ PBF by all *except:*
(a) Peripheral pruning
(b) End on prominence on hilum
(c) Arterial bronchus ratio > 1
(d) Right desc. PA > 15 in males

417. Shone complex A/E:

(a) Supravalvular membrane
(b) Subvalvular AS
(c) VSD
(d) COA

418. Pulmonary artery and aorta develop from:

(a) Truncus arteriosus (b) Bulbus cordis
(c) Sinus venosus (d) Primitive ventricle

419. Endocardial heart tube develops from which part of mesoderm?

(a) Somatic (b) Splanchnic
(c) Intermediate

420. Marfan's syndrome true *except:*

(a) All have fibrillin-1 mutation
(b) Beta blockers are DOC for aortic dilatation
(c) Spontaneous pneumothorax may occur
(d) Increase risk of aortic dissection

421. Morphology of RV A/E:

(a) Smooth apex
(b) Moderator band
(c) Septal attachment of leaflet
(d) Tricuspid valve more apical

422. TOF true A/E:

(a) Pink TOF have small restrictive VSD
(b) Due to anterior malalignment of aortopulmonary septum
(c) Association with chr. 22 deletion
(d) 25% association with right aortic arch

423. Young child (10 years) diminished left arm pulse operated for CHD in infancy. Operation is:

(a) Modified BT (b) Double aortic arch
(c) Right aortic acrh (d) COA

424. Goose neck deformity seen in:

(a) Endocardial AV canal defect
(b) TGA
(c) Parachute mitral valve

425. AP window pansystolic murmur decrease is due to:

(a) Pulmonary HTN (b) PS
(c) Increased aortic flow

426. Coarctation A/E:

(a) Associated with dissection
(b) Associated with BAV
(c) Rib notching seen in 3rd to 9th ribs in infancy
(d) SAH may occur

427. A 5 days old child with cyanosis with membranous subpulmonic PA with intact ventricular septum. Management to be done A/E:

(a) RVOT perforation (b) PDA stenting
(c) BT shunt (d) None

428. Subpulmonic VSD with pressure gradient of 90 mm Hg, all are expected in natural history of it *except:*

(a) AR
(b) I.E.
(c) Spontaneous closure
(d) None of above

429. Subpulmonic VSD–oximetric data: SVC-65%, RA-65%, RV–90%, PA-90%, PV-100%, LV-100, FA-100 Qp/Qs =:

(a) 0.5 (b) 1.5
(c) 2.5 (d) 3.5

430. Oxymetric data: SVC- 65%, RA- 65%, RV- 88%, PA-88%, PV- 98%, LV-88%, AO–88%. Diagnosis:

(a) TGA (b) TOF
(c) Tricuspid atresia (d) Supracardiac TAPVC

431. A man underwent corrective TOF surgery 25 years back, present with 1 episode of syncope. Least likely manifestations:

(a) PS (b) VSD
(c) Overriding of aorta (d) PR

432. All are indication of Fontan's surgery *except:*

(a) Balanced AVCD
(b) Single ventricle RV type
(c) Tricuspid atresia
(d) HLHS

433. Pulmonary and tricuspid valve separated by:

(a) Crista supraventricularis
(b) Crista terminalis
(c) Ligament of Marshall

434. False tendon A/E:

(a) Join two papillary muscles
(b) Join ventricular walls

(c) Join papillary muscle to septum
(d) Join papillary muscle to mitral valve

435. Premature baby with large PDA with CHF, TOC:
(a) Oral indomethacin (b) Surgical ligation
(c) PGE (d) Device closure

436. BT shunt in TOF indicated in A/E:
(a) Hypoplastic PA
(b) Cyanosis
(c) Absent pulmonary valve
(d) LAD from RCA

437. VSD + Eisenmenger, Hb –21 mg%, Hematocrit– 68%, asymptomatic treatment to be given:
(a) Phlebotomy as hematocrit > 64
(b) Nothing to be done
(c) Anticoagulant
(d) Repeat laboratory test after 1 month

438. Reversed differential cyanosis:
(a) TGA with COA with PDA
(b) Taussig-Bing syndrome + reversal
(c) PDA + reversal
(d) DORV

439. Infant with LVH + normal axis + cyanosis:
(a) DORV (b) Pulmonary atresia
(c) Tricuspid artesia (d) TAPVC

440. All true except in Marfan syndrome:
(a) Endocarditis
(b) Endofibroelastosis
(c) LV dysfunction without valvular involvement
(d) Arrhythmia

441. Coronary anomaly causing ischemia:
(a) RCA from left cusp
(b) RCA for right cusp
(c) Split RCA
(d) Coronary fistula

442. PFO associated with A/E:
(a) Atrial fibrillation
(b) Migraine
(c) Orthodexia-platypnea syndrome
(d) Decompression sickness

443. RA pressure-10, TR-Velocity 4/sec, RVSP=:
(a) 74 (b) 64
(c) 84 (d) 94

444. Noonan's syndrome A/E:
(a) Autosomal Dominant
(b) 45 X0 mutation
(c) PS
(d) HOCM

445. Square wave sign on valsalva all *except:*
(a) ASD (b) CHF
(c) HOCM (d) MS

466. Cyanosis + increase Qp + LV volume overload all *except:*
(a) TAPVC (b) TGA
(c) LCD (d) Truncus

447. Most common coronary anomaly:
(a) Separate LAD/LCX
(b) LCA from right
(c) RCA from left sinus
(d) LCX from RCA–20%

448. TGA at 2 weeks treatment:
(a) Arterial switch (b) Atrial switch
(c) Rastelli

449. TAPVC (obstructive) all *except:*
(a) Normal cardiac size
(b) Ground glass appearance
(c) Split S2
(d) M > F

450. Neonatal cyanosis seen in all *except:*
(a) TOF
(b) TGA
(c) HLHS
(d) TAPVC with obstruction

451. Accessory pathway not seen in:
(a) TGA (b) Ebstein
(c) MVP (d) TAPVC

452. Increase step up of O_2 at RA level not seen in:
(a) VSD with TR (b) Gerbode defect
(c) PAPVC (d) LSVC to RA

453. Chauusat's criteria are used in:
(a) Glenn's operation (b) Fontan's operation
(c) BT shunt (d) Ross procedure

454. All are cyanotic congenital heart disease *except:*
(a) Truncus arteriosus (b) TOA
(c) RSOV (d) TOF

455. Diastolic murmur is seen in all of the following *except:*
(a) Large VSD (b) Large PDA
(c) Small FDA (d) Severe MR

456. Pulmonary stenosis is associated with all *except:*
(a) Turner's syndrome (b) Noonan's syndrome
(c) Crest syndrome (d) Watson syndrome

457. Azygos vein drain into:
(a) SVC (b) IVC
(c) Right atrium (d) Right ventricle

458. Smallest valve is:
(a) Aortic valve (b) Mitral valve
(c) Tricuspid valve (d) Pulmonary valve

459. Following is the TOF palliative procedure:
(a) Kono procedure (b) Rastelli's procedure
(c) Nick's procedure (d) Brock's procedure

460. Probe patent foramen ovale is seen in:
(a) 0-5% (b) 0-10%
(c) 10-20% (d) 20-35%

461. Following seen in DORV:
(a) Sub pulmonic conus reabsorption
(b) Subsonic coitus reabsorption
(c) None of the above
(d) Both of the conus reabsorption

462. All are intrapericardial *except*:
(a) Pulm veins
(b) Main pulmonary artery
(c) Ductus arteriosus
(d) Asc aorta

463. Most common cause of death in PDA:
(a) CCF (b) IE
(c) Rupture

464. COA repair most common seen:
(a) Aneurysm (b) Dissection
(c) AS (d) AR

465. Central cyanosis:
(a) Sulphemoglobin > 0.5
(b) Methemoglobin > 0.5
(c) $SaO_2 < 94\%$
(d) Hb < 4 g%

466. Ejection click (early systolic) in A/E:
(a) TOF
(b) Severe PS with decompensation (seen in PS)
(c) Truncus arteriosus
(d) Ventricular aneurysm with wind socking effect

467. TOF inheritance A/E:
(a) 20% of father has conotruncal defect
(b) 10% of mother has conotruncal defect
(c) 1.4% if mother has TOF
(d) 2.5% if sibling has TOF

468. Cyanotic spell seen in A/E:
(a) Transposition (b) Eisenmenger's
(c) PS with PFO (d) Tricuspid atresia

469. Indication for PFO closure:
(a) Recurrent stroke/TIA despite adequate Anticoagulation
(b) Recurrent stroke/TIA
(c) Orthodeoxia platypnea syndrome
(d) Retractory migraine

470. Rubella A/E:
(a) Microcephaly
(b) Deafness
(c) Cataract
(d) Pulmonary artery stenosis
(e) None

471. Peripheral pulmonary artery stenosis seen in:
(a) William's syndrome (b) Noonan's syndrome
(c) Turner syndrome

472. Pulmonary vascular resistance fall early in:
(a) Full term babies (b) Preterm
(c) High birth weight (d) L-R shunt

473. Modified BT shunt:
(a) Done on side of aortic arch
(b) Done on side opposite of aortic arch
(c) End to side anastomosis both
(d) Peripheral pulse absent

474. Step up of O_2 saturation at RA level A/E:
(a) Ostium primum ASD
(b) VSD with TR
(c) RSOV
(d) PAPVR

475. CATCH 22 A/E:
(a) Cleft palate (b) Thymic hyperplasia
(c) Hypocalcaemia (d) TOF

476. RV identified by:
(a) Moderator band (b) Apical TV
(c) Trabeculations (d) Origin of PA

477. Bland white garland syndrome also known as:
(a) ALCAPA (b) VATER
(c) GEORGE

478. PFO indication for closure:
(a) Recurrent cryptogenic stroke
(b) Recurrent cryptogenic stroke after therapeutic INR
(c) Orthodeoxy platypnoea
(d) Refractory migraine

479. Shone complex A/E:
(a) Supravalvular AS
(b) Supramitral ring
(c) Parachute mitral valve
(d) COA

480. Turner A/E:
(a) Mental retardation (b) Webbed neck
(c) Short stature (d) Wide spaced nipple

481. Unoperated CHD survival in 2nd decade documented: (T/F)
(a) TGA (b) TAPVC–obstructive
(c) OS ASD (d) Small VSD
(e) VSD with Eisenmenger

482. Coanda effect seen in:
(a) Supravalvular AS (b) Valvular AS
(c) Severe AR

483. View for VSD:
(a) PA (b) AP
(c) RAO (d) LAO

484. LA appendage is:
(a) Tubular (b) Circular
(c) Triangular (d) Elliptical

485. Juxtaposed appendage:
(a) cc TGA (b) TOF
(c) TGA (d) TA

486. Murmur heard in first 48 hours of life:
(a) PDA (b) VSD
(c) ASD (d) PS

487. Marfan's syndrome pathology in aorta:
(a) CMD (b) Atherosclerotic
(c) Annuloaortic ectasia

488. Modified BT shunt:
(a) Aorto-pulmonary shunt with the use of poly tetra fluoroethylene (PTFE) grafts
(b) Left SCA to PA
(c) Desc. aorta to PA

489. TOF inheritance A/E:
(a) Mother having defect–10%
(b) Father having defect–20%
(c) Sibling–2.5%
(d) Father affected–1.5%

490. CATCH–22 A/E:
(a) Thymic hyperplasia (b) Hypocalcemia
(c) TOF

491. RFA complication, CHB least common in:
(a) AVNRT (b) WPW
(c) Atrial flutter (d) Left free wall pathway

492. CHB is associated with:
(a) cc -TGA (b) TGA
(c) TOF (d) TA

493. Cyanotic spell preceded by A/E:
(a) Anemia (b) Ephedrine
(c) SVT (d) Cold

494. Atrial pressure tracing A/E:
(a) LA pressure (mean) higher than RA
(b) a wave smaller than v wave in LA
(c) y descent is slower than fall of ventricular pressure during ventricular filling
(d) v wave is due to volume inflow in atrium during ventricular systole

495. Down syndrome A/E:
(a) Bruschfields spot in eye
(b) Mental retardation
(c) Hypertonicity

496. Clockwise rotation in ECG:
(a) TOF (b) DORV with PS
(c) AVSD (d) Single ventricle

497. Following is an extra pericardial structure:
(a) Ascending aorta
(b) 4 pulmonary veins
(c) Right and left pulmonary arteries
(d) Main pulmonary artery

498. Which of the following statement is true about mitral valve:
(a) Anterior mitral leaflet is rectangular and is divided into 3 scallops
(b) Posteromedial papillary muscle usually has multiple heads and is supplied by right coronary artery
(c) Dilatation of MV annulus primarily affects the anterior leaflet
(d) Anterolateral papillary muscle bas single blood supply

499. Regarding development of aortic arch, identify the false statement:
(a) Type B interrupted aortic arch results from disappearance of left dorsal aorta
(b) Right subclavian artery arises from right 4th aortic arch
(c) Absent left pulmonary artery is due to disappearance of proximal left 6th arch
(d) Left 6th arch persists as ductus arteriosus

500. Peripheral pulmonary artery stenosis is seen in all *except:*
(a) Poland syndrome (b) William's syndrome
(c) Rubella syndrome (d) Alagillae syndrome

501. Leopard syndrome results from:
(a) Mutation of 7 q 1I
(b) Deletion of 22 q 11
(c) Mutation in FBNI gene
(d) Deletion of PTPN 11 gene

502. Identify the moderate severity congenital heart disease in an adult:
(a) Pulmonary atresia
(b) VSD with AR
(c) Eisenmenger syndrome
(d) Double outlet right ventricle

503. All are cyanotic congenital heart diseases with increased pulmonary blood flow *except:*
(a) Double outlet right ventricle with pulmonary Stenosis
(b) Truncus arteriosus
(c) Common atrium
(d) Taussig-Bing anomaly

504. Identify the wrong statement in the management of a cyanotic patient:
(a) Phlebotomy is not indicated for asymptomatic patients
(b) Cyanotic patients should avoid iron deficiency which is associated with increased risk of stroke
(c) Aspirin and NSAIDs can be safely given
(d) Gouty arthritis can be treated with colchicin, probenecid or allopurinol

505. Pulmonary artery dilatation is not a feature in:
(a) TOF with absent pulmonary valve
(b) ASD with large L-R shunt
(c) VSD with Severe PH .
(d) Noonan's syndrome with severe PS due to dysplastic PV

506. Hereditary telangiectasia is associated with:
(a) ASD (b) VSD
(c) TOF (d) Pul AV fistula

507. In Loeys Dietz syndrome, all are true *except:*
(a) It is an autosomal dominant disorder
(b) Bifid broad uvula is a feature
(c) It is associated with arterial tortuosity and aortic aneurysms
(d) It has a less aggressive vascular phenotype than Marfan's syndrome

508. Congenital Heart Disease that can result in Eisenmenger's Syndrome include:
(a) ASD (b) VSD
(c) Univentricular Heart (d) All of the above

509. Oxygen step up in RV is seen in:
(a) PDA with PR (b) RSOV into LA
(c) Sinus venosus ASD (d) Cor triatriatum

510. Which of the following is NOT an Aorto-Pulmonary Shunt:
(a) Waterston (b) Potts
(c) Gott Shunt (d) Blalock-Taussig

511. Counterclockwise QRS is seen in all *except:*

(a) DORV (b) Tricuspid
(c) Pulmonary atresia (d) ECD

512. Valvular pulmonic stenosis is the most common defect in:

(a) Holt-Oram syndrome
(b) Noonan Syndrome
(c) Down syndrome
(d) Turner syndrome

513. Congenital heart defects that can result in Eisenmenger's syndrome include:

(a) ASD (b) VSD
(c) Univentricular heart (d) All of the above

514. "Atrialized Right Ventricle" is a feature of:

(a) Tricuspid atresia (b) Ebstein's anomaly
(c) Pulmonary atresia (d) Fallot's tetralogy

515. All of the following are features of Premature Ventricular Complexes *except:*

(a) Wide QRS complex
(b) Absent P wave
(c) Complete compensatory pause
(d) Prolonged PR interval

516. The boundaries of 'Triangle of Koch' does not include:

(a) Tendon of Todaro (b) Coronary sinus
(c) Tricuspid annulus (d) Crista terminalis

517. Which statement is false?

(a) Anterior mitral leaflet has a significantly larger surface area compared to posterior mitral leaflet
(b) Anterior mitral leaflet has close to double the width from annulus to its free margin, corn to posterior mitral leaflet
(c) Anterior leaflet occupies only half the circumference as compared to posterior leaflet
(d) Closure line of both mitral leaflets is not a margin of the leaflets but a few mm withal

518. When SVC O_2 saturation is 40% with arterial saturation 98% one must suspect:

(a) Hypoventilation
(b) Low cardiac output state
(c) High altitude physiology
(d) Variation in normal basal resting hemodynamics

519. A typical well defined left anterior descending artery is not a feature of:

(a) Double outlet RV
(b) Transposition of great vessels
(c) Single ventricle
(d) Corrected transposition of great vessels

520. In the fetus, amongst the following, blood snowing across has are highest oxygen saturation.

(a) Aortic isthmus
(b) The tricuspid valve
(c) The pulmonary veins into LA
(d) Right hepatic vein

521. In the infant, aorta to pulmonary artery shunt through PDA will result in stepdown in oxygen saturation in pulmonary artery in:

(a) Truncus arteriosus
(b) Tricuspid atresia
(c) Transposition of great vessels
(d) Obstructed TAPVC

522. The most important difference between a mild form of tetralogy and severe form of Tetralogy of Fallot is:

(a) Marked difference in RVOF gradient
(b) Marked difference in RVOF impedance
(c) Marked difference in RV systolic pressure
(d) Marked difference in RV filling pressure

523. A widely patent aortic valve may remain completely closed during the entire cardiac cycle after:

(a) Arterial switch surgery for TGA
(b) Double switch surgery for corrected TGA Damus Kaye Stansel procedure
(c) Post Fontan surgery

524. Cyanosis completely disappear with administra-tion of 100% oxygen in:

(a) Central hypoventilation
(b) Simple TGA
(c) Methemoglobinemia
(d) Sulfhemoglobinemia

525. Prostaglandin (PGE1) infusion to maintain ductal patency may not be useful in:

(a) Hypoplastic left heart syndrome
(b) Hypoplastic right heart syndrome
(c) Intern: red aortic arch
(d) Obstructed TAPVC

526. Which statement is false for sinus of valsalva aneurysm from right sinus, as compared to those from the non-coronary sinus?

(a) More commonly associated with VSD
(b) More likely to rupture into RA than RVOF
(c) More commonly associated with aortic incompetence
(d) Far more common than aneurysm from non-coronary sinus

527. Highest fatality to mother with pregnancy is associated with:

(a) Surgically corrected TOP
(b) Fontan repair
(c) Surgically corrected TGA
(d) Eisenmenger syndrome

528. Evaluation of pregnant lady with hypertension and aortic coarctation should include:

(a) Chest X-ray, electrocardiogram and echo Doppler studies
(b) Electrocardiogram, echo Doppler studies and CT angiogram
(c) Electrocardiogram, echo Doppler studies and MR angiogram
(d) Cardiac catheterization and assessment of hemodynamics

529. Association with 22q11 deletion is not a future of:

(a) TOF
(b) TGA
(c) Truncus arteriosus
(d) Type E aortic interruption

530. The Chest X-Ray of a 2 years old child with coarctation of aorta without CHF, is likely to show:

(a) Rib Notching (b) Cardiomegaly
(c) 'E' sign (d) Normal heart size

531. Interpret the following oxymetry data: IVC 55%, SVC 80%, RA 82%, RV 84%, Aorta 82%. The likely diagnosis is:

(a) TAPVC
(b) Sinus venosus ASD
(c) Double outlet right ventricle
(d) LV to RA shunt

532. Congenital complete heart block is associated with:

(a) Corrected Transposition of great arteries (c-TGA)
(b) Uncorrected TGA
(c) Coarctation of Aorta
(d) PDA

533. In a normal individual:

(a) Left atrium is less compliant than right atrium
(b) Right atrium is less compliant than left atrium
(c) Both LA and RA are equally compliant
(d) All of the above are wrong

534. The fontan procedure is:

(a) A corrective surgical procedure for patients with TGA
(b) A palliative procedure to redirect blood from aorta or its branches to the pulmonary artery
(c) A palliative procedure to redirect venous blood directly into the pulmonary arteries
(d) A corrective surgical procedure for patients with A-V canal defects

535. The term Taussig-Bing anomaly is used to describe:

(a) Double outlet right ventricle with sub-pulmonary VSD
(b) Double outlet right ventricle with sub aortic VSD
(c) Double inlet left ventricle with sub-pulmonary VSD
(d) Double inlet left ventricle with sub-aortic VSD

536. Common signs and symptoms of left atrial myxomas include all the following:

(a) Fever
(b) Anaemia
(c) Clubbing
(d) Mitral valve diastolic murmur

537. Blalock Taussig Operation connects:

(a) Subclavian A to PA (b) SVC to RPA
(c) RA to PA (d) IVC to LPA

538. The most common congenital heart disease is:

(a) Bicuspid aortic value (b) VSD
(c) ASD (d) Fallot's tetralogy

539. In LGL syndrome the PR interval is:

(a) Normal (b) Increased
(c) Decreased (d) Variable

540. Anatomic closure of PDA occurs at:

(a) Birth (b) 10-15 hours
(c) 2-3 weeks (d) 2-3 months

541. In Down's syndrome the most common congenital heart disease is:

(a) ASD (b) VSD

(c) A-V canal defect (d) Coarctation of aorta

542. Dose of IV propranolol in cyanotic spell is:

(a) 0.1 mg/kg (b) 1 mg/kg

(c) 10 mg/kg (d) 20 mg/kg

543. 45 years male present with LAD, which is most common cause?

(a) LVH (b) LAHB

(c) LPHB (d) Valvular heart disease

544. Which is not true regarding Allagille syndrome:

(a) It is AD and associated with JAG1 mutation

(b) Intrahepatic cholestasis

(c) Peripheral pulmonary artery stenosis

(d) Common atrium is the usual anomaly

545. Which congenital heart diseases is most common in Leopard syndrome?

(a) PS (b) ASD

(c) VSD (d) PDA

546. All are the X-ray changes in LA enlargement:

(a) Focal, posterior bulge in lateral X-ray

(b) Decreased carinal angle

(c) Straightening of left heart border

(d) Double atrial shadow in frontal view

547. A 7 days old child <0.45 kg weigh less than normal with decreased feeding and crying with ejection systolic murmur, bounding pulses, dilated biventricular, mild LV systolic dysfunction with dilated innominate vein so what is finding with bilateral normal UL/LL pulse?

(a) Continuous murmur over abdomen

(b) Costavertebral systolic bruit

(c) Continuous murmur over head

(d) Systolic abdominal bruit

548. Regarding RV anatomy which is not true?

(a) Presence of moderate band

(b) Presence of pectinate muscle

(c) Triparite morphology

549. Prophylaxis is given during dental extraction in which condition?

(a) PDA (b) Severe MR

(c) TOF with BT shunt

550. Unequal pulse is found in (Right and Left arm) in all condition *except:*

(a) Supravalvular AS

(b) Post ductal coartation of aorta

(c) Thoracic outlet compression

(d) Brachial artery external compression

551. During the strain phase of valsalva maneuver all are decreased *except:*

(a) VSD (b) MR

(c) HOCM (d) AR

552. Regarding Ebstein's anomaly which is not true?

(a) Wide split of S2

(b) Narrow spit of S1

(c) S1 has loud T1 component

(d) Presence of RV S3

553. Tricuspid stensosis: (T/F)

(a) Almost always stenotic

(b) Prominent a wave with steep y descent in JVP

(c) Mask MS

(d) Pulsatile liver presystolic

554. Fick method not used for CO:

(a) Hb

(b) PASP

(c) O_2 consumption

(d) Arteriovenous O_2 difference

555. Fontan operation A/E:

(a) Tricuspid atresia (b) DORV

(c) DOLV (d) HLHS

556. Ductus arteriosus develops from:

(a) Left 6th aortic arch

(b) Left 5th aortic arch

557. Bifid uvula seen in:

(a) Leoys Deitz syndrome

(b) Marfan syndrome

(c) Tangier's disease

(d) Wegener granulomatosis

558. PAPVC is common in which ASD:

(a) Sinus venosus ASD

(b) OS ASD
(c) Ostium primum ASD
(d) AVCD

559. Pulmonary venous obstruction seen in A/E:
(a) PAPVC
(b) Type III infracardiac
(c) Type I supracardiac
(d) Pulmonary vein stenosis

560. Infant at 4 weeks with weight of 0.45 kg less than birth weight, has sweating while feeding for > 30 min, has gallop rhythm with systolic murmur with normal cardiac anatomy, biventricular enlarge-ment with large innominate vein, which is most likely finding?
(a) Continuous abdominal bruit
(b) Continuous cranial bruit
(c) Systolic costovertebral bruit
(d) Systolic cervical bruit

561. Holt-Oram syndrome A/E:
(a) Autosomal recessive
(b) Foreman bone abnormality
(c) OS-ASD
(d) VSD

562. Pericardial patch closure of ASD not done in:
(a) OS–ASD
(b) OP–ASD
(c) SV–ASD
(d) ASD with cushion defect

563. Duration of intracardiac shunt at atrial level depends on:
(a) RA pressure
(b) Compliance of RV and LV
(c) Oxygen saturation
(d) VSD

564. Difference of BP in both upper limbs seen in A/E:
(a) Supravalvular AS
(b) Post ductal COA
(c) Thoracic outlet syndrome
(d) External brachial artery compression

565. Infant with large non restrictive VSD has heart failure commonly at what age?
(a) 2 days (b) 2 weeks
(c) 2 months (d) 6 months
(e) All true

566. Patient with neurofibromatosis–Most common cause of secondary hypertension:
(a) Pheochromocytoma
(b) Renal artery stenosis
(c) Cushing syndrome
(d) Polycystic kidney disease

567. All are component of TOF *except:*
(a) ASD
(b) VSD
(c) Dextroposition of aorta
(d) PS

568. Preterm baby with hyaline membrane disease on mechanical ventilation not able to wean, echo shows PDA, clinically what favours significant PDA?
(a) Continuous murmur
(b) Prominent precordial pulsation
(c) Reduced femoral pulses
(d) Jaundice

569. DORV A/E:
(a) Always associated with VSD
(b) Taussing-Bing anomaly has non committed VSD
(c) DORV with Taussing-Bing anomaly mimics TGA with VSD
(d) Subaortic VSD with PS is most common

570. Continuous murmur seen in:
(a) PDA
(b) Coronary cameral fistula
(c) Branch pulmonary stenosis
(d) All of the above

571. Mangement of tricuspid atresia in 1 month old infant:
(a) Observation
(b) Bidirectional cavopulmonary shunt
(c) Systemic artery to pulmonary shunting
(d) Pulmonary artery banding

572. Physical finding in COA in young adult:
(a) Peripheral cyanosis
(b) Systolic murmur in interscapular area
(c) Decreased femoral pulse
(d) Left arm BP > right arm

573. Optimal method of diagnosing PDA in infant:
(a) 2D echo with colour Doppler
(b) Retrograde aortography through umbilical artery
(c) Cardiac cath.

574. Survival of pulmonary atresia with intact ventricular septum depends on:
(a) Size of ASD (b) Size of RV
(c) RV

575. Most anterior valve:
(a) AoV (b) MV
(c) TV (d) PV

576. Most anterior structure in mediastinum:
(a) SVC (b) Hemiazygous vein
(c) Ascending Aorta (d) Thymus

577. Which of following drains into RA?
(a) Coronary sinus
(b) Thebesian vein
(c) Great vein of Marchall
(d) All of the above

578. Treatment of Eisenmenger syndrome A/E:
(a) Bosentan
(b) I/V prostaglandins
(c) Sildenafil
(d) Heart lung transplantation

579. Pulmonary Stenosis with gradient > 60 mm Hg treatment:
(a) BPV (b) Observation
(c) Surgery

580. PFO true A/E:
(a) 50% associated with cryptogenic stroke
(b) After closure recurrence rate is 0%
(c) Associated with platypnea orthodoexia, decompression sickness and migraine
(d) Diagnosed by contrast echo with TEE

581. In TOF boot shaped heart is due to:
(a) Transverse displacement of apex of RV as it dilates
(b) RVH
(c) Aortic override

582. LAMP2 Mutation associated with:
(a) Danon disease (b) HOCM
(c) Fabry

583. NFX 2.5 mutation associated with:
(a) ASD secundum with conduction block
(b) TOF with pulmonary Atresia
(c) HOCM

584. Anderson Tawil syndrome:
(a) Prominent U
(b) ↑ PR
(c) Notched upsloping QRS
(d) Notched ↓ s wave

585. JVP in Ebstein anomaly:
(a) Prominent 'a' wave (b) Prominent 'x' wave
(c) Prominent 'c' wave (d) Prominent 'v' wave

586. Diagnosis of Ebstein anomaly best by:
(a) Catheterization (b) Echoplaner MRI
(c) 4 chamber 2d echo (d) Angiography MDCT

587. Most common cause of SCD in Eisenmenger:
(a) Cerebral abscess with ↑ ICP
(b) Cerebral hemorrhage
(c) CHB
(d) Massive pulmonary haemorrhage

588. Ebstein anomaly associated with LV anomaly:
(a) Parachute MV
(b) Endocardial fibroelastosis
(c) Noncompaction LV
(d) LVOT obstruction

589. Cantrell syndrome associated with:
(a) Multiple peripheral PAS
(b) Aortic aneurysm
(c) Absent pericardium
(d) Fibroelastosis

590. Wide fixed and split S2:
(a) Ostium secundum ASD
(b) VSD
(c) Severe MR
(d) Small PDA

591. Baby discharged with normal neonatal exam. Presented on 3rd day with thread pulse, 180/min, liver 5 cm, capillary refill > 6 cm diagnosis:
(a) DORV (b) TA
(c) TGA (d) Pulmonary atresia

592. Cardinal symptoms of ASD and PFO:
(a) Platypnoea and orthodeoxia
(b) Dyspnoea
(c) Orthopnea
(d) Fatigue

593. TOF-Cyanotic spell characteristic:
(a) Hyperpnea (b) Pallor
(c) Bradycardia (d) ↑ systolic murmur

594. Boot shaped heart is due to:
(a) Transverse displacement of apex of RV as it dilates
(b) RVH

595. PDA uncomplicated true is:
(a) Upright T in V1 in pulmonary HTN
(b) Murmur ↑ on standing
(c) LVH on ECG

596. Berry aneurysm of coronary:
(a) PAN (b) Kawasaki disease
(c) COA

597. COA most common associated with:
(a) BAV (b) ASD
(c) VSD

598. Immediate tertiary referral in infants:
(a) Large VSD (b) Suspected COA
(c) Kawasaki disease (d) ASD

599. Cerebral abscess without IE in A/E:
(a) PDA (b) TOF
(c) TGA (d) TA

600. Associated with AVSD:
(a) RSR in V1
(b) Mild cyanosis from birth
(c) Wide variable S2
(d) Pansystolic murmur at apex

601. Congenital heart disease true is:
(a) 25–30% associated with extracardiac defects
(b) All can be diagnosed by antenatal echo
(c) Complex CHD requires staged procedure

602. Ostium secundum associated with A/E:
(a) LAD
(b) Treatment with Qp: Qs > 2
(c) Least common ASD

603. Large VSD A/E:
(a) Loud S2
(b) Pulmonary plethora with CT ratio > 60%
(c) Mild cyanosis at early stage
(d) CT

604. PAPVC with hypoplasia of right lung and right PA:
(a) Scimitar syndrome (b) DiGeorge syndrome
(c) Holt-Oram syndrome

605. The syndrome which includes childhood onset of Dilated Cardiomyopathy, neutropenia growth retardation which is related to mutations in tafazzin is:
(a) Turner's Syndrome
(b) Kearns-Sayre Syndrome
(c) Barth's Syndrome
(d) MELAS Syndrome

606. The "triangle of dysplasia" is:
(a) The Koch's triangle in complete heart block due to Lenegre's disease
(b) The Right Ventricular Outflow, Apex and Inflow in Arrhythmogenic Right Ventricular Cardiomyopathy
(c) The Right Atrium, Tricuspid Valve and the Right Ventricular Inflow in Ebstein's Anomaly
(d) The Right Atrium, Right Ventricular Inflow and Apex in Right Sided Endomyocardial Fibrosis

607. The tachycardia that arises from the aortic sinus of valsalva is:
(a) Atrial Fibrillation
(b) Fascicular ventricular tachycardia
(c) Repetitive Monomorphic Ventricular Tachycardia
(d) Idiopathic Left Ventricular Tachycardia

608. "Embryoid bodies" are:
(a) Cystic structures in culture of stem cells that contain foci of beating cardiomyocyte
(b) Bodies found in the cardiac jelly responsible for embryogenesis of the heart
(c) Embryoid remnants found in myocardium of Anomalous origin of Left Coronary Artery from the Pulmonary Artery (ALCAPA)
(d) Remnants of the valve found in the opening of the inferior vena cava to the right atrium

609. The Genetic Mutation NK × 2.5 in Atrial Septal Defect is associated with:

(a) Mitral valve prolapse
(b) A-V block
(c) Cleft mitral valve
(d) Earlier onset of the Eisenmenger syndrome

610. Children with prenatal exposure to anti-Ro or anti-La antibodies may have:
(a) Atrial Fibrillation
(b) Ventricular Tachycardia
(c) Sinus Node Disease
(d) Wolff-Parkinson-White Syndrome

611. The condition associated with an anomalous anterior atrioventricular node is:
(a) Congenitally, corrected transposition of the great arteries
(b) Ebstein's anomaly of the tricuspid valve
(c) Univentricular heart
(d) Endocardial cushion defects

612. Char syndrome an inherited disorder mapped to chromosome 6p12=p21 and characterized facial dysmorphism, abnormalities of the hand has:
(a) Secundum atrial septal defect
(b) Left Ventricle to Right Atrial Shunt (Gerbode's Defect)
(c) Total Anomalous Pulmonary Venous Connection
(d) Patent Ductus Arteriosus

613. Virtually all patients with Down's syndrome over 35 years of age will have:
(a) Endocardial Cushion Defects
(b) Alzheimer syndrome
(c) Eisenmenger's syndrome
(d) Chronic Obstructive Pulmonary Disease

614. The Electrocardiogram which has Right Bundle Branch Block (RBBB), Left Axis Deviation of P and QRS is characteristic of:
(a) Secundum Atrial Septal Defect
(b) IVC type of Atrial Septal Defect
(c) Common Atrium
(d) Primum Atrial Septal defects

615. Treatment of choice for postoperative junctional ectopic tachycardia (JET) in children is:
(a) Digoxin (b) Modest cooling
(c) Beta blockers (d) Calcium channel blockers

616. Which of the following condition has the lowest risk of post-operative sudden cardiac death on long term follow up?
(a) Tetralogy of Fallot
(b) Transposition of the great arteries
(c) Aortic stenosis
(d) Pulmonic stenosis

617. A single common pulmonary vein is seen with:
(a) Heterotaxy with asplenia
(b) Heterotaxy with polysplenia
(c) Truncus arteriosus
(d) Cor triatriatum

618. The lower limit of PR interval for an infant (less than 12 months of age) is:
(a) 0.075 sec (b) 0.080 sec
(c) 0.085 sec (d) 0.090 sec

619. All of the following promote closure of ductus arteriosus in newborns *except:*
(a) Increase in PaO_2 (b) Decrease in PGE2
(c) Increase in PGE1 (d) Indomethacin

620. The most common site of entry for the cardiac type of Total Anomalus Pulmonary Venous Connection (TAPVC) is:
(a) Left SVC (b) Coronary sinus
(c) Innominate vein (d) Right SVC

621. Marked male preponderance is seen in which type of Total Anomalous Pulmonary Venous Connection (TAPVC)?
(a) Supracardiac (b) Cardiac
(c) Infra Cardiac (d) Mixed

622. All of the following are cardiovascular malformation seen in asplenia syndrome *except:*
(a) Bilateral SVC (b) Interrupted IVC
(c) Common AV Valve (d) Absent coronary sinus

623. The most common vascular ring is:
(a) Double aortic arch
(b) Right aortic arch with left ligamentum arteriosum
(c) Anomalous innominate artery
(d) Anomalous left pulmonary artery

624. Anatomical landmark for the beginning of the coronary sinus from the great cardiac vein:
(a) Thebesian valve (b) Eustachian valve
(c) Tendon of Todaro (d) Valve of Vieussens

625. In the setting of PDA with aorta pulmonary artery shunting, which of these conditions is likely to has identical PA and Aortic oxygen saturation?

(a) Corrected TGA
(b) Single Ventricle with PS
(c) Simple TGA
(d) Teralogy of Fallot

626. A six years old deaf child with exercise related syncope and bradycardia had an abnormal T wave morphology in ECG. The most likely diagnosis is:
(a) Brugada syndrome
(b) Romano Ward syndrome
(c) Williams syndrome
(d) Lange-Nielsen syndrome

627. The most likely diagnosis in a 3 days old cyanotic neonate with respiratory distress and congestive failure is:
(a) Partially obstructed TAPVD
(b) Pulmonary A-V fistulae
(c) Pulmonary atresia with VSD
(d) Interruption hypoplastic left heart syndrome

628. Coil embolization is the most common procedure for:
(a) Pulmonary sequestration
(b) Aortopulmonary collaterals
(c) Congenital a-v malformation
(d) Systemic venous anomalies

629. Which one of the following pediatric dyarrythmias does not require treatment?
(a) Premature ventricular beats
(b) Wandering atrial pacemaker
(c) Ventricular tachycardia
(d) 3rd degree A-V block

630. Old with chest wall and spine abnormalities, the cardiac disorder to be examined for is:
(a) Coartation of aorta
(b) Cardiomyopathy
(c) Mitral valve prolapse
(d) Tetralogy of Fallot

631. Chromosome 7 microdeletion is associated with:
(a) ASD
(b) VSD
(c) Complete Heart Block
(d) Supravalvular aortic stenosis

632. Continuous murmur is not a feature of:
(a) PDA with severe PH
(b) Pulmonary AV fistula
(c) Small ASD with severe MS
(d) RSOV to RVOT

633. Ductus arterosus is embryologically derived from:
(a) Dorsal aorta
(b) 6th aortic arch
(c) 5th aortic arch
(d) 4th aortic arch

634. Regarding Paroxysmal Supraventricular Tachycardia (PSVT) one of the following statements is False:
(a) It is the most common abnormal tachyarrythmias in infants and children
(b) Its incidence is greater in newborns then in children of all ages
(c) Atrioventricular Reentrant Tachycardia (AVRT) is responsible for more than two third of childhood cases
(d) Wolff-Parkinson White (WPW) syndrome is included as an entity of AVRT

635. Carvallo's sign refers to:
(a) Systolic ejection click heard better in expiration in pulmonary valvular stenosis
(b) Continuous murmur heard over the back due to collaterals in Tetralogy of Fallot
(c) Wide, fixed splitting of second sound in atrial septal defect
(d) Increased intensity of pansystolic murmur during inspiration in tricuspid regurgitation

636. Regarding Lutembacher syndrome, one of the following statement is False:
(a) It is a predilection for males
(b) Mitral Stenosis (MS) is always of rheumatic origin
(c) Syndrome of mitral stenosis do not equate with severity of MS
(d) In nonrestrictive ADSs, left atrial enlargement is radiologically evident

637. The initial dose for synchronized electrocardio-version in cases of wide pulse is:
(a) 0.1–0.2 J/Kg
(b) 0.5–2.0 J/Kg
(c) 0.1–4.0 J/Kg
(d) 0.1–6.0 J/Kg

638. Regarding the auscultatory signs of total anomalous pulmonary venous drainage of non-obstructive type, one of the following statement is False:
(a) There is wide, variable splitting of second heart sound
(b) In pulmonary area, an ejection midsystolic murmur is heard
(c) Pulmonary systolic ejection sound is heard in pulmonary hypertension

(d) Over tricuspid area, there is often a mid diastolic flow murmur

639. With regard to Ventricular Septal Defect (VSD) associated with Aortic Reguragitation (AR) one of the following statements is NOT true:

(a) ASD with AR are more common in males

(b) AR is less common in subarterial infundibula type of VSD than in perimembranous VSD

(c) Prolapse of either right coronary cusp or no coronary or both results in AR

(d) Peak incidence of AR occurs with peak incidence between 5 and 9 years of age

640. Regarding Double Outlet Right Ventricle (DORV), one of the following statement is False:

(a) DORV describes hearts in which more than 50% of each semilunar valve arises from the morphological right ventricle

(b) DORV with subaortic VED is referred to as Taussig-Bing anomaly

(c) Posterior deviation of the outlet septum causes subpulmonic stenosis

(d) DORV with subpulmonary stenosis has with clinical features indistinguishable from those of Tetralogy of Fallot

641. One of the radiological features in Ebstein's anomaly is False:

(a) Marked cardiomegaly with "water bottle" appearance

(b) Conspicuous aortic and pulmonary trunk shadows

(c) Reduced pulmonary vasculature markings

(d) Marked convexity of right heart border beyond right sternal border

642. The most common type of atrioventricular septal defect (AVSD) associated with Down's syndrome is:

(a) Partial AVSD

(b) Type A complete AVSD

(c) Type B complete AVSD

(d) Type C complete AVSD

643. AV node:

(a) Right–sympathetic, right–vagal

(b) Left–sympathetic, left–vagal

(c) Right–sympathetic, left–vagal

(d) Left–sympathetic. right–vagal

644. X-linked cardiomyopathy:

(a) Friedreich ataxia

(b) Limb girdle myopathy

(c) Facio scapular humeral myopathy

(d) Barth's syndrome

645. Cyanotic congenital heart disease A/E:

(a) Pulmonary AV fistula

(b) Coronary AV fistula

(c) Ebstein anomaly

(d) TA

646. Werdig Hoffmann syndrome (SMA type 1) most common congenital heart disease:

(a) VSD (b) PDA

(c) TOF (d) ASD

647. True statement A/E:

(a) Septal attachment of MV

(b) Apical placement of TV

(c) RV trabeculated

648. Polysplenia most seen in:

(a) Interrupted aortic arch

(b) TAPVC

(c) ECD

649. Left sided rib notching in COA seen in:

(a) Right subclavian distal to coarctation

(b) Ascending aorta coarctation

(c) Coarctation involving left subclavian obstruction

(d) Coarctation distal to left subclavian

650. Most common tumour that metastasize to heart:

(a) Melanoma (b) Breast

(c) NHL (d) Hodgkin lymphoma

651. In septic shock inflammatory mediator:

(a) Adrenaline (b) Cortisol

(c) Glucagon (d) Proteases

652. Most common cause of neonatal mortality is:

(a) LBW

(b) Congenital anomalies

(c) Diarrhoeal disease

653. Type I chiari malformations A/E:

(a) Neck pain (b) Headache

(c) Hydrocephalous (d) Lower limb spasticity

654. Post concussion syndrome A/E:

(a) Headache (b) Vertigo
(c) Memory loss (d) Bell's palsy

655. Hypopituitarism in infancy A/E:

(a) Short birth length (b) Hypoglycemia
(c) Micropenis (d) Neonatal hepatitis

656. TOF physiology seen A/E: (T/F)

(a) DORV + VSD + PS
(b) Single ventricle + PS
(c) Truncus arteriosus
(d) Ebstein
(e) TGA +VSD+ PS

657. DORV true: (T/F)

(a) Aorta/PA arises from RV
(b) Aortomitral discontinuity
(c) DORV + subaortic VSD = TOF
(d) DORV + Subpulmonic VSD = TGA
(e) Ross procedure = DORV + subaortic VSD

658. DORV + VSD + PS false: (T/F)

(a) May have prolonged PR
(b) Counterclockwise rotation on ECG
(c) Left parasternal heave
(d) Aortomitral continuity

659. VSD shunt depends: (T/F)

(a) Small size VSD
(b) Large size VSD
(c) In large VSD shunt depends on SVR and PVR
(d) Does not depend on location of VSD

660. DORV vs VSD with PS, favouring DORV: (T/F)

(a) ↑ PR
(b) Counterclockwise loop on ECG
(c) Short ESM
(d) Grade III Rt PSH
(e) Wide split S2

661. Ebstein anomaly A/E: (T/F)

(a) Tall p wave
(b) RBBB
(c) WPW type A > WPW type B
(d) SVT common
(e) ↑ PR may be seen

662. Cc-TGA: (T/F)

(a) VSD in most
(b) VSD is restrictive
(c) Pulm. Atresia common
(d) Common in females
(e) Left AV regurgitation associated with long term outcome

663. CoA: (T/F)

(a) Balloon size at descending aorta at diaphragmatic level
(b) Surgery for localized disease
(c) Stenting for all
(d) Discontinue anti HTN post surgery in majority
(e) Successful by gradient < 10 mm Hg

664. Cyanotic spell treatment A/E: (T/F)

(a) Propranolol (b) ASA
(c) Physostigmine (d) Phenylephrine
(e) Nifedipine

665. ASD with cyanosis: (T/F)

(a) TAPVC
(b) Persistent LSVC
(c) Unroofing of coronary sinus
(d) Eisenmenger complex
(e) MR

666. Sinus veousus ASD: (T/F)

(a) RBBB on ECG
(b) Associated with PAPVC
(c) Best in bicaval on TEE
(d) TEE–inflow outflow view
(e) TEE–midoesophagus 4 chamber view

667. ALCAPA: (T/F)

(a) Also known as Bland white garland syndrome
(b) Can present prenatally
(c) Biventricular failure in neonatal period
(d) Coronary steal from RCA (left to right shunt)
(e) Papillary muscle dysfunction with MR

668. LAD in cyanotic heart disease with normal ventricular arterial connection: (T/F)

(a) TA (b) HLHS
(c) TOF (d) DORV
(e) PA

669. **Ductal dependent: (T/F)**
(a) TAPVC
(b) Interrupted aortic arch
(c) Critical AS
(d) HLHS
(e) PA with intact IVS

670. **SVC velocity > 1.2 cm/sec: (T/F)**
(a) Vertical vein (b) LSVC
(c) A-V fistula (d) RSOV
(e) SVC thrombosis

671. **Rupture of sinus valsalva: (T/F)**
(a) Most common right aortic sinus ruptures
(b) Usually childhood
(c) More common in winter
(d) 30% involves non coronary sinus

672. **DORV diagnosed by TEE: (T/F)**
(a) Both great vessel are parallel
(b) RV ejects into both great arteries
(c) Overriding of aorta > 50% in presence of VSD
(d) Hypoplastic LV
(e) Loss of aortomitral continuity

673. **Fetal echo A/E: (T/F)**
(a) PDA (b) Ebsten's anomaly
(c) HLHS (d) PS
(e) AS

674. **SCD: (T/F)**
(a) Incidence 1-2 per 10,000
(b) Incidence more till 6 months and then between 45-75 years
(c) CAD cause 1/4th of SCD
(d) Diabetes is not a risk factor for SCD
(e) HF with better functional capacity has increased risk of SCD

675. **RV enlargement in CXR: (T/F)**
(a) Boot shaped heart
(b) Splaying of carina
(c) CT ratio > 0.50
(d) Buldging of right upper mediastinal space
(e) In lateral view filling of retrosternal air spaces occurs

676. **Large PDA A/E: (T/F)**
(a) Paradoxical split S2
(b) RV S3
(c) LV S3
(d) Continuous murmur
(e) MDM at mitral area

677. **Cardiac anatomy: (T/F)**
(a) TV and PV not in continuity, separated by infundibulum
(b) MV more apical than TV
(c) LV false tendon apex to mitral valve
(d) AV has no chordae tendinea
(e) Morphological TV is almost always associated morphological RV

678. **DORV: (T/F)**
(a) Doubly committed DORV also known as Taussig-Bing anomaly
(b) DORV with VSD with PS similar to tricuspid atresia
(c) DORV with VSD without PS similar to TGA

679. **Figure of 8 on CXR: (T/F)**
(a) Supracardiac TAPVC in men
(b) TOF
(c) TGA
(d) Supracardiac TAPVC at 2 years
(e) Infracardiac obstructive TAPVC

680. **ECG in TOF: (T/F)**
(a) Abrupt transition to rS in V2
(b) Peaked P wave but amplitude not increased
(c) Counterclockwise rotation with LAD suggestive of ECD
(d) Wide QRS complex in neonates
(e) Associated with PR prolongation

681. **Eisenmenger associated with: (T/F)**
(a) Small VSD (b) Truncus arteriosus
(c) TAPVC (d) TGA
(e) TOF

682. **HF at 6 months duration with severe LV dysfunction: (T/F)**
(a) Hypocalcemia (b) Severe AS
(c) Severe COA (d) ALCAPA
(e) Myocarditis

683. PS with intact septum: (T/F)

(a) Ejection murmur (b) Loud P2
(c) Parasternal heave (d) Cardiomegaly
(e) Reverse split S2

684. Large VSD with Eisenmenger: (T/F)

(a) Pregnancy is safe
(b) SCD is common cause of death
(c) Cyanosis prominent in 2nd to 3rd decade
(d) Non cardiac surgery should be done
(e) < 25% survive by 10 years

685. TOF recurrence: (T/F)

(a) One sibling–2.5%
(b) Two sibling–8%
(c) Two sibling–5.5%
(d) Male affected–1.5%
(e) Female/mother–2.6%

686. TOF with absent pulmonary valve: (T/F)

(a) 2% patients of TOF
(b) Associated with dilatation of pulmonary artery
(c) To and fro murmur on right and upper mid stemal area
(d) Large VSD common
(e) Pulmonary complication most common cause of death

687. DORV A/E: (T/F)

(a) DORV with VSD = Taussig-Bing anomaly
(b) Pathophysiology depend on site of VSD and severity of PS
(c) Sub aortic VSD without PS resemble VSD with PHT with CCF
(d) Sub pulmonary VSD with PS resemble TOF
(e) DORV with sub pulmonary VSD with PS resemble tricuspid atresia

688. Fontan high risk: (T/F)

(a) PAP > 18 mm Hg (b) LVEDP > 12 mm Hg
(c) PVR < 2 unit/m^2 (d) AV regurgitation
(e) LVEF > 60%

689. CC-TGA: (T/F)

(a) Ventriculo arterial concordance
(b) Atrio-Ventricular concordance
(c) Coronary Artery concordance
(d) BB discordance
(e) 80% VSD

690. Cyanosis with ↑ PBF: (T/F)

(a) Truncus arteriosus
(b) TGA
(c) TAPVR
(d) Single Ventricle with PS
(e) DORV with PS

691. Rib notching: (T/F)

(a) May be unilateral
(b) Usually involved undersurface
(c) Anterior rib usually spared
(d) Usually neonates
(e) 3rd–8th Ribs

692. Eisenmenger ASD vs VSD (ASD favouring): (T/F)

(a) Parasternal Heave prominent
(b) Wide fixed S2 split
(c) Cardiomegaly absent
(d) Differential cyanosis
(e) TR

693. Holt-Oram syndrome: (T/F)

(a) TBX 5
(b) Shoulder hypoplasia
(c) 85% associated with cardiac defect
(d) Conduction defect may occur without structural heart disease
(e) LBBB

694. 2 weeks neonate, cyanosis, TGA with intact septum treatment: (T/F)

(a) Atrial switch after 3 months
(b) Atrial switch after 2 weeks
(c) Arterial switch after 2 weeks
(d) Rastelli operation after 3 months
(e) Arterial switch after 3 months

695. 6 years old TOF with normal pulmonary vasculature presented with excessive crying, cyanosis, requiring intubation next what? (T/F)

(a) Urgent ABGA
(b) Metoprolol, HCO_3, morphine IV
(c) Deepening of sedation by thiopental if required
(d) Hydration
(e) Emergency BT shunt if refractory cyanosis

696. Continuous murmur: (T/F)

(a) RSOV
(b) PDA

(c) Peripheral pulmonary branch Stenosis
(d) ALCAPA
(e) AS

697. LV: (T/F)
(a) More trabeculated than RV
(b) Anterolateral papillary musde from IVS
(c) Anterior mitral leaflet more apical than septal TV
(d) MV and AV in fibrous continuity
(e) False tendon common with LV

698. RV: (T/F)
(a) More trabeculated than LV
(b) Apex trabeculated
(c) Cristasupraventricularis separates TV and PV
(d) PV and TV fibrous continuity
(e) RV posterior structure

699. Eisenmenger correct: (T/F)
(a) ASD Eisenmenger worse prognosis than VSD Eisenmenger
(b) ASD Eisenmenger reverse splith
(c) LPH more prominent in ASD Eisenmenger
(d) VSD Eisenmenger should be closed early
(e) Down syndrome early Eisenmenger and less frequent

700. T/F:
(a) AVSD more common with trisomy 21
(b) Eisenmenger more common
(c) LVOT obstruction association with trisomy 21
(d) Operated at 3.4 years (preschool)
(e) Single valve mechanism more common in trisomy

701. cc-TGA: (T/F)
(a) Most common associated with VSD
(b) Subpulmonic obstruction–50%
(c) TV abnormal in almost all causes at autopsy
(d) CHB with TR increases with age in most
(e) COA is rearly associated

702. PDA: (T/F)
(a) Maternal rubella 1st trimester
(b) Holt-Oram syndrome
(c) Down's syndrome
(d) Valproate
(e) X linked incontinentia pigmenti

703. Cyanosis with normal heart size: (T/F)
(a) LSVC to LA
(b) Pulmonary A–V fistula
(c) Cerebral A–V fistula
(d) Peripheral A–V fistula
(e) Abnormal eustachian valve

704. True about coronary venous system: (T/F)
(a) Anterior inter-ventricular vein best for CRT
(b) Vein of marshall can be cauce of AF
(c) Left phrenic nerve is close proximity to obtuse marginal vein
(d) Dilated CS is seen with persistent left CS
(e) Right free wall pathway is associated with coronary sinus dilatation

705. Balloon atrial septostomy indicated in: (T/F)
(a) Tricuspid atresia (b) Severe PS
(c) TGA (corrected) (d) PPH
(e) In professional deep sea divers

706. Fontan surgery done in: (T/F)
(a) Tricuspid atresia
(b) Univentricular heart
(c) Pulmonary atresia with RV hypoplastic
(d) TGA
(e) TAPVC

707. LAD with counter clockwise rotation seen in: (T/F)
(a) ECD (b) Tricuspid atresia
(c) DORV (d) TGA
(e) PS with intact septum

708. ↑ pulm blood flow seen in: (T/F)
(a) Tricuspid atresia
(b) Common atrium
(c) Taussig-Bing anomaly
(d) Ebstein anomaly
(e) Eisenmenger syndrome

709. Cyanotic spells seen in: (T/F)
(a) Tricuspid atresia
(b) TOF
(c) TGA with VSD with PS
(d) ASD
(e) VSD

710. Adulthood survival is uncommon in: (T/F)
(a) Interrupted aortic arch
(b) TGA

(c) Ebstein anomaly
(d) Pulmonary atresia with intact septum
(e) PAPVC

711. Cyanotic spell–Management is: (T/F)
(a) Morphine (b) Normal Saline
(c) Esmolol (d) Ketamine
(e) $NaHCO_3$

712. Regarding conotruncal anomalies true is: (T/F)
(a) TOF most common
(b) TGA can be detected by fetal echo
(c) Pulm artery dilatation seen in TOF
(d) Aortomitral continuity seen in DORV

713. High risk for development of Eisenmenger: (T/F)
(a) TOF
(b) Truncus arteriosus
(c) Aortopulmonary window
(d) Restrictive PDA
(e) TAPVC

714. Coarctation of aorta A/E: (T/F)
(a) Aortic dissection
(b) Systemic HTN
(c) Mycotic aneurysm
(d) Bicuspid aortic valve

715. Coarctation of aorta–true are: (T/F)
(a) HTN is common association
(b) Surgery is treatment of choice in neonates
(c) Stenting is treatment of choice in neonates
(d) Prostaglandins used in neonatal period
(e) CT angiography useful in diagnosis

716. TGA-treatment in 2 weeks neonate with cyanosis and CHF: (T/F)
(a) Arterial switch within 2 weeks
(b) Atrial switch within 2 weeks
(c) Atrial switch after 3 months
(d) Rastelli after 3 months
(e) Atrial switch after 3 months

717. Neonate with cyanotic spell–emergency management–intubated and: (T/F)
(a) ABG
(b) Emergency BT shunt in refractory
(c) Metoprolol, $NaHCO_3$, I morphine
(d) Rehydration
(e) Thiopentone effect deepened if saturation fall further

718. Cyanotic spell: (T/F)
(a) Viral infection
(b) Present during sleep
(c) Commonly associated with cardiac catheterization
(d) Anaemia is common

719. MR is seen in A/E: (T/F)
(a) Congenital MS
(b) cc-TGA
(c) ALCAPA
(d) Septum primum ASD
(e) Vena cava associated with LA

720. Shunt lesions (R→L) SpO_2=100 PvO_2=88 MyO_2=64 shunt:
(a) 3 : 1 (b) 3 : 2
(c) 5 : 2 (d) 2 : 1

721. ASD with cyanosis: (T/F)
(a) Iatrogenic ASD following BMV
(b) Tricuspid atresia
(c) Persistent large eustachian valve
(d) Left SVC into LA
(e) Eisenmenger complex

722. 10 years old child with congenital PS pressure gradient 36 mm Hg, asymptomatic child treatment: (T/F)
(a) Valvotomy
(b) Diuretics
(c) Medical follow up
(d) Sports prescribed
(e) Balloon dilatation

723. Gross cardiomegaly on CAR: (T/F)
(a) Pericardial effusion
(b) Teratoma-posterior mediastinal
(c) TOF
(d) VSD with Eisenmenger
(e) Ebstein anomaly

724. TAPVC true: (T/F)
(a) Loud P2
(b) Narrow S2 split
(c) Infradiaphragmatic common
(d) Left axis on ECG
(e) 80% die within 1 year without treatment

725. cc-TGA true is: (T/F)
(a) 75% VSD
(b) Congenital CHB
(c) Subvalvular PS
(d) 10% left sided AV lesion
(e) q wave in left precordial lead and absent in right precordial lead

726. Cyanosis: (T/F)
(a) Met Hb > 0.5 g %
(b) Reduced Hb > 2 g %
(c) Reduced Hb > 4 g %
(d) O_2 saturation < 85 %
(e) O_2 saturation < 90 %

727. RV morphology: (T/F)
(a) Apex trabeculated
(b) RV > LV trabeculations
(c) RV is posterior
(d) Fibrous continuity is maintained between TV and PV
(e) Crista supraterminalis separate TV from PV

728. Single S_2: (T/F)
(a) ASD with Eisenmenger
(b) Pulmonary atresia
(c) Truncus arteriousus
(d) Mild PS
(e) MR

729. Reversed differential cyanosis in neonate: (T/F)
(a) COA
(b) PDA with Eisenmenger
(c) Interrupted aortic arch with PDA
(d) TGA with interrupted aortic arch with PDA
(e) Primary pulmonary HTN

730. Exertional angina in children: (T/F)
(a) Severe PS (b) PPH
(c) HOCM (d) ALCAPA

731. Ejection click in BAV: (T/F)
(a) Seen in severe AS only
(b) Better audible at apex
(c) Comes after ESM
(d) Intensity increases with increasing severity
(e) Non stenotic valve–gets increased S_1 EC gap

732. RSOV: (T/F)
(a) Congenital abnormality in aortic wall (media)
(b) Left coronary cusp (LCC) to RA and RV
(c) Never ruptures to pulmonary artery
(d) Device closure can be done
(e) Non coronary cusp to RA or RV
(f) Most common is LCC

733. Severity of pulmonary stenosis: (T/F)
(a) Prolonged murmur
(b) Left Pulmonary artery dilatation on X-ray
(c) Delayed ejection click
(d) Cyanosis in presence of PFO
(e) Soft/absent/delayed P_2

734. Visceral artery aneurysm: (T/F)
(a) Takayasu arteritis (b) Behcet's disease
(c) PAN (d) Giant cell arteritis
(e) None

735. Scimitar syndrome: (T/F)
(a) Aorta supplies Right Lower lung
(b) Right lung and right Pulmonary artery hypoplasia
(c) Right Lung drains to SVC
(d) PAH may occur
(e) Associated with valvular PS

736. Conotruncal anomaly: (T/F)
(a) Most common in TOF
(b) TOF–malalignment in muscular septum
(c) DORV–aortomitral continuity maintained
(d) TGA can be detected on fetal echo

737. TOF: (T/F)
(a) 25% have Right aortic arch
(b) Pink TOF–small restrictive VSD
(c) Left sided chamber usually small
(d) Dilated PA on X-ray
(e) Chronic hypoxia can cause LV dysfunction

738. RV morphology: (T/F)
(a) Apex trabeculated
(b) RV > LV trabeculations
(c) RV is posterior
(d) Fibrous continuity is maintained between TV and PV
(e) Crista supraterminalis separate TV from PV

739. LV morphology: (T/F)
(a) Aorto-mitral continuity is present
(b) Anterolateral papillary muscle is attached to IVS
(c) Septal leaflet of tricuspid valve is less superior to attachment of AML
(d) False tendon is a common finding
(e) More trabeculated

740. Peripheral PS seen in A/E: (T/F)
(a) William syndrome (b) Catch-22 syndrome
(c) Rubella (d) Allagille syndrome
(e) Down syndrome

741. Best outcome seen in: (T/F)
(a) Balloon Pulmonary Valve Dilatation
(b) Balloon Mitral Valvotomy
(c) Aortic Balloon Valve Dilatation
(d) Tricuspid Valve Balloon Dilatation
(e) COA–balloon dilatation

742. Fontan's operation not done/bad outcome: (T/F)
(a) Confluent good sized Pas
(b) PVRI = 6 WU
(c) Mild left AV valve regurgitation
(d) Bilateral SVC
(e) Malposed great arteries

743. Rastelli's repair done in: (T/F)
(a) d-TGA (b) DORV + VSD + PS
(c) SV + PS (d) Tricuspid atresia
(e) SV + PAH

744. 8 years old female with cyanotic spells, squatting, pulmonary oligemia, mesocardia, CHB: (T/F)
(a) d-TGA (b) cc-TGA
(c) TOF (d) TA
(e) DORV

745. 20 days old child with failure to thrive with dyspnea, normal CT ratio and ground glass appearance on CXR: (T/F)
(a) Hyaline membrane disease
(b) TGA
(c) Obstructed TAPVC
(d) Supracristal VSD
(e) Tricuspid atresia

746. Holt-Oram syndrome incorrect: (T/F)
(a) Thumb not involved
(b) Usually unilateral arm involvement
(c) Autosomal recessive
(d) Secundum ASD > primum ASD
(e) PTPN-11 gene is involved

747. Noonan's syndrome A/E: (T/F)
(a) Lymphatic dysplasia is common
(b) Tall stature
(c) Affects males only
(d) Valvular PS is the most common CVS abnormality
(c) Autosomal recessive

748. Down's syndrome incorrect: (T/F)
(a) PAH is rare
(b) AV canal defect common
(c) TGA is common
(d) MVP develops more commonly in elderly
(e) Ageing leads to early vascular changes

749. Incorrect about murmur: (T/F)
(a) PS murmur decreases with isometric murmur
(b) Rheumatic MR increases with post VPC
(c) VSD murmur increases with hand grip
(d) MVP murmur disappears with squatting
(e) Right sided murmur returned to baseline earlier after valsalva release than left side

750. Appropriate treatment of cyanotic spells: (T/F)
(a) O_2 (b) HCO_3 IV
(c) IV morphine (d) IV lasix
(e) Knee elbow position

751. Holt-Oram true: (T/F)
(a) AR
(b) Clavicular hypoplasia
(c) Unilateral limb involvement
(d) TBX5 gene
(e) Dermatoglyphyics

752. Teratogenicity: (T/F)
(a) Phenylalanine–TOF
(b) Ethanol–VSD
(c) Vitamin D–Valvular AS
(d) Erythromycin–ASD
(e) Valproate–coarctation

753. RV differentiated from LV: (T/F)
(a) Moderator bard
(b) Septal attachment of papillary muscle
(c) Basal attachment of AV valve
(d) Apical trabeculation
(e) Ellipsoid

754. Marfan mutation *except:* (T/F)
(a) Fibrillin I
(b) Trop T
(c) Trop I
(d) Tropomysin
(e) FGF

755. Marfan: (T/F)
(a) AS
(b) MVP
(c) AO dissection
(d) Myopia
(e) Splenomegaly

756. cc TGA: (T/F)
(a) 75% VSD
(b) CHB
(c) Subpulmonary stenosis
(d) 10% left AV valve abnormality
(e) q in lateral leads

757. TAPVC: (T/F)
(a) Left axis deviation
(b) Loud P_2
(c) S2 narrow and mobile split
(d) Infradiaphragmatic most common
(e) 80% mortality untreated in 1 year

758. ASD A/E: (T/F)
(a) AO knuckle prominent
(b) 2° ASD most common
(c) Children asymptomatic
(d) 1 year closure
(e) A wave > V wave in JVP

759. Autosomal dominant: (T/F)
(a) Noonan's syndrome
(b) HOCM
(c) MVP
(d) Fabry's disease
(e) Holt-Oram syndrome

760. Features of RV: (T/F)
(a) Moderator band
(b) Basal attachment of AV valve
(c) Septal attachment of papillary muscle
(d) Apical trabeculation
(e) Ellipsoid shape

761. cc-TGA: (T/F)
(a) 75% VSD
(b) 10% left AV valve abnormality
(c) Subpulmonary PS
(d) Congenital CHB
(e) Q absent in right precordial leads

762. ASD A/E: (T/F)
(a) Most common secundum
(b) Children usually asymptomatic
(c) Closes spontaneously in first year
(d) a > v wave in JVP
(e) Aortic knuckle prominent in CXR

763. TAPVC: (T/F)
(a) LAD
(b) Narrow split S2 and mobile
(c) P2 loud
(d) Most common is infradiaphragmatic type
(e) 80% mortality in first year in untreated

764. Central cyanosis: (T/F)
(a) $SaO_2 < 85\%$
(b) $SaO_2 < 90\%$
(c) Reduced Hb–2 g%
(d) Reduced Hb–4 g%
(e) Methemoglobin 0.5 g%

765. Lutembacher's syndrome consists of: (T/F)
(a) Congenital MS
(b) Acquired MS
(c) ASD
(d) VSD
(e) AS

766. Treatment of cyanotic spells in TOF include: (T/F)
(a) IV NTG
(b) IV morphine
(c) IV $NaHCO_3$
(d) O_2
(e) Knee-chest position

767. Clinical features of Eisenmenger's syndrome are: (T/F)
(a) Pulmonary ejection click
(b) Loud P_2
(c) Graham Steel murmur
(d) Widely split S_1
(e) TR murmur

768. Left axis deviation seen in: (T/F)
(a) TGA (b) TOF
(c) MS (d) DORV
(e) Tricuspid atresia

769. X-ray features of TOF include: (T/F)
(a) Boot shaped heart
(b) Pulmonary obigemia
(c) Left atria enlargement
(d) LV enlargement
(e) Prominent pulmonary artery

770. Coarctation of aorta: (T/F)
(a) Tubular hypoplasia most common
(b) Rib notching
(c) Near the attachment of ligament arteriosum
(d) Proximal to common carotid artery
(e) Distal to left subclavian artery

771. Gene mutations in Marfan's syndrome: (T/F)
(a) Trop-I (b) Trop-T
(c) p-MHC (d) Fibrillion-I
(e) FGF

772. Surgery C/I in PDA: (T/F)
(a) Aneurysmal PDA (b) Calcified PDA
(c) Large PDA (d) Dilated LV
(e) R-L shunt

773. C/F of ASD are A/E: (T/F)
(a) Wide fixed splitting of S_2
(b) Pulmonary oligemia
(c) Pulmonary plethora
(d) ESM at pulmonary area
(e) Diastolic murmur at tricuspid area

774. Prenatal exposure causes: (T/F)
(a) Alcohol–VSD (b) Erythromycin–ASD
(c) Valproate–COA (d) Phenylalanine–TOF
(e) Vit D–valvular AS

775. Cardioplegic solution ingredient causing diastolic arrest: (T/F)
(a) Ca (b) K
(c) Cl (d) Steroids
(e) Mannitol

776. Pulmonary AV fistula: (T/F)
(a) Congenital (b) Acquired
(c) Always multiple (d) Cyanosis
(e) L-R shunt

777. Palliative surgery in TOF A/E: (T/F)
(a) Brock's procedure (b) PA banding
(c) Closure of VSD (d) BT shunt
(e) WC shunt

778. DORV+VSD+PS seen in: (T/F)
(a) Lack of aorto-mitral contimity
(b) Side by side relation of great vessel
(c) No VSD
(d) Multiple VSD
(e) No cyanosis

779. Swan Ganz catheter directly measures: (T/F)
(a) PA pressure (b) CVP
(c) LA pressure (d) LV pressure
(e) Aortic pressure

780. ASD: (T/F)
(a) CHF in 1st year
(b) Most common presentation in 2nd year
(c) Most close by 1 year
(d) A wave prominent in JVP

781. AD: (T/F)
(a) Noonan's syndrome
(b) Holt-Oram syndrome
(c) HOCM
(d) Long QT syndrome

782. Marfan's syndrome clinical feature: (T/F)
(a) MVP (b) Aortic dissection
(c) AR (d) Myopia

783. RV morphology: (T/F)
(a) Moderator band
(b) Apex trabeculated
(c) Ellipsoid shape

784. Noonan's syndrome: (T/F)

(a) PS (b) PA stenosis
(c) ASD (d) HCM
(e) HLHS

785. L-TGA: (T/F)

(a) Congenital heart block
(b) 10% anomaly in left side

786. X-rays finding of LAE: (T/F)

(a) Straight left heart border
(b) Double density
(c) Elevation of MPA
(d) Acute convex border

787. Neonate CHF: (T/F)

(a) HLHS (b) TOF
(c) Myocarditis (d) Tachyarrhythmias

788. Holt-Oram syndrome A/E: (T/F)

(a) AD
(b) Unilateral upper limb defect
(c) Dermatoglyphics abnormal
(d) Clavicle hypoplastic

789. Diastolic murmur at MV A/E: (T/F)

(a) ASD (b) VSD
(c) AR (d) Rheumatic activity
(e) MR

790. High first month mortality in CHD: (T/F)

(a) TA (b) TGA
(c) TOF (d) Truncus arteriosus
(e) TAPVC

791. Central cyanosis with pulmonary edema due to: (T/F)

(a) Decreased diffusion capacity
(b) Increased H^+ conc.
(c) V/Q shunt mismatch
(d) Hyperventilation
(e) Increased circulation time in pulmonary circulation

792. P2 loud in:

(a) PS
(b) Pulmonary atresia
(c) Tricuspid atresia type Ib
(d) DORV with PS

793. Pulmonary atresia with Pott' s shunt, after few years presented with cath value with Hb-20g% of PA-75%, PV-95%, RA-60% and FA-90%, what is Qp/Qs?

(a) 1.25 (b) 1.75
(c) 0.33 (d) 1.50

794. SMA A/E:

(a) Type I and III, cardiac more involvement
(b) VSD most common defect
(c) DCMP in type III
(d) AF/AFI more common arrhythmias

795. Atrial septotomy A/E:

(a) TA with VSD with restrictive PFO
(b) PA with intact ventricular septum
(c) PA with VSD with TGA

796. Cor triatriatum false:

(a) Fibromuscular diaphragm separate LA into posterosuperior and anterioinferior chamber
(b) Diaphragm is just below LA appendage
(c) Can present with pulmonary edema
(d) Treatment is surgery

797. Pulmonary atresia which is not used:

(a) Pulmonary valve radioablation and dilatation
(b) Pulmonary valvotomy
(c) BT shunt
(d) Pulmonary valve replacement

798. Azygous vein drains into:

(a) Courses right of lumber spine into SVC
(b) Courses left of lumber spine into IVC

799. True about aortic arches:

(a) Left distal 6th–PDA
(b) 4th–right and left carotid
(c) 1, 2 and 6 regresses
(d) 4th left–left subclavian

800. Which surgery is not done in D-TGA?

(a) Nikadoah repair (b) Arterial switch
(c) Double switch (d) Rastelli repair

801. Sinus venosus ASD seen associated with:

(a) PAPVC (b) Down's syndrome

802. Watchman device used for:

(a) VSD (b) ASD
(c) LA appendage (d) Mitraclip repair

803. LV dominance without RV feature seen in:
(a) HLHS
(b) Tricuspid atresia
(c) Pulmonary atresia with VSD
(d) Taussing-Bing anomaly

804. Figure of 8 seen in:
(a) TAPVC

805. Ebstein anomaly:
(a) More than one accessory pathway in 6-36 % pts
(b) Complete heart block is rare

806. GOSES scoring:
(a) Ebstein's anomaly (b) TOF

807. Lithium causes:
(a) Ebstein's anomaly (b) Tricuspid atresia

808. Friedreich's ataxia A/E:
(a) AR
(b) Chromosome 6
(c) Frataxin gene
(d) Frataxin–mitochondrial enzyme and iron metabolism

809. William syndrome associated with:
(a) Chromosome 9 (b) Chromosome 21
(c) Chromosome 7 (d) Chromosome 10

810. Asplenia associated with A/E:
(a) AV canal defect (b) TGA
(c) Pulmonary atresia (d) LVOT obstruction

811. Tricuspid atresia severity correlation maximum with:
(a) Size of PDA
(b) Size of ASD
(c) Presence and size of VSD
(d) Presence of TGA

812. Gradient in catheterization in COA is significant:
(a) 20 mm Hg (b) 40 mm Hg
(c) 60 mm Hg (d) 50 mm Hg

813. 2 years child with VSD with recurrent chest infection. Gradient across VSD–40 mm Hg:
(a) Early VSD closure
(b) Cath. for reversibility before closure
(c) Decongest with ACE-I
(d) PA banding

814. Least O_2 in fetal circulation:
(a) Ductus venosus (b) Umbilical vein
(c) Ductus arteriosus (d) Pulmonary vein

815. LV non compaction A/E:
(a) Not associated with any cardiac abnormality
(b) Non compacted/compacted ratio > 4
(c) Blood in deep recesses on colour Doppler
(d) Trabeculation and deep recess

816. Tall R wave A/E:
(a) HOCM (b) PWMI
(c) Ebstein's anomaly (d) DMD

817. In cyanotic infant, ECG showing left axis deviation is suggestive of which condition?
(a) TAPVC (b) DORV without PS
(c) TGA (d) Tricuspid atresia

818. Dose of digoxin in premature infants is:
(a) 20 mg/kg (b) 30 mg/kg
(c) 40 mg/kg (d) 50 mg/kg

819. Which of the following statement is false about Taussig-Bing anomaly?
(a) Resembles corrected TGA with non restrictive VSD
(b) Reverse differential cyanosis may occur
(c) PA saturation always higher than aorta
(d) High incidence of aortic malformation associated

820. Leftward 'P' wave axis in ASD is suggestive of:
(a) Ostium primum ASD
(b) ASD with septal aneurysm
(c) IVC type of ASD
(d) Sinus venous ASD

821. Which of the following drug's intake during pregnancy is associated with Ebstein's anomaly in baby?
(a) Ethanol (b) Valproic acid
(c) Lithium (d) Thalidomide

822. Most common reported complication of arterial switch operation on follow up is:
(a) Ostial coronary artery disease
(b) Supra pulmonary artery stenosis
(c) Neo aortic valve regurgitation
(d) Ventricular arrhythmias

823. Supravalvular aortic stenosis is associated with which of the following condition?

(a) Down syndrome (b) Turner syndrome
(c) Williams syndrome

824. In which Eisenmenger syndrome, cardiomegaly is noted?

(a) ASD (b) VSD
(c) PSD (d) AP Window

825. "Figure of eight" appearance in chest X-ray is typically seen in:

(a) TAPVC (b) Tricuspid atresia
(c) TGA (d) Truncus arterosus

826. Coronary angiography may not be indicated in which of the following condition?

(a) Acute coronary syndrome
(b) Multivessel CAD
(c) CAD with left ventricular dysfunction
(d) CAD whose angina has responded to medical treatment

827. Congenital heart disease involving abnormal remodeling of the aortic arch arteries has been associated with maternal deficiencies of which vitamins?

(a) Vitamin A (b) Vitamin B
(c) Vitamin C (d) Vitamin D

828. Congenital heart disease involving the outflow tract can be associated with other defects if neural of neural crest, such as:

(a) Craniofacial defects (b) Nail defect
(c) Lower limb defect (d) Sterna defect

829. Differential cyanosis is seen in a patient with a:

(a) Large parent ductus arteriosus (PDA) and secondary pulmonary hypertension
(b) Large ventricular septal defect with secondary pulmonary hypertension
(c) Large atrial septal defect with secondary pulmonary hypertension
(d) Idiopathic Severe Pulmonary hypertension

830. Coronary sinus: (T/F)

(a) Middle cardiac vein running in posterior AV groove and draining into CS
(b) Coronary sinus opens into RA near SA node
(c) CS runs in anterior AV groove
(d) Unroofed CS can be associated with ASD
(e) SVC saturation more than coronary sinus saturation

831. Step up in RA: (T/F)

(a) ASD OS (b) PDA with PR
(c) RSOV to RV (d) PAPVC
(e) VSD with TR

832. Ebstein anomaly: (T/F)

(a) Grade III Left PSH
(b) TR murmur increases with inspiration
(c) Seccundum ASD often associated
(d) M > F
(e) Wide fixed S2

833. cc-TGA: (T/F)

(a) 90% conduction defect
(b) 95% situs solitus
(c) Most common left AV valve abnormality
(d) QRS prolongation is due to bundle of His inversion
(e) If no associated abnormality-normal life expectancy

834. Continuous murmur: (T/F)

(a) ALCAPA
(b) TOF with PR with PS
(c) Surgical shunt of TOF
(d) RSOV to PDA
(e) Leutember syndrome

835. T/F:

(a) Tricuspid septal leaflet–largest and mobile
(b) All aortic leaflet–equal in 80%
(c) RV is more trabeculated than LV

836. TAPVC: (T/F)

(a) 80% infradiaphragmatic TAPVC is obstructive
(b) Most of coronary sinus drainage is obstructive
(c) ASD is obligatory for survival
(d) Vertical vein forms left border of snowman heart
(e) Snowman is diagnostic in children

837. Shunt: (T/F)

(a) Shunt < 30% cannot be identified by oximetry
(b) Flamm equation for mixed venous oxygen saturation

(c) Van skyle formula for oxygen saturation because of simplicity
(d) Coronary fistula can lead to O_2 step up in RA, RV and PA
(e) Echo is not reliable for shunt estimation

838. Atrial septotomy: (T/F)
(a) Best done through Transjugular approach
(b) Umbilical vein can be used
(c) Brocken Brough needle used
(d) Reliable after 1 month
(e) Effective in RVF with PS
(f) Safely can be done echo

839. Anatomy: (T/F)
(a) RV is semilunar on cross section
(b) IVS function as a part of RV
(c) Chronic pressure overload of LV leads to spherical change
(d) RV adapts early to increase preload
(e) RV and LV both arise from primary heart field

840. Development: (T/F)
(a) Long conus leads to VSD
(b) Resorption of subpulm. conus rather than subaortic conus leads to DORV
(c) Failure of develop of pulm vessel or to develop connection with splanchic vessel leads to TAPVC
(d) Distal left 7th associated with PDA
(e) Development of septum primum with dorsal folding lead to VSD

841. Shunt: (T/F)
(a) Waterson = IVC–RPA
(b) Potts = ascending aorta–RPA
(c) Glenn = SVC–RPA
(d) Modified BT = direct SCA to RPA
(e) Classical BT = can be done on either side

842. Cyanosis in ASD: (T/F)
(a) Severe PAH
(b) TAPVC
(c) Surgical malformed connection of SVC
(d) Prominent eustachian valve directing blood to LA
(e) Child with TOF

843. Duct dependent: (T/F)
(a) Pulmonary atresia
(b) Mitral atresia
(c) Aortic atresia
(d) TAPVC
(e) Complete TGA

844. True or false: (T/F)
(a) Eisenmenger syndrome, single S2 is due to coincidence of A2 and P2
(b) Increased S2 OS gap widens in standing MS patient

845. Morphological RV: (T/F)
(a) Morphological RV has moderator band
(b) Crescent shaped cavity with fine trabeculations
(c) Left atrioventricular valve lower than right
(d) LV chordate has septal attachment
(e) Multiple irregular papillary muscles on RV

846. Ductal dependent lesions: (T/F)
(a) Mitral atresia
(b) Pulmonary atresia
(c) TAPVC
(d) Aortic atresia
(e) d-TGA

847. TOF–prominent PA seen in: (T/F)
(a) PDA
(b) AVCD
(c) Absent pulm valve
(d) Severe valvular stenosis
(e) Pink TOF

848. All are T/E:
(a) In PDA handgrip augments diastolic phase
(b) Standing decreases PS murmur
(c) Post PVC–VSD murmur decreases
(d) Squatting decreases HOCM murmur

849. Fetal circulation: (T/F)
(a) RV contribute 55% to CO
(b) Pulmonary Flow 7-10%
(c) PDA anatomical closure at birth
(d) In low birth < 1500 mg, PDA most common cone of CCF

850. Shunt in congenital disease: (T/F)
(a) Modified BT directly SCA to PA
(b) Pott shunt–ascending Aorta and RPA
(c) Waterson's shunt–IVC to RPA
(d) Glenn shunt–SVC to RPA
(e) Classical BT can be done on either side of Aortic arch

851. TOF with CHF: (T/F)
(a) Anaemia
(b) HTN
(c) Adult survival
(d) PR
(e) Severe RVOT obstruction

852. All condition can be presented in neonatal period: (T/F)
(a) CHB with low VR
(b) Severe PS
(c) PDA
(d) TOF
(e) Severe AV fistula

853. Atrial septostomy: (T/F)
(a) Can be done by umbilical vein
(b) Jugular vein–vein of choice
(c) In TAPVC to coronary sinus with restrictive ASD
(d) Better outcome in > 1 month
(e) In PAH it is done to ↓ cyanosis

854. Reading pathophysiology of heart: (T/F)
(a) TOF–neural crest defect
(b) COA–intracardiac blood flow defect
(c) TAPVC–due to targeted cell growth
(d) ECD–intracellular matrix defect
(e) Ebstein–due to cell death abnormality

855. T/F:
(a) Diabetic mother–d TGA
(b) Mother with lupus–d TGA

856. Embryology of heart: (T/F)
(a) At any time maximum 4 arches can be present
(b) Vessels derived from mesoderm
(c) PDA from 6th arch
(d) Total arches = 5
(e) Aortic arch–starts forming after 6th week IUL

857. T/F:
(a) RV cut section semilunar
(b) RV adapts to pressure changes quickly
(c) Septum function as part of RV
(d) RV, LV derived from a same linear tube
(e) Chronic pressure load–spherical DCMP

858. Balloon septal septostomy useful in: (T/F)
(a) TAPVC
(b) Mitral atresia
(c) TGA with VSD
(d) PS with suprasystemic RV pressure
(e) Pulmonary atresia with intact septum

859. Congenital Heart disease: (T/F)
(a) Cc–TGA–q wave inversion in precordial leads
(b) Primary ASD–RAD
(c) VSD–biventricular hypertrophy
(d) DORV–N-W Axis
(e) TOF–counter clockwise

860. T/F:
(a) Carbamazepine causes VSD and TOF
(b) Thalidomide–conotruncal anomaly
(c) Retinoic acid–conotruncal anomaly
(d) Triphalangeal thumb–ASD
(e) Noonan syndrome–supravalvular PS

861. Device closure: (T/F)
(a) Nitinol toxicity usual complication
(b) PDA most common cause
(c) Not used in cyanotic CHD
(d) Closes 12 hours after procedure
(e) Acquired defect can be treated after sometimes

862. DORV: (T/F)
(a) Subaortic VSD without PS is a common type
(b) Taussig-Bing anomaly has cyanosis at birth or in early infancy
(c) Great vessels have normal relationship
(d) Double committed VSD is common
(e) PR prolongation seen

863. Endocardial cushion defect: (T/F)
(a) PR prolongation common
(b) Defect in cleft mitral valve
(c) Associated with Down's syndrome in which PVOD is no early
(d) RAD is seen
(e) Goose neck deformity in LV angiography

864. PFO – indication of surgery: (T/F)
(a) Recurrent thromboembolism
(b) Decompression sickness
(c) Orthodexia and platypnea
(d) Severe PAH
(e) R to L shunt – leading to hypoxia

865. EDT < 120 and E/A > 1.5 – S/O severe pulm venous HTN: (T/F)
(a) Long MR not associated with cor triatriatum
(b) Atenolol shouldn't be used in renal failure
(c) BNP has got positive feedback causing ↑ BNP release
(d) Nitrate tolerance is because of ↑ free radicals
(e) Transplanted heart are supersensitive to adenosine if
(f) In aortic valve, the posterior and left valve leaflet are larger than other leaflet

866. PA: (T/F)
(a) > 1 mm diameter–elastic artery
(b) > 1 mm diameter = muscular artery
(c) After 1 year PA diameter is less than ½ of aorta
(d) Left bronchus passes over left PA artery
(e) Normal PVR <1-2 woods unit

867. Coronary anomalies: (T/F)
(a) 2% of live birth
(b) LCx from Rt simus is benign
(c) Most common anomaly is LCx from RCA
(d) Frequent cause of SCD
(e) MDCT–IOC

868. Continuous murmur: (T/F)
(a) Peripheral pulmonary artery stenosis
(b) VSD with AR
(c) Lutembacher syndrome
(d) Severe coarctation
(e) Pulmonary atresia with intact IVS

869. Cyanosis in first week seen in: (T/F)
(a) Pulmonary atresia with ASD
(b) TGA
(c) TOF
(d) Anomalous systemic venous connection to LA
(e) Hypoplastic right heart syndrome

870. Morphologic difference between LV and RV: (T/F)
(a) Crescent shape with fine apical trabeculation
(b) Chordal attachment of septum in LV
(c) Moderator band in LV
(d) Left atrioventricular valve inferior than right
(e) Multiple and irregular papillary muscles in RV

871. BT shunt: (T/F)
(a) Increased PBF
(b) Decreased PA pressure
(c) Equalization of pulmonary blood flow
(d) Decrease cyanosis in TOF
(e) Increased oxygenation of pulmonary blood

872. VSD versus papillary muscle rupture: (T/F)
(a) VSD most common in first MI
(b) Most common in AWMI
(c) Thrill more common in papillary muscle dysfunction than VSD
(d) Anterolateral PM dysfunction more than posterolateral PM dysfunction

873. About septum secundum and primun: (T/F)
(a) Septum secundum is anterosuperior to septum primum
(b) Limbus of fossa ovalis is made by septum primum
(c) Right horn of sinus venosus–give rise to coronary sinus
(d) Septum secundum is left of septum primum

874. Obligatory intracardiac mixing: (T/F)
(a) Corrected TGA
(b) Truncus arteriosus
(c) Pulmonary atresia
(d) D-TGA
(e) TAPVC

875. TOF surgery: (T/F)
(a) PA diameter measured at annulus
(b) Z-score 2 is better than z-score 3
(c) Pulmonary artery dilatation causes positive Z- score
(d) Z-score at pulmonary bifurcation is important
(e) Prebifurcation z-score defines right pulmonary artery

876. CHF at birth: (T/F)
(a) HLHS
(b) Tachyarrhythmias
(c) D-TGA with intact septum
(d) DORV with severe PS
(e) CHB
(f) TOF

877. Cyanosis at birth: (T/F)
(a) TOF (b) TAPVC
(c) DORV (d) DORV with PS
(e) Severe PS

878. COA least likely with: (T/F)
(a) DORV with PS
(b) Taussig-Bing anomaly
(c) Tricuspid atresia with VSD
(d) Multiple VSD
(e) TOF
(f) TGA with intact septum

879. Ductus dependent lesion: (T/F)
(a) Truncus arteriosus
(b) HLHS
(c) TGA with large VSD

880. LSVC: (T/F)
(a) Most common open in LA
(b) Cyanosis if only open in LA
(c) It connects invariably to LA
(d) Opening in coronary sinus associated with ASD
(e) Surgeon should be bearing in mind during open heart surgery

881. Post TOF surgery: (T/F)
(a) Increases in cyanosis
(b) Marked effort intolerance
(c) RBBB
(d) Regurgitant lesion

882. TOF clinical finding: (T/F)
(a) Split S2 with absent P2
(b) Murmur is proportional to degree of obstruction
(c) Palpable S2 frequent in malposition of great arteries
(d) Split S2 in adult TOF
(e) Constant ejection click indicate moderate PS

883. Dilated pulmonary artery with TOF: (T/F)
(a) TOF with absent pulmonary valve
(b) TOF with peripheral pulmonary artery stenosis
(c) Pink TOF with Branch pulmonary artery stenosis
(d) TOF with severe infundibular PS

884. Development of heart: (T/F)
(a) Heart development from splanchic mesoderm and endoderm
(b) Left sided looping is first sign of left right asymmetry
(c) Transverse axis rotates by 90° and pushed posteriorly
(d) IAS development from dorsocephalic invagination
(e) Dual origin of conduction system between cells of neuronal and muscular etiology

885. Cyanosis complications: (T/F)
(a) Iron deficiency causes hyperviscosity symptoms
(b) Cerebral artery thrombosis more common in adult CHD
(c) Increases erythropoietin causes progressive glomerular sclerosis
(d) Treatment of hyperuricemia prevent uric acid nephropathy and gout

886. Eisenmenger syndrome: (T/F)
(a) Associated with pulmonary haemorrhage with thrombosis

887. Step up in RV: (T/F)
(a) PDA with PR
(b) LSVC to RA

888. Congenital heart disease: (T/F)
(a) Trisomy 21 invariably associated with ECD
(b) Complete AV canal defect present late
(c) Noonan's syndrome associated with subpulmonic VSD
(d) Friedreich's ataxia causes DCMP
(e) Marfan's syndrome only with aortic annular dilatation

889. Adult CHD: (T/F)
(a) AF in adults as compared to VPC is in children
(b) Fontan can be done with PVR > 8 units/m^2
(c) Congenital PS gradually increases with age
(d) Progressive aortic root dilatation in bicuspid aortic valve irrespective of hemodynamic

890. T/F:
(a) Left 4th arch–arch of aorta
(b) Left 6th–left carotid artery
(c) Left 5th–Ductus
(d) 1st Aortic arch–CCA
(e) Rt 6th–RPA

891. Ebstein's anomaly: (T/F)

(a) Anterior leaflet of TV displaced
(b) On echo AML of TV > 20 mm/m^2
(c) TS occurs occasionally
(d) Prominent R in V1
(e) ASD/PFO in 50%

892. PS (pulmonary stenosis): (T/F)

(a) Mild PS > 50% have normal ECG
(b) Moderate PS > 90% have abnormal ECG
(c) Severe PS in infant, LVH with LAD more than expected
(d) Double level obstruction in infundibular PS
(e) In case of moderate PS, axis > 110° is more than 50% of patient

893. Hemodynamic finding of PS with VSD versus PS with intact septum: (T/F)

(a) Cyanosis is likely with intact septum
(b) With post extrasystolic beat, equal rise of systolic pressure in both ventricle
(c) Intensity of murmur in PS with VSD inversely proportional to degree of stenosis
(d) In infundibular PS, obstruction at 2 levels
(e) Height of R wave × 10= RV systolic pressure

894. TOF: (T/F)

(a) If sibling has TOF, then chance in other offspring is 2.5-3.5%
(b) If parents has TOF, then less chance as compared if sibling has TOF
(c) DiGeorge syndrome has association with TOF
(d) Retinoic acid ingestion in first trimester
(e) Infants of uncontrolled DM has high chance of having TOF

895. True of false:

(a) Schimitar syndrome – right upper pulmonary vein into IVC, ASD and right upper PA hypoplasia
(b) Portal vein drainage more common in females for TAPVC
(c) When drainage into umbili-vitelline obstruction is rare
(d) Single pulmonary vein drainage into right side not detected usually clinically
(e) Figure of 8 seen within first few months of life

896. Development of arch vessel: (T/F)

(a) 2nd–Common carotid artery
(b) 6th–PDA
(c) 5th–Pulmonary artery
(d) 1st –Maxillary artery
(e) Left 7th intersegmental–Left subclavian artery

897. Heart development: (T/F)

(a) Right horn of sinus venous form coronary sinus
(b) Ostium secundum is anterosuperior to ostium primum
(c) Septum secundum is on left of septum primum
(d) Limbus of fossa ovalis formed by ostium primum
(e) Ostium secundum defect is due to excessive absorption of septum primum

898. AS: (T/F)

(a) Calcific AS – no ejection click
(b) Under 15 years tricuspid valve is seen in 50%
(c) Bicuspid valve in infancy may cause obstruction
(d) In rheumatic AS, nodular thickening of commissure
(e) > 65 years tricuspid in 40%

899. Coarctation of aorta: (T/F)

(a) Biscuspid aortic valve in 25%
(b) In abdominal coarctation – RAS common
(c) Collateral seen in 2nd to 9th ribs after 5 years of age
(d) Rib erosion seen through out inferior margin of rib
(e) Collateral can cause erosion of ribs

900. Coarctation of aorta: (T/F)

(a) Collateral is due to muscular defect of media and posterior folding of wall
(b) Collateral can be seen occasionally along superior margin
(c) In Turner syndrome, COA seen in 70%
(d) LVOT obstruction associated in 30%

901. d- TGA: (T/F)

(a) 50% of cases associated with PFO or PDA
(b) VSD associated in 50%
(c) LVOT obstruction seen in 30%
(d) 2 years mortality is 50%
(e) Associated LVOT has more chance of having VSD

902. Vector cardiography: (T/F)

(a) Type A–ASD
(b) Type C–COPD
(c) Type C–clockwise
(d) Type A–clockwise, right and anterior
(e) Type B–clockwise, right and posterior

903. Coronary sinus: (T/F)
(a) O_2 saturation 55%
(b) O_2 content 5 ml/100 g/min
(c) PaO_2 = 15-20 mm Hg
(d) Coronary blood flow – 70-90 ml/100 g/min at rest
(e) O_2 consumption of heart = 15-20 ml/kg/min

904. ASD needed for: (T/F)
(a) Mitral atresia
(b) d-TGA
(c) Univentricular heart with PS
(d) TAPVC
(e) Pulmonary atresia with VSD

905. Torus of aorticus seen as:
(a) Indentation by non coronary sinus
(b) Indentation by right coronary sinus
(c) Indentation by left coronary sinus

906. Most common vascular ring:
(a) Double aortic arch
(b) Right aortic arch
(c) Pulmonary artery sling
(d) Retroduodenal descending aorta

907. PDA A/E:
(a) Small PDA have systolic murmur
(b) Surgery better than device for calcified PDA
(c) MDM in mitral area indicate > 2:1 shunt
(d) LVH earlier than RVH

908. COA associated commonly:
(a) BAV (b) PDA
(c) VSD (d) Cleft MV

909. Subaortic AS A/E:
(a) AR (b) Ejection click
(c) LVH

910. Ostium primum ASD > 2:1 A/E:
(a) Pulmonary murmur
(b) MDM at tricuspid area
(c) RAD + RBBB
(d) S2 split fixed

911. All true about TAPVC *except:*
(a) Figure of 8 in infracardiac TAPVC
(b) Saturation is same in all chambers

912. TOF true:
(a) ECG–no chamber enlargement
(b) Increased JVP
(c) All false

913. Least oxygen saturation:
(a) Single ventricle with PAH
(b) TGA with VSD with PS
(c) TAPVC

914. Norwood operation–all done in stage I repair *except:*
(a) Aortopulmonary shunt
(b) Anastomosis between pulmonary artery and aorta
(c) VSD closure
(d) PA banding

915. Taussig-Bing anomaly–Most common vascular artery:
(a) COA
(b) Interrupted Aorta
(c) Ao atresia

916. Most common cause of fetal hydrops:
(a) SVT (b) HLHS
(c) CHB (d) COA

917. DORV–least common great vessel associated:
(a) Normal great arteries (b) Left anterior
(c) Right anterior (d) Side by side

918. Rubella A/E:
(a) Valvular PS (b) COA
(c) ASD (d) PDA

919. TAPVC A/E:
(a) Figure of 8 is present in infracardiac type
(b) Continuous murmur
(c) RAD
(d) Equal saturation in all 4 chambers

920. VSD true:
(a) AR is seen in large VSD
(b) Pulmonary vascular disease is reversible in first year of life
(c) Large VSD produces murmur at birth
(d) Single S2 indicates large shunt

921. TGA A/E:

(a) Infant with normal body weight
(b) Common in male
(c) Extracardiac defect is common association
(d) May occur in diabetic mother

922. All four chambers enlarged in A/E:

(a) Gerbode defect (b) AVCD
(c) Aorta to LV tunnel (d) Systemic AV fistula

923. LAD A/E:

(a) AVCD (b) Tricuspid atresia
(c) Ebstein anomaly (d) Univentricular heart

924. TGA true:

(a) Cardiac cath. is the investigation of choice
(b) In patient with PS arterial switch is procedure of choice
(c) Common in female
(d) Normal split S2

925. Fontan circulation true:

(a) Univentricular heart circulation physiology
(b) Corrective surgery to prevent admixture of oxygenated and deoxygenated blood in univentricular heart
(c) Both true
(d) Both false

926. Paradoxical septal motion:

(a) Large VSD (b) MR
(c) TAPVC (d) PDA

927. TGA in neonate surgery of choice:

(a) Arterial switch (b) Atrial switch
(c) Rastelli (d) Fontan

928. TOF which is false:

(a) JVP not raised in children
(b) Gradient is proportionate to severity of disease
(c) Surgical outcome depends on RVOT
(d) Presence of LAD indicates association with AVCD

929. Continuous colour Doppler signal in PA seen in A/E:

(a) ALCAPA (b) Pulmonary AV fistula
(c) AP window (d) Coronary sinus to PA

930. RVSP = PASP without PS in A/E:

(a) ASD (b) VSD
(c) TGA (d) DORV

931. cc-TGA true A/E:

(a) 5% have congenital CHB
(b) Associated anomalies include VSD, subpulmonic stenosis, Left sided valve abnormality
(c) Recurrent atrial arrhythmias with ↑ age but no ↑ risk of acquired CHB
(d) Systemic valvular regurgitation ↑ with age

932. Ductus is called persistent when:

(a) After neonatal period (b) 2 months
(c) 6 months (d) 1 year

933. PA pressure–36 mmHg for all, highest PVR seen in:

(a) Primary PAH (b) MS
(c) ASD (d) VSD

934. Identical large L → R shunt in all, then PCWP least in:

(a) ASP (b) VSD
(c) PDA (d) AP window

935. Asplenia syndrome shows A/E:

(a) IVC interruption
(b) Anomalous pulmonary venous return
(c) RAA isomerism
(d) AV canal defect

936. Continuous murmur not seen in which PDA:

(a) Ductus dependent pulmonary circulation
(b) Ductus dependent systemic circulation
(c) TOF with PDA
(d) Adult with Calcific PDA

937. True in PS A/E:

(a) BPV curative
(b) Grade of murmur directly proportional to severity
(c) 50% have dysplastic valve

938. TOF true A/E:

(a) JVP not raised in children
(b) Severity proportional to gradient across PV
(c) Surgery result dependent of PV morphology
(d) LAD means AVSD

939. TOF physiology worst prognosis:

(a) TOF
(b) DORV with VSD with PS
(c) TGA with VSD with PS
(d) Single ventricle with PS
(e) TA with VSD with PS

940. VSD with Eisenmenger all C/I *except:*

(a) Nifedipine (b) Digitalis
(c) Diuretics (d) ACE-I
(d) Intravenous epinephrine

941. All A/E:

(a) Water fall appearance–Ebstein anomaly
(b) Egg on side–TGA
(c) Snowman appearance–TAPVC
(d) Figure of 3 sign–COA

942. All are cause of HF in 1st day *except:*

(a) COA (b) Large VSD
(c) Congenital CHB (d) AV malformation

943. Not forming left mediastinal contour on plain chest X-rays:

(a) MPA (b) LV
(c) LA (d) Aortic knob

944. Signs of impending of Eisenmenger's complex A/E:

(a) Increased intensity of tricuspid/pulmonary flow murmur
(b) P2 loud
(c) Development of single S2
(d) Appearance of Graham Steel murmur

945. 2 days old sick neonate was admitted to casuality in shock. The neonate significantly worsened on starting empirical prostaglandin infusion. Which of the following condition is likely?

(a) Pulmonary Atresia with IVS
(b) Aortic Atresia
(c) Interrupted aortic arch
(d) Obstructive supracardiac TAPVC

946. 15 years old girl present with HF and found to have significant Radiofemoral pulse delay. The most likely diagnosis is:

(a) Takayasu Arteritis (b) Coarctation of aorta
(c) Neurofibromatosis (d) Polyarteritis nodosa

947. Find the wrong match:

(a) Figure of '3' sign–COA
(b) Egg on side appearance–TGA
(c) Snowman appearance–supracardiac TAPVC
(d) Hilar waterfall sign– c-TGA

948. Ross procedure indications A/E:

(a) Young individual
(b) Bicuspid aortic valve stenosis
(c) Rheumatic AS
(d) Patient with C/I to anticoagulation

949. Rib notching sign on plain X-ray chest is characteristically seen in the following:

(a) Coarctation of aorta (b) Pheochromocytoma
(c) TOF (d) ASD

950. Noonan syndrome A/E:

(a) Autosomal recessive (b) PS with ASD
(c) Hypertelorism (d) Mental retardation

951. Infant preterm and term; ECG finding favoring preterm A/E:

(a) Short PR (b) Short QRS
(c) Prolonged QT (d) Less RV predominance

952. Crochetage sign is seen in:

(a) ASD (b) VSD
(c) PS (d) TOF

953. Which of the following is a cyanotic condition?

(a) Hemi anomalous pulmonary venous connection 36
(b) Post Hemi Fontan surgery
(c) Hernitruncus
(d) AV canal defect

954. One year old cyanosis with LVH diagnosis is:

(a) Tricuspid atresia (b) TOF
(c) ASD (d) PDA

955. Double chambered RV is associated with all *except:*

(a) Perimembranous VSD
(b) Aortic valve prolapse
(c) Tricuspid valve prolapse
(d) Subaortic stenosis

956. In CXR, narrow pedicle is found in:
(a) Tricuspid atresia (b) TOF
(c) D-TGA (d) L-TGA

957. In a preterm baby with L–R shunt regarding volume overload:
(a) Occur within 3 weeks
(b) Delayed
(c) Occurs early cyanosis
(d) Later than term baby

958. Which congenital heart diseases does not require antibiotic prophylaxis with tooth extraction?
(a) VSD (b) PDA
(c) ASD (d) COA

959. Left persistent superior vena cava drains to:
(a) Coronary sinus (b) Innominate vein

960. In DiGeorge syndrome which is seen:
(a) TGA (b) TOF
(c) Single ventricle (d) HLHS

961. Which is true regarding PDA:
(a) Seen in infants with increased birth weight
(b) Continuous murmur is typically heard over upper chest
(c) Prophylaxis for I.E. is not required

962. Regarding ASD which is true?
(a) Septum primum defect most commonly causes OS ASD
(b) Shunt is always left to right
(c) Pulmonary artery hypertension develops in adolesecence
(d) TTE better than TEE

963. Critical period during development of heart is:
(a) 25-50 days after fertilization
(b) 50-70 days after fertilization
(c) 70-90 days after fertilization
(d) 90-120 days after fertilization

964. Regarding coarctation of aorta all are true *except*:
(a) Male to female ratio is 1: 2
(b) Most common associated with tumour syndrome
(c) Berry aneurysm
(d) Gradient > 20 mm Hg is an indication for intervention

965. In a moderate VSD, which is seen?
(a) Increased blood flow in pulmonary circuit
(b) Increased blood flow in arterial circuit
(c) Decreased blood flow in pulmonary circuit
(d) Decreased blood flow in arterial circuit

966. In William syndrome all are seen *except:*
(a) Supravalvular AS (b) Hypercalcemia
(c) Mental retardation (d) Hyperthyroidism

967. Noonon's A/W A/E:
(a) Mental retardation (b) Branch PS
(c) MS (d) HCM

968. Continuous murmur louder in diastole A/E:
(a) Coronary AV fistula
(b) Pulmonary AV fistula
(c) RSOV to RV
(d) RSOV to PA

969. Most common CHD:
(a) VSD (b) PDA
(c) TOF (d) ASD

970. True in TOF:
(a) Overriding of aorta
(b) Most common VSD muscular
(c) Pulmonary arteries are normal

971. Apical variant of HOCM seen in:
(a) Japan (b) Italy
(c) India (d) Finland

972. All true *except* (about COA):
(a) Abdominal pulsation are always present
(b) High risk for intracerebral bleeding
(c) Rib erosion T3-T9 well develop in infancy

973. ASD–true:
(a) Most common CHD
(b) Always need of patch surgery
(c) Systolic murmur present in pulmonary area
(d) IVC opening is most common site

974. VSD:
(a) 25-40% of all CHD
(b) >75% spontaneous closure
(c) PHT presents by 1 year
(d) 8/10.000 incidence

975. Cyanotic HD with absence of q in V_6:
(a) Ventricular inversion (b) Situs inversus
(c) Atrial inversion (d) Dextroversion

976. Balloon angioplasty in COA most preferred:
(a) Restenosis after surgery
(b) Restenosis after angioplasty
(c) COA in adults
(d) COA in infants

977. In CCP, PV flow murmur:
(a) No atrial reversal
(b) Atrial reversal on inspiration
(c) Atrial reversal on expiration
(d) Triphasic response
(e) None

978. VSD true:
(a) > 75% spontaneous closure
(b) 8 in 10000 incidence
(c) 25-40% of all CHD
(d) PHT within 1 year in almost all patient
(e) Cyanotic HD

979. ASD true:
(a) Most common CHD
(b) Most common site near IVC orifice
(c) Systolic murmur at pulmonary area
(d) All to be closed with Dacron patch
(e) Clinical manifestation present in infancy

980. TOF true:
(a) Ao override
(b) VSD is muscular
(c) ASD for survival
(d) Most cases with normal pulmonary artery

981. PDA true:
(a) L→R shunt
(b) Between Ao to RPA
(c) First ligation by Ross
(d) Not present at birth in all patients
(e) All of above

982. Ideal I/V fluids in neoborn:
(a) Na =3 meq/l, K = 3 meq/l, Cl= 3 meq/l, glucose= 5 mg%
(b) 3.5, 2, 3, 5
(c) 3, 2, 2, 5
(d) 3, 2, 3, 5

983. Bulb of aorta is:
(a) Commencement of ascending aorta
(b) Ao at Ao valve
(c) Soft upper part of LV
(d) Shadow of Ao arch in PA view
(e) Junction of ascending Ao and arch

984. ASD:
(a) Sinus venosus mc
(b) Wide and fixed split S_2
(c) Diastolic murmur in mitral region
(d) Reversed split S_2

985. PDA:
(a) Male > Female
(b) Preantibiotic era most common cause of death was IE
(c) Deudaps from 4th aruh
(d) Most common in male

986. LV outlet VSD best view:
(a) RAO 30 cranial
(b) AP cranial
(c) LAO 65° 40° cranial
(d) LAO 40° 30° cranial

987. True about coarctation:
(a) > 50% personal in first week with CHF
(b) More in males
(c) Post ductal COA

988. PDA true:
(a) Continous machinery murmur
(b) More in males
(c) Arise from 9th arch
(d) Wide split 2

989. TOF A/E:
(a) LVH
(b) Overriding of aorta
(c) RVH

990. PDA true:
(a) Preantibiotic era most common cause of death was IE
(b) Deudaps from 4th aruh
(c) Most common in male

991. Most common CHD:
(a) ASD (b) VSD
(c) PDA (d) TOF

992. ASD-S2:
(a) Wide fixed split (b) Paradoxical split
(c) Single S_2 (d) Variable split

993. OS–ASD with 'a' wave = 10 cm of H_2O. What will be LVEDP?
(a) 10 (b) 15
(c) 20 (d) 25

994. Down syndrome is not associated with:
(a) Ostium primum ASD
(b) Sinus venosus ASD
(c) Common AV valve
(d) Absence of posterior part of ventricular septum

995. Asplenia/polysplenia is associated with:
(a) D-TGA
(b) Truncus arteriosus
(c) Mirror image dextrocardia
(d) Situs ambiguous

996. PDA not required for survival:
(a) Tricuspid atresia (b) Pulmonary atresia
(c) D-TGA (d) COA

997. Multiple peripheral Pulmonary artery Stenosis:
(a) Ellis-van Creveld syndrome
(b) Down syndrome
(c) Rubella
(d) Alagille syndrome

998. Increased step up at RA level:
(a) RSOV in RV (b) Gerbode defect
(c) PDA (d) COA

999. Ross procedure:
(a) In elderly with severe AS with non compliance
(b) Pulmonary valve transposition in aortic valve

1000. SVC to right PA shunt known as:
(a) Glenn's PA shunt
(b) B-T PA shunt
(c) Waterston's PA shunt
(d) Pott's PA shunt

1001. Open heart Surgery is:
(a) PA banding
(b) Modified BT shunt
(c) Arterial switch
(d) Surgical closure of PDA

1002. False negative myoscintigraphy:
(a) DCM
(b) Balanced hypoperfusion
(c) Micro vascular disease
(d) Conduction disease

1003. PFO A/E:
(a) Seen is 25% patients (adult)
(b) Associated with migraine and decompression sickness
(c) Coumarin derivatives are better than aspirin
(d) Contrast echo with TEE is most sensitive

1004. Cardiac anatomy true is A/E:
(a) Aortic valve tricuspid
(b) Pulmonary artery anterior to ascending aorta
(c) Entire ascending aorta is extrapericardial

1005. Cyanotic disease with increased PBF:
(a) Eisenmenger (b) Ebstein's anomaly
(c) Pulmonary atresia (d) Taussig-Bing anomaly

1006. Factors which doesn't decrease in cyanotic HD:
(a) V (b) VI
(c) VII (d) VIII

1007. 13 years webbed neck, short stature, decreased perfusion of lower extemities, rib notching likely cause:
(a) Post ductal CoA
(b) Preductal CoA
(c) Down syndrome

1008. Max. pulmonary artery pressure is seen in:
(a) ASD + Eisenmenger (b) Ebstein's anomaly

1009. AV discordance:
(a) Single ventricle (b) TGA
(c) Congenital CHB

1010. Pulmonary artery dilation are all *except:*
(a) Idiopathic pulmonary artery dilatation
(b) Dysplastic pulmonary artery
(c) TOF + absent pulmonary valve
(d) DORV

1011. Left atrial appendage enlargement in:
(a) MS (b) DORV
(c) ECD (d) AS

1012. Increase risk of LE with type of VSD:

(a) Small restrictive VSD (b) VSD + PS
(c) VSD + AR (d) LV → RA

1013. Non-pulmonary hypertensive:

(a) Holosystolic (b) Medium frequency
(c) Late systolic (d) Midsystolic

1014. Continuous murmur all *except:*

(a) PDA + PR
(b) TOF + Pulmonary atresia
(c) COA

1015. Pulmonary stenosis—all *except:*

(a) Pulmonary Ej. click increases on expiration
(b) Severity increases, murmur becomes longer and early peaking
(c) With non-restrictive VSD murmur becomes shorter with increasing severity
(d) Soft P2

1016. Central fibrous trigone is:

(a) Right fibrous trigone
(b) Left fibrous trigone
(c) Intervalvular trigone
(d) All of the above

1017. PFO all *except:*

(a) Indicated in decompression sickness and migraine
(b) 25% persist into adulthood
(c) Coumardin more effective than antiplatelet
(d) TEE with contrast is best for diagnosis

1018. Continuous murmur in all *except:*

(a) TOF with pulmonary atresia
(b) PDA with PR
(c) Pulmonary artery stenosis
(d) COA

1019. Cyanosis with normal heart examination A/E:

(a) ALCAPA
(b) Anomalous pulmonary venous drainage
(c) Pulmonary AV fistula
(d) Methemoglobinemia

1020. True for PS with intact IVS:

(a) Dysplastic valve most common cause of PS
(b) Inspiration increases PS ejection sound
(c) Surgery is only treatment
(d) Supravalvular PS is not usually progressive

1021. Pulmonary stenosis is associated with:

(a) Café au lait with mental retardation
(b) Hemorrhagic rash on palm and sole
(c) Swan Neck deformity of hand
(d) CREST syndrome

1022. Vascular development in human starts at:

(a) 3 weeks (b) 6 weeks
(c) 9 weeks (d) 12 weeks

1023. Cyanosis with increased PBF:

(a) Taussig-Bing anomaly

1024. PDA with diastolic murmur:

(a) Increases with isometric exercise
(b) Decrease with phenylephrine
(c) Increase with amylnitrate

1025. Straight left border A/E:

(a) Congenital absence of pericardium
(b) RV enlargement
(c) Ebstein anomaly
(d) TGA

1026. Factor deficient in CCHD A/E:

(a) 5 (b) 6
(c) 7 (d) 8

1027. RAA most common in:

(a) Truncus arteriosus (b) TOF
(c) TA

1028. Atrioventricular concordance A/E:

(a) Single ventricle (b) TGA

1029. Parachute Mitral valve A/E:

(a) TGA
(b) Endocardial fibroelastosis
(c) ECD

1030. PS–all true *except:*

(a) EC increases in inspiration
(b) Early peaking
(c) VSD associated
(d) Decrease murmur with increase severity

1031. Norwood procedure used in:

(a) HLHS (b) TGA

1032. Most unsaturated blood found in:

(a) Coronary sinus (b) SVC

(c) IVC

1033. All of the following are true for Ross procedure *except:*

(a) Preferred in younger patients

(b) Suitable for patients with rheumatic valve disease

(c) Long-term systemic anticoagulation is not required

(d) Pulmonary reconstruction is performed using pulmonary homograft

1034. The most common associated anomaly seen in a patient with Ebstein's anmoaly include:

(a) Patent ductus arteriosus

(b) Atrial septal defect

(c) Coarctation of aorta

(d) Pulmonary stenosis

1035. Which of the following coronary anomalies can interfere with the corrective surgery for Tetralogy of Fallot?

(a) LAD artery arising from the right aortic sinus

(b) Separate origin of LAD and LCX from left aortic sinus

(c) Separate origin of conus artery from right aortic sinus

(d) High origin of right coronary artery from right aortic sinus

1036. Higher valve of oxygen saturation (out of the given choices) will be observed under normal conditions in:

(a) Inferior vena cava (b) Superior vena cava

(c) Coronary sinus (d) Right atrium

1037. Which of the following congenital condition is associated with increased risk of complete heart block?

(a) Supravalvular aortic stenosis

(b) TOF with absent pulmonary valve

(c) c-TGA (corrected transposition of great arteries)

(d) Ebstein's anomaly

1038. Oblique vein of Marshall drains into:

(a) Right atrium (b) Coronary sinus

(c) Left atrium (d) Right ventricle

1039. All of the following are true regarding 'Fetal echocardiography' *except:*

(a) Should be done in the last trimester of pregnancy as the fetal heart is well developed

(b) Fetal arrhythmias can be diagnosed on echocardiography

(c) Hypoplastic left heart syndrome can be easily diagnosed

(d) Imaging of coarctation of aorta is difficult

1040. The triad of cyanosis, cardiomegaly and ischemic lung fields on chest X-ray suggests:

(a) ASD Eisenmenger

(b) TOF physiology

(c) Ebstein's anomaly

(d) Transposition physiology

1041. Which one of the following statements about a 40-year-old man presenting with upper limb hypertension and rib notching is true?

(a) Narrowing of the aorta is most likely to be proximal to the left subclavian artery

(b) An association with pulmonary stenosis would be an expected finding

(c) Marfan's syndrome is a recognized association

(d) There is likely to be an increased risk of cerebrovascular accidents

1042. Which of the following causes elevation of pulmonary capillary wedge pressure?

(a) Ebstein's anomaly

(b) Atrial septal defect

(c) Constrictive pericarditis

(d) Severe tricuspid regurgitation with low cardiac output

1043. Pulmonary capillary wedge pressure is lower than pulmonary artery diastolic pressure in all conditions stated below *except:*

(a) Primary pulmonary arterial hypertension

(b) Pulmonary artery embolism

(c) Pulmonary vein stenosis

(d) Tachycardia

1044. A 6-month-old child with recent pneumonia undergoes echocardiogram which shows 3 mm perimembranous VSD with maximum velocity of 4m/sec of VSD jet. Appropriate management includes:

(a) PA banding

(b) Medical follow up with diuretics
(c) Patch closure of VSD
(d) Cardiac catheterization to decide need of surgery

1045. One of the following is a palliative venous shunt:
(a) Potts shunt (b) Central shunt
(c) Glenn shunt (d) Blalock-Taussig shunt

1046. Continuous murmur is heard in one of the following condition:
(a) VSD with AR
(b) Lutembacher syndrome with restrictive ASD
(c) VSD with absent pulmonary valve
(d) Aortic stenosis with aortic regurgitation

1047. L loop is seen in:
(a) DTGA
(b) Isolated ventricular inversion
(c) TOF
(d) DORV

1048. True statement in asplenia syndrome:
(a) IVC interruption (b) Females
(c) PAPVC (d) Bilocular heart

1049. ECG features of corrected transposition of great arteries:
(a) Heart blocks
(b) Left axis deviation
(c) Septal Q wave inversion
(d) All of the above

1050. One of the following is not a feature of Williams syndrome:
(a) Supravalvular aortic stenosis
(b) Tall stature
(c) Coanda effect
(d) Pulmonary artery stenosis

1051. Steidele's complex refers to:
(a) Coarctation of aorta
(b) Aortopulmonary window
(c) Interruption of the aortic arch
(d) Truncus arteriosus

1052. CHB is seen in:
(a) TOF (b) CC-TGA
(c) PA (d) TA

1053. Tetralogy of Fallot:
(a) VSD + PS + RVH (b) ASD + PS + RVH
(c) Pink TOF (d) Adult TOF

1054. Taussig-Bing anomaly is:
(a) DORV with subpulmonary VSD
(b) DTGA
(c) LTGA
(d) TAPVC

1055. Syndromic associations with PDA:
(a) Rubella syndrome (b) Trisomy 18
(c) Char syndrome (d) All of the above

1056. ALCAPA refers to:
(a) Scimitar syndrome
(b) Bland-White-Garland syndrome
(c) Halfman syndrome
(d) Goldenhar syndrome

1057. Non-coronary sinus ruptures into:
(a) RA (b) RV
(c) RA + RV (d) LV

1058. Stereotyped QRS complexes are seen in:
(a) Tricuspid atresia (b) Single ventricle
(c) VSD (d) Pulmonary atresia

1059. Most commonly truncal valve is:
(a) Quadricuspid (b) Bicuspid
(c) Tricuspid (d) Pentacuspid

1060. Surgical treatment of DTGA + VSD + LVOT obstruction:
(a) Mustard operation (b) Senning operation
(c) Jatane operation (d) Rastelli ventricle

1061. Ross procedure is:
(a) Aortic homograft (b) Aortic autograft
(c) Pulmonary autograft (d) Pulmonary homograft

1062. Downs syndrome all *except*:
(a) TAPVC (b) AVSD
(c) VSD (d) PDA

1063. Straightening of left heart border, seen in all *except*:
(a) CC–TGA
(b) Ebstein anomaly
(c) Tricuspid atresia
(d) Absent left pericardium

1064. 2 years child, presently, with dyspeptic facies, ESM guide III/VI in anti acid regarding to carotids:

(a) William syndrome (b) 22
(c) 18 (d) 8

1065. Large ASD with polydactyly, finger nail dysplasisa:

(a) Ellis-Van Creveld
(b) Holt-Oram syndrome
(c) Alagille

1066. Type IV tricuspid atresia associated with:

(a) N placed heart arteries
(b) Transposed great arteries
(c) L-TGA
(d) Truncus arteriosus

1067. Apical HCM, all true *except*:

(a) Prevalence of 7% of all HCM cases in Japan
(b) Areas of spade configuration in Echo
(c) Relatively benign as compared to typical HCM
(d) Associated with deep T wave inversion

1068. Bicuspid aortic valve, most common defect:

(a) Fusion of right and non coronary cusp
(b) Fusion of right and left cusp
(c) Fusion of left and non coronary cusp
(d) Unicuspid valve

1069. Best view ortum securdum ASD:

(a) Subcostal view
(b) Parasternal long axes
(c) Parasternal short axes

1070. Correct about corchetage, all *except*:

(a) Notching of R wave in inferior leads
(b) Marker of plenty of ASD
(c) Present in ASD, patent foramen ovale, sinus venosus ASD
(d) New independent marker for ASD of thrombo-embolism in patient of PFO

1071. Pulmonary balloon valvotomy, RV pressure become equal to systemic pressure, mechanism:

(a) Infundibular septum
(b) Pulmonary HTN

1072. False statement:

(a) Situs inversus with dextrocardia associated with CHD in almost all cases
(b) Situs solitus with dextrocardia associated with CHD in almost all cases
(c) Situs solitus with dextrocardia associated with CC-TGA, USD

1073. Right and left atrium develops from:

(a) Common pulmonary vein and sinus venosus
(b) Premitive atrum and pulmonary veins
(c) Premitive atrum and sinus venosus

1074. Valve of coronary sinus:

(a) Thebesian valve

1075. False absent aortic arch derivatives:

(a) Maxillary artery from 1st arch

1076. Bicuspid aortic valve all *except*:

(a) SAH (b) AR
(c) AS (d) Aortic dissection

1077. Pulmonary artery derives from:

(a) 2nd arch (b) 4th arch
(c) 6th arch (d) 5th arch

1078. Tricuspid atresia have pulmonary obstructions most common at:

(a) Valvular
(b) Infundibular
(c) VSD
(d) Subvalvular level

1079. ASD with thrill in left 2nd ICS, all *except*:

(a) Eisenmenger
(b) Mitral regurgitation
(c) Mitral stenosis lenteineachea
(d) PS

1080. Atrial septostomy most commonly used for:

(a) TGA (b) Tricuspid atresia
(c) Truncus arteriosus (d) TOF

1081. Most common CHD at birth:

(a) VSD (b) ASD
(c) TOF (d) PDA

1082. Small VSD, velocity 2 m/sec, all can be true *except*:

(a) Gerbode defect
(b) Double chambered RV
(c) VSD with PAH
(d) Associated PS

1083. All *except*:

(a) LSVC–duct of cuvier
(b) Pulmonary vein–LA
(c) RA–right horn
(d) PDA left 6th aortic arch

1084. Nakata index favourable for fontan:

(a) > 100 (b) > 150
(c) > 200 (d) > 250

1085. B.P. difference in two arms, murmur radiating to carotids:

(a) Supravalvular AS (b) Subvalvular AS
(c) Valvular AS

1086. CXR – flask shaped heart, can be seen in all *except*:

(a) A.R. (b) A.V. regurgitation
(c) Ebstein anomaly (d) Cardiac tamponade

1087. CXR with snowman appearance (supracardiac TAPVC) all can be seen *except*:

(a) ASD (b) Dilated coronary sinus
(c) Dilated RV

1088. CXR of 10-year-old child, D/D all are true, *except*:

(a) Right phrenic palsy
(b) Situs solitus mesocardia
(c) N placed great vessels
(d) RV epicardial pacing

1089. What is incidence of right aortic arch in Tetralogy of Fallot ?

(a) 5% to 10% (b) 10% to 20%
(c) 20% to 30% (d) 30% to 40%

1090. Which one of the following is more specific view to diagnose MVP?

(a) Short axis view
(b) Apical four chamber view
(c) Subcostal view
(d) Parasternal long axis view

1091. Which one of the following type ASD is suitable for device closure?

(a) Ostium primum
(b) Ostium secundum
(c) Sinus venosus
(d) Unroofed coronary sinus

1092. Which one of the following genetic condition does not associated with aortic dissection?

(a) Marfan syndrome (b) Down syndrome
(c) Turner syndrome (d) Bicuspid aortic valve

1093. Ross procedure is used for:

(a) Diseased aortic valve
(b) Diseased mitral valve
(c) Diseased tricuspid valve
(d) Diseased pulmonary valve

1094. Which one of the following is not true for corrected transposition of great arteries?

(a) Atrioventricular discordance present
(b) Ventriculo arterial discordance present
(c) Cyanosis is common
(d) It produces loud second sound at left basal area

1095. What is incidence of complete heart block in patients with corrected transposition of great arteries?

(a) 10% (b) 5%
(c) 30% (d) 50%

1096. Particular for bicuspid aortic valve:

(a) Ejection click
(b) Late peaking ESM
(c) Carotid thrill
(d) Coanda effect

1097. Which of the following is the best echocardiographic view to diagnose coarctation of aorta:

(a) Suprasternal view
(b) Subcostal view
(c) Parasternal short axis view
(d) Parasternal long axis view

1098. Which one of the following is not a part of shone's complex?

(a) Subaortic stenosis
(b) Coarctation of aorta
(c) Parachute mitral valve
(d) Atretic aortic valve

1099. First trimester maternal rubella infection makes fetus vulnerable for:

(a) Supravalvular pulmonary stenosis
(b) Pulmonary artery stenosis
(c) Infundibular pulmonary stenosis
(d) Pulmonary atresia

1100. How much apical displacement of septal leaflet of tricuspid valve is used as a cut off limit for diagnosing Ebstein's anomaly in adults?

(a) 25 mm (b) 10 mm

(c) 15 mm (d) 20 mm

1101. Which one of the following is not common in ECG of patient with Ebstein's anomaly?

(a) Himalayan P wave

(b) Type A, WPW syndrome

(c) RBBB

(d) Prolonged PR interval

1102. Which one of the following is not true for Uhl's anomaly?

(a) Aplasia or hypoplasia of RV myocardium

(b) Ventricular arrhythmias are common

(c) RV is enlarged

(d) Paradoxical movement of septum

1103. Which one of the following is not true for total anomalous pulmonary venous connection?

(a) Right atrium and ventricle are significantly dilated

(b) ASD with left to right shunt

(c) Snowman appearance is common on X-ray

(d) Pulmonary hypertension is common

1104. What is the incidence of congenital heart disease in Down syndrome?

(a) 20% (b) 30%

(c) 70% (d) 50%

1105. Cleft mitral valve is common in:

(a) Ebstein's anomaly

(b) Cor triatriatum

(c) Atrioventricular septal defects

(d) Congenital mitral stenosis

1106. Most common ventricular septal defect is:

(a) Perimembranous VSD

(b) Muscular VSD

(c) Inlet VSD

(d) Subpulmonic VSD

1107. Spontaneous closure of VSD occurs up to:

(a) 1 year age (b) 4 years age

(c) 8 years age (d) 15 years age

1108. Which one of the following is not a component of Taussig-Bing anomaly?

(a) Double outer right ventricle

(b) Subpulmonic VSD

(c) Pulmonary stenosis

(d) Severe PAH

1109. Unequal unilateral pulse not seen in:

(a) Supravalvular (b) Subvalvular A5

(c) Takayasu (d) TAA dissection

1110. Differential cyanosis:

(a) PDA with postductal coarctation

(b) PDA with Secondary PAH

(c) PDA with Obstructive TAPVC

1111. Snowman's appearance:

(a) TAPVC (b) TGA

(c) TA (d) ToF

1112. Elfin facies is feature of:

(a) Supravalvular AS (b) Subvalvular AS

1113. Noonan's syndrome all *except*:

(a) HOCM (b) HS

(c) AS (d) ASD

1114. Infancy most common tumour:

(a) Rhabdomycoma (b) Myxoma

(c) Leyomyoma (d) Sarcoma

1115. VSD device closure not done in:

(a) Inlet (b) Subpulmonary

(c) PM (d) Muscular

1116. Foramen Ovale closure:

(a) LA pressure decrease

(b) RA pressure decrease due to ductus venous closure

(c) Constriction due to increase oxygenation

(d) All of the above

1117. Which of the following is false about ARVD (Arrhythmogenic Right Ventricular Dysplasia)?

(a) Mutation in genes encoding desmosomes

(b) Associated with sudden cardiac death

(c) Ventricular tachycardia is of LBBB morphology

(d) ECG shows epsilon wave

(e) All are true

1118. In cyanotic infant, if ECG shows left axis deviation which condition is probable?

(a) TAPVC (Anomalous pulmonary venous drainage)
(b) Transposition of great arteries
(c) Double outlet right ventricle with pulmonary stenosis
(d) Tricuspid atresia

1119. Which of the following is false statement about Taussig-Bing anomaly?

(a) Resembles CCTGA with large VSD
(b) Reverse differential cyanosis may occur
(c) PA saturation always higher than aorta
(d) Coarctation of aorta may be seen

1120. Which of the following drug intake in pregnancy is associated with Ebstein's anomaly in fetus?

(a) Ethanol (b) Valproic acid
(c) Lithium (d) Thalidomide

1121. Cardiomegaly is seen in which of the following Eisenmenger?

(a) Atrial septal defect Eisenmenger
(b) Ventricular septal defect Eisenmenger
(c) Patent ductus arteriosus Eisenmenger
(d) Aortopulmonary window Eisenmenger

1122. Supravalvular aortic stenosis is seen in which of the following syndrome?

(a) Down's syndrome (b) Turner's syndrome
(c) Williams syndrome (d) Rubella syndrome

1123. NHANES criteria to diagnose heart failure include all *except*:

(a) History
(b) Heart rate 91-110 beats/minute
(c) Abnormalities on echocardiography
(d) Abnormalities on chest X-ray

1124. All are true regarding Andersen Tawil syndrome, *except*:

(a) Long stature, low set ears, macrognathia and hypertelorism
(b) Weakness can be triggered by low, normal or high potassium levels
(c) Mutation of $KCNJ_2$ gene are responsible for the majority of cases
(d) It has been given a long QT syndrome 7 nomenclature

1125. Which of the following statements regarding anatomy of tricuspid valve is not correct?

(a) The anterior tricuspid leaflet is the largest
(b) The posterior leaflet is usually the smallest
(c) The septal leaflet is the most mobile
(d) The anterior tricuspid leaflet separates the inflow and outflow tracts of the right ventricle

1126. Persistent left superior vena cava results from failure of normal regression of:

(a) Left superior cardinal vein
(b) Right superior cardinal vein
(c) Left inferior cardinal vein
(d) Right inferior cardinal vein

1127. Knott-Craig approach is used in the treatment of:

(a) Transposition of great arteries
(b) Ebstein anomaly
(c) Tricuspid atresia
(d) Tetralogy of Fallot

1128. True about total anomalous pulmonary venous connection is:

(a) The anomalous connection is most often subdiaphragmatic
(b) ECG shows left axis deviation
(c) ECHO shows marked enlargement of right ventricle and left atrium
(d) In asymptomatic children without pulmonary hypertension, surgery can be deferred to 3–6 months of age

1129. All are more common in females than males *except*:

(a) HLHS
(b) TGA
(c) Pulmonary atresia
(d) None of the above

1130. Rash kinds procedure is done in all *except*:

(a) HLHS with restrictive ASD
(b) dTGA without ASD
(c) Tricuspid atresia
(d) ECMO with severe pulmonary oedema

1131. Manifestations of supraazygos SVC-obstruction includes all *except*:

(a) Distended arm and neck veins
(b) Congested mucous membrane (mouth)

(c) Dilatation of collateral vessels on anterior and posterior abdominal wall
(d) Edema of neck, face and arms

1132. All are ECG finding in Ebstein anomaly *except*:
(a) Peaked P waves in lead II and V_1 reflect RAE
(b) Low voltage is typical
(c) PR interval is generally prolonged
(d) LBBB is common in adults

1133. Correct match all *except*:
(a) PROSPECT–PFO device closure reduces risk of cryptogenic stroke significantly
(b) PROTECT AF–Watchmen device closure of LAA in AF patients is non-inferior to warfarin in reducing stroke in AF
(c) EVEREST–Mitraclip reduces morbidity in degenerative mitral regurgitation
(d) PARTNER – TAVR is superior to medical management

1134. Findings in congenital mitral stenosis include all *except*:
(a) Loud S_1
(b) MDM with presystolic accentuation
(c) No opening snap
(d) AF is rare in children

1135. Goal of phlebotomy in management of cyanosis is:
(a) Control of symptoms (b) Haematocrit < 65%
(c) Hb < 16 gm/dl (d) Normal MCV

1136. All are true about cardiac situs *except*:
(a) Situs solitus with dextro version is associated with congenital heart disease in more than 90% of cases
(b) Situs inversus with dextrocardia carries a high incidence of congenital heart disease
(c) Situs inversus with levocardia is associated with severe congenital disease in 100% of cases
(d) Up to 80% of patients of situs solitus with dextro version have c-TGA

1137. ECG in hypoplastic left heart syndrome shows all *except*:
(a) RAD (b) RAE
(c) RV enlargement (d) Q wave in V_6

1138. Protein loosing enteropathy following Fontan surgery is characterized by:
(a) High α1–antitrypsin stool clearance
(b) High serum albumin and protein
(c) High plasma lymphocyte
(d) 5-year survival rate of 25–30%

1139. Which of the following statement is false regarding echocardiography in post Fontan patient?
(a) Superior and inferior venae cava biphasic and pulmonary artery triphasic flow suggest unobstructed flow in the Fontan circuit
(b) Mean gradient between the Fontan circuit and the pulmonary artery should be 4 mm Hg or greater to represent significant obstruction
(c) Assessment of the pulmonary venous flow is important in detecting pulmonary venous obstruction caused by an enlarged right atrium
(d) TEE may be required if visualization of the Fontan anastomosis is inadequate

1140. Which of the following statement is false regarding device closure of an ASD?
(a) Patients should undergo echocardiography every 5 years or so following device closure because of the possibility of late issues like erosion
(b) Device closure is available only for patients with a secundum ASD of stretched diameter of less than 41 mm and adequate margins
(c) Patients should take aspirin and endocarditis prophylaxis for 1 year following device closure
(d) For patients with pulmonary hypertension, closure can be recommended if there is L-R shunt of at least 1.5:1 or evidence of pulmonary artery reactivity to pulmonary vasodilator

1141. Genetic loci for ARVD–5 is:
(a) Transforming growth factor–β3
(b) Ryanodine receptor–2
(c) Transmembrane protein–43
(d) Desmoplakin–3

1142. A 17 years old male is referred for evaluation of a mumur. Cardiac examination shows normal S1 and S2, no ejection sound with grade III/VI ejection systolic murmur at the right upper sternal border with radiation to the carotids. Blood pressure of the patient is 110/70, the carotid pulses are slightly delayed and the murmur softens with valsalva. Most likely diagnosis is:
(a) Bicuspid aortic valve
(b) Subvalvular aortic stenosis
(c) Hypertrophic cardiomyopathy
(d) None of the above

1143. Which of the following statements regarding RA anatomy is true?

(a) The venous component is located anteromedially and receives the systemic venous return from SVC, IVC and coronary venous return from the coronary sinus

(b) Vestibule is a coarsely trabeculated muscular wall around the tricuspid orifice and supports the leaflets of the TV

(c) The right atrial appendage lies over the antero-superior aspects of the right AV groove

(d) Right atrial appendage contains single pectinate muscle, which arise from the crista terminalis

1144. Which of the following derivatives of the aortic arches is correctly matched?

	Arch	Arterial Derivative
(a)	4th arch Left side	Left common carotid and first part of the internal carotid arteries
(b)	4th arch Right side	Arch of the aorta from the left common carotid to the left subclavian arteries
(c)	5th arch	Right and main pulmonary artery
(d)	6th arch Left side	Left pulmonary artery and ductus arteriosus

1145. X-ray suggestive of:

(a) TAPVC (b) PAPVC

(c) TGA (d) TOF

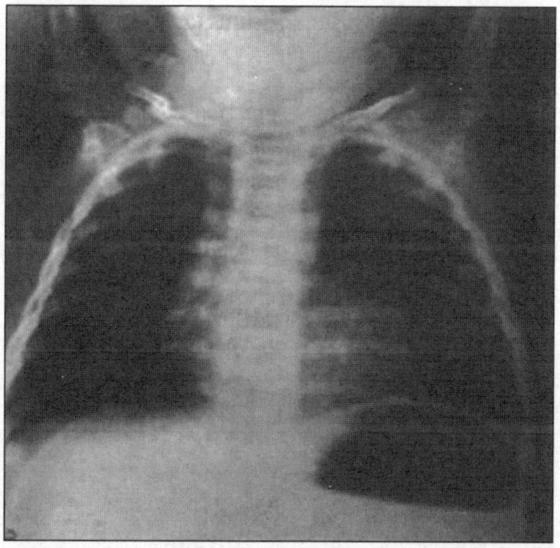

1146. All statements regarding autonomic innervations of atria are true, *except*:

(a) Sympathetic nerves originate inside the vertebral column and reach the stellate ganglion

(b) At the synapses within the ganglia, preganglionic neurons release acetylcholine

(c) Stimulatory beta adrenergic response is initiated via G protein subunit alpha complexes (Gα), leading to the activation of adenylcyclase

(d) Beta-1-receptors compose 20% to 30% of all beta receptors in the normal atrium

1147. Chest X-ray suggestive of:

(a) TOF (b) Ebstein

(c) TAPVC (d) PAPVC

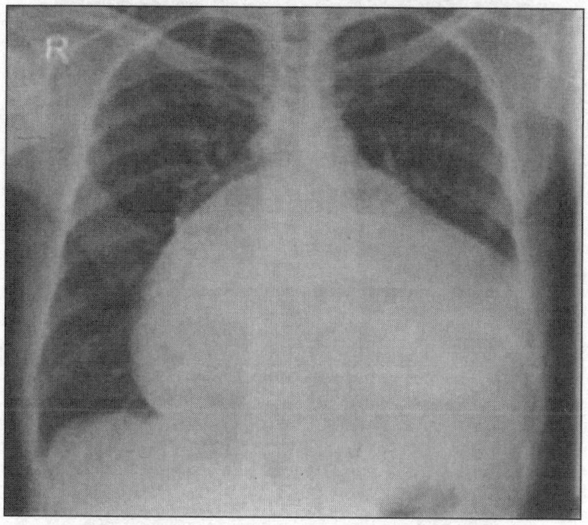

1148. Identify CHD:

(a) D-TGA (b) TAPVC

(c) L-TGA (d) TOF

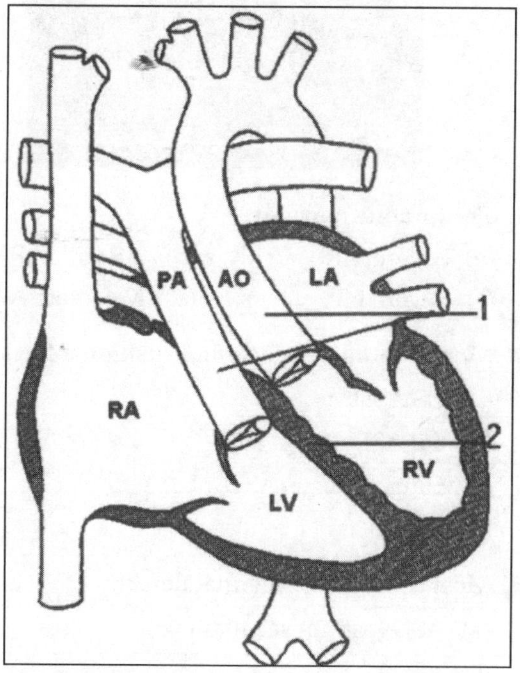

1149. Identify the structure:

(a) Ascending aorta

(b) Arch of aorta
(c) Descending aorta
(d) Pulmonary artery

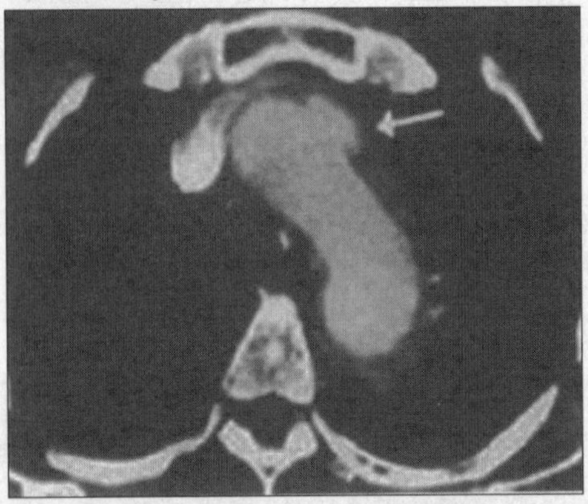

1150. Identify the lesion:

(a) PDA (b) COA
(c) AS (d) Aortic dissection

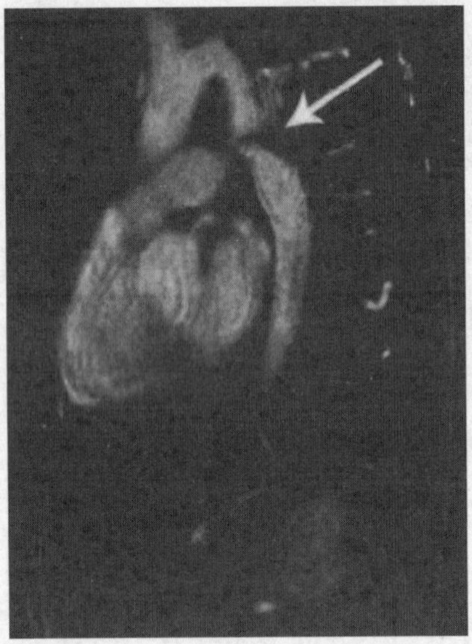

1151. Continuous murmur:

(a) Severe MR (b) AS with AR
(c) Severe PS (d) Moderate AR

1152. Most common endocardial cushion defect ASD is:

(a) OS ASD
(b) OP ASD
(c) Sinus venosus ASD
(d) AVCD

1153. Most common congenital defect:

(a) ASD (ostium secundum)
(b) VSD
(c) PDA
(d) TOF

1154. Which condition requires immediate intervention after birth?

(a) TOF (b) TGA
(c) Eisenmenger (d) ASD

1155. Williams syndrome is characterized by:

(a) Valvular AS
(b) Supravalvular AS
(c) Subaortic stenosis

1156. TAPVC–ECG presentation:

(a) Q in V5, V6 (b) RsR pattern
(c) LVH (d) LBBB

1157. Drug not to give for PDA closure:

(a) Prostaglandin E2 (b) Aspirin
(c) Indomethacin (d) Paracetamol

1158. Qp/Qs that requires surgery:

(a) >1 (b) >1.5
(c) >2 (d) >3

1159. Central cyanosis:

(a) Reduced cardiac output
(b) Cold exposure
(c) Redistribution of blood flow from extremities
(d) Decreased atmospheric pressure–high altitude

1160. ALCAPA ECG:

(a) Deep narrow q waves in leads I and aVL, LVH, left axis deviation
(b) Prolongation of PR
(c) RVH with strain, RAH
(d) LVH, Right axis deviation

1161. Alagille syndrome:

(a) Peripheral PA stenosis
(b) Hypercholesterolemia
(c) Butterfly-like vertebral arch defects
(d) All

1162. Noonan syndrome:

(a) PS (b) HCM
(c) Male (d) All

1163. Malaligned VSD is seen in A/E:

(a) TOF (b) IAA
(c) COA (d) Truncus arteriosus

1164. Infants increase cardiac output by:
(a) Increase in HR
(b) Increase in stroke volume
(c) Decrease in PVR
(d) Increase in preload

1165. In fetal circulation highest oxygen saturation is seen in:
(a) Ductus venosus (b) Ductus arteriosus
(c) Ascending aorta (d) Descending aorta

1166. Saturation data–IVC–65, SVC–62, MVO_2–62.5, RA–61, RV–65, MPA–65, LPA–80, aorta–95. What is Qp/Qs?
(a) 1 (b) 2
(c) 3 (d) 4

1167. All true, *except:*
(a) Holt-Oram syndrome–ASD
(b) Leopard syndrome–PS
(c) Rubella syndrome–PDA
(d) Tuberous sclerosis–AS

1168. All are true, *except*:
(a) Subcardinal vein–IVC
(b) Rt horn of sinus venosus–coronary sinus
(c) Rt common cardiac vein–SVC
(d) Lt horn of sinus venosus–oblique vein of LA

1169. In a patient with tricuspid atresia with VSD femoral artery saturation is 90%, jugular saturation is 60%. Qp/Qs is:
(a) 3 (b) 2
(c) 1 (d) Data not sufficient

1170. Homograft is not used in:
(a) Rastelli
(b) Arterial switch operation
(c) Ross procedure
(d) VSD with tricuspid atresia

1171. Cyanosis is present in A/E:
(a) Single atrium (b) Single ventricle
(c) AVSD (d) Truncus arteriosus

1172. DORV with restrictive VSD A/E:
(a) LVH on ECG
(b) No murmur on auscultation
(c) LV systolic pressure more than RV pressure
(d) Cyanosis is universal irrespective of PS

1173. Aorto-tricuspid continuity is seen in:
(a) Complete TGA
(b) DORV with malposition of vessels
(c) N heart
(d) Holmes heart

1174. Most common site of obstruction in TOF:
(a) Pulmonary valve (b) Infundibulum
(c) Aortic valve (d) All

1175. Most common CHD at birth:
(a) Muscular VSD (b) Inlet VSD
(c) Subarterial VSD (d) Perimembranous VSD

1176. PS with intact ventricular septum with normal ventricular function all true *except*:
(a) Suprasystemic pressure of RV
(b) Tall a wave in JVP
(c) Decreased cardiac output
(d) Height of R wave in V1 can estimate RVSP

1177. 60 hours after delivery baby becomes sick. SpO_2 less than 70%, not improving on 10 liters of O_2. DD are:
(a) d-TGA (b) PA
(c) CoA (d) PS
(e) HLHS

1178. TOF-PA, RVOT stenting–true is:
(a) Can be definitive procedure
(b) First perforation of membrane is required
(c) Same size used in all children
(d) It's a bridging procedure
(e) Very good outcomes

1179. Takotsubo cardiomyopathy all are T/E:
(a) RWMA is non territorial
(b) Always emotionally triggered
(c) Trop I may be elevated
(d) QT prolongation is seen

1180. Ebstein–true is:
(a) ASD in 80-95%
(b) Box shaped heart
(c) Displacement of tricuspid valve
(d) Left sided WPW
(e) RBBB

1181. Taussig-Bing anomaly–true is:
(a) A type of DORV

(b) Subaortic VSD
(c) May have multiple VSD
(d) May have abnormal pulmonary venous connection
(e) Similar to TGA

1182. Interventions to be used in diastolic heart failure:
(a) Atrial septostomy
(b) CRT
(c) Renal denervation
(d) CABG
(e) PCI

1183. Ebstein anomaly:
(a) SVT–rare
(b) Himalayan P wave
(c) Left sided accessory pathway
(d) Presents with palpitation in young most common
(e) Cardiothoracic ratio not increased

1184. Ruptured sinus of Valsalva true is:
(a) Most common is RCA cusp
(b) Most common presenting with dyspnea (sudden and progressive)
(c) Aneurysm is congenital
(d) Most common in males
(e) Most common in left coronary sinus

1185. Transient neonatal cyanosis–not seen in:
(a) Truncus arteriosus
(b) Classic TOF
(c) TOF without PS
(d) DORV with VSD with Subpulmonic stenosis
(e) TGA

1186. Neonatal circulation–true is:
(a) More connective tissue with decreased compliance
(b) Bradycardia decreases cardiac output
(c) Calcium sensitivity is low and increases later
(d) Fibres are arranged irregularly
(e) Cardiac output is rate dependent

1187. Fontan Ten Commandments include A/E:
(a) mPAP less than 25 mm Hg
(b) PVR less than 6 Woods
(c) Normal systemic venous return
(d) Age 4-15 years
(e) Competent mitral valve

1188. All are cyanotic heart diseases, *except*:
(a) C-TGA
(b) Mirror dextrocardia
(c) TAPVC
(d) D-TGA
(e) Common atrium

1189. Turner syndrome is associated with:
(a) PAPVC
(b) TAPVC
(c) COA
(d) TOF
(e) BAV

1190. CC–TGA true:
(a) 30% aortic valve regurgitation
(b) CHB is associated
(c) Not associated with CHB
(d) Q in V_5,V_6 and absent in V_1
(e) Q absent in V_5,V_6 present in V_1

1191. 47 years female with 40 mm ASD possible:
(a) Paradoxical embolism
(b) PAH
(c) Right heart failure due to decreased compliance
(d) Left heart failure due to increased RV load
(e) Atrial tachyarrhythmias

1192. Clubbing causes:
(a) Central right to left shunt
(b) Peripheral right to left shunt
(c) Infective endocarditis
(d) Rheumatic carditis
(e) RHD with multivalvular involvement

1193. Cardiothoracic ratio increased in A/E:
(a) Ebstein
(b) ASD
(c) Pulmonary AV fistula
(d) TOF
(e) AVSD

1194. Worst prognosis in a patient with operated TOF:
(a) Residual small VSD
(b) RBBB with QRS duration 110 ms young patient
(c) RBBB with QRS duration 80 ms in young
(d) RBBB with QRS duration 110 ms in old
(e) QRS duration >180 ms

1195. Carotid sinus morphology:
(a) Supplied by glossopharyngeal nerve

(b) Chemoreceptor
(c) Thin media, thick adventitia
(d) Increased glomus cells, sensory receptors, sinuse
(e) Central part of ICA

1196. ECHO is used as next step in:
(a) Systolic murmur 4/6
(b) Late systolic murmur
(c) Mid systolic
(d) Pansystolic
(e) Diastolic

1197. PDA true is:
(a) Practically closure occurs at less than 24 hours
(b) Practically closure occurs at less than 48 hours
(c) Practically closure occurs at less than 72 hours
(d) In preterm closure depends on birth weight
(e) In preterm PDA doesn't close in all infants

1198. Left atrium is derived from:
(a) Sinus venosus (b) Conus
(c) Pulmonary veins (d) All

1199. Sinus venosus develops into:
(a) Vein of Marshell (b) Left atrium
(c) SVC (d) IVC

1200. AV discordance is seen in:
(a) Situs inversus
(b) CC-TGA
(c) Truncus arteriosus
(d) D-TGA

1201. ECHO suggests:
(a) VSD (b) TOF
(c) DORV (d) TGA

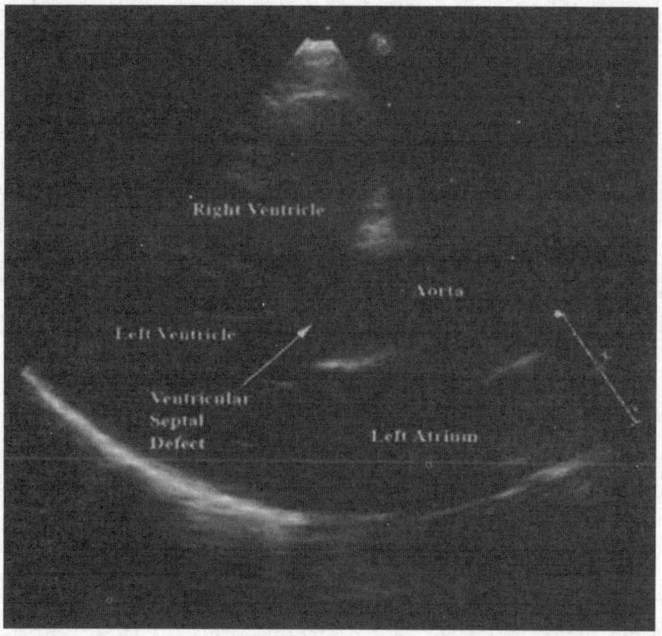

ANSWERS KEY

1. (b)	2. (c)	3. (d)	4. (b)	5. (b)	6. (d)	7. (b, d)	8. (c)
9. (d)	10. (b)	11. (a)	12. (b)	13. (c)	14. (a)	15. (a)	16. (a)
17. (a)	18. (a,c)	19. (b)	20. (a)	21. (b)	22. (b)	23. (d)	24. (c)
25. (d)	26. (b)	27. (a)	28. (d)	29. (a)	30. (d)	31. (b)	32. (d)
33. (b)	34. (b)	35. (d)	36. (a)	37. (d)	38. (a)	39. (b)	40. (d)
41. (a)	42. (a)	43. (c)	44. (c)	45. (c)	46. (c)	47. (a)	48. (b)
49. (a)	50. T	51. T	52. F	53. T	54. T	55. T	56. T
57. F	58. (a)	59. (d)	60. (b)	61. (d)	62. (a)	63. (b)	64. (a)
65. (a)	66. (c)	67. (a)	68. (d)	69. (c)	70. (d)	71. (d)	72. TTFFF
73. FTTFF	74. TTT?	75. FTFFT	76. TTTFF	77. FFTFT	78. TFTTF	79. FFFFT	80. FFFTT
81. TFTTT	82. (c)	83. (b)	84. (b)	85. (c)	86. (c)	87. (d)	88. (b)
89. (d)	90. (b)	91. (d)	92. (b)	93. (b)	94. (b)	95. (d)	96. (c)
97. (a)	98. (c)	99. (c)	100. (b)	101. (b)	102. (a,b,d)	103. (d)	104. (a)
105. (b)	106. (d)	107. (b)	108. (d)	109. (c)	110. (d)	111. (b)	112. (b)
113. (d)	114. (d)	115. (a)	116. (b)	117. (b)	118. (b)	119. (a)	120. (a)
121. (a)	122. (d)	123. (c)	124. (a)	125. (a)	126. (b)	127. (c)	128. (d)
129. (c)	130. (c)	131. (c)	132. (a)	133. (d)	134. (c)	135. (d)	136. (b)
137. (a)	138. (c)	139. (a)	140. (b)	141. (d)	142. (d)	143. (d)	144. (c)
145. (d)	146. (a)	147. (a)	148. (b)	149. (d)	150. (a)	151. (b)	152. (c)
153. (b)	154. (c)	155. (d)	156. (c)	157. (d)	158. (a)	159. (a)	160. (b)
161. (d)	162. (a)	163. (a)	164. (d)	165. (a)	166. (a)	167. (a)	168. (a)
169. (b)	170. (c)	171. (a)	172. (a)	173. (d)	174. (a)	175. (c)	176. (a)
177. (a)	178. (a)	179. (a)	180. (b)	181. (a)	182. (a)	183. (a)	184. (a)
185. (c)	186. (a)	187. (d)	188. (b)	189. (d)	190. (a)	191. (b)	192. (a)
193. (d)	194. (a)	195. (c)	196. (a)	197. (a)	198. (a)	199. (a)	200. (a)
201. (a)	202. (b)	203. (a)	204. (b)	205. (a)	206. (a)	207. (c)	208. (b)
209. (a)	210. (a)	211. (b)	212. (b)	213. (a)	214. (a)	215. (d)	216. (b)
217. (c)	218. (b)	219. (a)	220. (a)	221. (a)	222. (a)	223. (a)	224. (a)
225. (a)	226. (c)	227. (a)	228. (b)	229. (b)	230. (a)	231. (a)	232. (c)
233. (a)	234. (a)	235. (c)	236. (b)	237. (b)	238. (a)	239. (b)	240. (a)
241. (c)	242. (c)	243. (d)	244. (a)	245. (b)	246. (a)	247. (c)	248. (b)
249. (a)	250. (d)	251. (a)	252. (b)	253. (b)	254. (b)	255. (c)	256. (a)
257. (a)	258. (d)	259. (a)	260. (a)	261. (a)	262. (d)	263. (a)	264. (a)
265. (b)	266. (a,c)	267. (b)	268. (a)	269. (a)	270. (b)	271. (c)	272. (a)
273. (a)	274. (c)	275. (a)	276. (b)	277. (c)	278. (b)	279. (a)	280. (a)
281. (b)	282. (a)	283. (d)	284. (a)	285. (a)	286. (a)	287. (a)	288. (a)
289. (a)	290. (a)	291. (a)	292. (a)	293. (a)	294. (b)	295. (c)	296. (d)
297. (b)	298. (b)	299. (d)	300. (a)	301. (a)	302. (a)	303. (d)	304. TTT
305. TTTTF	306. (a)	307. (b)	308. (d)	309. (c)	310. (a)	311. (d)	312. (e)
313. (d)	314. (d)	315. (c)	316. TTTTT	317. (a)	318. (a)	319. (c,d)	320. (e)
321. (d)	322. (c)	323. (d)	324. TTFFT	325. (a)	326. (a,d)	327. (a)	328. TTTT
329. TTFF	330. (a,b)	331. (b)	332. (d)	333. (b)	334. (b)	335. (b,d)	336. (a)
337. (a)	338. (c)	339. (e)	340. (d)	341. (b,d)	342. (c,d)	343. (b,c)	344. (a,b,d)
345. (a,b)	346. (a,b,c)	347. (a)	348. (b)	349. (c)	350. (d)	351. (d)	352. (b)

353. (a)	354. (d)	355. (a)	356. (b)	357. (d)	358. (a)	359. (a)	360. (a)
361. (c)	362. (a)	363. (a)	364. (d)	365. (d)	366. (b)	367. (c)	368. (c)
369. (a)	370. (b)	371. (a)	372. (b)	373. (b)	374. (d)	375. (d)	376. (c)
377. (a)	378. (d)	379. (c)	380. (b)	381. (d)	382. (c)	383. (d)	384. TFFFF
385. (b)	386. (a)	387. (b)	388. (a)	389. (a)	390. (b)	391. (c)	392. (c)
393. (d)	394. (a)	395. (b)	396. (c)	397. (c)	398. (b)	399. (a)	400. (d)
401. (a)	402. (a)	403. (a)	404. (d)	405. (a)	406. (a)	407. (d)	408. (a)
409. (a)	410. (d)	411. (d)	412. (a)	413. (a)	414. (a)	415. (c)	416. (a)
417. (c)	418. (a)	419. (b)	420. (a)	421. (a)	422. (a)	423. (a)	424. (a)
425. (a)	426. (c)	427. (a)	428. (c)	429. (d)	430. (d)	431. (c)	432. (b)
433. (a)	434. (d)	435. (d)	436. (a)	437. (b)	438. (a)	439. (b)	440. (b)
441. (d)	442. (a)	443. (a)	444. (b)	445. (c)	446. (a)	447. (c)	448. (a)
449. (c)	450. (c)	451. (d)	452. (d)	453. (b)	454. (c)	455. (c)	456. (c)
457. (a)	458. (d)	459. (b)	460. (d)	461. (c)	462. (c)	463. (a)	464. (a)
465. (a)	466. (a)	467. (c)	468. (c)	469. (a)	470. (e)	471. (a)	472. (b)
473. (a)	474. (c)	475. (b)	476. (d)	477. (a)	478. (b)	479. (a)	480. (a)
481. FFTTT	482. (a)	483. (d)	484. (a)	485. (c)	486. (d)	487. (a,c)	488. (a)
489. (b)	490. (a)	491. (a)	492. (a)	493. (b)	494. (c)	495. (c)	496. (a)
497. (c)	498. (b)	499. (a)	500. (a)	501. (d)	502. (b)	503. (a)	504. (c)
505. (d)	506. (d)	507. (d)	508. (d)	509. (a)	510. (c)	511. (c)	512. (b)
513. (d)	514. (b)	515. (d)	516. (d)	517. (a)	518. (b)	519. (d)	520. (d)
521. (d)	522. (a)	523. (?)	524. (a)	525. (d)	526. (b)	527. (d)	528. (c)
529. (d)	530. (d)	531. (b)	532. (a)	533. (a)	534. (c)	535. (a)	536. (c)
537. (a)	538. (a)	539. (c)	540. (c)	541. (c)	542. (a)	543. (a)	544. (d)
545. (a)	546. (b)	547. (b)	548. (b)	549. (c)	550. (b)	551. (c)	552. (b)
553. TFTT	554. (b)	555. (d)	556. (a)	557. (a)	558. (a)	559. (a)	560. (c)
561. (a)	562. (b)	563. (b)	564. (b)	565. (e)	566. (c)	567. (c)	568. (b)
569. (b)	570. (d)	571. (b)	572. (c)	573. (a)	574. (b)	575. (c)	576. (d)
577. (d)	578. (b)	579. (a)	580. (b)	581. (a)	582. (a)	583. (a)	584. (a)
585. (d)	586. (b)	587. (d)	588. (c)	589. (c)	590. (a)	591. (d)	592. (a)
593. (a)	594. (a)	595. (a)	596. (b)	597. (a)	598. (c)	599. (a)	600. (c)
601. (a)	602. (b)	603. (c)	604. (a)	605. (c)	606. (b)	607. (c)	608. (a)
609. (b)	610. (c)	611. (a)	612. (d)	613. (a)	614. (d)	615. (b)	616. (d)
617. (a)	618. (a)	619. (c)	620. (b)	621. (c)	622. (b)	623. (a)	624. (a)
625. (b)	626. (d)	627. (d)	628. (b)	629. (b)	630. (c)	631. (d)	632. (a)
633. (b)	634. (b)	635. (d)	636. (a)	637. (b)	638. (a)	639. (b)	640. (b)
641. (b)	642. (b)	643. (a)	644. (d)	645. (b)	646. (d)	647. (a)	648. (a)
649. (c)	650. (a)	651. (d)	652. (c)	653. (c)	654. (d)	655. (d)	656. TTFFT
657. FTFTF	658. FFTT	659. FTTT	660. TTFTF	661. FFTFT	662. TFFFT	663. TTFTF	664. TFTTT
665. TTTTF	666. TTTFF	667. TFFFT	668. TFFFF	669. FTTTT	670. TFFFF	671. FFTF	672. TTTTT
673. FTTTT	674. TTTFF	675. TFTFT	676. TTFFF	677. FFFFT	678. FFT	679. TFFTF	680. TTTFT
681. FTTTF	682. TTTTT	683. TFTTF	684. FTTTF	685. TTFTF	686. TTFTT	687. FTTTF	688. TTFTF
689. FFTFT	690. TTTFF	691. TTTFT	692. FFFFT	693. TTTTF	694. FFTFF	695. TTTTT	696. TTTTF
697. FFFTT	698. FTTFT	699. FFTFF	700. TTTTF	701. TTTTT	702. TFTFF	703. TTFFT	704. FTTTF
705. TFFTF	706. TTTFF	707. TTTFF	708. FTTFF	709. TTTFF	710. TTFTF	711. TTTTT	712. TTFF
713. FTTFF	714. TTFT	715. TTFTT	716. TFFFF	717. TTTTT	718. FTTF	719. FFTTF	720. (a)
721. FTTTT	722. FFTFF	723. TTFTT	724. TTFFT	725. TTTFF	726. FFTTF	727. TTFFT	728. FTTFF
729. FFFTF	730. FTTFF	731. FTFFF	732. TFFFF?	733. TFTTT	734. TTTFF	735. TTFFF	736. TFFF
737. TFFFF	738. TTFFT	739. TFTTF	740. FFTFT	741. TFFFF	742. FTTTF	743. TTFFF	744. FTFFF

745.	TFTFF	746.	FTTFT	747.	FTTFF	748.	TFTFF	749.	TTFFF	750.	TTFFF	751.	FTFTT	752.	TTFFT
753.	TTFTF	754.	FTTTT	755.	FTTTF	756.	TTTFF	757.	FTFFT	758.	TFFFT	759.	TTTFT	760.	TFTTF
761.	TFTTF	762.	FFFTT	763.	FFTFT	764.	TFFTT	765.	FTTFF	766.	FTTTT	767.	TTTFT	768.	FFFTT
769.	TTFTF	770.	FTTFT	771.	FFFTF	772.	FFFFT	773.	FTFFF	774.	TFFTF	775.	FTFFF	776.	TTFTF
777.	FTTFF	778.	TTFFF	779.	TTFFF	780.	FTTF	781.	TTTT	782.	TTTT	783.	TTF	784.	TTTTT
785.	TF	786.	TFTF	787.	TFTT	788.	TFTT	789.	TFFFF	790.	TTFTT	791.	FFTFF	792.	(a)
793.	(d)	794.	(b)	795.	(c)	796.	(b)	797.	(b)	798.	(a)	799.	(a)	800.	(a)
801.	(a)	802.	(c)	803.	(b)	804.	(a)	805.	(a)	806.	(a)	807.	(a)	808.	(b)
809.	(c)	810.	(d)	811.	(d)	812.	(a)	813.	(a)	814.	(d)	815.	(b)	816.	(c)
817.	(d)	818.	(a)	819.	(a)	820.	(d)	821.	(c)	822.	(d)	823.	(c)	824.	(a)
825.	(a)	826.	(d)	827.	(a)	828.	(a)	829.	(a)	830.	TFFTT	831.	TFFTT	832.	TFFTT
833.	FFTTF	834.	TFTTF	835.	FTT	836.	TFTTT	837.	TT?TT	838.	FTTFTT	839.	FFFTT	840.	FFTFF
841.	FFTTT	842.	TTTTT	843.	TFTFT	844.	FF	845.	TFFFF	846.	TTFTF	847.	TTTFT	848.	(a)
849.	TTFT	850.	FFFTF	851.	TFTTF	852.	TTFTT	853.	TFTFF	854.	TFTTF	855.	TF	856.	FFTFF
857.	FFFTF	858.	TTFFT	859.	TFTTF	860.	TTTTT	861.	FFTFT	862.	TTFFT	863.	TTFFT	864.	TFFFT
865.	TFTTTT	866.	FF?FT	867.	TTFFF	868.	TFTTT	869.	TTTTT	870.	FFFFT	871.	TFFTT	872.	TTFF
873.	TFFF	874.	FTTTT	875.	TTTTT	876.	TTFFTF	877.	TTTTT	878.	TFFFTF	879.	FTF	880.	FTFFT
881.	FTTT	882.	FFTFF	883.	TFFF	884.	TTTFF	885.	TFTT	886.	T	887.	TF	888.	FFFFF
889.	TFFT	890.	TFFFT	891.	FFTTT	892.	TTTTT	893.	FFFFF	894.	TFTTF	895.	FFFTF	896.	FTFTT
897.	FTFTT	898.	TFTTF	899.	FTTFT	900.	TFFT	901.	FFTFT	902.	FTFTF	903.	FTTTF	904.	TTFTF
905.	(a)	906.	(a)	907.	(b)	908.	(a)	909.	(b)	910.	(c)	911.	(a)	912.	(c)
913.	(a)	914.	(c, d)	915.	(a)	916.	(a)	917.	(a)	918.	(b)	919.	(a)	920.	(a)
921.	(a)	922.	(c)	923.	(c)	924.	(b)	925.	(b)	926.	(c)	927.	(a)	928.	(b)
929.	(d)	930.	(c)	931.	(c)	932.	(c)	933.	(a)	934.	(a)	935.	(a)	936.	(c)
937.	(c)	938.	(c)	939.	(c)	940.	(a)	941.	(a)	942.	(b)	943.	(c)	944.	(a)
945.	(d)	946.	(a)	947.	(d)	948.	(d)	949.	(a)	950.	(a)	951.	(c)	952.	(a)
953.	(b)	954.	(a)	955.	(b)	956.	(d)	957.	(c)	958.	(d)	959.	(a)	960.	(b)
961.	(b)	962.	(d)	963.	(a)	964.	(b)	965.	(a)	966.	(d)	967.	(c)	968.	(c)
969.	(d)	970.	(a)	971.	(a)	972.	(c)	973.	(c)	974.	(c)	975.	(a)	976.	(b)
977.	(b)	978.	(a)	979.	(c)	980.	(a)	981.	(a)	982.	(d)	983.	(a)	984.	(b)
985.	(b)	986.	(a)	987.	(b)	988.	(a)	989.	(a)	990.	(a)	991.	(b)	992.	(a)
993.	(b)	994.	(b)	995.	(d)	996.	(d)	997.	(d)	998.	(b)	999.	(b)	1000.	(a)
1001.	(a)	1002.	(b)	1003.	(c)	1004.	(b)	1005.	(d)	1006.	(b)	1007.	(a)	1008.	(a)
1009.	(a)	1010.	(b)	1011.	(a)	1012.	(c)	1013.	(b)	1014.	(a)	1015.	(b)	1016.	(a)
1017.	(c)	1018.	(b)	1019.	(a)	1020.	(d)	1021.	(a)	1022.	(c)	1023.	(a)	1024.	(a)
1025.	(b)	1026.	(b)	1027.	(a)	1028.	(a)	1029.	(a)	1030.	(b)	1031.	(a)	1032.	(a)
1033.	(b)	1034.	(b)	1035.	(a)	1036.	(a)	1037.	(c)	1038.	(b)	1039.	(a)	1040.	(c)
1041.	(d)	1042.	(c)	1043.	(c)	1044.	(b)	1045.	(c)	1046.	(b)	1047.	(b)	1048.	(d)
1049.	(d)	1050.	(b)	1051.	(c)	1052.	(d)	1053.	(b)	1054.	(a)	1055.	(d)	1056.	(b)
1057.	(a)	1058.	(b)	1059.	(c)	1060.	(d)	1061.	(c)	1062.	(a)	1063.	(c)	1064.	(a)
1065.	(b)	1066.	(d)	1067.	(a)	1068.	(a)	1069.	(a)	1070.	(b)	1071.	(a)	1072.	(a)
1073.	(c)	1074.	(a)	1075.	(a)	1076.	(a)	1077.	(c)	1078.	(a)	1079.	(a)	1080.	(a)
1081.	(a)	1082.	(c)	1083.	(a)	1084.	(d)	1085.	(a)	1086.	(a)	1087.	(c)	1088.	(c)
1089.	(c)	1090.	(d)	1091.	(b)	1092.	(b)	1093.	(a)	1094.	(c)	1095.	(c)	1096.	(a)
1097.	(a)	1098.	(d)	1099.	(b)	1100.	(d)	1101.	(b)	1102.	(b)	1103.	(b)	1104.	(d)
1105.	(c)	1106.	(a)	1107.	(c)	1108.	(d)	1109.	(b)	1110.	(a)	1111.	(a)	1112.	(a)
1113.	(c)	1114.	(a)	1115.	(a)	1116.	(b)	1117.	(e)	1118.	(d)	1119.	(d)	1120.	(c)
1121.	(a)	1122.	(c)	1123.	(c)	1124.	(a)	1125.	(c)	1126.	(a)	1127.	(b)	1128.	(d)
1129.	(d)	1130.	(c)	1131.	(c)	1132.	(d)	1133.	(a)	1134.	(a)	1135.	(a)	1136.	(b)

1137. (d)	1138. (a)	1139. (b)	1140. (c)	1141. (c)	1142. (b)	1143. (c)	1144. (d)
1145. (d)	1146. (d)	1147. (b)	1148. (c)	1149. (a)	1150. (b)	1151. (b)	1152. (b)
1153. (a)	1154. (b)	1155. (b)	1156. (b)	1157. (a)	1158. (b)	1159. (d)	1160. (a)
1161. (d)	1162. (d)	1163. (d)	1164. (a)	1165. (a)	1166. (b)	1167. (d)	1168. (b)
1169. (d)	1170. (d)	1171. (c)	1172. (b)	1173. (c)	1174. (b)	1175. (d)	1176. (a)
1177. (a,b,e)	1178. (b,c,d)	1179. (b)	1180. (a,b,c,e)	1181. (a,c,d,e)	1182. (c,d,e)	1183. (b,d)	1184. (a,b,c,d)
1185. (a,c,e)	1186. (b,c,e)	1187. (a,b)	1188. (a,b)	1189. (a,c,e)	1190. (b,e)	1191. (a,b,c,e)	1192. (a,c)
1193. (a,b,e)	1194. (e)	1195. (a,c,d,e)	1196. (a,b,d,e)	1197. (c,d,e)	1198. (c)	1199. (a)	1200. (b)
1201. (b)							

CHAPTER SEVEN

CLINICAL CARDIOLOGY

1. **2° HT–all *except*:**
   (a) Liddle–NaCl mutation
   (b) Acromegaly–High renin
   (c) Bartter syndrome–High renin
   (d) All of the above

2. **Max. probability of mets to heart:**
   (a) Lung (b) Melanoma
   (c) Breast (d) Lymphoma

3. **Radiation induced cardiac injury A/E:**
   (a) LVD due to thrombosis of epicardial coronaries
   (b) Myocardial dysfunction most common m/f
   (c) Otial stenosis
   (d) Fibrosis seen

4. **(N) heart with pulmonary edema. Young male:**
   (a) Multivalvular HD with pulmonary edema
   (b) Bilateral pneumonia
   (c) Hypertensive HF
   (d) None of the above

5. **Mesocardia with right done of diaphragm elevated, pacing lead seen in ventricle. Which is not true?**
   (a) Great vessels normally related
   (b) Epicardial pacing
   (c) Mesocardia with situs solitus
   (d) (R) phrenic palsy

6. **Prevention of CIN not medicated:**
   (a) Steroid
   (b) NAC
   (c) H1 receptor blockers
   (d) H2 receptor blockers

7. **Prevention of radiation exposure to patient:**
   (a) Cine >> Fluro
   (b) Increase the frame count
   (c) Magnified view
   (d) Increase the distance from rediation

8. **Not true about pheochromocytoma:**
   (a) Salt restriction
   (b) Labetalol causes paradoxical hypertension
   (c) Preoperatively alpha blockade, followed by beta blockade
   (d) Echo screening for cardiomyopathy is done in all cases

9. **Rx of anaphylactic shock in a patient treated with beta blockers long term:**
   (a) Glucagon (b) Vasopressin
   (c) Dopamine (d) Salbutamol

10. **Mismatch:**
    (a) Pravastatin–Cyp3A4
    (b) Propafenone–Cyp2D6
    (c) Warfarin–Cyp2C9
    (d) Omeprazole–Cyp2C9

11. **Shock on inotropes, BP-90/70 mm Hg:**
    ABG pH 7.28. PaO_2-80 mm Hg, $PaCO_2$ 40 mm Hg, HCO_3 15 mEq/L, $NaHCO_3$ to be given in first 3 hours:
    (a) None (b) 30 ml
    (c) 50 ml (d) 20 ml

12. **Primary exertional headache A/E:**
    (a) Pheochromocytoma
    (b) Carotid stenosis
    (c) Myocardial ischemia
    (d) Methysergide

13. **Dabigatran monitoring best by:**
    (a) TT
    (b) PTT
    (c) Hept test
    (d) Prothrombinase induced clotting time

14. **Pregnancy–All T/E:**
    (a) ↑ CO
    (b) ↑ PCWP
    (c) ↓ PVR
    (d) ↓ colloidal osmotic pressure

15. Resistant HTN A/E:

(a) Renal outcome good
(b) Controlled by 4 drugs with diuretic
(c) Not controlled by 3 drugs
(d) 2° HTN – ↑ chances

16. Hypertensive crisis A/E:

(a) BP > 180/90
(b) BP > 220/130
(c) Immediate BP control
(d) End organ damage

17. Rate limiting step in RAAS:

(a) Renin–angiotensinogen–angiotensin I
(b) ACE–angiotensin I–AT II
(c) Renin–angiotensin I–AT I
(d) ACE–angiotensinogen–angiotensin I

18. Osler maneuver:

(a) White coat hypertension
(b) Pseudohypertension
(c) Auscultatory gap
(d) Masked hypertension

19. Collapsing pulse A/E in cyanotic heart disease:

(a) PDA with reversal (b) TA
(c) Ebstein (d) Fallot's with collaterals

20. Pregnancy changes:

(a) ↑ SVR
(b) ↑ PVR
(c) ↓ HR
(d) ↓ RBC Blood volume increases more than hematocrit mass

21. Pregnancy anticoagulation A/E:

(a) Warfarin discontinued between 6 and 12 W
(b) Low dose aspirin may be added
(c) LMWH can be used (anti xa monitoring not required)
(d) Warfarin stopped 36 W bridged with UFH infusion

22. Cardiac catheterisation, pregnancy test to be done before:

(a) 1 W (b) 2 W
(c) 3 W (d) 4 W

23. Hypertensive emergency true is:

(a) End organ damage
(b) BP 200/110 mm Hg
(c) Nitroprusside is drug of choice
(d) Target BP reduction 10% in first hour

24. Pulsus paradoxus may be seen in–all *except*:

(a) Positive pressure ventilation
(b) Obesity
(c) Massive pulmonary embolism
(d) Tension pneumothorax

25. HAART therapy in HIV did not reduce the incidence of following cardiac complication:

(a) Pericardial effusion
(b) Cardiomyopathy
(c) Kaposi sarcoma
(d) Pulmonary arterial hypertension

26. All are clinical clues to renovascular hypertension *except*:

(a) Abrupt onset of hypertension
(b) Recurrent flash pulmonary edema
(c) Advanced fundal changes
(d) Family history of hypertension

27. An "empty pericardial cavity" can be seen in:

(a) Gun shot wounds of the heart
(b) Stab injury to heart
(c) Blunt cardiac injury
(d) Electrical injury to the heart

28. Examples of drugs associated with withdrawal effects include the following *except*:

(a) Alcohol (b) Barbiturates
(c) Corticosteroids (d) Lofexidine

29. Coumarin–containing herbs include the following *except*:

(a) Horse chestnut (b) Red clover
(c) Fenugreek (d) Turmeric

30. Which one of the following drugs is less likely to cause erectile dysfunction?

(a) Beta blocker
(b) Alfa–adrenergic blocker
(c) Calcium channel blocker
(d) 5 Alfa–reductase inhibitor

31. Which of the following does not require dosage adjustment in renal impairment?

(a) Linezolid (b) Penicillin G
(c) Vancomycin (d) Daptomycin

32. **Hypercoagulation: (T/F)**
(a) Prothrombin mutation–arterial
(b) Protein C mutation–arterial
(c) Patient with thrombosis–usually multiple R/F
(d) Post OP pulmonary embolism–6 months anticoagulation sufficient
(e) APLA–thrombocytopenia with thrombosis iron def. anemia S/O–PNH

33. **Pregnancy–cholestasis: (T/F)**
(a) Cholestasis start in 3rd TM
(b) HEV–max. Prog.
(c) Acute fatty liver pregnancy 3rd TM
(d) Severe toxaemia of pregnancy can cause liver dysfunction
(e) Mild ↑ Bil. is normal

34. **Acute pericarditis: (T/F)**
(a) Markers can't difference between AMI and pericarditis
(b) ECG changes S/O endocardium involvement
(c) NSAIDs useful in viral pericarditis
(d) Pericardial rub–inspiration
(e) Pericardial rub–↑ specificity less sensitivity
(f) Acute pericarditis–Myocardial inflammation–perimyocarditis
(g) Chest pain–less common in acute pericarditis
(h) Pericardium–100-150 ml–normal
(i) Sitting and leaning forward ↑ pain

35. **Myopathy: (T/F)**
(a) CPK ↑ Hypothyroidism
(b) Osteomalacia painless proximal myopathy
(c) Steroid affect Type 1 fibre
(d) Statin induced myopathy shows antimyosin antibody
(e) Distal RTA present with acute flaccid paralysis

36. **HTN: (T/F)**
(a) < 60 years > 140/90 start drugs
(b) ACEI C/I in unilateral RAS
(c) Pregnancy induced HTN > 24 weeks
(d) Captopril screening (N) R/O renal stenosis
(e) Pheochromocytoma is the most common endocrine cause for HTN

37. **RAAS: (T/F)**
(a) Acute severe HF early activate of RAAS
(b) JGA cell secrete renin enzyme
(c) Aldosterone secrete by zona glomerulosa
(d) AT1 receptor mainly in kidney
(e) AT2 cause vasoconstriction and salt and wake retention

38. **Young female, diastolic HTN 160/110 mm Hg. No sweating, headache or palpitations: (T/F)**
(a) Pheochromocytoma should be ruled out
(b) Primary hyperaldosteronism should be ruled out by measuring serum potassium
(c) Takayasu arteritis is a diagnostic possibility
(d) Plasma cortisol level < 1.8 units on dexamethasone suppression test

39. **Pheochromocytoma: (T/F)**
(a) Hexagonal 1 chromaffin cells
(b) Labile HTN is invariable in all cases
(c) HTN is usually refractory
(d) 10% cases are bilateral
(e) MBG scan useful to detect metastases

40. **Kawasaki diseases: (T/F)**
(a) Most common in < 5 years of age
(b) Bilateral cervical lymphadenopathy
(c) Desquamative lesions occur early in the course of disease
(d) IVIG is the most definite therapy
(e) Coronary aneurysm is the major complication

41. **Which of the following drugs is renin inhibitor?**
(a) Ivabradine (b) Eplerenone
(c) Aliskiren (d) Satavaptan

42. **Which one of the following drugs has long half life?**
(a) Losartan (b) Irbesartan
(c) Telmisartan (d) Valsartan

43. **In Kawasaki disease, incidence of coronary aneurysms is:**
(a) Up to 50% (b) Up to 25%
(c) Up to 70% (d) Up to 90%

44. **Giant cell arteritis does not involve following artery:**
(a) Temporal artery (b) Internal carotid artery
(c) Subclavian artery (d) Axillary artery

45. **Newer oral anticoagulant drugs target thrombin or factor Xa. Select the true statement from the following in this context:**
(a) Dabigatranetexilate is an oral factor Xa inhibitor
(b) ROCKET AF study evaluated once daily dose of rivaroxaban in cases of atrial fibrillation compared to warfarin

(c) FDA has approved dabigatran for stroke thromboprophylaxis in patients of rheumatic heart diseases with atrial fibrillation
(d) Apixaban is a prodrug while rivaroxaban is not a prodrug

46. Pregnancy is contraindicated in which of the following cardiovascular conditions?

(a) Hypertrophic cardiomyopathy
(b) Repaired tetralogy of Fallot
(c) Fontan circulation
(d) Native severe coarctation

47. What is not true about cardiovascular disease in women?

(a) Women with MI have less comorbid conditions
(b) With PCI, women have more vascular complications than men
(c) With CABG, women have more postoperative depression
(d) Women have more atypical features

48. Blunt cardiac trauma with ventricular rupture most commonly involves:

(a) Right atrium (b) Left atrium
(c) Left ventricle (d) Right ventricle

49. HIV can cause A/E:

(a) Pulmonary HTN
(b) Pericardial effusion
(c) Construction pericarditis
(d) DCM

50. Neurocardiogenic syncope TT A/E:

(a) Diltiazem (b) Metaprolol
(c) Disopyramide (d) Sertaline

51. In Keith, Wagler staging for HTN all due to atherosclerosis *except*:

(a) ↑ Light reflex (b) AV nipping
(c) ↓ AV ratio (d) Silver wiring

52. Smoking cessation–Risk becomes same as non MI patients after:

(a) 3 months (b) 1 year
(c) 3.5 years (d) 7 years

53. Waist circumference above which risk of atherosclerosis ↑:

(a) F-33, M-40 (b) F-35, M-40
(c) F-37, M-44 (d) F-40, M-50

54. Heparin induced thrombocytopenia commonly present as:

(a) Bleeding (b) Clotting
(c) Patichae (d) Joint bleed

55. APLAS A/E:

(a) Thrombosis (b) Livedo reticularis
(c) Recurrent abortion (d) Thrombocytosis

56. Most common cause of hypercoagulation:

(a) Activated factor S resistance
(b) Factor C resistance
(c) Antithrombin III deficiency
(d) Factor S deficiency

57. Marfan's pregnancy–valve replacement decided by A/E:

(a) Aortic orifice > 4 cm
(b) Rapidly ↑ aortic orifice
(c) History of aortic dissection in family
(d) Severity of AR

58. All are true about heart rate turbulence (HRT) *except*:

(a) HRT is an index of changes in the sinus discharge rate after a PVC that is followed by a compensatory pause
(b) HRT is a measure of reflex vagal control of the heart, whereas heart rate variability is more indicative of overall vagal tone
(c) Beta blocker is an absolute contraindication in patients with HRT
(d) Abnormal HRT is a strong independent predictor of mortality in patients with CAD and DCMP

59. Lyme carditis is characterized by all, *except*:

(a) It is caused by Borrelia burgdorferi
(b) It usually begins in winter month with a characteristic rash
(c) 10% of untreated patients with Lyme disease demonstrated transient cardiac disease
(d) The most common manifestation is atrioventricular block of variable degree

60. All are important aspects of blood pressure measurement *except*:

(a) Cuff length and width should be 80% and 40% of arm circumference respectively
(b) Column or dial should be read to nearest 2 mm Hg
(c) Cuff should be deflated at < 3 mm Hg/sec
(d) None of the above

61. **Diagnostic criteria for POTS include all *except*:**
(a) Orthostatic tachycardia (> 30 BPM increase)
(b) Transient decrease in SBP of more than 20 mm Hg, with recovery after the first minute of tilt
(c) Standing plasma NE levels higher than 600 pg/ml
(d) Severe orthostatic symptoms

62. **Each of the following statements regarding age related valve changes are true, *except*:**
(a) In normal hearts, the thickness of the aortic and mitral leaflets increases progressively with each decade, particularly along their closure margins
(b) The circumferences of all four cardiac valves decrease with age in normal hearts
(c) Age-related thickening can be associated with the formation of whisker-like projections called Lam excrescences
(d) Mitral annular calcification almost invariably involves only the posterior annulus and forms a C-shaped ring of annular and subannular calcium

63. **All of the following are biochemical characteristics of metabolic syndrome, *except*:**
(a) Elevated cholesteryl ester transfer protein
(b) Hyperinsulinemia
(c) Low lipoprotein lipase
(d) Low hepatic lipase

64. **A 50-year-old male with type 2 DM and gouty arthritis has multiple office BP readings > 150/90 mm Hg despite being on lifestyle modifications for last months. His ambulatory BP monitoring reveals average sleep time BP of 126/74 mm Hg. Which of the following statements regarding management of this patient is not false?**
(a) Patient does not require pharmacotherapy for management of hypertension as he has only white coat hypertension should continue with lifestyle modifications
(b) Chlorthalidone is suitable first line drug for this patient
(c) ACEI + CCB is suitable combination therapy for hypertension in this patient
(d) Target BP should be <125/75 mg Hg if patient is proteinuric

65. **All are true regarding complications of radiation therapy *except*:**
(a) Premature cardiovascular disease accounts for 25% of non oncological deaths in long-term survivors
(b) It increases risk of significant valvular disease especially involving mitral valve
(c) Systolic dysfunction is relatively infrequent
(d) Conduction system is the least commonly involved of all cardiac structures

66. **Immediate blood pressure reduction is advised in all *except*:**
(a) Hypertensive encephalopathy
(b) Acute coronary syndrome
(c) Hypertensive crisis with acute renal insufficiency
(d) Acute aortic dissection

67. **HASBLED score includes all *except*:**
(a) Hypertension
(b) Stroke
(c) Elderly > 60 years
(d) Labile INR

68. **All are true about quitting of smoking *except*:**
(a) Decrease risk of CAD to that of non-smokers in 3-8 years
(b) Decrease risk of stroke to that of non-smokers in 5-15 years
(c) Decrease risk of CAD is not appreciable within 1 year of quitting smoking
(d) Risk of lung cancer falls to about half of non-smoker at 10 years

69. **All statements regarding cardiovascular pharmacogenetics are true, *except*:**
(a) A prerequisite for pharmacogenetics is heterogeneity in drug response
(b) Genetic variants in the hepatic transporter, SLCO1B1, influence the risk of adverse events
(c) Carriers of *5 variant of SLCO1B1 leads to higher plasma statin concentrations
(d) Risk for myopathy with *5 variant of SLCO1B1 depends on the statin type: the risk is greatest for fluvastatin

70. **Most potent endogenous cardio stimulatory peptide is:**
(a) Asopressin (b) Endothelin
(c) Urotensin (d) Apelin

71. **ENGAGE – AF:**
(a) Edoxaban (b) Rivaroxaban
(c) Dabigatran

72. **Kawasaki A/E:**
(a) Common in Europe (b) < 5 years
(c) Coronary aneurysm 25%

73. **ROX coupler used:**
(a) HT (b) Syncope vasovagal
(c) Paroxysmal AF (d) PPHT

74. **CHADS$_2$–VASC score risk close to 0 if:**
(a) 0 (b) 1
(c) 2 (d) 3

75. **HIT A/E:**
(a) Platelet fall to < 1 lac
(b) Venous > arterial thrombosis
(c) Medical > Surgery
(d) Common if heparin given for > 4 days

76. **Cocaine causes A/E:**
(a) MI
(b) Postural hypotension
(c) Heart block
(d) Aortic dissection

77. **Continuous murmur A/E:**
(a) Mammary souffle
(b) VSD with AR
(c) Peripheral PAS
(d) Coronary cameral fistula

78. **Which of the following requires fasting sample?**
(a) HBA1C (b) TSH
(c) Apolipoprotein A (d) C-peptide

79. **Most riding graphic result:**
(a) At PCWP = 18–25 mm Hg in patient of mitral stenosis, lower zone vessel more prominent then upper zone
(b) At PCWP 12–18 mm Hg- haziness and blurring of vascular markings
(c) In patient of myocarditis at PCWP 12-18 mm Hg, lower zone vessel equal or more than upper zone vessel
(d) In patient of MI, PCWP > 25 mm Hg, batwing distribution and pulmonary edema

80. **True about cardiac injuries A/E:**
(a) Tricuspid valve most commonly involved
(b) Bullet injury more lethal than stab injury
(c) Pericardiac tear can lead to cardiac strangulation
(d) Mortality > 50% when coronary artery is involved

81. **DOC for cocaine induced accelerated HIN:**
(a) Phentolamine (b) Labetolol
(c) Urapidil (d) Nicardipine

82. **I.V. drug having immediate onset of action:**
(a) Nitroprusside (b) NTG
(c) Labetolol (d) Nicardipine

83. **True about cardiac manifestation of HIV A/E:**
(a) Pulmonary HTN develops in 10%
(b) LV dysfunction found in 25% at autopsy
(c) Pericarditis resolves in 40% of patient spontaneously
(d) Pericarditis increase 6 months mortality

84. **Pre cardiac surgery high risk A/E:**
(a) C I <4
(b) Prior TA
(c) Pancreaticoduodenectomy
(d) DM on insulin therapy

85. **Pansystolic murmur all *except*:**
(a) PPH (b) Post MI VSD
(c) MVP (d) Ebstein's anomaly

86. **Accelerated HTN with renal ischemia DOC:**
(a) Fenoldopam (b) Enalaprilat
(c) Nitruprusside (d) Nifedipine

87. **Renal sympathetic denervation true:**
(a) Drug naive patient effect
(b) Effect not persist beyond 2 years
(c) Ablation near renal artery intima
(d) Contraindicated in significant RAS

88. **Pseudoxanthoma elasticum A/E:**
(a) Calcium intake mitigate effect
(b) Increases coronary atherosclerosis
(c) Present and life threatening GI bleeding
(d) Retina-angiod streak

89. **Exercise ST elevation in AVL lead in stress:**
(a) Signifies MI (b) Worse prognosis
(c) Regional wall motion (d) Sensitivity

90. **Pregnancy A/E:**
(a) Coronary dissection (b) Decreased SVR
(c) Increased creatinine (d) Increased ESR

91. **HIT A/E:**
(a) Thrombin inhibitors are used
(b) Associated with paradoxical thrombosis
(c) Antibodies against PF-4
(d) Type 1 has poor prognosis

92. First line therapy in HTN A/E:
(a) Amlodipine (b) CTD
(c) Lisnopril (d) Atenolol

93. Angioedema A/E:
(a) Non dependent areas
(b) ARBs cannot be used
(c) Spironolactone can be used
(d) Incidence 0.1-0.7%

94. Best epidemiological study for risk factor:
(a) RCT (b) Cohort study
(c) Case control study (d) Cross sectional study

95. ACC lipid guidelines true:
(a) High dose statin for all PVD patients
(b) DM irrespective of LDL level – statin
(c) Statin in LDL > 190 mg/dl to reduce by 50%
(d) Medium to high dose statin in 5 years risk > 7.5%

96. Hyperdynamic shock with tachyarrhythmias DOC:
(a) Epinephrine (b) Phenylephrine
(c) Dobutamine (d) Milrinone

97. High risk for non cardiac surgery A/E:
(a) Whipple disease
(b) TIA
(c) Creatinine > 2.1 mg/dl
(d) Syncope

98. NSAIDs causing HTN A/E:
(a) Aspirin (b) Celecoxib
(c) Piroxicam (d) Indomethacin

99. Trial all true *except*:
(a) Aspirin associated with reduced bleeding–POISE-2
(b) Spirinolactone have beneficial role in HFpEF–TOPCAT
(c) Renal denervation has no role in resistant HTN–SIMPLICITY-3

100. Pregnancy contraindicated A/E:
(a) PTU (b) Spironolactone
(c) Losartan (d) ACE-I

101. Locus heterogenicity (multiple foci with similar phenotype) A/E:
(a) Marfan's syndrome (b) HOCM
(c) Long QT (d) Muscular dystrophy

102. CYP- 2D6 all *except:*
(a) Simvastatin (b) Clopidogrel
(c) Codeine (d) Metoprolol

103. High risk individual for non cardiac surgery all *except:*
(a) EF < 40%
(b) Pancreato duodenectomy
(c) DM on insulin
(d) TIA

104. Postural syncope treatment:
(a) Midodrine
(b) B blockers
(c) Tilt training
(d) Isometric compressive manoeuvre

105. Renal denervation true:
(a) C/I in RAS (b) Done on intima
(c) In drug naïve patient

106. HTN emergency with renal involvement:
(a) NTG (b) Nitoprusside
(c) Fenoldopam (d) Hydralazine

107. Pregnancy all *except:*
(a) ACE inhibitor–oligohydramnios
(b) B blockers–teratogenic
(c) Amiodarone–neonatal thyroid disease

108. Transfatty acids all *except:*
(a) 1%↑= 23% ↑ mortality
(b) WHO-< 1% overall energy intake in diet
(c) Induces inflammation
(d) Causes insulin resistance

109. Mismatch in drugs during pregnancy:
(a) β blockers–teratogenic
(b) Aspirin–premature ductal closure
(c) Amiodarone–neonatal goiter
(d) ACE inhibitor–oligohydramnios

110. (A-a) O_2 gradient is decreased in all *except:*
(a) VP mismatch
(b) Hypoventilation
(c) Amiodarone induced lung toxicity
(d) Left to right shunt

111. Cardiac amyloidosis true *except:*
(a) Cardiac transplantation may be curative in transthyretin deposits

(b) Beta blockers and ACE-I are poorly tolerated in CHF of cardiac amyloidosis
(c) Cardiac MRI is not specific in picking up amyloid deposits before it is seen in echocardiography
(d) ICD may not be useful in secondary prevention of arrhythmias

112. OCT all *except:*
(a) Has higher resolution but better penetration than IVUS
(b) Needs RBC's devoid field
(c) Cannot differentiate between red and white thrombi
(d) Advential visualization is suboptimal

113. Acute CVS changes all *except:*
(a) EF increases
(b) Right mean pressure increases
(c) Renal blood flow decreases
(d) Splanchnic blood flow decreases

114. High cardiac risk for non cardiac surgery all *except:*
(a) DM on insulin
(b) Pancreaticoduodenectomy
(c) Ejection fraction =40%
(d) History of TIA

115. Mixed venous O_2 decreased in all *except:*
(a) Traumatic shock
(b) Hypoadrenal shock
(c) Septic shock
(d) Neurogenic shock

116. Periprocedural MI most commonly occurs during non cardiac surgery:
(a) Intraoperatively
(b) Within 4 hours of surgery
(c) 24-48 hours of surgery
(d) 7 days of surgery

117. Primary hypoaldosteronism true is:
(a) Adrenal adenoma is most common cause
(b) Edema present usually due to fluid retention
(c) LVH disproportionate to degree of hypertension in comparison to essential HTN
(d) Associated with metabolic acidosis

118. Hemodynamic changes in pregnancy all *except:*
(a) Blood volume increases y 40-50%
(b) HR increases by 10-20%
(c) PVR increases by 10-15%
(d) Leg veins pressure increases

119. Renal denervation true is:
(a) Ill sustained effect
(b) Renal vein ablation
(c) Multiple bilateral circumferential ablation is necessary for successful result
(d) Useful in naïve HTN

120. Dabigatran all *except:*
(a) Prodrug
(b) Amiodarone ↑ ses level by inhibiting P-Glycoprotein
(c) More absorbed in low pH
(d) Prevents more MI as compared to warfarin

121. All usual for HIT *except:*
(a) Dalteparin (b) Bivalirudin
(c) Fondaparinux (d) Lepirudin

122. Non cardiac surgery not a high risk:
(a) BP-160/100
(b) Creatinine–2.1mg/dl
(c) Vascular surgery
(d) Insulin use in T2 DM

123. All *except:*
(a) HTN majority low or normal renin activity
(b) ACE-I not effective in low PRA
(c) Local RAA–causes remodeling independent of PRA
(d) Elderly–low renin activity

124. Cardiac indication for cardiac surgery *except:*
(a) Patient on warfarin INR>2
(b) Marfan aortic root >4 cm
(c) AR
(d) MS (severe) with PAH

125. Muller's manoeuvre all *except:*
(a) ↓ed RV filling (b) ↑ed LV after load
(c) ↓ed SV (d) ↓ed EF

126. Rhabdomyoma all *except:*
(a) 90% tumor of children
(b) ↑es size with growth
(c) Associated tuberous sclerosis
(d) Can produce conduction abnormality

127. Most common primary cardiac malignant tumour:
(a) Hemangiosarcoma (b) Rhabdomyosarcoma
(c) Lymphoma

128. Pain of pericarditis:
(a) Due to pleura involvement
(b) ANS innervation of pericardium
(c) Pain receptors

129. All true *except* (for Women):
(a) Vascular complication less
(b) Normal coronaries most common
(c) Atypical chest pain most common
(d) Thrombolysis equally effective

130. Calculate CO in severe AS, Hb-10 g%, O_2 consumption-136 ml/min, pulmonary artery saturation-75%, systemic saturation-95%:
(a) 4 (b) 5
(c) 10 (d) 2

131. Prehypertension in children defined as:
(a) B/W 90-95th percentile N for age and sex
(b) B/W 85-90th percentile N for age and sex
(c) B/W 80-85th percentile N for age and sex
(d) B/W 95-99th percentile N for age and sex

132. True or false match:
(a) Prasugrel–ADP receptor inhibitor
(b) Congrelor–I/V ADP inhibitor
(c) Ticagrelor–Reversible ADP inhibitor
(d) Cilostazol–Adenosine reuptake blocker

133. Risk of non cardiac surgery all *except:*
(a) BP 180/104
(b) Creat.-2.5 mg%
(c) TIA history
(d) Insulin for NIDDM

134. Aliskiren:
(a) Not approved for HTN
(b) Inhibit Ang I to Ang II
(c) With losartan further ↓ proteinuria in DM
(d) No angioedema

135. All CI in pregnancy all *except:*
(a) Losartan (b) Torsemide
(c) Bosentan (d) Statin

136. Isolated ↑ BP in old age:
(a) Peripheral arterial resistance ↑
(b) Peripheral arteriolar resistance ↑
(c) ↑ SV
(d) ↓ Parasympathetic activity—normal phenomenon

137. All *except* about anthracycline toxicity:
(a) Cumulative dose ↑ toxicity
(b) Dilatation and hypertrophy of myocardium
(c) Diagnosed by biopsy
(d) Non proportional ↑ adrenergic activity

138. ↑ pulmonary artery blood flow all *except:*
(a) Peripheral prunning
(b) Artery to bronchus ratio > 1
(c) ↑ end on appearance of vessel on hilum
(d) Right desc. PA >15 mm is males

139. Heparin not to be given:
(a) LV thrombus
(b) Septic thrombophlebitis
(c) Before elective cardioversion
(d) Within 24 hours of rt-Pa in stroke

140. DMD all *except:*
(a) Cardiac inv. < 25%
(b) Female carrier cause DCMP
(c) R in V_1 in typical but not often seen
(d) Verapamil I.V. cause respiratory arrest

141. Aspirin not used:
(a) BT shunt
(b) ASD closure (< 6 months)
(c) Kawasaki disease
(d) Post coarctation dilatation

142. Pregnancy absolute C/I all *except:*
(a) Marfan (b) COA
(c) PA pr > 50 (d) Takayasu arteritis

143. Changes in pregnancy true:
(a) CO ↑ 100%
(b) BP 140/90
(c) GFR and Cr Cl ↑
(d) CO normalizes 3-6 days

144. Preoperative evaluation all *except:*
(a) Prophylactic revascularization not effective
(b) Preoperative PCI doesn't ↓ risk
(c) FEV1 <50% is not absolute C/I
(d) Smoking to be stopped 2 weeks before

145. All true about pulse *except:*

(a) Exaggerated anacrotic notch in AS
(b) 2:1 Wenkebach block leads to bigeminus pulse
(c) Dicrotic in cardiac tamponade
(d) RVF causes alternans in pulmonary artery tracing

146. Normal Split S_2:

(a) cc-TGA (b) ASD closure
(c) MS with PAH (d) PPI

147. Reverse pulsus paradoxus A/E:

(a) Cardiac tamponade (b) HOCM
(c) IPPV (d) CCP

148. Rytand's murmur:

(a) MDM with CHB (b) MDM with TR
(c) With AR (d) With MS

149. Myxoma syndrome:

(a) Holt-Oram syndrome
(b) Carney complex
(c) Naxo's syndrome

150. Systolic murmur in pulmonary area abolished on full inspiration:

(a) Straight back syndrome
(b) Pulmonary stenosis
(c) HOCM
(d) Aortic stenosis

151. Lithium in pregnancy causes abnormality of:

(a) Tricuspid Valve (b) Mitral Valve
(c) Aortic Valve (d) Pulmonary Valve

152. Korotkoff's 4th sound found in A/E:

(a) AR (b) Children
(c) Pregnancy (d) Hypertension

153. Wide pulse pressure seen in A/E:

(a) PDA with flow reversal
(b) AR
(c) Fever
(d) AV fistula

154. Paradoxical pulse seen in:

(a) PPV (b) Malignant effusion
(c) HOCM (d) RCMP

155. Dose decrease in renal failure:

(a) Verapamil (b) Metoprolol
(c) Atenolol (d) Carvedilol

156. During valsalva if Korotkoff's sounds in all phases:

(a) Decrease EF (b) Increase afterload
(c) Increase filling pressure

157. Korotkoff's sound in which phase of valsalva is normal?

(a) I and IV (b) I and III
(c) III and IV (d) All phases → I/IV

158. HTN goal JNC 7 in HTN + CRF:

(a) 140 and 90 (b) 130 and 80
(c) 120 and 80 (d) 130 and 85

159. Bleeding time is ↑ ed in A/E:

(a) Classical hemophilia
(b) ↓ Platelet count
(c) Qualitative platelet defect
(d) vWD

160. ↑ PT due to:

(a) Vitamin K deficiency
(b) Fibrinogen deficiency
(c) Factor XII deficiency

161. Doxorubicin is:

(a) Alkylating agent
(b) Antimetabolite
(c) Antibiotic (antitumour)
(d) Antimitotic

162. Essential HTN due to:

(a) Insulin deficiency (b) Insulin resistance
(c) ↑ endothelin

163. Before EPO→the measurement of which is essential?

(a) Serum iron (b) TIBC
(c) EPO

164. Rheumatoid arthritis associated with:

(a) AR (b) MS
(c) MR (d) PR

165. Orthostatic Hypotension—Definition:

(a) Decrease in SBP by 10 mm Hg within 3 min
(b) Decrease in DBP by 10 mm Hg within 3 min
(c) Both A+B
(d) Decrease in SBP by 20 mm Hg within 3 min

166. Catheter pull back with ↑ of 5 mm Hg in systolic peripheral BP in:

(a) Mild AS
(b) Aortic sclerosis
(c) Aortic value area < 0.5 cm^2
(d) HOCM

167. Worst prognosis in pregnancy:

(a) TOF with Hematocrit > 60%
(b) COA
(c) Ebstein's Anomaly
(d) Severe PS

168. AF with severe renal dysfunction DOC:

(a) Propafenone (b) Dofetilide
(c) Sotalol (d) Flecainide

169. Lymphatic vessels A/E:

(a) Scanty cytoplasm
(b) Interrupted basement membrane
(c) Tightly adherent pericytes

170. Hyperkinetic pulse in A/E:

(a) PDA (b) Acute MI
(c) Anemia (d) Hypovolemia

171. Isosmotic contrast:

(a) Iodixanol (b) Iohexol
(c) Diatriazoate

172. Which of the following not used in treatment of pheochromocytoma?

(a) Propranolol (b) Torsemide
(c) Phentolamine

173. Most vulnerable period of teratogenicity to heart:

(a) 15 to 50 days (b) 5 to 15 days

174. Least common manifestation of ARF:

(a) Carditis
(b) Arthritis
(c) Erythema marginatum
(d) Subcutaneous nodules

175. Most common CVS disease in India:

(a) HTN (b) RHD
(c) CHD (d) Cardiomyopathy

176. Not a cause of secondary HTN:

(a) ↓ Na (b) ↑ Ca
(c) Renovascular HTN

177. Which is not ACE-I trial:

(a) SAVE (b) BHAT
(c) SOLVD (d) AIRE

178. Most useful anti HTN in insulin requiring DM:

(a) Captopril (b) CCB
(c) B Blocker

179. Best anti-hypertensive in BPH:

(a) Prazosin (b) CCB
(c) B Blocker

180. Mixed venous sampling best site:

(a) PA (b) RA
(c) RV (d) PV

181. Drug with renoprotection in renal parenchymal disease:

(a) B Blockers (b) CCB
(c) ACE I

182. Normal upper limit of BP:

(a) 140/90 (b) 120/80
(c) 150/90

183. PCWP=12, PAP= 60/25:

(a) Pulmonary embolism (b) MS
(c) LV dysfunction

184. Primary cardiac tumour in children:

(a) Myxoma (b) Fibroma
(c) Rhabdomyoma

185. Antihypertensive treatment decreases mortality by:

(a) 10% (b) 14%
(c) 30% (d) 60%

186. Pregnancy all seen *except:*

(a) Increased blood volume
(b) Increased peripheral resistance
(c) Increased HR

187. Most innocent murmur are:

(a) Mid diastolic (b) Mid systolic
(c) Early systolic (d) Pansystolic

188. BP difference > 5 mm Hg seen in A/E:

(a) Subvalvular AS
(b) PDA
(c) Right subclavian artery from descending aorta

189. AV nodal artery arises from:

(a) RCA (b) LCx

190. Cardiac trauma least likely:

(a) VSD

(b) ASD

(c) Free wall rupture

(d) Coronary artery thrombosis

191. Neurocardiogenic syncope A/E:

(a) Mydriasis (b) Tilt table testing

(c) Bradycardia (d) Hypotension

192. RV all *except:*

(a) Tendon of tadaro (b) Trabecular septum

(c) Moderator band (d) Papillary muscle

193. Pregnancy all can be seen *except:*

(a) ACE-I (b) Metoprolol

(c) Amlodipine

194. Kawasaki's A/E:

(a) Cutaneous lesion common

(b) Seen in young adult

(c) CAD seen

195. Acute pericarditis A/E:

(a) Global ST elevation

(b) Convex ST elevation

(c) Pericardial pain aggravates on lying

(d) PR depression

196. Acute pericarditis A/E:

(a) T wave inversion comes down before ST reaches baseline

(b) ESR raised

197. Most common benign tumour in child:

(a) Rhabdomyoma (b) Angiosarcoma

198. All of the following decreases BP *except:*

(a) Mg supplement

(b) Reduce diet to 1000 calorie/day

(c) Hyponatremia

(d) Alcohol to < 1 oz/day

199. In HTN all following decreases BP *except:*

(a) Alcohol supplement (b) K supplement

(c) Ca supplement (d) Mg supplement

200. Pregnancy C/I A/E:

(a) Heparin (b) Fibrinolytic

(c) Beta blocker

201. Non cardiac surgery which is more important?

(a) Ejection fraction

(b) Exercise functional capacity

(c) NYHA class

(d) History of HTN

202. Gordon's syndrome A/E:

(a) Cause metabolic alkalosis

(b) Pseudohypoaldosteronism II

(c) Thiazides DOC

(d) Low salt sensitive HTN

203. Case series—28 years old female with mild HTN with pregnancy had 2 hours of retrosternal chest pain.

1. **On echo:**

   (a) RWMA (b) LVH

   (c) Normal

2. **First investigation:**

   (a) ECG (b) Stress test

   (c) CT (d) Biomarker

3. **Cause of chest pain:**

   (a) Atherosclerosis (b) Coronary dissection

   (c) Trauma

204. Case series—patient of HTN on irregular treatment, presents with altered sensorium, HR –45/min, BP–180/ 100 mm Hg.

1. **Diagnosis:**

   (a) Acute coronary syndrome

   (b) Acute renal failure

   (c) CVA

2. **Ion impaired:**

   (a) Na (b) K

   (c) Cl (d) Ca

3. **Immediate treatment:**

   (a) Correct hyperkalemia

   (b) TPI

205. Case series—Obese female with HTN presents with dyspnea on exertion, CATH–LVEDP–25 mm Hg PA–40/28/34 mm Hg, BP–140/90:

1. **Best drug option:**

   (a) CCB (b) Diuretics

   (c) ACE-I (d) Beta blockers

2. **On cath LVSP:**
   (a) 140 mm Hg (b) < 200 mm Hg
   (c) >400 mm Hg (d) 200-400 mm Hg
3. **True:**
   (a) Dyspnea due to raised LVEDP

206. Patient on radiotherapy for CA breast 10 years back, came with dyspnea, JVP increases with inspiration, *expect:*
(a) Ventricular interdependence
(b) No prominent y wave

207. Case series—28 years female asymptomatic before present with dyspnea after weight lift:
1. **Which parasternal murmur?**
   (a) Continuous (b) Systolic
   (c) Pan systolic (d) Diastolic
2. **Diagnosis:**
   (a) RSOV
   (b) Aorta to RV tunnel
   (c) COA
3. **Treatment:**
   (a) Percutaneous closure
   (b) Surgical correction
   (c) Medical
   (d) None

208. 16 years female symptomatic till 10 years improved after that, clubbing present:
1. **Murmur:**
   (a) Early diastolic (b) Continuous
   (c) Systolic (d) Mid diastolic
2. **If differential cyanosis:**
   (a) PDA Eisenmenger
   (b) ASD Eisenmenger
   (c) VSD Eisenmenger
   (d) TOF
3. **Treatment option:**
   (a) Immediate device closure
   (b) Surgery
   (c) Medical treatment
   (d) None

209. Pregnancy changes:
(a) Decreased SVR
(b) Increase HR
(c) Increased PVR
(d) Increased venous pressure

210. Drugs in pregnancy: (T/F)
(a) Labetalol (b) Clonidine
(c) Aliskiren (d) Nifedipine
(e) Hydralazine

211. In pregnancy true is:
(a) HR ↑
(b) No change
(c) HR ↓
(d) In third trimester volume increase is because of SV, not HR

212. CSS true:
(a) Should be done in all > 40 years with syncope
(b) In upright position positive
(c) Massage below angle of jaw
(d) > 3 secs pause and ↓ BP > 50 mm Hg

213. HT crisis all *except:*
(a) Papilloedema
(b) Oliguria
(c) Microangiopathic haemolytic anemia
(d) CHF
(e) DBP > 110

214. Drug safe in pregnancy (multiple options):
(a) Clonidine
(b) Nifedipine extended release
(c) Labetalol
(d) Hydralazine
(e) Aliskerin

215. HIT: (T/F)
(a) Diagnosed by serotonin release assay most specific
(b) Diagnosed by ELISA against PF4
(c) Platelet rich plasma given
(d) Warfarin not given till platelet reach baseline
(e) DTI are DOC

216. Orthostatic hypotension all *except:*
(a) Ranolazine (b) Diuertic
(c) Alcohol (d) Prazosin
(e) MAO-I

217. Rhabdomyoma T/F:
(a) No recurrence recorded as yet

(b) Spider cell on histolgy
(c) Most common site is LA
(d) Poor prognosis
(e) Most common tumour of childhood

218. Myxoma: (T/F)
(a) Carney's syndrome most common familial
(b) RA most common site
(c) 75% of primary cardiac tumour
(d) Carney no predilection for age/gender
(e) 90% are single

219. OSA all *except:*
(a) Severe with AHA > 20
(b) I in 20 symptomatic
(c) ↑ risk of CVA, hypertension/Stroke
(d) Associated with obesity
(e) ↑ risk of CHF

220. High risk pregnancy:
(a) Mechanical valve
(b) DCMP with EF <40%
(c) Marfan's syndrome with aortic dilatation >40 mm
(d) Pulmonary HTN
(e) All of the above

221. Takayasu arteritis: (T/F)
(a) F:M–5:1
(b) Stenosis 3 times less common than aneurysm
(c) ESR normal in 50%
(d) Coronary artery involvement in < 5%
(e) LV dysfunction in 18%

222. Anaerobic threshold all *except:*
(a) 40-60% of maximum oxygen uptake
(b) Below it proportional CO_2 and O_2 uptake
(c) Above it exponential increase in CO_2
(d) Below it metabolism switches to completely anaerobic

223. Pregnancy C/I in:
(a) Eisenmenger (b) COA
(c) HOCM

224. Xa:IIa ratio more in:
(a) Daltaparin (b) Enoxaparin
(c) Raviparin (d) Tinzaparin
(e) Danaparoid

225. Warfarin in pregnancy:
(a) Should be stopped in 1st trimester
(b) No anticoagulation
(c) Elective CS at 38 weeks
(d) Should be stopped in 2nd trimester

226. On OCP 34 years female had 4 baby no family history of HT, headache, fatigue had history of UTI:
(a) Essential HT
(b) Renal parenchymal disease
(c) Renal vasculitis
(d) OCP induced
(e) All of the above

227. DVT:
(a) Provoked X 6 months
(b) Better in 48 hours but can be for 14 days
(c) Catheter embolization > Surgery embolectomy in selected cases
(d) Thrombolysis if C. shock

228. OSA high risk all *except:*
(a) P edema (b) > 75 years
(c) T ↓ > 0.2 (d) Tachycardia
(e) S_3

229. Transbronchial lung biopsy: (T/F)
(a) C/I in pneumocystic carinii
(b) Indicated for histological evaluation of pulmonary fibrosis
(c) Indicated for sarcoidosis
(d) Pneumothorax is complication

230. Hyperthyroidism true is:
(a) SVR 700-1200
(b) Blood volume 85% of normal
(c) CO < 4.5 L
(d) All of the above

231. Carney complex diagnostic criteria:
(a) 3 out of 12 clinical criteria
(b) 8 out of 10
(c) 1 clinical + 1 genetic
(d) 1 major + 2 minor

232. Commotio cordis:
(a) SCD due to blow to chest wall

(b) AV node conduction is cause
(c) Chest and cardiac is reason
(d) Age > 30 years

233. Papillary muscle fibroelastoma:
(a) More common in female
(b) Mean age < 20 years
(c) MRI is diagnostic procedure of choice
(d) Gross appearance sea anemone
(e) All of the above

234. Transbronchial biopsy true:
(a) C/I in PCP
(b) Useful to see prognosis of idiopathic pulmonary fibrosis
(c) Can cause pneumothorax
(d) Useful for sarcoidosis

235. Pleural effusion amylase increased:
(a) Esophageal rupture (b) Pancreatitis
(c) Metastasis (d) TB

236. Fibromuscular dysplasia in all *except:*
(a) Distal 2/3 usually affected
(b) All layers affected
(c) Older women
(d) Branches can be affected
(e) Ballooning without stenting TOC

237. Lesion well tolerated in pregnancy true:
(a) MS (b) AS
(c) PS (d) COA
(e) HCM

238. Syndrome–X: (T/F)
(a) Antidepressants are useful in some cases
(b) Prognosis is worse than CAD
(c) Microvascular dysfunction can be seen in some patients
(d) CAG is normal

239. HT in elderly false is:
(a) Antihypertensive ↓es dementia
(b) Tolerate antihypertensives poorly
(c) SBP goal is generally not <150
(d) Mortality benefit less in young
(e) Case fatality rate higher in elderly

240. ISH true is:
(a) Most common cause of diastolic HF in elderly
(b) Arises de novo after 60 years age
(c) It occurs less commonly in those who have high normal BP at <60 years age
(d) DBP ↑es till age 55 years of age and then progressively falls

241. Pregnancy and TOF: (T/F)
(a) Due to ↓ peripheral resistance hemodynamics improve
(b) Palliative BT shunt done earlier have better oxygenation dut to ↑ed cardiac output

242. T/F:
(a) HR ↑ses in IIIrd trimester
(b) HR ↓ses in IIIrd trimester
(c) Cardiac output ↓ses due to stroke volume and not HR
(d) HR does not vary

243. Epidemiology true is:
(a) Precipitous tall in infant and child mortality in degenerative phase
(b) CVS mortality overtaken infections in receding pandemic
(c) Age adjusted CVD mortality rate ↓ing in degenerative
(d) Inactivity and obesity phase more evident in children

244. Neural syncope all *except:*
(a) Isotonic exercise
(b) Moderate isometric exercise
(c) Head tilt downward while sleeping
(d) Tilt training
(e) Isometric leg and arm counter pressure maneuver

245. Homocystinuria all *except:*
(a) CVD risk due to platelet dysfunction
(b) Pyridoxine rich diet to be given
(c) Heterozygosity associated with ↑CVD
(d) Mental retardation is seen

246. Central obesity associated with all *except:*
(a) DM-2
(b) Metabolic syndrome
(c) Female sex
(d) Insulin resistance
(e) CVS complication

247. Radiation induced heart injury true:
(a) Myocardium is most commonly involved
(b) Can affect 5-20 years after exposure

248. Normal hip waist ratio:
(a) 0.85 (b) 0.90
(c) 0.75

249. Hoffmann rigler sign:
(a) LVH (b) RVH
(c) RBBB (d) LBBB

250. Drugs used in vasovagal syncope all *except:*
(a) Scopolamine (b) Dipyridamole
(c) Ephedrine (d) Beta blocker
(e) Edrophonium

251. Familial myxoma, true is:
(a) Elderly age (b) Autosomal dominant
(c) Usually unilateral (d) None

252. Leptospirosis affects heart by:
(a) Myocardial necrosis
(b) First degree heart block
(c) Bradycardia
(d) All

253. Chagas disease:
(a) LV wall thickened and aneurysmal
(b) Apex necrosis and aneurysm
(c) Right heart failure
(d) Patient with apical presentation at high risk of death

254. Hypokalemia with HTN causes:
(a) Diuretics
(b) Malignant hypertension
(c) Pheochromocytoma
(d) RAS

255. Regarding myxedema:
(a) Minimal correction done after CABG
(b) Beta blockers causes severe bradycardia
(c) Correction of hypothyroidism relieves angina
(d) Acute correction required for surgery

256. Patient with syncope, EF<40% ECG shows conduction defect EPS-N study next step:
(a) Amiodarone (b) Sotalol
(c) AICD (d) All

257. NTG to be given in AMI patient till:
(a) SBP–105
(b) SBP decrease 15 mm Hg from standing
(c) SBP–90
(d) Large anterior infarct

258. Angiotensin II causes hypertension by:
(a) AT I (b) AT II
(c) Endothelin (d) All

259. Cocaine causes:
(a) Hypertension
(b) Sudden death
(c) ↑ Atherosclerosis
(d) Contraction necrosis
(e) All

260. Amyloidosis:
(a) LV wall thinning (b) Low voltage ECG

261. Lithium causes:
(a) Sinus node dysfunction
(b) VF
(c) T wave inversion

262. In pregnancy:
(a) Heart rate ↑ in 3rd trimester
(b) Heart rate ↓ in 3rd trimester
(c) Stroke volume ↑ in 3rd trimester

263. Acute intermittent porphyria:
(a) Pregnancy tolerated
(b) Remain latent upto puberty in majority
(c) Males more common
(d) Corticosteroids exacerbate it

264. BP recording all true *except:*
(a) Reduce @2 min/sec
(b) Readings near 2 mm Hg
(c) Minimum 2 readings
(d) CSA of cuff > 50% of arm circumference

265. Homocystinuria treatment A/E:
(a) Pyridoxine 25-500 mg/day
(b) Betaine given when pyridoxine non responsive
(c) Folate given in its deficiency
(d) Protein restricted diet with methionine and cystine

266. Obesity in females intervention advised *except:*
(a) Jogging 10 miles/week
(b) Wine reduce to 2/day
(c) Mediterranean diet

267. All true *except:*
(a) Marfan's syndrome–Dural ectasia
(b) Mulberrynanism–CP
(c) Neurofibromatosis–renal artery stenosis
(d) Moya moya disease–aortic aneurysm

268. Ground glass appearance in interventricular septum is seen in:
(a) HOCM (b) Hemochromatosis
(c) Amyloidosis

269. Which is not a prodrug?
(a) Captopril (b) Enalapril
(c) Ramipril (d) Lisnopril

270. All the following agents are used as an anticoagulant in a patient with heparin induced thrombocytopenia *except*:
(a) Bivalirudin (b) Argatroban
(c) Fond aparinux (d) Dalteparin

271. The comparator agents in Paradigm-HF trial are:
(a) Ramipril Vs neprilysin inhibitor
(b) Enalapril Vs neprilysin inhibitor
(c) Valsartan Vs neprilysin inhibitor
(d) Valsartan + sacubitril Vs Enalapril

272. With the current available evidence, all of the following diuretics may be used as a first line agent in essential hypertension *except*:
(a) Hydrochlorthiazide (b) Chlorthalidone
(c) Indapamide (d) Spiranolactone

273. All of the following conditions may be associated with a mass lesion inside the heart *except:*
(a) Glioma of brain
(b) Wilm's tumour
(c) Tuberculosis
(d) Wegener's granulomatosis

274. All of the following conditions are likely in this patient *except*:
(a) Papillary muscle rupture following myocardial infarction
(b) Multivalvular heart disease
(c) Hypertensive pulmonary oedema
(d) Acute myocarditis

275. The appropriate treatment for this 26 years old woman is:
(a) Pericardiectomy
(b) Balloon dilatation
(c) Alcohol septal ablation
(d) Pacemaker implantation

276. Following are true about hemodynamic changes during pregnancy *except*:
(a) Plasma volume increases by 50% above baseline by second trimester
(b) Heart rate increase 10-20% above baseline
(c) There may be slight fall in B.P. due to fall in peripheral resistance
(d) Asymptomatic severe mitral regurgitation is poorly tolerated lesion

277. Regarding anticoagulation during pregnancy, all are true *except*:
(a) Wearing exposure during 1st trimester causes embyropathy
(b) Risk is low if warfare dose < 5 mg
(c) Warfare increases the risk of fetal loss and spontaneous shorting
(d) Heparin is as effective as warfare in preventing valve thrombosis

278. About peripartum cardiomyopathy, all are true *except*:
(a) LV dysfunction occurring in last month of pregnancy or within 5 months of delivery
(b) Incidence is 1 in 3000
(c) Risk factors–black race, multiparity, pre-eclampsia
(d) Spontaneous recovery of LV function occurs in <25% of patients

279. Blue sclera are most likely to be associated with:
(a) Peripheral vascular disease
(b) Hypertrophic Cardiomyopathy
(c) Aortic regurgitation
(d) Heart Blocks

280. Osler Sign is:
(a) Non palpable brachial artery after its obliteration with BP cuff
(b) Is indicative of high intra arterial pressure
(c) Associated with radio femoral delay
(d) None of the above

281. Resistant hypertension is defined as high BP that remains uncontrolled:
(a) After intensive treatment for 6 weeks
(b) On a 4 drug regime
(c) After optimal doses of three drugs and a diuretic

(d) After optimal dose of three drugs including a diuretic

282. Treatment of resistant hypertension was addressed in which trial:

(a) Beautiful (b) Simplicity 2
(c) Stitch (d) Allahat

283. All are true about cilastozol except that it:

(a) Increases claudication distance
(b) Is a PDE-III inhibitor
(c) Inhibits platelets
(d) Decreases HdL levels

284. Drugs given for prevention of HAPE A/E:

(a) Subcutaneous morphine
(b) Acetazolamide
(c) Salmetrol
(d) Nifedipine

285. Kissing vegetation:

(a) APLA (b) Rheumatic fever
(c) Infective endocarditis

286. Accrochage:

(a) Acquired CHB (b) Congenital CHB
(c) Takotsubo CMP

287. Trials:

(a) Aliskiren–ALTITUDE
(b) Telmisartan–ONTARGET
(c) Rosvastatin–ASTRONOMER
(d) Irbesartan–ROADMAP

288. Osmolality of iodixanol:

(a) 290 mOsm/kg (b) 280 mOsm/kg
(c) 300 mOsm/kg (d) 310 mOsm/kg

289. Heparin side effect A/E:

(a) Osteoporosis
(b) Bilateral adrenal hyperplasia
(c) Hyperkalemia
(d) Skin necrosis

290. Anticoagulation given in renal failure:

(a) Apixaban (b) Rivaroxaban
(c) Warfarin (d) Dabigatran

291. True about fondaparinux *except:*

(a) Indirect Xa inhibitor
(b) Can be used in place of heparin in PCI
(c) Can be used as anticoagulant after STEMI
(d) Causes less bleeding than enoxaparin

292. Peripartum CMP true is:

(a) Maximum incidence in second trimester
(b) More common in developed countries
(c) Subsequent pregnancy risk of heart failure decreases
(d) Bromcriptine may be helpful

293. All are age related changes *except:*

(a) Increased HR variability
(b) Increased LA size
(c) Reduced sensitivity to beta receptors

294. True is:

(a) Risk of stroke only to raised DBP
(b) Risk of HTN and stroke specific to elderly
(c) HTN level is linearly correlated to risk of stroke
(d) HTN linked more to CAD than HTN linked to stroke

295. Rhabdomyoma A/E:

(a) Arises from ventricles
(b) Arises from cardiac myocyte
(c) Solitary lesion causing obstruction
(d) Rhabdomyoma regression

296. D-dimer true A/E:

(a) Test of choice in high probability patients
(b) Negative d-dimer rules out disease in low probability patients
(c) ELISA
(d) Useful for emergency screening

297. Most characteristic of Friedreich's ataxia true:

(a) Asymmetric septal hypertrophy with myocardial disarray
(b) Conc. LVH with dilated cavity
(c) DCMP common

298. ACE-I true is:

(a) Started after 3-5 days
(b) Decreases infarct expansion
(c) ACE-I + ARB given together

299. True about HIT is:

(a) LMWH do not cause it

(b) Warfarin is DOC for thrombosis
(c) Occurs within 2-3 hours if prior exposure has occur
(d) Continue LMWH even if HIT occurs

300. Lipoprotein (a) true A/E:
(a) Diet and exercise modify Lp(a)
(b) Statin donot lower Lp(a)
(c) Lp(a) high correlation with family history
(d) Lp(a) done in selective group of high risk patient

301. Takayasu arteritis A/E:
(a) Aneurysm may occur
(b) PA is involved
(c) Predominantly involved vascular endothelium
(d) High aldosterone level may be found

302. K/C/O HTN on thiazide, new anti-hypertensive added, now C/O sleeplessness and fatigue during exercise, which drug is culprit?
(a) Metoprolol (b) Nifedipine
(c) Clonidine (d) α–blocker

303. Patient of hypertension put on treatment, develops swelling around lips and periorbital edema:
(a) Lisnopril (b) Nifedipine
(c) Furosemide (d) Clonidine

304. Patient on ACE-I with mild renal dysfunction. New drug is added which caused hyperkalemia:
(a) Digoxin (b) Salbutamol
(c) NSAIDs

305. Risk factor for non cardiac surgery are A/E:
(a) High grade AV block
(b) Unstable angina
(c) LBBB
(d) Severe valvular heart disease

306. Molecules used in PET A/E:
(a) Rubidium–82 (b) Carbon–11
(c) Fluorine–18 (d) Tc–99

307. 70 years old male type 2 DM has normal ECG and LV function, going for hernia surgery under G(a) Next evaluation:
(a) No further test
(b) TMT
(c) Stress thallium
(d) CT coronary angiography

308. Pregnancy C/I A/E:
(a) Bosentan (b) ACE-I
(c) Hydralazine (d) Statin

309. Dose reduction in renal failure:
(a) Atenolol (b) INH
(c) Rifampicin (d) Pravastatin

310. $CHADS_2$ A/E:
(a) Age > 65 years (b) CHF
(c) HTN (d) DM

311. Wrong match:
(a) ABCD–CPR
(b) SYNTAX–Complex coronary artery in CAD
(c) HAS- BLED–Bleeding with anticoagulation
(d) TIMI–Unstable angina

312. Cirrhosis with cyanosis diagnosed by:
(a) Contrast echo (b) TEE
(c) CT chest (d) Intracardiac echo

313. Cyclosporine induced HTN DOC:
(a) Diuretic (b) CCB
(c) ACE-I (d) Beta blocker

314. Supine to standing, compensatory changes occur is:
(a) Decreased HR
(b) PVR decreased
(c) Increased contractility
(d) Decreased CO

315. Carotid sinus massage causes:
(a) Increased ERP of AV node
(b) Decreased baroreceptor firing rate
(c) Ventricular myocardium

316. 70 years old male; supine HR-65 bpm, BP-160/90; standing HR-70 bpm, BP- 80/60 A/E:
(a) Parkinsonism
(b) Paraneoplastic
(c) Shy Dragger syndrome
(d) Sick sinus syndrome

317. Postpartum cardiomyopathy new modality found to be effective:
(a) Depot medroxyprogesterone
(b) IVIG
(c) Oral prednisolone
(d) Bromcriptine

318. IVIG useful in which myocarditis?

(a) Giant cell myocarditis
(b) Lymphocytic myocarditis
(c) Postpartum CMP
(d) Pediatric myocarditis

319. Aliskiren A/E:

(a) Effective more than 24 hours
(b) Reactive increase in renin after treatment
(c) Most common side effect is dry cough
(d) Inhibit conversion of angiotensinogen to angiotensin

320. Anti-hypertensive vaccine uses:

(a) Renin (b) Angiotensinogen
(c) Calmodulin (d) Angiotensin–III

321. Pharmacodynamic therapy A/E:

(a) Warfarin + clopidogrel
(b) Warfarin + amiodarone
(c) Warfarin + metronidazole
(d) Warfarin + digoxin

322. Amiodarone increases effect of A/E:

(a) Metoprolol (b) Pravastatin
(c) Simvastatin (d) Warfarin

323. Induction of CYP3A4:

(a) Rifampicin (b) Grape fruit juice
(c) Cyclosporine

324. Bone marrow mononuclear stem cell:

(a) Not arrhythmogenic
(b) CD 133^{+} cells increases restenosis risk
(c) Not useful if used < 4 days of MI
(d) All of the above

325. Postpartum–least preferred antihypertensive:

(a) Ramipril (b) Methyldopa
(c) Amlodipine (d) Metoprolol

326. 55 years old male with chest pain for 3 days now asymptomatic, normotensive, non-diabetic, ECG and ECHO - normal, next investigation:

(a) Trop-T
(b) Reassurance and NSAIDS
(c) Rule out cervical spondylitis
(d) TMT

327. Perioperative risk stratification, least useful:

(a) Dobutamine echo (b) ECHO
(c) MPI (d) Thallium scan

328. Kawasaki's disease, third day fever, ectasia in proximal LA(d). Likely course is:

(a) Slowly progresses over next 4 weeks
(b) More chance of regression because of proximal involvement
(c) 100% normalization over next 10 years
(d) Does not regress

329. 28 weeks pregnancy advised rest because of obstetric reasons develops breathlessness with BP=90/60 mm Hg:

(a) D-dimer false positive in pregnancy
(b) CT angiography should be avoided because of fetal radiation risk
(c) STK–DOC
(d) Heparin preferred over STK for risk of fetal toxicity

330. 16 hours air travel, lady develops DVT, duration of anticoagulant:

(a) 3 months (b) 6 months
(c) 2 weeks (d) 4 weeks

331. HIV all are manifestation *except:*

(a) Autonomic dysfunction
(b) LQTS
(c) Isolated RV dysfunction
(d) None

332. Prehypertension—A male with office reading 135/84, 136/88, 138/84. Evidence based indication:

(a) Life style modification arrest progression of BP
(b) > 50% chances of developing BP
(c) Antihypertensives is cost effective

333. Migraine association:

(a) PFO
(b) ASD
(c) Pulmonary AV malformations
(d) All of the above

334. Drugs contraindicated in pregnancy:

(a) Flecainide (b) Losartan
(c) Hydralazine (d) Digoxin

335. Renin in ↑ ed in A/E:

(a) OCP
(b) Primary hyperaldosteronism
(c) Secondary hyperaldosteronism
(d) Malignant HTN

336. HIV not seen:
(a) High grade AV block
(b) Torsade de pointes
(c) Isolated RVH
(d) Accelerated atherosclerosis

337. HIV not seen:
(a) Constrictive pericarditis
(b) Cardiac lymphoma
(c) Pulmonary HTN
(d) DCMP

338. 2nd day platelet count ↓es from 2 lakh to 1,60,000/ml after starting UFH, next strategy:
(a) UFH to continue as it is transient
(b) LMWH
(c) Lipirudin
(d) GP II b/IIIa

339. Pregnancy risk most in:
(a) Severe PAH (b) AR
(c) MR (d) Unoperated ASD

340. Multiple myeloma, 40-year-old female + echo – EF=50%, E/a < 1, scintillating appearance, no LVH, HR–80/min, present with HF, next to be done:
(a) Endomyocardial biopsy
(b) Diuretics
(c) Digoxin
(d) Verapamil

341. Most common cause of renovascular HTN in young Indians:
(a) Aorto-arteritis
(b) Atherosclerosis
(c) Intimal fibro muscular dysplasia
(d) Medial fibro muscular dysplasia

342. HTN in urban Indian:
(a) 22 % (b) 25.5%
(c) 29% (d) 10.2%

343. Which is not affected by liver disease?
(a) Pravastatin (b) Simvastatin
(c) Atorvastatin (d) Lovastatin

344. Metabolic injury to heart, A/E:
(a) DKA (b) Multiorgan trauma
(c) Sepsis (d) Burns

345. Highest cardiac risk of surgery:
(a) Intrathoracic
(b) Carotid endarterectomy
(c) Intra-peritoneal
(d) Peripheral vascular surgery

346. Competitive sports are contraindicated:
(a) Marfan with aortic diameter > 40 mm
(b) Non-obstructive HOCM
(c) DCMP with EF < 35% (stage II)
(d) Myocarditis (recent)

347. Most common metastasis to heart:
(a) CA lung (b) Ca breast
(c) Lymphoma (d) Leukemia

348. 1 year old infant asymptomatic with multiple rhabdomyoma - prognosis:
(a) Repeated arrhythmia
(b) Spontaneous regression
(c) Progress to rhabomyosarcoma
(d) No progression

349. Drug with 1st order kinetic achieve steady stage in ___ $t^{1/2}$.
(a) 10 (b) 2
(c) 5 (d) No relation

350. Risk factor for HTN A/E:
(a) Sleep apnea (b) Low birth-weight
(c) Obesity (d) None of the above

351. Diet in cardiovascular disease least effect:
(a) ↓ Fatty diet
(b) ↑ PUFA
(c) ↑ Omega-3 fatty acids
(d) Whole diet

352. CIN all useful A/E:
(a) Low dose of dopamine
(b) Iso-osmotic contrast
(c) Aminophylline
(d) Ascorbic acid

353. Mismatch toxic:
(a) Mercury–CAD
(b) Arsenic–Pericardial effusion
(c) Lead–AV block
(d) Cobalt–DCMP

354. Cardiac atrophy seen in A/E:
(a) K^+ deficient diet (b) Anorexia
(c) Addison's disease (d) Astronaut's

355. **OSA cardiac manifestation A/E:**
(a) AV block (b) Systolic dysfunction
(c) HTN (d) Atherosclerosis
(e) All true

356. **POTS A/E:**
(a) ↓ SBP >20 mm Hg for > 1min
(b) Severe orthostatic symptom
(c) Standing NE > 600 pg/ml
(d) HR ↑ es > 30/min

357. **Hyperhomocysteinemia all *except:***
(a) HRT (b) CRF
(c) Statin (Fenofibrate)

358. **Least common in AIDS:**
(a) Kaposi (b) IE
(c) Myocarditis (d) Atherosclerosis

359. **Anti-arrhythmic of choice in pregnancy:**
(a) IA (b) IC
(c) BB (d) DC cardioversion

360. **Selective beta-blocker without ISA are all *except:***
(a) Acebutalol (b) Betaxolol
(c) Esmolol (d) Bisoprolol

361. **Parenteral vasodilator drugs for hypertensive emergency are all *except:***
(a) Phentolamine (b) Enalapril
(c) Nicardipine (d) Fenoldopam

362. **Hypertensive emergency like conditions are:**
(a) Encephalitis
(b) Hypercalcemia
(c) Anxiety with hyperventilation
(d) AD

363. **Contrast nephropathy prevented by all *except:***
(a) NAC (b) Saline
(c) Ionic solution (d) Theophylline

364. **All are seen in RA *except:***
(a) Eustachian
(b) Thebasian
(c) Ligament of Marshall

365. **Secondary prevention trial in IUD all *except:***
(a) CAD (b) Maveric
(c) AVID (d) CIDS

366. **Geneva risk score are all *except:***
(a) Hypertension (b) Prior DVT
(c) Cancer (d) HF

367. **Which of the following is WHO criteria added to definition of metabolic syndrome?**
(a) Hyperalbuminemia
(b) Impaired glucose tolerance
(c) Decreased HDL
(d) Obesity

368. **All are true about hypereosinophilic syndrome *except:***
(a) Increased eosinophils in peripheral blood
(b) Lymphadenopathy is seen
(c) Heart involvement is uncommon
(d) Can cause restrictive lung disease

369. **Metabolic syndrome is associated with:**
(a) Hypothyroidism (b) Acromegaly
(c) PCOD (d) Cushing's disease

370. **All are indicators of inappropriate hypertension *except:***
(a) Age between 30 and 40 years
(b) BP > 180/110
(c) Presence of LVH in ECG
(d) Abdominal bruit

371. **Giant coronary artery aneurysm is seen in:**
(a) SLE (b) Syphilis
(c) PAN (d) Sarcoidosis

372. **All are seen in metabolic syndrome *except:***
(a) Increased fibrinogen
(b) Increased fibrin
(c) Impaired glucose tolerance
(d) Obesity

373. **Renovascular hypertension is seen in all of the following conditions *except:***
(a) Fibromuscular hyperplasia
(b) Takayasu artertitis
(c) Renal artery embolization
(d) Atherosclerosis

374. **Control of hypertension decreases the incidence of all of the following *except:***
(a) Sudden cardiac death
(b) Stroke
(c) CAD
(d) Heart failure

375. All of the following are criteria for diagnosis of metabolic syndrome *except:*
(a) Obesity
(b) BP > 130/85
(c) LDL > 200
(d) Impaired glucose tolerance

376. Which of the following drug Is contraindicated in pregnancy?
(a) Hydralazine (b) Enalapril
(c) Beta blockers (d) Methyl dopa

377. In HIV patient incidence of all of the following are increased *except:*
(a) Lymphoma
(b) Kaposi's sarcoma
(c) Infective endocarditis
(d) Dilated cardiomyopathy

378. For the prevention of contrast nephropathy best is:
(a) Mannitol (b) IV saline
(c) Furosemidc (d) Soda bicarbonate

379. All of the following are true about renew vascular hypertension *except:*
(a) Renal bruit is heard
(b) Flash pulmonary edema is seen
(c) Retinopathy is uncommon
(d) Aorta arthritis is one of the causes

380. Least common in SLEs:
(a) Pericardial effusion
(b) Pericarditis
(c) Myocardial infarction
(d) Pulmonary artery hypertension

381. 20 years boy most common cause of HTN:
(a) Renovascular HTN
(b) CRF
(c) Takayasu arteritis with renal artery involvement
(d) Essential HTN

382. False +ve RA factor in A/E:
(a) HbSAg (b) VDRL
(c) Coomb's test (d) IBD

383. Rivaroxaban A/E:
(a) Oral Xa inhibitor
(b) More bleeding than standard treatment (LMWH followed by oral Vit K antagonist)
(c) No need to monitor
(d) For management of DVT

384. Smoking causes A/E:
(a) SCLC (b) BOOP
(c) Acute bronchiolitis (d) Emphysema

385. Monogenic cause of HTN with AD inheritance:
(a) 17 α hydroxylase deficiency X
(b) 11 β hydroxylase deficiency X
(c) Conn's disease (Familial)
(d) Glucocorticoid remedial aldosteronism

386. Accelerated hypertension metabolic change:
(a) Hypomagnesemia
(b) ↑ anion gap acidosis
(c) Normal anion gap acidosis
(d) Metabolic alkalosis

387. Marfan's syndrome most specific:
(a) Myopia
(b) Dural ectasia
(c) Hyperextensible joints
(d) MVP

388. True vs pseudoaneurysm A/E:
(a) Myocardium forms wall
(b) ↑ ed chance of rupture
(c) Wide base

389. Carcinoid commonly involves (most commonly):
(a) RV inflow tract (b) RV outflow tract
(c) Pulmonary valve (d) Bifurcation of PA

390. Reserpine:
(a) α 2 agonist
(b) α 2 antagonist
(c) Pan adrenergic blocker
(d) Imidazole receptor antagonist

391. Blunt chest trauma causes:
(a) AR (b) MR
(c) TR (d) PR

392. Rivaroxaban is:
(a) DTI (b) Xa inhibitor
(c) ADP blockers

393. B blocker not hepatic excretion:
(a) Propranolol (b) Sotalol
(c) Nadolol (d) Bisoprolol

394. Pheochromocytoma A/E:

(a) Low cortisol
(b) Orthostatic hypotension
(c) Flushing of face

395. Hypertension seen in A/E:

(a) Bartter's syndrome
(b) Liddle's syndrome
(c) Conn's syndrome

396. Phenylephrine ↓ murmur of:

(a) AS (b) AR
(c) TOF

397. Renal sympathetic denervation is a recent modality of treatment for:

(a) Resistant HTN
(b) Bilateral RAS
(c) Unilateral RAS
(d) Hypertensive nephropathy

398. Maternal risk of pregnancy is very high in all *except:*

(a) VSD with severe pH
(b) Marfan syndrome with aortic root > 40 mm
(c) Dilated cardiomyopathy with EF < 40%
(d) Pulmonary stenosis with GRDT 50 mm Hg

399. Identify the wrong statement regarding hemodynamic changes during pregnancy:

(a) Plasma volume increases by about 50% above baseline
(b) Heart rate increase by 20%
(c) Pulmonary vascular resistance increases
(d) Venous pressure in lower limbs increases

400. Identify the wrong statement in rhabdomyoma of the heart:

(a) Probably hamatomas
(b) Can mimic restrictive cardiomyopathy
(c) Most often require resection
(d) 90% are multiple

401. All of the following are common manifestations of bleeding caused by von Willebrand disease *except:*

(a) Epistaxis
(b) Menorrhagia
(c) Postpartum hemorrhage
(d) Spontaneous

402. A 24 years old woman is newly diagnosed with systemic lupus erythematosis. Which of the following organ system complications is she most likely to have over the course of her lifetime?

(a) Cardiopulmonary (b) Cutaneous
(c) Hematologic (d) Musculoskeletal

403. All of the following hormones are produced by the Anterior pituitary *except:*

(a) Adrenocorticotropic Hormone
(b) Growth hormone
(c) Oxytocin
(d) Prolactin

404. Isolated systolic hypertension in young adults (between 17-25 years age) is due to:

(a) Stiff Aorta
(b) Increased cardiac output
(c) Overactive sympathetic nervous system
(d) All of the above

405. The following cardiovascular drug is contraindicated in pregnancy:

(a) Beta blocker (b) ACE inhibitor
(c) Digoxin (d) Methyldopa

406. All of the following cause prolongation of the activated partial thromboplastin time that does not correct with the 1:1 mixture with pooled plasma *except:*

(a) Lupus anti-coagulant (b) Factor VIII inhibitor
(c) Heparin (d) Factor VII inhibitor

407. Which of the following is drug of choice in low BP and high cardiac situation:

(a) Inotropes (b) Vasodilator
(c) Vasopresser (d) Inodilator

408. ACE-inhibitor is contraindicated in:

(a) Unilateral renal artery stenosis
(b) Bilateral renal artery stenosis
(c) Renal failure with 2-3 mg%
(d) Diabetic nephropathy

409. Least lipid soluble beta blockers:

(a) Metoprolol (b) Atenolol
(c) Propranolol (d) Timolol

410. All of the following are risk factors for chronic obstructive pulmonary disease *except:*

(a) Airway hyper responsiveness
(b) Coal dust exposure
(c) Passive cigarette smoke exposure
(d) Recurrent respiratory infections

411. Which of the following cardiovascular conditions is a contraindication to pregnancy?

(a) Arterial septal defect without Eisenmenger syndrome
(b) Idiopathic pulmonary arterial hypertension
(c) Marfan syndrome
(d) Mitral regurgitation

412. A patient is evaluated in the emergency department for peripheral cyanosis. All of the following are potential etiologies *except:*

(a) Cold exposure
(b) Deep venous thromobosis
(c) Methemoglobinemia
(d) Peripheral vascular disease

413. In an elderly patient with hypertension with diabetes, proteinuria without renal failure, the Anti-hypertensive of choice is:

(a) Furosemide (b) Methyldopa
(c) Enalapril (d) Propranolol

414. Drug of choice in case of Aspirin allergy is:

(a) Dipyridamole (b) Ticlopidine
(c) Sulfinpyrazone (d) Clopidogrel

415. Isolated systolic hypertension in young adults (between 17 and 25 years of age) is due to:

(a) Stiff aorta
(b) Increased cardiac output
(c) Overactive sympathetic nervous system
(d) All of the above

416. The following cardiovascular drug is contra-indicated in pregnancy:

(a) Beta Blocker (b) ACE inhibitor
(c) Digoxin (d) Methyldopa

417. All of the following are predisposing factors to urinary Tract Infections in children, *except:*

(a) Vesicoureteric Reflux (b) Circumscised males
(c) Spina bifida (d) Antibiotic treatment

418. A neonatologist, during routine rounds, finds a few hours old baby which is otherwise healthy and feeding well. On auscultation, there is a loud, harsh, pansystolic mumur best heard over the sternal border with a thrill. Chest X-ray shows mild cardiomegaly and slight increase in pulmonary vascularity confirmed with Doppler and Colour flow mapping. Which is true of this condition?

(a) It is one of the rare congenital cardiac defects
(b) It commonly results in heart failure in the first week of life
(c) Surgical repair is recommended in all cases
(d) Prophylaxis against endocarditis is required

419. Earliest radiological sign of pulmonary venous Hypertension in Chest X-ray is:

(a) Cephalization of pulmonary vascularity
(b) Pleural effusion
(c) Kerley B lines
(d) Alveolar pulmonary edema

420. In CHF, angiotensin receptor blockers are a reasonable alternative to ACE inhibitors in ACEI intolerant patients due to the following reasons *except:*

(a) Angioedema (b) Irritant cough
(c) Renal insufficiency (d) Skin rash

421. Initial drugs of choice, for a young black American with essential hypertension when compared to whites:

(a) Beta blocker and diuretics
(b) ACEI and diuretics
(c) Calcium channel blockers and beta blockers
(d) Diuretics and calcium channel blocker

422. Which of these statements is not true for arterio-sclerosis of hypertension?

(a) It has diffuse distribution along the course of the vessel
(b) It affects the arterial media
(c) It is primarily due to collagen fragmentation and loss of collagen
(d) It is one cause of age related rise in arterial systolic pressure

423. Beta-blocker with beta 1 selectivity and intrinsic partial agonist activity:

(a) Pindolol (b) Nadolol
(c) Acebutalol (d) Esmolol

424. The most useful information with regard to autonomic nervous system function is obtained during and phases of valsalva maneuver.

(a) Phase I and III (b) Phase II and III
(c) Phase I and IV (d) Phase III and IV

425. When blood pressure elevation during pregnancy is noted at 12-16 weeks of gestation, one must suspect:

(a) Gestational hypertension
(b) Chronic/essential hypertension
(c) Pre eclampsia
(d) Eclampsia

426. Thiazide diuretic cause the following changes in serum/blood:

(a) Increase HCO_3 (b) Increase Cl
(c) Increase Na^+ (d) Increase Mg^{++}

427. Drug of choice for cyclosporine induced hypertension:

(a) Beta-blocker
(b) Calcium channel blocker
(c) ACE inhibitors
(d) Diuretics

428. Hemodynamic changes in pregnancy include:

(a) Increase in systematic vascular resistance
(b) Increase in cardiac output
(c) Maximal increase in left atrial pressure in mitral stenosis in first trimester
(d) Non-tolerance of regurgitant lesion

429. The disorder where you would consider pregnancy to be contraindicated is:

(a) Mini regurgitation
(b) Aortic regurgitation
(c) Atrial septal defect
(d) Pulmonary arterial hypertension

430. Which of the following is not a predictor of sudden death in an otherwise healthy individual with no structural heart disease or metabolic dearrangement?

(a) Markedly prolonged PR interval of 0.36 ms
(b) QTc 0.245 ms
(c) QTc 580 ms
(d) Epsilon wave in right precordial leads

431. Preparation for surgery for patients with pheochromocytoma include:

(a) Alpha-blockade (b) Volume expansion
(c) High salt diet (d) All of the above

432. Cardiac Amyloidosis presents as:

(a) Restrictive cardiomyopathy
(b) Congestive heart failure
(c) Orthostatic hypotension
(d) All of the above

433. Hirudin and Bivaluridin:

(a) Act by inhibiting antithrombin III
(b) Potentiate the action of antithrombin III
(c) Are direct thrombin inhibitors
(d) Require frequent a PTT monitoring

434. The optimal INR with warfarin therapy in patients with atrial fibrillation and underlying heart disease is between:

(a) 1.5–2.0 (b) 2.0–3.0
(c) 2.5–3.5 (d) 3.0–4.0

435. Esmolol is a:

(a) Long acting beta blocker
(b) Ultra short acting bet blocker
(c) Selective beta-2 antagonist
(d) Has intrinsic sympathomimetic activity

436. Carvedilol is most useful in presence of:

(a) Hypertension (b) Angina
(c) LV dysfunction (d) Arrhythmia

437. A 75 years old hypertensive male came with AF so what is true?

(a) Calculate risk score for starting anticoagulation
(b) No need to score start directly anticoagulation
(c) Check fasting blood sugar

438. A 50 years old diabetic hypertensive came to you with AF, so what is her CHADS2 score?

(a) 2 (b) 3
(c) 4 (d) 5

439. Regarding HIT which is not true?

(a) Platelet count is usually > 20,000
(b) There is significant bleeding risk
(c) Occur more than 5 days after starting heparin
(d) Occur with both heparin and LMWH

440. Best method to prevent contrast induced nephropathy is:

(a) Give N-acetyleysteine
(b) Give 0.9% NaCl 3-12 hr before procedure
(c) Give low and isoosmolar visipaque and <100 ml volume
(d) Give NaHCl3 before and after procedure

441. Regarding malignancy (metastasis) which is true?

(a) Most common malignancy is breast carcinoma
(b) RCC reaches to heart via venous route
(c) ST T changes does not occur with metastases
(d) Metastasis most commonly involved myocardium than pericardium

442. Which suggest neurally medicated syncope?

(a) Presence of aura

(b) Nausea and diaphoresis prior to episode
(c) Duration > 5 min
(d) Post episodic confusion

443. Heart rate turbulence true:
(a) Reflect vagal tone
(b) Overall vagal tone
(c) No prognostic value
(d) No drug to control heart rate

444. PVR in pregnancy:
(a) Unchanged (b) Increased
(c) Decreased (d) Variable

445. Syndrome X A/E:
(a) Most common in post menopausal female
(b) EF reduced on exercise
(c) Sunlingual nitroglycerine improves symptoms
(d) Variable response with beta blockers/CB

446. Pregnancy contraindicated in:
(a) HCM
(b) Peripartum CMP
(c) Eisenmenger syndrome
(d) Marfan's aortic dissection

447. Pregnancy true A/E:
(a) Loud S1
(b) S3 very common
(c) JVP increased
(d) Diastolic murmur at apex

448. Sudden HTN control required in A/E:
(a) Acute ischemic stroke (b) SAH
(c) Papilledema (d) Aortic dissection

449. Fabry's disease A/E:
(a) AR (b) α-galactosidase A
(c) Block (d) MI

450. Hypercoagulable state A/E:
(a) Factor V leiden
(b) Chronic liver disease
(c) Myeloproliferative disease
(d) Postpartum state

451. DOC in HTN with DM:
(a) ARB (b) ACE inhibitor

452. Rhabdomyoma:
(a) 50% atria
(b) Poor prognosis
(c) Resection is curative and recurrence common

453. All are parts of metabolic syndrome *except:*
(a) LDL (b) TG
(c) HDL (d) HTN

454. Jupiter trial A/E:
(a) Rosvastatin dose used was 20 mg
(b) Increased incidence of myopathy
(c) LDL < 130 mg%, CRP > 2 mg% patients included
(d) No increase in incidence of new onset diabetes and dyslipidemia

455. Beta blockers with α blocking prosperity A/E:
(a) Labetlol (b) Carvediol
(c) Bucindolol (d) Alprenolol

456. D-dimer all true *except:*
(a) Negative test has high NPV
(b) Positive test is highly specific
(c) Increased in pregnancy
(d) Is a product of fibrin breakdown

457. Lead poisoning most common cardiac feature:
(a) Cardiomyopathy (b) CAD
(c) Hypertension (d) AV block

458. All of these should be evaluated for secondary cause of HTN *except:*
(a) 55 years old male with family history of HTN, BP= 150/100
(b) 70 years old male with no past history of HTN BP= 190/110
(c) 20 years old female with hematuria with family history renal disease, BP= 150/100
(d) 30 years old female with DM, dyslipidemia BP= 150/110

459. Most effective measure to prevent CIN:
(a) Preload with 0.9% saline 3-12 hours before CAG
(b) NAC 600 mg bd
(c) Sodium bicarbonate
(d) Low or isoosmolar contrast with < 100 ml

460. Absolute C/I for pregnancy:
(a) AS
(b) TOF
(c) Eisenmenger syndrome
(d) COA

461. JNC VII ACC to NHLBI BP 142/92 is classified in:
(a) Prehypertension (b) Stage I
(c) Stage II (d) Normal

462. Treatment of HTN true:
(a) Loop's Diuretics preferred
(b) ACE I are first choice in < 50 years
(c) In diabetic target is 140/85 mng

463. Pregnancy C/I A/E:
(a) Severe obstructive lesion
(b) PPH
(c) HOCM
(d) Marfan with Aortic root >40 mm

464. SPAF trial for AF, 4 risk factors were followed which is not among these 4 risk factors:
(a) DM (b) Recent stroke
(c) HTN (d) HF

465. Pheochromocytoma true:
(a) Arise from adrenal cortex rarely
(b) Persistent hypertension in 50%
(c) Familial more common
(d) MIBG confirm diagnosis

466. Which is used to ↓ doxorubicin toxicity?
(a) Dexrazoxane (b) Saline
(c) Mannitol (d) Colchicine

467. Drug used in hypertensive emergency A/E:
(a) Fenoldopam (b) IV NTG
(c) Labetalol (d) S/L nifedipine

468. APLA true A/E:
(a) Livedo Reticularis (b) Rash
(c) Peripheral gangrene (d) Venous ulcer

469. Most common tumour metastasize to heart:
(a) Ca breast (b) Malignant melanoma
(c) NHL (d) Ca lung

470. Fetal effect of vitamin D given in pregnancy:
(a) Aortic Valve stenosis (b) IHSS
(c) Supravalvular AS

471. Isoosmolar contrast agent:
(a) Iohexol (b) Iopamidol
(c) Iodixanol (d) Ioxagalate

472. Maximum chance of Pulmonary edema in pregnancy with MS:
(a) At peak of labour
(b) 6-7 hours of delivery
(c) 24-36 hours of delivery
(d) 36 weeks of pregnancy

473. Mumps vaccination associated with:
(a) Endocardial fibroelastosis
(b) Myocarditis
(c) I.E.
(d) Pericarditis

474. HAART treatment lipid change:
(a) ↑ TG (b) ↓ HDL
(c) ↑ LpA (d) ↓ LDL

475. Factor V leiden associated with:
(a) Venous thromboembolism
(b) MI
(c) CVA
(d) PAD

476. Recurrent abortion, venous and arterial thrombosis:
(a) APLA
(b) Homocysteinemia
(c) Factor V leiden deficiency

477. Anti Ro, Anti La associated with:
(a) Congenital CHB
(b) TGA
(c) Ebstein anomaly

478. Central α2 antagonist A/E:
(a) Methyl dopa
(b) Nimodipine
(c) Guanfacine

479. Systolic HTN in child A/E:
(a) > 99 percentile definition
(b) DMSA usually detects defect
(c) Headache is most common presentation
(d) Nitroprusside long term treatment

480. Angiotensin II MOA for HTN:
(a) Systemic vasoconstriction
(b) Na retention due to ↑ aldosterone
(c) Renin mediated feedback

481. Labial HTN due to impaired baroreflex function:

(a) Severe retinal changes
(b) Multiple lacunar infarct
(c) LVH
(d) Gradual renal dysfunction

482. Primary HTN due to ↑ SVR:

(a) Endothelial dysfunction with vascular remodeling
(b) Smooth muscle hypertrophy
(c) Impaired vascular relaxation
(d) ↑ vasoconstriction

483. The classic "add-on-therapy" syndrome is:

(a) Ischemic Heart Disease
(b) Atrial Fibrillation
(c) Hypertension
(d) Heart Failure

484. The following drugs are effective in Neuro-Cardiogenic syncope *except:*

(a) Metoprolol (b) Escitalopram
(c) Erythropoietin (d) Clonidine

485. Mutation in PTPN11 gene is seen in:

(a) Noonan syndrome (b) Williams syndrome
(c) Alagille syndrome (d) Hall-Hittner syndrome

486. Among the six signs that compose the principal clinical features of Kawasaki Disease the least common is:

(a) Rash
(b) Conjunctivitis
(c) Changes in the hands and feet
(d) Cervical lymph node enlargement

487. The superficial femoral artery becomes the popliteal artery on exiting the adductor canal through the tendinous opening in:

(a) Adductor longus (b) Adductor brevis
(c) Adductor magnus (d) Quadriceps muscle

488. Which statement is false with respect to hemodynamics and pregnancy?

(a) Maximal hemodynamic changes peak by 36 weeks of pregnancy
(b) Stroke volume, increases during pregnancy
(c) There is increase in preload and afterload during uterine contraction
(d) Marked increase in preload immediately after delivery

489. Common cardiac finding in children with Lyme's disease is:

(a) Pericarditis
(b) Global myocarditis
(c) Varying degrees of A-V block
(d) Endocarditis

490. In Ehler-Danlos syndrome all are true *except:*

(a) Variable involvement of skin and joints
(b) Aortic root dilatation is seen in majority of patients
(c) Spontaneous rupture of medium and large caliber arteries can occur
(d) Pregnancy is hazardous

491. Identify the drug which has cardiovascular teratogenic effect:

(a) Propranalol (b) Ramipril
(c) Retinoic acid (d) Digoxin

492. Pregnancy is contraindicated in all *except:*

(a) Marfan's syndrome with dilated aortic root
(b) Mechanical prosthetic valves
(c) Peripartum cardiomyopathy
(d) Eisenmenger's syndrome

493. Homocysteine level is reduced by:

(a) Folic acid (b) Vitamin A
(c) Vitamin C (d) Atorvastatin

494. Carcinoid heart disease may present with all the following *except:*

(a) Hypertension
(b) Hypotension
(c) Mitral regurgitation
(d) Tricuspid regurgitation

495. ECG of hypothyroid patient may have all the features *except:*

(a) Low Voltage
(b) Short QT interval
(c) Prolonged AV conduction
(d) Decreased 'P' wave voltage

496. Regarding anticoagulant therapy for prevention of systemic thromboembolism in mitral stenosis patients, all of the following statement are true *except*:

(a) Anticoagulant therapy is indicated in patients with mitral stenosis with paroxysmal or persistent atrial arrhythmias

(b) It is indicated in severe mitral stenosis in sinus rhythm but with severe enlargement of left atrial appendage
(c) Anticoagulant therapy must be initiated in all mitral stenotic patients with previous embolic events
(d) Anticoagulant therapy must be aimed at maintaining the International Normalized Ratio (INR) between 2 and 3

497. Maternal vitamin D ingestion:
(a) William syndrome (b) Peripheral PS

498. HIC causes A/E:
(a) DCMP (b) Pericardial effusion
(c) AR (d) Pulmonary HTN

499. Salt restriction decrease adrenergic response:
(a) High renin HTN
(b) Low renin HTN
(c) Non modulating HTN
(d) Essential HTN

500. Pregnancy causes A/E:
(a) SV increases 40-45%
(b) HR increases 10-20%
(c) SBP increases
(d) Lower extremities venous pressure increases

501. Absolute C/I to thrombolysis A/E:
(a) Pregnancy (b) Aortic dissection
(c) ICH (d) Stroke 3 months old

502. Sinus bradycardia A/E:
(a) Leptospirosis
(b) Brucellosis
(c) Advanced liver disease
(d) Hypothyroidism

503. Whipple disease seen in:
(a) CHB (b) Atrial flutter
(c) AF (d) VT

504. Congested pharyngitis and conjunctiva–cause:
(a) Kawasaki disease (b) Adenovirus

505. Hyperthyroidism A/E:
(a) AF is 13.8%
(b) Anticoagulation very useful
(c) Pulmonary HTN common
(d) 90% return to sinus rate

506. Rebound HTN:
(a) Clonidine (b) α methyl dopa
(c) CCB

507. Cough induced by ACE-inhibitor treatment:
(a) Colchicine (b) Icaliditide

508. Metabolic syndrome all except:
(a) Increase HDL (b) Increase LDL
(c) Increase TG (d) Increase BP

509. Non-cardiac surgery in >40-year-old male increase risk except:
(a) Class II CSA
(b) S3
(c) AMI < 3 months
(d) VPC > 5/min in preoperative ECG

510. Cyt P 450 is inhibitory effect on:
(a) Pantoprazole
(b) Esomeprazole
(c) Omeprazole
(d) Rabeprazole

511. Fabry's disease true: (T/F)
(a) AR
(b) Alpha-glucosidase
(c) LVH
(d) Female carrier same disease
(e) Angina without vessel obstruction

512. Cardiac manifestation of neurologic diseases false: (T/F)
(a) DMD causes DCM after 18 years
(b) Limb girdle–DCM more in IIe than IId
(c) Friederich ataxia–manifestation of LVH increases with age and GAG repeats

513. JNC-8 true: (T/F)
(a) < 60 years=< 140/90
(b) > 60 years=<150/90
(c) Diabetes, CKD= target 130/85
(d) Preferred first line thiazide less than 60 years
(e) ACE- I not used in CKD

514. Incorrect: (T/F)
(a) Rhabdomyoma most common cardiac tumour in adult
(b) Myxoma most common cardiac tumour in adult

(c) Angiosarcoma MC sarcoma in adult

(d) RA > LA involvement in myxoma

(e) Myxoma more common in male

515. Drug in pregnancy A/E: (T/F)

(a) Losartan (b) Methyldopa
(c) Hydralazine (d) Enalapril
(e) Nifedipine

516. Positive pressure ventilation during inspiration: (T/F)

(a) ↑ preload RV (b) LV ↑ preload
(c) LV ↓ preload (d) LV ↑ afterload
(e) LV ↓ afterload

517. HTN: (T/F)

(a) White coat HTN in 20%
(b) In DM goal < 120/80
(c) In ALLHAT, lisnopril + chlorthalidone + amlodipine only in DM
(d) Renal sympathetic denervation in all
(e) DASH diet

518. Hypothermia ECG manifestations: (T/F)

(a) Increased PR (b) Bradycardia
(c) Tachycardia (d) Increased QT
(e) Decreased PR

519. Hypothermia post cardiac surgery (CABG):

(a) 50% ↓ metabolic requirement/10 ºC
(b) ↑ RBC deformity
(c) Inhibition Na^+ K^+ ATPase
(d) Right shift of curve
(e) ↓ coronary vascular resistance

520. HIV: (T/F)

(a) Increased PAH 5%
(b) Accelerated CAD
(c) Pericardial effusion most common
(d) HAART increased effusion
(e) Commonly progress to CP

521. Cardiac manifestations in COPD A/E: (T/F)

(a) MAT (b) RVF
(c) LVF (d) CAD
(e) PAH

522. Life long anticoagulation A/E: (T/F)

(a) Lone AF 50 years
(b) Bioprosthetic with AF
(c) Double bioprosthetic valve
(d) Mechanical valve
(e) AF with CVA

523. Fabry's A/E: (T/F)

(a) Enzyme defect- α- glucosidase
(b) More severe in females
(c) Short PR
(d) LVH may be seen
(e) SCD is most common cause of death

524. PEEP: (T/F)

(a) ↑ total lung water content
(b) ↑ CVP
(c) ↑ mean arterial pressure
(d) ↑ LV distensibility
(e) ↑ CO in LV dysfunction

525. Drugs C/I in pregnancy: (T/F)

(a) Furosemide (b) Telmisartan
(c) Ramipril (d) Amlodipine
(e) Digoxin

526. Resistant HTN–renal sympathetic denervation: (T/F)

(a) Afferent grows earlier than efferent fibres
(b) Sustained effect upto 2 years
(c) Also used in CRF and sleep apnea
(d) Decreased stroke, MI, cardiac death and CKD
(e) Lumbar sympathectomy done earlier was very effective for HTN control

527. Syncope causes: (T/F)

(a) Alcohol (b) Hyperglycemia
(c) Cough (d) Hypoxia
(e) Pulmonary embolism

528. Thyroid hormones: (T/F)

(a) Hyperthyroidism causes HTN with increased renin
(b) Thyroid hormones causes phosphorylation of phospholamban
(c) In hyperthyroidism reduced catecholamines in blood
(d) In hyperthyroidism IVRT increased
(e) CO in hyperthyroidism increases 2 times

529. Metabolic syndrome A/E: (T/F)

(a) FBG > 110 mg%
(b) Male waist circumference > 40 inch

(c) In female HDL < 40 mg%
(d) TG > 150 mg%
(e) BP > 130/85 mm Hg

530. True or False:
(a) Iodixanol is useful in renal failure
(b) Osmolality is 400 mosm/kg
(c) Recurrent contrast reaction is > 50%
(d) Contrast reaction difficult to manage in patient in beta blockers
(e) Iodixanol is better anticoagulation action than urograffin

531. Fabry's disease: (T/F)
(a) LV wall thinning
(b) F > M
(c) AR inheritance
(d) Angina and MI with normal coronary system

532. Marfan's syndrome–Ghant major criteria: (T/F)
(a) Dural ectasia and lumbar erosion
(b) Ectopic lentis
(c) MVP
(d) Aortic dissection
(e) Myopia

533. Pulmonary AV fistula: (T/F)
(a) Brain abscess
(b) Paradoxical emboli
(c) Complicates Glenn shunt
(d) Contrast appear earlier
(e) Bronchiectasis associated with Osler Weber Rendu syndrome

534. Cardiac tumours: (T/F)
(a) Most common primary cardiac malignant tumour is lymphoma
(b) Most common primary cardiac tumour is myxoma
(c) Myxoma most common in LA
(d) Rhabdomyoma most common in valves
(e) Metastasis most common than primary cardiac tumour

535. HIV: (T/F)
(a) PPH less common
(b) KS rarely symptomatic
(c) Most common primary malignancy – lymphoma
(d) Accelerated atherosclerosis is more common without risk factors
(e) QT prolongation

536. Odd's ratio: (T/F)
(a) Less useful than relative risk
(b) Indicates association
(c) Useful in clinical research
(d) Indicates probability of having disease versus bone disease
(e) Does not indicate relative sample size

537. Transfatty acids: (T/F)
(a) Decreases LDL
(b) Decreases HDL
(c) Increased LP (a)
(d) Occurs in milk
(e) Contains double bonds

538. HIT: (T/F)
(a) LMWX never cause HIT
(b) Never seen with fondaparinux
(c) Platelet transfusions treatment
(d) Bivalirudin can be used
(e) UFH not to be stopped

539. All true about epidemiology *except:* (T/F)
(a) Receding pandemic stage I
(b) Stage II – cardiac mortaliy–< 10%
(c) Inc receding pandemic mortaliy: 10-35%
(d) Famine and pestilence stage – predominant cause of mortality is RHD
(e) Stage IV degenerative and man made

540. 65 years female, radical mastectomy, presurgical TMT Normal, no c/o angina starting adriamycin, advice: (T/F)
(a) Baseline and serial MUGA during chemotherapy
(b) Repeat post surgical TMT
(c) Do stress thalium
(d) Prescribe ramipril
(e) Treat with carvedilol

541. 65 years HT on treatment, non DM, Normal lipid, 4-5 cigarettes/day, going for cataract surgery, jogging for 40 min without chest pain advice that is essential: (T/F)
(a) ECG
(b) TMT
(c) Dobutamine echo
(d) Stress thalium
(e) CXR

542. Endocardial fibroelastosis false: (T/F)
(a) Incidence increasing in India
(b) Predilection for outflow tracts
(c) Corticosteroids curative
(d) Calcification of endocardium may be associated
(e) Age mean–60 years

543. Fabry's disease: (T/F)
(a) α-glucosidase deficiency
(b) AR
(c) Renal involvement common
(d) Angiokeratoma most common on face
(e) Cardiac–LVH most common type

544. True regarding metabolic syndrome: (T/F)
(a) Waist in female > 102 cm
(b) TG > 150 mg%
(c) HDL < 50 mg% in males
(d) BP > 130/85 mm Hg
(e) FBG > 110 mg%

545. Normal BP: (T/F)
(a) SBP < 120 mm Hg (b) SBP < 130 mm Hg
(c) SBP < 140 mm Hg (d) DBP < 80 mm Hg
(e) CBP < 90 mm Hg

546. Poorly tolerated syndrome in pregnancy: (T/F)
(a) PPH (b) Eisenmenger
(c) Severe MS (d) COA
(e) TOF

547. Pregnancy safe durgs are: (T/F)
(a) Statins (b) Digoxin
(c) Dilzem (d) ACE-I
(e) Clopidogrel

548. ATP–III, LDL < 100 mg% indication is A/E: (T/F)
(a) Post MI
(b) Metabolic syndrome
(c) HTN
(d) Atherosclerotic abdominal aortic aneurysm
(e) DM

549. Metabolic syndrome includes: (T/F)
(a) Hyperuricemia (b) HTN
(c) Insulin resistance (d) Abdominal obesity

550. ACE C/I in: (T/F)
(a) U/L RAS (b) S. Creat. = 2 mg%
(c) Pregnancy (d) Severe AS
(e) Proteinuria

551. Cardiac tumour true is a: (T/F)
(a) Primary > secondary tumours
(b) Angiosarcoma most common primary sarcoma in adults
(c) Rhabdomyosarcoma most common primary sarcoma in children
(d) Lymphoma most common primary tumour
(e) Most common site of metastasis is endocardium

552. Patient going for cataract surgery, smoker with HTN controlled on metoprolol 25 mg SR, non diabetic, non dyslipidemic, jogging for 40 min without pain: (T/F)
(a) ECG (b) Echo
(c) TMT (d) Stress thallium
(e) Stress echo

553. ARBs: (T/F)
(a) Inhibit AT-1
(b) Causes cough equivalent to ACE-I
(c) Does not increase bradykinin
(d) Equivalent to ACE-I in HTN
(e) Can be used in pregnancy

554. HELLP syndrome: (T/F)
(a) Can be seen in gestational HTN
(b) Poor prognosis
(c) Hemolysis, low platelet count and raised liver enzymes
(d) Erythrocytosis

555. Cardiac tumours: (T/F)
(a) Most common angiosarcoma–malignant
(b) Metastatic > primary
(c) Rhabdomyosarcoma has good prognosis
(d) Sarcomas are most common variety
(e) RA tumour most common

556. Prazosin: (T/F)
(a) α1–antagonist
(b) C/I in prostate hypertrophy
(c) Negative effect on lipid profile

557. Clonidine: (T/F)
(a) Central sympatholytic
(b) Side effect–sedation
(c) On stoppage–tachycardia
(d) Withdrawal HTN

558. IVC filter–indications are: (T/F)
(a) Repeated episode of VTE despite therapeutic anticoagulation
(b) C/I for anti-coagulation

(c) Floating thrombus
(d) Pre-op after >1 month if anti-coagulants to be stopped temporarily
(e) As adjunct to fibrinolysis

559. Cardiac myxoma: (T/F)
(a) RA > RV
(b) Usually pedunculated
(c) Can be multicentric
(d) Can be AD in some
(e) Usually multiple bony metastasis

560. Fabry disease: (T/F)
(a) F > M
(b) Deficiency of α-galactosidase enzyme
(c) Autosomal recessive
(d) LVH on echo
(e) Angiokeratoma may occur on buttock

561. Cardiac tumours: (T/F)
(a) Most common angiosarcoma–malignant
(b) Metastatic > primary
(c) Rhabdomyosarcoma has good prognosis
(d) Sarcomas are most common variety
(e) RA tumour most common

562. Changes with ageing in cardiac valves: (T/F)
(a) Lambi's excrescence
(b) Inceased annular circumference
(c) Thinning of leaflets
(d) Mitral annular calcification
(e) Aortic sclerosis

563. Fabry's disease true: (T/F)
(a) AR (b) Angiokeratoma
(c) Deafness (d) CHB
(e) LV thinning

564. Clonidine true: (T/F)
(a) Centrally acting
(b) Sedative
(c) Long half life–2 weeks
(d) Rebound HTN
(e) Withdrawal tachycardia

565. Tumours: (T/F)
(a) 75% malignant
(b) Most common maligant–angiosarcoma
(c) Sporadic myxoma–10 years age presentation
(d) Most common valve tumour–lipoma
(e) Recurrence rate= 2-19%

566. Myxoma: (T/F)
(a) Most common–freewall LA
(b) Recurrence post op–30%
(c) Neuroendocrine markers common +
(d) IL-6 Constitutional symptom
(e) Familial at younger age

567. Amyloidosis: (T/F)
(a) IAS thickening
(b) Cardiac valves thickening
(c) S4 common
(d) Pericardial effusion
(e) Pre-excitation

568. AD: (T/F)
(a) HCM (b) MVP
(c) Noonan (d) Fabry's disease
(e) Holt-Oram syndrome

569. Pregnancy Normal A/E: (T/F)
(a) EDM (b) Loud S1
(c) Wide S_2 (d) S4
(e) Continuous murmur

570. Primary tumor of heart: (T/F)
(a) 75% malignant
(b) Myxoma common in RA
(c) Most common tumour on AV valve is lipoma
(d) Most common tumour in adult is angiosarcoma
(e) Sporadic myxoma–mean age 10 years

571. Heparin adverse effect: (T/F)
(a) Alopecia (b) Hepatitis
(c) Neuritis (d) Thrombocytopenia
(e) Osteopenia

572. Clonidine: (T/F)
(a) Centrally acting sympatholytics
(b) Sedation
(c) T ½ - 2 weeks
(d) Withdrawal causes tachycardia
(e) HTN, restlessness and sweating

573. Drugs used in pregnancy in HTN: (T/F)
(a) Methyl dopa (b) Hydralazine
(c) ARB (d) ACE-I
(e) Diuretics

574. HELLP: (T/F)
(a) Seen in pregnancy
(b) Seen in obstructive jaundice
(c) Hemolysis, elevated liver enzymes, low platelet
(d) Erythrocytosis, low platelet, hepatitis
(e) Poor prognosis

575. Hs CRP: (T/F)
(a) Predicts CAD in all age groups
(b) Even in women
(c) Predicts mortality in MI
(d) Mediates innate immunity
(e) Mostly produced in muscle

576. ARB: (T/F)
(a) Acts on AT1
(b) Does not increase bradykinin
(c) Cough same evidence As ACE-I
(d) Given in pregnancy
(e) As effective as ACE-I

577. JNC VI: (T/F)
(a) ≥ 18 years person
(b) Optimal BP group in addition to normal and high normal
(c) 3 stages–I, II and III
(d) No specific status for DM
(e) Drug only in stage III, irrespective of risk factor

578. Clinical features of pregnancy are A/E: (T/F)
(a) Early diastolic murmur
(b) Loud S_1
(c) Wide splitting of S_2
(d) Venous hum
(e) S_4

579. Myxoma: (T/F)
(a) Most common on free wall of LA
(b) IL-6 for systemic manifestations
(c) Younger age presentation in familial form
(d) Angiosarcoma most common malignancy in adult

580. Clonidine: (T/F)
(a) Central acting
(b) Sedation
(c) Withdrawal HTN
(d) Withdrawal tachycardia
(e) Biological half life > 2 weeks

581. Neurocardiogenic syncope A/E: (T/F)
(a) Flecainide (b) Amiodarone
(c) Fludrocortisone (d) SSRI
(e) Beta blocker

582. Na nitroprusside: (T/F)
(a) Increased compliance of aorta
(b) Dilate arteries and vein
(c) DOC in HTN with IHD
(d) CN and NO released quickly

583. Peripartum CMP: (T/F)
(a) < 25 years
(b) 3rd or 4th baby increased risk
(c) Increased with twins
(d) Maximum in 2nd trimester

584. Amyloidosis: (T/F)
(a) Interatrial septal hypertrophy
(b) Pericardial effusion
(c) S_4 commonly seen

585. ACE-I C/I in:
(a) Aortic stenosis (b) COPD
(c) Dehydration (d) Left RAS stenosis

586. Marked increase in BP is normal in: (T/F)
(a) Pregnancy (b) Exercise
(c) Alcohol ingestion (d) None

587. HTN is most common cause of A/E: (T/F)
(a) CAD
(b) Stroke
(c) Renal failure
(d) Abdominal saccular aneurysm

588. Feature of mild HTN:
(a) No specific symptoms
(b) Tachycardia
(c) Loss of circadium rhythm
(d) Increased pulse pressure
(e) Increased stroke volume

589. High risk marker in essential HTN: (T/F)
(a) Glycosuria (b) Grade II retinopathy
(c) Alcohol (d) LVH

590. Drugs used in CHF with NSR: (T/F)

(a) LMWH (b) Digoxin
(c) ACE-I (d) Amiodarone

591. Drug interaction of methyl dopa: (T/F)

(a) Haloperidol (b) Lithium
(c) Amlodipine

592. Drug interaction with statin: (T/F)

(a) Gemfibrozil (b) Erythromycin
(c) OHA (d) Warfarin
(e) Digoxin

593. HTN as most common cause of: (T/F)

(a) CCRF (b) CVD
(c) Stroke (d) Aortic aneurysm

594. ACE-I C/I: (T/F)

(a) Dehydration
(b) COPD
(c) Left renal artery stenosis
(d) Dissection of aorta

595. Kawasaki Disease A/E:

(a) Coronary aneurysm in > 25% if untreated
(b) Common in < 5 year of age
(c) IVIG and apheresis is the treatment
(d) Common in Africa

596. Which does not decrease risk of CIN?

(a) ISO osmolar contrast
(b) Intravenous saline
(c) Less dose of contrast
(d) Prophylactic NAC

597. Myxoma—Sporadic vs Familial:

(a) Recurrence more common
(b) Occur in multiple sites
(c) Occur in middle age female
(d) Associated with hormonal imbalance

598. Not dependent on antithrombin III:

(a) Argatroban (b) Fondaparinux

599. Prodrug is:

(a) Prasugrel (b) Clopidogrel
(c) Cangrelor

600. Anticoagulation in pregnancy A/E:

(a) Warfarin C/I in 6-12 weeks
(b) Warfarin replaced by heparin in 2-3 weeks prior to delivery
(c) LMWH can be used in place of UFH without Xa monitoring
(d) Aspirin added in 3rd trimester with warf/heparin

601. Most adverse outcome in pregnancy:

(a) PPH
(b) AR
(c) MR
(d) Severe MS with moderate PAH

602. Central sleep apnea associated A/E:

(a) HTN (b) AF
(c) Acute MI (d) Prinzmental angina

603. All causes peripheral edema *except:*

(a) Cyclosporine (b) OKT 3
(c) Leflonamide (d) Sulfonamide

604. Rhabdomyoma A/E:

(a) Most common cardiac tumour in paediatric population
(b) Multiple sites
(c) RV free wall most common
(d) Tuberous sclerosis > 50% association

605. JNC–VII A/E:

(a) DM–138/82, needs drug therapy
(b) 158/98–requires thiazide diuretics
(c) > 160/>100–stage 2
(d) Normal < 120 systolic

606. Metabolic syndrome A/E:

(a) FBS > 126
(b) TG > 150
(c) Waist circumference 88 cm (F), 102 (M)
(d) BP ≥ 130/85 mm Hg

607. Cilastozol A/E:

(a) PDE5 inhibitor
(b) Quinolone derivative
(c) Proven mortality benefit in PVD
(d) ↓es restenosis in stent

608. Child fever > 5 days all *except* for Kawasaki disease:

(a) Bilateral conjunctional injection
(b) Strawberry tongue

(c) Cervical LAP
(d) Oliguria

609. Maximum blood volume in pregnancy:
(a) Term pregnancy (b) 12–14 weeks
(c) 24–27 weeks (d) 32–34 weeks

610. CHADS2 A/E:
(a) Female gender (b) DM
(c) Recent CHF (d) HTN

611. Osteogenesis imperfecta A/E:
(a) Produced by collagen type III disorder
(b) AR
(c) Minimal trauma causes fracture
(d) Scoliosis > 50%

612. Angiotensinogen → Ang I:
(a) Renal renin (b) ACE
(c) Tissue kinase (d) Chymase

613. Following are the true statements regarding hyperthyroidism *except*:
(a) Is commonly seen in elderly
(b) Is commonly associated with bradycardia
(c) Is associated with atrial fibrillation
(d) Could be one of the cause of unexplained heart failure

614. Following is the typical cardiac manifestation of lyme disease:
(a) Fluctuating AV block
(b) Inappropriate sinus tachycardia
(c) Ventricular tachycardia
(d) Supraventricular tachycardia

615. Following cardiac lesion is typically seen in ankylosing spondolytis:
(a) Aortic stenosis (b) Aortic regurgitation
(c) Mitral stenosis (d) Mitral regurgitation

616. Which of the following anti arrhythmic drug can cause lupus erythematous like syndrome?
(a) Amlodarone (b) Fleicanide
(c) Procainamide (d) Mexilltine

617. Pregnancy changes: (T/F)
(a) SVR increases (b) CO increases
(c) SV increases (d) HR increases
(e) HTN increases

618. T/F:
(a) Multiple myeloma—hyperviscosity
(b) Amyloidosis most common in kappa
(c) Osteosclerotic changes in IgG
(d) β2 M-prognosis good
(e) Melphalan/prednisolone treatment

619. AKI in CIN: (T/F)
(a) Increases in 0.3 mg% creatinine in 24-48 hours
(b) Decrease renal output 0.5 ml/kg/hour for 6 hours
(c) Fraction excretion of Na > 1

620. T/F:
(a) Kidney–20% cardiac output
(b) 20% filtered by bowman capsule
(c) 30% water absorbed in PCT
(d) Macula densa–tubulaglomerular feedback

621. CHD: (T/F)
(a) Hyperviscosity increases iron deficiency
(b) Lipomatous hypertrophy of inter atrial septum lead to AV conduction defect

622. Syncope: (T/F)
(a) After strenous exercise–neurocardiogenic
(b) During exercise–cardiac cause
(c) NTG is relative contraindication in HUTT
(d) Long term recurrent syncope suggestive of cardiac cause
(e) > 50 mm Hg decreases in SBP hypersensitive carotid sinus

623. True or false:
(a) Mediterranean diet–good compliance
(b) Almond contain PUFA
(c) Fast food–trans fatty acids
(d) Omega 3 fatty acids decreases LDL

624. Takayasu arteritis: (T/F)
(a) Lt SCA– 90%
(b) Pulmoanary Artery–50%
(c) HTN in India > Japan
(d) Aneurysm is not a feature
(e) 2nd/3rd decade most common

625. Rhabdomyoma: (T/F)

(a) Associated with tuberous sclerosis
(b) More common in male
(c) Atria more common
(d) Regression below 6 years
(e) 80% cases in < 1 year

626. Endomyocardial fibrosis: (T/F)

(a) LV involvement > 80%
(b) Associated with eosinophilia
(c) Middle age and elderly
(d) Diagnostic–apex obliteration
(e) Systolic function preserved

627. Mediterranean diet: (T/F)

(a) Only fat source–sunflower oil
(b) Red meat and eggs allowed
(c) Moderate wine allowed
(d) Poor compliance
(e) Contains 35-40% calories fat

628. Contrast nephropathy: (T/F)

(a) Duration of procedure
(b) Dose of contrast
(c) DM
(d) LV dysfunction
(e) No. of vessels with > 70% stenosis

629. Pregnancy physiological changes: (T/F)

(a) Plasma volume ↑ since 10 weeks
(b) Plateau in 2 trimester
(c) ↑ CO upto 30-50% in 2nd trimester
(d) ↓ VR immediately after birth
(e) Diastolic murmur is abnormal

630. Metabolic syndrome: (T/F)

(a) Waist circumference in men < 100 cm
(b) TG=145 mg%
(c) BP–140/90
(d) HDL in female=45 mg%
(e) Fasting glucose=115 mg%

631. BP: (T/F)

(a) Sibutramine ↓ses BP
(b) Alcohol withdrawal ↑ses BP
(c) Cyclosporin ↓ses BP
(d) EPO ↑ses BP
(e) Licorice ↑ HTN

632. Pregnancy: (T/F)

(a) HR ↑ses 20%
(b) Systemic and pulmonary pressure ↓ses
(c) Venous pressure in lower limb ↓ses
(d) Eisenmenger death–50%

633. Myxoma: (T/F)

(a) Carney's complex–Autosomal recessive
(b) Carney's–Most common in males
(c) Carney's recurrence–10%
(d) Fibroelastoma–aortic valve
(e) Fibroma–IVS and LV

634. JNV VIII: (T/F)

(a) Grade I–164/84
(b) DM–Goal–130/94
(c) PreHTN–130/94
(d) Normal BP life style modification–no role

635. Preoperative Non cardiac Surgery: (T/F)

(a) Aortic surgery is high risk in young
(b) Severe AS is high risk surgery
(c) AF is low risk
(d) Prior LBBB–at always high risk
(e) Regional anesthesia ↑ses L–R shunt

636. T/F:

(a) Smoking ↑ses hs CRP
(b) Statin ↓ses fibrinogen
(c) Thiazolidiones ↓ses hs CRP
(d) Fenofibrate ↑ses homocysteine level
(e) Hs CRP is better than LDL for atherosclerotic CAD

637. T/F:

(a) Inflammation has role in CHF
(b) Inflammation has role in stroke
(c) TLC S/O CAD risk
(d) Estrogen ↑ CRP
(e) HRT ↓ses fibrinogen

638. T/F:

(a) Psychiatric illness in mother–dysplastic PS
(b) DM in mother–CCTGA

(c) DM in mother–d TGA
(d) Epilepsy in mother–IAA
(e) Hb > 16 gm% in CHD mother–live birth 70%
(f) Eisenmenger–50% mortality
(g) Lupus in mother–d-TGA

639. CIN: (T/F)
(a) Patient requiring dialysis–24 hours mortality is high
(b) Anemia ↑ ses risk of CIN
(c) Low osmolar agents have osmolarity < plasma
(d) Antithrombotic effect is more in low osmolar agents
(e) Non ionic low osmolar–does not cause hypocalcemia

640. Metabolic syndrome: (T/F)
(a) Fasting glucose > 100 mg%
(b) Diastolic BP > 90 mm Hg
(c) Asian women > 88 cm
(d) TG> 175 mg%
(e) HDL < 45 mg%

641. Hypertensive emergencies: (T/F)
(a) Hyperadrenergic states–nitroprusside
(b) Post renal transplant–CCB
(c) Accelerated HTN–retinal exudates and haemorrhage
(d) Malignant hypertension–papilledema
(e) Labetalol in liver failure

642. Hypertensive emergencies: (T/F)
(a) CCB in Raynaud phenomenon
(b) ARB in pregnancy
(c) CCB in ARF
(d) HTN with osteoporosis–thiazides

643. Renal dysfunction: (T/F)
(a) 30-60 ml/min–moderate renal failure
(b) < 15 ml/min–end stage renal failure
(c) PCI is not beneficial as medical treatment
(d) Mild increase in creatinine in hypotension need ACE- I
(e) Even mild renal dysfunction increases mortality

644. Pheochromocytoma: (T/F)
(a) Causes MI (b) HOCM
(c) DCMP (d) SCD

645. Polygenic and monogenic: (T/F)
(a) Hyperlipidemia–polygenic
(b) Marfan's syndrome–polygenic
(c) Polygenic present in mid late life
(d) HOCM–polygenic
(e) LQTS3–polygenic

646. Tumour heart: (T/F)
(a) Melanoma has high likelihood for cardiac metastasis
(b) Osteosarcoma has cardiac metastasis
(c) Myxoma arises from endocardium
(d) IL-6–constitutional symptoms
(e) RCC can present as mass in IVC

647. Hypertension: (T/F)
(a) Raynaud phenomenon–CCB
(b) Osteoporosis–thiazides
(c) Hepatic disease–labetalol
(d) Pregnancy–ARB
(e) Cyclosporine induced HTN–CCB

648. CIN: (T/F)
(a) Typically occurs immediately after procedure and early peaking of creatinine
(b) Almost complete recovery within 1 week
(c) Direct toxicity of contrast or vasoconstriction
(d) Urine–active sediments with granular cast
(e) Sometimes may require HD

649. Carney complex: (T/F)
(a) Multicentric in heart
(b) Endocrine involvement
(c) Lentigenes
(d) Cardiac and mucocutaneous myxoma
(e) Cushings
(f) All are true

650. DMD: (T/F)
(a) ↑ R in V1
(b) Q-long and deep in II, III, AVF
(c) MR is common in late stages
(d) Extensive septal fibrosis
(e) Primary ventricular arrhythmia common

651. Muscular Dystrophy: (T/F)
(a) CHB common
(b) SVT uncommon
(c) Arrhythmia causes death in 1/3th cases
(d) Barth syndrome is isolated noncompaction
(e) F. ataxia CMP and severe arrhythmia

652. Marfan: (T/F)
(a) Malar hypoplasia
(b) Arm span < 150% of ht.
(c) Pes planus
(d) Pectus carinatum
(e) Wrist/thums sign +ve

653. Cardiac syndrome X: (T/F)
(a) Cardiac syndrome X and metabolic syndrome are synonymous
(b) More common in males
(c) Subendocardial ischemia is cause
(d) Can be presence of perfusion defect
(e) Doesn't affect prognosis in comparison to N population
(f) Half cases show coronary flow abnormality

654. Trial's of ACE-I: (T/F)
(a) AIRE
(b) Consensus
(c) ISIS-I
(d) MADIT
(e) V- HEFT

655. Atrial myxoma: (T/F)
(a) Familial preponderance
(b) Histological diagnosis by emboli
(c) Tumour plop in systole
(d) Arises from posterior wall
(e) MR and TR

656. Renovascular HTN: (T/F)
(a) Aortoarteritis involves distal third of renal artery
(b) Atherosclerosis proximal third of renal artery
(c) FMD most common in elderly female
(d) FMD distal 2/3rd
(e) Atherosclerosis > 50%

657. Physiological changes in pregnancy: (T/F)
(a) Blood volume increased at least by 50%
(b) Max. CO by mid second trimester
(c) Max. decrease in peripheral resistance in first trimester
(d) Increased CO in third trimester because of increased SV and HR
(e) CO increased by 30-50%

658. DASH diet: (T/F)
(a) Rich in vegetables and fruit
(b) Rich in potassium and calcium
(c) Milk and egg only animal product included
(d) Decreases BP by 4–6 mm Hg
(e) 1600 mg Na reduction = 1 antihypertensive drug

659. Cocaine related to: (T/F)
(a) Acute myocarditis
(b) Sudden severe hypotension
(c) Acute MI
(d) Ventricular tachyarrhythmias
(e) Dissection of aorta

660. Major criteria of Marfan's syndrome: (T/F)
(a) Dural ectasia
(b) Positive family history in first degree relatives
(c) MVP
(d) High arched palate
(e) Tall and thin habitus

661. Metabolic syndrome: (T/F)
(a) Waist circumference > 35 inches in males
(b) HDL < 40 mg% in males
(c) TG > 200 mg%
(d) FBS > 120 mg%
(e) ≥ 130/85 mm Hg

662. Mediterranean diet: (T/F)
(a) 35-40% of fat allowed
(b) Red meat and egg allowed
(c) Moderate quantity of red wine allowed
(d) Poor compliance
(e) Sunflower oil source of cholesterol

663. True or false:
(a) Coconut is a rich source of cholesterol
(b) Olive oil–MUFA
(c) Nuts–PUFA
(d) All transfatty acids harmful
(e) Increase in dietary cholesterol causes hepatic cholesterol synthesis

664. T/F:
(a) Plant sterol and stanol compete with cholesterol for absorption
(b) Excess plant sterol causes fat malabsorption
(c) High absorption occur in excess
(d) High cholesterol absorption decreases LDL production

665. Obesity: (T/F)
(a) QT prolongation
(b) Increase CO and blood volume to suuply increase adipose tissue
(c) Causes concentric LVH with diastolic dysfunction

(d) Marked obesity have more LV systolic dysfunction
(e) Diastolic dysfunction is more important

666. Pregnancy contraindicated in: (T/F)
(a) Eisenmenger's syndrome
(b) Moderate PAH
(c) Moderate MR with normal LV function
(d) Mafan's syndrome with normal aortic root
(e) Uncorrected TOF

667. Changes in pregnancy: (T/F)
(a) CO and blood volume increases as early as 5 weeks
(b) In twin pregnancy CO increases by 30%
(c) Stroke volume starts increasing by 8 weeks
(d) Postpartum HR increases upto second stage and then decreases by 10 days
(e) CO reverted to preterm levels by 10-30 days

668. HIV: (T/F)
(a) Acute pericarditis
(b) CCP
(c) Myxoma
(d) Chronic pericardial effusion
(e) Lymphoma

669. APLA: (T/F)
(a) Arterial thrombosis
(b) Thrombocytosis
(c) Infectious disease
(d) Recurrent abortions
(e) Livedoreticularis

670. T/F:
(a) Persistent handgrip decreases HR
(b) Valsalva phase II associated with increased LV volume
(c) Squatting decreases LV volume
(d) Squatting decreases BP
(e) Amyl nitrate initiation decreases LV volume

671. Hyperhomocysteinemia: (T/F)
(a) Increased CRF
(b) Hyperthyroidism
(c) APLA
(d) Chronic barbiturate therapy
(e) Psoriasis

672. Cardiac trauma: (T/F)
(a) RA rupture most common seen
(b) Mitral valve rupture most common
(c) Aortic valve rupture most common
(d) Blow to LVOT during diastole causes mitral valve rupture
(e) Ascending aorta trauma most common

673. Thyrotoxicosis: (T/F)
(a) Means Lerman scratch is characteristic
(b) Sinus tachycardia is less in young as compared to adults
(c) Amiodarone causes it
(d) CHF resistant to cardiac glycoside
(e) Persistent AF < 5%

674. Thiazide diuretics: (T/F)
(a) ↑ LDL and TG
(b) Effective on GFR < 20 ml/min
(c) Acts on DCT
(d) Ethachrynic and spironolactone are non sulphur drugs
(e) Triamterene acts on DCT and CT as Na exchanger

675. Marfan's syndrome: (T/F)
(a) Dural ectasia–major criteria
(b) Aortic dissection distal to SCA
(c) Valsalva aneurysm since birth
(d) MR in children and AR in adults
(e) Elastin gene mutation

676. Radiation damage: (T/F)
(a) Coronary vasospasm
(b) MR
(c) CCP
(d) Atherosclerosis
(e) HOCM

677. Atheroembolism: (T/F)
(a) Distal pulses absent in LL in 70%
(b) Usually from aorta
(c) Livedo reticularis seen in 50% of cases
(d) Depends on plaque size

678. Heparin: (T/F)
(a) LMWH mol. wt. 4000-6000
(b) LMWH inhibits platelets more than heparin
(c) LMWH excretion by liver
(d) LMWH more protein binding
(e) LMWH has less anti IIa activity than UFH
(f) LMWH no effect on platelets

679. HIT: (T/F)

(a) Incidence–5%
(b) HIT incidence more with bovine heparin
(c) Thrombocytopenia improves within 2-3 weeks
(d) Thrombus seen in artery
(e) Diagnosed by fragmantation test

680. True or false:

(a) Factor V leiden mutation in 15%
(b) Antithrombin III deficiency autosomal dominant
(c) Protein C is cofactor for protein S
(d) Protein C deficiency due to factor V leiden mutation
(e) Protein C or protein S deficiency–single gene mutation

681. True or false:

(a) Coconut oil–linolenic acid
(b) Olive oil–oleic acid
(c) Linolenic and linoleic acid are essential fatty acids
(d) A step II recommends cholesterol < 100 mg/day

682. Myxoma:

(a) Chance of recurrence after excision is 10%
(b) Arises from posterior wall
(c) Can lead to mitral valve destruction
(d) Systemic effect can cause clubbing
(e) Leimyosarcoma aparts from myxoma is most common

683. HIV:

(a) Can cause lymphoma
(b) Decreases atherosclerosis
(c) Pulmonary HTN
(d) Myopericarditis
(e) Marantic endocarditis

684. JNC-VII: (T/F)

(a) ARB are first line drug
(b) Upto stage III
(c) In renal failure target is 140/80 mm Hg
(d) Old age systolic HTN is important as diastolic HTN
(e) Microalbuminuria major risk factor

685. SCN 5A mutation causes:

(a) Familial AF
(b) Short QT syndrome
(c) Progressive conduction defect
(d) Sinus node disease

686. HTN true:

(a) Dietary modification in pre-HTN

687. Diastolic HTN common in:

(a) Young age (b) Middle age
(c) > 55 years (d) Children

688. Red wine contain:

(a) Arginine (b) Berberine
(c) Resveratrol

689. Both renal and hepatic metabolism:

(a) Azathioprine (b) Digoxin
(c) Flecainide (d) 6-MP

690. Pregnant lady with ACE-I:

(a) Coronary dissection
(b) APLA
(c) Paradoxical Embolism
(d) Vasculitis

691. In pregnancy all are normal *except:*

(a) Diastolic murmur (b) Raised JVP
(c) Loud S2 (d) LV S3
(e) Continuous murmur

692. Renin levels ↓ed by:

(a) Aliskiren (b) Metoprolol
(c) Ramipril (d) Hydrochlorthiazide

693. HTN–Na restriction not required in:

(a) Pheochromocytoma
(b) Primary HT–essential HT
(c) Conn's syndrome
(d) COA

694. C/I in pregnancy:

(a) Bosentan (b) Epoprostenal
(c) Nifedipine (d) Sildenafil

695. Most common cause of syncope:

(a) Cardiac (b) Neurogenic
(c) Vascular (d) Metabolic

696. Warfarin acts by ↓sing:

(a) II (b) VII
(c) I (d) XI

697. **HTN with COA in pregnancy:**
(a) Cardiac cath, ECG, Doppler echo
(b) ECG, echo, Doppler MRI
(c) CXR, ECG, Doppler, MRI
(d) ECG, Doppler CT angio

698. **Most common tumour in infant cardiac:**
(a) Rhabdomyoma (b) Myxoma
(c) Fibroma (d) Lipoma

699. **Pregnancy normal hemodynamics:**
(a) Raised SVR
(b) Raised CO
(c) Regurgitation less tolerated
(d) LA pressure increase to maximum in third trimester

700. **Pregnancy C/I:**
(a) PHT (b) AR
(c) MR (d) ASD

701. **INR-3.5 Post MVR Patient develop new onset AF started on amiodarone:**
(a) ↓ Warfarin dose (b) ↓ Warfarin dose
(c) ↓ Amiodarone dose (d) Nothing

702. **Amyloidosis true is A/E:**
(a) Biventricular dilatation common
(b) Present with RCM commonly
(c) Low voltage complexes on ECG
(d) Abnormal fat pad aspirate is best diagnosis

703. **Amyloidosis true A/E:**
(a) Secondary Amyloid is AA
(b) TTAR amyloid is most common in Alzheimer disease
(c) Skin manifestation more common in primary amyloidosis
(d) Carpal Tunnel syndrome can occur in many types of amyloidosis

704. **AD A/E:**
(a) Friedreich ataxia (b) Von-Recklinghausen
(c) Tuberous sclerosis (d) AIP

705. **Calcification in cardiac mass:**
(a) Myxoma
(b) Fibroma
(c) Rhabdomyoma
(d) Papillary fibroblastoma

706. **Prodrug:**
(a) Enalaprilat (b) Lisnopril
(c) Ramipril (d) Captopril

707. **True about hemodynamic changes in pregnancy A/E:**
(a) ↑ venous pressure in legs
(b) HR ↑ 10-20%
(c) Blood volume ↑ 40%
(d) Pulm. Vascular resistance ↑ 10-20%

708. **Worst prognosis:**
(a) Giant cell myocarditis
(b) EBV myocarditis
(c) HIV myocarditis
(d) Lyme's myocarditis

709. **Most common cause of metastasis to heart:**
(a) Ca Breast
(b) Lymphoma
(c) Malignant melanoma
(d) Osteosarcoma

710. **Masked HTN:**
(a) Clinical BP lower than home BP
(b) Clinical BP higher than home BP
(c) HTN due to coarctation of aorta
(d) HTN with Acute LVF

711. **Papillary fibroelastoma A/E:**
(a) Commonly single
(b) Commonly young age
(c) Most common involved aortic valve
(d) Commonly presents with embolic phenomenon

712. **Noncardiac surgery with high risk for cardiac events A/E:**
(a) Renal dysfunction
(b) LVEF–40%
(c) Age > 75 years
(d) Pancreatoduodenectomy

713. **Pregnancy change in CVS A/E:**
(a) ↑ Pulmonary vascular resistance
(b) ↓ BP
(c) ↑ 50% blood volume
(d) ↑ HR by 10-20%

714. Risk peripartum cardiomyopathy A/E:

(a) Multiparity (b) Preeclampsia

(c) Black Race (d) Young age

715. Blue sclera is associated:

(a) AV block (b) AR

(c) HOCM

716. Hypocalcemia causes:

(a) Prolonged PR (b) Prolonged ST

(c) ST depression (d) Atrial stand still

717. Myasthenia gravis True A/E:

(a) 15% thymoma

(b) Pre-synaptic Ach receptors antibody

(c) Autoimmune disease

(d) Anti-musk positive in anti-Ach R and negative in bulbar myasthenia

718. High risk pregnancy is A/E:

(a) Critical AS

(b) Eisenmenger syndrome

(c) Marfan syndrome

(d) TGA with atrial switch done

719. Commotio cordis causes death by VF due to sport injury. The critical period during which injury occur is:

(a) QRS

(b) P wave

(c) Ascending limb of T wave

(d) TP segment

720. Takayasu arteritis is an:

(a) Aorto arterial occlusive disease

(b) Aorto arterial connective tissue disease

(c) Aorto arterial atherosclerotic

(d) Aorto arterial sporadic

721. 65 years old elderly male with BP=160/90 mm Hg and no other comorbidities, which of the following is the anti-hypertensive of choice?

(a) Amlodipine (b) Atenolol

(c) α blocker (d) ACE-I

722. Dalteparin, enoxaparin are:

(a) LMWH (b) DTI

(c) GP IIb IIIa inhibitor

723. Orthostatic hypotension indicates fall in:

(a) 5 mm Hg of systolic BP

(b) 10 mm Hg of systolic BP

(c) 20 mm Hg of systolic BP

(d) 20 mm Hg of diastolic BP

724. Familial myxoma A/E:

(a) No gender predilection

(b) LA most common site

(c) Recurrence after surgery

(d) Similar histology

725. Diuretics in treatment of HTN in elderly A/E:

(a) Cause lipid abnormalities

(b) Cause less electrolyte abnormal than in treatment of CHF

(c) Loop diuretics preferred

(d) ACEI TOC in < 50 years age

726. Secondary HTN suggested by A/E:

(a) Onset < 20 or > 50 years age

(b) Failure to respond to > 2 days

(c) Strong family history of HTN

(d) Recurrent flash pulm edema

727. ACE I A/E:

(a) Should not be given to patients with MI and CRF

(b) Prevents remodelling

(c) Should be started as early in MI

(d) ↑ Survival after MI

728. Long standing HTN risk factor A/E:

(a) CAD (b) Stroke

(c) PVD (d) Diastolic HF

729. Evaluation of syncope A/E:

(a) HUTT (b) Loop recorder

(c) Holter (d) Nuclear imaging

730. Regarding long standing HT true is:

(a) ACEI are drug of choice in age < 55 years

(b) It is a strong risk factor for ICH

(c) Diuretics are not effective in old age

(d) In DM the target BP 140/85 mm Hg (Nephropathy)

731. NAC best used for:

(a) To prevent CIN in high risk patient

(b) CCF with hypervolumia

(c) CRF

(d) To treat CIN
(e) To prevent acute renal shut down

732. BP cuff width:
(a) 40% of arm circumference
(b) 80% of arm diameter
(c) 1/3rd of diameter
(d) 2/3rd of covered arm

733. Fever + cardiovascular collapse + hypoperfusion +generalized edema:
(a) Water syndrome
(b) SIRs
(c) Conn's syndrome
(d) Adrenal haemorrhage syndrome
(e) Hepatorenal syndrome

734. Neonatal hypoglycemia:
(a) 100 g/dl (b) 80
(c) 60 (d) 40
(e) 20

735. 5 days child with strawberry tongue, conjunctival congestion, edema and aneurysm of coronary on echo:
(a) Kawasaki disease (b) Sjögren disease
(c) PAN (d) Takayasu arteritis

736. Antihypertensive not effective as monotherapy in blacks:
(a) CCB (b) Diuretic
(c) α blockers (d) Beta blocker

737. Heart muscle uses at rest:
(a) FFA (b) Glucose
(c) Ketones

738. B blocker decreasing manifestation of metabolic syndrome:
(a) Bisoprolol (b) Carvedilol
(c) Metoprolol (d) Nebivolol

739. Metabolic syndrome A/E:
(a) Insulin resistance (b) Obesity
(c) Normal or ↑ HDL (d) HTN

740. Acute corpulmonale A/E:
(a) S1Q3T3
(b) 'T' prominent in V1-V4
(c) RAD
(d) Poor progression of 'R' wave

741. Radiation A/E:
(a) Lead apron should be > 5 mm
(b) 150 time more exposure with CAG compared to X-ray chest
(c) Anyone with fluoroscopy > 60 mins should be counselled for radiation
(d) Most lesion are above upper back and infraaxillary

742. Radiation true is:
(a) Fluoroscopy more radiation > angio (cine)
(b) Biplane associated with less exposure
(c) Permissible limit 3 REM for 3 months
(d) Oblique view has least exposure

743. ARDS with direct injuring A/E:
(a) CPB
(b) Pneumonia
(c) Aspiration of gastric contents
(d) Contusion

744. True about cardiac tumours:
(a) Most common primary lymphoma
(b) Metastatic tumors are more common than primary
(c) Most common malignant is leiomyosarcoma
(d) Rhabdomyosarcoma has a good prognosis

745. Heparin S/E all *except:*
(a) Alopecia (b) Osteoporosis
(c) Hyperaldosteronism (d) Rash

746. Marfan syndrome seen:
(a) MVP (b) MS
(c) AS (d) HOCM

747. Pregnancy worst outcome:
(a) PPH (b) Ostium secundum AD
(c) COA (d) MR

748. Beta blocker may improve some feature of metabolic syndrome:
(a) Bisoprolol (b) Carvedilol
(c) Nebivolol (d) Metoprolol

749. Fabry disease true *except:*
(a) Deficiency α-galatoside A

(b) AR
(c) ↓ LV thickening
(d) LVH

750. Most common cardiac tumour in infancy:
(a) Rhabdomyoma (b) Myxoma
(c) Fibroma

751. True about cardiac tumour is:
(a) Rhabdomyosarcoma has good prognosis
(b) Metastatic malignant tumour > primary
(c) Lymphomas most common primary tumour

752. All proven to ↓ contrast nephropathy *except:*
(a) NAC (b) Statin
(c) Ascorbic acid (d) PGE-2

753. Least common is amyloidosis:
(a) RCM (b) CCP
(c) Systolic dysfunction

754. About radiation true is all *except:*
(a) Thickness of lead apron is 5 mm
(b) Patient subjected to fluoroscopy > 60 min should be counseled about long term radiation toxicity
(c) PCI causes 150 time than exposure of X-ray
(d) Radiation injury most common upper back and axilla

755. HTN crisis true all *except:*
(a) Azotemia and proteinuria
(b) Normal mental status
(c) Microangiopathic hemolytic anemia
(d) Retinal haemorrhage

756. Drug interaction with potential toxicity A/E:
(a) Simvastatin and erythromycin
(b) Pravastatin and ketoconazole
(c) Digoxin and verapamil
(d) Sildenafil and nitrates

757. Digoxin concentration:
(a) Increased by verapamil
(b) Increased by cyclosporine
(c) Decreased by quinidine
(d) Increased by rifampicin

758. Pregnancy C/I in A/E:
(a) Eisenmenger
(b) MVP with severe MR
(c) Asymptomatic severe AS
(d) Marfan's with aortic root of 45 mm without AR

759. Thiazide all true *except:*
(a) Hypouricemia
(b) Hypercalcemia
(c) Hypercholesterolemia
(d) Decreased wall thickness

760. Radiation causes A/E:
(a) Pericarditis (b) Valvular stenosis
(c) Conduction defect (d) ASH

761. Regarding blood pressure measurement true is:
(a) In children diastolic pressure is recorded at korotkoff phase IV
(b) Auscultatory gap is between phase II and III
(c) Sounds become crisp and increase in intensity in phase II
(d) Good correlation in arm BP between direct and indirect

762. Metabolized in liver A/E:
(a) Adenosine (b) Digoxin
(c) Polypill (d) Amiodarone

763. Obesity – maximum increase seen in:
(a) Chylomicrons (b) LDL
(c) VLDL (d) HDL

764. Poorest prognosis in pregnancy:
(a) PPH (b) MS
(c) AS

765. Normal physiologic changes during pregnancy include:
(a) Fall in systemic blood pressure occurs predominantly during the last trimester
(b) Increase in cardiac output predominantly occurs due to increase in stroke volume which occurs during last trimester
(c) Pulmonary artery systolic and diastolic pressures remain normal
(d) Physiological anaemia during pregnancy reduces the placental perfusion

766. All of the following statements are true for cardiac amyloidosis *except:*

(a) Atrial septal thickening on echocardiography is a specific finding
(b) Diltiazem is useful for improving diastolic dysfunction
(c) Hypertension is an unusual finding
(d) Low-voltage complexes are seen in the limb leads of ECG

767. A 50-year-old male was recently started on anti-hypertensive therapy with multiple drugs. He reported 3 months later with skin lesions diagnosed as psoriasis. Which drug is most likely responsible?
(a) Atenolol (b) Amlodipine
(c) Olmesartan (d) Spironolactone

768. All are true about management of hypertension in black patients *except:*
(a) Multiple drug combinations are often required
(b) ACE inhibitors are less effective
(c) Thiazide diuretics have high BP lowering efficacy
(d) Sinificantly low incidence of angioedema with ACE inhibitors

769. Rare finding in preeclampsia:
(a) Left ventricular hypertrophy
(b) Proteinuria
(c) Elevated plasma uric acid
(d) Sudden weight gain

770. Clinical characteristics of hypertensive crisis:
(a) Diastolic BP > 140 mm of Hg
(b) Congestive heart failure
(c) Microangiopathic hemolysis
(d) All of the above

771. Coconut oil contains:
(a) Saturated fatty acids
(b) Monounsaturated fatty acids
(c) Polyunsaturated fatty acids
(d) Trans fatty acids

772. Hypertensive retinopathy is a feature of:
(a) Coarctation of aorta
(b) Takayasu arteritis
(c) HOCM
(d) MVP

773. Carcinoid heart disease manifest as:
(a) Tricuspid regurgitation
(b) Pulmonic stenosis
(c) Both of the above
(d) None of the above

774. Cocaine causes:
(a) Myocardial infarction (b) Arrhythmias
(c) Aortic dissection (d) All of the above

775. Papillary fibroelastoma occurs on:
(a) Heart valves (b) Inter atrial septum
(c) Atrium (d) Ventricle

776. Electrical injury produces:
(a) QT prolongation
(b) Atrial fibrillation
(c) Ventricular fibrillation
(d) All of the above

777. Hemodynamic changes during pregnancy:
(a) Heart rate increases
(b) Blood volume increases
(c) Pulmonary vascular resistance decreases
(d) All of the above

778. False statement about cardiovascular effects of hypothyroidism:
(a) Systemic vascular resistance decreases
(b) Heart rate decreases
(c) Cardiac output decreases
(d) Blood volume decreases

779. (PCWP) in RHC–True:
(a) At wedge, Mean art. pr. suddenly falls
(b) In left pneumonitis, catheter in left PA SpO_2 < 95% always
(c) Swan Ganz catheter in wedge position–high top excursions
(d) 'a' and 'v' waves of PCWP, Rag behind v

780. Peritoneal dialysis–A/E:
(a) Hypoglycemia (b) Hyperglycemia
(c) Weight gain (d) Peritonitis

781. Hyperprolactinemia–A/E:
(a) Hypoglycemia (b) Hyperglycemia
(c) Weight gain (d) Peritonitis

782. Counter regulatory mech. of hypoglycemia:
(a) Decrease glucagon (b) Increase insulin
(c) Increase epinephrine (d) Decrease cortisol

783. DVT–best initial IOC:
(a) D-dimer (b) MR venography
(c) Compressive USG (d) Invasive venography

784. **Rheumatic fever age 8 years secondary pro-phylaxis:**
(a) Not years
(b) Life long
(c) 5 years to 18 years whichever is long
(d) 10 years to 70 years whichever is long

785. **Rheumatic fever most common:**
(a) Polyarthritis (b) Carditis
(c) Chorea (d) Erythema marginatum

786. **8 years child post ARF incidence of carditis:**
(a) 50% (b) 30%
(c) 80% (d) 90%

787. **Downward ectopia lentis + aortic dissection:**
(a) Marfan syndrome
(b) Homocysteinemia with early CAD
(c) Osteogenesis imperfecta

788. **Cocaine can cause, all *except*:**
(a) Postural hypotension
(b) MR
(c) Aortic dissection
(d) CHB

789. **↑ murmur of HOCM by:**
(a) Isometric hand grip (b) Amyl nitrate
(c) Squating (d) β-blocker

790. **Paradoxical split, all *except:***
(a) DCMP (b) VSD
(c) PDA (d) Aortic stenosis

791. **Most specific for HCM:**
(a) SAM
(b) LV thickness > 14 mm
(c) LVOT gradient 30 mm Hg at rest and 50 mm Hg with exercise
(d) Brockenborgh–Brauwald phenomenon

792. **Stress induced MI/apical ballooning syndrome, true all *except*:**
(a) Most common in young Asian females
(b) Inotropes C/I
(c) Recovery in 1-2 months

793. **Can cause pulmonary HTN:**
(a) Schistosomiasis (b) Ascaris

794. **HIT:**
(a) Susceptibility after 4 days of heparin use
(b) Venous thrombosis more common than arterial
(c) More common in medical than surgical patients

795. **Incorrectly mentioned:**
(a) DABIGATRAN–RELY
(b) AVEROSS–edoxasan
(c) ARISTOTLE–APIXABAN
(d) ROCKET AF–RIVOROXABAN

796. **CHAS, VAS score 1, when risk of stroke is about zero:**
(a) 0 (b) 1
(c) 2 (d) 3

797. **Most cost effective investigation for screening and prognosis in PAD:**
(a) Duplex USG (b) ABI
(c) CT (d) MRI/Angio

798. **1% reduction in LDC, decrease in event late by:**
(a) 10% (b) 3%
(c) 1% (d) 2%

799. **Which of the following have equal efficiency in AF RHD as compared to warfarin?**
(a) Dabigatran (b) Apixaban
(c) Rivoroxaban (d) None

800. **CACS scoring in asymptomatic patient for prognosis:**
(a) I (b) IIa
(c) IIb (d) III

801. **60 years old male with exertional syncope not common:**
(a) LQT (b) HOCM
(c) Coronary anomaly (d) CAD

802. **Cardiac disease without any symptoms, stage:**
(a) A (b) B
(c) C (d) D

803. **False statement regarding RHD:**
(a) Macrolide can be used for prophylaxis when penicillin C/I
(b) Infective endocarditis prophylaxis not indicted for procedure like GI endoscopy
(c) Lifelong prophylaxis after valve replacement

804. **Athletic heart vs HOCM can be differentiated by, all *except*:**
(a) Bizarre ECG
(b) LV septal thickness < 18 mm

(c) LV cavity < 45 mm
(d) Late gadolinium enhancement

805. Safe in cirrhosis:
(a) Lisinopril (b) Captopril
(c) Losartan (d) Enalapril

806. In elderly which is not seen normally?
(a) Orthostatic hypotension
(b) S4
(c) ↑ pulse pressure
(d) Murmur of aortic stenosis can be heard

807. SPRINT trial correct statement:
(a) Azilsartan used in intensive arm
(b) Similar outcome in intensive and control arm
(c) Major complications same in both arm
(d) GFR increased in intensive arm

808. Methemoglobinemia in all *except*:
(a) Furosemide (b) Cocaine
(c) Lidocaine (d) Dapsone

809. Secondary HTN all *except*:
(a) Acromegaly–increase renin
(b) Liddle syndrome–AD with amiloride sensitive channel
(c) Congenital adrenal hyperplasia–deoxycortisone effects of mineralocorticosteroids
(d) Renovascular HTN may be due to obstruction at any level

810. Decreased radiation exposure by:
(a) Cineangiography in place of fluoroscopy
(b) Increasing framecount rate
(c) Closer image intensified to patient
(d) Using magnifying image

811. Most reliable sign of return of spontaneous circulation (ROSC):
(a) Palpable pulse (b) Sinus rhythm
(c) ET CO_2 > 35 (d) SpO_2 >94%

812. Contrast anaphylaxis can be prevented by, all *except*:
(a) H_2 blocker (b) H_1 blocker
(c) NAC (d) Dexamethasone

813. Which is incorrect?
(a) NF–RAS
(b) Marfan–abdominal aortic aneurysm
(c) Tuberoeruptive–type II
(d) Adenoma sebaceum rhabdomyoma

814. All are minor criteria for rheumatic fever according to Recent guidelines in Indian scenario *except*:
(a) ESR > 60 (b) Fever
(c) Polyarthralgia (d) 1° AV block

815. HIT all *except*:
(a) Platelet transfusion
(b) Antibody against PF-4
(c) Thrombocytopenia with paradoxical thrombosis
(d) Early HIT better prognosis

816. Renal artery stenosis seen in:
(a) NF (b) Refsum's
(c) Turner syndrome (d) Marfan's

817. Female, 42 years, with sudden onset dyspnea, BP 90 mm Hg Abg - Ph - 7.48 PO_2 55, PCO_2 - 38, HCO_3 -16 investigation:
(a) Pulmonary CT angio (b) Coronary angio
(c) Trop I (d) Echo

818. Greatest probability for metastasis to heart:
(a) Melanoma (b) Breast
(c) Lung (d) Ovary

819. 45-year-old female, with pregnancy, Echo normal, BP normal, next investigation:
(a) EPS (b) Angiography
(c) Pacemaker (d) Head tilt test

820. 22-year-old male, with exercise text had following BIs (2 CPVT), all *except*:
(a) Risk of SCD
(b) Due to coronary spasm
(c) Echo revealed N heart

821. 14-year-old child:
(a) A-S (b) Supracarinal VSD
(c) Valvular PS

822. Which is seen?
(a) Bistenius pulse
(b) Ejection click
(c) ESM increased on standing

823. Which of the following drug is renin inhibitor?
(a) Ivabradine (b) Eplerenone
(c) Aliskiren (d) Satavaptan

824. Which one of the following is not true for Bivalirudin?

(a) It is direct thrombin inhibitor
(b) It has half life of 3 hours
(c) It does not cause thrombocytopenia
(d) It is used in percutaneous coronary interventions

825. Cross sectional area of normal mitral valve is:

(a) 1 to 2 cm square (b) 2 to 4 cm square
(c) 4 to 6 cm square (d) 6 to 8 cm square

826. Which beta blocker from following is excreted through kidney?

(a) Propranolol (b) Atenolol
(c) Carvedilol (d) Metoprolol

827. Verapamil does not increase blood level of following drug:

(a) Digoxin (b) Atorvastatin
(c) Aspirin (d) Ketoconazole

828. Which one of the following drug has long half life?

(a) Losartan (b) Irbesartan
(c) Telmisartan (d) Valsartan

829. Cutoff limit for maternal warfarin dose to minimize risk of fetal embryopathy in the first trimester is:

(a) 2 mg (b) 5 mg
(c) 7 mg (d) 10 mg

830. Which of the following is not useful to prevent contrast induced acute kidney injury?

(a) Hydration with intravenous normal saline prior to procedure
(b) Hydration with intravenous isotonic bicarbonate prior to procedure
(c) Use of nonionic isoosmolar contrast Iodixanol
(d) Ace inhibitors 6 hours prior to procedure

831. Which one of the following statement is not true for inferior vena cava filters?

(a) It is used in patients in whom anticoagulants are contraindicated
(b) It is used in patients recurrent pulmonary embolism despite therapeutic levels of anticoagulation
(c) It is used in patients with massive pulmonary embolism with very poor cardiopulmonary reserve
(d) Anticoagulants are must

832. In Kawasaki disease, incidence of coronary aneurysms is:

(a) Up to 50% (b) Up to 25%
(c) Up to 70% (d) Up to 90%

833. Giant cell arteritis does not involve following artery:

(a) Temporal artery (b) Internal carotid artery
(c) Subclavian artery (d) Axillary artery

834. Which one of the following ECG abnormality is uncommon in amyloidosis?

(a) Low voltage in limb leads
(b) Left bundle branch block
(c) First degree AV block
(d) Pseudo infarction pattern in inferior and septal leads

835. Which one of the following is not true for ECG in hypokalemia?

(a) Depression of ST segment
(b) Prominent U wave
(c) P wave becomes small and narrow
(d) T wave becomes small or inverted

836. Stage 6 of Bruce protocol is eqivalent to:

(a) 15.8 METs (b) 16.5 METs
(c) 16.9 METs (d) 17.1 METs

837. For dobutamine stress echo, maximum dose of dobutamine is used up to:

(a) 20 micogram/kg/minute
(b) 30 micogram/kg/minute
(c) 40 micogram/kg/minute
(d) 50 micogram/kg/minute

838. To assesses viability of myocardium following test is not useful:

(a) PET imaging
(b) MRI imaging
(c) Dobutamine stress echo
(d) Coronary angiography

839. Not a CT Angio trial in:

(a) CT stat (b) ACRIN-CT
(c) ACCURATE

840. Not a Prime prevention trial:

(a) CARE (b) Jupiter
(c) Voscope (d) AFCAB

841. Square root sign–True:

(a) MS (b) CCP
(c) Restrictive CMP (d) Cardiac Tamponade

842. Valsalva Maneuver–True:

(a) Phase 2–Increase venous return
(b) Phase 3–bradycardia

(c) Phase 3–A2–P2 widens
(d) Phase 3–BP decrease abruptly

843. Squatting decrease murmur:
(a) MR (b) HOCM
(c) VSD (d) PDA

844. Pregnancy–Physiological changes false:
(a) C.O. increase (b) PVR increase
(c) PVR decrease (d) HR increase

845. Syncope:
(a) Pulm embolism (b) Tanponade
(c) AV block (d) All

846. Left ventricular S_3 is least likely to be seen in:
(a) Mitral stenosis (b) Mitral regurgitation
(c) Aortic stenosis (d) Aortic regurgitation

847. Which statin was used in ASTRONOMER trial?
(a) Atarvastatin (b) Simvastatin
(c) Rosuvastatin (d) Pitavastatin

848. Regarding trans fatty acids all are true *except*:
(a) Increases LDL, decreases LDL size, increases TG and LPA
(b) Repeated cooking in same oil decreases trans fat intake
(c) Associated with increased risk of sudden cardiac death
(d) Even low levels (1–3% of total calories intake) of consumption increases risk

849. According to latest lipids guidelines you will prescribe statins to:
(a) Any person of age more than 25 years with LDL more than 150 mg/dl
(b) Any one with age between 40 and 75 years with diabetes and LDL between 70 and 189 mg/dl
(c) Any one with age between 40 and 75 years without diabetes and LDL between 70 and189 mg/dl with estimated 10 years risk of ASCVD >5%
(d) All current smokers with age >40 years

850. Which of the following drug used in patient with HIT with renal insufficiency?
(a) LMWH (b) LEPURIDIN
(c) ARGATROBAN (d) UFT

851. All are true regarding IMPROVE–IT trial *except*:
(a) Ezetimibe was added to baseline SIMVASTATIN therapy
(b) Study did not show any incremental benefit of additional Ezetimibe therapy
(c) Involved ACS patients only
(d) Ezetimibe further reduced LDL cholesterol levels when added to simvastatin

852. Following statements are true about contrast induced nephropathy (CIN) *except*:
(a) Patients at highest risk are those with DM and an estimated GFR below 60 ml/min
(b) IV saline at 1 ml/kg/hr to 1.5 ml/kg/hr for 3–12 hours before the procedure and 6–12 hours after the procedure should be given to prevent CIN
(c) N-Acetylcysteine is no longer recommended for prevention of CIN
(d) Low osmolarity or iso osmolar contrast media should be used judicially with a contrast volume to Cr clearance ratio lesser than 3.7 as a ceiling for contrast load

853. All are important aspects of blood pressure measurement *except*:
(a) Cuff length and width should be 80% and 40% of arm circumference respectively
(b) Column or dial should be read to nearest 2 mm Hg
(c) Cuff should be deflated at < 3 mm Hg/sec
(d) None of the above

854. Diagnostic criteria for POTS include all *except*:
(a) Orthostatic tachycardia (>30 BPM increase)
(b) Transient decrease in SBP of more than 20 mm Hg, with recovery after the first minute of tilt
(c) Standing plasma NE levels higher than 600 pg/ml
(d) Severe orthostatic symptoms

855. All of the following match *except*:
(a) CYP2D6–WARFARIN
(b) CYP2C9–PHENYTOIN
(c) CYP2C19–CLOPIDOGREL
(d) CYP2C19–OMEPRAZOLE

856. Each of the following statements regarding age related valve changes are true *except*:
(a) In normal hearts, the thickness of the aortic and mitral leaflets increases progressively with each decade, particularly along their closure margins
(b) The circumferences of all four cardiac valves decrease with age in normal hearts
(c) Age-related thickening can be associated with the formation of whisker-like projections called Lambi excrescences
(d) Mitral annular calcification almost invariably involves only the posterior annulus and forms a C-shaped ring of annular and subannular calcium

857. All of the following are biochemical characteristics of Metabolic syndrome, *except:*

(a) Elevated cholesteryl ester transfer protein
(b) Hyperinsulinemia
(c) Low lipoprotein lipase
(d) Low hepatic lipase

858. Which of the following pair is not correctly matched?

(a) Elinogrel–reversible, direct-acting P2Y 12- receptor inhibitor
(b) Vorapaxar–selective, PAR-1 inhibitor that blocks thrombin-mediated platelet activation
(c) Terutroban–thromboxane A2 synthase inhibitor
(d) Ridogrel–dual inhibitor of thromboxane A2 synthase and Thromboxane-receptor

859. Which of the following statements is not correct?

(a) The commonly used units of radiation are the Rad (radiation absorbed dose) and the Gray (Gy)
(b) 100 rad = 1 Gy, while 1 Gy is equal to 1 joule/kg
(c) The Sievert (Sv) is the SI unit that refers to the equivalent radiation dose in biologic tissues
(d) Sievert (Sv) and Gray (Gy) are interchangeable units of the radiation, both refer to the biologic effect of the radiation

860. 32 years premenopausal married female presented with rheumatic heart disease and severe aortic stenosis (LVEF 40%) with 2 early abortions due to APLA syndrome. True statement is:

(a) AVR: only if symptoms present
(b) Must undergo CAG followed by AVR with metallic valve CABG
(c) CAG not required before AVR
(d) AVR with bioprosthetic valve preferred over metallic valve

861. A 50 years old male with type 2 DM and gouty arthritis has multiple office BP readings 150–90 mm Hg despite being on lifestyle modifications for last 3 months. His ambulatory BP monitoring reveals average sleep time BP of 126/74 mm Hg. Which of the following statements regarding management of this patient is not false?

(a) Patient does not require pharmacotherapy for management of hypertension as he has only white coat hypertension should continue with lifestyle modifications
(b) Chlorthalidone is suitable first line drug for this patient
(c) ACEI + CCB is suitable combination therapy for hypertension in this patient
(d) Target BP should <125/75 mm Hg if patient is proteinuric

862. All are true regarding complications of radiation therapy *except*:

(a) Premature cardiovascular disease accounts for 25% of non-oncological deaths in long-term survivors
(b) It increases risk of significant valvular disease especially involving mitral valve
(c) Systolic dysfunction is relatively infrequent
(d) Conduction system is the least commonly involved of all cardiac structures

863. Abdominojugular reflux is characterized by all, *except*:

(a) It requires firm pressure over upper abdomen preferably right upper quadrant for 10 seconds
(b) A sustained rise of > 3 cm in venous pressure during continued compression
(c) Patient should avoid holding of breath
(d) It can predict heart failure and pulmonary artery wedge pressure higher than 25 mm Hg

864. Immediate blood pressure reduction is advised in all *except*:

(a) Hypertensive encephalopathy
(b) Acute coronary syndrome
(c) Hypertensive crisis with acute renal insufficiency
(d) Acute aortic dissection

865. Most common finding in myxoma is:

(a) Loud P_2
(b) Diastolic murmur
(c) Systolic murmur
(d) Tumor polyp

866. HASBLED score includes all *except*:

(a) Hypertension
(b) Stroke
(c) Elderly >60 years
(d) Labile INR

867. All are true about quitting of smoking *except*:

(a) Decrease risk of CAD to that of non-smokers in 3–8 years
(b) Decrease risk of stroke to that of non-smokers in 5–15 years
(c) Decrease risk of CAD is not appreciable within 1 year of quitting smoking
(d) Risk of lung cancer falls to about half of non-smoker at 10 years

868. All are true regarding EVOLOCUMAB *except*:

(a) It is a PCSK9 inhibitor
(b) It is approved by FDA

(c) Decreases LDL cholesterol levels

(d) None of the above

869. A 79 years old retired service man with known aortic stenosis (AS) comes for his annual check-up. He remains physically active with no symptoms but his blood pressure is 180/110 mm Hg. Following echo findings were obtained: Severe AS-peak velocity has increased from 3.8 m/sec a year ago to 4.0 m/sec at present, mean gradient 40 mm Hg, aortic valve area 1 cm^2, mild LVH and good overall LV systolic function:

Which one of the following statement is correct?

(a) A statin should be prescribed to reduce the rate of AS progression

(b) An antihypertensive drug should be prescribed

(c) The increase in peak velocity of $\geq$ 0.2 m/s/year suggests that surgery should be considered

(d) An exercise tolerance test (ETT) is unsafe in asymptomatic severe AS

870. Which one of the following patient characteristics is ideal for performance of a good quality coronary CT angiogram?

(a) Atrial fibrillation with a low ventricular response

(b) High body mass index

(c) Ability to breath hold for 2 seconds to 3 seconds maximum

(d) Ability to hold arms straight above the head

871. Which of the following is a normal response during exercise test on ECG?

(a) Horizontal ST depression

(b) Down sloping ST depression

(c) ST segment elevation

(d) Rapid up sloping ST depression

872. The weakest predictor of prognosis on exercise testing is:

(a) BP response (b) Exercise induce angina

(c) ST depression (d) Exercise capacity

873. Tei index for LV is:

(a) <0.5 (b) <0.4

(c) <0.3 (d) <0.1

874. False positive regional wall motion abnormality on 2D echo is seen in all *except*:

(a) Hypertensive response to stress

(b) Left circumflex disease

(c) Localized basal inferior wall abnormalities

(d) LBBB

875. The tracer used for ischemic memory in patient with restored perfusion after ischemia:

(a) C^{11} palmitate

(b) C^{11} acetate

(c) F^{18} flurtage

(d) ^{123}I-beta methyl iodopepentadecanoic acid (BMIPP)

876. The tracer approved by FDA for sympathetic innervations of heart:

(a) ^{99}TC sestamibi (b) ^{99}TC DTPA

(c) ^{123}I MIBG (d) ^{123}I BMIP

877. Which of the following statements regarding the cardiac fibrosis is not true?

(a) Myofibroblasts are derived from cardiac fibroblasts

(b) Myofibroblasts have 2-fold higher capacity to synthesize collagen

(c) TGF β stimulates transformations of myofibroblasts to fibroblasts

(d) Among the numerous regulatory factors, angiotensin II and transforming growth factor beta-1 are the most potent stimulators of collagen synthesis by cardiac fibroblasts

878. Which of the following statement is not true?

(a) Arterial baroreceptors (high-pressure receptors) are located in the carotid sinus and the aortic arch

(b) Cardiopulmonary baroreceptors (volume receptors) are located in the great veins and the cardiac chambers

(c) Cardiopulmonary baroreceptors (volume receptors) detect changes in the filling of the central venous circulation and are essential for short term orthostatic cardiovascular homeostasis

(d) Veno-arteriolar axon reflex, results in constriction of arterial flow to the muscles, skin, and adipose tissue, leading to the increase in vascular resistance in the limbs upon standing

879. Adexanet is a:

(a) PCSK9 inhibitor

(b) Novel antidote to the anticoagulation effects of Factor XA inhibitors

(c) Novel antidote to the antiplatlet effects of P2Y12 receptor antagonists

(d) Novel drug for Transthyretin induced cardiac amyloidosis

880. All are deterministic effects of radiation *except*:

(a) Skin necrosis (b) Hair loss
(c) Neoplasm (d) Cataract

881. Maximum lifetime allowable whole body radiation dose for those working with radiation is:

(a) 10 REM (b) 50 REM
(c) 40 REM (d) 5 REM

882. Which of the following drugs acts solely in factor Xa?

(a) UFH (b) Fondaparinux
(c) LMWH (d) Bivalirudin

883. Argatroban acts through inhibitor of:

(a) Factor II (b) Factor V
(c) Factor VII (d) Factor I

884. 70 years old male with home BP <140/75 at clinic 155/95, already on hydrochlorothiazide 25 mg OD, next line:

(a) ↑ dose of hydrochlorothiazide
(b) Add second anti HTN agent
(c) No ..... as she has white coat HTN
(d) Evaluate for 2° HTN

885. Patient with 40 years age has a BP 115/75 mm Hg few years ago. Now has a BP 155/75 mm Hg, risk of cardiovascular risk:

(a) No change (b) 2 times
(c) 4 times (d) 10 times

886. Patient already on clinidine for HTN, left medical for 2 days now has BP 175/80 mmHg, management:

(a) Restart clonidine (b) Nitroprusside
(c) Esmolol (d) Hydrochlorothiazide

887. Stains trial, all *except*:

(a) Proveit TIMI-22–in ACS patients, high dose pravastation ↓ mortality by 16%
(b) ASCOTT LLA-10% mg atorvastatin cause ↓ cardiovasc mortality and not all cause in 1% risk prevention
(c) US/CARE/LIPID–2% trial
(d) JUPITER trial UL trial with LDL–108, hsCRP >2 Vs <2

888. CT scan photo–30 years male dyspnea on standing, standing saturation–90%, supine–96%:

(a) Bilateral pulmonary embolism
(b) Pulmonary artery aneurysm
(c) IE due to septic abortion (in pulm art)
(d) ILD

889. ECHO:

(a) Severe MS (b) MVP
(c) HCM with SAM

890. ECHO:

(a) AF with aberrancy
(b) Junctional tachycardia with accessory pathway
(c) Pre excitation with aberrancy
(d) Sinus tachycardia with LBBB

891. S/e of statins all *except*:

(a) Headache
(b) Renal insufficiency
(c) Hepatic dysfuntion
(d) ↑ muscular dysfunction

892. Dabigatran should be stopped in a patient planned for surgery before:

(a) 24 hours (b) 48 hours
(c) 5 days (d) 36 hours

893. CETP deficiency is associated with:

(a) Slight increase in HDL
(b) Marked increase in HDL
(c) Slight decrease in LDL
(d) Slight increase in LDL

894. Apo C_2 is a cofactor for:

(a) LPL (b) Lipoprotein a
(c) HDL (d) LDL

895. CETP is associated with:

(a) LDL (b) LCAT
(c) VLDL (d) Chylomicron

896. Risk factors for sudden death in HOCM are A/E:

(a) History of sudden cardiac arrest
(b) LV thickness more than 30 mm Hg
(c) SVT on holter
(d) Spontaneous nonsustained VT

897. Treatment of HOCM all are T/E:

(a) Septal ablation is done
(b) Myomectomy is useful
(c) MVR is always required
(d) ICD for secondary prevention advised

898. Myxoma all T/E:
(a) Associated with Carney complex
(b) Left IAS is most common site
(c) Common in females
(d) CAG and cath is must for every patient

899. Common tumors of cardiac valves:
(a) Myxoma
(b) Rhabdomyoma
(c) Papillary fibroelastoma
(d) Fibroma

900. All are true about rhabdomyoma *except*:
(a) Associated with tuberous sclerosis
(b) Multiple in 90% cases
(c) Most common cardiac tumor of children
(d) Surgery is required

901. Hepatojugular reflex true is:
(a) Firm pressure over upper abdomen for more than 15 sec
(b) Deep inspiration is required
(c) Tensing of abdominal muscles is acceptable
(d) Immediate fall in JVP

902. Hepatojugular reflex estimates PCWP as:
(a) 5 mm Hg (b) 10 mm Hg
(c) 15 mm Hg (d) 20 mm Hg

903. Peripheral vascular resistance is accurately determined by:
(a) DBP
(b) Pulse pressure
(c) Mean arterial pressure
(d) SBP

904. CHADSVASC all T/E:
(a) CCF (b) Age
(c) DM (d) Male

905. Aortic dissection most common site of tear:
(a) Ascending aorta (b) Arch
(c) Descending aorta (d) Abdominal aorta

906. Valsalva maneuver changes in first phase:
(a) Increase in BP and fall in HR
(b) Fall in BP increase in HR
(c) Fall in BP fall in FR
(d) Raise in BP raise in HR

907. True is:
(a) Essential hypertension is isolated systolic hypertension
(b) Isolated diastolic hypertension is more common in female
(c) Isolated systolic hypertension in females and elderly
(d) DHF common in males

908. Mortality of PHT is maximum in:
(a) Eisenmenger (b) IPAH
(c) Scleroderma (d) COPD

909. Elevated CVP is suspected but venous pulsations cannot be appreciated, the patient should be asked to:
(a) Inspire and hold
(b) Sit upright with the feet dangling
(c) Lay supine
(d) Bend forward

910. S4 absent in:
(a) MR (b) AF
(c) HCM (d) AS

911. Kussmaul sign positive in:
(a) Severe LV dysfunction
(b) Pericardial effusion
(c) RV failure
(d) Severe AS

912. HOCM–triple ripple is due to:
(a) S1, S2, S3 (b) S2, S3, S4
(c) S1, S2, S4 (d) S4, pulses bisferiens

913. HOCM:
(a) AS+MR murmur (b) AR+MS murmur
(c) TR+MR murmur (d) PS+AS murmur

914. HOCM–risk factor of sudden death all *except*:
(a) Family history of sudden death due to HCM
(b) Unexplained recent syncope
(c) Multiple/repetitive nonsustained VT (on ambulatory ECG tracing)
(d) Hypertensive blood pressure response to exercise

915. Slow "Y" descent seen in:
(a) Acute pericarditis (b) Hypovolemia
(c) Tamponade (d) None

916. Most common cardiac tumor in children:
(a) Rhabdomyosarcoma (b) Sarcoma
(c) Rhabdomyoma (d) Lipoma

917. Kussmaul's sign seen in:
(a) Cardiac temponade (b) Acute pericarditis
(c) Right heart failure (d) All of the above

918. **Pulse oximetry affected by A/E:**
(a) Nail polish (b) High altitude
(c) Stable COPD (d) None of the above

919. **Palpitations (Pathological):**
(a) Regular (b) Accelerated
(c) Anxiety (d) Skipping

920. **Austin Flint murmur:**
(a) AR (c) MR
(b) TR (d) PR

921. **HTN caused by:**
(a) BNP (b) ANP
(c) Endothelin (d) All of the above

922. **Masked HTN:**
(a) Office BP abnormal
(b) Office BP normal
(c) Ambulatory BP normal
(d) None of the above

923. **40 years with low HDL Rx:**
(a) Niacin (b) Omega fatty acids
(c) Exercise (d) All of the above

924. **Pulsus paradoxus:**
(a) Exacerbation of normal phenomenon
(b) Fall in BP on expiration
(c) Fall in HR on inspiration
(d) None of the above

925. **Newer oral anticoagulants–true is:**
(a) More effective than vitamin K antagonists
(b) More GI bleeding
(c) Needs INR monitoring
(d) Antidotes not available

926. **All are high risk patients in HOCM *except*:**
(a) Unexplained recent syncope
(b) Hypotensive response on exercise
(c) Hypertensive response on exercise
(d) History of cardiac arrest

927. **SPRINT trial–all are T/E:**
(a) Intensive group had BP control to less than 120 mm Hg
(b) Antihypertensives to BP more than 130 mm Hg
(c) Diabetics were included
(d) No difference in the incidence of orthostatic hypotension among the groups

928. **All have end holes *except*:**
(a) Eppendrof (b) Cournaud
(c) Grollman (d) Sones

929. **Diagnosis is:**

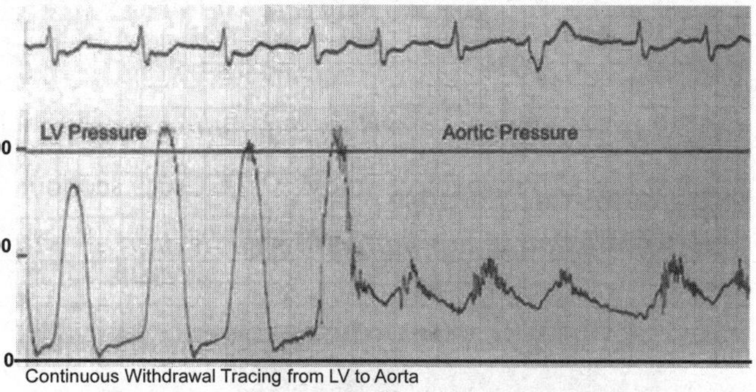

(a) AS (b) HOCM
(c) Supravalvular AS (d) AR

930. **Diagnosis for B image is:**

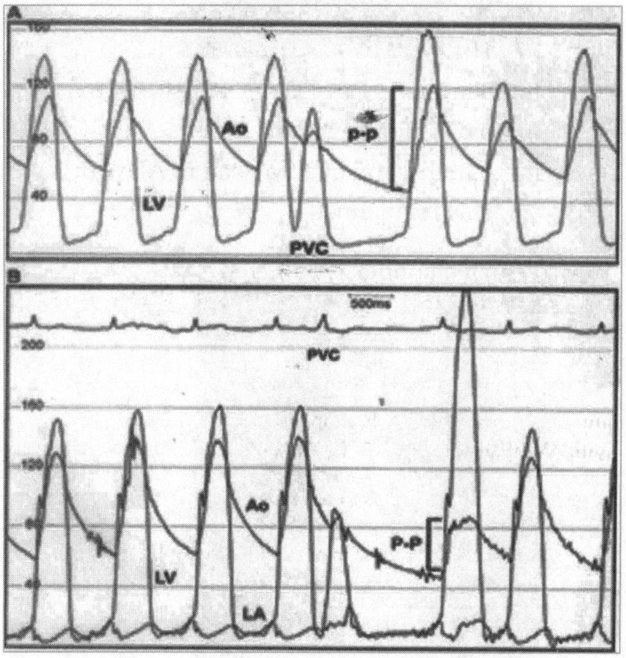

(a) AS (b) HOCM
(c) PS (d) MS

931. **Tracing suggests:**

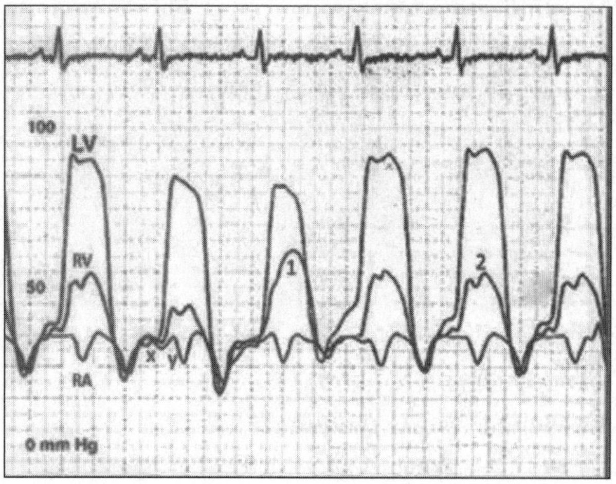

(a) Cardiac temponade
(b) Constrictive pericarditis
(c) RCM
(d) HOCM

932. Indication for this:

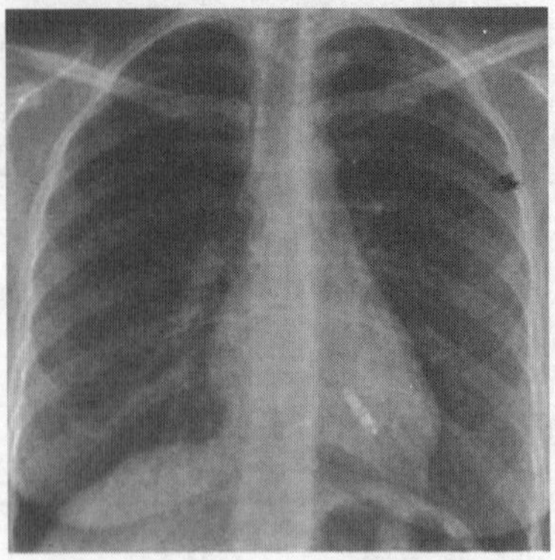

(a) Simultaneous ICD or CRT is required
(b) Implanted vena cava filter
(c) Inability to put atrial lead in AF with AV block
(d) DDD is planned

933. Which chamber is enlarged?

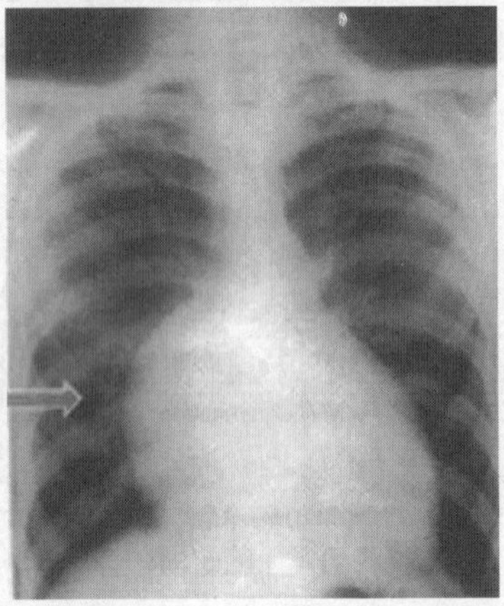

(a) RV (b) RA
(c) LV (d) LA

934. Indication for this:

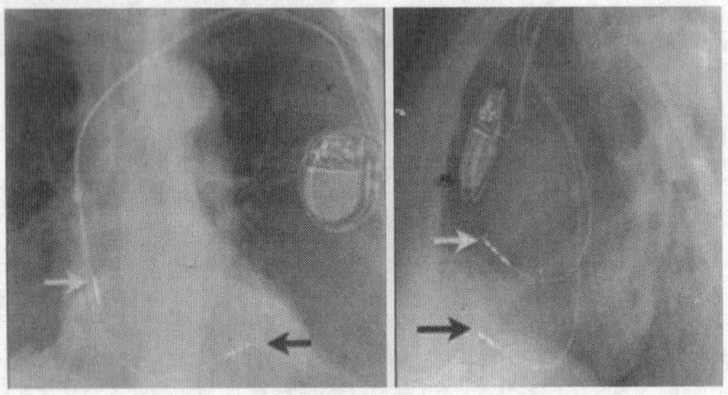

(a) Ventricular pacing required
(b) Old age with AV block
(c) Sick sinus syndrome
(d) AV synchrony needed

935. Diagnosis is:

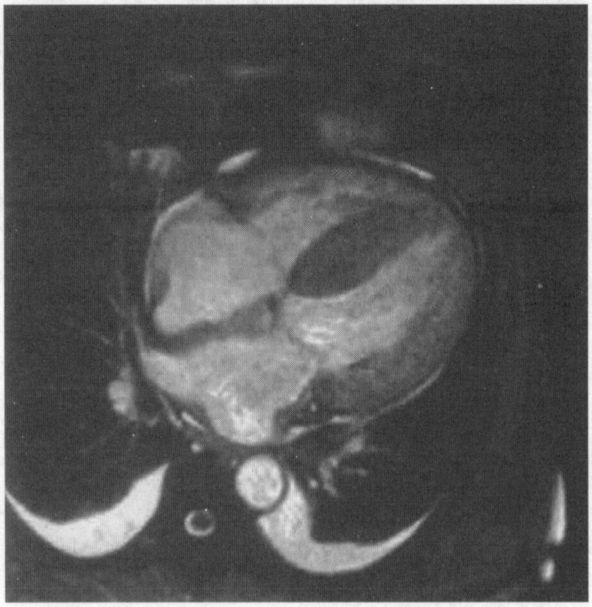

(a) MI (b) LVH
(c) Amyloidosis (d) Pericarditis

936. Diagnosis is:

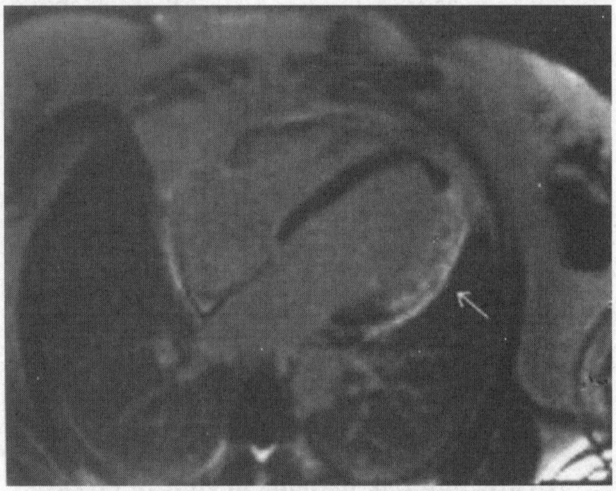

(a) Lateral wall MI (b) Pericarditis
(c) Pericardial effusion (d) RCM

937. Young male with breathlessness. What is the next step?

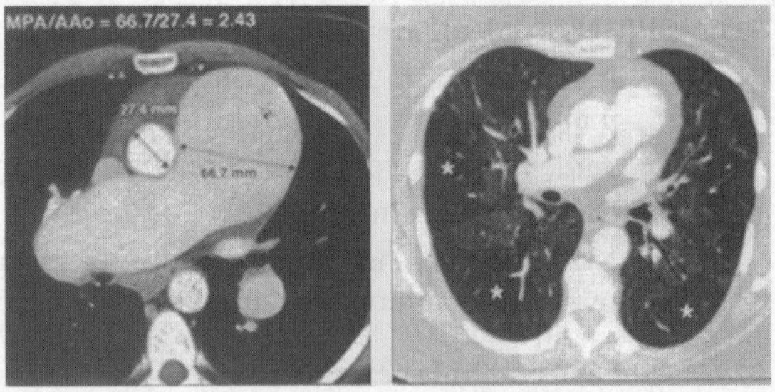

(a) Diuretics (b) PDE inhibitors
(c) Atrial septostomy (d) Thrombectomy

938. Diagnosis is:

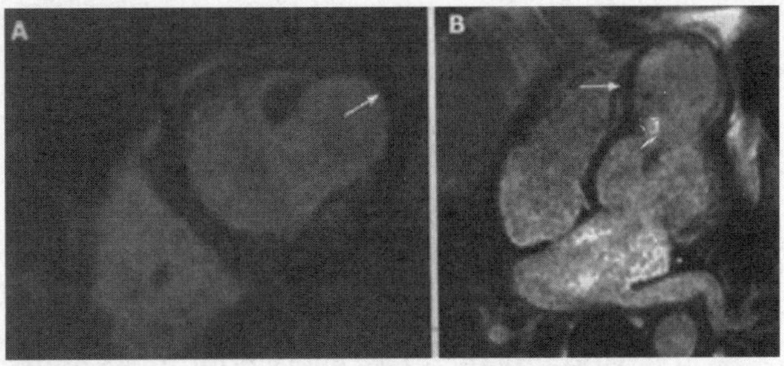

(a) LV aneurysm (b) Pericardial effusion
(c) CP (d) HOCM

939. Pansystolic murmur A/E:

(a) Traumatic TR (b) MVP
(c) VSD (d) Primary PAH

940. Wrong match:

(a) CVD–QRISK 2 score
(b) PAH–WHF counting
(c) CAD population–Rose questionnaire
(d) Pediatric CHF–Ross score

941. Most common finding with embolism during cardiac catheterization is:

(a) V1-V6–ST elevation
(b) ST depression in aVR
(c) ST elevation in II, III, aVF
(d) RBBB

942. Cardiovascular changes with acute exercise A/E:

(a) Increase in RA pressure
(b) Decrease in renal perfusion
(c) Decrease in splanchnic perfusion
(d) Increase in EF

943. Patient presented with chest pain, BP in right arm –180/90 mm Hg, left arm 100/80, ECG shows ST elevation in II, III, aVF, 1 cm of pericardial effusion. Next step is:

(a) CT angio
(b) MR angio
(c) Cardiac catheterization
(d) Doppler of upper limbs

944. True are:

(a) CO at rest is more in supine than erect
(b) During exercise in supine position CO increases mainly due to HR
(c) In the upright posture, the increase in cardiac output results from a combination of elevations in stroke volume and heart rate
(d) Change in supine to erect position causes increase in venous return
(e) EF increases on getting up from supine position

945. Type of TEVAR leaks–true is:

(a) Type I–Distal graft site leaks
(b) Type II–Retrograde flow into aneurismal sack
(c) Type IV–Graft porosity
(d) Type III–Defect in the graft
(e) Type V–Graft rupture

946. For pulmonary hypertension in children all are used *except:*

(a) Steroids (b) Sildenafil
(c) Bosentan (d) Digoxin
(e) CCB

947. Pre-eclampsia defined by:

(a) BP more than 140 systolic after 20th week of pregnancy
(b) Proteinuria
(c) Pedal edema
(d) Anemia
(e) Seizures

948. Pulmonary artery diastolic pressure calculated by:

(a) Based on Bernoulli equation
(b) PAEDP = End diastolic PR gradient + RVEDP
(c) PR gradient is required
(d) Continuous wave Doppler used
(e) RAP is not required

949. PCWP more than LVEDP in:

(a) LA Myxoma
(b) Decreased ventricular compliance
(c) MS
(d) Cor triatrium
(e) Severe LV dysfunction

950. Chest X-ray true is:

(a) Figure of eight–TAPVC
(b) Snowman–TGA
(c) Pericardial effusion–Margin blurred
(d) Batwing–Pulmonary edema
(e) "3" like appearance–Coarctation of aorta

951. Heart sounds–true is:

(a) S3 is associated with early rapid filling
(b) S4 has worse prognosis as compared to S3
(c) S4 associated with severe AS

(d) Split S1–suspect ejection click
(e) A2 is loudest at apex

952. CRT true is:
(a) Reverse remodeling
(b) Nonresponders are 30%
(c) Nonresponders are 25%
(d) Nonischemic DCM is more responsive than Ischemic DCM
(e) Useful in DCM

953. Heparin induced thrombocytopenia–true is:
(a) Common in medical patients
(b) Absolute CI of platelet transfusion
(c) Warfarin is given
(d) Long term antibody
(e) PF-4 antibody

954. Atrial myxoma–not true:
(a) Primary is more common than secondary
(b) Rhabdomyoma is most common pediatric tumor
(c) LA myxoma is common in females
(d) Associated with CAD in 1/3rd patients
(e) RA myxoma is most common

955. Discrepancy between PCWP and LVEDP is seen in:
(a) Increased PEEP
(b) COPD
(c) AR
(d) Very low pulmonary vascular resistance
(e) MS

956. CCP A/E:
(a) RVSP > 50 mm Hg
(b) PAH
(c) Right heart failure
(d) 25% increase in mitral inflow velocity during inspiration
(e) Expiratory reversal in hepatic flow

957. Lipoprotein a:
(a) Statin use decreases levels
(b) Resembles LDL and plasminogen
(c) Independent CAD risk factor
(d) Diet decreases Lipoprotein a levels
(e) Varies among ethnic and racial background

958. Noncompaction:
(a) Rarely associated with thromboembolism
(b) ECHO shows no blood flow into trabecular recess
(c) Optimal medical therapy same as others
(d) Jenni and chin echo criteria is used
(e) Rare cardiomyopathy

959. Case scenario: BP–220/110 mm Hg, Stanford A dissection:
(a) First drug of choice is beta blockers
(b) NTG is given as first drug
(c) Mortality increases every hour till 48 hours
(d) Medical stabilization before surgery
(e) Surgery is delayed

960. If BP is 140/180 mm Hg, what is mean arterial pressure?
(a) 80 (b) 90
(c) 100 (d) 110

961. PPH–true is:
(a) BMPR 2 mutation (b) BMPR-1
(c) BMPR-3 (d) BMPR-4

962. Signs of severe AR:
(a) Holodiastolic reversal in aorta
(b) Vena contracta greater than 3 mm
(c) AR PHT less than 400 ms
(d) All of the above

963. Aortic dissection type B A/E:
(a) Thoracic aorta (b) Abdominal aorta
(c) Arch (d) All of the above

964. CT in pericardial effusion true is:
(a) Attenuation coefficient will not help to differentiate types of PE
(b) Thickness of more than 4.1 mm on CT points to metastatic involvement
(c) CT will not help in pericardial diseases
(d) None of the above

965. ECHO suggests:
(a) Pericarditis (b) DCM
(c) Pericardial effusion (d) Pulmonary embolism

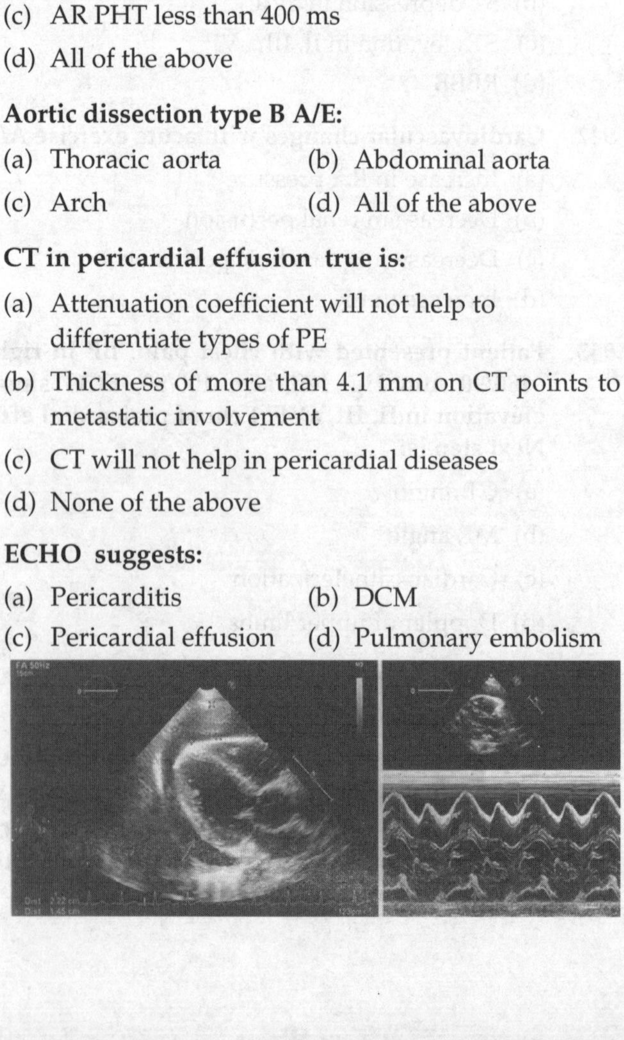

966. JVP signs of TR:
(a) Prominent a wave
(b) CV wave
(c) Prominent v wave
(d) Deep X descent

967. Pulsus paradoxus seen in A/E:
(a) COPD
(b) Constructive pericarditis
(c) PE
(d) Hypervolemia

968. Cardiac temponade:
(a) Raised JVP with prominent x descent
(b) Raised JVP with prominent y descent
(c) Normal JVP with prominent x descent
(d) None of the above

969. Dicrotic notch is due to:
(a) Interruption of blood flow due to sudden closure of aortic valve
(b) Arrival of impulse generated by LV
(c) Echo from upper part of body
(d) Echo from lower part of body

970. Corneal microdeposits are seen in:
(a) Propafenone (b) Ibutalide
(c) Amiodarone (d) Flecainide

971. CI formula is:
(a) SV × HR/BSA
(b) SV/HR × BSA
(c) BSA/HR × SV
(d) None of the above

972. A2-OS interval decreases with:
(a) Bradycardia (b) Short cycle of AF
(c) Low LAP (d) All of the above

973. Marfan criteria is:
(a) Jones (b) Dukes
(c) Bekey (d) Ghent

974. S_4 is due to:
(a) Ventricular contraction
(b) Flow across mitral valve
(c) Atrial contraction
(d) Mitral valve closure

975. Chronic hypoxia causes:
(a) Peripheral vasoconstriction
(b) Peripheral vasodilatation
(c) Pulmonary vasoconstriction
(d) Pulmonary vasodilatation

976. All are tolerated in pregnancy except:
(a) Marfan syndrome (b) ASD
(c) VSD (d) CoA

977. Myxoma all except:
(a) 50% of cardiac tumors
(b) Recurrence is 20%
(c) Prone for malignancy

978. Combined peripheral + central cyanosis without dyspnoea:
(a) Methylene blue (b) Cyanide poisoning
(c) CO poisoning (d) Anemia

979. Syndrome X all except:
(a) Good prognosis
(b) With LBBB worse prognosis
(c) 20% TMT +ve
(d) Generally typical angina

980. True about AV node conduction:
(a) Atropine + CSM–decrease both
(b) Atropine increase + CSM decrease

ANSWERS KEY

1. (b)	2. (b)	3. (a)	4. (c)	5. (b)	6. (?)	7. (d)	8. (a)
9. (a)	10. (a)	11. (a)	12. (d)	13. (a)	14. (b)	15. (a)	16. (b)
17. (a)	18. (b)	19. (c)	20. (d)	21. (c)	22. (b)	23. (a)	24. (a)
25. (d)	26. (d)	27. (c)	28. (d)	29. (d)	30. (b)	31. (a)	32. TTTTT
33. FTTTT	34. TTTTT FTFF	35. TFFFT	36. TFFFF	37. TTTFF	38. TFTT	39. TFTTT	40. TFTTT
41. (c)	42. (c)	43. (b)	44. (b)	45. (b)	46. (d)	47. (a)	48. (c)
49. (c)	50. (a)	51. (a)	52. (c)	53. (a)	54. (b)	55. (d)	56. (b)
57. (d)	58. (c)	59. (b)	60. (d)	61. (b)	62. (b)	63. (d)	64. (c)
65. (d)	66. (c)	67. (c)	68. (c)	69. (d)	70. (c)	71. (a)	72. (a)
73. (a)	74. (a)	75. (c)	76. (b)	77. (b)	78. (c)	79. (a)	80. (a)
81. (a)	82. (a)	83. (a)	84. (c)	85. (d)	86. (a)	87. (d)	88. (a)
89. (c)	90. (c)	91. (d)	92. (d)	93. (b)	94. (b)	95. (c)	96. (b)
97. (d)	98. (a)	99. (a, b)	100. (a)	101. (a)	102. (a)	103. (a)	104. (d)
105. (a)	106. (c)	107. (b)	108. (b)	109. (a)	110. (d)	111. (a)	112. (c)
113. (?)	114. (d)	115. (c)	116. (c)	117. (d)	118. (c)	119. (d)	120. (d)
121. (a)	122. (a)	123. (b)	124. (c)	125. (a)	126. (b)	127. (a)	128. (c)
129. (a)	130. (b)	131. (a)	132. (d)	133. (a)	134. (c)	135. (b)	136. (a)
137. (b)	138. (a)	139. (d)	140. (c)	141. (d)	142. (d)	143. (c)	144. (d)
145. (b)	146. (a)	147. (a)	148. (a)	149. (b)	150. (a)	151. (a)	152. (d)
153. (a)	154. (b)	155. (b)	156. (c)	157. (a)	158. (b)	159. (a)	160. (a)
161. (c)	162. (b)	163. (a)	164. (a)	165. (d)	166. (c)	167. (a)	168. (a)
169. (a)	170. (b)	171. (a)	172. (b)	173. (a)	174. (c)	175. (a)	176. (a)
177. (b)	178. (a)	179. (a)	180. (a)	181. (b)	182. (a)	183. (a)	184. (c)
185. (a)	186. (b)	187. (b)	188. (a)	189. (a)	190. (b)	191. (a)	192. (a)
193. (a)	194. (b)	195. (b)	196. (a)	197. (a)	198. (b)	199. (a)	200. (a)
201. (b)	202. (a)	203. 1(a)2(a)3(b)	204. 1(b)2(b)3(b)	205. 1(?)2(?)3(a)	206. (a)	207. 1(a)2(a)3(b)	208. 1(c)2(a)3(c)
209. (c)	210. (c)	211. (a)	212. (d)	213. (a)	214. (a,b,c,d)	215. TTFFT	216. (a)
217. TTFFT	218. TFTTT	219. (b)	220. (e)	221. TFTTT	222. (d)	223. (a)	224. (e)
225. (a)	226. (b)	227. (a)	228. (c)	229. FTTF	230. (d)	231. (c)	232. (a,b)
233. (d)	234. (b,d)	235. (d)	236. (c)	237. (e)	238. (b)	239. (d)	240. (b,d)
241. TT	242. TFTF	243. (d)	244. (c)	245. (c)	246. (d,e)	247. (a)	248. (a)
249. (a)	250. (b)	251. (d)	252. (d)	253. (d)	254. (c)	255. (a)	256. (c)
257. (c)	258. (a)	259. (e)	260. (b)	261. (a)	262. (c)	263. (b)	264. (c)
265. (d)	266. (b)	267. (d)	268. (c)	269. (d)	270. (d)	271. (d)	272. (d)
273. (a)	274. (b)	275. (b)	276. (d)	277. (d)	278. (d)	279. (c)	280. (d)
281. (d)	282. (b)	283. (d)	284. (a)	285. (c)	286. (a)	287. (d)	288. (a)
289. (b)	290. (c)	291. (b)	292. (d)	293. (a)	294. (c,d)	295. (c)	296. (a)
297. (a)	298. (b)	299. (c)	300. (a)	301. (c)	302. (a)	303. (a)	304. (c)
305. (c)	306. (d)	307. (a)	308. (c)	309. (a)	310. (a)	311. (a)	312. (a)
313. (b)	314. (c)	315. (a)	316. (d)	317. (a)	318. (c)	319. (a)	320. (d)
321. (b)	322. (a)	323. (b)	324. (a)	325. (b)	326. (c)	327. (b)	328. (b)
329. (b)	330. (a)	331. (a)	332. (c)	333. (b)	334. (b)	335. (b)	336. (a)
337. (a)	338. (a)	339. (a)	340. (a)	341. (a)	342. (b)	343. (a)	344. (a)

345. (d)	346. (d)	347. (a)	348. (b)	349. (c)	350. (d)	351. (a)	352. (a)
353. (a)	354. (a)	355. (e)	356. (a)	357. (a)	358. (a)	359. (d)	360. (a)
361. (b)	362. (d)	363. (c)	364. (c)	365. (b)	366. (a)	367. (a)	368. (c)
369. (c)	370. (a)	371. (a)	372. (b)	373. (c)	374. (c)	375. (c)	376. (b)
377. (c)	378. (b)	379. (c)	380. (c)	381. (a)	382. (d)	383. (b)	384. (a)
385. (d)	386. (d)	387. (b)	388. (b)	389. (a)	390. (c)	391. (a)	392. (b)
393. (b)	394. (a)	395. (a)	396. (a)	397. (a)	398. (d)	399. (c)	400. (c)
401. (d)	402. (d)	403. (c)	404. (d)	405. (b)	406. (d)	407. (c)	408. (b)
409. (b)	410. (d)	411. (b)	412. (c)	413. (c)	414. (d)	415. (d)	416. (b)
417. (b)	418. (a)	419. (a)	420. (c)	421. (d)	422. (c)	423. (c)	424. (d)
425. (b)	426. (a)	427. (a)	428. (b)	429. (d)	430. (d)	431. (d)	432. (d)
433. (c)	434. (b)	435. (b)	436. (c)	437. (a)	438. (a)	439. (c)	440. (b)
441. (b)	442. (b)	443. (a)	444. (c)	445. (b)	446. (c)	447. (d)	448. (c)
449. (a)	450. (a)	451. (b)	452. (c)	453. (a)	454. (c)	455. (d)	456. (b)
457. (b)	458. (a)	459. (a)	460. (c)	461. (b)	462. (b)	463. (c)	464. (a)
465. (d)	466. (a)	467. (d)	468. (d)	469. (b)	470. (c)	471. (c)	472. (a)
473. (a)	474. (a)	475. (a)	476. (a)	477. (a)	478. (b)	479. (d)	480. (b)
481. (d)	482. (d)	483. (d)	484. (d)	485. (a)	486. (d)	487. (c)	488. (a)
489. (c)	490. (b)	491. (c)	492. (c)	493. (a)	494. (a)	495. (b)	496. (c)
497. (a)	498. (c)	499. (b)	500. (c)	501. (a)	502. (a)	503. (a)	504. (a)
505. (b)	506. (a)	507. (b)	508. (b)	509. (a)	510. (c)	511. FTTFF	512. TFT
513. TTFFF	514. FFTFT	515. FTTTF	516. FFTFT	517. FTTTT	518. TTFTF	519. TFFFF	520. FTTFF
521. TTFTT	522. FTFTT	523. FFTTT	524. FFFTT	525. FTTFF	526. FTFTT	527. TTTTT	528. TTFFT
529. FFTFF	530. FTTTF	531. FFFT	532. TTFTF	533. TTTFT	534. FTTTT	535. TTTTT	536. TTTTT
537. FTTFT	538. FTFTF	539. FFTTF	540. TFFFF	541. FFFFF	542. FTTFF	543. FFTFT	544. FTFTF
545. TFFTF	546. FFFFF	547. FTTFT	548. FTTFF	549. TTTT	550. TTFF	551. FTTFF	552. TFFFF
553. TFTTT	554. FTTF	555. TTTFF	556. TTT	557. FTFT	558. TTFFF	559. TTFTF	560. FTFFF
561. TTTFF	562. TTFTT	563. FTFFF	564. TTFTT	565. FTTTF	566. TFTTT	567. TTTTF	568. TTTFT
569. TFFTF	570. FFFFF	571. TFFTT	572. TTFTF	573. TTFFF	574. TFTFT	575. TTFTF	576. TTFFT
577. TTTFF	578. TFFFT	579. FTTT	580. TTTTF	581. FFTTT	582. FTFT	583. FTTF	584. TTF
585. (c)	586. (b)	587. (d)	588. (a)	589. TTTT	590. FTTF	591. TFF	592. TFTT
593. FFTF	594. TFFF	595. (d)	596. (d)	597. (c)	598. (a)	599. (b)	600. (d)
601. (a)	602. (d)	603. (d)	604. (c,d)	605. (b)	606. (a)	607. (a)	608. (d)
609. (d)	610. (a)	611. (a)	612. (a)	613. (b)	614. (a)	615. (b)	616. (c)
617. FTTTF	618. TTFTT	619. FTF	620. TFTT	621. TT	622. FTFFT	623. TTFF	624. TTTFT
625. TFFTT	626. FTFTT	627. FTTFT	628. FTTTF	629. FFTFT	630. FFFFF	631. FTFTT	632. TFFT
633. FFFTT	634. FFFF	635. TTTFF	636. TFTTT	637. TTTTT	638. TFTTTTF	639. TTFFT	640. TFFFF
641. FTTTF	642. TFTT	643. TTFTT	644. TFTT	645. TFTFT	646. TFFTT	647. TTFFT	648. TTTTT
649. TTTTTT	650. TFTFT	651. TFTTT	652. FFTTT	653. FFTTFT	654. TTFFF	655. TTFFT	656. FTFTT
657. TFFFT	658. TTFFT	659. TFTTT	660. TTFFF	661. FTFFT	662. TTTFF	663. FTTTF	664. TTFT
665. TTFTT	666. TTFFT	667. TTTFT	668. TFFTT	669. TFFTT	670. FFFFT	671. TFTTT	672. TFTFF
673. TFTTF	674. TTTTT	675. TFTTF	676. TTTTF	677. FTTT	678. TFFFTF	679. TTTTT	680. FTFFT
681. FTTF	682. FFFTF	683. TFTTT	684. FFFFT	685. (b)	686. (a)	687. (b)	688. (c)
689. (b)	690. (a)	691. (a)	692. (b)	693. (a)	694. (a)	695. (b)	696. (a)
697. (b)	698. (a)	699. (b)	700. (a)	701. (a)	702. (a)	703. (b)	704. (a)
705. (c)	706. (c)	707. (d)	708. (a)	709. (a)	710. (a)	711. (b)	712. (b)
713. (a)	714. (d)	715. (a)	716. (b)	717. (d)	718. (d)	719. (b)	720. (a)
721. (a)	722. (a)	723. (c)	724. (b)	725. (d)	726. (c)	727. (a)	728. (c)
729. (d)	730. (b)	731. (a)	732. (a)	733. (d)	734. (d)	735. (a)	736. (d)

737. (a)	738. (b)	739. (c)	740. (b)	741. (a)	742. (d)	743. (d)	744. (b)
745. (c)	746. (a)	747. (b)	748. (b)	749. (b)	750. (a)	751. (b)	752. (d)
753. (b)	754. (a)	755. (b)	756. (b)	757. (a)	758. (b)	759. (a)	760. (d)
761. (a)	762. (a)	763. (c)	764. (a)	765. (c)	766. (b)	767. (a)	768. (d)
769. (a)	770. (d)	771. (a)	772. (b)	773. (c)	774. (d)	775. (a)	776. (d)
777. (d)	778. (a)	779. (d)	780. (a)	781. (d)	782. (c)	783. (a)	784. (c)
785. (b)	786. (a)	787. (b)	788. (a)	789. (d)	790. (a)	791. (b)	792. (c)
793. (a)	794. (b)	795. (b)	796. (a)	797. (a)	798. (b)	799. (c)	800. (a)
801. (d)	802. (a)	803. (c)	804. (b)	805. (c)	806. (b)	807. (c)	808. (a)
809. (a)	810. (c)	811. (c)	812. (c)	813. (c)	814. (d)	815. (a)	816. (a)
817. (a)	818. (a)	819. (a)	820. (b)	821. (b)	822. (a)	823. (c)	824. (b)
825. (c)	826. (b)	827. (d)	828. (c)	829. (b)	830. (d)	831. (d)	832. (b)
833. (b)	834. (b)	835. (c)	836. (c)	837. (c)	838. (d)	839. (c)	840. (a)
841. (b)	842. (d)	843. (d)	844. (b)	845. (d)	846. (a)	847. (c)	848. (c)
849. (b)	850. (b)	851. (b)	852. (b)	853. (d)	854. (b)	855. (a)	856. (b)
857. (d)	858. (c)	859. (d)	860. (b)	861. (c)	862. (b)	863. (d)	864. (c)
865. (c)	866. (c)	867. (c)	868. (d)	869. (b)	870. (d)	871. (d)	872. (c)
873. (b)	874. (b)	875. (d)	876. (c)	877. (c)	878. (c)	879. (b)	880. (c)
881. (b)	882. (b)	883. (a)	884. (b)	885. (b)	886. (a)	887. (c)	888. (b)
889. (a)	890. (c)	891. (a)	892. (b)	893. (b)	894. (a)	895. (b)	896. (c)
897. (c)	898. (d)	899. (c)	900. (d)	901. (a)	902. (c)	903. (a)	904. (d)
905. (a)	906. (a)	907. (c)	908. (c)	909. (b)	910. (b)	911. (c)	912. (d)
913. (a)	914. (d)	915. (c)	916. (c)	917. (c)	918. (c)	919. (d)	920. (a)
921. (c)	922. (b)	923. (d)	924. (a)	925. (b)	926. (c)	927. (c)	928. (a)
929. (a)	930. (b)	931. (b)	932. (c)	933. (b)	934. (d)	935. (c)	936. (a)
937. (b)	938. (a)	939. (a)	940. (b)	941. (d)	942. (d)	943. (a)	944. (a,b,c)
945. (a,b,c,d)	946. (b,c,d,e)	947. (a,b)	948. (a,b,c,d)	949. (a,c,d)	950. (a,c,d,e)	951. (a,c,d)	952. (a,c,d,e)
953. (b,e)	954. (e)	955. (a,b,c,e)	956. (a,b,c)	957. (b,c,e)	958. (c,d,e)	959. (a,c)	960. (c)
961. (a)	962. (a)	963. (c)	964. (b)	965. (c)	966. (b)	967. (d)	968. (a)
969. (a)	970. (c)	971. (a)	972. (b)	973. (b)	974. (c)	975. (c)	976. (d)
977. (c)	978. (b)	979. (c)	980. (b)				

CHAPTER EIGHT

PREVENTIVE CARDIOLOGY

1. **Patient with diabetic nephropathy posted for angioplasty, drug to be stopped:**
(a) Chlorthalidone (b) Metformin
(c) Insulin (d) Ramipril

2. **SPRINT trial:**
(a) Intensive therapy have better results than moderate control
(b) Done in diabetic patients
(c) BP maintained at 150/80
(d) All are true

3. **Cardiomegaly (Gross):**
(a) Tamponade
(b) Ebstein
(c) AV regurgitation
(d) AR with LV dysfunction

4. **Fibrates–mechanism of action–all *except*:**
(a) LPL stimulation
(b) Induction of hepatic fatty acid uptake
(c) Reverse cholesterol transport
(d) Mildly inhibits MHG CoA reductase

5. **Cherry red staining is in:**
(a) Diabetic CMP (b) Chagas
(c) EMF (d) Amyloid

6. **Injectable drug to ↓ LDL:**
(a) Toracetabid (b) Ricaniguat
(c) PCSK-9 inhibitor (d) Cangrelor

7. **DM patient with HTN 1st line–A/E:**
(a) Beta blocker (b) Thiazide
(c) ACE (d) CCB

8. **1% LDL–mortality benefit:**
(a) 1% (b) 2%
(c) 4% (d) 6%

9. **Aspirin in diabetic patients is the risk is:**
(a) Higher than 10% in 10 years
(b) Higher than 10% in 20 years
(c) Lower than 5% in 5 years
(d) Lower than 5% in 20 years

10. **Following is not a cause of "Type 2" MI according to universal MI classification:**
(a) Coronary artery spasm
(b) Coronary embolism
(c) Coronary dissection with intra luminal thrombus
(d) Endothelial dysfunction

11. **Palmar crease xanthomas are specific for:**
(a) Type IV hyperlipoproteinemia
(b) Type III hyperlipoproteinemia
(c) Type II hyperlipoproteinemia
(d) Type I hyperlipoproteinemia

12. **Annual surveillance procedures for diabetic patients include the following *except*:**
(a) Eye examination
(b) Blood pressure record
(c) Medical nutrition therapy
(d) Patient education

13. **Lipid–all are 2° prevent trial *except*: (T/F)**
(a) WOSCOPS (b) 4S
(c) CARE (d) LIPID
(e) JUPITER

14. **DM-ACS:**
(a) Hyperglycemia per se ↑ CAD risk
(b) Albuminuria–risk 10 times
(c) Type 1 DM genetic susceptibility is more responsible to diabetic nephropathy than the duration of diabetes
(d) Insulin level independently correlated with CAD

(e) Type 2 DM hyperglycemia control CAD risk manifestation corrected

15. **Which of the following is not useful to prevent contrast induced acute kidney injury?**

(a) Hydration with intravenous normal saline prior to procedure

(b) Hydration with intravenous isotonic bicarbonate prior to procedure

(c) Use of nonionic isoosmolar contrast Iodixanol

(d) Ace inhibitors 6 hours prior to procedure

16. **Lipids have proven to be the best substantiated risk factors for coronary artery disease. Select the false statement from the following:**

(a) Most patients with familial hypertriglyceridemia have corneal arcus, xanthoma or xanthelesma

(b) Familial defective apo B 100 is clinically indistinguishable from familial hypercholesterolemia

(c) Apo B 100 is major apoprotein in LDL

(d) Dysbetalipoproteinemia develops in patients who are homozygous for ApoE2 allele

17. **Regarding fibrates all are true *except*:**

(a) Good efficacy in lowering fasting as well as postprandial triglyceride levels

(b) HDL-C-raising effects are modest

(c) Antagonists of peroxisome proliferator-activated receptor (PPAR)

(d) Reported to raise both serum creatinine and homocysteine in both short-term and long-term studies

18. **Effects of exercise on lipid profiles demonstrates greatest effect on:**

(a) LDL (b) HDL

(c) Triglycerides (d) Small dense LDL

19. **Statin A/E:**

(a) ↓ Lipid content in plaque

(b) ↓ Fibrous cap

(c) ↓ Metalloproteinases

(d) Causes arterial remodeling

20. **C-RP level in JUPITER associated 1 bad prognosis:**

(a) >1 (b) >2

(c) >3 (d) >4

21. **Statin–true A/E:**

(a) ↓ MI

(b) ↓ All cause mortality

(c) Reverses stenosis

(d) ↓ CVA/TIA

22. **Antidiabetic causing pedal edemal CCF:**

(a) MF (b) Rosiglitazone

(c) Glimeperide (d) Acarbose

23. **↑ Cholesterol seen in:**

(a) PVFA

(b) MUFA

(c) Omega 3 fatty acids

(d) Coconut oil

24. **All are true regarding IMPROVE-IT trial *except*:**

(a) Ezetimibe was added to baseline SIMVASTATIN therapy

(b) Study did not show any incremental benefit of additional Ezetimibe therapy

(c) Involved ACS patients only

(d) Ezetimibe further reduced LDL cholesterol levels when added to simvastatin

25. **Following statements are true about contrast induced nephropathy (CIN) *except*:**

(a) Patients at highest risk are those with DM and an estimated GFR below 60 ml/min

(b) IV saline at 1 ml/kg/hr to 1.5 ml/kg/hr for 3-12 hours before the procedure and 6-12 hours after the procedure should be given to prevent CIN

(c) N-acetylcysteine is no longer recommended for prevention of CIN

(d) Low osmolarity or iso osmolar contrast media should be used judicially with a contrast volume to Cr clearance ratio lesser than 3.7 as a ceiling for contrast load

26. **All of the following pairs are matched, *except*:**

(a) Ezetimibe–epithelial cell–Niemann-Pick Cl-like protein

(b) Mipomirsen–antisense oligonucleotide that targets apoB-100 mRNA

(c) Eprotirome and sobetirome–Thyroid mimetics

(d) Lomitapide–HDL-bound enzyme cholesterol ester transfer protein inhibitor

27. **REWIND trial includes:**

(a) Empagliflozin (b) Canagliflozin

(c) Dulaglutide (d) Sitagliptin

28. **Which of the following is not a feature of atherosclerosis in diabetics?**

(a) Increased apoptosis of smooth muscle cells
(b) Vascular cell adhesion molecule (VCAM) expression is increased
(c) Increased expression of matrix metalloproteinases (MMPs) 1, 2 and 9
(d) Increased adopkines

29. **Which of the following is not true about omega 3 fatty acids?**
(a) High dose omega 3 fatty acids have shown modest but significant reduction in BP
(b) DHA more effective than EPA in BP reduction
(c) Diastolic BP is reduced by about 6-8 mm Hg
(d) May lead to decreased secretion of aldosterone

30. **All are true regarding SPRINT trial *except*:**
(a) Involved diabetic patients
(b) Target blood pressure level in intensive treatment group is systolic <120 mm Hg
(c) Target blood pressure level in standard treatment group is systolic <140 mm Hg
(d) Incidence of AKI was higher in intensive treatment group

31. **All are true regarding EVOLOCUMAB *except*:**
(a) It is a PCSK9 inhibitor
(b) It is approved by FDA
(c) Decreases LDL cholesterol levels
(d) None of the above

32. **Adexanet is a:**
(a) PCSK9 inhibitor
(b) Novel antidote to the anticoagulation effects of factor X_A inhibitors
(c) Novel antidote to the antiplatelet effects of P2Y12 receptor antagonists
(d) Novel drug for transthyretin induced cardiac amyloidosis

33. **1% ↓ LDL associated with ↓ CV risk by:**
(a) 2% (b) 5%
(c) 10% (d) 1%

34. **AKI true statement:**
(a) AKI has no relation with blood flow
(b) Creatinine increases immediately after AKI
(c) Both reduces urine output and increased creatinine must for diagnosing AKI
(d) Tissue inhibitor of metalloproteinase is marker for impending AKI

35. **Trans fatty acids *except*:**
(a) <1% recommended
(b) >2% increase mortality by 23%
(c) Replacement by linoleic acid increase insulin sensitivity
(d) Fatty acids replacement by sat. Fatty acids-no change in TC/HDL ratio

36. **As cholesterol enter into cell induces enzyme:**
(a) LCAT
(b) HMG COA synthetase
(c) HMG COA reductase
(d) LDL receptor

37. **Hyperuricemia false:**
(a) Febuxastat-non purine selective inhibitor of X-oxidase
(b) Target < 6 mg/dl
(c) Allopurinol < 300 mg in CKD patient
(d) APEX trial-majority of patient on febuxastat achieved target early as compared to allopurinol

38. **SSA:**
(a) Transthyretin (b) ANP

39. **Which of the test require fasting:**
(a) TSH (b) Apolipoprotein
(c) HbA1c (d) C-peptide

40. **Cholesterol into cell induces:**
(a) ACAT
(b) HMG COA synthase
(c) HMG COA reductase
(d) LDL receptor

41. **TTR (time in therapeutic range) all *except:***
(a) For warfarin
(b) Decreases mortality
(c) Decreases CAD
(d) Increases bleeding

42. **All are diabetogenic *except:***
(a) Ranolazine (b) Atenolol
(c) Hydrochlorthiazide (d) Atorvastatin

43. **Low HDL all *except:***
(a) Cigarette smoking
(b) Hypo α-apolipoproteinemia
(c) Hypertriglyceridemia
(d) Estrogen supplements

44. In diabetes all *except:*
(a) PCI increase mortality
(b) PCI increases MI
(c) CABG decreased incidence of stroke
(d) CABG decreases rate of revascularization

45. Lp (a) true *except*:
(a) Statins lower Lp (a)
(b) Lp (a) > 30 mg/dl–doubles the CHD risk
(c) Mild transient acute phase reactant
(d) 2% increase in Lp (a) leads to increase in 23% CHD risk

46. All are true *except:*
(a) Niacin in AIM HIGH trial ↓ mortality
(b) ↑ ed TG related to ↓ ed HDL
(c) Tangier disease–low/absent HDL
(d) CETP inhibition–high CVD mortality

47. Weight gain in DM:
(a) Chlorpropamide (b) Pramilinide
(c) Rosiglitazone (d) Glimipride

48. Pitvastatin all *except:*
(a) ↑ HDL also
(b) Metabolised by CYP 3A4
(c) Less drug interaction
(d) Less myositis

49. Niacin induced flushing ↓ all *except:*
(a) Aspirin (b) Gemfibrozil
(c) Laparobant (d) Inositol hexacetamide

50. Statin prevents formation of:
(a) Squalene
(b) Mevalonate
(c) Farnesyl pyrophosphate
(d) HMG pyrophosphate

51. Lp (a) ↓ by:
(a) Atorvastatin (b) Rosvastatin
(c) Gemfibrozil (d) Fenofibrate

52. Post femoropopliteal bypass asymptomatic LDL goal:
(a) < 100 (b) < 130
(c) <160 (d) < 190

53. Level of hs-CRP denotes ↑ cardiac risk:
(a) >1 (b) >3
(c) > 10 (d) > 0-1

54. HDL true:
(a) Smoking cessation ↑ es HDL
(b) Nicotinic acid is most effective in ↑ HDL
(c) Good cholesterol
(d) All are true

55. LDL goal:
(a) No risk factor < 130 mg/dl
(b) 2 risk factor and cholesterol > 200, start treatment
(c) 10 years risk >20%, start treatment

56. Mechanism of action of fibrates through inhibition of:
(a) PPAR-(alpha) (b) PPAR-(gamma)
(c) HMG CoA

57. Type II hyperlipidemia all *except*:
(a) Tendon xanthoma
(b) Corneal arcus
(c) Increase atherosclerosis
(d) Pancreatitis

58. Familial hypertriglyceridemia all *except*:
(a) AD
(b) Acute pancreatitis
(c) Increase by alcohol
(d) Increase atherosclerosis

59. DM with increase TG treatment goal is:
(a) 100 mg% (b) 150 mg%
(c) 200 mg% (d) 125 mg%

60. Gestational DM treatment:
(a) Incertin (b) Insulin
(c) Thiazolidiones (d) Metformin

61. Incertin→ euglycemia by:
(a) Direct stimulation of insulin
(b) ↓ DPP-4
(c) Peripheral utilization of glucose
(d) ↑ adiponectin

62. Homocystenuria A/E:
(a) Heterozygotes → atherosclerosis
(b) MR common
(c) Vascular complication is due to platelet dysfunction
(d) Pyridoxine diet advised

63. CABG–LDL level target:

(a) < 100 mg % (b) < 150 mg %
(c) < 200 mg %

64. Most common lesion seen in ankylosing spondylitis:

(a) AR (b) CHB
(c) Myocarditis

65. Metabolic syndrome A/E:

(a) Abdominal (central) obesity
(b) Elevated fasting plasma glucose
(c) High serum triglycerides
(d) High LDL

66. CARE/4S/ WOSCOPS trial for:

(a) Antiatherogenic (b) To correct lipid levels
(c) Antidiabetic

67. Metformin stopped during radioiodine contrast studies because:

(a) Radio contrast agents interact with metformin
(b) To prevent lactic acidosis

68. All are true *except*:

(a) Torcetrapib increases HDL
(b) Niacin increases HDL
(c) Fibrates increases HDL
(d) Omega 3 fatty acids increases TG

69. CIN: (T/F)

(a) Felbamate is used for treatment
(b) NS used
(c) Theophylline is useful
(d) Na HCO_3 is used

70. CIN: (T/F)

(a) 12-20% may develop CIN
(b) NAC for prevention
(c) DM, CHF risk factor for CIN
(d) Iodixanol is low osmolar
(e) Low + high osmolar less deleterious

71. LDH as cardiac marker: (T/F)

(a) Least sensitive and least specific
(b) LDH1 more in heart
(c) CPR more in female
(d) CPK less in males

72. CIN False is:

(a) 10% ↑ in creatinine in 48 hours definition
(b) I/V fluid isotonic 1 ml/kg/hr class I indication
(c) Contrast/GFR > 3.7 – high risk
(d) Haemofiltration before PCI is recommended in CKD

73. ATP III for lipid to start treatment:

(a) Treatment if TC > 200 mg with 1-2 risk factor
(b) ≥ 2 r/f < 10% - 160 mg
(c) < 10% start treatment at 160 mg

74. HDL:

(a) Smoking cessation increases HDL
(b) Nicotine best
(c) 10% ↓ wt ↑ HDL
(d) Low carbohydrate ↑HDL

75. Incidence of CIN after angiography:

(a) 1-6% (b) 6-12%
(c) 12-20% (d) >20%

76. Contrast nephropathy:

(a) Definition - > 0.5 mg/dl or > 25% rise in 24 hours in Serum creatinine
(b) Started before + continued for 48 hours after–AC
(c) Isosmolar, nonionic-iodixanol
(d) Stage III CKD–eGFR<60 ml
(e) Showing of microemboli–IABP
(f) All are true

77. Type-2 DM with CVD:

(a) FPG > 126
(b) BP goal < 130/80
(c) No use of statin if lipids normal
(d) Fibrate is DOC in TG /↓HDL
(e) Rigorous life style prevents onset of DM

78. Xanthema stratum palmaris seen in:

(a) Type I (b) Type II
(c) Type III (d) Type IV
(e) Type V

79. All statements regarding hypercholesterolemia are true *except*:

(a) Heterozyous develops increased atherosclerosis
(b) Platelet dysfunction
(c) Caused by cystathione deficiency
(d) Treated by pyridoxine

80. **CIN beneficial effect of drug shown in recent trials:**
(a) NAC (b) Fenoldopam
(c) Furosemide

81. **Apoproteins:**
(a) VLDL= B-100
(b) LDL= B-100
(c) HDL= Apo AII
(d) Chylomicron= Apo CII

82. **All are diabetogenic *except:***
(a) Atorvastatin (b) Losartan
(c) Hydrochlorthiazide (d) Beta blockers

83. **Statin therapy reduce mortality by 33%, control arm–12%, treatment arm–8%, how many patients required to be treated to save one death?**
(a) 25 (b) 33
(c) Insufficient data

84. **All of the following are true about PCSK9 *except*:**
(a) PCSK stands for-Proprotein cholesterol surface kinases
(b) PCSK 9 binds to LDL receptors
(c) Major action of PCSK9 is degradation of LDL receptors
(d) Evolocumab is a following is antibody that inhibits the action of PCSK9

85. **As per the current lipid guidelines, which one of the following patients would require a high intensity statin?**
(a) 40-year-old diabetic, LDL 100 mg/dL, calculated risk-1%
(b) 30-year-old normotensive, non-diabetic with LDL 195
(c) 75-year-old with LDL 130 mg/dL
(d) 25-year-old, normotensive, non-diabetic

86. **Statis induced myopathy may be more common in all of the following *except*:**
(a) Elderly
(b) Patients on fibrates
(c) Renal failure and diabetes
(d) Obese males

87. **Contrast induced nephtopathy, all are true *except*:**
(a) Common if eGFR <60 ml/min/1.73 m^2
(b) Lowest with iodixanol
(c) I.V. hydration with normal saline is most effective preventive strategy
(d) Pretreatment with NAC is very effective in prevention

88. **All are Trials of statins in ACS/MI except:**
(a) A to Z (b) Prove-IT TIMI 22
(c) Miracle (d) TNT

89. **Current recommendation for statin therapy is:**
(a) Treat to target
(b) Lowest is best
(c) Treat populations at risk
(d) All of the above

90. **Which of the following is correct for new onset diabetes with statins?**
(a) Reduce statin dose
(b) Discontinue statins
(c) Start insulin/Oral anti diabetic
(d) Advise dietary and lifestyle changes

91. **NIACIN use has fallen out of grace following which trial:**
(a) AIM HIGH (b) ACCORD
(c) CARDS (d) ASCOT

92. **Statin inhibit conversion of HMG to:**
(a) Mevalonate (b) Squalene
(c) Acetyl COA

93. **Anti-hypertensive causing dyslipidemia:**
(a) ACE-I (b) Thiazide
(c) CCB (d) α blockers

94. **Statins act on HMG-COA by inhibiting formation of:**
(a) Farnesyl pyrophosphate
(b) Geranyl pyrophosphate
(c) Mevalonic acid
(d) Squalene

95. **ACCORD/ADVANCE trial:**
(a) HbA1c < 5%
(b) Tight glycemic control has no effect on total mortality
(c) Tight glucose control decreases microvascular complication
(d) Tight glucose no effect on macrovascular complication

96. **Treatment of CIN *except:***
(a) NAC 600 mg 2 days before and then for 1week
(b) Forced I/V diuresis
(c) Intravenous saline
(d) None of the above

97. Female CAD versus male CAD A/E:

(a) LDL (b) TG
(c) Smoking (d) DM

98. Prevalence of DM in urban India:

(a) 3.5% (b) 10%
(c) 5% (d) 20%

99. In thiazides, DM development over 4 years is:

(a) 12% (b) 16%
(c) 20% (d) 25%

100. 42 years NIDDM + acute pancreatitis + no cardio-vascular risk factors + no clinical abnormality. Initial triglycerides – 2800 mg%, T. Chol.–360 mg%.

2nd valve = Triglycerides–1200 mg%, T. Chol. 250 mg%, HDL–22 mg%, diagnosis.

(a) Type-I
(b) Type-V
(c) Type-III
(d) Familial hyper lipoproteinemia

101. Torcetrapib (CETP inbititor) A/E:

(a) ↑ Transaminase
(b) ↑ Abdominal symptom
(c) ↑ Cholesterol influx by increasing macro – HDL
(d) HTN

102. DM + dyslipidemia A/E:

(a) ↑ LDL (b) ↓ HDL
(c) ↑TG (d) ↑ Small dense LDL

103. Statin trial in ACS all *except:*

(a) Prove it (b) Miracle
(c) A to Z (d) Prosper

104. Cardiac MRI:

(a) Endomyocardial fibrosis
(b) Tuberculosis
(c) Sarcoidosis
(d) Amyloidosis

105. Tangier disease all *except:*

(a) Autosomal recessive
(b) Increase HDL
(c) Peripheral lipid deposition
(d) Risk of CAD lo

106. Following is true about ezetimibe:

(a) 10 mg atorvastatin + 10 mg ezetimibe = 80 mg simvastatin
(b) Inhibit cholesterol absorption
(c) Inhibit biliary cholesterol formation
(d) Inhibit triglyceride absorption

107. All are true about non-ionic contrast *except:*

(a) Less tendency to form clots
(b) Less nephrotoxic
(c) Preferred in patients with deranged kidney function test
(d) Less chances of arrhythmia

108. Best preventive treatment for contrast-induced nephropathy is:

(a) N-acetyl cysteine (b) Theophylline
(c) Saline hydration (d) Mannitol

109. Which drug is withdrawn from the market because of its side effects causing rhabdo myolysis?

(a) Rosvastatin (b) Simvastatin
(c) Pravastatin (d) Cerivastatin

110. All are secondary prevention trial *except:*

(a) Care (b) Lipid
(c) 4S (d) AFCAPS

111. AIM HIGH trial drugs used A/E:

(a) Niacin (b) Atorvastatin
(c) Simvastatin (d) Ezetimide

112. Torcetrapib:

(a) ↑ HDL (b) ↓ LDL
(c) ↓ HDL

113. Apo B-48 is constituent of:

(a) Chylomicron (b) LDL
(c) TG (d) HDL

114. Modifiable risk factor A/E:

(a) Insulin resistance
(b) Obesity
(c) Socioeconomic status
(d) Elevated homocysteine level

115. Treatment goals for adults with diabetes include all of the following *except:*

(a) LDL–C < 70 mg/dl
(b) HbA1C < 7%
(c) Peak postprandial capillary plasma glucose < 180 mg/dl
(d) Blood pressure <130/80

116. Valvular pulmonic stenosis is the most common defect in:

(a) Holt-Oram syndrome (b) Noonan syndrome
(c) Down syndrome (d) Turner syndrome

117. The goal for LDL-cholesterol lowering in patients with coronary artery disease is:

(a) <100 mg/dl (b) <115 mg/dl
(c) <130 mg/dl (d) <160 mg/dl

118. Tendinous exanthomas are most commonly associated with hyperlipoproteinemia:

(a) Type-I (b) Type-II
(c) Type-III (d) Type-IV

119. Ideal drug for isolated hypertriglyceridemia:

(a) Statins (b) Resins
(c) Fibric and derivatives (d) Nicotinic acid

120. In obesity weight reduction is better than physical activity:

(a) Stroke (b) Osteoporosis
(c) Sleep apnea

121. Contrast induced nephropathy A/E:

(a) Saline hydration (b) Bicarbonate
(c) IV furosemide (d) Acetyl cysteine

122. Not a lipid trial:

(a) PROSPER (b) CARE
(c) WOSCOPS (d) ALLHAT–LLT

123. MIRACL trial:

(a) Atorvastatin 80 mg
(b) Atorvastatin 10 mg
(c) Pravastatin 20 mg

124. HCRP high risk in:

(a) >1 (b) >2
(c) >3 (d) >6

125. Lp(a) A/E:

(a) It must be done in all patient with ACS to predict prognosis
(b) Niacin ↓ Lp (a)
(c) Standardization is difficult
(d) LpA predicts risk in non linear manner

126. Xanthoma on palmer creases seen in which hyperlipoproteinemia?

(a) I (b) II
(c) III (d) IV

127. Macrovascular complication of DM decreased by A/E:

(a) ACE–I (b) Tight glucose control
(c) Genfibrozil (d) BP < 130/85 mm Hg

128. Xanthelesma—Most common cholesterol abnormality:

(a) Increased HDL (b) Decreased HDL
(c) Reduced LDL (d) Raised LDL

129. Metabolic syndrome A/E:

(a) Hypertriglyceridemia (b) Increased LDL
(c) Reduced HDL (d) Abdominal obesity

130. Familial hypercholesterolemia A/E: (T/F)

(a) AR
(b) Arcus senilis < 45 years
(c) Tendon xanthomas
(d) Mutation at 19q6 (LDL receptor)

131. Primary prevention lipids trial: (T/F)

(a) 4S (b) CARE
(c) WOSCOPS (d) PROSPER
(e) LIPID

132. Nicotinic acid causes A/E: (T/F)

(a) Hyperuricemia (b) Acanthosis nigricans
(c) Flushing (d) Hepatoxicity
(e) Nephrotoxicity

133. LP (a) (T/F):

(a) Non-linear association
(b) Level best decreased by fibrate
(c) LDL reduction ameliorate the risk associated with increased LP (a)
(d) Standardization of laboratory is problematic
(e) Homologous with plasminogen

134. Familial hypercholesterolemia: (T/F)

(a) AD
(b) Tendon xanthoma
(c) Heterozygous form–TC= 700-900 mg%
(d) Homozygous form–resistant to drug treatment
(e) LDL apharesis

135. Effects of statins: (T/F)

(a) ↑ suicide
(b) ↓ CV mortality

(c) ↓ stroke incidence
(d) ↑ osteoporosis
(e) Plaque stabilization

136. Familial hypercholesterolemia: (T/F)
(a) AD
(b) Tendon xanthoma common
(c) Heterozygotes LDL—800—900 mg%
(d) Homozygotes show poor responds to therapy
(e) Leukopheresis play a role in treatment

137. Dyslipidemia *except:* (T/F)
(a) HDL > 35 mg% negative risk factor
(b) HDL < 35 mg% positive risk factor
(c) Total cholesterol < 200 mg%
(d) HRT improves lipid profile in post menopausal female

138. Familial hypercholesterolemia: (T/F)
(a) AD
(b) Heterozygotes–700-900 gm total cholesterol
(c) Homozygotes–Poor drug response
(d) LDL appresis treatment
(e) Tendon xanthoma +

139. Dyslipidemia: (T/F)
(a) HDL < 35 mg% negative risk factor
(b) HDL > 35 mg% positive risk factor
(c) TG should be less than 200 mg%
(d) Estrogen improves lipid profile
(e) LDL-C goal in CAD < 160 mg%

140. Statins–True are: (T/F)
(a) High COA reductase inhibitors
(b) Fibric acid derivatives
(c) ↑ QT
(d) ↓ LDL
(e) Myopathy and ↑ liver enzymes

141. Hs CRP: (T/F)
(a) Major role in innate immunity
(b) Applied in female
(c) Applied in all age groups (young and old)
(d) Apparent healthy people with raised hs CRP shows risk of MI

142. Decrease in LDL by 1% decreases CV risk by:
(a) 5% (b) 10%
(c) 1% (d) 2%

143. A/E:
(a) Type I: Eruptive xanthoma
(b) Type II: Tendinous xanthoma
(c) Type III: Tuberoeruptive
(d) Type IV: Xanthoma Palmaris

144. Statin with least protein binding:
(a) Pravastatin (b) Simvastatin
(c) Lovastatin (d) Atorvastatin

145. Palmer xanthoma seen in dyslipidemia:
(a) Type IV (b) Type IIa
(c) Type III (d) Type IIb

146. HDL–lipoprotein A/E:
(a) A II (b) C II
(c) D (d) J

147. Not associated with pravastatin:
(a) ALLHAT–LLT (b) Lipid
(c) HPS (d) Prosper

148. True A/E:
(a) Eruptive xanthoma–type I
(b) Tendon xanthoma–type II
(c) Tendonous xanthoma–type VI
(d) Xanthoma straitum palmaris–IV

149. Palmar crease xanthomas are specific for which type of hyperlipoproteinemia?
(a) Type 1 (b) Type 2
(c) Type 3 (d) Type 4

150. Regarding trans fatty acids all are true *except*:
(a) Increase LDL, decrease LDL size, increase TG, and LPa
(b) Repeated cooking in the same oil decreases trans fat intake
(c) Associated with increased risk of sudden cardiac death
(d) Even low levels (1-3% of total calorie intake) of consumption increases risk

151. According to latest lipid guidelines, you will prescribe statins to:
(a) Any person of age more than 25 years with LDL more than 150 mg/dl
(b) Anyone with between 40-75 years with diabetes and LDL between 70-189 mg/dl

(c) Anyone with age between 40-75 years without diabetes and LDL between 70-189 mg/dl with estimated 10 year risk of ASCVD > 5%
(d) All current smokers with age > 40 years

152. Which statin was used in ASTRONOMER trial?
(a) Atorvastatin (b) Simvastatin
(c) Pitavastatin (d) Rosuvastatin

153. T/F:
(a) T1DM 90% in monozygotic twin
(b) T2DM screening start immediately for microvascular involvement
(c) Intensive glycemic control decreases macro-vascular complication
(d) Metformin is first drug
(e) Type 1 islet cell are pathogenic

154. Hypetriglyceridemia: (T/F)
(a) Apo B 100 major LP in LDL
(b) Xanthalesma more common in hyper-triglyceridemia
(c) Apo E2 homozygous mutation in dysbetalipoproteinemia
(d) Apo b 100 MUTATION NOT clinically different from familial hyperholestrolemia
(e) PBC- lipoprotein X

155. Lipid lowering drugs: (T/F)
(a) Side effect is ↑ TG of cholestyramine
(b) Ezetimibe–act on PPARα
(c) Acanthosis nigricans is side effect of niacin
(d) Fish rich in MUFA

156. T/F:
(a) Stearic acid is a saturated FA and it increases LDL
(b) Plant sterols decrease LDL and fat soluble vitamins
(c) High carbohydrate with low fat diet ↓s HDL
(d) MUFA decreases LDL
(e) Plant stands ↓ CAD risk by 25%

157. Dyslipidemia: (T/F)
(a) FCHL is most common dyslipidemia
(b) Palmar striae are s/o dysbetaliprotenemia
(c) Arcus and xanthelesma commonly seen in FCHL
(d) Famitral hyperchylomicronemia treatment for long chain FA
(e) Apo B is associated with HDL

158. Statin myopathy: (T/F)
(a) More in younger patients
(b) Verapamil and niacin increases myopathy
(c) Coenzyme Q10 is useful
(d) Diabetic nephropathy increase chances
(e) > 10 times CPK is diagnostic for myocytes

159. Adiposity: (T/F)
(a) Inflammatory cytokines are increased
(b) Adiponectin increased in DM
(c) Adiponectin increases mortality
(d) Adiponectin increases obesity
(e) Adiponectin anti-inflammatory and antiatherogenic

160. Adiposity: (T/F)
(a) Liposuction decreases visceral fat
(b) Adiponectin decreases DM and CVD risk

161. T/F:
(a) Atorvastatin = 10 mg (A)
Gemfibrofil = 600 mg (B)
Cholestyramine = 800 mg (C)
↓ LDL = A>B>C
(b) Drug t ½ doesn't depend on absorption and clearance

162. Primary treatment trials of statins: (T/F)
(a) AFCAPS (b) BIP
(c) V-HIT (d) 4S
(e) LIPID

163. Omega-3 fatty acid: (T/F)
(a) Decrease incidence of MI and stroke
(b) Decreased SCD
(c) Decrease homocysteine
(d) Decreases monocyte recruitment

164. Complication of DM: (T/F)
(a) Complication of CAD can be correlated with hyperglycemic phase
(b) Development of nephropathy increases chance of CAD
(c) Type 1 DM nephropathy partly by hyperglycemia and duration of DM and partly by genetic mechanisms
(d) Insulin levels consistent by related to CAD
(e) Increased catabolism of HDL

165. **Oxidized LDL: (T/F)**
(a) –ve charge
(b) Cytotoxicity
(c) ↑ vitamin E level
(d) ↑ es atherosclerosis
(e) Malenoaldehyde ↑es

166. **T/F:**
(a) FCH is polygenic
(b) Broad beta disease suggestive of remnant LDL
(c) Incidence is 1 : 500
(d) Obesity is not secondary cause of hyperlipidemia
(e) Absence of CETP causes ↓ HDL

167. **Statins were not used in which trials? (T/F)**
(a) CARE (b) STAR
(c) AVERT (d) CLAS-I
(e) CLAS-II

168. **Primary prevention trials of statin: (T/F)**
(a) AFCAPS (b) VA- HIT
(c) BIPS (d) LIPID
(e) 4S

169. **Lipoprotein (a)–apo lipoprotein:**
(a) Apo A (b) Apo B 100
(c) Apo B 48 (d) Apo E

170. **Post-stenting, statin for 4 months at 20 mg, lipids TC-150 mg%, TG-180 mg%, HDL-28 mg% –add:**
(a) Ezetimibe (b) Niacin
(c) ↑ Statin 40 mg (d) No change

171. **50 years diabetic male-target BP:**
(a) 130/80 mm Hg (b) 130/85 mm Hg
(c) 140/90 mm Hg (d) 160/100 mm Hg

172. **Drug to be avoided in a diabetic with border line RFT pre-cath:**
(a) Metformin (b) Dilzem
(c) Nicorandil (d) Dipyridamole

173. **Xanthoma without hypercholesterolemia:**
(a) Palmer xanthoma
(b) Tendinous xanthoma
(c) Palmer and planter xanthoma
(d) Tuberous

174. **All the following drugs are diabetogenic *except:***
(a) Atenolol (b) Hydrochlorthiazide
(c) Rosvastatin (d) Ranolazine

175. **Dyslipidemia caused by A/E:**
(a) Diuretics (b) Cyclosporine
(c) Glucocorticoid (d) ACE inhibitors

176. **Bivalirudin is used for:**
(a) DVT treatment
(b) Pulmonary embolism treatment
(c) AF treatment
(d) HIT

177. **The lipid profile in Indian differs from western population by:**
(a) Low LDL
(b) High TG, Low HDL
(c) Low HDL, raised LDL
(d) High non HDL cholestrol

178. **Friedwald formula used for calculation of:**
(a) HDL (b) LDL
(c) Total cholesterol (d) TG

179. **ACS patient underwent PCI on ideal antiplatelet and anticoagulant support, post procedure developed hypoxia, lung infiltrates and hemoptysis. Cause is:**
(a) Abciximab induced pulmonary hemorrhage
(b) Pneumonia
(c) Pulmonary edema
(d) Cardiac temponade

180. **A 75 years old male non diabetic, non smoker and no history suggestive of CAD with BP 150/94 mm Hg after one month of lifestyle modification with lipid profile of total chol. – 190 mg/dl, LDL–110 mg/dl, HDL–42 mg/dl so what will be next management?**
(a) Amlodipine (b) ACE-I
(c) Diuretics (d) No treatment

181. **Action of insulin in hyperkalemia is:**
(a) Movement of K from intracellular to extracellular
(b) Movement of K from extracellular to intracellular
(c) Movement of K from intravascular to extravascular

182. **Protective apolipoprotein:**
(a) A1 (b) B1
(c) B (d) E

183. Cardio-protective lipoprotein:

(a) A (b) B1
(c) B2 (d) E

184. Old age–better prognosis:

(a) Low CRP, ↑ LCL (b) ↑ CRP, ↓ LDL
(c) ↑ TG, ↓ HDL (d) ↓ LDL, ↓ HDL

185. Better combination in 55 years old male:

(a) High LDL low CRP
(b) High LDL high CRP
(c) Low LDL high CRP
(d) High TG low HDL
(e) High TG high CRP

186. TG in LDL:

(a) < 10% (b) > 50%
(c) 33% (d) 25%

187. ↓ TG least effective:

(a) Fish oil (b) Resin
(c) Niacin (d) Ezetimibe

188. 1% ↑ in HBAC associated with ↑ glucose:

(a) 70 (b) 90
(c) 50 (d) 30

189. Skin manifestations of type III hyperlipidemia:

(a) Eruptive xanthoma
(b) Tendon xanthoma
(c) Palmer crease xanthoma

190. Characteristic dyslipidemia in blacks:

(a) ↓ Total cholesterol, ↑ Lp-a, ↓ LDL
(b) ↓ Total cholesterol, ↑ Lp-a, ↑ HDL
(c) ↓ Total cholesterol, ↑ Lp-a, ↓ HDL
(d) ↓ Total cholesterol, ↑ TG, ↓ LDL

191. Statin trials A/E:

(a) 4S (b) WOSCOPS
(c) CARE (d) DIAS

192. I. Fibrates target:

(a) TG (b) LDL
(c) ApO (a) (d) HDL

193. HDL antiatherogenic:

(a) I (b) II
(c) III (d) IV

194. All true about dietary fats *except:*

(a) Fish consumption decreases SCD
(b) Olive oil is MUFA
(c) Nuts have PUFA
(d) All transfatty acids are not harmful

195. True statement is A/E:

(a) Statin decreases hs CRP in proportional to LDL decrease
(b) Hs CRP > 3 times bad prognostic factor in USA
(c) Aspirin decreases mortality in case of increased Hs CRP
(d) Hs CRP is associated with development of diabetes

196. Lipid lowering drug associated with QT prolongation include:

(a) Ezetimibe (b) Probucol
(c) Gemfibrozil (d) Niacin

197. Metabolic syndrome is typically associated with all of the following *except:*

(a) Increased waist circumference
(b) Elevated LDL–Cholesterol
(c) Impaired fasting glucose
(d) Low HDL–Cholesterol

198. Which of the following therapy has conclusively shown to increase HDL and decrease cardio-vascular mortality?

(a) Anacetrapib (b) Niacin
(c) Fibrates (d) None of the above

199. One of the following lipoprotein is not secreted from liver:

(a) VLDL (b) HDL
(c) Chylomicrons (d) Lipoprotein (a)

200. Tangier disease is:

(a) Familial hypercholesterolemia
(b) Familial HDL deficiency
(c) Lipoprotein lipase deficiency
(d) Abetalipoproteinemia

201. Patient comes in emergency with breathlessness chest vein dilation, fecal puffiness; male smoker:

(a) SVC syn. (b) CT
(c) CCP

202. Which is not activated X inhibitor?

(a) Dabigatran
(b) Rivaroxaban
(c) Apixaban
(d) Edoxaban

203. True about H/T all *except*:

(a) Clinical dignity, suspected when platelet < 1 lakh

204. Radiation induced cardiotoxicity all *except:*

(a) Myocardial dysfunction most common
(b) Capillary endothelial damage can lead to fibrosis
(c) LV dysfunction can present late
(d) Coronary ostial stenosis

ANSWERS KEY

1. (b)	2. (a)	3. (a)	4. (d)	5. (d)	6. (c)	7. (d)	8. (b)
9. (a)	10. (c)	11. (b)	12. (c)	13. FTTTF	14. TTTTF	15. (d)	16. (a)
17. (d)	18. (c)	19. (b)	20. (b)	21. (c)	22. (b)	23. (d)	24. (b)
25. (d)	26. (d)	27. (c)	28. (a)	29. (c)	30. (a)	31. (d)	32. (b)
33. (a)	34. (d)	35. (d)	36. (c)	37. (d)	38. (a)	39. (b)	40. (a)
41. (c)	42. (a)	43. (d)	44. (c)	45. (b)	46. (a)	47. (b)	48. (b)
49. (b)	50. (b)	51. (d)	52. (a)	53. (b)	54. (d)	55. (a)	56. (a)
57. (d)	58. (a)	59. (b)	60. (b)	61. (a)	62. (a)	63. (a)	64. (a)
65. (d)	66. (b)	67. (b)	68. (d)	69. FTFT	70. TTTFF	71. TTFF	72. (a)
73. (c)	74. (b)	75. (c)	76. (f)	77. (c)	78. (c)	79. (c)	80. (a)
81. (a)	82. (b)	83. (a)	84. (a)	85. (b)	86. (d)	87. (d)	88. (d)
89. (c)	90. (d)	91. (a)	92. (a)	93. (b)	94. (c)	95. (a)	96. (b)
97. (a)	98. (a)	99. (a)	100. (b)	101. (c)	102. (a)	103. (d)	104. (a)
105. (a)	106. (b)	107. (a)	108. (c)	109. (d)	110. (d)	111. (b)	112. (a)
113. (a)	114. (d)	115. (a)	116. (b)	117. (a)	118. (b)	119. (c)	120. (c)
121. (c)	122. (c)	123. (a)	124. (c)	125. (a)	126. (c)	127. (b)	128. (b)
129. (b)	130. TTTT	131. FFTFF	132. FFFFT	133. TFTTT	134. TTFTT	135. FTFFT	136. TTFTT
137. FTFF	138. TFTTT	139. FFFTF	140. TFFTT	141. TTTT	142. (d)	143. (d)	144. (a)
145. (c)	146. (b)	147. (c)	148. (c)	149. (c)	150. (b)	151. (c)	152. (d)
153. TTTTT	154. TFTTT	155. TFTF	156. FTTTF	157. TTFFF	158. FTTTT	159. TFFFT	160. FT
161. TF	162. TFFFF	163. TTTT	164. TTTTT	165. TFTFF	166. TFTFF	167. TFTFF	168. TFFFT
169. (b)	170. (b)	171. (a)	172. (a)	173. (d)	174. (d)	175. (d)	176. (d)
177. (b)	178. (b)	179. (a)	180. (c)	181. (a)	182. (d)	183. (d)	184. (a)
185. (a)	186. (c)	187. (d)	188. (d)	189. (c)	190. (a)	191. (d)	192. (a)
193. (b)	194. (d)	195. (a)	196. (b)	197. (b)	198. (d)	199. (c)	200. (b)
201. (a)	202. (a)	203. (a)	204. (a)				

CHAPTER NINE

NON INVASIVE CARDIOLOGY

1. **Adverse finding on exercise stress test A/E:**
   (a) Dizziness
   (b) Early HR acceleration in 1st min
   (c) Hypotension exercise induced
   (d) Pallor

2. **RVH criteria A/E:**
   (a) $S_1S_2S_3$
   (b) S_1Q_3
   (c) QR in V_1
   (d) Rsr in V_1 with R > 0.5 mV

3. **Young male with TMT/CPVT A/E:**
   (a) Risk of SCD
   (b) Syncope with exertion
   (c) Structurally normal heart
   (d) Coronary spasm as cause

4. **Echo→M mode tamponade, clinically not seen:**
   (a) Arterial hypotension
   (b) Friedreich's sign
   (c) Pulsus paradoxus
   (d) Absent × Descent

5. **Snowman sign–not seen in Echo:**
   (a) Dilated coronary sinus
   (b) ASD
   (c) Dilate LA
   (d) Dilated RA

6. **CT showing asplenia which is seen?**
   (a) Sickle cell
   (b) Howell-Jolly
   (c) Spherocytes
   (d) Lymphocytes

7. **MRI showing endocardial enhancement with apical sparing:**
   (a) EMF
   (b) Sarcoid
   (c) Amyloidosis
   (d) TB

8. **Lung uptake on MPI, not true is:**
   (a) Better with Thallium than Tc 99 m
   (b) More with low EF
   (c) Rapid transit
   (d) More in multivessel disease

9. **Lung uptake during nuclear scan–all *except*:**
   (a) Indicative of multivessel decrease
   (b) Increased LVEDP
   (c) Due to slow transit of tracer
   (d) Better identified in technetium than thallium

10. **Spectral Doppler of PR. Early diastolic velocity 4 m/s, RAP=6 mm Hg peak PAP would be:**
    (a) 70 mm Hg
    (b) 30 mm Hg
    (c) 36 mm Hg
    (d) 64 mm Hg

11. **Optical coherence tomography–A/E:**
    (a) Doesn't differentiate between white and red thrombus
    (b) It has good resolution but poor penetration
    (c) It needs blood free space
    (d) Does not visualize adventitia

12. **60 years with insidious on set CCF-ECG shows–other findings may be: (See below figure)**

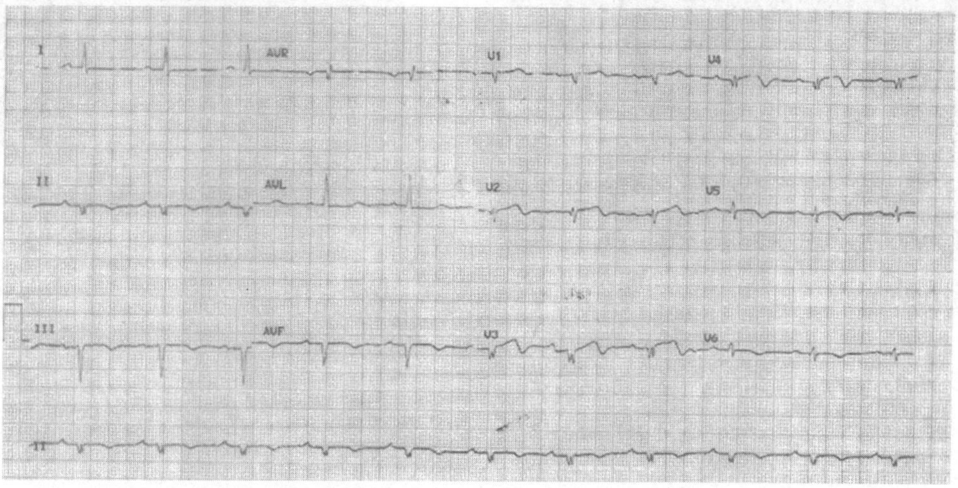

(a) Atrial septal hypertrophy
(b) Normal BNP
(c) Trolated circumflex block
(d) Atrial myxoma

13. **CT angio shows:**

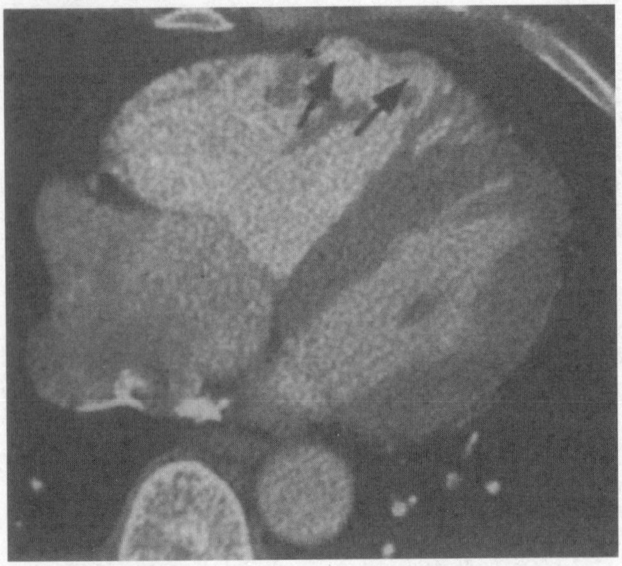

Intervention is:
(a) Pericardiocentesis
(b) Biopsy
(c) Bentall procedure

14. **MRI cardiac shows:**

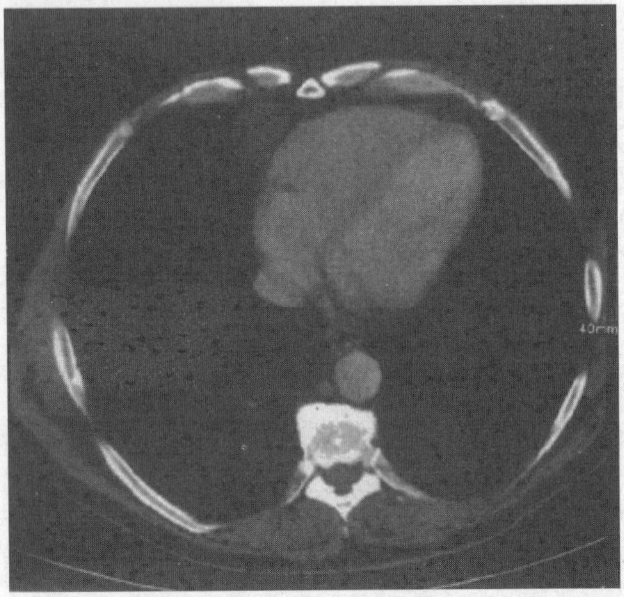

(a) Submitral aneurysm
(b) Pericardial cyst
(c) Effusion

15. **Renal CT angio:**

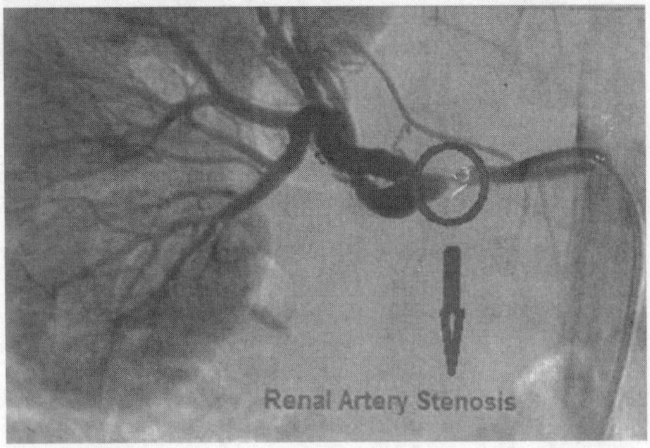

(a) FMD
(b) Aortoarteritis
(c) Atherosclerosis
(d) Post stent block

16. **ECG shows A/E:**
(a) AF
(b) RBBB pattern in VPC
(c) It is supraventricular origin
(d) Predisposed for idiopathic VF

17. **ECHO tracing shows PR:**

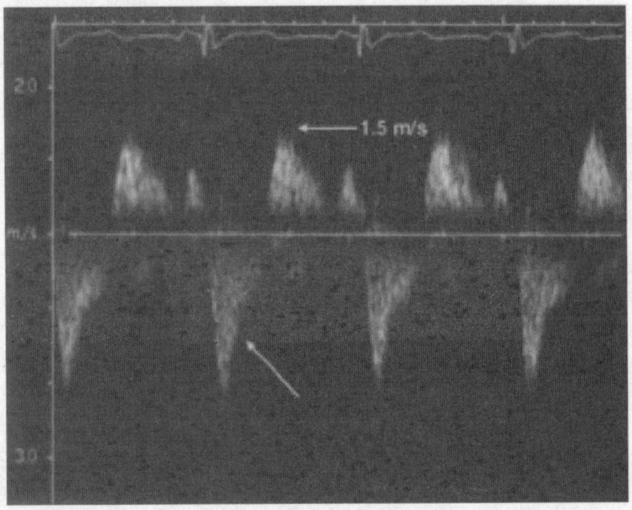

(a) Ebstein anomaly
(b) Bilateral pulmonary stenosis

18. ECHO shows:

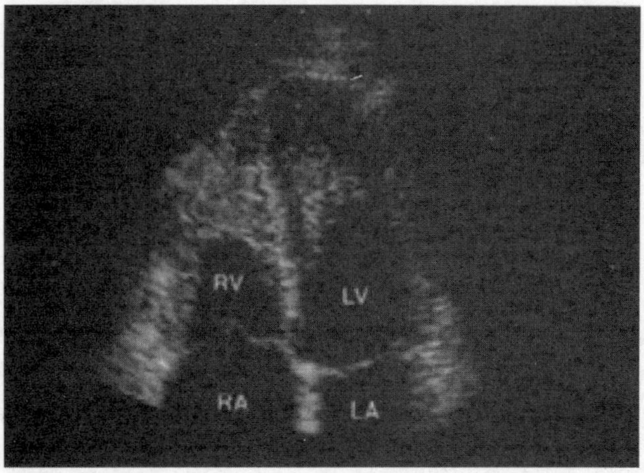

(a) Lymphoma (b) Thymoma
(c) Eosinophilia

19. A 14 years female with cyanosis, X-ray shows Rx is:

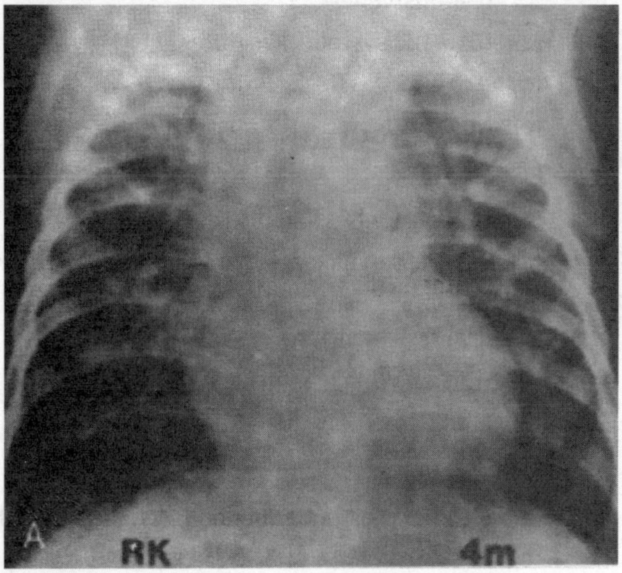

(a) Cardiac surgery (b) ICD
(c) Biopsy

20. LA hypertrophy A/E:

(a) P axis 0 to 60 (b) P axis –30 to –45
(c) VI depth ↑ (d) II-Notching

21. In TMT –A/E:

(a) Less false positive in male
(b) Baseline RBBB–C/I
(c) ST ↓ don't localize lesion
(d) Sensitivity and specificity ~ 60-70 and 70-80%

22. Aspirin A/E:

(a) Clopitab + warf < asp + warf for bleeding
(b) Decreased cancer in low dose
(c) DM > 45 years – given
(d) Primary prevention always useful

23. Nuclear scan shows–Rx is:

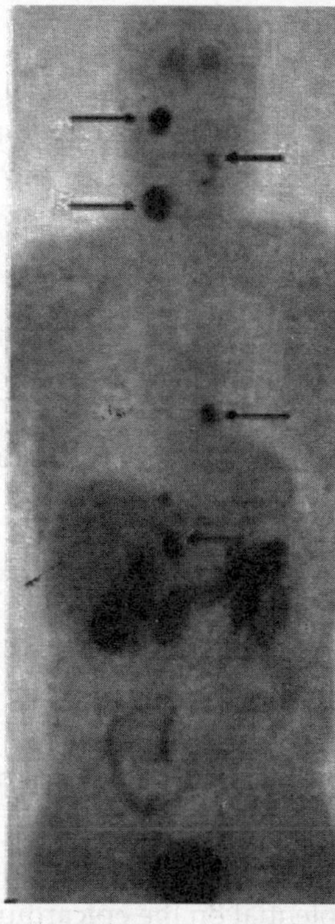

(a) Amlodipine + Spironolactone
(b) Prazocin + Propranolol
(c) Metoprolol + Spironolactone
(d) Enalapril + Spironolactone

24. Criteria for LVH A/E:

(a) Bazet (b) Cornell
(c) Romhilt–Estes (d) Talbot

25. True about TMT in presence of LBBB:

(a) Abnormal septal motion in LAD territory can occur in absence of ischemia
(b) Adenosine/dipyridamole can be used
(c) Specificity 33%
(d) Permanent LBBB seen in approx. 50% with transient LBBB

26. Contrast echo used in all *except*:

(a) VSD
(b) ASD
(c) Myocardial perfusion
(d) PFO

27. Himalayan 'P' waves:

(a) Ebstein's anomaly (b) TOF
(c) TGA (d) Bicuspid aortic valve

28. **Myocardial viability:**
(a) PET (b) MRI
(c) SPECT (d) Echo

29. **Low voltage QRS A/E:**
(a) Anemia (b) Obesity
(c) Extensive MI (d) Anasarca

30. **Hyperkalemia causes–all *except*:**
(a) Shortening of QT interval
(b) Shortening of PR interval
(c) ST elevation
(d) Tall peaked T waves

31. **Most sensitive technique to study early transplant vasculopathy:**
(a) IVTJS
(b) FFR
(c) Coronary angiography
(d) OCT

32. **Regarding 'J' wave on ECG–all are true *except*:**
(a) It has same polarity as the preceding QRS
(b) Its origin is corrected with a prominent notch in phase 2 of action potential on the epicardium
(c) Prominent J wave is a normal variant
(d) Prominent J wave is a feature of Brugada pattern

33. **Identify the wrong statement in LBBB:**
(a) Left axis deviation in LBBB suggests dilated cardiomyopathy
(b) LBBB can cause "false positive" reversible myocardial perfusion defects during exercise stress testing
(c) 10% of patients with LBBB have no clinically demonstrable heart disease
(d) LBBB is associated with higher risk of mortality

34. **Following is not a limitation for CT coronary angiography:**
(a) Atrial fibrillation
(b) Coronary bypass grafts
(c) BMI > 40 kg/M^2
(d) Coronary stents

35. **During myocardial perfusion imaging for CAD, specificity may be enhanced by:**
(a) Using thallium-201
(b) ECG gated SPECT imaging
(c) Exercise SPECT imaging
(d) Dipyridamole stress imaging

36. **The earliest ECG change with hyperkalemia is:**
(a) QRS complex widen
(b) Decrease in P wave amplitude
(c) Peaking of T waves
(d) Sine-wave pattern

37. **Thallium scan: (T/F)**
(a) Tc emit 80 kev photon
(b) Th. shorter half life than TC
(c) Early uptake is associated with rapid wash out from myocardium–normal
(d) Tetrofosmin minimal redistributed than thallium
(e) MPI graded in 0-5

38. **TMT: (T/F)**
(a) Symp. severe AS–can be done for risk stratification
(b) Cong. HB–required for assessment of rate responsiveness
(c) BP > 180 systolic–absolute C/I
(d) Acquired CHB–C/I for exercise
(e) Mission-Icon used for stress ECG

39. **ECG: (T/F)**
(a) PR segment–AV conduction
(b) Sgarbossa–max. point to concordant ST Elevation in V_5-V_6
(c) P-mitrale–amplitude > 2.5 in lead II
(d) Cornell voltage–S in V_1 and R in V_5
(e) LAHB–axis 0 to–30

40. **Echo: (T/F)**
(a) Normal diastolic function E/A > 1 E/E′ > 10
(b) Myocardial tissue velocity e′↓ in CCP
(c) Bernheim effect RV effect due to LVH
(d) PHT is useful in AR and MS
(e) Continuity equation for severity of AS

41. **Nyquist frequency: (T/F)**
(a) Intensity of brightness of color correlates with severity of velocity
(b) Nyquist frequency < 1/3 or CW
(c) PW Doppler frequency <Nyquist limit
(d) CW Doppler not related to Nyquist
(e) Strain rate–strain velocity (differ)

42. **ECG: (T/F)**
(a) Amplifier gain 5000
(b) Last area of LV activates inferobasal part of LA
(c) Anterobasal part of LV last activated

43. Which one of the following ECG patterns is not true for left anterior fascicular block?

(a) rS pattern in leads I and aVL
(b) qR pattern in lead aVL
(c) Time to peak r wave in aVL 45 msec
(d) Frontal plane mean QRS axis is 45 to 90 degrees

44. Which one of the following pressure half time of AR Doppler signal is suggestive of severe AR?

(a) > 800 ms (b) 400 to 800 ms
(c) 251 to 399 ms (d) < 250 ms

45. Inverted Mercedes Benz sign on echocardiography is used for following valve:

(a) Tricuspid (b) Aortic
(c) Pulmonary (d) Mitral

46. Which one of the following is more specific view to diagnose MVP?

(a) Short axis view
(b) Apical four chamber view
(c) Subcostal view
(d) Parasternal long axis view

47. To define severe AR, vena contraction echo should be more than:

(a) 0.5 cm (b) 0.4 cm
(c) 0.6 cm (d) 0.7 cm

48. Cross sectional area of normal mitral valve is:

(a) 1 to 2 cm square (b) 2 to 4 cm square
(c) 4 to 6 cm square (d) 6 to 8 cm square

49. Mechanism of balloon mitral valvuloplasty is:

(a) Chordal separation
(b) Commissural separation
(c) Leaflet stretch
(d) Papillary muscle separation

50. Which one of the following echo findings is suggestive of severe MR?

(a) Effective regurgitant orifice 0.40 cm square
(b) Vena contracts 0.30 cm
(c) Central jet MR area > 50% la area
(d) Regurgitant fraction 40%

51. Which of the following is the best echocardiographic view to diagnose coarctation of aorta?

(a) Suprasternal view
(b) Subcostal view
(c) Parasternal short axis view
(d) Parasternal long axis view

52. Which one of the following is not true for left posterior hemiblock in ECG?

(a) North west axis deviation (usually 120 degree)
(b) Small q in 2, 3 and aVF
(c) Increased QRS voltage in limb leads
(d) No evidence of right ventricular hypertrophy

53. Which one of the following is not true Osborn waves in ECG?

(a) It is seen in hypothermia
(b) It is an elevated j waves
(c) It represents distortion of the earliest stage of repolarisation
(d) QT interval shortens

54. Which one of the following is not true for ECG in hypokalemia?

(a) Depression of ST segment
(b) Prominent U wave
(c) P wave becomes small and narrow
(d) T wave becomes small or inverted

55. Which one of the following is not true for Sino ventricular rhythm in ECG?

(a) It is seen in hyperkalemia
(b) Absent P wave
(c) It is common after heart transplant
(d) Conduction between SA node and AV node persists

56. Which one of the following is true for electrical alternans in ECG?

(a) It is common in patients with cardiac tamponade
(b) It is ventricular bigeminy pattern
(c) It is atrial bigeminy pattern
(d) It is common in patients with rheumatic heart disease

57. Stage 6 of Bruce protocol is equivalent to:

(a) 15.8 METs (b) 16.5 METs
(c) 16.9 METs (d) 17.1 METs

58. Which one of the following is not true for echo finding in patients with severe diastolic dysfunction?

(a) E/A > 1.5
(b) Deceleration time of E wave > 220 msec
(c) E/e′ > 10
(d) e′ < 5 cm/sec

59. TAPSE (tricuspid annular plane systolic excursion) is determined by:

(a) M mode echo (b) 2 dimension echo
(c) 3 dimension echo (d) Doppler

60. If inferior vena cava diameter is <2.1 cm and show >50% collapse with inspiration, than estimated RA pressure is:

(a) 5 mm of Hg (b) 10 mm of Hg
(c) 15 mm of Hg (d) 20 mm of Hg

61. For dobutamine stress echo, maximum dose of dobutamine is used up to:

(a) 20 micogram/kg/minute
(b) 30 micogram/kg/minute
(c) 40 micogram/kg/minute
(d) 50 micogram/kg/minute

62. To assesses viability of myocardium following test is not useful:

(a) PET imaging
(b) MRI imaging
(c) Dobutamine stress echo
(d) Coronary angiography

63. Presence of ST elevation and Q waves in the ECG are markers of transmural infarction and necrosis. Select the false statement amongst the following:

(a) LBBB conduction abnormality may have Q wave not secondary to myocardial infarction
(b) Generally, an amplitude of Q wave more than 25% of R wave represents a necrosis Q wave
(c) Brugada syndrome and hypothermia may cause ST segment elevation in absence of ischemic heart disease
(d) In cases of inferior wall MI, ST segment elevation in lead III more than lead II is suggestive of occlusion of proximal left circumflex artery

64. SV3 + SaVL > 2.8 mV (for men) and 2.0 mV (for women) is a diagnostic criteria for diagnosing left ventricular hypertrophy. This ECG criteria is known as:

(a) Romhilt Estes score system
(b) Sokolow-Lyon Index
(c) Cornell voltage criteria
(d) None of the above

65. Mason Likar modification of standard 12 lead ECG requires that extremity electrodes be moved to torso to reduce motion artefact. This medication results in:

(a) New q waves in inferior leads
(b) Loss of q waves in aVL
(c) Right axis shift
(d) Decreased voltage in inferior leads

66. Regarding Duke TM score, choose the wrong statement:

(a) Calculated as exercise time – (5 × ST deviation) – (4 × TM angina index)
(b) TM score of –11 or less had a 5 years survival rate of 72%
(c) TM score of +5 or more had a 5 years survival rate of 97%
(d) Duke TM score is as effective in elderly more than 75 years of age as in young individuals

67. Incorrect about normal diastolic filling pattern:

(a) E/A > 1.5
(b) DT (septal) = 160-240 ms
(c) Ea > 10 cm/sec
(d) E/Ea > 8

68. Not true regarding the properties of SPECT tracers:

(a) Half-life of thallium–201 is 73 hours
(b) Differential washout is minimal for thallium–201 and Tc 99m teboroxime
(c) Half-life of Tc 99m sestamibi is 6 hours
(d) Uptake for thallium is active while that for technetium tracers is passive

69. Which is not perfusion tracer for cardiac imaging?

(a) Nitrogen–13 (b) Rubidium–82
(c) Fluorine–18 (d) Oxygen–15

70. Which of the following attenuation values is correct for non-contrast CT?

(a) Air: 0-10 (b) Bone: 1000
(c) Water: 3000 (d) Blood: 35-65

71. An ankle brachial index (ABI) >1.40 signifies what of the following?

(a) Stiff (calcified) arteries
(b) May be observed in the case of diabetes, ESRD, and in the very elderly
(c) A substantial proportion of patients with an elevated ABI actually do have occlusive artery disease
(d) All of the above

72. Severe tricuspid stenosis is diagnosed at a mean gradient of:

(a) > 2 mm Hg (b) > 5 mm Hg
(c) > 10 mm Hg (d) > 20 mm Hg

73. Echocardiographic criteria for severe AR includes all *except*:
(a) Effective regurgitant orifice area > 30 mm^2
(b) Vena contracta width > 3 mm
(c) Regurgitant volume > 60 ml/beat
(d) Pressure half time < 200 ms

74. Enhanced expiratory flow reversal in hepatic veins is a feature of:
(a) Constrictive pericarditis
(b) Restrictive cardiomyopathy
(c) Both
(d) None

75. ↑ flow across mitral valve I expiration A/E:
(a) Constrictive pericarditis
(b) Cardiac tamponade
(c) COPD
(d) Restrictive cardiomyopathy

76. SVT favored in:
(a) Fusion beat
(b) 2:1 Ventriculoatrial conduction
(c) RP < 100 m
(d) AV dissociation

77. Best for LV and RV–EF calculation:
(a) Thallium scan (b) MRI
(c) CT (d) MUGA

78. Critical ABI:
(a) ABI <0.9 (b) <1.2
(c) <0.3 (d) Pedal edema

79. 'Cabrera' sign is seen in:
(a) New MI I LBBB (b) Old MI I LBBB
(c) MI I RBBB (d) HOCM

80. Osborn waves seen in:
(a) Hypokalemia (b) Hypocalcemia
(c) Hypothermia (d) Hyponatremia

81. QT-interval response to exercise in long QT syndrome-I is:
(a) Normal QT during exercise but with exaggeration of QT-hysteresis
(b) Attenuated QTc shortening and an exaggerated QTc prolongation during early and peak exercise
(c) Supernormal QT-shortening
(d) No change in QT-interval

82. Which one of the following patient characteristics is ideal for performance of good quality coronary CT angiogram?
(a) Atrial fibrillation with a low ventricular response
(b) High body mass index
(c) Ability to breath hold for 2 seconds to 3 seconds maximum
(d) Ability to hold arms straight above the head

83. Which of the following is a normal response during exercise test on ECG?
(a) Horizontal ST depression
(b) Down sloping ST depression
(c) ST segment elevation
(d) Rapid up sloping ST depression

84. The weakest predictor of prognosis on exercise testing is:
(a) BP response (b) Exercise induce angina
(c) ST depression (d) Exercise capacity

85. Tei index for LV is:
(a) < 0.5 (b) < 0.4
(c) < 0.3 (d) < 0.1

86. False positive regional wall motion abnormality on 2D echo is seen in all *except*:
(a) Hypertensive response to stress
(b) Left circumflex disease
(c) Localized basal inferior wall abnormalities
(d) LBBB

87. The tracer used for ischemic-memory in patient with restored perfusion after ischemia:
(a) C^{11} palmitate
(b) C^{11} acetate
(c) F^{18} flurtage
(d) ^{123}I beta methyl iodide pentadecanoic acid (BMIPP)

88. The tracer approved by FDA for sympathetic innervations of heart:
(a) ^{99}TC sestamibi (b) $^{99}TCDTPA$
(c) ^{123}I MIBG (d) ^{123}I BMIP

89. Early repolarization is present if all of the following criteria are met *except*:

(a) There is an end-QRS notch or slur on the downslope of a prominent R-wave

(b) If there is a notch, it should lie entirely above the baseline. The onset of a slur must also be above the baseline

(c) J peak is > 0.1 mV in 2 or more contiguous leads of the 12-lead ECG, excluding leads V_1 to V_3

(d) QRS duration is > 120 ms

90. Which of the following statements regarding the transcranial Doppler is not true?

(a) It is useful for diagnosis of acute occlusion of middle cerebral artery

(b) Valsalva maneuver helps in detection of patent foramen ovale on transcranial Doppler

(c) Transcranial Doppler studies can differentiate between a shunt at atrial, ventricular and pulmonary level

(d) Transcranial Doppler with contrast has a greater sensitivity than transthoracic echocardiography with contrast at identifying PFO

91. Maximum HR on b-blocker by EST in 60 years old:

(a) 160 (b) 112

(c) 166 (d) 180

92. Asymptomatic patient as per ACC/AHA level for coronary calcium score:

(a) I (b) IIa

(c) IIb (d) III

93. Most cost effective clinically useful for PVD?

(a) Doppler (b) ABI

(c) Angiography

94. Thallium acts by:

(a) Redistribution

(b) Mitochondrial metabolism

(c) Glucose metabolism

95. ECHO in MR → False:

(a) Eccentric jet underestimates severity

(b) Vena contracta > 6 mm

(c) 3D Echo can be used to measure regurgitant orifice area

96. Tei Index:

(a) $\frac{ICT+IRT}{ET}$ (b) $\frac{ET+JRT}{JIT}$

(c) $\frac{JCT+ET}{JRT}$

97. Einthoven law:

(a) I + III = II (b) I+II=III

(c) I+II+III=I

98. >10 METs can do:

(a) Walh at 4 mph (b) Doubles Tennis

(c) Swimming (d) Sweeping floor

99. Coronary calcium score in asymptomatic patient for CAD risk assessment:

(a) I (b) IIa

(c) IIb (d) III

100. ECG abnormality in Atrial enlargement A/E:

(a) P wave duration > 0.12 sec in LA enlargement

(b) ECG more specific than sensitive for atrial enlargement

(c) P wave abnormality does not lead to QRS changes

(d) P wave has RAD in RA enlargement

101. True about J-point elevation A/E:

(a) Upper limit of normal value, 0.1 mm < 40 year

(b) Predispose to VF

(c) Same polarity of QRS

(d) Signifies notch in phase 1

102. Pulmonary vein systolic wave (S wave) decreased in A/E:

(a) Severe MR (b) AF

(c) CCP (d) Pulm vein stenosis

103. Myocardial imaging true A/E:

(a) Free gadolinium ions causes fibrosis

(b) Gadolinium has first pass metabolism time of 10 mins

(c) MRA images acquired in phase 1

(d) Allergic reaction to gadolinium incidence <1%

104. True about hibernating myocardium:

(a) Myocardial O_2 demand is reduced

(b) Abnormal response

(c) Decreased in myocardial cell volume, preservation of contractile protein

(d) SPECT thallium investigation of choice for detection

105. Elderly-confusion:

(a) Holterstudy (b) ICD

(c) Pacemaker (d) PCI

106. Tall R in V1 A/E:

(a) DMD (b) HOCM
(c) RBBB (d) WPW right sided

107. Hypermagnesium all *except:*

(a) Hypercalcemia (b) CHB
(c) CKD (d) ↓ tendon reflexes

108. ECG regarding limb leads all *except:*

(a) Lead I–LA and RA
(b) Lead II–left foot and left arm
(c) Lead III–left foot and right arm
(d) Lead III–lead I + lead II voltage amplitude

109. TID all true *except:*

(a) Suggests intense myocardial damage
(b) May can be seen after several hours
(c) Corelates with ↑ lung uptakes
(d) LV preexercise/post exercise diameter > 1.22

110. MRI least useful in diagnosing:

(a) Acute myocarditis (b) CTE-PAH
(c) Ebstein's anomaly (d) Amyloidosis

111. RAE finding on ECG all *except:*

(a) P wave in II > 0.25 mV
(b) P wave amplitude duration ratio > 1.6
(c) qR in right precordial lead in absence of MI
(d) P wave initial phase > 0.15 seen in V1

112. Drug used in pharmacological stress testing *except:*

(a) Adenosine (b) Dipyridamole
(c) Aminophylline (d) Regadenoson

113. Dyspnoea indication of cardiac disease in TMT *except:*

(a) FEVI unchanged
(b) Vmax > 80% of predicted
(c) Sat O_2 > 90%
(d) CO ↓ ed

114. Poor prognosis in SPECT all *except:*

(a) LV dilatation
(b) ↑ Lung uptake
(c) Diffusion homogenous myocardial uptake
(d) Summation score high

115. Mismatch:

(a) Th-sarcoplasmic memb
(b) Tc mitochondrial integrity
(c) Tissue Doppler-tissue characteristic
(d) Contrast echo-micro vascular integrity

116. RV function best investigation of choice:

(a) MRI (b) PET
(c) CT angio (d) 3D echo

117. Myocardial contrast echo:

(a) Agitated saline (b) Perfluoro carbon
(c) Gadolinium (d) Liposomal iodine

118. TEE better than TTE all *except:*

(a) Aortic dissection
(b) Acute MI
(c) MR to know cause etiology
(d) Before elective cardioversion

119. ECG findings in SAH:

(a) Hypokalemia (b) T wave ↓
(c) Osborn wave (d) Prolonged TdP

120. TR velocity > 4 m/sec, all *except:*

(a) TOF (b) PS
(c) PPH (d) MS with PAH

121. TMT all *except:*

(a) In asymptomatic routinely
(b) Diabetic before exercise programming
(c) First line non-invasive test for female
(d) Can be done 7 days after MI for risk stratification

122. All about echo *except:*

(a) Pulmonary vein flow systole > diastole
(b) Hepatic vein flow systole > diastole
(c) Mitral valve flow– E>A
(d) Tricuspid valve flow–A > E on TDI

123. All *except:*

(a) U wave inversion specific for LAD (Prox)
(b) T Pseudonormalization doesn't occur in absence of CAD
(c) Upsloping of ST may be due to atrial repolarisation
(d) ST ↑ in Q wave indicates severe ischemia

124. All about ECG *except:*

(a) P wave upright in II, III, aVF in situs inversus
(b) Shorter PR in infants
(c) Upper limit of QU in 460 msec
(d) QT measured best in V_2–V_4

125. All *except*:

(a) Q wave in LBBB in V_5–V_6 ↑ septal infarction
(b) VPC of qR indicative of MI (other than V_1 and aVR)
(c) Thrombolysis not effective if Q wave develops in AMI
(d) Q wave can occur in amyloidosis

126. Dart and dome 'P' wave seen in:

(a) LA (b) RA
(c) Sinus rhythm (d) Junctional rythym

127. Epsilon wave seen in:

(a) ARVD (b) CPVT
(c) Brugada syndrome (d) Digitoxicity

128. Mason likar modification:

(a) Non Q wave in avL
(b) Disappearance of Q in inferior leads
(c) ↑sed voltage in inferior leads
(d) LAD

129. May Turner syndrome:

(a) Subclavian vein–subclavian artery compression
(b) Iliac vein–Iliac artery compression
(c) Aberrent subclavian artery compression by esophagus
(d) Vertebral erosion in aortic aneurysm

130. TEE long axis view:

(a) 180° (b) 45°
(c) 135° (d) 270°

131. ↑ ed frequency of Doppler:

(a) ↑ed resolution, ↓ed penetration
(b) ↓ed - resolution, ↑ed - penetration
(c) ↓ed - resolution, ↓ed - penetration

132. Maximum heart rate:

(a) 220–age
(b) 110+age
(c) 200–age

133. Most accurate gold standard for myocardial viability:

(a) SPECT
(b) PET
(c) Dobutamine echocardiography
(d) MRI

134. Himalayan 'P' waves:

(a) Ebstein's syndrome
(b) Eisenmenger's syndrome
(c) Pericardial effusion

135. RVH most specific criteria:

(a) R/S > 1 in is (b) SI QIII T3
(c) RAD > 90°

136. LVH criteria A/E:

(a) Cornell (b) Romhilt Estes
(c) Sokolow-lyon (d) Bazett's criteria

137. Reverse split S_2:

(a) RBBB (b) LBBB
(c) MR (d) LV pacing

138. On TMT good (best) predictor of survival:

(a) SBP × HR >24000
(b) MET > 13
(c) Absence of ST depression

139. PR interval alternans seen in:

(a) Dual A-V node pathway
(b) AVRT
(c) Pulmonary embolism

140. MRI C/I in all *except*:

(a) Electronic pump infusion
(b) Cochlear implant
(c) Neurovascular clips
(d) Prosthetic implants

141. Pulmonary flow velocity 120 cm/sec and acceleration time 60 sec. What is PASP?

(a) 40 (b) 50
(c) 60 (d) 70

142. Class 1 indication for Holter monitoring (ambulatory):

(a) Routine post MI
(b) Silent ischemia
(c) Malfunction pacemaker
(d) Vasovagal syncope

143. Maximum conduction velocity seen in:

(a) SA Node (b) AV Node
(c) Purkinje fibre (d) Ventricle

144. Mason Likar modification is:
(a) LAD
(b) Q in aVL
(c) Q in inferior lead
(d) Decrease in inferior lead

145. Atrial infarction all *except*:
(a) More in RA
(b) <20% cases
(c) Atrial arrhythmias uncommon
(d) Atrial rupture can occur

146. Purkinje fibre–True:
(a) Less resistant to ischemia
(b) Innervates inner 2/3rd of endocardium
(c) More in papillary muscle tip
(d) More rapid repolarisation time

147. Thallium sensitivity and specificity for CAD:
(a) 90, 90 (b) 95, 95
(c) 90, 70 (d) 80, 50

148. PET:
(a) Stunned and hibernating differentiation
(b) Calcium score
(c) Plaque

149. Calcium level correlate with:
(a) QT
(b) QaT
(c) Q wave to peak of T wave
(d) PR

150. Mason likar modification:
(a) Decrease QRS in inferior leads
(b) Absent Q wave in inferior leads
(c) Absent Q wave in aVL
(d) LAD

151. Supernormal conduction:
(a) Conduction with sub threshold
(b) May be seen with normal myocardium
(c) Seen with relative refractory period
(d) With depressed conduction

152. Negative S in V1 & inferior Leads which pathway?
(a) Right postero septal (b) Right free wall
(c) Left postero septal (d) Right anteroseptal

153. Fastest conduction of APD:
(a) Sinus atrial node (b) AV node
(c) Purkinje fiber (d) His Bundle

154. True about EAD:
(a) ↑ by EAD
(b) ↓ by catecholamine
(c) ↑ by large cycle length

155. Doppler peak velocity of PR is indicative of:
(a) PASP (b) PADP
(c) RVSP

156. BP measurement invention:
(a) Riva Rocci (b) Stephen Hales
(c) Laennac

157. ECG invented by:
(a) Einthoven (b) Stephen Hales

158. Primordial prevention applies to:
(a) Development of risk factor
(b) Community with low prevalence
(c) 1st relatives of CAD patients

159. Irreversible thallium scan, which indicates hibernating myocardium:
(a) Redistribution (b) Cold spot
(c) Hot spot

160. TEE is used in diagnosis of:
(a) LA thrombosis (b) LA myxoma
(c) PV endocarditis (d) All

161. Pulsus paradoxsus not seen in:
(a) PTE
(b) Cardiac tamponade + IPPV
(c) Br. Asthma
(d) Shock

162. In TMT impaired LV function indicated by:
(a) Failure to rise BP (b) Failure to rise HR
(c) NSVT

163. Contrast echo:
(a) Useful in left to right shunt
(b) Useful in right to left shunt
(c) Both
(d) None

164. Normal Echo Doppler pattern on mitral valve:
(a) M pattern seen (b) E/A < 1
(c) DT–150-220 ms

165. EPSS normal:
(a) < 6 mm (b) < 10 mm

166. EFSLP normal:
(a) < 15 (b) 20-30
(c) 30-50

167. Normal PVR:
(a) 20-250 (b) 800-1600

168. Radiation in CXR:
(a) 0.1 rad (b) 0.3 rad
(c) 0.5 rad (d) 1 rad

169. Radiation causes A/E:
(a) Valvular stenosis
(b) CAD
(c) AV conduction disturbances
(d) Myocarditis

170. TMT–which of the following does not show poor prognosis?
(a) 1 mm ST deviation (b) Ventricular ectopic
(c) NSVT (d) Hypotension

171. In PSAX which is not seen:
(a) ASD (b) Coronary artery
(c) LV (d) Pulmonary artery

172. Eccentric hypertrophy classical seen in:
(a) AR (b) AS
(c) HOCM

173. Myocardial viability best by:
(a) PET (b) Thallium

174. Hyperkalemia changes in ECG A/E:
(a) Loss of 'p' wave (b) Tall T wave
(c) Sine wave pattern (d) QT prolongation

175. Stress test–all are indicator of pulmonary involvement *except:*
(a) Failure to achieve expected saturation
(b) No ECG ST changes
(c) Failure of THR achievement
(d) Dyspnea without chest pain

176. LVH: S in I + R in III–true:
(a) 10 mm (b) 25 mm
(c) 5 mm (d) None of above

177. MRI used for A/E:
(a) LVEF
(b) Myocardial tissue imaging
(c) Coronary stenosis

178. OCT detects A/E:
(a) Plaque composition
(b) Thrombus
(c) Transplant vasculopathy

179. IVUS for A/E:
(a) Plaque burden
(b) To access stent size for lesion
(c) Intracoronary drug delivery
(d) Coronary stenosis

180. Hyperkalemia: (T/F)
(a) Decreased QT
(b) PR prolonged
(c) Decreased J point
(d) Narrow based large T wave

181. qR in V1: (T/F)
(a) LA abnormality (b) RA abnormality
(c) Accurate in AF (d) 99% specificity

182. HUTT all *except:*
(a) > 90% reproducibility
(b) 60-80% at 20-45°
(c) 10-15% false positive
(d) β blocker ↓ hypotensive response

183. QT true all *except:*
(a) From origin of QRS to onset of T wave
(b) Represent total ventricular activity
(c) More in female

184. U wave:
(a) Normal < 0.1 mm
(b) Mid precordial leads
(c) Polarity same as preceding T wave
(d) Seen in hypokalemia

185. Gold standard of viability:
(a) PET (b) SPECT
(c) MRI (d) Dobutamine
(e) 3D Echo

186. Functional assessment by all *except:*
(a) CT angio (b) Dobutamine stress
(c) SPECT (d) MRI
(e) FFR

187. U wave all *except:*
(a) Prominent in mid precordial lead
(b) Polarity same as preceding T wave
(c) Prominent in hypokalemia
(d) Prominent in slow HR
(e) Amplitude usually < 0.1

188. Noninfarction Q wave:
(a) Hyperkalemia (b) LBBB
(c) WPW (d) Dextrocardia
(e) All of the above

189. Non coronary cause of ST↓ all *except:*
(a) Glucose load (b) ↑ ICT
(c) Hypoxia (d) Hypotension
(e) Kawasaki

190. Absolute C/I of TMT:
(a) High risk USA
(b) MI < 7 days
(c) High degree AV block
(d) Acute pulmonary edema
(e) Systemic illness (fever)

191. High risk for TMT all *except:*
(a) ST ↑ in AVR
(b) Attain < 4 MET
(c) BP < 120 mm Hg or > 10 mm Hg fall
(d) Angina pectoris at any stage
(e) ST ↓ ≥ 5 mm/Persist ≥ 5 min of recovery

192. Paradoxical split S_2: (T/F)
(a) Complete RBBB (b) LV ischemia
(c) RVapex pacing (d) AS
(e) HOCM

193. Severe TR all *except:*
(a) Vene contracta > 6.5
(b) Regurgitation volume > 45 ml
(c) Doppler width >30% in RA
(d) Annulus > 4 cm
(e) ERO > 0.6 cm

194. False statements:
(a) qR in V_1 transition to S in V_6
(b) Ta has inverse polarity to P wave
(c) Septal q wave in inferior leads

195. Most specific inertia of RVH:
(a) R/S > 1, R>0.5 msec in V_1
(b) S1 Q3 (c) RAD
(d) r in V_6 > 7 (e) s in V_6

196. Pseudoinfarct pattern in: (T/F)
(a) WPW (b) LBBB
(c) HCM (d) PWMI
(e) Cerebral thrombosis

197. LBBB with stress testing: (T/F)
(a) Adenosine/Dipyridamole can be used
(b) At ↑ ed HR produces defects in septal area in LAD territory
(c) Specificity 33% with adenosine

198. Contrast echo not useful:
(a) ASD (b) RSOV
(c) VSD (d) Myocardial perfusion
(e) PFO

199. Gold standard for viability:
(a) SPECT (b) MRI
(c) PET (d) None

200. Electromagnetic interference seen in all *except:*
(a) MRI (b) USG
(c) RFA (d) Therapeutic radiation

201. Low amplitude ECG all *except:*
(a) Anemia (b) Chest thick
(c) Anasarca (d) Adrenal insufficiency
(e) Extensive MI

202. RBBB type VT: (T/F)
(a) qR and qS in V_6 (b) Axis 60 to 90
(c) rSr in V_1 (d) QRS in V_1

203. ST/HR slope: (T/F)
(a) < 2.6 abnormal
(b) Cornell needed
(c) Bruce may be used
(d) ST/HR index has low cutoff
(e) Indicate post infarction prognosis

204. Normal pericardial thickness upper reference in MRI:
(a) 1 mm (b) 2 mm
(c) 3 mm (d) 4 mm

205. 15 years girl with recurrent syncope underwent HUTT shows asystole for 12 sec followed by: Polymorphic VT. ECG, echo, Holter–Normal:

(a) ICD for VT
(b) Fluids saline, exercise training advice
(c) Treatment to be decided after MRI
(d) HUTT may be false positive

206. Patient with infrequent syncope. 1 episode in 1 years inv. With prodrome without injury:

(a) Holter
(b) Implantable loop recorder
(c) Event recorder

207. ECG repeat in patient with suspected MI and normal ECG:

(a) 5-10 min (b) 30 min
(c) 1 hour

208. Exercise tolerance true:

(a) Upsloping ST depression is +ve sign
(b) Intensity and extent of ST depression related to severity of exercise
(c) TMT less accurate/predictive in women

209. Phase 4 depolarisation:

(a) If (b) Na
(c) K (d) Ca-T
(e) Ca-L

210. Strain velocity and strain rate used in:

(a) Echo (b) MRI
(c) Invasive evaluation

211. True about U waves:

(a) Inverted U wave in a normal ECG is abnormal
(b) Inverted U wave is seen in hypertension

212. Resting membrane potential is due to which current?

(a) I Na (b) I Ca
(c) $I K_1$ (d) $I K_R$

213. Screening method used for coronary calcification is:

(a) MRI (b) EBCT
(c) Fluroscopy (d) Coronary angiography

214. Smoker developed dyspnoea, investigations to rule out IPF:

(a) HRCT (b) Biopsy
(c) PFT (d) CXR

215. Infant with LVH, least dangerous:

(a) Pompe's disease
(b) Infant of diabetic mother

216. True A/E:

(a) Late enhancement of scar in MRI
(b) Re-injection of thallium in hibernating myocardium
(c) Dobutamine stress echo in hibernating myocardium
(d) Akinetic segment no benefit after revascularization

217. All are true *except:*

(a) TIA can have infarct on CT
(b) Infarct constitute 50% of stroke
(c) Syncope is unusual presentation of TIA

218. Investigation used for assessment of myocardial viability after MI *except:*

(a) MRI
(b) Dobutamine stress echo
(c) Stress thallium
(d) TMT

219. Cardic MRI is very useful in assessment of all of the following *except*:

(a) Myocardial viability
(b) Ebstein's anomaly
(c) Periphiral pulmonary ARTERIAL stenosis
(d) Myocarditis

220. Which one of the following indicates abnormal RV systolic function in echocardiography?

(a) TAPSE > 1.6 cm
(b) Pulse Doppler peak velocity at annulus > 10 cm/sec
(c) Tissue Doppler MPI <0.53
(d) Fractional area change <35

221. All of the following findings on non-invasive testing indicate a high risk for death or MI *except*:

(a) Exercise induced ST segment elevation
(b) Resting perfusion defect involving 70% of myocardium
(c) A drop of > 10% of LVEF with exercise
(d) CAC score > 400 Agatston units

222. The OCT picture shows:

(a) Thrombus and plague repture
(b) Subacute stent thrombosis
(c) Flushing artifact
(d) In-stent restenosis

223. Most common short RP tachycardia is:

(a) AVRT (b) Atypical AVNRT
(c) Typical AVNRT (d) None of the above

224. Following ECG changes are give a score of 3 in Romhilt Estes criteria *except*:

(a) R or S in limb leads >–20 mm
(b) S in V1-V2 >–30 mm
(c) Left atrial abnormality
(d) Left axis deviation of >–30 degrees

225. All can be used for myocardial viability estimation in normal regular sinus rhythm *except*:

(a) Left ventricular angiography
(b) Contrast enhanced cardiac MRI
(c) Dobutamine stress echocardiography
(d) Thallium Perfusion scan

226. The presence of Pseudo r in VI suggests:

(a) Posterior MI
(b) Type 1 WPW
(c) AV Nodal reentry Tachycardia
(d) Ventricular tachycardia

227. The duration of the QRS is:

(a) Longer in the precordial leads
(b) Is equal in the limb and precordial leads
(c) More than 0.16 sees in Orthodromic aVRT
(d) Is less than 0.08 sees in Incomplete RBBB

228. Diagnosis of LAHB in Inferior MI can be made by:

(a) The QRS axis more than minus 60 degrees
(b) Absent of a terminal r in aVR
(c) Presence of a terminal r in inferior leads
(d) ST ELEVATION in aVR

229. In Sgarbossa's criteria maximum points are given to:

(a) Concordant ST elevation
(b) Discordant ST elevation
(c) Discordant ST depression
(d) Concordant ST depression

230. All are Methods to calculate QTc *except*:

(a) Bazett's formula
(b) FRIDERICIA'S formula
(c) Goodwin's formula
(d) Framingham formula

231. Uncomplicated LBBB may have all these findings *except*:

(a) Q in L2 (b) Q in AVF
(c) Q in VI (d) Q in V6

232. TAPSE used in A/E:

(a) LV function (b) Pulmonary embolism
(c) TR (d) RV dysfunction

233. FFR true is:

(a) Specific index for epicardial stenosis
(b) 0.9–signifies functional severe stenosis
(c) Dopamine used
(d) Variation due to SBP and HR

234. OCT true is:

(a) Normal saline used for flush
(b) It is very good for adventitia
(c) Useful for ostial lesion
(d) Useful for bioabsorable vascular stent

235. OCT used for:

(a) Intima (b) External elastic lamina
(c) Adventitia (d) Media

236. Duke's criteria in TMT A/E:

(a) ST depression (b) Angina
(c) Exercise duration (d) Double product

237. LAHB true is:

(a) qR in avL
(b) QRS > 120 msec
(c) q wave in II, III and avF
(d) RAD

238. Large a wave on M mode echo on pulmonary valve:

(a) PAH (b) PS
(c) TR (d) MS

239. Half life of thallium:

(a) 73 hours (b) 20 hours
(c) 10 days (d) 15 min

240. LVH: SV1 + RV5 > 35:

(a) Sokolow lyon (b) Cornell voltage
(c) Romhilt estes criteria (d) Cornell regression

241. Adverse factors in exercise testing A/E:

(a) Upsloping ST segment

(b) Flat ST depression
(c) Ventricular arrhythmias
(d) ST elevation

242. ST segment alternans A/E:
(a) Variant angina (b) TMT
(c) SAH (d) Digoxin toxicity

243. True statement is:
(a) Phase 0 upstroke of ventricular myocardium is due to Na
(b) Phase 0 upstroke of purkinje fibre is due to Na
(c) Phase 0 upstroke of SA node due to Na
(d) Plateau phase due to Na

244. ST alternans seen in all *except*:
(a) TMT (b) SAH
(c) Variant angina (d) LQTS

245. Prominent R wave in V1:
(a) RBBB
(b) Left accessory pathway
(c) Right accessory pathway
(d) Posterior wall MI

246. CT index true A/E:
(a) Adults upto 40% normal
(b) Neonates upto 60% normal
(c) 1-24 months upto 50% normal
(d) Neonates upto 70% normal

247. Severity of stress thallium A/E:
(a) Diffuse homogenous uptake suggest severe ischemia
(b) LV dilatation suggest severe ischemia
(c) LBBB is associated with severe CAD
(d) Adenosine is often used for pharmacological stress test

248. Increased QT A/E:
(a) Hypermagnesium (b) Hypomagnesium
(c) Hypocalcemia (d) Hypokalemia

249. Angiographic assessment of AVA:
(a) Continuity equation (b) Gorlin formula
(c) Counard (d) Starr equation

250. HUTT at 10 min asystole with BP < 60 mm Hg, which type of response response?
(a) Mixed type (b) Cardioinhibitory 2a
(c) Cardioinhibitory 2b (d) Vasodepressor

251. Continuity equation is for:
(a) Stenotic lesion (b) Regurgitant lesion
(c) Mixed

252. Optical coherence tomography can detect A/E:
(a) Macrophage (b) Lipid core
(c) Fibrous cap (d) Thrombus

253. 3D-ECHO *except:*
(a) No geometrical assumption
(b) Better in AF patients
(c) To diagnose dyssynchrony for CRT suitability
(d) LV volume, mass and EF correlate with MRI

254. LVH criteria, most sensitive:
(a) Cornel's voltage
(b) Sokolo–lyon criteria
(c) Novocode–regression
(d) Tolbot

255. Pressure ½ time, T ½ - 110 msec. MVA is:
(a) 2 (b) 1
(c) 15 (d) 0.5

256. P wave alternans:
(a) PTE
(b) AVRT
(c) Right pneumothorax
(d) Digoxin toxicity

257. 5 years survival in Duke's treadmill (-11) mortality:
(a) 13% (b) 97%
(c) 72% (d) 32%

258. CXR–Lateral view, border not formed:
(a) RA Appendage (b) LA
(c) RV (d) Aorta

259. PET–Metabolic tracer:
(a) F_{18} (b) O_{15}
(c) N_2 (d) Rubidium

260. Cardiac MRI A/E:
(a) Differential diagnosis of MI
(b) For systolic dysfunction

(c) Accurate estimation of coronary stenosis
(d) Myocardial viability

261. CT angiography:
(a) Increased positive predictive valve
(b) Increased negative predictive valve
(c) Accurate diagosis of CABG graft
(d) Over estimate of coronary stenosis

262. Reverse redistribution on thallium:
(a) CAD (b) Amyloidosis
(c) Sarcoidosis (d) Fabry's

263. C/I of TMT all *except:*
(a) M1 > 5 days (b) Advanced HB
(c) Symptomatic AS (d) Uncontrolled HTN

264. Myocardial viability all *except:*
(a) Contrast echo (b) PET
(c) Stress echo (d) TDI

265. TMT to be done in:
(a) MI (<5 days)
(b) Evaluation of CAD in valvular HD
(c) Routine evaluation of asymptomatic young
(d) Routine evaluation of post PCI

266. False negative ABI in all *except:*
(a) PVD of upper limb
(b) Calcific and non-compressible AS
(c) Small cuff
(d) HTN LVF

267. All are non-coronary causes of ST depression during TMT *except:*
(a) WPW syndrome (b) Glucose overload
(c) Excessive exercise (d) Long QT syndrome

268. Echo finding in patients of MS is:
(a) Anterior motion of the posterior leaflet
(b) Posterior motion of the posterior leaflet
(c) Immobile posterior leaflet
(d) Anterior motion of the anterior leaflet

269. Which of the following investigation is most sensitive and specific for myocardial viability test?
(a) Treadmill test
(b) Doppler echocardiography
(c) SPECT scan
(d) PET scan

270. U wave is seen in all *except:*
(a) AR (b) CAD
(c) Hypothermia (d) Hypokalemia

271. All are true about TMT *except:*
(a) SVT is relative indication to stop
(b) 2/4 angina is absolute indication to stop
(c) Sinosis and pallor is absolute indication to stop
(d) Inability to measure BP is an absolute indication to stop

272. All are absolute indication to stop the TMT *except:*
(a) Hypertensive response
(b) Patient desire to stop
(c) Ataxia and palor
(d) Sustained VT

273. Agitated saline useful in A/E:
(a) Persistent left SVC
(b) PFO
(c) Intrapulmonary shunt
(d) Coronary AV fistula

274. True about grade 3 diastolic dysfunction A/E:
(a) Pseudonormalization
(b) DT < 160 msec
(c) Ea < 7
(d) ↑ ed LV filling pressures

275. Hyperkalemia ECG A/E:
(a) Peaked tall T waves (b) Sine wave pattern
(c) Absent P wave (d) U wave

276. Earliest sign in ECG hyperkalemia:
(a) Tall and tented T waves
(b) PR prolongation
(c) Sinusoidal QRS wave

277. RVH + RBBB:
(a) R in V1 > 7 mm (b) 10 mm
(c) 15 mm (d) R/S > 1 + RV1 > 5 mm

278. Lewis lead used for:
(a) ↑ atrial amplitude
(b) SA–ECG
(c) Ventricular contour
(d) ↑ ventricular amplitude

279. Thallium physiology is similar to:

(a) Na (b) Ca

(c) K

280. Ideal HR for cardiac CT:

(a) 60 (b) 70

(c) 80 (d) 75

281. TMT relative indication to terminate A/E:

(a) SVT (b) Fatigue

(c) Patient desire to stop (d) HTN response

282. QT dispersion associated with:

(a) Bazzett's formula (b) Risk of VT

283. Diastolic properties on echo suggested by A/E:

(a) –dp/dt

(b) Tau index

(c) Peak rate of LV thinning

(d) IVRT

284. Following is not a limitation of cardiac MRI:

(a) Need for iodinated contrast agents

(b) Risk of developing nephrogenic systemic fibrosis (NSF) in patients with renal disease receiving gadolinium

(c) Significant arrhythmias

(d) Cerebral aneurysm clips

285. In which of the following clinical scenario, ST depression during TMT increases diagnostic probability of significant CAD?

(a) 65 years old diabetic female with recent onset exertional dyspnea and normal LV function

(b) 45 years old premenopausal women with atypical chest pain

(c) 60 years old male with HTN, angina and LVH on ECG

(d) 55 years old male diabetic with pre-excitation

286. The ECG finding in acute pericarditis:

(a) ST depression

(b) PR segment elevation

(c) PR segment depression

(d) Bundle branch block

287. LBBB is a marker of one of the 4 underlying conditions, associated with increased risk of cardiovascular mortality and morbidity. Among the options given below, which one is not true?

(a) CAD with LV dysfunction

(b) Hypertensive heart disease

(c) Arrhythmogenic right ventricular dysplasia

(d) Aortic valve disease

288. Identify the correct statement regarding metabolic and drug effects on ECG:

(a) Digitalis glycosides prolong QT interval

(b) Hypercalcemia shortens QT interval

(c) Prominent 'U' waves are a feature of Hyper-Kelmia

(d) "Sino ventricular rhythm" may be seen in hypokalemia

289. Regarding CT coronary angiogram, all are true *except:*

(a) It has a sensitivity and specificity of >90% for detecting CAD

(b) Heavy calcification and artifacts from stents preclude accurate assessment of severity of stenosis

(c) It has highest accuracy for RCA

(d) Atrial fibrillation with fast ventricular rate limits accuracy

290. Regarding echo true is:

(a) In adults transducer frequency used is 8-10 MHz

(b) In color Doppler, blue is blood flow away from transducer

(c) In color Doppler red is blood flow away from transducer

(d) In children transducer frequency used is 10-20 MHz

291. In Mason-likar modification, all are true *except:*

(a) Q waves appears in aVL

(b) Voltage increases in inferior leads

(c) Absent q waves in inferior

(d) There is left axis deviation

292. Left bundle branch block is indicative of which of the following sets of conditions?

(a) Atrial septal defect, coronary heart disease, aortic valve disease

(b) Coronary heart disease, aortic valve disease, hypertensive heart disease

(c) Coronary heart disease, aortic valve disease, pulmonary hypertension

(d) Pulmonary embolism, cardiomyopathy, hypertensive heart disease

293. Diagnostic criteria commonly used to diagnose right atrial abnormality include all *except:*

(a) Peaked P waves with amplitude in lead II > 0.25 mv (P pulmonale)

(b) Prominent notching of the P wave, usually most in lead II, with an interval of >40 between the notches (P mitrale)

(c) Rightward shift of the mean P wave axis to above +75 degrees

(d) Increased area under the initial positive portion of the P wave in lead V1 to > 0.06 mm sec

294. TMT is used in all *except:*

(a) Diagnosis of unstable angina

(b) Post CABG

(c) Males with atypical symptoms

(d) Post MI with Stent implantation

295. According ACC/AHA guidelines: Absolute contraindication to exercise testing include all *except:*

(a) Acute myocardial infarction (within 2 days)

(b) Left main coronary stenosis

(c) High risk unstable angina

(d) Symptomatic severe aortic stenosis

296. MI in presence of LBBB is Diagnosed by all *except:*

(a) > 3 mm ST elevation in V_1 V_2

(b) q wave in I, avL, V_5 V_6

(c) Slurring upstroke in V_3 V_4

(d) Primary ST-T changes in V_5 V_6

297. Romhilt-Estes point score system of 3 points common diagnostic criteria for left ventricular hypertrophy include all *except:*

(a) Any limb lead R wave or S wave ≥ 2.0 mV

(b) SV1 or SV2 ≥ mV

(c) RV5 to RV6 ≥ 3.0 mV

(d) Intrinsicoid deflection in V_5 or V_6 > 50 m.sec

298. Regarding Echo following is true:

(a) In adults transducer frequency used is 8–10 MHz

(b) In colour Doppler, red is blood flow away from transducer

(c) In color Doppler red is blood flow away from transducer

(d) In children transducer frequency is 10–20 MHz

299. TMT:

(a) RBBB decreases sensitivity

(b) Digoxin can induce ST-T changes even with normal resting ECG

(c) ST depression in I, aVL, diagonal disease

(d) Hypotension increases severity risk

(e) ECG changes in preexcitation are not interpretable

300. According to ACC/AHA Guidelines: Absolute indications for terminating exercise testing include all *except:*

(a) Moderate to severe angina

(b) Fatigue, shortness of breath, wheezing, leg cramps, or claudication

(c) Sustained ventricular tachycardia

(d) Subject's desire to stop

301. Highly specific for IW hypertrophy in a neonate:

(a) Tall 'R' with inverted waves in VI beyond first week of life

(b) Deep 'S' with upright 'T' waves in VI within 7 days of life

(c) Tall 'R' waves with upright 'T' waves in VI beyond first week of life

(d) Tall 'R' waves with upright 'T'· waves in the VI at birth

302. Sinus node artery, AV nodal artery and acute marginal artery, all three can arise from:

(a) Dominant right coronary artery

(b) Dominant left circumflex artery

(c) From either

(d) From neither

303. Is not included as a feature of IAHB:

(a) QRS axis between -45 and -90

(b) RS pattern in IL III and aVF

(c) QRS duration 120 ms

(d) Persistent '5' waves in V_6

304. Paradoxical movement of the IVS is seen in all *except:*

(a) Pulmonary artery hypertension

(b) Pulmonary embolism

(c) Cardiac tamponade

(d) Right ventricular MI

305. The best way of diagnosing CAD in a patient with LBBB is:

(a) Treadmil Test

(b) Nuclear imaging

(c) Dobutamine stress testing

(d) Contrast Echocardigraphy

306. E-point Septal Separation (EPSS) is markedly increased in:

(a) Hypertrophic cardiomyopathy
(b) Cardiac Tamponade
(c) Dilated Cardiomyopathy
(d) Corrected Transposition of great vessels

307. Adult echocardiography is performed by a 2.5 MHz transducer because:

(a) Resolution is better with a low frequency transducer
(b) Low frequency ultrasound penetrates adult chest wall better than high frequency ultrasound
(c) Higher frequency ultrasound damages tissues
(d) Resolution is better with high frequency transducer

308. Exercise induced disappearance of delta wave in ECG of WPW syndrome patient helps in predicting:

(a) Prognosis
(b) Type of WPW syndrome
(c) All of the above
(d) None of the above

309. The following are the ECG manifestations of hyperkalemia *except:*

(a) ST elevation (b) Loss of P wave
(c) Tall T wave (d) Prolonged QRS duration

310. TMT is absolute CI in all *except*:

(a) Severe MS (b) Severe symptomatic AS
(c) Acute MI (d) Acute pericarditis

311. All are ECG finding in ARVD *except*:

(a) T wave inversion V_1-V_3
(b) PR prolongation
(c) In complete RBBB
(d) Epsilon wave

312. All are ECHO criteria for severe AR *except*:

(a) PHT < 150 msec
(b) Regurgitation ejection fraction 50%
(c) Regurgitant volume 60 ml
(d) Regurgitant area/LVOT area > 65%

313. CMR contraindicated in:

(a) Cochlear implant
(b) Mechanical valve
(c) Dental implant
(d) Sternal wire

314. Disadvantage of MRI:

(a) High cost limit availability
(b) Assess microvascular integrity
(c) Cannot be used for real time imaging
(d) Claustrophobic patient not done

315. Epicardial hyperenhancement in MRI A/E:

(a) Amyloidosis
(b) Chagas
(c) Sarcoidosis
(d) Anderson Fabry disease

316. Thallium 201 vs Technetium:

(a) Active uptake
(b) Longer half life
(c) Minimal differential washout
(d) Clearance

317. Calcium scoring:

(a) Agatstson score (b) Rentrop score

318. Stress test–post exercise significant ST depression:

(a) 65 years old normal ECG
(b) Pre excitation
(c) LVH
(d) LBBB

319. ST elevation A/E:

(a) Hypothermia (b) Hypocalcemia
(c) Pericardial effusion (d) None

320. QT dispersion:

(a) 24 hours ECG recording
(b) 12 lead ECG
(c) Varies with time and season
(d) Varies with age

321. LBBB A/E:

(a) Can be seen in normal heart
(b) 1/3rd HF
(c) Has role in long term morbidity
(d) LBBB + RAD indicate biventricular enlargement

322. TTE sensitivity in aortic dissection:

(a) 40-60% (b) 50-60%
(c) 80-85% (d) 90-95%

323. Echo RA not visible:
(a) Chiari network (b) Crista terminalis
(c) Coumadin ridge (d) Eustachian valve

324. Einthoven's equation:
(a) I + III = II (b) I + II = III
(c) II + III= I

325. ST elevation causes A/E:
(a) Brugada syndrome
(b) Hypokalemia
(c) Pulmonary embolism
(d) Class – Ic antiarrhythmias

326. Absolute C/I for TMT A/E:
(a) Acute MI (7th day)
(b) High risk unstable angina
(c) Severe symptomatic AS
(d) Advanced AV block

327. ECG feature of hypercalcemia:
(a) Increased QT
(b) Decreased QT
(c) Increased PR

328. ST depression on TMT which is most significantly associated:
(a) LBBB on ECG
(b) Preexcitation on ECG
(c) Hypertensive heart disease with normal ECG
(d) Normal baseline ECG with HTN, DM and dyslipidemia

329. Subtle sign of ischemia on ECG:
(a) U wave inversion
(b) Coplane T wave inversion
(c) Upsloping ST depression
(d) Discordant QRST

330. Nonviable infracted myocardium best on MRI by:
(a) Delayed enhancement of gadolinium
(b) Echo planar MR
(c) Cine MRI with breath holding 10-15 sec
(d) T2 W imaging

331. Radionuclide image feature in MR suggestive of poor prognosis:
(a) Exercise EF decreased
(b) Increased RWMA from rest to exercise
(c) Decreased maximum CO
(d) Decreased MHR

332. Long QT by A/E:
(a) Hypokalemia (b) Hypomagnesemia
(c) Hypocalcemia (d) Rheumatic carditis

333. Hypocalcemia prolong QT by affecting:
(a) Prolong ST segment (b) Prolong QRS
(c) Prolong T wave (d) Prolong QU segment

334. Inverted U wave in anterior precordial leads:
(a) Prox. LAD lesion (b) RCA lesion
(c) LCX lesion

335. ABI rest pain:
(a) <0.7 (b) <0.6
(c) <0.5 (d) <0.4

336. Drugs used in HUTT A/E:
(a) Esmolol (b) Edrophonium
(c) I/V NTG (d) IV isoproterenol

337. Speckle tracking used for:
(a) Quantify myocardial motion in various plane
(b) Measurement of RWMA
(c) LVEF
(d) LV mass

338. Fastest MRI:
(a) FLAIR
(b) SSFP
(c) Echo planer

339. Sympathetic innervations is seen by:
(a) MIBG scanning (b) Tc scan
(c) SPECT

340. Normal diastolic function:
(a) E/A < 1 (b) IVRT < 70
(c) DT < 160 (d) E/Ea > 15

341. ECG assess A/E:
(a) SA node
(b) AV node
(c) Bundle branches
(d) Ventricular Myocardium

342. LBBB in CAD A/E:
(a) 30% of HF have LBBB
(b) 12% of LBBB have no heart disease
(c) Does not have high mortality

343. True about MRI imaging A/E:

(a) TPI absolute C/I of MRI
(b) After 2000 pacemaker compatible with 1.5 T MRI
(c) It cause electromechnical interference
(d) All pacemakers are incompatible with MRI

344. During phase 3 of Action Potential which event occur in ECG:

(a) ST segment (b) T wave
(c) QRS (d) QT

345. J wave:

(a) At the end of QRS epicardial origin
(b) At the end of QRS endocardial origin
(c) At the end of R wave epicardial origin
(d) At the end of R wave endocardial origin

346. AD inheritance with WPW:

(a) Holt Oram (b) Noonan disease
(c) Pompe syndrome (d) Fabry disease

347. MRI:

(a) Ionized radiation with iodinated contrast is used
(b) Used in thalassemia for iron overload assessment
(c) To evaluate stenosis and regurgitant lesion
(d) Has replaced echo for assessing LV ejection

348. Ashmann phenomenon:

(a) Cycle length dependent refractoriness
(b) Deceleration dependent RBBB or LBBB
(c) Acceleration dependent RBBB

349. METS:

(a) 3.5 ml/kg/min (b) 5 ml/kg/min
(c) 10 ml/kg/min (d) 15 ml/kg/min

350. The scan that can provide direct evidence of a recent severe ischemia at a time when perfusion had returned to normal is:

(a) ^{201}Thallium-SPECT scan
(b) ^{123}Iodine SPECT scan
(c) BMIPP-SPECT scan
(d) PET scan

351. An abnormal speckled pattern or ground glass appearance of the myocardinm has been described on 2D echocardiography in:

(a) Amyloidosis (b) Chagas Disease
(c) Kawasaki Disease (d) Lyme carditis

352. Identify the wrong statement:

(a) Damage to left anterior fascicle is very common because of its delicate nature
(b) Left posterior fascicle is thicker and is protected near the LV in low
(c) ECG features of left septal fascicular block is absence of septal Q waves
(d) QRS duration is prolonged in fascicular block

353. All are causes of tall R in V1 *except:*

(a) Duchenne muscular dystrophy
(b) Type B WPW syndrome
(c) Hypertrophic cardiomyopathy
(d) Posterior wall MI

354. During stress testing all are true *except:*

(a) In about 10% of patients ischemic response may appear only in the recovery phase
(b) ST ↑ in leads with abnormal Q waves is a marked of more extensive CAD
(c) 'U' wave inversion is relatively specific for CAD
(d) PseudonormalisationTb waves is non diagnostic finding

355. P wave inversion in lead 1 is not seen in:

(a) Limb lead reversal (b) Situs inversus
(c) Right trial rhythm (d) Left atrial rhythm

356. Pericardial invasion by tumors is best visualized by:

(a) USG (b) CT
(c) MRI (d) PET

357. IRH (Intrinsic heart rate) is calculated by which formula?

(a) 117 (Constant × age)
(b) 117 (Constant × weight)
(c) 117 (Constant × height)
(d) 117 – (Constant × BMI)

358. MAT is characterized by everything *except:*

(a) Normal isoelectric baseline
(b) Normal looking 'p' waves
(c) Abnormal PR interval
(d) Absence of normal sinus beat

359. Pericardial knock is absent in all *except:*

(a) Cardiac tamponade
(b) Constrictive pericarditis
(c) Restrictive cardiomyopathy
(d) RV myocardial infarction

360. All are true Echocardiographically regarding cardiac tamponade *except:*
(a) Small right ventricle
(b) Right atrial collapse
(c) Increased mitral flow
(d) Exaggerated respiratory variation

361. Acute hyperkalemia ECG change is:
(a) Prolong QRS
(b) Short PR
(c) ST segment prolongation
(d) U waves

362. Duke tread mill score include A/E:
(a) ST deviation (b) Exercise duration
(c) Angina (d) Fall in BP

363. EST—all indicates ischemia *except:*
(a) ST elevation in leads with pathological Q waves
(b) J point depression is normal
(c) U wave inversion is specific of CAD
(d) Pseudonormalisation of T waves is non-specific finding

364. Agaston score is for:
(a) CT coronary calcification

365. Midesophageal echo long axis: (T/F)
(a) LV (b) Aortic valve
(c) Mitral valve (d) Aorta
(e) Tricuspid valve

366. ECG changes in hyperkalemia: (T/F)
(a) Early stage reduces QT
(b) Tall and wide T wave
(c) ST Elevation in V_1-V_3
(d) PR prolongation
(e) Reduces P wave amplitude

367. CT angiography versus CAG, CT angiography better in: (T/F)
(a) Critical ostial stenosis of LMCA
(b) Vessel distal to complete occlusion
(c) Congenital coronary anomalies
(d) Coronary collaterals
(e) Stent < 3 mm

368. LBBB: (T/F)
(a) Widely split S2
(b) Paradoxical S2
(c) Early systolic multiphasic anterior septal motion with decrease septal thickness
(d) Presystolic transient (<50 msec) with preserved septal thickening with septal motion
(e) Abrupt stoppage of pulmonary venous flow

369. ST elevation is seen in: (T/F)
(a) WPW syndrome (b) Takatsubo CMP
(c) LV aneurysm (d) Myocarditis
(e) Hypocalcemia

370. ST elevation in LBBB: (T/F)
(a) > 1 mm in concordant leads
(b) > 5 mm in disconcordant leads
(c) q in V_1–V_4
(d) q in I, avL, V_5, V_6
(e) s wave notching of mid precordial leads

371. LBBB in TMT A/E: (T/F)
(a) Incidence 0.8%
(b) Increases risk of cardiovascular events (MACE)
(c) High degree of AV block is rare
(d) 50% develop permanent LBBB
(e) ST segment depression not diagnostic or prognostic of CAD

372. Myocardial perfusion imaging: (T/F)
(a) Indicated in LVH
(b) Rubidium 82–metabolic tracer
(c) F-18: Perfusion tracer
(d) In female sestamibi Tc is less useful than thallium 201
(e) Multiple perfusion abnormality is more suggestive of CAD than DCM

373. Viability of myocardium: (T/F)
(a) TMT (b) PET
(c) CT (d) Cardiac MRI
(e) Dobutamine stress echo

374. QT interval: (T/F)
(a) Longest in V_2–V_3
(b) Start of QRS to start of T wave
(c) PR segment–end of P wave to start of R wave
(d) QT correlates with ventricular repolarisation
(e) U wave–repolarisation of Purkinje's fibres

375. Q in V1: (T/F)

(a) AWMI (b) ALCAPA
(c) Severe AS (d) Severe PS
(e) cc-TGA

376. LAHB: (T/F)

(a) Mean axis–45 to 90
(b) qR–avF
(c) S–slurred in V5-V6
(d) avL–Q to R duration $\geq$ 45 ms
(e) QRS > 120 ms

377. Septal q waves are seen in leads:

(a) V_1, V_2 (b) V_3, V_4
(c) V_5, V_6 (d) I, II

378. Absolute C/I of TMT: (T/F)

(a) Heart failure
(b) High risk UA
(c) Acute myopericarditis
(d) Severe AS

379. LBBB correct: (T/F)

(a) 20% in acute MI
(b) 3% general population
(c) Increases morbidity and mortality
(d) Acute has less mortality than previous present
(e) LBBB in MI has worse prognosis

380. MSCT: (T/F)

(a) Complex congenital heart disease
(b) Coronary anomalies
(c) BMI > 40
(d) Alternative to CAG for prior CABG
(e) Exclude CAD as a cause of early HF

381. Paradoxical septal motion on echo: (T/F)

(a) LBBB
(b) RBBB
(c) Left free wall pathway
(d) His bundle pacing
(e) Atrial pacing

382. Cardiac neuronal imaging with PET true is: (T/F)

(a) Primary target for hydroxyephedrine is NET/Uptake-1 system
(b) HED rapidly metabolised by MAO/COMT
(c) HED commony used for post synaptic sympathetic neuronal evaluation
(d) F-18 fluorodopa identifies cardiac and extracardiac sympathetic system
(e) t ½ of C-11 phenylephrine is 110 min

383. RVH seen in all *except* (T/F):

(a) Severe MS (b) Adult AS
(c) Neonatal AS (d) Hypertension
(e) Acute MI

384. MI one week mid LAD best treatment with normal LC function and asymptomatic:

(a) Stress imaging (b) PCI with BMS
(c) PCI with DES (d) Medical treatment

385. 65 years for adriamycin used chemotherapy, preop TMT negative, before starting chemo-investigation: (T/F)

(a) MUGA baseline and serial
(b) TMT repeat
(c) Stress thallium
(d) Ramipril
(e) Carvedilol

386. ECG ST ↑ right precordial lead all *except*:

(a) Hypercalcemia (b) Friedreich ataxia
(c) Thiamine deficiency (d) LQT syndrome

387. Hyperkalemia ECG changes: (T/F)

(a) Broadbased T wave (b) PR prolongs
(c) Absent P wave (d) Broad QRS
(e) Broad QT

388. All true *except* for exercise test: (T/F)

(a) Peak activity for routine work–5 MET
(b) Resting–3 MET
(c) For elite athlete, max. is 11 MET
(d) CAD patient exercising to 10 MET, progonosis equal for medical Rx + CABG
(e) 2 mile/hour= 9 MET

389. Hyperkalemia ECG changes: (T/F)
(a) Broad based T wave
(b) PR prolongs
(c) Absent P wave
(d) Broad QRS
(e) Broad QT

390. Diastolic function on echo: (T/F)
(a) IVRT
(b) Tau
(c) Transmitral flow
(d) Fractional shortening
(e) Strain

391. Hyperkalemia ECG: (T/F)
(a) Tall tented T (b) Narrow QRS
(c) ↑ PR (d) T ↓
(e) P↓

392. Pericarditis ECG: (T/F)
(a) Tall P (b) ST ↑ in aVR
(c) LBBB (d) RBBB
(e) PR ↓

393. Tall R in V_1: (T/F)
(a) IWMI (b) PWMI
(c) Apical MI (d) Duchenne's dystrophy
(e) RVH

394. Hyperkalemia ECG, ST elevation in right leads V_1 > V_2: (T/F)
(a) Long PR (b) Tall T wave
(c) Flat p wave (d) Narrow QRS
(e) T wave disappear

395. ECG features of hyperkalemia: (T/F)
(a) Narrow, peaked t waves
(b) Flattened T waves
(c) Increased U wave
(d) Absent P waves
(e) Decreased QT interval

396. Tall R wave in V1: (T/F)
(a) DMD (b) PWMI
(c) RVH (d) IWMI

397. Hyperkalemia: (T/F)
(a) Tall T wave (b) Narrow QRS
(c) Long PR (d) Absent p wave
(e) Diminished T wave

398. Post MI TMT indicated at: (T/F)
(a) 2 weeks
(b) 3 weeks
(c) VT
(d) Persistent ST elevation
(e) Angina

399. Thallium in ischemic segment work on principle of:
(a) Redistribution
(b) Mitochondrial function
(c) Glucose metabolism

400. Early repolarisation A/E:
(a) > 2 mm J point elevation
(b) 6-13% incidence
(c) Tall T wave
(d) Concavity upwards

401. Echo finding in MS A/E:
(a) DE slope decrease
(b) A wave absent
(c) EF decrease
(d) Posterior motion of PML reduced

402. Romhilt Estes criteria A/E:
(a) V5 or V6 > 30 (b) LAD
(c) Long QT (d) Morris index > 0.04

403. RVH – most specific:
(a) RAD > 90°
(b) S1 Q3
(c) R/S ratio >1 with R > 0.05 mV in V1
(d) P pulmonale

404. Left posterior hemiblock:
(a) QRS axis < 120 (b) QRS < 120 msec
(c) RS in I, aVL (d) QR in inferior leads

405. Multislice CT is maximum useful in:
(a) Bypass graft
(b) Stenosis in stent
(c) Bifurcation lesion
(d) Evaluation of LCx and distal RCA

406. NADAS criteria in neonates A/E:
(a) Cyanosis (b) Diastolic murmur
(c) Abnormal ECG (d) CHF

407. Adverse prognosis on TMT:
(a) Angina in low workload
(b) ST ↑ except avR
(c) < 5 METS
(d) NSVT on exercise and recovery

408. Right ventricular systolic dysfunction is suggested when tricuspid annular systolic excursion (TAPSE) is:
(a) < 12 mm (b) <14 mm
(c) <16 mm (d) <18 mm

409. E/A ratio 1.3, DT 160 msec, E/e′ 15; findings on ECHO are suggestive of:
(a) Normal diastolic function
(b) LV diastolic dysfunction grade 1
(c) LV diastolic dysfunction grade 2
(d) LV diastolic dysfunction grade 3

410. Which of the following statement is false regarding Chronotropic incompetence?
(a) Defined as failure to reach 85% of predicated maximal heart rate at exercise
(b) Defined as failure to teach 50% of predicted maximal heat rate > 100 beats/min with exercise
(c) Defined as failure to achieve a hear rate > 100 beats/min with exercise
(d) Defined as maximal heart rate with exercise less than two standard deviations below that of an age-matched control population

411. Epicardial hyperenhancement in Cardiac MRI is not seen in:
(a) Sarcoidosis
(b) Anderson fabry disease
(c) Amyloidosis
(d) Chagas disease

412. With regards to routine treadmill test:
(a) Development of 1 mm or more of J point depression with a relatively flat ST-segment slope (< 0.7 to 1 mV/sec), at 80 ms after the j point (ST80) is considered to be an abnormal
(b) If ST-segment depression is 0.1 mV or greater at rest the exercise ECG become more specific
(c) ST-segment depression localizes the coronary artery involved
(d) Exercise-induced ST-segment elevation is relatively non-specific as compared to depressions

413. Measures of LV systolic function of heart: (T/F)
(a) EF (b) MPI
(c) ESPVR (d) Fractional shortening
(e) TAPSE

414. Pregnancy changes: (T/F)
(a) 50% increase in PVR
(b) HR in third trimester maintain CO
(c) Postpartum decrease Blood volume due to various losses
(d) Decrease in BP in early gestation
(e) RAD

415. ECG: (T/F)
(a) ARVD-RBBB VT
(b) Monomorphic BBB rentry tachycardia is seen in DCM most commonly
(c) Isolated fascicular VT, reentry is mech. and resistant to verapamil
(d) CHADS2 in non valvular AF–bleeding assessment

416. TMT: (T/F)
(a) MAP increases, SBP increases, DBP static
(b) Supine position increases CO due to increases SV
(c) SV/ CO more in supine than standing
(d) O_2 dept during recovery
(e) Lactic acid accumulation occur after 75% of aerobic threshold

417. Diastolic HF: (T/F)
(a) Grade I = A> E, E: A < 1, DT decreased
(b) Grade II – E:A -1-1.5, with normal DT
(c) Grade III, IV E>A; E:A >2 and DT < 160, IVRT> 70
(d) Myocardial systolic ratio– IVRT+ IVCT/ PEP
(e) If the velocity < nyquist frequency – alasing occur

418. PISA: (T/F)
(a) In eccentric MR better than central MR
(b) Also used for stenotic valve area
(c) Best measured in midsystole below the flow convergence
(d) PHT –velocity decreases to vel/V_2
(e) Dp/dt > 600

419. ECG: (T/F)
(a) III = II + I
(b) Amplification–1000
(c) AHA frequency band width 0.05–150 Hz

(d) PR interval measured with shortest PR

(e) POSTEROBASAL LV is last to be activated

420. ECG localization: (T/F)

(a) q RBBB–distal to diagonal

(b) avR ST elevation–prox LAD

(c) AWMI with STE in inf lead–mid LAD

(d) IWMI with reciprocal right precordial STE rule out RVMI

(e) STE II > III is LCX involvement

421. True or false:

(a) Tau = 160 msec

(b) E/e < 15 normal

422. True or false:

(a) q RBBB marker of proximal LAD before D1 branch

(b) ST elevation in lead II more than lead III–LCx involvement

(c) ST elevation in inferior lead in AWMI–mid LAD

(d) IWMI with ST depression in V_1 to V_3 rule out RVMI

423. Mason likar modification: (T/F)

(a) RAD

(b) Increased voltage in inferior lead

(c) Q in inferior lead

(d) Loss of q wave in inferior lead

(e) Presence of R/s wave in precordial leads

424. ECG: (T/F)

(a) V9–left of spine

(b) V7–on posterior scapular line

(c) AvR–right arm reference with negative in other two leads

(d) Wilson lead–average of two leads

425. TMT absolute C/I: (T/F)

(a) Age < 75 years

(b) High risk UA

(c) Acute MI < 7 days

(d) High grade AV block

(e) WPW syndrome

426. TMT and PET: (T/F)

(a) Inability to achieve 85% of THR poor prognosis

(b) < 10 min exercise poor prognosis

(c) Severe asymptomatic AS absolute C/I

(d) Transient LV dilatation poor prognosis

(e) Decreased lung and heart uptake poor prognosis

427. True or false: (T/F)

(a) Palpography for temperature in atherosclerosis

(b) OCT revealing after revascularisation

(c) FFR is investigation of choice for effectiveness of stent placement

(d) CAG Investigation of choice for mechanism of occlusion

(e) FFR and temperature for microvascular integrity

428. TMT poor prognosis: (T/F)

(a) MET < 6

(b) Typical chest pain

(c) No ↑ in BP, DBP to 120 mm Hg or sustain ↓ for > 10 mm Hg

(d) Reproducible sustained VT

(e) ST ↑ in all leads except avR

429. TMT absolute C/I: (T/F)

(a) Age < 75 years

(b) High risk UA

(c) Acute MI < 7 days

(d) High grade AV block

(e) WPW syndrome

430. Thallium: (T/F)

(a) Thallium short half life than Tc

(b) For viability sestamibi better than thallium

(c) Redistribution less with sestamibi and thallium tetraphosmin

(d) Normal myocardium–early uptake and early redistribute

(e) MPI – 0 to 4 grade for each segment

431. T/F:

(a) Notch in p wave in lead II > 40 mm – LAE

(b) Initial P in VI >0.06 = LAE

(c) P axis > 75 + = RAE

(d) P duration/PR segment < 1.6 = LAE

(e) P wave in lead II > 120 m sec = RAE

432. TMT: (T/F)

(a) Sev AS–Absolute contraindication

(b) Severe HOCM–Absolute contraindication

(c) Delta wave disappearance – s/o Left accessory pathway
(d) RBBB – ↓ses sensitivity
(e) Exercise induced LBBB – 50% chances of developing permanent LBBB

433. CT: (T/F)
(a) Heavy calcification–cause difficulty in assessment
(b) Absence of calcification practically rule out significant CAD
(c) Heavy Ca ++ s/o significant obstructive CAD
(d) Very well images distal anastomoses and run off vessels
(e) Instent restenosis–well imaged
(f) Dual head CT scan give better image even at HR of 90/min

434. Efflex of potassium through K^+ channels causes:
(a) Depolarization (b) Repolarization
(c) Hyperpolarization (d) All of the above

435. T/F:
(a) E/E′ > 15 is sensitive marker of diastolic dysfunction
(b) Doppler bean should be parallel to tissue
(c) Severe hyponatremia in 25-30%
(d) E/E′ correlate wall with LV invasive filling pressure
(e) BNP indeed therapy improve surgery
(f) PCWP < 16 mmHg is goal
(g) BNP > 100 in DHF

436. Stress ECHO: (T/F)
(a) Biphasic response is specific and sensitive for viability
(b) Wall thickness < 5 mm at rest is non viable
(c) > 50% segment is more sensitive for viable
(d) Adenosine is better than dobutamine
(e) Dobutamine negative test excludes viability
(f) Atropine can be given if target HR not reached

437. Voltage criteria ECG: (T/F)
(a) More sensitive and less specific for LVH
(b) More specific and less sensitive for RVH
(c) qR in V1 denotes RVH suggest suprasystemic pressure
(d) Type A RVH is seen in V1 R wave
(e) Tall T wave in V1 with early V_1/V_2 transition suggestive of RVOT with VSD

438. CT angiography: (T/F)
(a) Not used for CABG graft
(b) Used in asymptomatic individuals
(c) It can be used in COPD
(d) Severly calcific arteries

439. Echo used in all these indication as IOC which is better alternative investigation for the assessment of these indication *except:* (T/F)
(a) MS (b) TGA
(c) CT (d) A-dissection
(e) Cardiac contusion

440. Romhilt estes criteria: (T/F)
(a) Intrinscoid deflection–2 points
(b) LAD–3 points
(c) Digoxin with ST change–no point
(d) Cornell criteria–gender dependent
(e) QRS duration > 0.9 = 2 points

441. QRS voltage: (T/F)
(a) After septal activation–RV free wall next activated
(b) Intrinscoid deflection S/O depolarization of epicardium below electrode
(c) QT indicates AP duration
(d) Septal activation from apex to base
(e) U wave more imp in tachycardia

442. TMT in WPW: (T/F)
(a) WPW invalidates stress test
(b) Abrupt disappearance of delta wave–short accessory pathway
(c) Disappearance of delta wave is commoner in type A than B
(d) Disappearance of delta wave in 20-50%
(e) Does not affect physical activity

443. PET scan: (T/F)
(a) Normal blood flow with increase glucose in stunning

(b) Decrease blood flow with decrease glucose in scar
(c) Decrease blood flow with normal glucose in hibernating myocardium
(d) Minimal blood flow with decrease glucose in fibrosis
(e) Improved contractility associated with decrease O^2 uptake

444. PET: (T/F)
(a) Rb^{82} for myocardial oxygen consumption
(b) C^{11} palmitate for fatty acid
(c) NH_3 is used for blood flow
(d) FDG for fatty acid uptake
(e) O_{15} for perfusion

445. TMT: (T/F)
(a) Angle between flat ground and TMT is 10 degree
(b) Stage 2 = 6 – 8 METS of Bruce protocol
(c) Height of elevated end of TMT is 10 degree
(d) Height of elevated end of TMT is 10 degree for every 100″ horizontal length of table

446. False negative stress perfusion study: (T/F)
(a) Balanced hypoperfusion
(b) Cardiomyopathy
(c) Microvascular disease
(d) Collateral circulation
(e) Conduction defect

447. TMT–not true is:
(a) Positive if desaturation, ST elevation, angina occurs
(b) Less than–11 is low risk
(c) More sensitive for women
(d) Changes in aVR not included
(e) ST elevation is more specific for territory involved

448. Noninvasive testing: (T/F)
(a) Noninvasive testing is best in intermediate risk group
(b) Exercise dobutamine better than dipyridamole and adenosine in LBBB
(c) Dipyridamole can be given in bilateral carotid artery stenosis
(d) Dobutamine not to be given in serious arrhythmias

449. Lewis lead: (T/F)
(a) Unipolar and esophageal leads
(b) Bipolar with right 2nd and 4th left ICS
(c) Most common used for p wave
(d) Best for T wave
(e) Placement of limbs leads on central chest

450. Mason likar modification: (T/F)
(a) RAD
(b) Increases voltage in inferior leads
(c) ↑ voltage in anterior leads
(d) Absent q wave in aVL
(e) q in inf. leads

451. TMT: (T/F)
(a) Asymptomatic males have abnormal test= 15-20%
(b) Rate pressure product 20000-35000 mm Hg
(c) After acute MI, achievement of 5-6 MET signifies low risk
(d) In WPW, abrupt disappearance of delta wave means longer RP of anterograde pathway
(e) Disappearance of delta wave more common with right sided pathway as compared to left

452. Head up tilt test: (T/F)
(a) Done at 60-80° angle for 20-40 min
(b) Increasing angle increases the chance of false positive
(c) Drugs increasing sensitivity but decreases specificity
(d) Sensitivity depends on population (standard)
(e) < 40° angle decreases sensitivity

453. 40 years old male history of repeat syncope, ECG, echo, Holter normal, patient has weakness and nausea before syncope, next IOC:
(a) EPS
(b) Head up tilt test
(c) Signal average ECG
(d) Implantable arrhythmia monitor

454. Frank lead system used in:
(a) Vector cardiography
(b) Exercise stress test
(c) Holter monitoring

455. ECG LVH criteria—least specific:
(a) R in V6 > V5
(b) R in avL > 7.5 mm
(c) S in V1 + R in V6 > 35 mm
(d) R in I + S in III > 25 mm

456. Sonicated albumin used for:

(a) Ventricular delineation and function
(b) Doppler flow study
(c) Plaque morphology (surface study)
(d) Ventilation perfusion study

457. Exercise testing false statement:

(a) In sedentary person on exercise CO increases 4 times
(b) Stroke volume increases in isometric exercise
(c) LVH regress after stopping exercise

458. Inravascular USG strongly recommended in all *except:*

(a) Primary angioplasty
(b) Transplant vasculopathy
(c) Stent restenosis
(d) Left main disease

459. Cardiac MRI distinguished ischemic and non-ischemic CMP because of presence of:

(a) No enhancement
(b) Mid myocardial enhancement
(c) Epicardial enhancement
(d) Subendocardial enhancement

460. U wave A/E:

(a) Opposite polarity as preceding T wave
(b) Prominent is mid precordial lead
(c) Indicates Purkinje fiber repolarization
(d) Indicates late repolarization potential

461. Frank lead system used in:

(a) Vector electrocardiography
(b) Exercise TMT
(c) Holter monitoring
(d) Telemetry

462. RVH in neonate:

(a) In V1 R/S > 1 (b) RAD
(c) Sin V6 (d) Upright T in V1

463. 1.5 Tesla MRI A/E:

(a) Severe MS
(b) Ebstein with severe tricuspid deformity
(c) Severe PHT
(d) ASD

464. Tilt table testing A/E:

(a) NTG (b) Isoprenaline
(c) Atropine (d) Edrophonium

465. ECG A/E:

(a) Speed of paper 50 mm/sec
(b) In adult frequency 0.05 to 150 Hz
(c) 1 small square – 40 msec
(d) I mV = 10 mm

466. QRS negative in I, avR, avL, frontal axis is:

(a) + 90 to +120 (b) +60 to + 90
(c) +60 to +150 (d) +120 to + 150

467. Negative M1 T1:

(a) Severe MS
(b) Ebstein anomaly with severe tricuspid deformity
(c) Severe PHT
(d) ASD

468. Largest acting SPECT tracer with active myocardial uptake seen with:

(a) Tc tetrofosmin (b) Thallium-201
(c) Tc Sestamibi (d) Tc Teboroxime

469. ECG leads at some horizontal plane:

(a) V_1 and V_2 (b) V_2 and V_3
(c) V_3 and V_4 (d) V_3 and V_1

470. 45 years old presents with lone AF. Echo show normal cardiac valves and chamber:

(a) Start aspirin
(b) Start aspirin + warfarin
(c) Start aspirin + warfarin only if LV thrombus present
(d) Start aspirin + warfarin with history of embolic event

471. LBBB with MI A/E:

(a) q in I, avL and V_5
(b) ST elevation 1mm in V_5
(c) Slurring of wave in V_2, V_3
(d) ST elevation V_1–V_3

472. ECG changes of hyperkalemia and depolarization, DOC is:

(a) Metoprolol (b) Calcium
(c) Procainamide (d) Lidocaine

473. Which of the following is represented in a standard ECG?

(a) SA node depolarization
(b) AV node depolarization
(c) His bundle depolarization
(d) Atrial muscle depolarization

474. Which of the following is false of the below mentioned statements?

(a) TR velocity is used to calculate mean pulmonary artery pressure
(b) Bernoulliequation is used to calculate gradient across AV valve
(c) Colour Doppler estimation of regurgitation of the TR is semiquantitative
(d) Cardiac output is assessed by square of radius of aorta

475. A 50 years old male by echo LV mass has been calculated as 200 gm/m^2, the LVH is:

(a) Mild (b) Moderate
(c) Severe (d) Normal LVH

476. About ECG which is true?

(a) PR interval = 0.12 to 0.2 sec
(b) Earliest change in MI = ST elevation
(c) QT interval is initiation of QRS to initiation of T wave
(d) Axis is commonly +30 to +90

477. TMT is contraindicated in A/E:

(a) Severe HOCM
(b) Acute myocarditis
(c) Critical AS
(d) Intra-abdominal aneurysm > 5.5 cm

478. Hexa axial system in ECG is:

(a) Standard lead
(b) Augmented lead
(c) Standard + augmented lead

479. Which is true regarding PR *except*?

(a) Presence of PR in ECHO is prolonged
(b) Associated with Grahm Steel murmur if PASP > 60 mm Hg
(c) Wide split S2
(d) Associated with collagen vascular disease

480. Hyperkalemia ECG:

(a) Loss of P with wide QRS
(b) ST depression
(c) Prominent U
(d) Prolonged QT

481. TMT absolute CI A/E:

(a) Severe asymptomatic AS
(b) Uncontrolled HTN
(c) Advanced AV block
(d) Acute pericarditis

482. Cardiac CT for CAD:

(a) High sensitivity (b) Highly specific
(c) High PPV (d) High NPV

483. Tall R in V1 A/E:

(a) WPW type B
(b) Mirror image dextrocardia
(c) Post MI
(d) RBBB

484. TMT, false +ve can occur A/E:

(a) Digitalis
(b) LVH
(c) ST ↓ at baseline
(d) High pretest probability of CAD

485. Stress echo not used:

(a) Adenosine (b) Ivabradine
(c) Ergonovine (d) Mental stress

486. CMP – dobutamine stress test best predictor for surgery outcome:

(a) Improve with low and high dose
(b) Improve with low, no improve in high dose
(c) Improves with low and further ↑ in high dose

487. Tissue doppler in diastolic dysfunction false:

(a) EM < AM–good prognosis
(b) Cut off is 3 cm/s
(c) EM doesn't ↑ preload
(d) EM ↑ es with diastolic dysfunction

488. TMT absolute indication to stop:

(a) Patient desires to stop
(b) BP > 250
(c) ↑ ing chest pain
(d) ST change > 2 mm depression

489. True is:

(a) LBBB in AMI denotes prox LAD
(b) WPW type A mimicks lateral WMI
(c) WPW B masks ant. WMI
(d) LAHB mimicks inf. WMI

490. 36 years male, with palpitations, dizziness QRS 120, RBBB with LAD echo N, rate 200/mm–Treatment long term:

(a) Amiodarone (b) BB
(c) Flecainide (d) Quinidine

491. True about ECG:
(a) LBBB in STEMI S/O prox LAD
(b) Type A WPW mimics lateral MI
(c) Type B WPW masks AWMI
(d) LAFB mimics IWMI
(e) WPW cellularity prolongs PR

492. Absence of q wave in V_6 S/O in cyanotic CHD:
(a) Ventricular inversion (b) Dextrocardia
(c) Situs inversus (d) RVH
(e) Intact IV septum

493. Absolute indication to stop TMT:
(a) Increasing chest pain
(b) ST deviation > 2 mm
(c) Patients desire to stop
(d) SBP > 250 mm Hg
(e) Pulse rate > 120 bpm

494. Multislice CT in CAD S/O:
(a) High sensitivity
(b) Low sensitivity with high specificity
(c) High PPV
(d) High NPV
(e) None

495. Application of 4v2 on Doppler echo in AS is S/O:
(a) Peak to peak gradient
(b) Mean pressure gradient
(c) Peak pressure gradient
(d) Peak instantaneous gradient
(e) All of the above

496. TAPSE is used for:
(a) RV systolic dysfunction
(b) RV diastolic dysfunction
(c) RV systolic dysfunction with TR
(d) RV diastolic dysfunction with EMF

497. HDL not decreased by:
(a) CETP inhibitor
(b) PPAR α and γ activator
(c) $NCP_1 L_1$ antagonist
(d) Niacin

498. Hyperkalemia ECG A/E:
(a) Tall T wave
(b) Short PR
(c) Wide QRS
(d) Disappearance of 'P' wave

499. Stress TMT—ST elevation in non-Q wave MI suggests:
(a) Subendocardial severe ischemia
(b) Specific for coronary artery localization
(c) Normal in 10%
(d) Always due to vasopressin

500. Hyperkalemia ECG all *except:*
(a) Increase PR (b) Increase QRS
(c) Increase QT (d) Asystole

501. Low voltage ECG all *except:*
(a) Normal variant (b) Myocarditis
(c) Pericarditis (d) COPD

502. TMT absolute C/I all *except:*
(a) Acute pericarditis
(b) USA with recent chest pain
(c) Advanced AV block
(d) AS

503. PET scan for:
(a) Viability in CAD
(b) For arrhythmias
(c) Pericardial disease
(d) Cardiac tumour detection

504. CT is done for:
(a) Pericardial cyst (b) LA myxoma
(c) CMP (d) Intracardiac tumour

505. Diastolic depolarization is seen in:
(a) SA node (b) AV node
(c) Purkinje fibres (d) Myocytes

506. TMT not to be done A/E:
(a) Severe AS (b) Mild AS
(c) USA

507. TMT true is:
(a) TMT done to check effect of antiarrhythmics
(b) To differentiate arrhythmias of structural heart disease versus autonomic involvement
(c) To trigger atrial arrhythmias

508. **Echo of cardiac tamponade A/E:**
(a) RVOT collapse in early diastole
(b) Exaggerated mitral velocity decreases on inspiration
(c) Exaggerated tricuspid flow on inspiration
(d) Increased E/A of mitral valve

509. **CCP hallmark in ECHO:**
(a) Respiratory variation in velocity
(b) Septal bounce

510. **Fluoro view for ventricular septum:**
(a) LAO 60 (b) RAO 30

511. **A statistical analysis test which is used to compare the survival distributions of two sets of data is:**
(a) Chi-square test
(b) Linear regression analysis
(c) Logistic regression analysis
(d) Log-rank test

512. **The strongest prognostic variable during treadmill testing is:**
(a) Ventricular ectopics during exercise
(b) LBBB during exercise
(c) Exercise duration
(d) 3 mm ST segment depression during exercise

513. **All of the following are true regarding carotid duplex ultrasound for measuring the severity of carotid artery stenosis *except:***
(a) It is less precise in determining stenosis of less than 50 percent compared with higher percent stenosis
(b) Can accurately distinguish between subtotal and total occlusion of carotid artery
(c) Contralateral stenosis results in overestimation of ipsilateral stenosis
(d) The measurement is dependent on the cardiac output

514. **Which of the following is true regarding the measurement of pressure gradient across the aortic valve for assessing the severity of aortic stenosis?**
(a) Peak-to-peak gradients are more than peak instantaneous gradients
(b) Peak-to-peak gradients are assessed using Doppler echocardiography
(c) Peak-to-peak gradient reflect the true physiologic gradient
(d) Mean gradient across the aortic valve correlates well as assessed using Doppler echocardiography and cardiac catheterization

515. **Which of the following is true regarding Intravascular ultrasound (IVUS) and Optical coherence tomography (OCT) imaging of coronary arteries?**
(a) IVUS has better axial resolution than OCT
(b) IVUS detects thrombus better than OCT
(c) IVUS is better for detection of far-field signals than OCT
(d) IVUS detects vulnerable plaque better than OCT

516. **Drug which is used for pharmacologic provocation during upright tilt table test includes:**
(a) Esmolol (b) Nifedipine
(c) Isoproterenol (d) Nikornadil

517. **A 55-year-old male patient has exercised on treadmill for 6 minutes using standard Bruce protocol. He developed 2 mm maximum ST segment depression and non-limiting angina at peak exercise. The Duke Treadmill score will be:**
(a) –8 (b) –6
(c) –4 (d) –10

518. **A 55-year-old male underwent CT coronary angiography in view of a midly positive treadmill test on routine health checkup. Anomalous left main coronary artery from noncoronary sinus coursing retro aortic between aorta and left atrium was reported. He should be advised:**
(a) No therapy
(b) Restricted physical activity
(c) Stenting of the retro aortic portion to prevent systolic compression
(d) Surgical implantation of left main coronary artery to left coronary sinus

519. **Which of the following food/nutrients has convincing effect on lowering hypertension?**
(a) Dark chocolate (b) High calcium intake
(c) Vitamin D (d) Soy foods

520. **Global myocardial enhancement on MRI is seen in all *except:***
(a) Idiopathic dilated cardiomyopathy
(b) Post cardiac transplant
(c) Amyloidosis
(d) Systemic sclerosis

521. In presence of normal systolic function criteria of severe AS by Doppler haemodynamics, all are true *except:*

(a) Peak aortic valve velocity of ≥ 4.5 m sec
(b) Mean pressure gradient of ≥ 50 mmHg
(c) LVOT/AV TVI of 0.25 or less
(d) Aortic valve area of 1 cm^2 or less

522. All of the following are echo cardiographic indicators of severe mitral stenosis *except:*

(a) Mean gradient at rest of > 10 mmHg across mitral valve
(b) MVA < 1 cm^2
(c) PHT of > 240 msecs
(d) Mean gradient after exercise of > 15 mm across mitral valve

523. Following statements are true about 'hang out' interval *except:*

(a) Duration is related to the impedance of the vascular bed into which blood is being received
(b) Normal intervals is <15 msecs in systemic circulation
(c) Normal interval in pulmonary circulation is 43 to 86 milli seconds
(d) Decrease in impedance in systemic vascular bed alters hand out interval and causes wide splitting of 2nd heart sound

524. Which of the following ECG feature is typical of LAHB?

(a) Q wave in inferior leads
(b) Mean QRS axis between 0 and –30 degree
(c) rS pattern in inferior leads and qR pattern in lateral leads
(d) Marked right axis deviation

525. True statement about late potentials:

(a) Filtered QRS duration 114-120 msec
(b) <20 mV of root mean square signal amplitude in the last 40 msec of filtered QRS complex
(c) Terminal filtered QRS complex remains below 40 mV for >39 msec
(d) All of the above

526. Crochetage sign in ECG is seen in:

(a) ASD (b) VSD
(c) PDS (d) Coronary AV fistula

527. Macruz index is:

(a) 'P' duration/PR segment in L-II is > 1.6
(b) Duration X depth of 'P' terminal force in V_1 is >0.04 mm. sec
(c) Bifid 'P' waves
(d) P duration > 120 m. sec

528. The following criteria is not applicable for left ventricular hypertrophy:

(a) Sokolow-Lyon (b) Romhilt-Estes
(c) Schomroth (d) Cornell

529. 1 MET =

(a) 2 ml O_2/kg/min of body weight
(b) 3.5 ml O_2/kg/min of body weight
(c) 5 ml O_2/kg/min of body weight
(d) 7.5 ml O_2/kg/min of body weight

530. Mason-Likar modification is useful during:

(a) Holter analysis
(b) Coronary angiography
(c) Ambulatory blood pressure recording
(d) Treadmill test

531. LV Ejection Fraction (LVEF) is calculated by all of the following methods *except:*

(a) [(LVEDV-LVESV)/LVEDV]×100
(b) [($LVEDD^2$-$LVESD^2$)/$LVEDD^2$]×100
(c) (S.V/LVEDV)×100
(d) (LVEDD-LVESD)/LVEDD

532. False statement about Tei Index:

(a) (IVCT+IVRT)/LVET
(b) Myocardial performance index
(c) (IVCT-IVRT)/LVET
(d) Global ventricular function

533. ECG changes particular to COPD other than RVH include A/E:

(a) Reduced amplitude of the QRS complex
(b) Right axis deviation in the frontal plane
(c) Delayed transition in the precordial leads
(d) S1Q3T3 pattern

534. One of the following SPECT tracers has long half life:

(a) ^{99}Tc-Sestamibi (b) Thallium-201
(c) ^{99}Tc-Tetrafosmin (d) ^{99}Tc-Teboroxime

535. One of the following is metabolism tracer in PET imaging:

(a) Fluorine–18
(b) Oxygen–15
(c) Nitrogen–13
(d) Rubidium–82

536. Cardiac magnetic resonance imaging is useful for the diagnosis of:
(a) ARVD
(b) Sarcoidosis
(c) Amyloidosis
(d) All of the above

537. Deceleration time:
(a) Decreases
(b) Increases
(c) Increase then decrease
(d) Decrease then increase

538. Prominent U waves are seen with:
(a) Procainamide
(b) Dofetalide
(c) Lidocaine
(d) Mexiletine

539. ST elevation seen in A/E:
(a) Acute pulmonary embolism
(b) Acute MI
(c) Hyperthermia
(d) Hypercalcemia

540. Radionuclide used in SPECT are A/E:
(a) Technetium
(b) Thallium
(c) MIBG
(d) Rubidium

541. Exercise stress test relative contraindications are A/E:
(a) Moderate aortic stenosis with uncertain relation to symptoms
(b) Acquired complete heart block
(c) Hypertrophic cardiomyopathy with severe resting gradient
(d) RBBB

542. Triple rule out test:
(a) ECHO
(b) USG abdomen
(c) CT angio
(d) CT chest

543. Causes of ST elevation are A/E:
(a) MI
(b) Constrictive pericarditis
(c) Coronary spasm
(d) Ventricular aneurysm

544. ST elevation seen in A/E:
(a) Hyperkalemia
(b) Hypocalcemia
(c) Hypercalcemia
(d) Hypothermia

545. All true about ECG leads *except*:
(a) Lead I is potential difference between RA and LA
(b) Lead II is potential difference between RA and LL
(c) Lead III is potential difference between LA and LL
(d) III = II+I

546. TEE mid esophageal view, all are seen *except*:
(a) 4 chamber
(b) 5 chamber
(c) 2 chamber
(d) Short axis papillary muscle level
(e) Short axis mitral valve level

547. Gated MPI–correct is:
(a) NH3 may be used
(b) FDG-18 for perfusion
(c) Adenosine
(d) EF can be calculated
(e) Incorporates perfusion and function

548. If stroke volume is 60 ml and end-diastolic volume is 120 ml, what is ejection fraction?
(a) 40
(b) 50
(c) 60
(d) 70

549. IVC measuring 2 cm with no collapsing, RA pressure is:
(a) 3
(b) 8
(c) 12
(d) 15

550. What is the RVSP if VSD gradient is 94 mm Hg and systolic BP is 120 mm Hg:

(a) 10 (b) 20

(c) 26 (d) 30

551. ECG suggests: (See Figure 1)

(a) Hypercalcemia (b) Hypocalcemia

(c) Hypokalemia (d) Hyperkalemia

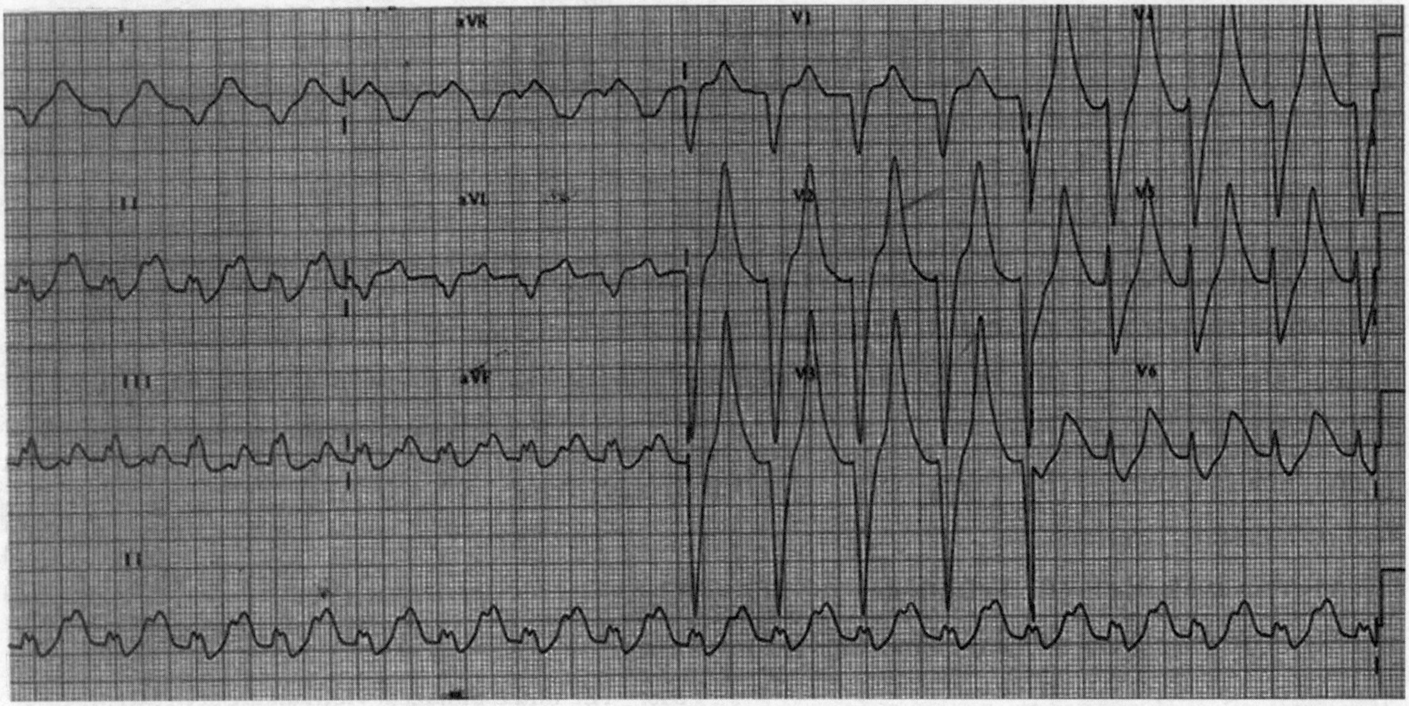

Figure 1

ANSWERS KEY

1. (b)	2. (d)	3. (d)	4. (b)	5. (c)	6. (b)	7. (a)	8. (c)
9. (d)	10. (a)	11. (a)	12. (a)	13. (b)	14. (b)	15. (a)	16. (c)
17. (a)	18. (c)	19. (a)	20. (b)	21. (b)	22. (d)	23. (b)	24. (a)
25. (d)	26. (a)	27. (a)	28. (a,b)	29. (a)	30. (b)	31. (a)	32. (b)
33. (a)	34. (b)	35. (b)	36. (c)	37. FFTTF	38. FTFTT	39. TTFFF	40. FFTTT
41. TFTTF	42. FFF	43. (a)	44. (d)	45. (b)	46. (d)	47. (c)	48. (c)
49. (b)	50. (a)	51. (a)	52. (a)	53. (d)	54. (c)	55. (c)	56. (a)
57. (c)	58. (b)	59. (a)	60. (a)	61. (c)	62. (d)	63. (d)	64. (c)
65. (c)	66. (d)	67. (d)	68. (b)	69. (c)	70. (d)	71. (d)	72. (b)
73. (b)	74. (a)	75. (d)	76. (c)	77. (d)	78. (c)	79. (b)	80. (c)
81. (b)	82. (d)	83. (d)	84. (c)	85. (b)	86. (b)	87. (d)	88. (c)
89. (d)	90. (c)	91. (b)	92. (b)	93. (b)	94. (a)	95. (b)	96. (a)
97. (a)	98. (c)	99. (b)	100. (c)	101. (c)	102. (d)	103. (b)	104. (a)
105. (a)	106. (d)	107. (b)	108. (d)	109. (c)	110. (b)	111. (b)	112. (c)
113. (b)	114. (c)	115. (c)	116. (a)	117. (b)	118. (b)	119. (b)	120. (a)
121. (a)	122. (d)	123. (d)	124. (c)	125. (c)	126. (a)	127. (a)	128. (d)
129. (b)	130. (c)	131. (a)	132. (a)	133. (c)	134. (a)	135. (c)	136. (d)
137. (b)	138. (b)	139. (b)	140. (d)	141. (b)	142. (c)	143. (c)	144. (a)
145. (c)	146. (a)	147. (c)	148. (a)	149. (a)	150. (a)	151. (a)	152. (a)
153. (c)	154. (c)	155. (b)	156. (a)	157. (a)	158. (a)	159. (a)	160. (d)
161. (b)	162. (a)	163. (a)	164. (c)	165. (a)	166. (?)	167. (a)	168. (c)
169. (c)	170. (b)	171. (a)	172. (a)	173. (a)	174. (d)	175. (c)	176. (a)
177. (a)	178. (a)	179. (c)	180. TTFT	181. FTFT	182. (d)	183. (a)	184. (b)
185. (a)	186. (e)	187. (a)	188. (e)	189. (d)	190. (e)	191. (a)	192. FFTTT
193. (d)	194. (a)	195. (c)	196. TTTFT	197. TTF	198. (b)	199. (c)	200. (b)
201. (a)	202. FFFF	203. FTFTF	204. (d)	205. (a)	206. (b)	207. (a)	208. (b)
209. (d)	210. (a)	211. (a)	212. (d)	213. (d)	214. (c)	215. (b)	216. (a)
217. (c)	218. (d)	219. (c)	220. (d)	221. (b)	222. (d)	223. (c)	224. (d)
225. (a)	226. (c)	227. (a)	228. (a)	229. (a)	230. (c)	231. (d)	232. (a)
233. (a)	234. (a)	235. (a)	236. (d)	237. (a)	238. (a)	239. (a)	240. (a)
241. (a)	242. (d)	243. (a)	244. (d)	245. (c)	246. (a)	247. (a)	248. (a)
249. (b)	250. (c)	251. (a)	252. (a)	253. (c)	254. (a)	255. (a)	256. (a)
257. (c)	258. (a)	259. (a)	260. (c)	261. (b)	262. (a)	263. (a)	264. (d)
265. (b)	266. (d)	267. (d)	268. (a)	269. (d)	270. (b)	271. (b)	272. (a)
273. (d)	274. (a)	275. (d)	276. (a)	277. (c)	278. (a)	279. (c)	280. (a)
281. (c)	282. (b)	283. (c)	284. (a)	285. (a)	286. (c)	287. (c)	288. (b)
289. (c)	290. (b)	291. (d)	292. (b)	293. (b)	294. (a)	295. (b)	296. (a)
297. (d)	298. (b)	299. (b,d)	300. (b)	301. (c)	302. (a)	303. (d)	304. (a)
305. (b)	306. (c)	307. (b)	308. (c)	309. (a)	310. (a)	311. (b)	312. (a)
313. (b)	314. (a)	315. (a)	316. (b)	317. (a)	318. (a)	319. (d)	320. (a)
321. (d)	322. (b)	323. (a)	324. (a)	325. (b)	326. (a)	327. (b)	328. (d)
329. (a)	330. (a)	331. (c)	332. (d)	333. (a)	334. (a)	335. (c)	336. (a)
337. (a)	338. (c)	339. (a)	340. (a)	341. (a)	342. (c)	343. (d)	344. (a)

345.	(a)	346.	(c)	347.	(b,c)	348.	(a)	349.	(a)	350.	(c)	351.	(a)	352.	(d)
353.	(b)	354.	(b)	355.	(c)	356.	(c)	357.	(a)	358.	(b)	359.	(b)	360.	(c)
361.	(a)	362.	(d)	363.	(a)	364.	(a)	365.	TTTFT	366.	FTFTT	367.	FTTFF	368.	FTFTF
369.	FTTTF	370.	TTFTT	371.	TTTTT	372.	TFFFT	373.	FTFTT	374.	TFTFT	375.	TTFTT	376.	TFTTF
377.	(c)	378.	FTTF	379.	TTTFF	380.	TTFFT	381.	TFFFF	382.	TFTFF	383.	FTTTT	384.	(a)
385.	TFFFF	386.	(b)	387.	FTTTF	388.	TTFFF	389.	FTTTF	390.	FTFFF	391.	TFTFF	392.	FFFFT
393.	FTFTT	394.	TTTFF	395.	TFFTT	396.	TTTF	397.	TFTTF	398.	TTFFF	399.	(a)	400.	(b)
401.	(c)	402.	(b)	403.	(c)	404.	(a)	405.	(a)	406.	(c)	407.	(d)	408.	(c)
409.	(c)	410.	(b)	411.	(c)	412.	(a)	413.	TFFTF	414.	FTTTT	415.	TTFT	416.	TFFTF
417.	TTFFF	418.	FFFTT	419.	FTTTT	420.	TFFFT	421.	FF	422.	TTFF	423.	TTFTF	424.	TFTF
425.	FTFFF	426.	TFFTF	427.	FTFFF	428.	FTTTT	429.	FTFFF	430.	FFTTT	431.	TFTFF	432.	FFTTT
433.	TTFTTT	434.	(c)	435.	TTFTTTT	436.	TTTFFT	437.	FTTTT	438.	FFFF	439.	TFTFF	440.	FFFTF
441.	FTTTF	442.	TFTTT	443.	TTTFF	444.	FTTFT	445.	TTFT	446.	TFTTF	447.	(b,c,d)	448.	TFFT
449.	FTTFT	450.	TTFFF	451.	FTTTF	452.	TTTFT	453.	(d)	454.	(a)	455.	(c)	456.	(a)
457.	(b)	458.	(a)	459.	(d)	460.	(a)	461.	(a)	462.	(d)	463.	(a)	464.	(c)
465.	(a)	466.	(a)	467.	(a)	468.	(a)	469.	(a)	470.	(a)	471.	(b)	472.	(b)
473.	(d)	474.	(d)	475.	(c)	476.	(a)	477.	(d)	478.	(c)	479.	(c)	480.	(a)
481.	(a)	482.	(a)	483.	(a)	484.	(d)	485.	(b)	486.	(b)	487.	(c)	488.	(a)
489.	(d)	490.	(c)	491.	(d)	492.	(a)	493.	(c)	494.	(d)	495.	(b)	496.	(a)
497.	(b)	498.	(b)	499.	(b)	500.	(c)	501.	(c)	502.	(d)	503.	(a)	504.	(b)
505.	(a)	506.	(b)	507.	(a)	508.	(d)	509.	(b)	510.	(a)	511.	(d)	512.	(c)
513.	(b)	514.	(d)	515.	(c)	516.	(c)	517.	(a)	518.	(a)	519.	(a)	520.	(a)
521.	(d)	522.	(c)	523.	(d)	524.	(c)	525.	(d)	526.	(a)	527.	(a)	528.	(c)
529.	(b)	530.	(d)	531.	(d)	532.	(c)	533.	(d)	534.	(b)	535.	(a)	536.	(d)
537.	(c)	538.	(b)	539.	(c)	540.	(d)	541.	(d)	542.	(c)	543.	(b)	544.	(b)
545.	(d)	546.	(e)	547.	(c)	548.	(b)	549.	(b)	550.	(c)	551.	(d)		

CHAPTER TEN

MEDICINE

1. **ROSC most reliable:**
   (a) $ETCO_2 > 35$ (b) Pulses palpable
   (c) ECG (d) $SPO_2 > 95\%$

2. **Heuristic:**
   (a) Occam's razor (b) Sulton law
   (c) Sulli's law (d) Murphy's law

3. **Desmosomal mutation:**
   (a) ARVC (b) DCM
   (c) RCM

4. **HIT, which is not true?**
   (a) Platelet transfusion in asymptomatic
   (b) Paradoxical thrombosis
   (c) PF_4 immune complex
   (d) Type I HIT has better prognosis

5. **Amyloidosis – all are true *except*:**
   (a) Isolated atrial amyloid – SAA
   (b) Familial–mutant transthyretin
   (c) Senile–transthyretin
   (d) Primary amyloidosis–AL

6. **Evolocumab–true is:**
   (a) Oral PCSK9 inhibitor
   (b) AST/ALT > 3 ULN common
   (c) PCSK9 mutation cause AD hypercholesterolemia
   (d) PCSK9 decreases LDL by increasing its clearance

7. **Not true is:**
   (a) Café au lait spots–RAS
   (b) Alagille syndrome–peripheral PS
   (c) Cardiac fibroma–Angiofibroma
   (d) Noonan syndrome–HCM

8. **Term 'Risk factor' was coined by:**
   (a) Braunwald (b) William B. Cannel
   (c) Rose (d) Lauer

9. **Primary hyperaldosteronism–all *except*:**
   (a) Alkalosis (b) Hypomagnesemia
   (c) LV hypertrophy (d) Systemic congestion

10. **Identify the graph: (See table below)**
    (a) Farrest-plot (b) Kaplan Meir curve
    (c) ROC curve

Study of subgroup	Experimental			Control			St. Mean difference		Std. Mean difference
	Mean	SD	Total	Mean	SD	Total	Weight	IV Fixed 95% CI	IV Fixed 95% CI
Evans 2011	0	1	90	0.5	1	90	29.8%	–0.50 [–0.79, –0.20]	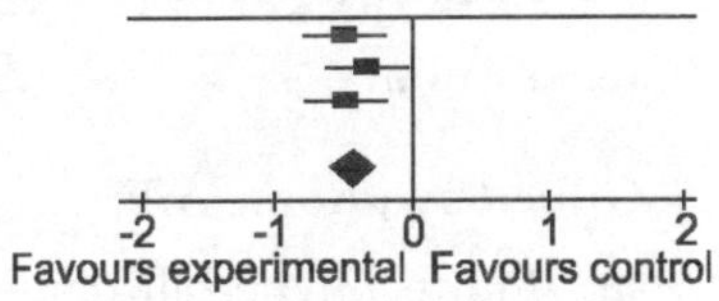
Jones 2010	0	1	110	0.3	1	110	37.1%	–0.30 [–0.56, –0.03]	
Smith 2013	0.5	1	100	1	1	100	33.1%	–0.50 [–0.78, –0.22]	
Total (95% CI)			300			300	100.0%	–0.42 [–0.59, –0.26]	

Heterogeneity: $Chi^2 = 1.35$, df = 2 (P = 0.51); $I^2 = 0\%$
Test for overall effect Z=5.13 (P < 0.00001)

11. **A-a O_2 gradient is normal in:**
(a) Hypoventilation (b) V-Q mismatch
(c) Pulmonary edema (d) Pneumonia

12. **X-ray show–pacemaker inserted with pneumothorax, Immediate intervention:**
(a) Intercostal drainage (b) IV fluids
(c) Repositioning of lead

13. **Drug t 1/2=5 hours. Steady state achieved in:**
(a) 25 hours (b) 4 hours
(c) 7 hours (d) 70 hours

14. **Direct thrombin inhibitor A/E:**
(a) Hirudin (b) Argatroban
(c) Dabigatran (d) Apixaban

15. **All T/E:**
(a) B blockers–lipolysis on chronic therapy
(b) Omarcintisc–myosin receptor activator
(c) B. arrestin–antiopoptotic receptor
(d) B2 receptors, upregulated in ventricle–heart failure

16. **Least cardiac side effect:**
(a) Diclofenac (b) Naproxin
(c) Celecoxib (d) Rofecoxib

17. **Becker muscular dystrophy:**
(a) Heart failure may be the first symptom
(b) Marked improvement with steroids in early phase
(c) Dystrophin length deletion does not correlate with severity
(d) Facial weakness less common

18. **High anion gap metabolic acidosis A/E:**
(a) Starvation (b) Antifreeze
(c) Type IV RTA (d) Methanol

19. **Hypokalemia A/E:**
(a) Licorice abuse (b) Salbutamol
(c) Insulin (d) Theophylline toxicity

20. **Gilbert syndrome A/E:**
(a) Indirect hyperbilirubinemia
(b) Female–common
(c) 3-5% incidence
(d) Icterus increased by stress, fever

21. **B_{12} decreased in:**
(a) Renal failure
(b) Cirrhosis
(c) Myeloproliferative disease
(d) Eosinophilia

22. **All are true in critical illness Px *except*:**
(a) Brain–glucose utilization–90 gm
(b) Benedict equation for colorial requirement
(c) Protein atleast 0.7 gm/kg
(d) On ventilator calorie requirement 1.5 times

23. **Hereditary nephrogenic DI All T/E:**
(a) Indomethacin (b) Salt restriction
(c) Thiazide (d) Vasopressin

24. **Peptic ulcer A/E:**
(a) Clopidogrel (b) Misoprostol
(c) Helicobacter (d) Annular pancreas

25. **HIT all T/E:**
(a) Fondaparinux used in normal renal function
(b) Warfarin for 3 months if thrombus present
(c) More in surgical than medical patient
(d) PF. 4 antibodies are diagnostic

26. **Vitamin D A/E:**
(a) Atherosclerosis (b) Heart failure
(c) Bradyarrhythmia

27. **Intestinal microbes degrade:**
(a) DCM
(b) Atherosclerosis
(c) RHD
(d) Neural tube defect and CHS

28. **Giant all arteritis A/E:**
(a) Can cause ischemic optic neuropathy
(b) Complement decreased
(c) Panarteritis medium and large–vessel
(d) Aortic dissection in late stage

29. **Wegener–All T/E:**
(a) Medium and small vessel
(b) MMC complex deposition in kidney
(c) Necrotizing glomerulus involvement
(d) >90% upper airway involvement

30. **Hypothermia–A/E:**
(a) Alcohol (b) Dinitrophenol
(c) Hypoglycemia (d) Shapiro syndrome

31. **Epidemiological tool for risk factor assessment:**
(a) Cross sectional (b) RCT
(c) Cohort study (d) Case series

32. **Normal diet contains:**
(a) Long chain fatty acids
(b) MCFA
(c) SCFA
(d) USCFA

33. **A/E:**

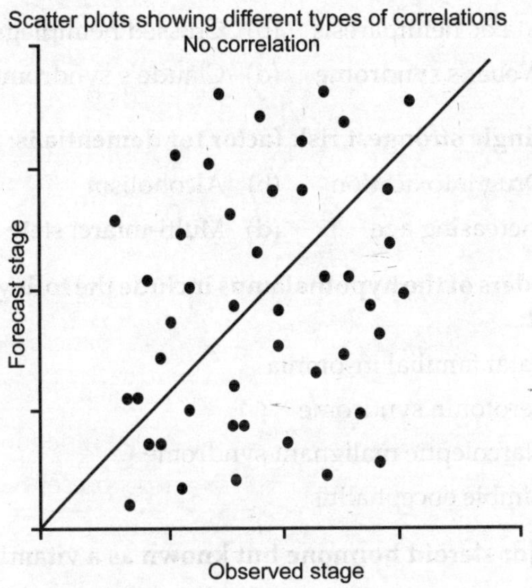

(a) X and Y linearly related
(b) 'r' varies from – +1 to –1
(c) Coefficient of correlation variance/product of SD
(d) > 0.55 high correction

34. **HIT not done:**
(a) Bivalirudin of anticoag. required
(b) Platelet transfer
(c) Stop all heparin
(d) DVT evaluation

35. **Exudative pleural effusion in:**
(a) SVC obstruction (b) Pulm. infarction
(c) CCP (d) HF

36. **Which has less likely hypokalemia?**
(a) Hypothyroid (b) Pheochromocytoma
(c) Eclampsia (d) Renovascular HTN

37. **Predictive value includes:**
(a) Only null hypothesis
(b) Specificity only
(c) Sensitivity only
(d) Both null hypothesis and prevalence

Exudative pleural effusion (T/F) (38 to 41)

38. **LDH > 250**

39. **S. gravity > 1.121**

40. **Plot > 2.6**

41. **Glucose of pleural fluid > 1.5 times serum**

42. **INR cut off for radial catheterization:**
(a) < 1.8 (b) < 2.2
(c) 2.2 (d) 2.8

43. **Immune mediated manifestation in I/E all *except*:**
(a) Roth spots (b) Osler nodes
(c) Janeway lesion (d) Rheumatoid factor

44. **Hypermagnesemia A/E:**
(a) PR, QT, QRS ↑ when Mg 2.5-5 mEq
(b) ↓ Tendon reflex, muscle weakness 2-2.5 mEq
(c) Cardiac arrest and bradycardia Mg 6-10 mEq
(d) Renal failure–less dose toxicity

45. **Embolic stroke risk:**
(a) CHA_2DS-Vasc (b) HAS BLED
(c) ATRIA (d) CHADS

46. **Needs dental extraction. What to do his warfarin?**
(a) Continue warfarin
(b) Stop warfarin
(c) Start LMWH
(d) Stop for 3 days and then restart

47. **Heart is not affected in:**
(a) AL amyloidosis
(b) Familial (ATTR) amyloidosis
(c) AA amyloidosis
(d) Senile systemic amyloidosis

48. **Regarding cardiac complications of radiation therapy all are true *except*:**
(a) Many patients with radiation induced CAD do not experience "angina warning symptoms"
(b) Systolic LV dysfunction is more common than diastolic dysfunction
(c) Anthracycline therapy further increases the risk of CAD and aortic valve disease
(d) Bundle branch block and CHB may occur

49. **Variegate porphyria is due to deficiency of:**
(a) Ferrochelatase
(b) Coproporphyrinogen oxidase
(c) Protoporphyrinogen oxidase
(d) Uroporphyrinogen synthase

50. **The antidote for yellow oleander poisoning is:**
(a) Atropine
(b) IV magnesium
(c) Digoxin-specific antibody fragments
(d) Beta blocker

51. **The speculative etiology of idiopathic pulmonary fibrosis include the following *except*:**
(a) Epstein-Barr virus (b) Occupational dusts
(c) Antidepressants (d) Cigarette smoking

52. **The abnormal level of serum testosterone levels in women is:**
(a) More than 5 nmol/L (b) 2-5 nmol/L
(c) Less than 2 nmol/L (d) Less than 1 nmol/L

53. **The parathyroid hormone resistance is found in:**
(a) Chronic kidney disease
(b) Pseudo hypoparathyroidism
(c) Autoimmune disorders
(d) Inherited disorders

54. **The function of immunoglobulin D (IgD) is:**
(a) Unknown
(b) Opsonisation
(c) Complement activation
(d) Defence against parasitic infections

55. **Scott's syndrome is:**
(a) Defect of platelet adhesion
(b) Defect of platelet coagulant activity
(c) Defect of platelet secretion
(d) Defect of platelet aggregation

56. **In a case of polycythemia C.T. of head is done to detect:**
(a) Secondaries
(b) Intracerebellar hemorrhage
(c) Cerebellar hemangioma
(d) Berry aneurysms

57. **Presence of palpable spleen in a patient which sickle cell disease after age five suggests:**
(a) Thalassemia (b) Splenosis
(c) Ectopic spleen (d) Marrow failure

58. **Conditions that mimic stroke include the following *except*:**
(a) Seizure (b) Intracranial tumour
(c) Migraine (d) Conversion reaction

59. **A third nerve palsy with contralateral ataxia is known as:**
(a) Ataxic hemiparesis (b) Crossed hemiplegia
(c) Weber's syndrome (d) Claude's syndrome

60. **The single strongest risk factor for dementia is:**
(a) Drug intoxication (b) Alcoholism
(c) Increasing age (d) Multi-infarct state

61. **Disorders of the hypothalamus include the following *except*:**
(a) Fatal familial insomnia
(b) Serotonin syndrome
(c) Narcoleptic malignant syndrome
(d) Limbic encephalitis

62. **A major steroid hormone but known as a vitamin is:**
(a) Vitamin D (b) Vitamin A
(c) Vitamin K (d) Vitamin E

63. **Katayama fever is associated with:**
(a) Leishmaniasis
(b) Acute schistosomiasis
(c) Chronic schistosomiasis
(d) Praziquantel therapy

64. **The drug of choice for U parvum infection is:**
(a) Azithromycin (b) Clarithromycin
(c) Doxycycline (d) Gemifloxacin

65. **Nervous system manifestation of SLE include all *except*:**
(a) Cognitive dysfunction
(b) Psychosis
(c) Seizures
(d) Dementia

66. **Which type of lymphoma is most common in RA?**
(a) Diffuse large "B" cell lymphoma
(b) Lymphoblastic lymphoma
(c) Mantle cell lymphoma
(d) Follicular lymphoma

67. Flowing wax sign in spinal X-ray is seen:

(a) Pott's spine
(b) Klippel-Feil anomaly
(c) Diffuse idiopathic skeletal hyperostosis (DISH)
(d) Rheumatoid arthritis

68. Conditions that mimic diffuse parenchymal lung disease include the following *except*:

(a) Bronchogenic carcinoma
(b) Lymphangitic carcinomatosis
(c) Bronchoalveolar carcinoma
(d) Leukemia

69. Total energy requirement in a term neonate is:

(a) 150-170 kcal/kg/day
(b) 130-150 kcal/kg/day
(c) 199-120 kcal/kg/day
(d) 80-100 kcal/kg/day

70. The causes of hypergonadotropic hypogonadism include the following *except*:

(a) Kallmann's syndrome
(b) Autoimmune gonadal failure
(c) Hemochromatosis
(d) Klinefelter's syndrome

71. An important component to define pediatric sepsis is:

(a) Increase in respiratory rate
(b) Increase in heart rate
(c) Change in core temperature
(d) Fall in hemoglobin

72. The blood volume in a 2 years old child in mL/kg is:

(a) 120 (b) 100
(c) 80 (d) 60

73. Post-diarrhea complications of Ac infections diarrheal illness include the following *except*:

(a) Hemolytic–Uremic syndrome
(b) Guillain-Barré syndrome
(c) Irritable bowel syndrome
(d) Rectal prolapse

74. Which of the following is the least common among children with cerebral palsy?

(a) Spasticity (b) Seizure
(c) Ataxia (d) Hearing impairment

75. Mixed T and B cell deficiency/dysfunction defects are associated with the following *except*:

(a) Ataxia-Telangiectasia
(b) Wiskott-Aldrich syndrome
(c) AIDS
(d) X-linked hyper-IgM syndrome

76. The infant's head forms....% of the total body surface.

(a) 9% (b) 15%
(c) 20% (d) 30%

77. 'Relapsing fever' is caused by:

(a) Leishmaniasis (b) Brucellosis
(c) Malaria (d) Borrelia

78. With regard to hyponatremia in children, all are true *except*:

(a) Children can develop hyponatremic encephalopathy at higher sodium levels than adults because they have a lower brain-skull ratio
(b) Symptomatic hyponatremic encephalopathy can lead to death or permanent neurological disability
(c) Problems can arise if hypotonic maintenance fluids are given to resuscitate or replace losses
(d) Hyponatremia can also happen if maintenance fluids have been given in excess

79. In a surgical setting most common cause of hyponatremia is:

(a) Insufficient sodium infusion
(b) Excess free water
(c) Increased renal loss
(d) Nasogastric aspiration

80. Rickettsialpox is transmitted by:

(a) Tick bite (b) Mite bite
(c) Flea (d) Louse feces

81. Iron deficiency anemia: (T/F)

(a) 10-15% iron is absorbed
(b) S ferritin < 50 is diagnostic
(c) Iron glucose is safer than iron dextrose
(d) Daily iron 200-300 mg is given per day in IDA
(e) Heparin ↑ iron absorption

82. Aphasia: (T/F)

(a) Speech therapy more useful in Brocha's as comp. Wernicke

(b) Anomic aphasia–Most common presentation
(c) Anomic aphasia–Comprehension is present
(d) Wernicke's–Comprehension–impaired, fluency–preserved
(e) Pure ataxia–Comprehension of spoken language impaired

83. Acute ischemic stroke: (T/F)
(a) Thrombolysis beneficial within 6 hours
(b) Dual antiplatelet within 4 hours reverses neurological deficit
(c) Aspirin useful within 24 hours
(d) BP should be reduced to < 120/80
(e) Anticoagulant beneficial in embolic stroke

84. OP poisoning: (T/F)
(a) Irrev. inhi. of anticholinesterase
(b) Slowly excreted by kidney
(c) Muscarinic effect–salivation, sweating, lacrimation
(d) Atropine–DOC
(e) Pralidoxime reverse CNS effect

85. Psychiatric minor disorder: (T/F)
(a) SSRI used in generalized anxiety disorder
(b) Long term B2P therapy useful in panic disorder
(c) B blocker useful in social anxiety disorder
(d) Antidep. respond in OCD in 30-60%
(e) Buspirone doesn't cause sedation

86. Immunization–adult: (T/F)
(a) Diphtheria and tetanus given every 5 years
(b) Varicella vaccine can be given even after infection
(c) Pneumococcal vaccine should be given atleast 2 weeks before splenectomy
(d) Rota virus vaccine–inactivated vaccine
(e) HPV–inactivated virus vaccine

87. True are: (T/F)
(a) HBV vaccination in HIV
(b) HAV in I/V drug abuser
(c) HBV–subunit vaccine
(d) BCG–live bacteria
(e) Measles–live attenuated vaccine

88. Immunosuppression: (T/F)
(a) Steroid given in evening
(b) 100 mg Hydrocortisone – 15 mg Prednisolone
(c) Deflazocort–less metabolic side effect than prednisolone
(d) In RA–sustained release preparation of prednisolone given at night
(e) Alternate day steroids–less bacterial infection

89. Cohort study: (T/F)
(a) Case control study, followed over time
(b) In cohort–exposed with non exposed divided randomly
(c) Cohort always prospective
(d) For diet study, a complete family can be randomized for 1 group for single diet
(e) Blinding is more useful when result of study is quality of life rather than death

90. HCV: (T/F)
(a) 20% chances of infectivity of needle injury
(b) IP–Max. 8 weeks
(c) Chronicity rate 20-30%
(d) Infection is recovered, no reinfection occurs
(e) Acute infection asymptomatic mostly

91. Nutrition: (T/F)
(a) Mid aim circumference–fat
(b) BMI–India–18.5-22.9
(c) Severe acute malnutrition albumin < 2.8
(d) Starvation malnutrition maintains immunocompetency
(e) Folic acid def – dose 1 mg/day

92. TEN: (T/F)
(a) Involve > 10% BSA
(b) Immunosuppression with IVIG decreases mortality
(c) Mortality rate–20-30%
(d) Malignancy underlying has decreased risk in TEN
(e) Allopurinol induced TEN has genetic link

93. Community acquired pneumonia: (T/F)
(a) Levoflox DOC in DM
(b) Macrolide if good response, can be used within 3 months
(c) Culture from pleural effusion required therapeutic drainage
(d) Recurrent pneumonia in same lobe S/O–malignancy
(e) Pneumococcal resistance solely due to altera of beta lactam binding plot

94. Acid base: (T/F)

(a) Normal AG-20
(b) Nephrotic syndrome – ↓ AG
(c) Salicylic toxicity – ↑ AG
(d) –K-associated with metabolic alkalosis
(e) Alkalinization done to maintain pH–7.35

95. ATT: (T/F)

(a) Rifampicin – ↑ bleeding with anticoagulants
(b) Hyperuricemia–pyrazinamide
(c) Cyclosporine–CI in seizure patients
(d) Isoniazid–optic neuritis
(e) Rifampicin–flue like symptom

96. Osteoporosis: (T/F)

(a) Bisphosphonate–PTH analogue
(b) Calcitonin (nasal)–↓ osteoclast activity
(c) Denosumab–RANK legend
(d) Teriperatide–25%–Hypercalcemia
(e) Zoledronate–given every 1 year

97. HIV in rheumatoid: (T/F)

(a) Septic arthritis–more common
(b) Psoriatic arthritis is most common presentation
(c) Reactive arthritis is less seen
(d) Arthralgia more common than arthritis
(e) H2AB27 same in reactive arthritis as HIV

98. Stone: (T/F)

(a) Calcium most common constituent
(b) Uric acid are radio opaque
(c) Uric acid precipitate in alkaline urine
(d) Thiazide diuretic ↓ Recurrence of uric acid stones
(e) > 2.5 L water ↓ stone recurrence in 50%

99. Peripheral smear: (T/F)

(a) Microsporocyte S/O heredity spherocytosis
(b) Target and microcyte in thalassemia
(c) Schiztocyte in MAHA
(d) Iron deficiency anemia in PNH
(e) Nucleated RBC and ↑ WBC in myelopathies

100. Rash with fever: (T/F)

(a) Parvovirus–slapped check
(b) Varicella–1st day of fever
(c) Koplik spot–rubella
(d) Rash after 6 days of fever–measles
(e) Roseola–Rash disappearance of fever

101. Primary amyloidosis: (T/F)

(a) RCM is cardiac manifestation
(b) Macroglossia is uncommon
(c) Raccoon sign is dft factor X deficiency
(d) Serum immunofixation is useful
(e) It is a disease of heavy chains

102. Anemia of chronic disease: (T/F)

(a) Iron deficiency anemia is imp DD
(b) Hepcidin is decreased
(c) Red cell survival may be reduced
(d) May have normocytic normochromic picture
(e) Hyperplastic bond narrow

103. Chronic fatigue syndrome (CFS): (T/F)

(a) Symptoms not alleviated by rest
(b) Childhood inactivity is a risk factor
(c) Pregnancy precipitates CFS
(d) Antidepressants may be useful
(e) Sore throat

104. Side effects: (T/F)

(a) Zidovudine–Anemia
(b) Stavudine–Pancreatitis
(c) Lamivudine–Neuropathy
(d) Nevirapine–SJS
(e) Raltegravir–Abnormal fat distribution

105. ARDS: (T/F)

(a) Lung protective ventilation–using high PEE
(b) HFOV started early–improves mortality
(c) Prone position ventilation–improves mortality
(d) Low tidal volume ventilation worsen mortality compared to conventional ventilation

106. Fungi: (T/F)

(a) Mycetia are the infective forms in histoplasma
(b) Progressive histoplasmosis–duration of treatment 6 months
(c) Mucormycosis causes angio invasion
(d) Cryptococcal antigen in sputum–high sensitivity and high specificity for pulmonary Cryptococcus
(e) Yeast detection in CSF India ink preparation–indicates poor prognosis

107. Corticosteroids: (T/F)

(a) Receptors are present on surface
(b) Acts through 'transcription'
(c) Inhibition of phospholipase A_2 (Inhibits arachidonic acid metabolism by inhibiting PLA_2)
(d) HTN is rennin-angiotensin mediated

108. Acid peptic disease: (T/F)

(a) Duodenal ulcer symptoms occur 90 min. after taking meals
(b) Gastric ulcers associated with increased acid production
(c) NSAID ulcers–10% risk of perforation
(d) NSAID ulcers–80-90% complication previously asymptotic cases

109. Lupus nephritis: (T/F)

(a) Children had lesser prevalence of lupus nephritis
(b) Wire loop lesions are characteristic
(c) Subendothelial deposits in membranous glomerulitis
(d) Presence of thrombotic microangiopathy – suspect APLAS
(e) Renal transplantation–25% recurrence

110. About glucose homeostasis: (T/F)

(a) C-peptide differentiates endogenous and exogenous insulin
(b) Brain needs 50 G glucose per day for its metabolic needs
(c) Response to hypoglycemia–low insulin and anti-insulin hormones
(d) Gluconeogenesis

111. Regarding diarrhea: (T/F)

(a) Small volume and less frequent–in small bowel diarrhea
(b) Secretory diarrhea improves with fasting
(c) Stool osmolality is useful to detect factitious diarrhea
(d) Steatorrhea–pancreatic exocrine insufficiency

112. UTI: (T/F)

(a) Asymptomatic bacteriuria needs antibiotic to prevent symptomatic UTI
(b) Asymptomatic bacteria–5% prevalence in 20-40 years women
(c) E. coli–Most common organism in lower UTI
(d) E. coli–Most common organism in upper UTI
(e) Nitrofurazone coating of catheter prevents UTI

113. Joints: (T/F)

(a) Cranial bone sutures are cartilaginous joints
(b) Symphysis pubis is fibrous joint
(c) Synovium covers articular surfaces of joints
(d) Synovium attached at the junction of bony and cartilaginous parts
(e) Normal synovium has 5-6 layers of cells

114. Arthritis (Psoriatic): (T/F)

(a) Skin lesions can precede arthritis
(b) DIP joint involvement is invariably associated with nail dystrophy
(c) RF is negative in majority of cases
(d) Uveitis–acute
(e) Marginal erosions with adjacent bony proliferation

115. SAH: (T/F)

(a) After head trauma, most common cause of SAH is ruptured of saccular aneurysm
(b) Aneurysm, most common on anterior circulation
(c) Vasospasm occurs within 24 hours
(d) Hyponatremia of SAH should not be treated with fluid restriction
(e) Rerupture peak in the first 7 days

116. Regarding DNA: (T/F)

(a) No. of genes 50,000
(b) 10% of DNA is functionally encoding
(c) Cytosine methylation – silences gene expression
(d) Mitochondrial disorders follow maternal inheritance
(e) Fragile X–trinucleotide repeats

117. Immunoglobulins: (T/F)

(a) Heavy chain and light chains are encoded on different chromosomes
(b) Heavy chain has V.J.C. segments only
(c) Light chain recombination occurs earlier than heavy chain recombination
(d) Allelic exclusion–responsible for specific antibody production by B cells

118. Sarcoidosis: (T/F)

(a) Peribronchial infiltrates are characteristic
(b) ACE levels are useful screening test

(c) Plaque indicates chronic skin lesions

(d) 50% cases granulomas with asymp cases

(e) FVC–decreased–30% cases

119. Regarding normal Gaussian distribution: (T/F)

(a) Mean and mode are same

(b) Median and mode are different

(c) Most frequent is median

(d) Interquartile range comprises mean ± I SD

(e) ± 2.5 SD covers all values

120. Statistics: (T/F)

(a) Interquartile range 25-75%

(b) Intention to treat analysis–subjects analysed as per randomization irrespective of treatment received (or) adherence to protocol

(c) Phase 2 clinical trials studied for effectiveness and short term side effects

121. Regarding allergy: (T/F)

(a) Skin prick testing useful in food allergy

(b) Eczema lesions are not itchy

(c) Chronic urticaria is associated with–IgE levels

(d) Patients with atopy have more urticaria than eczema

(e) Aspirin sensitive patients can have anaphylaxis

122. Insulinomas: (T/F)

(a) Majority of insulinomas are large and unresectable by the time of diagnosis

(b) Hypoglycemia in hepatoma is because of secretion of IGF-2

(c) Symptoms due to excess catecholamine release

(d) 5-15% are malignant

(e) Family history of MEN-1

123. Nutrition: (T/F)

(a) Proteins →20-25% of total calorie intake

(b) Fats →30% of total calorie intake

(c) Serum prealbumin is good marker of protein deficiency

(d) Saturated fat and trans-fat should be limited to <10% of calories

(e) 55% of total calories should be derived from carbohydrates

124. Verapamil does not increase blood level of following drug:

(a) Digoxin (b) Atorvastatin

(c) Aspirin (d) Ketoconazole

125. Cutoff limit for maternal warfarin dose to minimize risk of fetal embryopathy in the first trimester is:

(a) 2 mg (b) 5 mg

(c) 7 mg (d) 10 mg

126. Which one of the following ECG abnormalities is uncommon in amyloidosis?

(a) Low voltage in limb leads

(b) Left bundle branch block

(c) First degree AV block

(d) Pseudo infarction pattern in inferior and septal leads

127. Examples of normal anion gap metabolic acidosis include all *except*:

(a) Diarrhea

(b) Potassium sparing diuretics

(c) Diabetic ketoacidosis

(d) Renal tubular acidosis

128. Kearns Sayre syndrome is associated with all *except*:

(a) Progressive external ophthalmoplegia

(b) Corneal involvement

(c) Atrioventricular block

(d) None of the above

129. Set of traits that combine anxious and depressive feelings and tendency towards social inhibition and isolation and associated with higher mortality rates is:

(a) Type A personality (b) Type B personality

(c) Type C personality (d) Type D personality

130. Select the true statement for sarcoidosis:

(a) There is predilection for granulomatous infiltration to upper septal area

(b) Conduction disturbance is more common than pump dysfunction

(c) Both of the above

(d) None of the above

131. Not a feature of Kawasaki syndrome:

(a) Strawberry tongue

(b) Vesicular eruptions

(c) Coronary artery aneurysms

(d) Cervical lymphadenopathy

132. Cardiovascular manifestations of acromegaly include all *except*:

(a) Accelerated atherosclerosis

(b) Secondary hypertension with dramatic response to ARBs

(c) Four-fold increase in ventricular arrhythmias
(d) Late potentials in SAECG

133. Most common game associated with commotio-cordis is:

(a) Football (b) Baseball
(c) Cricket (d) Ice hockey

134. Patient has after 100% O_2 administration, arterial saturation –100%, P α O_2–300, O_2 1.5% diagnosis in:

(a) Methemoglobinemia
(b) Congenital heart disease
(c) Hypoventilation
(d) None of the above

135. Amyloidosis A/E:

(a) Interstitial deposit
(b) Plasmapheresis may help
(c) Atrial septal hypertrophy
(d) Cardiac amyloid from albumin

136. Drug–half life–4 hours, given every 4 hours – steady state reached at:

(a) 10 hours (b) 20 hours
(c) 48 hours (d) 72 hours

137. Half life of drug mainly determined by:

(a) Clearance (b) Lipid solubility
(c) Absorption (d) Receptor adhesion

138. BMI–Obesity:

(a) >25 (b) >30
(c) >35 (d) >40

139. Patient on ketoconazole–statin of choice:

(a) Atorvastatin (b) Preventation
(c) Fluvastatin (d) Simvastatin

140. Sleep apnea:

(a) 10 sec (b) 20 sec
(c) 30 sec (d) 40 sec

141. Noncardiogenic pulmonary edema A/E:

(a) RAS
(b) High altitude pulmonary edema
(c) Post CABG
(d) Sedative overdose

142. Laboratory findings consistent with atheroembolism include all *except*:

(a) Elevated ESR (b) Eosinophilia
(c) Polycythemia (d) Azotemia

143. All of the following math *except*:

(a) CYP2D6 – Warfarin
(b) CYP2C9 – Phenytoin
(c) CYP2C19 – Clopidogrel
(d) CYP2C19 – Omeprazole

144. Which of the following statements is not correct?

(a) The commonly used units of radiation are the Rad (radiation absorbed dose) and the Gray (Gy)
(b) 100 rad = 1 Gy, while 1 Gy is equal to 1 joule/kg
(c) The Sievert (Sv) is the SI unit that refers to the equivalent radiation, dose in biologic tissues
(d) Sievert (Sv) and Gray (Gy) are interchangeable units of the radiation, both refer to the biologic effect of the radiation

145. All are points of ABCD² Score *except*:

(a) Age > 65 years
(b) Unilateral weakness
(c) Blood pressure > 140/90 mm Hg
(d) Diabetes

146. Regarding cardiac amyloidosis, all statements are true, *except*:

(a) Two types of amyloid commonly infiltrate the heart: AL or primary systemic and transthyretin (TTR) amyloid
(b) Transthyretin (TTR) related amyloid cardiomyopathy is slowly progressive and clinically well tolerated
(c) I-SAP (Serum amyloid P) can assess the amyloid burden affecting the heart, permitting its use for diagnosis or serial quantification of cardiac amyloidosis
(d) Tafamidis is a TTR stabilizing drug

147. Which of the following statement regarding receiver operating characteristic curves is true?

(a) Obtained by plotting a test's true positive rate (sensitivity) against its false positive rate (100 minus specificity)
(b) A test that discriminates perfectly between the presence and absence of disease would have an ROC curve that passes exactly through the centre
(c) The closer the curve is to the lower right corner, the higher the overall accuracy of the test

(d) A completely random test would have an ROC curve that passes through the upper left corner

148. The microRNAs (miRNAs) play a role in several diseases and are advancing to clinical application in acute coronary syndromes, acute myocardial infarction, cardiomyopathies, type 2 diabetes, hypertension and heart failure. Which statement is true about miRNAs?

(a) miRNAs interfere with transcription through degradation of the message RNA

(b) miRNAs are usually 2-10 nucleotides in length

(c) miRNAs are also known as small interfering RNAs

(d) miRNA act through a silencing complex and inhibit gene expression by binding to complementary 32 untranslated regions of target mRNA

149. Each of the following statements regarding Genome Wide Association Studies (GWASs) are true, *except*:

(a) These studies provide information on common DNA variants associated with complex phenotypes

(b) The total number of loci for coronary artery disease now exceeds 46

(c) Together, these variants account for 90% of the heritability of CAD

(d) Region on chromosome 9 near the genes CDKN2A/CDKN2B – represent truly novel risk variants

150. All are deterministic effects of radiation *except*:

(a) Skin necrosis (b) Hair loss

(c) Neoplasm (d) Cataract

151. Maximum lifetime allowable whole body radiation dose for those working with radiation is:

(a) 10 REM (b) 50 REM

(c) 40 REM (d) 5 REM

152. Intention to treat analysis A/E:

(a) Non compliance (b) Protocol

(c) Cross-over design (d) Type II error

153. Class II, LOE C S/O:

(a) Evidence benefit on basis of general consensus

(b) Multiple RCT

154. All are true about pregnancy *except*:

(a) Pulmonary edema develops 24-72 hrs after labour

(b) Blood loss is more in vaginal delivery as compared to cesarean

(c) Cesarean delivery preferred for patient on warfarin

(d) Cardiac output increased by 50% during delivery

155. True about contrast reaction:

(a) Premedication to be given in patents having history of anaphylout reaction

(b) Low dose contrast should be given all patients suspected of having contrast redtops

156. True regarding drug integration all *except*:

(a) Warfarin dose has to be reduced with amiodarone

(b) Amoxicillin reduces bioavailability

(c) NSAIDs block antihypertensive action of CCB

(d) Rifampicin reduces dose of verapamil

157. If X is suspected to be causing a disease, best study to determine relation:

(a) Cohort (b) Nested case control

(c) Case control

158. Method to determine results of meta-analysis and systemic review:

(a) Forrest graph (b) Funnel graph

(c) Peto method

159. Most unbiased result with:

(a) Intention to treat

(b) Modified intention to treat

(c) Pre protocol

160. Micro RNA true statement A/E:

(a) Found in nucleus of plants

(b) Rise in Post translational modification

(c) M-RNA 712 mutation leads to increased atherogenesis in mice

(d) Function along with m-RNA

161. Hypermagnesia A/E:

(a) CHB

(b) Decrease tendon reflexes

(c) CKD with anasarca

(d) Cardiac conduction defect due to increase Ca

162. Wrong:

(a) H1N1–Parotid enlargement

(b) Mg–tetany

(c) Hypergeusia–Zn

(d) Thalamus–confabulation

163. Wrong match:
(a) Cardiac danon disease–LAMP
(b) Fabry's disease–X GLA
(c) Barth syndrome–Tafazin gene
(d) Haptoglobin–Diencephalon

164. Dabigatran vs warfarin A/E:
(a) Decrease bleeding
(b) Increase thromboembolic
(c) Decrease mortality
(d) <50 ng/ml–trough level

165. Drug metabolism by CYP 2D6 A/E:
(a) Metoprolol (b) Clopidogrel
(c) Codeine (d) Ivabradine

166. TTR (Time in therapeutic range) A/E:
(a) Increase TTR–increase bleeding
(b) Increase TTR–reduces mortality
(c) Increases TTR–reduces stroke

167. Following hyperalimentation true:
(a) Currently has volume overload with edema
(b) Patient has hypokalemia with hyperaldosternism
(c) Mild acidosis
(d) Disproportionate LVH with increased PP as compared to essential HTN

168. Hypothyroidism *except*:
(a) Diastolic HTN
(b) Decrease PP
(c) Increase PVR
(d) High renin hypertension

169. Wrong match:
(a) Catheterisation–frossman
(b) Angiography–sones
(c) Stent–pault sebert
(d) ICD–brown

170. Wrong match:
(a) T Arteriosus–REV procedure
(b) TOF and PS–BT shunt
(c) ALCAPA–Takeuchi repair
(d) Single ventricle with obstructed IVC–kawashima

171. Most important determinant of risk factor:
(a) RCT (b) Cohort
(c) Cross section (d) Case registry

172. Wrong match:
(a) ACEI–oligohydroamnios
(b) Amiodarone–neonatal goitre
(c) BB–teratogenicity
(d) Aspirin–premature ductal closure

173. Acanthosis nigricans A/E:
(a) Vitamin D supplementation aggravates it
(b) Signs of insulin resistance
(c) Can be seen as paraneoplastic manifestation
(d) Can be seen in PCOD female

174. Hepatitis C A/E:
(a) Indinavir (b) Telepravir
(c) Bocipravir (d) Sofubovir

175. Hypophosphatemia A/E:
(a) Vitamin D deficiency (b) Hyperventilation
(c) Fanconi syndrome (d) DKA

176. APLA A/E:
(a) Recurrent arterial thrombosis
(b) Thrombocytopenia
(c) SLE in 50%
(d) Increased APTT

177. All are true *except* in cancer screening for ACS of > 55 years asymptomatic:
(a) PSA every 1 year
(b) CXR every 5 years
(c) Fecal occult blood every 1 year
(d) Colonoscopy every 10 years

178. Hypothyroidism which can be seen?
(a) CHB (b) Cardiac tamponade
(c) Pretibial myxedema (d) Carotenemia

179. Non anion gap acidosis A/E:
(a) DKA
(b) RTA
(c) Hyperalimination
(d) Pyroglutamic acid toxicity

180. Folate deficiency A/E:
(a) CHF (b) Tropical sprue
(c) Sulfasalazine (d) Excess melon intake

181. Linked angina A/E:
(a) Increases on bending
(b) Normal coronaries
(c) Due to acid stimulation
(d) Increased by food intake

182. All are true *except*:

(a) Thiamine deficiency–diuretics

(b) Vitamin C–tryptophan deficiency

(c) Vit. B_{12}–iron treatment for iron deficiency anemia

(d) Vit. D deficiency–blacks

183. All are true *except*:

(a) Broca area–converts laxical information to conversation

(b) Wernicke area–converts heard information to laxical

(c) Limbic–memory storage

(d) Prefrontal cortex–emotions

184. Antibiotic used A/E:

(a) Febrile dysentery

(b) Severe traveller diarrhea

(c) Antibiotic induced diarrhoea

(d) Non typhoidal salmonella

185. Primary hyperaldosteronism true:

(a) Hypokalemia common in bilateral involvement

(b) Edema because of fluid retention

(c) M>F

(d) Aldosterone secretion not changing with posture

186. Hypothyroid all *except:*

(a) Increase SVR

(b) Increase renin level

(c) Pulse pressure decreases

(d) Diastolic HTN

187. Procedure decreasing mortality on long term:

(a) Pap smear 18-64 years

(b) Stop smoking at 34 years

(c) PSA at 50 years

188. AAA expansion decreased by all *except:*

(a) B blockers (b) Losartan

(c) Doxycycline (d) Colchicine

189. Study for risk factors:

(a) Cohort study (b) RCT

(c) Use history (d) Cross sectional study

190. P-glycoprotein all *except:*

(a) By ABCB1 Gene

(b) Ritonavir induces

(c) Amiodarone inhibits

(d) Seen in blood brain barrier

191. False:

(a) Magnesium–tetany

(b) Zinc–hypogeusia

(c) Vit A–parotid enlargement

(d) Thiamine–confabulation

192. Dabigatran vs warfarin for mechanical valves all *except:*

(a) Oral DTI (b) Decreases bleed

(c) Non inferior to warf (d) Increases thrombosis

193. Anaphylactic reactions in beta blocking best agents:

(a) Dopamine (b) Vasopressin

(c) Glucagon (d) Salbutamol

194. Low anion gap found in all *except:*

(a) Multiple myeloma (b) Hyperlipidemia

(c) Methanol poisoning (d) Hypoalbuminemia

195. Hypertonic solution is:

(a) 0.9% NS (b) 5% dextrose

(c) 2.5% dextrose (d) 5% dextrose + 0.9% NS

196. Mismatch: (T/F)

(a) Boron toxicity–testicular atrophy

(b) Fluoride toxicity–osteoporosis

(c) Manganese toxicity–progressive parkinsonism

(d) Chromium toxicity–impaired glucose tolerance

197. Ankylosing spondylitis true *except:*

(a) Only 20% of HLA B-27 patients have AS

(b) Coronary arteritis is common

(c) AR in children may precede joint manifestations

(d) Ophthalmic involvement includes anterior uveitis

198. Type I error is:

(a) False positive (b) False negative

(c) True positive (d) True negative

199. Best study for risk assessment:

(a) Cohort study (b) Case control study

(c) Cross sectional study (d) RCT

200. CHD-prevalence in community best assessed by:

(a) TMT

(b) Stress echo

(c) Coronary calcium
(d) Rose angina questionnaire

201. Chronic duplication syndrome associated with:
(a) Prader-Willi syndrome
(b) Angelman syndrome
(c) Charcot-Marie-Tooth syndrome
(d) Digeorge's syndrome

202. ABG: PH-7.18, PCO_2-72, PaO_2- 63, SaO_2- 80%, least likely is:
(a) CHF
(b) Narcotic overdose
(c) Flail chest
(d) Guillain-Barrè syndrome

203. Antidote mismatch:
(a) Paracetamol–N-acetyl cysteine
(b) Methemoglobinemia–amyl nitrate
(c) Isoniazid–pyridoxine
(d) Ethylene glycol–fomepizole

204. Active charcoal useful in:
(a) Ethanol (b) Phenobarbitone
(c) Arsenic (d) Liquid ammonia

205. Acute hypercalcemia treatment all *except:*
(a) Calcitonin (b) Oral phosphate
(c) IV magnesium (d) IV saline

206. Radiation all *except:*
(a) RCMP (b) CCP
(c) Premature CAD (d) Aortitis

207. Conn's syndrome:
(a) M>F
(b) Hypokalemia in majority
(c) Edema in majority
(d) Aldosterone secretion not changing with posture

208. Specificity:
(a) TN/TN+FP (b) TP/TP+FN
(c) =TP/TP+FP (d) TN/FN+TN

209. Pheochromocytoma:
(a) T2 W-MRI–differentiate functionally active from inactive
(b) NE secretion–flushing and headache
(c) MIBG–to localise
(d) Clonidine suppression test for borderline catecholamine

210. Air hunger of acute pulmonary edema:
(a) J receptors
(b) Muscle metaboreceptors
(c) Chemoreceptors
(d) Alveolar receptors

211. pH=7.19, PCO_2-72, PO_2-62, SO_2-84%, male—what is true:
(a) CHF (b) Narcotic overdose
(c) Myasthenia gravis (d) Flail chest

212. Neurocardiogenic syncope in young female on prolonged standing, not recommended:
(a) Physical counterpressure manoeuvre
(b) Epinephrine
(c) Tilt training
(d) B blockers

213. All *except:*
(a) More perfusion at lung base and more ventilation at apex
(b) Dead space 30% of TV
(c) PAO_2-PaO_2 = < 30 in healthy adult
(d) Residual capacity determined by helium dilution method

214. Creatnine clearance age-68, weight-50, creat=2, female:
(a) 42.5 (b) 50
(c) 21.5 (d) 25

215. Normal values all *except:*
(a) LV mass–76 gm/m^2 in male
(b) Pump–6-12 mm Hg
(c) PVR–6-7 wood unit
(d) AV O_2 differences : 40

216. True/False:
(a) Noonan–Lymphedema
(b) HHT endothelial receptor defect
(c) Carney–lentigine
(d) LQT 3–Na Channel

217. Risk marker of apoptosis:
(a) Annexin V (b) Taxol-n
(c) Intergrin (d) Q dot

218. Hypothyroidism *except:*

(a) ↑ SVR

(b) ↑ Micro circulation time

(c) ↓ Blood volume

(d) ↓ Mixed AV O_2 diff

219. Subclinical hypothyroidism all *except:*

(a) Elderly M:F-1:1

(b) Associated with ↑ chol

(c) Odd ratio for MI risk is twice

(d) ↓ Isovolumic relaxation time

220. Flashes of light (Phosphene) all *except:*

(a) Sildenafil (b) Tadafil

(c) Nicorandil (d) Ivabradine

221. Liver toxicity drugs all *except:*

(a) Bosentan (b) Dabigatran

(c) Dronedarone (d) Statin

222. COPD all *except:*

(a) Most common cause of death is IHD

(b) MAT = Treatment with digoxin

(c) Diuretic induced metabolic alkalosis causes respiratory depression

(d) Cardio selective B blockers may be used if required

223. Neurocardiogenic syndrome all *except:*

(a) Headup tilt training

(b) β blocker

(c) Isometric exercise on prodrome

(d) PPM for cardio inhibition

224. Epidemiology true *except:*

(a) 30% death of CAD

(b) DM highest no. of cases in China

(c) Japanese highest life expectancy

(d) Mediterranean people have ↓ CAD risk than other

225. Best epidemiological tool for risk factor:

(a) Case control (b) Cohort study

(c) Case registry (d) Cross sectional study

226. Met acidosis with Na-132, K-4.6, chloride-100, HCO_{3-} 20 all *except:*

(a) Spironolactone (b) Addison disease

(c) DKA (d) TPN

227. PCO_2-50, PO_2-40, (A-a) O_2 diff.-12, SPO_2-89% most likely:

(a) Resp ms paralysis (b) Atelectasis

(c) Pulmonary edema (d) TOF

228. Multifocal myoclonus A/W:

(a) Acute vertebral occlusion

(b) Acute ACA occlusion

(c) Metabolic encephalopathy

(d) IC bleed

229. Efficacy of HBV vaccine hemodialysis patients:

(a) 50% (b) 20%

(c) 80% (d) 30%

230. Seen in hypomagnesemia:

(a) Muscle weakness (b) Tremors

(c) Diminished reflexes (d) Somnolence

231. UA level ↑ in all *except:*

(a) Losartan (b) Furosemide

(c) Levodopa (d) Contrast agent

232. Angina prevalence in population:

(a) Rose questionnaire (b) Ca score

(c) Stress echo (d) Stess thallium

233. Postpartum DVT all *except:*

(a) d dimer physiologically ↑ in all stages of pregnancy

(b) ↑ in postpartum most common

(c) Anticoag atleast for 2 years

(d) UFH/LMWH primarily used

234. Newer drug with less hemorrhage all *except:*

(a) Prasngrel Vs clopidogrel

(b) Dabigatran Vs warf

(c) Fondaparinux Vs Enoxaparin

(d) Bivalirudin Vs Gp IIb IIIa heparin

235. Bromcriptine effective all *except:*

(a) Type II DM (b) IPF

(c) NMS (d) PPCMP

236. Biphasic shock:

(a) More effective

(b) Phase reversal in last part of shock

(c) Dampen sine wave pattern used
(d) Automatic adjustment of ↓ energy according to measured impedance

237. Syncope all *except:*
(a) Left MCA infarct (b) Short QT syndrome
(c) Non-obstructive HOCM

238. Prolonged exposure to zero gravity all *except:*
(a) Facial puffiness
(b) Fluid retention
(c) Postural hypotension as shift to gravitational area
(d) As shift of fluid to upper body

239. Ph-7.34, PCO_2-62, HCO_3:
(a) Compensated respiratory acidosis–chronic
(b) Respiratory alkalosis
(c) Metabolic acidosis

240. Na 135, K-4.8, HCO_3- 12, Cl- 100, diagnosis:
(a) DKA (b) Proximal RTA
(c) Addison (d) TPN

241. All normal *except*:
(a) LVEDP > 18 mm Hg
(b) PASP = 25 mm Hg
(c) SVR = 1100 dyne cm–5
(d) MV gradient = 2 mm Hg

242. Mismatch:
(a) Ryanodine–Ca release channel
(b) Calseqestrin–Ca storage protein
(c) Titin–Ca binding proteim in contractile apparatus
(d) L type–Ca dependent Ca release

243. Match all *except:*
(a) CHADS–anticoagulation
(b) Bleeding–HASBLEED
(c) ABCD–CPR score of successful resuscitation
(d) Syntax–angio score

244. 2011 census counting:
(a) Population 140 crore
(b) 15% surface area, 20% population
(c) Gender ratio in 0-6 year better than adult
(d) Decline of total population is largest in this decade since 97

245. Less known and unknown bias:
(a) RCT (b) Clinical consensus
(c) Systematic review (d) Case report

246. Best for studying risk factor:
(a) Case control (b) Cohort
(c) Cross sectional study (d) Case registry

247. Volume control ventilation all *except:*
(a) ↓ Barotrauma
(b) Fixed minute ventilation
(c) Independent of lung compliance
(d) Useful in variable pulmonary compliance

248. PEEP in pulmonary edema:
(a) PEEP ↑ PAP (b) Hyperinflation ↑ PVR
(c) ↓ O_2 consumption (d) ↓ Venous return

249. Hyponatremia in all *except:*
(a) DM with ketosis
(b) SIADH
(c) Cushing causes hypovolumic hyponatremia
(d) Rapid correction cause ODS in chronic hyponatremia

250. All are C/I in stroke (tpa) *except:*
(a) Lumbar puncture (<7 days)
(b) MI < 3 months
(c) Rapidly improving symptom
(d) Oral anticoagulate

251. Wrong match:
(a) Vaso vagal syncope–promatin
(b) Meniere disease–fludrocortisone
(c) Carotid sinus syndrome–pacemaker
(d) Glossopharyngeal neuralgia–carbamazepine

252. ph-7.55, PO_2-92, PCO_2-40, Na^+ 130, k^+-2.5:
(a) Hyperemesis gravidarum
(b) Crohn's disease
(c) Panic attacks
(d) Pulmonary embolism

253. Fundus–Hollenhorst plaque transient vision loss in right eye diagnosis:
(a) Carotid stenosis
(b) Temporal arteritis
(c) LA myxoma

254. All *except* (for statins):

(a) ↓ Non fatal MI in CSA

(b) ↓ New onset DM

(c) ↓ Stroke

(d) ↓ Periprocedural MI in stable angina

255. PT/INR not useful in all *except:*

(a) Pregnant female on anticoagulants

(b) Polycythemia

(c) Hypothermia

(d) LMWH

256. All *except:*

(a) Normal O_2 content in mild anemia

(b) Alkalosis ↑ ed O_2 releases to further

(c) >10,000 feet, PaO_2- 60 mm Hg

257. All about COX *except:*

(a) COX-1 constitutive

(b) COX-2 less nephrotoxic than COX-1

(c) Paracetamol COX-3 inhibition

(d) Fish oil acts via COX pathway

258. All true about elderly *except:*

(a) Hyperthyroidism presentation–AF without goitre

(b) Acute confusional states less commons due to new brain lesion than young

(c) Law of parsimony not applicable

(d) Frontal releases reflexes not normal

259. All favour pulmonary pathology on cardiopulmonary testing *except:*

(a) Maximum ventilation capacity achieved

(b) THR not achieved

(c) Low anaerobic threshold

(d) Significant desaturation

260. Venous return ↑ses tachycardia:

(a) Bezold Jarish reflex (b) Bainbridge reflex

(c) Branham effect (d) Marie

261. Calcium sign seen in:

(a) CP (b) MS

(c) AS (d) Dissection of aorta

262. Metabolic modulators are:

(a) Ranolazine (b) Perhexilene

(c) Fasudil (d) Ivabradine

263. HLA association in Type 1 DM:

(a) HLA - DRB *404 (b) HLA-DRB

(c) HLA - DR3 (d) DR4

264. Hyperthermia seen in all *except*:

(a) Enteric fever (b) Fluoxetine

(c) Thyrotoxicosis (d) Phatothiazine

265. Donovani infection finding most common:

(a) Asymptomatic (b) Splenomegaly

266. NCC not a minor criteria is:

(a) + cigar shaped

(b) Antibodies in CSF

(c) Antibodies ELISA (Serum)

(d) MRI finding suggestive of NCC

267. Nazar criteria all *except*:

(a) Albumin (b) Bilirubin

(c) AST (d) PT

268. Acute pancreatitis all *except*:

(a) Hemochromatosis

(b) Hypercalcemia

(c) Parathyroid adenoma

(d) Cushing's syndrome

269. ARDS treatment true all *except*:

(a) Corticosteroids (b) Decrease LAP

(c) Surfactant (d) Low tidal volume

270. Absent pain and temperature on one side/loss of proprioception/loss of motor:

(a) Brown-Sequard syndrome

(b) Harlequine sensory loss

271. Category A – Bioterrorism:

(a) Smallpox (b) Anthrax

(c) Brucellosis

272. Case of viral infection:

(a) Adult T-cell leukemia

(b) Burkitt's lymphoma B

(c) Hairy cell leukemia

(d) Mycosis fungoides

273. Congenital erythropoietic porphyria :

(a) HMB synthase (b) URO synthetase

(c) ALA dehydratase

274. HIV– toxoplasma seen at ___ CD_4 count.

(a) >350 (b) <350

(c) <100 (d) <50

275. SLE criteria are all *except*:
(a) ANA (b) APLA
(c) Elevated AST/ALT

276. RA in rheumatic arthritis:
(a) Has high predictive value
(b) 75% cases +ve, can be used for screening
(c) Can be used as screening test

277. Abnormal organization of cells:
(a) Dysplasia (b) Disruption
(c) Malformation (d) Deformation

278. Auto immune hepatitis all true *except*:
(a) Amenorrhoea
(b) Hypogammaglobulinemia
(c) Thyroiditis

279. Most common immunodeficiency:
(a) IgA deficiency (b) CVID
(c) SCID

280. Treatment of uncomplicated P. vivax:
(a) Chloroquines (b) Proguanil
(c) Quinidine (d) Metloquine

281. Patient on follow up of methotrexate treatment:
(a) Hemogram + urine exam
(b) Hemogram + liver enzymes
(c) Urine exam
(d) Hemogram

282. Deberine-Sotto syndrome all *except*:
(a) Ant. cranial artery involvement
(b) Pain in opposite side

283. Apoptosis all *except*:
(a) CD 95 is required (b) Inflammation is seen
(c) DNA cleavage

284. POTS all true *except*:
(a) NE > 300
(b) SBP transiently decrease by 20
(c) Tachycardia >30 b/min
(d) Severe orthostatic symp

285. Pseudoseizure vs seizure differentiated by:
(a) Increase prolactin (b) Increase lactate
(c) Decrease glucose (d) Increase IGF

286. CREST syndrome associated with:
(a) PSS
(b) PAN
(c) SLE
(d) Churg-Strauss syndrome

287. Radiation induced cardiac injury all *except*:
(a) Valvular stenosis (b) CAD
(c) Pericarditis (d) Pericardial effusion
(e) All

288. Lung rarely involved in:
(a) PAN (b) PSS
(c) SLE

289. Warfarin level increase in:
(a) Phenobarbitone (b) Allopurinol
(c) Rifampicin (d) Sucralfate

290. Ramsay Hunt Syndrome most characteristic:
(a) Blister on pinna
(b) Infranuclear VII nerve palsy
(c) Loss of taste sensation in anterior 2/3rd of tongue
(d) Bell's phenomena

291. BCR ABL gene is seen in:
(a) CML (b) ALL
(c) AML (d) Follicular lymphoma

292. Significant hematuria (No. of RBCs in single HPF):
(a) 3 - 100 (b) 5 - 50
(c) 10 - 100 (d) 20 - 100

293. SIRS all *except*:
(a) Polytrauma
(b) Sepsis
(c) Immune mediated origin
(d) Cytokine infusion

294. TNF-α causes true:
(a) Cachexia (b) Weight gain

295. Human genome no. of genes are:
(a) 30-4000 (b) 10-20,000
(c) 20-3000 (d) 50-60

296. High anion gap all *except*:
(a) Diarrhoea (b) Renal failure
(c) Ethylene (d) Methanol

297. Anti-retroviral–nephrocalcinosis is seen in:

(a) Indinavir (b) Saquinavir

(c) Retonavir (d) Tenofovir

298. Leptin true:

(a) Act on Hypothalamus (b) Increase appetite

(c) Decrease appetite (d) Decrease in obese

299. Parvovirus B_{19}:

(a) Erythema infectiosum

(b) Persistent anaemia

(c) Both

300. Hepatitis C:

(a) 90% in hemophilia (b) DNA virus

(c) Rare chronic liver disease

301. Lacrimation + miosis + blurring of vision:

(a) Nerve gas (b) Phosgene

(c) Nitrogen mustard

302. Desquamative interpruritis all *except*:

(a) Common in 2nd decade

(b) Exclusive in smoker

(c) Haziness in chest X-ray and CT

(d) Increase macrophage in alveolar space

303. P_{53} true:

(a) Decrease apoptosis

(b) Prevents entering cells in S phase

(c) 1st event is inactivation in colonic carcinoma

304. APC:

(a) Dendritic cell (b) Monocyte

305. I-131 antidote:

(a) KOH (b) KI

(c) Ca DTPA (d) Zn DTPA

306. Decrease complement level seen in all *except*:

(a) Acute PSGN

(b) Anti GBM disease

(c) Mesangioproliferative type II

(d) Lupus nephritis

307. Cardiac dyspnoea all *except*:

(a) Decrease FRC

(b) Decrease VC

(c) Decrease diff. capacity

(d) Decrease compliance

308. Oral cyanosis + asymptomatic with SaO_2— 100%:

(a) Alveolar decrease affinity Hb%

(b) Alveolar ventilation ventil decrease

(c) Decrease diffusion

309. Obesity all *except*:

(a) Decrease CO

(b) Eccentric hypertrophy

310. Absolute contraindication to exercise plan:

(a) DM

(b) DCM

(c) IHD

(d) No pace advance AV block

(e) No

311. Which acts by cell surface receptor?

(a) Opioid (b) Thyroid hormone

(c) Androgen (d) Glucocorticoids

312. Familial Parkinson's disease:

(a) Autosomal Dominant

(b) Autosomal Recessive

(c) X-Linked Dominant

(d) X-linked autosomal recessive

313. SCA (spino cerebellar ataxia):

(a) AD (b) AR

(c) X-Linked Recessive (d) X-Linked Dominant

314. Retinoblastoma due to:

(a) Microdeletion of gene

(b) Translocation of gene

(c) Non-dysjunction of gene

(d) Non-deletion of chromosome

315. Phenobarbitone coma used for:

(a) Intracranial HTN

(b) Status epilepticus

(c) Intracranial bleed

(d) Hyperventilation syndrome

316. Bartter's present with:

(a) ↓ K due to ↑ K excretion

(b) Metabolic Acidosis

(c) Hyperparathyroidism

(d) ↑ Na

317. Aldosterone causes:
(a) ↑ Na retention (b) K retention
(c) Na excretion

318. Metabolic cause of acute pain abdomen:
(a) DKA (b) Porphyria
(c) Lead poisoning (d) Addison disease

319. Hypoglycemia in paraneoplastic syndrome due to:
(a) ↑ utilization of glucose by tumour cells
(b) ↓ glucagon
(c) ↓ cytokine production
(d) ↑ IGF-II

320. CMT due to:
(a) Inversion of gene (b) Microduplication
(c) Linkage disequilibrium

321. P_{53} ↑ es by A/E:
(a) UV-radiation (b) γ-radiation
(c) Oncogene (d) Chemotherapy

322. Tumor suppressor gene present with:
(a) Point mutation (b) Clonal expression
(c) Gene activation (d) Clonal selection

323. Tumor cell vaccine:
(a) ↑ CD-4 count (b) ↑ T-cell immunity
(c) ↑ Ig by B-cell

324. Sickle cell disease presents with:
(a) MGN (b) FSGS
(c) RDGN

325. Cyclosporine causes renal toxicity with:
(a) Intrarenal vasoconstriction induced ARF
(b) PCT damage
(c) Pigment induced damage

326. FENa⁺ > 1:
(a) ATN (b) Prerenal ARF
(c) Conn's syn.

327. Rifampin causes:
(a) Tubulointerstitial disease
(b) FSGS
(c) MPGN

328. Osteitis fibrosa cystica:
(a) Paget's disease
(b) Tertiary hyperthyroidism
(c) Primary hypoparathyroidism
(d) Hyperparathyroidism

329. Hypophosphatemia causes:
(a) Convulsions
(b) Bradyarrhythmia
(c) Tachypnea
(d) Episodic muscle weakness

330. Stiff person syndrome due to:
(a) Hodgkin's Disease (b) Neuromyotonia
(c) Breast Ca (d) Small cell lung Ca

331. Pemphigus antibody against:
(a) Desmoglein glycoprotein
(b) Dermal lipoprotein
(c) BM antigen
(d) Keratin

332. Linear IgA disease responds to:
(a) Corticosteroids (b) Dapsone
(c) Plasmapheresis (d) Monoclonal antibodies

333. GFR measured by A/E:
(a) Inulin (b) Creatine
(c) Phenol red (d) Mannitol

334. Vesicoureteral reflux causes:
(a) HTN (b) ↑ Phosphate
(c) ↑ Ca^{+2} (d) RTA

335. Emphysematous cholecystitis:
(a) Clostridium perfringens
(b) Proteus
(c) Pseudomonas

336. Desquamative interstitial pneumonitis associated:
(a) Psoriasis (b) Smoking
(c) Rheumatoid arthritis (d) Sarcoidosis

337. Hypoxia with VQ/P mismatch:
(a) Alveolar collapse (b) Pulmonary edema
(c) Intracardiac shunt (d) IPF

338. COPD associated with TLC:
(a) ↑ (b) ↓
(c) Variable

339. Drabopoietin alpha used in:
(a) Renal failure induced anaemia
(b) CHF

(c) DVT
(d) Seizures

340. Ring sideroblasts:
(a) MDS (b) Iron deficiency
(c) MPS

341. Sickle cell anaemia presents with:
(a) Hemolytic anaemia (b) Splenomegaly
(c) Lymphadenopathy

342. Beta-thalassemia presents with:
(a) Microcytic hypochromic
(b) Dimorphic anemia
(c) Macrocytic

343. Iron store absent if S. ferritin level is:
(a) <15 μg/l (b) 25 μg/l
(c) 50 μg/l (d) 75 μg/l

344. HSP → counterpart in renal disease:
(a) IgA nephropathy (b) MPGN
(c) Nephrotic syndrome (d) MGN

345. Dermatitis herpetiformis:
(a) HLA-B27 (b) HLA-B8 with DR-W3
(c) B-27 with DRW3

346. Neutrophil marker → in all stages:
(a) CD 31 (b) CD 33
(c) CD 4 (d) CD 8

347. Respiratory burst during phagocytosis due to:
(a) Oxidase (b) Hydrolase
(c) Peroxidase (d) Dehydrogenase

348. PPI→long term use causes:
(a) Carcinoid (b) Multiple polyposis
(c) Metabolic acidosis

349. Procidentia is seen with:
(a) Rectal prolapse (b) Volvulus
(c) UC

350. H. pylori→newer treatment option:
(a) PAS (b) Ethambutol
(c) Rifabutin

351. Multifocal atrophic gastritis:
(a) Pernicious anaemia (b) Adenocarcinoma
(c) Gastric perforation (d) Hemorrhage

352. HBeAg +ve indicates:
(a) Multiplication of HBV
(b) Chronic infection
(c) After vaccination

353. Lamivudine treatment in chronic HBV given:
(a) IgM anti Hbc +ve
(b) Anti HBS
(c) Anti HBeAg
(d) HBV DNA after 3 months of infection

354. AIH–treatment:
(a) Steroids (b) IVIG
(c) Interferon

355. HCV treatment:
(a) RNA detectable (b) >60 years age
(c) Normal ALT

356. NASH:
(a) Metabolic Alkalosis (b) Metabolic Acidosis
(c) Hyperuricemia (d) ↑ Anion gap

357. Cullen's sign:
(a) Acute pancreatitis (b) Ischemic colitis
(c) Intestinal perforation

358. Extraintestinal manifestation of UC:
(a) Exfoliative dermatitis
(b) Eczematous dermatitis
(c) Pyoderma gangrenosum

359. Prolonged TPN–Alopecia with acrodermatitis diagnosis:
(a) Zinc deficiency
(b) EFA deficiency
(c) Iron excess

360. Tumor lysis syndrome treatment:
(a) Hydration with allopurinol
(b) Forced diuresis
(c) Mg^{+2} repletion

361. Left parasternal lift due to:
(a) RV displacement because of ↑ ed LA
(b) RVE
(c) LVH
(d) LAE

362. Normal anion gap acidosis due to:
(a) Severe diarrhoea (b) Starvation
(c) DKA (d) Renal failure

363. Olanzepine:
(a) Orthostatic hypotension
(b) Anticholinergic effect
(c) Agranulocytosis
(d) ↑ prolactin

364. Drug causing hyperthermia:
(a) Phenothiazine (b) Amiodarone
(c) B blocker (d) CCB

365. True about EPO:
(a) ↓ in RCC
(b) ↑ in polycythemia vera
(c) ↑ed due to inflammatory cytokines
(d) ↓ed due to IL-1

366. Apraxic gait due to:
(a) Frontal lobe lesion
(b) Corpus callosal lesion
(c) Parasagittal lobule lesion
(d) Substantia nigra

367. Graphesthesia is a test for:
(a) Cortical sensory function
(b) Motor function
(c) Cerebellar function

368. CREST syndrome:
(a) ↑ anticentromere Antibody
(b) ↑ anti disease DNA
(c) Anti-Smith Antigen

369. Northern-blot used for:
(a) Gene expression
(b) RFLP
(c) Nucleic acid hybridization

370. Drug with antiangiogenic effect act by:
(a) ↓ replication of endothelium
(b) ↓ replication of vascular BM
(c) ↓ migration of tumor cells into blood vessels
(d) ↓ Attachment of tumor cells to blood vessels

371. Erythema infectiosum due to:
(a) Parvovirus-B_{19} (b) Coxsackie-A virus
(c) Roseola virus

372. Lithium used in:
(a) Cluster headache (b) Migraine
(c) Trigeminal neuralgia (d) Neurosis

373. Steroids used in lymphoma, mechanisms of action may be:
(a) ↑ apoptosis of tumor cells
(b) ↓ TNF-α
(c) Lympholytic effect

374. Mosaicism:
(a) > 2 different cell lines
(b) Chromosomal aberration
(c) Non-disjunction of chromosomes

375. Koplik spot True is:
(a) Typhoid (b) Measles
(c) Chickenpox

376. Most common space occupying lesion in HIV:
(a) Tuberculosis (b) Toxoplasmosis
(c) NHL (d) Hodgkin

377. Ataxia with peripheral neuropathy A/E:
(a) Refsum's Disease
(b) Abetalipproteinemia
(c) Ataxia Telangiectasia
(d) Leigh's disease

378. Amyloidosis associated with hemodialysis due to deposition of:
(a) B 2 microglobulin (b) ATTR
(c) ANP (d) Light chain

379. Potassium – 2.1 meq/l, least likely in:
(a) Rhabdomyolysis (b) Amphotericin-B
(c) Hyperaldosteronism (d) Diuretics

380. Hepatitis E, best described as:
(a) Acute hepatitis enteral transmission with poor prognosis in pregnancy
(b) Chronic hepatitis
(c) Fulminant hepatitis
(d) Acute hepatitis, sexual transmission

381. ↑ Na^+ and Cl^- excretion with fluid diuresis and no effect on HCO_3:

(a) Furosemide (b) Bumetanide
(c) Ethacrynic Acid (d) Acetazolamide

382. Rheumatoid nodule not seen in:

(a) Pericardium (b) Pleura
(c) Subcutaneous tissue (d) Epidermis

383. Anti-TNF human-mouse antibody:

(a) Etanercept (b) Infliximab
(c) Anakinra (d) Adalimumab

384. Proximal myopathy A/E:

(a) Statin (b) Vitamin E
(c) Artesunate (d) Snake Venom

385. Rain drop pigmentation:

(a) Lead (b) Arsenic
(c) Mercury (d) Cobalt

386. AIDP characterized by:

(a) Albumino cytological dissociation
(b) Sensory loss
(c) Highly responsive to steroids
(d) Similar to myopathy

387. Systemic mastocytosis diagnostic criteria A/E:

(a) Detection of codon 816 mutation
(b) Aberrant mast cell surface phenotype
(c) Abnormal mast cell morphology
(d) Tissue infiltration

388. ABPA true is:

(a) Normal CXR
(b) DOC is Amphotericin-B
(c) Central bronchiectasis
(d) Restrictive physiology

389. Friedreich's ataxia true is:

(a) Presentation age > 25
(b) Skin lesion common
(c) Repeat GAA

390. Duchenne muscular dystrophy (DMD) characterized by:

(a) Common presentation- 2nd decade
(b) Autosomal dominant
(c) CRK always raised
(d) Prenatal Diagnosis

391. Autosomal recessive disorder characterized by A/E:

(a) Double dose of gene required
(b) 25% chance including disease
(c) Consanguineous marriage
(d) Vertical transmission

392. Wimberger's sign:

(a) Rickets (b) Survey
(c) Osteomalacia

393. McConnel's sign:

(a) Pulmonary Embolism
(b) Cardiac tamponade
(c) Pneumothorax
(d) Pericarditis

394. PTH related peptide induced hypercalcemia A/E:

(a) Squamous cell CA (b) Lung Ca
(c) Renal cell Ca (d) Ca ovary

395. Ulcerative colitis true A/E:

(a) Antibiotic not useful
(b) ASA used for maintenance
(c) Infliximab used in acute phase
(d) Azathioprine in steroid resistant

396. Down beat nystagmus in:

(a) Labyrinthine (b) Cerebellum
(c) Posterior fossa (d) Cerebral

397. Increased residual volume in:

(a) COPD (b) Sarcoidosis
(c) ILD (d) Cystic fibrosis

398. Drug causing HUS:

(a) Mitomycin-C (b) D-Actinomycin
(c) Paracetamol (d) Aspirin

399. Adalimumab mechanism of action:

(a) TGF-β blocker (b) IL-2 Activation
(c) TNF-α blocker (d) IGF-1 Agonist

400. Hormone acting through receptor as enzyme:

(a) Insulin (b) Cortisol
(c) Vitamin-D3 (d) Thyroxine

401. Antiobesity drug modulating cannabinoid receptor:

(a) Rimonabant (b) Fengluramine
(c) Orlistat (d) Sertaline

402. **Bronchial asthma true A/E:**
(a) Viral induced type is always responsive to steroid
(b) TH-2 cell important in pathogenesis
(c) Can be associated with atopic dermatitis

403. **About HIV all true *except*:**
(a) Ig ↓
(b) CD-4 ↓
(c) CD-8 normal or increased
(d) Dysfunction of NK cells

404. **Infectious mononucleosis:**
(a) Atypical cell >10%
(b) Positive monospot test
(c) Rash with amoxicillin
(d) Deranged LFT

405. **Parvovirus B-19 A/E:**
(a) Causes aplastic crisis in hemolytic anemia
(b) Causes myocarditis
(c) Hydrops foetalis
(d) Erythema infectiosum

406. **EBV mononucleosis:**
(a) Acyclovir in oral hairy cell leucoplakia
(b) Monospot more sensitive than IgM serology
(c) Transmitted through body secretions
(d) Pulmonary involvement common

407. **PRCA A/E:**
(a) Parvo B_{19}
(b) Diamond-Blackfan
(c) Swachman-Diamond syndrome
(d) Thymoma

408. **Urinary incontinence and ↑ chances of hydronephrosis:**
(a) Alzeimer (b) GBS
(c) NPH

409. **Tremor in parkinsonism A/E:**
(a) To and tro
(b) Pronation and supination
(c) ↑ es on voluntary action
(d) Head and Hand

410. **↑ Gonadal estrogen:**
(a) PCOD
(b) CAH
(c) Testicular feminization
(d) Arrhenoblastoma

411. **Normal in child A/E:**
(a) Bed wetting at 3 years in female
(b) Moro's reflex after 3 months
(c) Flatfoot at 1 year
(d) Parachute after 9 months

412. **Aqueductal stenosis in:**
(a) CMV (b) Mumps
(c) Rubella (d) Toxoplasmosis

413. **HIV drugs A/E:**
(a) Lamivudine (b) Didanosine
(c) Zidovudine (d) Stavudine
(e) All of the above

414. **↑ Staph. aureus infection seen in A/E:**
(a) Bloom syndrome
(b) Chediak-Higashi
(c) Job's syndrome

415. **Generalized osteoporosis A/E:**
(a) Down's syndrome (b) Adrenal insensitive
(c) RA (d) Acromegaly

416. **Kocher Debré Semelaigne syndrome:**
(a) Congenital hypothyroidism
(b) Hypoparathyroidism
(c) GH deficiency
(d) Hyperthyroidism

417. **OSA true:**
(a) M=F
(b) Initial presentation can be personality disorder
(c) Estrogen can be effective in treatment
(d) Corpulmonale present but not hypertension

418. **Drug inhibiting CYP-3A:**
(a) Clarithromycin (b) Tacrolimus
(c) Quinidine

419. **First reported case of SARS in Asia:**
(a) Feb. 2003 (b) Dec. 2003
(c) April 2004 (d) March 2004

420. **Prenatal asphyxia, indicated are all *except*:**
(a) Hypoxanthine (b) Adenosine
(c) CPK (d) Erythropoietin
(e) All of the above

421. Mechanism of stroke in extra cranial stenosis is:
(a) Embolism (b) Atherosclerosis
(c) HTN (d) Hemorrhage

422. Saline infusion used for diagnosis of:
(a) Hyperaldosteronism
(b) Pheochromocytoma
(c) Renovascular HTN
(d) Renal parenchymal disease

423. Not a cardiac teratogen:
(a) Hydralazine (b) Phenytoin
(c) Alcohol (d) Lithium

424. All seen in myxedema *except:*
(a) Hypotension (b) Bradycardia
(c) Raised QT (d) Pericardial effusion

425. Amyloidosis A/E:
(a) Biventricular failure
(b) Arrhythmias commonly seen
(c) Orthostatic hypotension
(d) Constrictive pericarditis

426. Large tongue seen in A/E:
(a) Hyperthyroidism (b) Anderson syndrome
(c) Amyloidosis (d) Down's syndrome

427. Life span of platelet:
(a) 3 days (b) 7 days
(c) 10 days (d) 14 days

428. RA factor:
(a) IgM (b) IgG
(c) IgA

429. Platelet storage temperature:
(a) 22-25°C (b) 2-5°C
(c) 5-10°C

430. Migraine acute attack treatment:
(a) Sumatriptans (b) NSAIDs
(c) Regular use of anticonvulsant

431. Lactic acidosis type A A/E:
(a) Liver failure (b) Hypoxia
(c) Septic shock (d) CO poisoning

432. NASH A/E:
(a) Gall stones (b) Obesity
(c) DM 2

433. Peptic ulcer A/E:
(a) ZE syndrome
(b) Plummer Vinson syndrome
(c) Cirrhosis

434. Delayed skeletal maturity A/E:
(a) CKD
(b) Congenital adrenal hyperplasia
(c) Hypothyroidism
(d) PEM

435. Risk factors for CA stomach:
(a) A+ve blood group (b) Duodenal ulcer
(c) Atrophic gastritis (d) Partial gastrectomy

436. E. Coli enterotoxigenic secretory diarrhea caused by inhibition of:
(a) c AMP (b) c GMP
(c) NO (d) Ach

437. Primary TB A/E:
(a) Pleural effusion
(b) Phylectangular conjuctivitis
(c) Cavitatory lesion
(d) Fibrocaseous

438. Child with multiple bee stings, treatment to be given:
(a) Adrenaline (b) Hydrocortisone
(c) Soda bicarb

439. What present in blood is safe:
(a) Anti HBsAg (b) HBsAg
(c) IgM Anti HBc

440. Cavitatory lesions are seen in:
(a) Wegener's granulomatosis
(b) PAN
(c) SLE
(d) Sarcoidosis

441. Most common chronic hepatitis:
(a) Hepatitis A (b) Hepatitis B
(c) Hepatitis C (d) Hepatitis D

442. Patient having acute viral hepatitis, what test to be done?
(a) Hepatitis A, B, C, E (b) HIV related options
(c) Toxoplasmosis

443. Quadriparesis in young male followed by loose stool:
(a) GBS (b) H. pylori
(c) Campylobacter

444. Patient having paraplegia, upgoing planters lesion at:
(a) T 10 (b) T 12
(c) T 8

445. Cyclophosphamide induced hemorrhagic cystitis prevented:
(a) MESNA (b) Saline
(c) Furosemide

446. Hb=7 g/dl, monoovalocytes, hypersegmented neutrophils:
(a) Folate (b) Niacin
(c) Thiamine

447. Isolated unilateral 7th nerve palsy (Ramsay Hunt syndrome):
(a) EBV (b) Adenovirus
(c) Arbovirus (d) Polio

448. Macrocytosis caused by:
(a) NFT (b) Zidovudine
(c) Warfarin (d) Vancomycin

449. S/E Rifampicin:
(a) Flu like syndrome (b) Anemia
(c) Renal dysfunction

450. IDA A/E:
(a) Decreased TIBC (b) Decreased ferritin
(c) Low serum iron

451. Hemophilia B true:
(a) APTT increased (b) BT prolonged
(c) CT prolonged

452. ITP:
(a) BT prolonged (b) CT prolonged
(c) APTT increased

453. Cryoprecipitate contain A/E:
(a) Factor VII (b) Factor VIII
(c) VWF (d) Fibrinogen

454. Intravascular hemolysis A/E:
(a) $CuSO_4$ (b) Snake bite
(c) Thalassemia

455. Burn ulcer also known as:
(a) Curling ulcer (b) Cushing ulcer

456. Succinyl choline causes:
(a) Malignant hyperthermia
(b) Hemolysis
(c) Renal failure

457. Ulcerative colitis A/E:
(a) Does not predispose to malignancy
(b) Toxic mega colon
(c) Episcleritis
(d) Pyoderma gangrenosum

458. Asthma patient with chest pain diagnosis:
(a) ACS (b) Acid peptic disease
(c) Bronchial spasm

459. Female delayed menarche:
(a) Systolic murmur + edema feet+ cubitus valgus
(b) Tall stature + diastolic murmur + pneumothorax
(c) Club foot + cyanosis + simian crease

460. History of NSAIDs intake for 5 years presented with anasarca:
(a) Nephrotic syndrome (b) GI complication
(c) Anemia

461. X-linked disorder A/E:
(a) ADPKD
(b) Marfan syndrome
(c) Familial hypercholesterolemia
(d) HOCM

462. Diabetic patient with fatty density and calculi on USG:
(a) Xanthogranulomatosis pyelonephritis
(b) Renal papillary necrosis

463. Rash on trunk and limbs, family history positive:
(a) Sacroptes scabies
(b) Streptococcal infection
(c) Measles

464. Male patient with jaundice and splenomegaly:
(a) Hereditary spherocytosis
(b) Thalassemia
(c) ALL

465. Acute liver failure precipitated in cirrhosis by:
(a) UGI bleed
(b) Intravenous albumin
(c) High carbohydrate diet

466. Patient with 10 days of chills and rigors along with cola coloured urine:
(a) Cerebral malaria
(b) Alkaptonuria
(c) Rifampicin induced

467. Vesiculobullous eruption with buccal mucosa involved A/E:
(a) Drug induced (lamotrignine)
(b) Pemphigus vulgaris
(c) Erythema multiforme
(d) Stevenson Johnson syndrome

468. A child having chickenpox, grandfather having lesions in one dermatome:
(a) Herpes zoster (b) Eczema
(c) Atopic dermatitis (d) Psoriasis

469. Japanese encephalitis involves:
(a) Frontal lobe (b) Temporal lobe
(c) Cerebellar lobe (d) Basal ganglia

470. Polycythemia A/E:
(a) Pancreatic carcinoma (b) Gastric carcinoma
(c) Hepatoma (d) VHL

471. Methemoglobinemia A/E:
(a) Methylene blue used for treatment
(b) May be caused by dapsone
(c) O_2 saturation might be normal
(d) Cause of cyanosis

472. ↓FSH, ↓LH, ↑Prolactin diagnosis:
(a) Pituitary stalk syndrome
(b) Bromcriptine induced
(c) Sheehan syndrome
(d) Turner syndrome

473. BISAP score A/E:
(a) BUN > 22
(b) Age > 65
(c) Impaired mental status
(d) Pleural effusion

474. Exudative pleural effusion:
(a) Bronchogenic carcinoma
(b) CCF
(c) Renal failure
(d) Pulmonary embolism

475. Budd Chiari syndrome due to occlusion:
(a) Hepatic vein
(b) Portal vein
(c) Intrahepatic obstruction
(d) Bile duct

476. Anti LKM-3:
(a) Hepatitis B
(b) Hepatitis D
(c) Autoimmune hepatitis
(d) Sjogren syndrome

477. Fat embolism treatment:
(a) Dextran (b) Oral anticoagulant
(c) Oxygen (d) Heparin

478. Carcinoma tongue on lateral 1/3rd—treatment:
(a) Irradiation (b) Chemotherapy
(c) IBRT (d) Surgery

479. Acute lung injury A/E:
(a) $FiO_2/PaO_2 < 200$
(b) Hypoxia
(c) Pulmonary infiltrates
(d) Intrapulmonary shunting

480. D-dimer:
(a) High positive predictive value
(b) High negative predictive value
(c) Sensitivity
(d) Specificity

481. Class III recommendation:
(a) May be useful
(b) May be harmful
(c) In favour of effectiveness

482. APLA true:
(a) Recurrent syncope
(b) Recurrent pregnancy loss uncommon
(c) Limited period of anticoagulation
(d) β2-gp antibodies associated with increased thrombosis

483. All are type II contrast allergy *except:*
(a) Hives (b) Chills
(c) Vertigo (d) Fever

484. St. John's Wart true A/E:
(a) Induces CYP3A4
(b) Induces P- glycoprotein
(c) Increases cyclosporine level
(d) Decreases verpamil

485. Maximum CYP activity in intestine and liver:
(a) CYP 3A4 (b) CYP 2C9
(c) CYP 2C19 (d) CYP 2D6

486. Which is metabolized by CYP 3A4?
(a) Propranolol (b) Losartan
(c) Verapamil (d) Codeine

487. hs CRP A/E:
(a) Treatment if > 2 mg/dl
(b) Has circadian rhythm
(c) Synthesized in liver
(d) Trial goal < 1 and LDL < 70 mg/dl

488. Patient has no disease and test is normal:
(a) Sensitivity (b) Specificity
(c) Predictability (d) PPV

489. Hyper magnesium:
(a) 2-2.5 mg%=severe Ms weakness, loss of tendon reflex
(b) 6-10 mg%=c. arrest
(c) 2.5-5= all prolong PR, QRS, etc
(d) Renal failure=Toxicity, ppt early

490. Bronchial carcinoid: (T/F)
(a) Mostly symptomatic
(b) Surgery indicated
(c) Chemotherapy given
(d) Multicentric

491. Lymphangiomatosis: (T/F)
(a) Most premenopausal women
(b) Hemoptysis due to hypertrophied bronchial
(c) Atypical smooth muscle hyperplasia

492. Bronchial carcinoid:
(a) Multicentric
(b) Surgery is required
(c) Chemotherapy is recommended
(d) Usually present with carcinoid syndrome

493. Inoperability of bronchogenic Ca:
(a) Hyper Ca
(b) Cerebellar syndrome
(c) Skin metastasis
(d) Hypertrophic osteoarthropathy

494. Linezolid adverse effect:
(a) Thrombocytopenia (b) Leucopenia
(c) Anemia (d) Hemolysis

495. Regarding thyroid radioiodine all true *except:*
(a) One month before treatment–start antithyroid drugs
(b) 3 days before treatment–stop antithyroid drugs to increase uptake
(c) Young male early relapse
(d) Retreatment–extra dose after 3 months

496. Lithium induced nephrotoxicity treatment:
(a) Amiloride (b) Chlorpropamide
(c) Thiazide (d) Spironolactone

497. All are autosomal dominant all *except:*
(a) α1–antitrypsin deficiency
(b) Marfan's syndrome
(c) ADPKD

498. Increased anion gap all *except:*
(a) Diarrhea (b) Metabolic acidosis
(c) DKA (d) Alcohol

499. Type I lepra reaction:
(a) Type IV hypersensitivity reaction
(b) Steroid treatment
(c) Thalidomide in refractory cases
(d) Seen in borderline cases

500. Syphilis–late change is:
(a) Interstitial keratitis (b) Bone change
(c) Syphilis pemphigus (d) Snuffles

501. Anion gap:
(a) Na–(Cl + HCO_3) (b) (Na + K) - (Cl + HCO_3)
(c) Na - HCO_3

502. Tuberous sclerosis brain tumour:
(a) Meningioma (b) Acoustic neuroma
(c) Subglial astrocytoma

503. Fulminant hepatic failure by overdose of:
(a) Niacin (b) Vitamin A
(c) Vitamin B_6 (d) Vitamin E

504. Folic acid daily requirement:
(a) 1 mg (b) 50 μg
(c) 50 mg (d) 1 μg

505. SLE not cause by:
(a) Propafenone (b) Disopyramide
(c) Procainamide (d) Mexilitine

506. Polycythemia vera all *except:*
(a) Hypoxia present
(b) EPO decreased
(c) Myeloproliferative disorders

507. Aldosteronism:
(a) Female more than male
(b) Unilateral adenoma most common
(c) LVH absent

508. Isolated hematuria all *except:*
(a) Thin GBM disease (b) Hereditary nephritis
(c) MPGN (d) IgA nephropathy

509. Glycemic disturbances caused by:
(a) Gatifloxacin (b) Ofloxacin
(c) Ciprofloxacin

510. Sensitivity:
(a) TP/ TP+FN (b) TN/ TN+ FP
(c) TN/ FP+TP (d) TP/ TP+ TN

511. Y. pestis is:
(a) Gram negative coccobacilli
(b) Gram positive coccobacilli
(c) Gram negative bacilli
(d) Gram positive bacilli

512. Tubercular pleural effusion uncommon finding is:
(a) Decreased sugar
(b) Abundant mesothelial cell
(c) AFB

513. Germ cell tumour seen in Klinefilter's syndrome:
(a) Mediastinum
(b) Retroperitoneum
(c) Testis

514. Ankylosing spondylitis all *except:*
(a) HLA- B27 essential for diagnosis
(b) Bamboo spine
(c) Square vertebra
(d) Osteoporosis

515. Pulmonary nodule (metastatic) resection done in:
(a) Colon Ca (b) Thyroid Ca
(c) Nephroblastoma (d) Osteosarcoma

516. Sarcoidosis all *except:*
(a) Lung involvement common
(b) Hemoptysis rare
(c) BAL is normal in most cases

517. Sarcoidosis all *except:*
(a) Hemoptysis common
(b) Paratracheal LN commonly involved
(c) Generalized lymphadenopathy

518. Goodpasture syndrome:
(a) Bimodal age of presentation
(b) Elderly
(c) Lung haemorrhage common
(d) Collagen α3 chain (antigen)

519. Cerebellar involvement in:
(a) Dimethyl mercury (b) Cadmium
(c) Tetraethyl lead (d) Arsenic

520. OSA and CAD–treatment:
(a) CPAP (b) Fluoxetine
(c) Sertaline

521. PGA type II all *except:*
(a) HLA association
(b) AR
(c) Female more than male
(d) Graves' disease can be present

522. Hyper magnesium all *except:*
(a) DTR increased
(b) Intravenous Ca in treatment
(c) CRF
(d) Excess Mg can be excreted by kidney

523. Broadcast seen in:
(a) CRF (b) CHF
(c) RTA (d) RPGN

524. Brush border loss and flat necrosis:
(a) Whipple's disease (b) Abetalipoproteinemia
(c) Lymphangiectasia (d) Agammaglobinemia

525. Anticipation seen in:
(a) Trinucleotide repeat disorder
(b) Mosacism

526. Increased paternal age not a risk factor in:
(a) Mafan's syndrome (b) Neurofibromatosis
(c) Achondroplasia (d) Huntington's disease

527. Classic complement pathway mediated by:
(a) IgG (b) IgA
(c) IgM (d) IgD

528. Molluscum contangiosum like lesion in HIV seen in:
(a) HSV-1 (b) CMV
(c) Cryptococci

529. Radiation to brain characteristic late sign:
(a) Lhermitte's sign (b) Sun downing sign

530. Purpura fulminans:
(a) Meningococci
(b) Pneumococci
(c) Gonococci

531. Chancroid DOC:
(a) Azithromycin (b) Penicillin
(c) Tetracycline (d) Amikacin

532. Pheochromocytoma treatment all *except:*
(a) Alpha blockade followed by beta blockade
(b) Beta blockade followed by alpha blockade
(c) Only alpha blockade

533. Bone resorption marker all *except:*
(a) N-telopeptide
(b) C-telopeptide
(c) TRAP
(d) Bone specific alkaline phosphatase

534. Heaptitis A:
(a) DNA virus
(b) Once jaundice occurs, viral shedding stops
(c) Asymptomatic in adults
(d) Incubation 4 months

535. K^+ infusion by both central or peripheral vein:
(a) 20 mmol/hour (b) 40 mmol/hour
(c) 60 mmol/hour (d) 80 mmol/hour

536. Oxygen carried by serum:
(a) 0.03 ml/dl (b) 0.3 ml/dl
(c) 1.34 ml/dl (d) 13.4 ml/dl

537. Sarin gas is a derivative of:
(a) Organophosphorus compounds
(b) Organochlorine compounds
(c) Carbamates
(d) Nitrous oxide

538. When there is no need for investigation of thrombophilic conditions:
(a) Thrombosis in less than 50 years age group
(b) Thromboembolism after major surgery
(c) Recurrent thromboembolism

539. Drug that can be given safely in porphyria is:
(a) Carbamazepine (b) Alcohol
(c) Aspirin (d) Barbiturate

540. Left parietal infact, anticoagulation indication in 75 years old:
(a) AF (b) MI
(c) HTN

541. Patient had acute MR. After 4 days, he developed cyanosis, ABG pH = 7.2, PO_2 = 90 mmHg, treatment:
(a) MVR (b) I.V. methylene blue

542. HbA1c units by IFCC:
(a) % age (b) mmol/mol
(c) Mole (d) μg

543. Low anion gap A/E:
(a) Lithium (b) Iron overdose
(c) Hypoalbuminemia (d) Multiple myeloma

544. ACCORD and ADVANCE trial all true *except:*
(a) HbA1c < 5%
(b) Does not affect macrovascular
(c) Effects microvascular
(d) Excessive glycemic control does not affect mortality

545. 50 years male of AS, did exercise till 11 minutes gradient was 60 mmHg, treatment:
(a) AVR (b) Follow up
(c) Balloon dilatation

546. Stem cell precursor:
(a) CD 34 (b) CD 134
(c) CD 59

547. Antidote of ethylene glycol:
(a) Fomepizole (b) Soda bicarb
(c) Methanol

548. All true *except:*
(a) Sotalol C/I in renal failure
(b) Nifedipine C/I in liver failure
(c) Metoprolol C/I in renal failure
(d) Lignocaine C/I in CHF

549. HDL ↑ by A/E:
(a) Transfatty acids
(b) CETP inhibition–Torcetapib
(c) Fibrates
(d) Pravastatin

550. After 3rd day MI all of following raised *except:*
(a) HDL (b) CPK–MB
(c) CRP (d) TLC

551. Pulmonary artery HTN:
(a) PA pressure > 25 mm Hg at rest
(b) PA pressure > 30 mm Hg on exercise
(c) Pulmonary wedge pressure > 16 mm Hg
(d) PA pressure > 3 wood units

552. Method of measuring aortic valve area in cardiac cath:
(a) Gorlin formula (b) Cournard equation
(c) Continuity equation

553. Antibiotic all true *except:*
(a) Cefepime–4th generation
(b) Ceftazidine–3rd generation
(c) Cefotan–2nd generation
(d) Cefoxitin–1st generation

554. Heart block which can be treated with antibiotic therapy:
(a) Lyme's disease (b) Diphtheria
(c) Rheumatic fever (d) Congenital syphilis

555. Myasthenia gravis worsened by all *except:*
(a) Quinolones (b) Mg
(c) Cephalosporin (d) Botulinum toxin

556. All are acute effects of cocaine *except:*
(a) Hypothermia (b) Seizures
(c) Hypertension (d) MI

557. Elderly patients all are true *except:*
(a) Bacteriuria does not mean UTI
(b) Digoxin at normal serum level can cause toxicity
(c) Law of parsimony may be present
(d) Physiological anemia may exist

558. Type II error all true *except:*
(a) False negative
(b) Due to small study population
(c) Null hypothesis is rejected
(d) Difference is present but does not reach statistical significance

559. Wilson's disease–neurological manifestation treatment:
(a) Penicillamine (b) Zinc and trientine
(c) Tetrathiomolybdate

560. Patient of CKD stage IV, BP= 140/90, S. Ferritin- 275 ng/ml, iron saturation=26%, treatment of choice:
(a) Oral iron (b) Intravenous iron
(c) EPO

561. Which has definite role?
(a) Myocarditis–immunoglobin
(b) Bosentan–Eisenmenger syndrome
(c) Prasugrel–chronic stable angina
(d) Low dose dopamine–renal failure

562. Erythema nodosum seen in A/E:
(a) ITP
(b) Takayasu arteritis
(c) Infective endocarditis
(d) APLA

563. pH- 7.2, Na- 135, K- 3.0, Cl- 80, HCO_3- 25, PCO_2- 42, possible explanation:
(a) Chronic diarrhea
(b) DKA
(c) CHF on diuretics use
(d) Compensated RTA

564. Diabetic patient, mild renal failure, on ACE-I, chances of hyperkalemia increased by:
(a) Digoxin (b) NSAID
(c) Salbutamol (d) Alkalosis

565. Marfan's syndrome:
(a) Myopia
(b) Slow retardation of aortic aneurysm
(c) All are due to fibrillin mutation
(d) Inguinal hernia

566. GBS A/E:
(a) Duration < 2 weeks
(b) Exclusion of other diseases
(c) Areflexia
(d) Progressive weakness of more than 2 limbs suggestive of neuropathy

567. Primary TB after exposure:
(a) 10% (b) 20%
(c) 30% (d) 40%

568. Explanatory variable:
(a) Any factor that can influence the response variable
(b) Dependent variable

569. Post hypoxia effect earliest:
(a) Mamillary body
(b) Hippocampus
(c) Reticular formation in pons
(d) Cerebellum

570. Lyme's disease:
(a) Facial palsy (b) Conduction block
(c) Human louse is vector

571. Maximum resistance in airways at level of:
(a) Large airways (b) Small airways
(c) Bronchioles (d) Alveoli

572. Reactive enteropathic arthritis not seen with:
(a) Salmonella infection
(b) Shigella boydii
(c) Campylobacter jejuni
(d) Streptococci

573. Psoriatic arthritis not seen:
(a) Associated with HLA CD 55/59
(b) M > F
(c) Nail involvement
(d) All of the above

574. SLE is not associated with which antibody?
(a) Anti-ds DNA (b) Anti histone antibody
(c) Anti-Smith (d) Anti RNP antibodies

575. Scleroderma crisis what is true?
(a) ACE- I to be used if creatinine is normal
(b) Steroids to be started at once
(c) ACE-I also lead to regression of skin lesion

576. Primary Sjogren syndrome is:
(a) Not seen in children
(b) Associated with HLA DR-52
(c) Females more than males
(d) Carries good prognosis

577. Medium vessel vasculitis is:
(a) Takayasu's arteritis
(b) PAN
(c) Wegener's granulomatosis
(d) Kawasaki's disease

578. HLA B-27 what is not true?
(a) Necessary for diagnosis of Ankylosing Spondylitis
(b) Seen in 90% of patients of Ankylosing Spondylitis
(c) Only 1-2% of patient with HLA B-27 develop Ankylosing Spondylitis

579. Sunitinib is used in:
(a) Renal cell carcinoma
(b) Myeloleukemia
(c) Angiokeratoma

580. Treatment for stage I cutaneous sezary syndrome:
(a) PUVA
(b) Radiation and predicort
(c) CHOP

581. Pseudomyxoma peritonei what is not true?
(a) M > F (b) Arises from appendix
(c) LN spread (d) Extraperitoneal spread

582. Hb A2 not true is:
(a) Most abundant in fetus
(b) Increased in beta thalassemia
(c) Hb Bart disease severe form beta thalassemia

583. Not found in human is:
(a) Hb $\alpha 2\ \beta 2$ (b) Hb $\alpha 2\ \gamma 2$
(c) Hb $\alpha 2\ \delta 2$ (d) Hb $\alpha 2\ \varepsilon 2$

584. Not seen in minor thalassemia:
(a) Anemia (b) Spleen
(c) Jaundice (d) Dactylitis

585. Pancytopenia with splenomegaly not seen in:
(a) Aplastic anemia
(b) Hemophagocytic syndrome
(c) Lymphoma
(d) Myelodysplasia

586. Paroxysmal cold hemoglobinuria is associated with:
(a) Ig G (b) Ig M
(c) Ig A (d) Ig D

587. Intravascular hemolysis not seen in:
(a) Paroxysmal cold hemoglobinuria
(b) Thalassemia
(c) Snake bite

588. Factor VIII half life is:
(a) 6 hours (b) 7 hours
(c) 8 hours (d) 12 hours

589. Factor VIII should be increased by.....in hemophilia:
(a) 20% (b) 50%
(c) 80% (d) 100%

590. Monogenic inheritance seen with:
(a) Sickle cell anemia (b) CHD
(c) Rheumatoid arthritis (d) Marfan's syndrome

591. Pancreatic mucinous cystadenoma is associated with:
(a) Pancreatitis
(b) Pancreatic pseudocyst
(c) Extrahepatic neoplasm
(d) All of the above

592. Not seen with lung cancer:
(a) Cushing's syndrome (b) Hypernatremia
(c) Hypercalcemia (d) SIADH

593. Maximum velocity of height in prepubertal boy is:
(a) 6.5 (b) 7.5
(c) 8.5 (d) 10

594. In HS purpura renal involvement is seen in:
(a) 30% (b) 50%
(c) 60% (d) 80%

595. Which is not prothrombotic?
(a) Glanzmann's sick thrombocytes
(b) Homocystinemia
(c) OCP
(d) Buerger's disease

596. What is not a proinflammatory cytokine?
(a) IL-6 (b) IL-12
(c) TNF-α

597. In patient with factor VII deficiency treatment:
(a) Platelet (b) FFP
(c) Cryoprecipitate

598. Hemochromatosis–not used for iron chelation:
(a) Penicillamine (b) Desferrioxamine
(c) Hexaten

599. Subaortic stenosis not seen in:
(a) AR (b) Ejection click
(c) Systolic murmur (d) LVH

600. Creation of IV chamber and replacement of pulmonary artery is known as:
(a) Senning's operation (b) Mustard's operation
(c) Blalock's shunt (d) Reink's shunt

601. Fluctuating AV block is seen with:
(a) Myocarditis (b) Rheumatic carditis
(c) Congenital (d) Degenerative

602. Drug used for AF is all *except:*
(a) Dilzem (b) Digoxin
(c) Metoprolol (d) Ivabradine

603. Which drug doesn't prevent AF?
(a) Digoxin (b) Losartan
(c) Statins

604. Drug not affected by rifampicin is:
(a) CMZ (b) Amiodarone
(c) Protease inhibitor (d) Warfarin

605. What is pressure gradient across aortic valve if velocity is 4 m/s:
(a) 16 (b) 32
(c) 64 (d) 24

606. GIST not true is:
(a) Stomach is common site
(b) Treatment is surgery
(c) Involves 5th to 6th decade
(d) Tyrosine kinase inhibitor no role

607. Heat stroke is not associated with:
(a) Anti parkinsonism drugs
(b) Antihypertensives
(c) Bed-ridden status
(d) Heat wave

608. Thermoregulatory system for heat loss is:
(a) Conduction (b) Evaporation
(c) Convection (d) All of the above

609. Cooing/seagull murmur is heard in:
(a) Papillary muscle rupture
(b) Chordae tendonae rupture
(c) Rheumatic valvulitis
(d) Perforation of aortic cusp

610. IVIG is used in AIDP, mechanism of action is all *except:*
(a) Immune complex inhibition
(b) Immunomodulation
(c) Complement activation

611. Not associated with high steppage gait is:
(a) L5 radiculopathy (b) Sciatica
(c) Peripheral neuropathy

612. Charcot's joint is not associated with:
(a) DM (b) Syringomyelia
(c) Friedreich's ataxia (d) Leprosy

613. Spondylosis means:
(a) Degeneration of facet's joints
(b) Protrusion of disc
(c) Osteosclerosis of nerve

614. Anti parkinsonism associated with valvular lesion is:
(a) L-dopa (b) Pergolide
(c) Ropinrole

615. Not seen in NPH:
(a) Dementia (b) Ataxia
(c) Incontinence of urine (d) Diplopia

616. Patient with intractable pain in right lower limb, benefitted by:
(a) Morphine (b) NSAID
(c) TCA

617. Pigmented retinal degeneration is seen in:
(a) SCA 1 (b) SCA 6
(c) SCA 7 (d) SCA 10

618. Which drug causes parkinsonism?
(a) Gabapentin (b) Losartan
(c) Metoclopramide (d) Digoxin

619. Lepromatous leprosy is associated with:
(a) Severe HS reaction to lepromin's test
(b) Few skin lesion
(c) Anaesthetic patch
(d) Thickening of nerves

620. Commonly associated with catheter induced infection:
(a) S. aureus
(b) Coagulase negative S. aureus
(c) Gram negative bacilli
(d) Fungi

621. Mechanisms of resistance of linezolid is:
(a) Protein change (b) Plasmid mediated
(c) Cell wall change

622. Aminoglycosides true is:
(a) Inhibit cell wall
(b) Active against S. aureus
(c) Contraindicated in renal impairment
(d) Cause blindness in elderly

623. Hypophosphatemia is seen in:
(a) Primary hyperparathyroidism
(b) Rickets
(c) Refeeding syndrome
(d) All of the above

624. Tumour lysis syndrome not associated with:
(a) Hypercalcemia (b) Hypokalemia
(c) Hypophosphatemia (d) Hypomagnesemia

625. In pregnancy change not seen in bile:
(a) ↑ Cholesterol
(b) ↑ cholic acid
(c) ↓ deoxycholic acid
(d) Decreased glycine/taurine bile acid ratio

626. LES pressure is ↑ sed by all *except*:
(a) Gastrin (b) Secretin
(c) Serotonin (d) Histamine

627. **ABG in a patient of chronic bronchitis with cyanosis is:**
(a) pH -7.15, PCO_2-80 mm Hg, PO_2-70 mm Hg
(b) pH -7.35, PCO_2-40 mm Hg, PO_2-80 mm Hg
(c) pH -7.40, PCO_2-80 mm Hg, PO_2-70 mm Hg

628. **Lung scan is done with all *except:***
(a) Gallium (b) Technetium
(c) Thallium

629. **Drug used in second trimester of pregnancy is:**
(a) Carbimazole (b) Propyl thiouracil
(c) Radioiodine (d) Methimazole

630. **Difficulty in spelling or muttering words of grammar is:**
(a) Alexia
(b) Agraphia
(c) Gertsmann syndrome

631. **Legionnaire disease is associated with all *except:***
(a) Nausea, vomiting and diarrhoea
(b) Marked clinical signs with clear lungs
(c) Man to man transmission not seen
(d) Recovers within a week

632. **Statistics–median square test is done by:**
(a) Chi square test (b) t-test
(c) Mc-Nemer test

633. **Drug not associated with K+ channel is:**
(a) Glimepride (b) Glubyride
(c) Sitagliptin

634. **Which is not 'B' category in bioterrorism?**
(a) Anthrax
(b) Cl. botulism
(c) Viral hemorrhagic fever
(d) Polio

635. **Hallmark of glomerular proteinuria:**
(a) Granular casts (b) Acanthocytes
(c) Bifid RBCs

636. **FENa is used to distinguish:**
(a) Ischemic ARF (b) Nephrotoxic ARF
(c) Pre-renal azotemia

637. **Which is not a negative acute phase reactant?**
(a) Albumin (b) Ferritin
(c) Transthyretin (d) Transferrin

638. **What is not associated with Fe absorption?**
(a) Fe reductase (b) Acidic medium
(c) Erythropoietin (d) Hemosiderin

639. **Reciprocal inhibition of eye muscle:**
(a) Sherrington's law (b) Herring's law
(c) Laplace law

640. **Amaurosis fugax:**
(a) Binocular vision loss
(b) Associated with Hollenhorst's plague
(c) Retinal haemorrhages

641. **Anosmia is mostly seen with:**
(a) Inferior frontal tumour
(b) Parietal tumour
(c) Temporal tumour

642. **Actinomycosis most common infection:**
(a) Pulmonary (b) Cervicofacial
(c) Abdominal

643. **Amphotericin B is not effective in:**
(a) Nocardiosis (b) Histoplasmosis
(c) Coccidoidomycosis (d) Aspergillosis

644. **Which ovarian tumour are bilateral?**
(a) Dysgerminoma
(b) Fibroma
(c) Brenner tumour
(d) Endodermal sinus tumour

645. **Sensitivity means:**
(a) Less false +ve (b) Less false -ve
(c) More false +ve (d) More false -ve

646. **Which is a non-narcotic analgesic:**
(a) Ketorolac (b) Bupropion
(c) Mepredine

647. **A lady comes with thigh mass attached to muscle but overlying skin is free, which best treatment?**
(a) Radiotherapy (b) Incisional biopsy
(c) Excisional biopsy (d) Surgical removal

648. **Plummer Vinson syndrome:**
(a) More in females
(b) Symptoms disappear with correction of anemia
(c) Premalignant condition
(d) All are correct

649. Alien hand syndrome seen in:
(a) Balint's syndrome (b) Gerstmann syndrome

650. TB reactivation is due to:
(a) Perfusion
(b) High oxygen saturation
(c) Genetic factors

651. Eggs of helminthes not found in stool:
(a) Strongyloides (b) Ankylostoma
(c) Fasiola bushki (d) Trichuris trichiura

652. Tropical pulmonary eosinophilia caused by:
(a) Brugaya malayi (b) Ascariasis
(c) Strongyloidosis (d) Schistosoma

653. Enteric gram negative bacilli A/E:
(a) E. coli (b) Klebsiella
(c) Pseudomonas (d) Proteus

654. Imatinib used in:
(a) GIST (b) Sarcoma
(c) Lipoma (d) Leiomyoma

655. Hypokalemia with HTN seen in:
(a) Primary aldosteronism
(b) Barter's syndrome
(c) Hyporeninimic hypoaldosteronism
(d) Pheochromocytoma

656. Hypokalemic periodic paralysis channel:
(a) Na (b) Ca
(c) K (d) Mg

657. Episodic paralysis generalized in:
(a) Myasthenia
(b) LEMS
(c) Hypokalemic periodic paralysis
(d) All of the above

658. Kidney increase excretion of all of the following with decreased GFR *except:*
(a) Urea (b) K^+
(c) Phosphate (d) H^+

659. Carcinogenic in lungs A/E:
(a) Nickel (b) Chromium
(c) Benzene (d) Arsenic

660. Most common site of actinomycosis:
(a) Craniofacial actinomycosis
(b) Thoracic actinomycosis
(c) Abdominal actinomycosis
(d) Pelvic actinomycosis

661. Most common branch of abdominal aorta involved in Takayasu arteritis:
(a) Iliac artery (b) Renal artery
(c) SMA (d) Celiac trunk

662. GFR starts decreasing after age of:
(a) 30 (b) 40
(c) 50 (d) 60

663. Thick GBM is seen in:
(a) MPGN (b) FSGS
(c) MCD

664. Urothelial carcinoma is associated with:
(a) Renal stones
(b) Analgesic nephropathy
(c) Chronic interstitial nephritis

665. Treatment of FSGS is:
(a) Prednisolone (b) Cyclosporine
(c) Azathiopurine (d) Cyclophosphamide

666. H. pylori causes:
(a) Chronic superficial gastritis
(b) Gastric cancer
(c) All of the above

667. All are used for myocardial viability A/E:
(a) PET (b) MRI
(c) MDCT (d) Dobutamine echo

668. Cardiac hemochromatosis diagnosis:
(a) MRI (b) CT
(c) Radionuclide study (d) ECHO

669. Most common cardiac complication in SLE:
(a) Pericarditis
(b) Libmann sack endocarditis
(c) Myocarditis
(d) AR

670. Most common route for entry of organisms for native valve endocarditis:
(a) Oral cavity (b) Intravenous cannula
(c) Genital tract (d) Hemodialysis

671. **Most common cause of I.E. in intravenous drug abuser:**
(a) Staph. aureus (b) Pseudomonas
(c) Pneumococci (d) Enterococci

672. **Shift of K^+ in ICF is seen in:**
(a) Metabolic acidosis (b) Hypoglycemia
(c) Metabolic alkalosis (d) Ca gluconate

673. **Short QT is caused by A/E:**
(a) Digoxin (b) Hypercalcemia
(c) Hypothermia (d) Acidosis

674. **All are monogenic disorder *except:***
(a) Essential HTN
(b) HOCM
(c) Congenital QT syndrome
(d) Marfan's syndrome

675. **True about S1–ejection click interval in PS is:**
(a) Increased interval with severity
(b) Decreased interval with severity
(c) No variability with respiration

676. **Aortic continuous Doppler velocity-4 m/s, then gradient is:**
(a) 64 (b) 74
(c) 84 (d) 54

677. **Rifampicin do not decrease the level of:**
(a) Amiodarone
(b) Protease inhibitor
(c) OCP
(d) Anticonvulsant

678. **Which of the following is not prodrug?**
(a) Lisnopril (b) Captopril
(c) Ramipril (d) Enalapril

679. **Which of the following do not prevent against AF?**
(a) Digoxin (b) ACE-I
(c) Amiodarone (d) Statin

680. **OC pills increase A/E:**
(a) Uterine cancer (b) Stroke
(c) Cervical cancer (d) DVT

681. **Which of the following is not evaluated while looking at risk for DVT?**
(a) Surgery under GA (b) Malignancy
(c) Estrogen (d) Pelvis fracture

682. **Absolute contraindication for thrombolysis:**
(a) Hemorrhagic stroke any time in past
(b) Surgery in past 3 months
(c) Oral anticoagulants
(d) Pregnancy

683. **t-PA absolute contraindication:**
(a) Stroke 1/3rd of MCA territory
(b) Age > 18 years
(c) Presentations < 3 hours

684. **Pulmonary renal syndrome seen in A/E:**
(a) Buerger's disease
(b) Wegener's granulomatosis
(c) Goodpasture syndrome
(d) Microscopic polyangitis

685. **Goodpasture syndrome A/E:**
(a) M > F yong age
(b) Nephrotic range proteinuria
(c) Lung haemorrhage–50-70%
(d) Plasmaphresis improves outcome

686. **Sundowning syndrome A/E:**
(a) Delirium (b) Myasthenia
(c) Dementia

687. **Granuloma seen in:**
(a) Giant cell arteritis
(b) Wegener's granulomatois
(c) Microscopic polyangitis
(d) Churg Strauss syndrome

688. **False positive ANA seen in:**
(a) Qunidine (b) Interferon–α
(c) INH

689. **Tetany seen in A/E:**
(a) Diltiazem (b) Hyperventilation
(c) Malabsorption

690. **Single dose penicillin curative in:**
(a) Gonorrhoea
(b) I.E.
(c) Non gonococcal arthritis

691. **All are negative phase reactants *except:***
(a) Ferritin (b) Albumin
(c) Transferrin

692. Category A organisms in bioterronism:
(a) Small pox + anthrax
(b) Anthrax + C. burnetti

693. Cushing reflex A/E:
(a) Irregular breathing (b) Bradycardia
(c) HTN (d) Altered sensorium

694. Dopa decarboxylase inhibitor used in:
(a) Involuntary movements
(b) Psychiatric disturbances
(c) Postural HTN
(d) Nausea and vomiting

695. Snowflake deposits in outer cornea is seen in:
(a) Chalcosis (b) Loa loa
(c) Onchocerciasis (d) Chagas disease

696. Most dangerous bite in splenectomy is:
(a) Dog bite (b) Cat bite
(c) Human bite (d) Rat bite

697. Lymphocytosis is seen in A/E:
(a) Steroids (b) CMV
(c) Sarcoidosis (d) Lymphoma

698. Most common infections in renal transplant:
(a) HBV (b) HIV
(c) CMV (d) VZV

699. Which of the following virus does not cause malignancy?
(a) HPV (b) HIV
(c) EBV (d) HAV

700. Protective titre of Hbs Ag:
(a) 0.1 IU/ml (b) 10 IU/ml
(c) 1 IU/ml (d) 100 IU/ml

701. First manifestation of autoimmune neuropathy in DM is:
(a) Erectile dysfunction (b) Gastroparesis
(c) Postural HTN (d) Nocturnal diarrhea

702. Anemia with reticulocytosis seen in A/E:
(a) Aplastic anemia
(b) Hemorrhage
(c) Vitamin B_{12} deficiency
(d) PNH

703. Increased breast cancer seen in:
(a) Gorlin's syndrome
(b) Ataxia telangiectasia
(c) Cowden's syndrome
(d) Lifraumani's syndrome

704. Acquired defect in grammar spelling of written language:
(a) Alexia
(b) Agraphia
(c) Semantic paraphasia
(d) Phenomic paraphasia

705. Sodium deficit to increase Na from 105 to 115 in 60 kg women:
(a) 100 (b) 200
(c) 300 (d) 400

706. DOC in 2nd trimester pregnancy is:
(a) Propylthiouracil (b) Methimazole
(c) Radioiodine

707. Valve covering coronary sinus:
(a) Thebesian valve (b) Eustachian valve
(c) Crista terminalis

708. Acrodynia seen in (pink disease):
(a) Arsenic (b) Mercury
(c) Lead

709. Best documentation of renal dementia is with:
(a) Aluminium (b) Lead
(c) Arsenic

710. VII nerve involvement is seen in:
(a) Sarcoidosis
(b) Miller Fischer syndrome
(c) Diphtheria
(d) Tabesdorsalis

711. Charcot joint is caused by A/E:
(a) Tabes (b) DM
(c) Syringomyelia (d) Friedreich's ataxia

712. Foot drop is seen in A/E:
(a) Distal neuropathy
(b) Sciatica
(c) LS radiculopathy
(d) Common peroneal neuropathy

713. Kidney produces all hormones *except:*
(a) ANP (b) EPO
(c) Vitamin D (d) Renin

714. **Vitamin D deficiency all are seen *except:***
(a) Rachitic rosary (b) Joint effusion
(c) Bow legs

715. **Down's syndrome A/E:**
(a) Neck webbing (b) Single palmer crease
(c) Mental retardation (d) Short stature

716. **Macrophage activation syndrome is associated with:**
(a) Systemic JRA (b) Systemic sclerosis

717. **Thalassemia is:**
(a) AR
(b) AD
(c) X-linked recessive
(d) Autosomal co dominant

718. **Which is not seen due to genetic mutation?**
(a) Hyperhomocystemia

719. **Which is not caused due to phenytoin?**
(a) Ataxia (b) Nystagmus
(c) Anemia due to vitamin B_{12} deficiency

720. **Antibody seen in Miller Fischer syndrome:**
(a) Anti G21b antibodies
(b) Anti G1b antibodies

721. **Which is not seen in scarlet fever *except:***
(a) Streptococcal infection
(b) Septic shock
(c) Pharyngitis
(d) Rash

722. **All can be used to treat mania *except:***
(a) Carbamazepine (b) Lithium
(c) Chlorpromazine (d) Valproate

723. **Pheochromocytoma secretes A/E:**
(a) Norepinephrine (b) Dopamine
(c) Epinephrine

724. **False about GIST is:**
(a) Most common location is stomach
(b) Histology cannot prove malignancy definitely
(c) Submucosal location is most common
(d) Lymphatic spread is common

725. **All are seen in subaortic stenosis *except:***
(a) Ejection click (b) LVH
(c) AR

726. **Hirsutism seen in A/E:**
(a) Hypothyroidism (b) PCOD
(c) CAH (d) Cushing's syndrome

727. **Short acing insulin A/E:**
(a) Lispro (b) Glulisine
(c) Aspartate (d) Detemir

728. **Spondylosis is:**
(a) Defect in pars interarticularis
(b) Slippage of one vertebra over one another

729. **Treatment of cystitis in women given for:**
(a) 1 day (b) 3 days
(c) 7 days (d) 14 days

730. **Pulmonary fibrosis is seen in A/E:**
(a) Amiodarone (b) Bleomycin
(c) Methotrexate (d) Azathiopurine

731. **Pancreatic mucinous tumour A/E:**
(a) Most common type mucinous cystic carcinoma
(b) Increased vascularity helps to differentiate from pseudocyst
(c) Calcification of tumour on CT is seen in PCIN

732. **Physiological changes in bile in pregnancy:**
(a) Supersaturation of bile
(b) Decreased chemodeoxycholic acid
(c) Increased cholic acid
(d) Decreased bile acid pool

733. **In exercise true *except:***
(a) O_2 dissociation curve shift to left
(b) Increased O_2 extraction by tissue
(c) Increased blood flow
(d) Increased stroke volume

734. **Pseudomyxoma peritonei true *except:***
(a) More common in females
(b) Source is appendix
(c) Lymphatic spread is common
(d) Extraperitoneal spread seen

735. **Diverticular true A/E:**
(a) Most common cause of occult blood loss
(b) Inflammation is causative factor
(c) Bleeding uncommon manifestation
(d) Bleeding stops spontaneously

736. Drugs used in obesity A/E:
(a) Rimonabant (b) Orlistat
(c) Amphetamines (d) Metformin

737. Which do not act on ATP sensitive K channel?
(a) Sitagliptans (b) Glitazones
(c) Glimepride (d) Repaglinide

738. Drugs used to prevent postmenopausal osteoporosis A/E:
(a) Estrogen (b) Calcitonin
(c) Raloxibene (d) Bisphosphonates

739. True regarding portal vein A/E:
(a) Length is constant
(b) Forms behind head of pancreas
(c) No major branch in last 5 cm
(d) Major branches seen

740. Epidemiology of HEV A/E:
(a) 25-30% death in pregnancy
(b) Most common route is fecooral
(c) No evidence of blood or sexual transmission
(d) Highest susceptibility seen in children and adults

741. Electric shock like sensation in neck flexion:
(a) Barbar chair sign (b) Fobe's sign
(c) Lasegue's sign

742. True LV aneurysm A/E:
(a) Most common at inferobasal wall
(b) All three layers of LV present
(c) Common after transmural infarct
(d) Can be source of inferobasal infarct

743. Bronholm disease is seen in:
(a) Coxsackie virus disease (b) Adeno virus
(c) Herpes virus

744. Increased PCWP is indicated by:
(a) Loud S1 (b) MDM
(c) A2 – OS gap

745. Which is least likely in small cell lung Ca?
(a) Hypercalcemia (b) Cerebellar ataxia
(c) ACTH

746. Acute cerebellar involvement is most common in:
(a) Anoxia (b) Viral
(c) Autoimmune (d) Trauma

747. Peripheral neuropathy in CRF:
(a) Lower limb more than upper limb
(b) No improvement after transplantation
(c) Proximal muscle weakness seen

748. Risk factor for NSAID induced PUD A/E:
(a) Elderly
(b) Ethanol
(c) Smoking
(d) Past history of PUD
(e) All are true

749. Which contrast can be used in CRF?
(a) Iodixanol (b) Omnipaque

750. Tone of LES is decreased by:
(a) Gastrin (b) Secretin
(c) Motilin (d) Substance P

751. Travellor's diarrhea caused by A/E:
(a) Giardia (b) E. histolytica
(c) Rota virus (d) All of the above

752. Alcoholic liver disease true is:
(a) GGT is exclusively seen in liver
(b) AST is more specific for liver disease
(c) GGT/ ALP ratio < 2 is specific for alcoholic liver disease
(d) ALT > 1000 is seen in ALD

753. Which is non narcotic analgesic?
(a) Ketorlac (b) Fentanyl
(c) Morphine (d) Mepridine

754. ICF is how much of TBW?
(a) 1/3rd (b) ½
(c) 2/3rd

755. Low complement seen in A/E:
(a) MPGN (b) SLE
(c) PSGN (d) FSGN

756. Which causes anemia in chronic inflammation?
(a) IFN – γ (b) TNF – α
(c) IL-1

757. Which is not proinflammatory cytokine?
(a) IL-8 (b) TNF
(c) IL-11

758. Patient with severe bleeding level of factor VIII in hemophilia to be increased by:

(a) 50% (b) 100%
(c) 10% (d) 30%

759. In liver disease treatment for coagulopathy:

(a) FFP (b) Whole blood
(c) Cryoprecipitate (d) Platelets

760. True regarding Plummer Vinson syndrome:

(a) Predisposes to adenomacarcinoma
(b) Web disappear after treatment with iron deficiency
(c) More common in females
(d) Associated celiac sprue

761. Rectal temperature is more than oral temp. by:

(a) 0.3°C (b) 1°C
(c) 0.5°C (d) 0.8°C

762. Which is not seen in apoptosis?

(a) Inflammatory cells seen
(b) Nuclear condensation
(c) Chromatin breakage

763. Pericardial friction rub true is:

(a) Presystolic, systolic and early diastolic component

764. Finer criteria is for:

(a) Good research question
(b) Evaluation of new therapies
(c) Withdrawal studies
(d) Fractional design

765. Hypermagnesemia is associated with all of the following *except*:

(a) Hypercalcemia
(b) Decreased tendon reflexes
(c) Chronic renal failure
(d) Complete heart block

766. Negative predictive value is a ratio of:

(a) True negative and true positives
(b) True negatives to all negatives
(c) True negatives and false negatives
(d) True negatives and false negatives plus false positives

767. Wilson disease:

(a) ATP 7B gene
(b) Microscopic hematuria
(c) Muscular and sensory abnormalities
(d) 99% patients who have neurological manifestations have k-y rings

768. TB test in IFN – γ quantiferon gold test:

(a) TB 7.7 (b) ESAT–4
(c) ESAT–7 (d) P–10

769. Donath Landsteiner Ab:

(a) Anti-I (b) Anti-P
(c) Anti-K (d) Anti-J

770. Cholestasis:

(a) Erythromycin (b) INH
(c) Methyl dopa

771. All drug causes exudative pleural effusion *except:*

(a) Bromocriptine (b) Dantrolene
(c) Diltiazem (d) Nitrofurantoin

772. PSRA all *except:*

(a) Asymmetric
(b) Latent period 1 week
(c) Small joints
(d) Slow response to salicylates

773. Alcohol dependence treatment used A/E:

(a) Disulfiram (b) Acamprosate
(c) Chlordiazepoxide (d) Naltrexone

774. Opiod toxicity true:

(a) Mydriasis
(b) Therapeutic effect of naloxone
(c) Diarrhea with rhinorrhea
(d) High anion gap metabolic acidosis

775. MEN1 most common is:

(a) Parathyroid hyperplasia
(b) Pheochromocytoma
(c) Enteropancreatic tumour

776. Acute hepatitis B A/E:

(a) Ig G anti HBcAg (b) HbsAg positive
(c) Anti HbsAg negative (d) Anti HbeAg negative

777. Gastric acid secretion increases by A/E:

(a) PG (b) Histamine
(c) Muscarianic (d) Gastrin

778. Gastric ulcer least common in:
(a) Chronic COPD (b) Cushing syndrome
(c) CRF (d) Systemic mastocytosis

779. H. pylori A/E:
(a) Gastritis (b) Gastric ulcer
(c) Curling ulcer (d) Gastric carcinoma

780. Pseudo – Cushing syndrome A/E:
(a) Alcoholism (b) Obesity
(c) Starvation (d) Diabetes

781. Cushing syndrome A/E:
(a) Bruising (b) Hypotension
(c) Hirsutism (d) Obesity

782. All are side effects of mitoxantrone *except:*
(a) Amenorrhoea (b) Cardiomyopathy
(c) Malignancy (d) ARF

783. Which is not a complication of dialysis?
(a) Fever (b) Hyperglycemia
(c) Cramps (d) Aluminium toxicity

784. CPIS:
(a) Fever (b) Leucocytosis
(c) ↓ O_2 saturation (d) Altered sensorium

785. Most common cause of hypercalcemia:
(a) Parathyroid hyperplasia
(b) Malignancy
(c) Iatrogenic
(d) Milk alkali syndrome

786. Zenker's diverticulum:
(a) Halitosis (b) Lung abscess
(c) Mid oesophagus (d) Dysphagia

787. Achalasia symptoms A/E:
(a) GERD (b) Dysphagia
(c) Chest pain (d) Weight loss

788. SIRS A/E:
(a) Tachypnea (b) Hypothermia
(c) Bradycardia (d) Leucocytosis

789. Most common indication for lung transplant:
(a) COPD (b) IPF
(c) Pulmonary HTN (d) Cystic fibrosis

790. Familial hypocalcemic hypocalciuria:
(a) AD (b) AR
(c) X-dominant (d) X-recessive

791. Gene associated with hypophosphatemic rickets:
(a) PHEX (b) FGF-23

792. Exenatide A/E:
(a) GLP-1 analogue
(b) Weight gain
(c) Pancreatitis
(d) Delays gastric emptying

793. Fecal route of excretion:
(a) Vildagliptan (b) Saxagliptan
(c) Linagliptan

794. Safe in renal failure:
(a) Vildagliptan (b) Saxagliptan
(c) Linagliptan

795. Bloody diarrhoea A/E:
(a) Entamoeba (b) Cryptosporidium
(c) Shigella (d) C. jejuni

796. Automatism seen in:
(a) Partialis continua
(b) Absence of seizures
(c) Myoclonus
(d) Mesial temporal lobe epilepsy

797. Hypokalemic periodic paralysis A/E:
(a) Provoked by high Na diet
(b) Calcium channelopathy
(c) Hypothermia worsen myotonia
(d) Na mutation

798. Eculizumab act on which complement?
(a) C3 (b) C5
(c) C8

799. Phenylketonuria, diet prescribed:
(a) High phenylalanine diet
(b) Low phenylalanine and high tyrosine diet
(c) Low phenylalanine diet
(d) Low tyrosine diet

800. Cognitive dysfunction with typical EEG with multiple type seizures:
(a) Lennou x-Gestaut syndrome
(b) Upshaw Shulmann syndrome
(c) Shiender

801. WADA test:
(a) CNS (b) CVS
(c) GIT

802. Polycythemia vera – enzyme involved:
(a) Pyruvate dehydrogenase
(b) Tyrosine kinase
(c) Co-Q
(d) None of the above

803. Loss of consciousness without loss of muscle tone:
(a) Absence seizure (b) Tonic clonic seizure
(c) Myoclonic epilepsy

804. Hemolytic anemia A/E:
(a) ↑ haptoglobin (b) Reticulocytosis

805. Hartnup disease due to deficiency:
(a) Histidine (b) Neutral aminoacids
(c) Methionine (d) Carnitine

806. Evan's syndrome:
(a) Thrombocytopenia (b) Lymphadenopathy
(c) Splenomegaly

807. Anorexia nervosa versus Bulimia nervosa A/E:
(a) Binge eating (b) Weight loss
(c) Induced vomiting (d) Electrolyte imbalance

808. Earliest change in DM-2:
(a) Hyperfiltration (b) Proteinuria
(c) Hypertension

809. Vitamin D intoxication measures:
(a) 1,25- OH_2 D3
(b) 1,25 – OH_2 vitamin D2
(c) 25- OH vitamin D

810. X-linked SMA:
(a) Bulbospinal SMA (b) SMA-I
(c) SMA-II (d) SMA-III

811. Low complement found in:
(a) HSP
(b) IgA
(c) Wegener's granulomatosis
(d) MPGN

812. PSGN treatment A/E:
(a) Antibiotic for streptococcus
(b) Anti-hypertensives
(c) Immunosuppressant
(d) 1-3 weeks after pharyngitis

813. Scorpion sting DOC:
(a) Prazocin (b) Dexazocin
(c) Diazepam (d) Anti-snake venom

814. Broadbent's sign see in:
(a) CCP (b) Cardiac tamponade
(c) RCMP

815. Rule of 'ten' seen in:
(a) Pheochromocytoma
(b) Wilm's tumour
(c) Nephroblastoma

816. Most common brain herniation seen in:
(a) Transtentorial (b) Transfalcine
(c) None of the above

817. Acute kidney injury markers A/E:
(a) Cystatin-C (b) N-GAL
(c) KIM-1 (d) α 2-macroglobulin

818. ADPKD associated with A/E:
(a) Splenic cyst (b) Saccular aneurysm
(c) Colonic diverticulum (d) All of the above

819. New vessels in tumour without endothelium called:
(a) Neovascularisation (b) Oncovasculogenesis
(c) None of the above

820. Tumour lysis syndrome A/E:
(a) Hypercalcemia (b) Hyperphosphatemia

821. Not a cause of reversible CMP:
(a) Selenium (b) Hypercalcemia
(c) Hypophosphatemia (d) Thiamine deficiency

822. Fever with peripheral eruption:
(a) Rocky mountain spotted fever
(b) Epidemic typhus
(c) Rubella
(d) Herpes virus

823. Vesicular eruption A/E:
(a) HSV
(b) VZV
(c) Pseudomonas ↑ hot tub eruption
(d) Scarlet fever folliculitis

824. Blood vessel in stomach just under mucosa cover:
(a) Dilefauy's lesion
(b) Mallory Weiss's syndrome

825. Vinyl chloride causes cancer:
(a) Bladder Ca (b) Angiosarcoma liver
(c) Hepatoma

826. BOAA causes:
(a) Lathyrism (b) Epidemic dropsy

827. Tropical spastic paraplegia caused by:
(a) HTLV-I (b) HTLV-II
(c) Both of the above (d) None of the above

828. Transcortical motor aphasia, what is maintained?
(a) Repetition (b) Fluency
(c) Naming (d) None of the above

829. Liddle's syndrome channel mutation:
(a) Na channel (b) Na-K-2Cl

830. Hypothyroid A/E:
(a) Decreased CO
(b) Increased peripheral oxygen consumption
(c) Increased PVR
(d) Normal pulmonary artery pressure

831. Urinary retention associated with:
(a) Propafenone (b) Disopyramide
(c) Amiodarone (d) Procainamide

832. Most common source of primary for cardiac mets:
(a) Lung (b) Breast
(c) Stomach (d) Thyroid

833. Target of SPRINT trial:
(a) SBP <120 (b) SBP <140
(c) DBP <85 (d) DBP <90

834. Uric acid:
(a) Sudden weight loss can increase
(b) Has antioxidant property
(c) Losartan increases uric acid level
(d) Radiocontrast uricosuric

835. Histoplasmosis, Amp–B, patient experiencing weakness and palpitations, ECG-frequent VPC's cause:
(a) Renal tubular dysfunction
(b) Cardiac muscle damage

836. Anion gap true all *except:*
(a) ↑ in AG n uremia
(b) Hypoalbuminemia ↓ AG
(c) Addison disease ↓ AG
(d) Na, Cl, HCO_3, K used for anion gap

837. Non-parametric tests *except:*
(a) Mann-Whitney U test
(b) ANOVA test
(c) Spearman's coefficient
(d) Pearson's coefficient

838. Cosynactrin assay used in:
(a) Pituitary apoplexy
(b) Adrenocortical reserve
(c) Hypogonadism
(d) 11- hydroxylase deficiency

839. Erythema nodosum in A/E:
(a) Sarcoidosis (b) Pregnancy
(c) I.E. (d) ITP

840. Oral hairy leukoplakia DOC:
(a) Podophyllin
(b) Ketokonazole
(c) Doxycycline

841. Bromcriptine in A/E:
(a) Type 2 DM
(b) NMS
(c) Peripartum CMP
(d) Idiopathic pulmonary fibrosis

842. NMS characterized by:
(a) Lead pipe rigidity

843. VEGF inhibitor in A/E:
(a) Retinoblastoma
(b) Colon CA
(c) Hemangioblastoma

844. Drug useful for prevention of colonic CA:
(a) Lycopene (b) α-tocopherol
(c) High dose celecoxib (d) Isoretinoin

845. Ca 19-9 increased in:

(a) Ovarian CA (b) Choriocarcinoma
(c) Colonic CA (d) Hepatoma

846. Decreased expression of VEGF causes:

(a) Pulmonary fibrosis (b) Emphysema
(c) Cystic fibrosis

847. Largest diameter Aβ fibre responds to:

(a) Crude touch (b) Pain
(c) Vibration (d) Fine touch

848. Painful stimuli abolished by damage to:

(a) $A\delta + C$ (b) $A\beta + \theta$
(c) $A\beta + C$

849. Clinical finding in congenital MS:

(a) Very loud S1
(b) Absence of OS
(c) Absence of diastolic murmur
(d) LA hypoplasia

850. MELAS is associated with:

(a) Seizure disorder (b) Dementia
(c) Parkinsonism

851. Familial hemiplegic migraine true:

(a) Hemiplegia with aura
(b) Hemiplegia after migraine

852. Kerley B line due to:

(a) Cephalization (b) Straight line
(c) Costophrenic angles

853. Osteosclerosis is a prominent finding in:

(a) Paget's disease

854. Tinel's sign diagnostic in:

(a) Carpal tunnel syndrome
(b) MND

855. Imatinib besides CML is useful in:

(a) Hairy cell leukaemia
(b) Lymphoma
(c) Glioblastoma
(d) Multiple myeloma

856. Lyme's disease A/E:

(a) Tick borne
(b) Caused by T. cruzi
(c) Treated by antibiotic

857. Leptospirosis TOC:

(a) Intravenous penicillin
(b) Vancomycin
(c) Metronidazole
(d) Imipenem

858. DOC for microsporidium:

(a) I/V ketoconazole (b) Metronidazole
(c) Albendazole (d) Cotrimoxazole

859. Viral hemorrhagic fever DOC:

(a) Ribavirin (b) Adenavir
(c) Xidovudine (d) Acyclovir

860. Retrobulbar hemorrhage can present as A/E:

(a) Dilated pupil (b) Proptosis
(c) Optic atrophy (d) Vision loss

861. Paraphasia is:

(a) Inability to find correct word
(b) Inability to comprehend word
(c) Inability to comprehend written language

862. Argyll Robertson pupil in:

(a) Neurosyphilis (b) Lead poisoning
(c) Weber syndrome

863. Allelic heterogenecity:

(a) Non dysjunction of chromosome
(b) One allele involved
(c) Two alleles involved
(d) Heterogenous phenotypic expression

864. Genomic imprinting:

(a) Mosaicism
(b) Selective expression of parental origin

865. AL amyloidosis TOC:

(a) Melphalan + prednisolone
(b) Vincristine + prednisolone
(c) High dose of vit OC + Mtx
(d) Adriamycin

866. Pancreatic divisum:

(a) Ventral and dorsal duct fusion absent
(b) Head of pancreas double
(c) Anomalous drainage of duct

867. Systolic murmur of TOF depends on:
(a) VSD (b) PS
(c) Aorta

868. Gordon syndrome:
(a) Hypokalemic periodic paralysis
(b) Increased Cl absorption
(c) Increased Mg absorption
(d) Decreased absorption of K

869. Increased renin A/E:
(a) Conn's syndrome (b) Cushing's syndrome
(c) Cirrhosis (d) Accelerated HTN

870. Fecal nitrogen excretion:
(a) Kwashiokar
(b) Patient nutritional status
(c) Exocrine function of pancreas
(d) Intestinal amyloidosis

871. Hyporenin hypoaldosteronism:
(a) Hypernatremia (b) Hypokalemia
(c) Hyperkalemia (d) Hypochloridemia

872. Walled of necrosis:
(a) Necrotizing fasciitis
(b) Pancreatic necrosis
(c) Wegener's granulomatosis

873. ANCA + small vessel vasculitis:
(a) Churg strauss syndrome
(b) Takayasu arteritis
(c) Microscopic polyangiitis
(d) Wegener's granuomatosis

874. 10 kg weight loss causes:
(a) Decrease SBP by 40 mm Hg
(b) Decrease SBP by 20 mm Hg
(c) Decrease DBP by 20 mm Hg
(d) Decrease DBP by 10 mm Hg

875. Drug induced lupus:
(a) Sulfasalazine (b) TNF alpha inhibitor
(c) Leflunamide (d) Ankarin

876. Desquamative interstitial pneumonitis:
(a) Cigarette smoking (b) ILD

877. Sibogluconate toxicity causes:
(a) Hypocalcemia (b) Hyperglycemia
(c) SIADH (d) Hypothyroid

878. PEP prophylaxis TOC:
(a) Lamivudine (b) Ritonavir
(c) Tinofovir (d) Abacavir

879. Insulin resistant by:
(a) Ritonavir (b) Zidovudine
(c) Nevirapine

880. Fractional excretion of sodium < 1, diagnosis:
(a) Prerenal (b) ATN
(c) RPGN

881. Bleomycin causes:
(a) CMP (b) HTN
(c) Pericarditis (d) Myocardial infarct

882. Autoimmune disease mechanisms:
(a) Sequestration of superantigen
(b) Increased expression of superantigen
(c) Change in autoantigen

883. Ataxia telangiectasia caused by:
(a) Defect in DNA repair
(b) Deletion of DNA

884. Optic ataxia:
(a) Infarct between MCA and PCA
(b) Occipital artery involvement
(c) Vertebral artery thrombus

885. Muscle bridging seen in:
(a) LAD (b) RCA
(c) LCx

886. HNF1 α mutation
(a) MODY 1 (b) Type 2 DM
(c) Gestational DM

887. Glycemia index:
(a) Increase in blood glucose at 2 hours after 50 g of glucose
(b) Increase in blood glucose at 2 hours after 75 g of glucose
(c) Increase in blood glucose at 1 hour after 75 g of glucose

888. Erythema nodosum leprosum:
(a) Type I reaction

(b) Immune complex mediated
(c) Delayed hypersensitivity
(d) Cell mediated

889. Pulmonary embolism diagnostic test:
(a) Increased d–dimer (b) Increased FDP
(c) Increased factor IX (d) Increased INR

890. Dubin Johnson syndrome:
(a) Mutation in TATA-UDP
(b) Mutation in 5′ promoter–UDP
(c) Mutation in MDR transporter
(d) Mutation in UDP glucornyl transferase

891. Pig is reservoir in:
(a) Japanese B encephalitis
(b) SARS

892. Stochastic effects:
(a) Radiation induced leukaemia
(b) Lymphoma

893. S2 paradoxical split A/E:
(a) LBBB
(b) Paced rhythm
(c) Right accessory pathway
(d) PDA

894. Middle systolic click A/E:
(a) AS (b) PS
(c) MVP (d) Atrial septal aneurysm

895. Fontan's procedure:
(a) Palliative operation in CHD
(b) Closed mitral valvotomy

896. Sirolimus MOA:
(a) Cytosolic inhibition of growth factors
(b) Blocks attachment of VCAM
(c) Antagonizes the effect of PDGF
(d) Blocks endothelial proliferation

897. SIADH:
(a) Iso-osmolar hyponatremia
(b) Hypoosmolar
(c) Hyperosmolar
(d) Isotonic

898. Ebstein's anomaly:
(a) Atrialized right ventricle
(b) Atrialized left ventricle
(c) PS

899. AVNRT:
(a) Inverted p wave (b) Bifid p wave
(c) p buried in QRS (d) Tall p wave

900. LEMS:
(a) Demyelinating
(b) Autoimmune
(c) Immune complex disease
(d) Axonal degeneration

901. Algid malaria:
(a) Encephalopathy (b) Hepatic involvement
(c) Pulmonary edema (d) Shock

902. Myocarditis A/E:
(a) Coksackie (b) Diphtheria
(c) Syphilis (d) Lyme's disease

903. Folic acid deficiency prevent:
(a) Anencephaly
(b) Microcytic hypochromic anemia
(c) Achondroplasia

904. DOC of psoriasis:
(a) Infliximab (b) Rituximab
(c) Basiliximab (d) Efalizumab

905. Macrocytic anemia:
(a) Hypothyroidism
(b) Hyperthyroidism
(c) Hyperparathyroidism
(d) Addison's disease

906. Sleep apnea most common associated with:
(a) Hypothyroidism (b) Hypoparathyroidism
(c) Adrenal insufficiency

907. Pseudotumour cerebri:
(a) Idiopathic intracranial HTN

908. HIT patients, what to be given?
(a) Bivalirudin

909. Hoover's sign:
(a) Paradoxical diaphragmatic movement
(b) Inward movement of rib cage

910. Co-prescription in acute pulmonary edema:
(a) Intravenous GTN (b) Intravenous digitalis

911. Pulsus parvus et tardus:
(a) AS (b) MS
(c) MR (d) HOCM

912. Opening snap seen in:
(a) AS (b) TS
(c) PS (d) Atrial septal aneurysm

913. Polmyalgia rheumatic:
(a) High ESR (b) High hs- CRP
(c) High CK

914. Culture negative endocarditis (afebrile):
(a) T. whippelli (b) Bartonella
(c) Coxiella

915. Familial breast CA gene:
(a) BRCA 2

916. Nitrate MOA:
(a) Decrease preload and afterload
(b) Decrease afterload

917. Ammonium chloride (acid loading test) done in:
(a) RTA
(b) Metabolic acidosis
(c) Metabolic alkalosis
(d) Respiratory acidosis

918. Seligman's disease:
(a) Presents with diarrhoea and weight loss
(b) Respond to chemotherapy and Ab
(c) Lymphadenopathy
(d) Light chains in blood and urine

919. Rolfing related to:
(a) Papez circuit
(b) New drug in depression
(c) None of the above
(d) Alternative medicine

920. Sequoiosis:
(a) Fertilizers (b) Red wood
(c) Saw dust (d) Cork

921. Ataxia telangiectasia:
(a) Low IgA
(b) Abnormal IgA
(c) High IgG
(d) Low IgM

922. Palinopia:
(a) Balint syndrome
(b) Foster-Kennedy syndrome
(c) Down syndrome
(d) Goldenhar syndrome

923. Myotonia dystrophica - chromosome:
(a) 19 (b) 20
(c) 21 (d) 12

924. Caisson's disease A/E:
(a) Paraplegia (b) Myonecrosis
(c) Joints pain (d) Lymphedema

925. Dent's disease A/E:
(a) Medullary Ca
(b) AR
(c) Proteinuria
(d) Affect proximal renal tubules

926. Xanthogranulomatosis pyelonephritis:
(a) Proteus (b) Klebsiella
(c) TB (d) Pseudomonas

927. PSVT with asthma:
(a) Adenosine (b) Verapamil
(c) Esmolol (d) Amiodarone

928. MELD score A/E:
(a) PT/INR
(b) Serum protein
(c) S. creatinine
(d) S. bilirubin

929. CJD:
(a) 12% familial
(b) ↑ Protein in CSF
(c) Periodic muscle spikes
(d) May cause cortical blindness

930. Pellagra treatment and duration (niacin):
(a) 100-200 mg TID × 5 days
(b) 100-200 mg OD × 5 days
(c) 100-200 mg TID × 1 month
(d) 10-20 mg TID × 5 days

931. Which vitamin does not cause toxicity?
(a) B_5 (b) B_6
(c) B_3 (d) Vit C

932. Sarcoidosis least common site:
(a) Lung (b) Spleen
(c) Heart (d) Brain

933. Prolactin t ½:
(a) 20 min (b) 50 min
(c) 180 min (d) 120 min

934. Asymptomatic DM reliable and most convenient:
(a) HbA_1c (b) Fasting BS > 120
(c) RBS>200 (d) GTT

935. Trigeminal neuralgia A/E:
(a) Pain in gums
(b) Duration—seconds to min
(c) Objective sensory loss
(d) Ophthalmic division less involved

936. POEMS syndrome:
(a) Lymphadenopathy (b) Thrombocytopenia
(c) Type 2DM (d) Ascitis

937. SAPHO syndrome A/E:
(a) Synovitis (b) Acne
(c) Pneumonitis (d) Hyperostosis

938. Metastasis to brain least common from:
(a) Lung (b) Breast
(c) Git (d) Malignant melanoma

939. NF type-1 A/E:
(a) Tibial pseudo arthrosis
(b) AR
(c) Hydrocephalus
(d) Lisch nodules

940. Depression (major):
(a) 2 weeks (b) 4 weeks
(c) 6 weeks (d) 8 weeks

941. Prolonged fasting A/E:
(a) Gluconeogenesis (b) ↑ urine nitrogen
(c) ↑ed-lipolysis (d) None of the above

942. Thyrotoxicosis in pregnancy A/E:
(a) PTU DOC
(b) Methimazole lead to aplasia cutis
(c) Difficult to manage in 3rd trimester
(d) β blocker in emergency

943. CHARGE A/E:
(a) Coloboma (b) TOF
(c) Genital abnormality (d) Alopecia

944. Mumps A/E:
(a) Aseptic meningitis
(b) Sterility rare
(c) Fetal malformation in pregnancy
(d) None of the above

945. Aprosodia is due to lesion in:
(a) Peri sylvian (b) Frontal
(c) Occipital (d) Temporal

946. Arterial oxygen pressure:
(a) 95 ± 5 kpa (b) 40 ± 5
(c) 12.7 ± 7 (d) 5.9 ± 7

947. Most sensitive to hypoxia:
(a) Hippocampus (b) Cerebellum
(c) Pons (d) Thalamus

948. Bone marrow transplant, lung infection in 1 month:
(a) CMV (b) Toxoplasma
(c) Pneumocystis (d) Herpes

949. Class IB antiarrhythmic:
(a) Procainamide (b) Flecainide
(c) Tocainide (d) Encainide

950. Paradoxical bradycardia:
(a) PE (b) Anterior wall MI
(c) PHT (d) Sarcoidosis

951. Granulomatous lung disease A/E:
(a) Churg Strauss
(b) Sarcoidosis
(c) Pulmonary eosinophilia
(d) Wegener's granulomatosis

952. Tumour in tuberous sclerosis:
(a) Giant cell astrocytoma
(b) Medulloblastoma
(c) Meningioma

953. Most common subependymal astrocytoma:
(a) 4th ventricle
(b) Trigone of 3rd ventricle
(c) Foramen of Monro
(d) Horn of lateral ventricle

954. Insulinoma A/E:
(a) Multiple (b) 40-50 years age
(c) Asymptomatic (d) 5-15% malignant

955. Treatment of Shy-Drager syndrome:
(a) Fludrocortisone (b) Prazosin
(c) B-blocker (d) None of the above

956. Type of emphysema in a1 anti trypsin deficiency:
(a) Panacinar (b) Centriacinar
(c) Paraseptal

957. Pheochromocytoma after adrenal gland:
(a) Gland of Zuckerkandl
(b) Urinary bladder
(c) Hilum of kidney
(d) Neck

958. Guardian of genome:
(a) P 53 (b) Bcl 2
(c) BMP

959. Fever of unknown origin with neutropenia all *except:*
(a) ANC 500
(b) 5 days hospital stay–inconclusive
(c) Culture negative in 2 days
(d) Fever > 38°C on several occasion

960. Corrected platelets count not include:
(a) Body weight
(b) BSA
(c) Pre transfusion count
(d) Post transfusion count

961. Cryoprecipitate A/E:
(a) VWF
(b) F VIII
(c) Cold precipitate plasma protein
(d) Fibrinogen

962. Pseudotumour syndrome:
(a) Hyperparathyroidism
(b) Thalassemia
(c) Luekaemia
(d) Hemophilia

963. Wrong match:
(a) aPL = Venous thrombosis
(b) Homocysteinemia = both arterial and venous
(c) Antithrombin III def. = venous
(d) Protein C = venous

964. Pseudohermophrodite in female:
(a) 21 α def. (b) 17 α def.
(c) 11 β def. (d) 13 β def.

965. Liddle syndrome:
(a) AR (b) HTN
(c) Metabolic alkalosis (d) ↑ renin

966. Not corrected by hemodialysis:
(a) Hyperkalemia (b) Pericarditis
(c) Asterixis (d) Leucocytopenia

967. Digoxin not seen:
(a) ST elevation (b) PR prolongation
(c) QT ↓sed (d) T ↓ inversion

968. Dangerous dehydration:
(a) Hyponatremia (b) Hypernatremia
(c) Non diarrhoeal (d) Isonatremia

969. Takatsubo CMP true:
(a) Young male (b) Stress induced
(c) ↑ Catecholamines (d) Acute chest pain

970. Post traumatic cardiac injury:
(a) Recurrence is rare
(b) Can present after 1 month
(c) Fibrous pericarditis

971. Primary myocardial involvement:
(a) FA
(b) Hemochromocytosis
(c) Eosinophilic endomyocardial fibrosis
(d) SLE

972. Fat distribution in HIV:
(a) Chick (b) Abdomen
(c) Temple (d) Hip

973. False channelopathies:
(a) AD
(b) Hyperkalemic to due to Na^+ channel
(c) Pseudomyotonia ↓ with cold
(d) Episodic weakness in Anderson's syndrome

974. Wells scoring used in:
(a) Pulmonary embolism (b) Ascitis
(c) Pleural effusion (d) Cirrhosis

975. **GOLD COPD FEV1/ FVC < 70%, FEV1< 50%:**
(a) Stage I (b) Stage II
(c) Stage III (d) Stage IV

976. **D-xylose test:**
(a) Chronic pancreatitis (b) Ileal disease
(c) Celiac (d) All of the above

977. **Roma II criteria:**
(a) Pain relieved after defecation
(b) Altered frequency
(c) Altered form/consistency
(d) >12 weeks in a year

978. **Ulcerative colitis:**
(a) ANCA +ve (b) Continuous disease
(c) Massive bleeding (d) Antibiotic treatment

979. **GBS A/E:**
(a) Areflexia (b) > 6 weeks
(c) 2 or more limb involvement

980. **CT scan A/E:**
(a) Spine CT- Bony lesion
(b) S. creat= 1 mg/dl ↑ in 48 hours
(c) 3-5 Gray exposure in CT
(d) Sensitive to iodine than to gadolinium

981. **Acquired loss of pituitary hormones:**
(a) TSH (b) LH-FSH
(c) ACTH (d) LH

982. **GH secretion A/E:**
(a) Pulsatile secretion in night
(b) Protein ↑ GH
(c) Depends on nutritional state
(d) Secretion from anterior pituitary

983. **Small vessel stroke with dementia:**
(a) CADASIL (b) Moya Moya
(c) Binswanger

984. **Not seen in Steel Richardson syndrome:**
(a) Seizures (b) Dementia
(c) PSP (d) Ataxia

985. **Exercise induced asthma A/E:**
(a) Exercise running > walking
(b) Long term sequelae
(c) No airway hyperresponsiveness

986. **Proximal + distal weakness/handgrip:**
(a) IBM (b) PM
(c) DM

987. **Oseltamavir:**
(a) 50 mg BD (b) 50 mg TDS
(c) 75 mg BD (d) 7 mg TDS

988. **Most common tumour of lung:**
(a) SCLC (b) LCLC
(c) Bronchoalveolar (d) Carcinoid

989. **Wrong in antiepileptic drug:**
(a) Saturation kinetics in phenytoin
(b) Skin reaction in lamotrigine
(c) Valproate ↓es t ½ of lamotrigine
(d) Valproate cause reversible bone marrow toxicity

990. **Wallenberg syndrome cranial nerve A/E:**
(a) IX (b) X
(c) XI (d) XII

991. **Metabolic syndrome A/E:**
(a) ↑ TG (b) ↑ LDL
(c) HTN (d) ↑ waist circumference

992. **Incidental adrenal mass A/E:**
(a) > 90% asymptomatic
(b) Size > 4 × 6 cm ↑ risk of Ca
(c) FNAC can differentiate between benign and malignant

993. **HCC–staging:**
(a) Bilirubin (b) Albumin
(c) SGOT/SGPT (d) Ascitis

994. **Hyperventilation causes:**
(a) ↑ed resistance to PBF
(b) ↓ed blood flow to brain
(c) ↓ PH
(d) Stimulate chemoreceptors

995. **SIRS:**
(a) > 38 °C (b) < 36 °C
(c) HR > 90 (d) BP < 100/60

996. All increases effect of simvastatin and rosvastatin *except:*

(a) Cyclosporine (b) Verapamil
(c) Diltiazem (d) Sotalol

997. Hyperparathyroidism A/E:

(a) Increased QT (b) Normal LV function
(c) HTN (d) None of the above

998. Rat bite:

(a) Cleaning
(b) Cleaning +TT +antibiotics
(c) Cleaning + TT+ antibiotics + Anti Rabies Vaccine
(d) Cleaning + TT+antibiotics + Anti Rabies Vaccine + serum

999. Clindamycin in:

(a) Babesiosis (b) Giardiasis
(c) Cryptosporoidosis (d) Trypanosomiasis

1000. Nephropathy in malaria:

(a) P. Malariae (b) P. Ovale
(c) P. Falciparum (d) P. Vivax

1001. Massive splenomegaly A/E:

(a) Sickle cell anemia (b) Sarcoidosis
(c) Hairy cell leukemia (d) CML

1002. Friedreich's ataxia A/E:

(a) Most common inherited ataxia
(b) Associated with musculoskeletal deformity
(c) < 50% cardiac involvement
(d) Females better prognosis

1003. GVHD not seen in:

(a) Autologous Stem Cell Transplantation
(b) Blood transfusion
(c) Allogenic Stem Cell Transplantation
(d) Cord blood SCT

1004. Channelopathies false:

(a) Episodic Ataxia-2 = Ca^{++}
(b) Episodic Ataxia-1 = Na^{+}
(c) Congenital myotonia– Cl
(d) Hypokalemic periodic paralysis =Na^{+}

1005. Stored blood after 48 hours ↓ in A/E:

(a) Factor-V (b) Factor-VII
(c) WBC (d) Platelets

1006. Rheumatoid arthritis most common involvement (axial)

(a) Lumbar (b) Upper Cervical
(c) Lower cervical (d) Thoracic

1007. Drug not used in rheumatoid arthritis:

(a) HCQ's (b) Adriamycin
(c) Methotrexate (d) Rituximab

1008. Side effect of rituximab in SLE:

(a) Aseptic meningitis
(b) Mucormycosis
(c) Progressive multifocal leucoencephalopathy
(d) Vasculitis

1009. Essential cryoglobulinemia vasculitis is:

(a) Large vessels (b) Medium vessels
(c) Small vessels (d) Aneurysm

1010. Antibodies in celiac disease A/E:

(a) Antigluten (b) Anti TTG
(c) Antigliadin (d) Antiendomysin

1011. Ifosfamide toxicity treatment:

(a) Methylene blue (b) Penicillin
(c) Calcium (d) Magnesium

1012. QT prolongation A/E:

(a) Digitalis toxicity (b) TCA (antidepressant)
(c) CVA (d) Mg^{+2}

1013. Digoxin toxicity in A/E:

(a) Hypocalcemia
(b) Coadminister of propafenone
(c) Hypomagnesemia

1014. Tumor lysis syndrome A/E:

(a) Hypocalcemia
(b) Hypercalcemia
(c) Hyperphosphatemia
(d) Hyperkalemia

40-year-old female with fever, Hb = 8 g%, temp= 103°F, RR=40, TLC=20000, HR=110/min, BP=80/60, Platelet count=60000, pH=7.2, PCO_2=20, PO_2=60, HCO_3=10

1015. Investigation of choice:

(a) Blood culture (b) Urine culture
(c) USG (d) CT chest

1016. ABG diagnosis:
(a) Metabolic alkalosis (b) Metabolic acidosis
(c) Respiratory acidosis (d) Respiratory alkalosis

1017. Initial treatment to be given:
(a) Intravenous saline (b) Dopamine
(c) Norepinephrine (d) 5% Dextrose

1018. Treatment all *except:*
(a) Activated Protein C
(b) PCM
(c) Antibiotics
(d) Insulin to keep RBS – 80 mg%

1019. Prognostic marker for sepsis:
(a) GH (b) Prolactin
(c) Thyroxine (d) Procalcitonin

1020. HBc Ag-ve, HBV DNA +ve:
(a) Core/precore mutant
(b) Easily Rx
(c) Not exist
(d) Non progressive

1021. Cord blood stem cell:
(a) ↓ Telomere length (b) ↓ Clonigenecity
(c) ↓ Number of cells (nucleated)

1022. Marker of hematopoeitic stem cell:
(a) CD 34^+/CD38^+ (b) CD 34^+/CD 138^+
(c) CD 34^+/CD 38^- (d) CD 34^+/CD 138^-

1023. MRI T1 image - hyperintensity:
(a) CSF (b) Edema
(c) Fat (d) Brain

1024. Prion disease A/E:
(a) Kuru (b) CJD
(c) GSS (d) Exotic encephalopathy

1025. Whipple's disease A/E:
(a) Caused by T. whippeli
(b) Dementia late mainfestation
(c) Cotrimoxazole for 14 days
(d) Migratory arthropathy

1026. Echo in cardiac tamponade:
(a) LA collapse (b) LV collapse
(c) RV dilated (d) IVC dilated

1027. Chikungunya fever A/E:
(a) Abrupt onset
(b) Aedes mosquito
(c) Maculopapular rash common
(d) Multiply in RBC

1028. Ig D:
(a) Marker of B cell maturity
(b) Bind to basophil
(c) Bind to lymphocyte
(d) Bind to macrophage

1029. Functional evaluation of B cell assessed by:
(a) Ig G subclass evaluation
(b) Growth response to mitogen
(c) Delayed hypersensitivity reaction
(d) Cytokine assay

1030. ATN:
(a) Red cell casts (b) Muddy brown casts
(c) Eosinophilia (d) Hyaline cast

1031. Atheroembolism true:
(a) Eosinophilia
(b) Red cell cast in urine
(c) Massive proteinuria
(d) History of pulmonary embolism

1032. Myalgia + eosinophilia + scleroderma rash
(a) L-tryptophan ingestion
(b) Nicotine
(c) Rifampicin

1033. IPPV A/E:
(a) ↓ Afterload (b) ↑ Afterload
(c) ↑ Preload (d) ↓ Work of ventilation

1034. Virchow's triad A/E:
(a) Epithelial injury
(b) ↓ Blood flow
(c) Endothelial injury
(d) Mismatch between procoagulant and anticoagulants

1035. Lecithin acyl transferase deficiency (LCAT) deficiency nephropathy:
(a) MCD (b) FSGS
(c) MPGN (d) Membranous GN

1036. Calciphylaxis:
(a) Chronic renal failure
(b) Multiple myeloma
(c) Angioneurotic edema
(d) Anaphylaxis

1037. P. carini pneumonia chest X-ray picture:
(a) Lung abscess
(b) Pleural effusion
(c) Midzone infiltrations
(d) Pneumothorax

1038. 30 years old female with otitis media, lung cavitation, renal involvement investigation:
(a) ANA (b) c-ANCA
(c) ASO (d) Complement

1039. Mesial temporal lobe epilepsy A/E:
(a) Most common cause of partial seizures
(b) Good response to surgery
(c) Good response to anticonvulsants
(d) MRI-Hippocampal sclerosis

1040. Metabolic encephalopathy A/E:
(a) Bilateral plantars extensors
(b) Multifocal myoclonus
(c) Focal neurodeficit
(d) Fluctuating sensorium

1041. Truncal growth mediated by:
(a) GH (b) IGF-1
(c) Estrogen (d) 1-25 OH–vitamin D

1042. Ghrelin by:
(a) Stomach (b) Intestinal L-cells
(c) Pituitary (d) Islet cells

1043. Heat stroke A/E:
(a) DIC (b) Panhypopituitarism
(c) Low platelet count (d) Rhabdomyolysis

1044. Hyperthermia caused by:
(a) Anticholinergic drugs
(b) Nicotine withdrawal
(c) Opioid withdrawal
(d) Ciprofloxacin administration

1045. TPN-can be given by peripheral vein:
(a) 20% Lipids
(b) 50% Dextrose water + 20% lipids
(c) 20% Proteins
(d) 50% Dextrose water

1046. Peripartum cardiomyopathy A/E:
(a) Very high mortality
(b) Common in Multiparous
(c) Last trimester to 6 months postpartum
(d) Recurrence in subsequent pregnancies

1047. Hirsutism caused by:
(a) Vincristine (b) α- methyl dopa
(c) Cyclosporine (d) Hydroxyurea

1048. Drug contraindicated in pregnancy:
(a) Hydralazine (b) Losartan
(c) Flecainide (d) Digoxin

1049. Metabolic syndrome A/E:
(a) Abdominal obesity (b) ↑ LDL
(c) ↑ FBS (d) ↑ TG

1050. Drug used in treatment of orthostatic hypotension:
(a) Fludrocortisone (b) Clonidine
(c) Esmolol (d) Phenylephrine

1051. Prebiotic A/E:
(a) Pectin (b) Inulin
(c) Lactobacillus (d) Raffinose

1052. Virus causing malignancy A/E:
(a) H. pylori (b) Hepatitis-G virus
(c) Papilloma virus (d) EBV

1053. Specificity:
(a) True positive (b) True negative
(c) False positive (d) False negative

1054. Most effective treatment in COPD to change course of disease:
(a) Smoking cessation
(b) Inhaled steroids
(c) Inhaled beta-agonists
(d) Oxygen therapy

1055. D-Dimer true:
(a) High negative predictive value
(b) Highly specific
(c) Tube agglutination
(d) Positive after 48 hours

1056. Thrombocytopenia in chronic liver disease A/E:
(a) Hepatorenal syndrome
(b) DIC

(c) Hypersplenism
(d) Thrombopoietin deficiency

1057. Hormone acting through Janus kinase pathway
(a) GH (b) TSH
(c) ACTH (d) PTH

1058. CVP measurement done in:
(a) Mid expiration (b) End expiration
(c) Mid inspiratory (d) End inspiratory

1059. Glucocorticoid remediable HTN:
(a) Strong family history
(b) ↑ Renin angiotensin system
(c) Onset in middle age
(d) ↑ Aldosterone in upright position

1060. Most specific marker of iron deficiency anemia:
(a) ↓ Serum ferritin
(b) ↓ Serum iron
(c) ↓ MCV
(d) Microcytic hypochromic picture on PBF

1061. Most important for CPR:
(a) Defibrillation
(b) ET intubation
(c) Intravenous adrenaline
(d) Intravenous soda bicarb

1062. Not an indicator of myocardial O_2 demand supply:
(a) Cardiac output
(b) SVO_2
(c) Serum lactate (arterial)
(d) O_2 consumption measurement

1063. Incretins A/E:
(a) GIP inhibit gastric emptying
(b) GIP secreted by K-cells from proximal gut
(c) GIP-1 secreted by L–cells from distal gut
(d) GLP levels ↑↑ in DM

1064. Intrathecal vincristine used in:
(a) Primary CNS lymphoma
(b) AML
(c) ALL
(d) Is fatal

1065. Fetal alcohol syndrome A/E:
(a) PS (b) PR
(c) PDA (d) VSD

1066. Acquired hemophilia (Factor VIII) positive investigation is:
(a) PT (b) INR
(c) APTT (d) Thrombin time

1067. Blindness, papillary reflex present, denies blindness:
(a) Bilateral Posterior Cerebral Artery thrombosis
(b) Bilateral Posterior Inferior Cerebeller Artery thrombosis
(c) Hysteria
(d) Basilar artery embolism

1068. 30 years postpartum female paraparesis with generalised seizures and headache:
(a) Cortical venous thrombosis
(b) Acute meningitis
(c) ADEM
(d) LGB syndrome

1069. Most common cause of adrenal insufficiency in India:
(a) Tuberculosis
(b) Kala azar
(c) Autoimmune
(d) 21-α hydroxylase deficiency

1070. Best method for control of infection:
(a) Hand washing (b) Isolation
(c) Bleaching (d) Fumigation

1071. BP in diabetic (target BP):
(a) 130/85 mm Hg (b) 120/80 mm Hg
(c) 130/80 mm Hg (d) 120/85 mm Hg

1072. Endotoxin A/E:
(a) Gram positive bacteria produces it
(b) Gram negative bacteria produces it
(c) Needed for bacteria survival
(d) Is a lipopolysaccharide

1073. Drug of choice in aortic dissection:
(a) Esmolol (b) NTG
(c) Nitroprusside (d) CCB

1074. Hematopoietic growth factors are:
(a) Glycoprotein (b) Carboprotein
(c) Carbohydrates (d) Protein

1075. Glucocorticoid deficiency:
(a) Normovolumic hyponatremia
(b) Hypovolumic hyponatremia
(c) Euvolumic hypernatremia
(d) Hypervolumic hyponatremia

1076. Metal toxicity A/E:
(a) Hg–CAD
(b) Pb–CHB
(c) Cabalt–DCM
(d) Arsenic–pericardial effusion

1077. HIV transmission least is:
(a) Semen (b) Blood
(c) Tears (d) Pleural fluid

1078. Bayes theorem A/E:
(a) Disease prevalence
(b) Likelihood ratio
(c) Probability of disease
(d) Predictive valve of test

1079. Type - D personality disorder:
(a) Competitive + aggressive
(b) ↓ Cardiovascular disease prevalence
(c) Social isolation
(d) ↓ Tension

1080. Which is seen in left pneumothorax?
(a) T wave inversion (b) Height of R wave ↓ed
(c) Left axis deviation (d) ST ↑

1081. Recovery from anesthesia what is seen?
(a) Hypotension and bradycardia
(b) Hypotension and hypercoagulability
(c) Hypertension and tachycardia
(d) Bradycardia and hypercoagulability

1082. Joint erosion seen in A/E:
(a) SLE (b) RA
(c) Psoriasis

1083. Normal anion gap metabolic acidosis:
(a) Diarrhea
(b) RTA
(c) Alcoholic ketoacidosis
(d) DKA

1084. P-ANCA sensitive and specific for:
(a) Post streptococcal GN
(b) Idiopathic crescentic GN
(c) Diffuse glomerulosclerosis
(d) Diabetic glomerulosclerosis

1085. Most common changes in kidney after septic shock:
(a) Papillary necrosis
(b) ATN
(c) Acute glomerulonephritis
(d) Cortical necrosis

1086. Sickle cell A/E:
(a) LV systolic dysfunction
(b) ↓ LV compliance
(c) Pulmonary HTN
(d) Proliferative vascular arteriopathy in systemic circulation

1087. Shock lung seen is:
(a) Diffuse alveolar damage
(b) Organizing phenomossics
(c) Usual interstitial pneumonia

1088. Lung to lung mets seen with:
(a) Adeno Ca
(b) Squamous Ca
(c) SCLC
(d) Neuroendocrine tumour

1089. Phocomelia seen with:
(a) Thalidomide (b) Dilantin
(c) Alcohol

1090. Recurrent respiratory infection seen in A/E:
(a) Kartagener's
(b) Single ventricle with PS
(c) TOF with absent pulmonary valve
(d) TOF (severe) with large MAPCA

1091. Lung volume calcification in emphysema with bulla best with:
(a) Transdiaphragmatic pr. gradient
(b) DLCO
(c) Plethysmography
(d) Helium dilution

1092. Rheos device for treatment of:
(a) Retractory HTN (b) Incessant VT
(c) Retractory HF (d) Retractory angina

1093. Calmodulin acts by:
(a) Ca^{++} dependent
(b) c AMP adenylate cyclase
(c) c GMP adenylate cyclase
(d) $Na^{+}K^{+}$ ATPase

1094. Charcot's joint A/E:
(a) DM (b) Leprosy
(c) AML (d) Syringomyelia

1095. Pseudoxanthoma elasticum A/E:
(a) Coronary artery disease
(b) PVD
(c) MVP
(d) Angioid streaks in retina
(e) All of the above

1096. Drug induced lupus by:
(a) Anti ds DNA (b) Anti histone
(c) Anti sm

1097. Primary hyperaldosteronism A/E:
(a) Low renin levels (b) Hyponatremia
(c) Metabolic acidosis (d) Hypokalemia

1098. SIADH:
(a) Small cell ca (b) Adeno ca
(c) Squamous ca (d) Mixed

1099. Gene therapy treatment in:
(a) Ischemic CMP
(b) PVD
(c) Familial hypercholesterolemia
(d) HOCM

1100. Conn's syndrome most common cause:
(a) Adrenal adenoma (b) Adrenal hyperplasia
(c) Carcinoma

1101. HLA associated DM:
(a) DM 1
(b) DM 2
(c) Pregnancy associated
(d) Malnutrition associated

1102. Addison disease A/E:
(a) Low renin (b) Weight loss
(c) Hypotension

1103. Acute hepatitis B marker:
(a) DNA polymerase (b) HBcAg
(c) IgG HBc (d) Anti HBs

1104. Portal pressure (mm Hg):
(a) 3-5 (b) 5-10
(c) 10-20 (d) 20-40

1105. Autosomal recessive:
(a) Wilson disease (b) Tuberous sclerosis
(c) Huntington disease (d) Schizophrenia

1106. Hypoglycemia seen in:
(a) Hypopituitarism (b) Hypothyroidism
(c) Acromegaly (d) Cushing's syndrome

1107. Early finding in congenital syphilis:
(a) Microcephaly (b) Interstitial keratitis
(c) Vesicular bullae over palm

1108. Salt losing nephropathy:
(a) Interstitial nephritis
(b) Amyloidosis
(c) PSGN

1109. Papillary necrosis A/E:
(a) DM (b) Salicylates
(c) PNH (d) Renal vein thrombosis

1110. HIV affects:
(a) CD 4 cells (b) CD 8 cells
(c) Macrophages

1111. AIDS defining illness A/E:
(a) CMV retinitis
(b) PCP
(c) Cryptogenic meningitis
(d) Hodgkin's lymphoma

1112. Renal pathology seen in A/E:
(a) Hyaline cast (b) Broad cast
(c) Coarse granular (d) Epithelial

1113. Pickwickian syndrome A/E:
(a) Obesity (b) Cyanosis
(c) Clubbing (d) Somnolence

1114. Refractory migraine not used:
(a) Verapamil (b) Ethosuximide
(c) Valproate (d) Topiramate

1115. Tabes dorsalis A/E:
(a) Ataxia
(b) Argyll Robertson pupil
(c) Hyperreflexia

1116. Cushing's syndrome A/E:
(a) Hypoglycemia (b) Frank psychosis
(c) Diastolic HTN (d) Hypokalemia

1117. All of the following cancers commonly metastasize to liver *except:*
(a) Breast (b) Lung
(c) Colon (d) Prostate

1118. All of the following are complications during hemodialysis *except:*
(a) Anaphylactoid reaction
(b) Fever
(c) Hyperglycemia
(d) Hypotension

1119. Kidney size may be normal in the face of CKD, in all of the following *except:*
(a) Diabetes mellitus (b) HIV nephropathy
(c) Amyloidosis (d) Sarcoidosis

1120. Which of the following is not a physiological response to hypoxia?
(a) Erythrocytosis
(b) Hyperventilation
(c) Systemic arterial vasoconstriction
(d) Increased cardiac output

1121. In the absence of prophylactic antiretroviral therapy to the mother during pregnancy, and to the fetus following birth, the probability of transmission of HIV from mother to infant/fetus in developing countries ranges from:
(a) 15-25% (b) 25-35%
(c) 40-50% (d) 60-70%

1122. Characteristics of Immune Reconstitution Syndrome in HIV include all of the following *except:*
(a) Frequently seen in the setting of tuberculosis
(b) Improvement of clinical condition following the initiation of antiretroviral therapy
(c) Common in patients starting therapy with a CD4+ T cell count under 50/ml experience a precipitous drop in viral load
(d) Can be fatal

1123. Most cases of neonatal sepsis in the community are caused by:
(a) E Coli (b) Salmonella
(c) Pseudomonas (d) Streptococcus

1124. All of the following are components of polysomnography *except:*
(a) Electrocardiography
(b) Electromyography
(c) Pulseoxymetry
(d) Arterial carbon dioxide monitoring

1125. The cutoff for a positive tuberculin skin test for close contacts of infectious cases is an area of induration:
(a) $\geq$ 5 mm (b) $\geq$ 10 mm
(c) $\geq$ 15 mm (d) $\geq$ 20 mm

1126. Drugs that carry definitive risk of clinical hemolysis in persons with G6PD deficiency are all of the following *except:*
(a) Dapsone (b) Primaquine
(c) Cotrimoxazole (d) Chloramphenicol

1127. In French-American-British (FAB) Classification of AML, which subtype has the highest incidence:
(a) M1 (b) M2
(c) M3 (d) M4

1128. All of the following are included under CDC Category A agents under microbial bioterrorism, *except:*
(a) Anthrax (*Bacillus anthracis*)
(b) Brucellosis (*Brucella spp.*)
(c) Tularemia (*Francisella tularensis*)
(d) Plague (*Yersinia pestis*)

1129. All are potentially reversible causes of dementia, *except:*
(a) Chronic subdural hematoma
(b) Pernicious anemia
(c) Normal-pressure hydrocephalus
(d) HIV

1130. In adults with viral hepatitis, progression to chronicity is maximum with which of the following viral infections?

(a) Hepatitis A (b) Hepatitis B

(c) Hepatitis C (d) Hepatitis E

1131. All of the following are useful in Multidrug-Resistant Enteric fever in adults, *except:*

(a) Azithromycin (b) Ceftriaxone

(c) Ciprofloxacin (d) Amoxicillin

1132. All of the following conditions are associated with increased incidance of cancer *except:*

(a) Down's syndrome (b) Fancoy's anemia

(c) Neurofibromatosis (d) Fragile X syndrome

1133. Which of the following drugs for HIV is incorrectly matched with their side effect?

(a) Indinavir–kidney stones

(b) Nelfinavir–lipodystrophy

(c) Didanosine–pancreatitis

(d) Efavirenz–lactic acidosis

1134. CPR guidelines 2010:One of the following statements is false:

(a) Sequence of steps in Basic Life Support: "C-A-B" (Chest compression, Airway, Breathing)

(b) Ventilations with advanced airway (8-10 breaths/min)

(c) Compression to ventilation ratio of 30:2 in adults

(d) Routine use of atropine during asystole is likely to have therapeutic benefit

1135. Which of the following does not cause small vessel vasculitis?

(a) Churg-Strauss syndrome

(b) Essential mixed cryoglobulinemia

(c) Takayasu's arteritis

(d) Henoch-Schönlein Purpura

1136. Postmenopausal hormonal replacement therapy bas been shown to increase a female's risk of all of the following *except:*

(a) Breast cancer

(b) Myocardial infarction

(c) Venous thromboembolism

(d) Hip fracture

1137. All of the following are effects of hypercalcemia *except:*

(a) Diarrhoea (b) Confusion

(c) Nephrolithiasis (d) Shortened QT interval

1138. The most common cause of a cerebral embolism is:

(a) Cardiac prosthetic valves

(b) Dilated cardiomyopathy

(c) Endocarditis

(d) Atrial fibrillation

1139. The frequency of intravascular ultrasound catheter:

(a) 2-5 MHz (b) 7-10 MHz

(c) 20-45 MHz (d) 10-15 MHz

1140. Cryoprecipitate can be used to treat all *except:*

(a) Hemophilia A

(b) Hemophilia B

(c) Afibrinogenimia

(d) Von Willebrand disease

1141. All are seen in SLE *except:*

(a) Oral ulcers (b) Malar rash

(c) Erosive arthritis (d) Vasculitis

1142. Nine months old baby can do all the following *except:*

(a) Pivoting (b) Pincergrasp

(c) Speak by syllables (d) Wave bye bye

1143. Kawasaki disease criteria includes all *except:*

(a) Fever > 5 days

(b) Lymphadenopathy

(c) Suppurative conjunctivitis

(d) Skin desquamation

1144. Polyuria is a feature of all *except:*

(a) Renal tubular acidosis

(b) Bartter's syndrome

(c) Diabetes insipidus

(d) Polycystic kidney

1145. Complications of nephrotic syndrome are all *except:*

(a) Peritonitis

(b) Pneumonia

(c) Renal failure

(d) Renal vein thrombosis

1146. Which of the following statements regarding gastric decontamination for toxin ingestion is true?

(a) Activated charcoals most common side effect is aspiration
(b) Syrup of ipecac has no role in the hospital setting
(c) There are insufficient data to support or exclude a benefit when gastric decontamination is used more than 1 hour after a toxic ingestion
(d) All of the above are true

1147. Which of the following has been demonstrated to reduce mortatility in patients with ARDS?

(a) High frequency mechanical ventilation
(b) Inhaled nitric oxide
(c) Low tidal volume mechanical ventilation
(d) Surfactant replacement

1148. Which of the following treatments is recommended to improve mortality in Septic Shocks:

(a) Activated protein C (drotrecogin alpha)
(b) Administration of Antibiotics within 1 hour presentation
(c) Bicarbonate therapy for severe acidosis
(d) Erythropoietin

1149. Which of the following viral cause of acute hepatitis is most likely to cause Fulminant hepatitis in a pregnant woman?

(a) Hepatitis B (b) Hepatitis C
(c) Hepatitis D (d) Hepatitis E

1150. Which of the following phenomena is classically associated with herniation of the brain through the foramen magnum:

(a) Catatonia (b) "Locked-in" state
(c) Miotic pupils (d) Respiratory arrest

1151. What is the optimal percentage of daily caloric intake derived from carbohydrates?

(a) <25% (b) 25 – 35%
(c) 45 – 55% (d) 65 – 75%

1152. Which of the following is the most common cause of hypothyroidism worldwide?

(a) Graves' Disease
(b) Hashimoto's thyroiditis
(c) Latrogenic hypothyroidism
(d) Iodine deficiency

1153. All of the following syndromes are associated with obesity *except:*

(a) Acromegaly (b) Cushing's syndrome
(c) Hypothyroidism (d) Insulinoma

1154. In general which of the following is the greatest risk factor for the development of cancer?

(a) Age (b) Alcohol Use
(c) Cigarette Smoking (d) Female Sex

1155. Among women younger than sixty years of who die from cancer, which of the following is the most common primary organ of orign?

(a) Breast (b) Cervix
(c) Colon (d) Lung

1156. What is the most common side effect of Chemo-therapy?

(a) Alopecia
(b) Diarrhea
(c) Febrile Neutropenia
(d) Nausea with or without vomiting

1157. A primary tumor of which of these organs is the least likely to metastasize to bone:

(a) Breast (b) Colon
(c) Lung (d) Prostrate

1158. All the following are suggested of iron-deficiency anemia *except:*

(a) Koilonychia
(b) Pica
(c) Decreased serum ferritin
(d) Decreased total iron-binding capacity (TIBC)

1159. Which of the following carries the best disease prognosis with appropriate treatment:

(a) Burkitt's lymphoma
(b) Diffuse large B-cell lymphoma
(c) Follicular lymphoma
(d) Nodular sclerosing Hodgkin's disease

1160. All of the following neurologic disease are matched correctly with the neurotransmitter system that is dysfunctional *except:*

(a) Lambert-Eaton syndrome: acetylcholine
(b) Myasthenia gravis: acetylcholine
(c) Orthostatic tachycardia syndrome: serotonin
(d) Parkinson's disease: dopamine

1161. In food poisoning caused by Staphococcus aureus all of the following characteristics would be common feature of food poisoning due to this organism *except:*

(a) Abdominal Cramping (b) Diarrhea
(c) Fever (d) Vomiting

1162. **Which of the following antibiotics inhibit cell wall synthesis?**

(a) Ciprofloxacin, metronidazole and quinupristin/dalfopristin
(b) Rifampin, sulfamicin and clindamycin
(c) Tetramycin, deptomycin, azythromycin
(d) Vancomycin, bacitramycin and penicillin

1163. **Helicobacter pylori canonization increases the odds ratio of developing all of the following conditions *except:***

(a) Duodenal ulcer disease
(b) Esophagel adenocarcinoma
(c) Gastric adenocarcinoma
(d) Gastric mucosa-associated lymphoid tissue (MALT) lymphoma

1164. **HIV related dilated cardiomyopathy was strongly associated with a CD4 count of:**

(a) Less than 100 cells/ml
(b) Less than 150 cells/ml
(c) Less than 200 cells/ml
(d) Less than 250 cells/ml

1165. **A 42-year-old man with heme-positive stools and a history epigastric pain is found to have a duodenal ulcer that is biopsy-proven positive for H. Pylori. All of the following are effective eradication regimens *except:***

(a) Amoxicillin and levofloxacin for 14 days
(b) Omeprazole, clarithromycin and metronidazole for 14 days
(c) Omeprazole, clarithromycin and amoxicillin for 14 days
(d) Omeprazole, Bismuth, tetracycline and metronidazole

1166. **Which of the following is a major reservoir for anaerobic organisms in the human body?**

(a) Duodenum (b) Female genital tract
(c) Gallbladder (d) Lung

1167. **All of the following factors influence the likelihood of transmitting active tuberculosis *except:***

(a) Duration of contact with an infected person
(b) Presence of extra pulmonary tuberculosis
(c) Presence of laryngeal tuberculosis
(d) Probability of contact with an infectious person

1168. **Drug of choice for aspirin allergy is:**

(a) Dipyridamole (b) Ticlopidine
(c) Sulfinpyrazone (d) Clopidogrel

1169. **A 50-year-old man is admitted to the hospital for active pulmonary tuberculosis with a positive sputum acid-fast bacilli smear. He is HIV positive with CD4 count of 85/UL and is not on highly active antiretroviral therapy. In addition to pulmonary disease, he is found to have disease in the L4 vertebral body. What is the most appropriate initial therapy?**

(a) Isoniazed, rifampin, ethambutol and pyrazinamide
(b) Isoniazed, rifampin, ethambutol and pyrazinamide; initiate antiretroviral therapy
(c) Isoniazed, rifampin, ethambutol and pyrazinamide and streptomycin
(d) Isoniazed, rifampin, ethambutol

1170. **Which of the following concept prove particularly useful in cardiovascular genetics?**

(a) Genotyping (b) Genomics
(c) Proteomics (d) All of the above

1171. **All of the following viruses have been implicated as a cause of human cancer *except:***

(a) Dengue fever virus
(b) Hepatitis B virus
(c) Hepatitis C virus
(d) Human papilloma virus

1172. **All of the following statements regarding the drug mefloquine are true *except:***

(a) Dose adjustment is necessary in patients with renal insufficiency
(b) It is only available in oral form
(c) It is the preferred drug for prophylaxis of chloroquine-resistant malaria
(d) Psychiatric side effects limit it use in certain patients

1173. **All of the following are clinical manifestations of Ascaris lumbricoides infection *except:***

(a) Asymptomatic carriage
(b) Fever, headache, photophobia, nuchal rigidity and eosinophilia
(c) Nonproductive cough and pleurisy with eosinophilia
(d) Small bowel obstruction

1174. **Acute hyperkalemia is associated with which of the following electrocardiographic charges?**

(a) Decrease in the PR interval
(b) Prominent U waves
(c) QRS widening
(d) T-wave flattening

1175. Which of the following is the most common cause of diffuse bronchiectasis worldwide?

(a) Cystic fibrosis
(b) Immunoglobulin deficiency
(c) Mycobacterium tuberculosis infection
(d) Rheumatoid arthritis

1176. Which of the following is the best definition of evidence based medicine?

(a) A type of research that compares the results of one approach to treating a disease with another approach to treating the same disease
(b) Clinical decision making support tools developed by professional organizations that include expert opinions and data from clinical trials
(c) Clinical decision making supported by data, preferably from randomized controlled clinical trials
(d) One physician's clinical experience in caring for multiple patients with a specific disorder over many years

1177. In stage 5 chronic kidney disease the glomerular filtration rate is below:

(a) 50 ml/min per 1.73 m^2
(b) 25 ml/min per 1.73 m^2
(c) 15 ml/min per 1.73 m^2
(d) 0 ml/min per 1.73 m^2 (anuria)

1178. Which of the following classes of medicines has been linked the occurrence of hip fractures in elderly?

(a) Benzodiazepines
(b) Opiates
(c) Angiotensin-converting enzyme inhibitors
(d) Beta-blockers

1179. Which of the following organisms has been used in the treatment of inflammatory bowel disease (IBD)?

(a) Campylobacter Spp. (b) Clostridium diffcile
(c) Escherichia Spp. (d) Lactobacillus Spp.

1180. All of the following cause definitive hemolysis in G6PD deficiency *except:*

(a) Methylene blue (b) Ciprofloxacin
(c) Primaquine (d) Nalidixic acid

1181. Childhood phase of Atopic dermatitis involves:

(a) Flexural area (b) External area
(c) Palm and soles (d) Facial area

1182. Disproportionate growth is seen in all *except:*

(a) Achondroplasia (b) Hypopituitarism
(c) Cretinism (d) Rickets

1183. The immunoglobulin is actively transported across the placenta is:

(a) IgG (b) IgM
(c) IgA (d) IgE

1184. The ratio of US to LS in a 3 years old baby is:

(a) 1:8 (b) 1:5
(c) 1:3 (d) 1:10

1185. Increase in the Airway resistances is seen in:

(a) Bronchial asthma
(b) In 80% people, increase in work load
(c) Bronchitis
(d) All of the above

1186. Toxic shock syndrome diagnostic criteria include all *except:*

(a) Hyperthermia
(b) Mucosal involvement
(c) Squamous-skin erosions
(d) Hypotension

1187. All of the following are true about Baritosis *except:*

(a) It involves the lower lobes
(b) It is due barium sulfate dust
(c) Resolution after the cessation of exposure dust
(d) Later diffuse

1188. The following constituent of laxatives that cause constipation is:

(a) Magnesium chloride
(b) Aluminium hydroxide
(c) Selenium
(d) Calcium carbonate

1189. A child can draw a square and a triangle, but not able to draw a diamond. Appropriate age of child could be:

(a) 4 years (b) 5 years
(c) 6 years (d) 3 years

1190. Acute Fulminant Hepatitis in a child is most commonly associated with infection of:

(a) Herpes simplex
(b) Varicella

(c) Paramxovirus

(d) Infectious mononucleosis

1191. Most common cause of Thyrotoxicosis in infants is:

(a) Thyrotoxicosis facticia

(b) Graves' disease

(c) Multinodular goiter

(d) Toxic adenoma

1192. Most common cause of pneumonia in 3 months to 3-year-old children is:

(a) Streptoccoccus pneumoniae

(b) E. coli

(c) H. influenzae

(d) Klebsiella

1193. Transient loss consciousness; precipitated by hyper-ventilation, frequent episodes through the day, are all features characterizing which seizure?

(a) Absence (b) Atonic

(c) Simple Partial (d) Complex Partial

1194. Incorrect about filgrastim:

(a) Produces initial transient neutropenia

(b) Causes bone pain

(c) Used in chemotherapy CML

(d) Increases granulocyte count

1195. The drug of choice in severe complicated falciparum malaria:

(a) Chloroquine (b) Quinine

(c) Artesunate (d) Artemether

1196. All of the following statements are true about Benedict's syndrome, *except:*

(a) Contralateral tremor

(b) 3rd nerve palsy

(c) Involvement of the penetrating branch of the basilar artery

(d) Lesion at the level of the pons

1197. Which one of the following is NOT commonly seen in polycythemia vera?

(a) Thrombosis

(b) Hyperuricemia

(c) Prone for acute leukemia

(d) Spontaneous severe infection

1198. Coombs' positive hemolytic anemia associated with:

(a) TTP (b) PAN

(c) SLE (d) HUS

1199. Which of the following is common in the children of pregnant woman whose age is above 40 years of age?

(a) Klinefelter's syndrome

(b) Turner's syndrome

(c) Marfan's syndrome

(d) Down's tetralogy

1200. Clinical manifestations of Congenital Rubella Syndrome in children following Maternal Rubella include all *except:*

(a) Nerve deafness

(b) Psychomotor retardation

(c) Patent Ductus Arteriosus

(d) Aortic stenosis

1201. All of the following drugs are used in the remission induction in a case of all *except:*

(a) Vincristine (b) Prednisone

(c) L-asparaginase (d) Cytosine arabinoside

1202. Drug of choice for Neurogenic Shock:

(a) Methoxamine (b) Norepinephrine

(c) Adrenaline (d) Dopamine

1203. Which match is NOT correct?

(a) SLE–APL

(b) Kawasaki disease–Aneurysms

(c) Behcet's–Venous thrombosis

(d) Wegener's–ANCA

1204. The principal causes of death in Hemochromatosis include all, *except:*

(a) Hepatocellular failure of Portal hypertension

(b) Congestive cardiac failure

(c) Diabetes mellitus

(d) Hepatocellular carcinoma

1205. A person suffering from fever, with truncal rash started over abdomen with peripheral distribution for one week with chill following Louse bite, possible diagnosis is:

(a) Epidemic typhus (b) Endemic typhus

(c) Scrub typhus (d) Rickettsial pox

1206. HIV related dilated cardiomyopathy was strongly associated with a CD4 count of:

(a) Less than 100 cells/ml

(b) Less than 150 cells/ml

(c) Less than 200 cells/ml

(d) Less than 250 cells/ml

1207. WHO estimates that 60 percent of the world's cardiac patients will be from the following country by 2010:
(a) China (b) America
(c) Japan (d) India

1208. Which of the following concept prove particulary useful in cardiovascular genetics?
(a) Genotyping (b) Genomics
(c) Proteomics (d) All of the above

1209. True statement about pulmonary Lymphangio-leiomyomatosis:
(a) Is common in males < 45 years
(b) Hemoptysis is life threatening
(c) Does not cause pneumothorax
(d) Responds to steroids

1210. Which of the following is a natural compound which causes increased risk of hepatocellular carcinoma?
(a) Thorostat
(b) Arsenic
(c) Aflatoxin B
(d) Ophisthotonus sinensis

1211. GFR was measured to be between 60-89 in a patient with chronic renal failure. Which stage is he in?
(a) Stage 1 (b) Stage 2
(c) Stage 3 (d) Stage 4

1212. Which one of the following is least expected to precipitate hepatic encephalopathy in a liver cirrhosis patient?
(a) Peritoneal tap (b) Antibiotic treatment
(c) Variceal bleed (d) Hypokalemia

1213. All of the following are WHO classified Myelodysplastic Syndromes *except:*
(a) CML
(b) Refractory anemia with excess blasts
(c) Refractory anemia with ringed sideroblasts
(d) Refractory anemia

1214. The most sensitive test for Diabetic nephropathy is:
(a) Urine albumin (b) Creatinine clearance
(c) Serum creatinine (d) Glucose tolerance

1215. The gold standard test for the diagnosis of Paroxysmal Nocturnal Hemoglobinuria (PNH) is:
(a) Flow cytometry (b) Sucrose hemolysis test
(c) Ham's test d) None of the above

1216. Neurasthenia is associated with all *except:*
(a) Depressed mood (b) Easy fatiguability
(c) Anxiety (d) Loss of libido

1217. NOT a criteria for Allergic Broncho Pulmonary Aspergillosis (ABPA):
(a) Serum precipitates for Aspergillus fumigatus
(b) Bronchial asthma
(c) Positive culture of aspergillus from sputum
(d) Pulmonary infiltrates

1218. A patient presents with headache for one hour on awakening, associated with nasal stuffiness and reddening of eye. Suggestive of:
(a) Cluster headache (b) Tension headache
(c) Migraine (d) All of the above

1219. Flow murmur of across the mitral valve is not a feature of:
(a) Anemia
(b) Pulmonary arteriovenous fistula (pulmonary)
(c) Thyrotoxicosis
(d) Systemic arteriovenous fistula

1220. Kearns Sayre syndrome is characterized by the triad which includes the following *except:*
(a) Cardiomyopathy
(b) External ophthalmoplegia
(c) Pigmentary degeneration of the retina
(d) Cardiac conduction blocks

1221. First heart sound can be constant in intensity in complete heart block, when associated with the following, *except:*
(a) On DDD pacing (b) On VDD pacing
(c) VVIR pacing (d) Atrial fibrillation

1222. The body organ with the most adverse ratio of oxygen consumption to blood supply:
(a) Kidney (b) Heart
(c) Liver (d) Brain

1223. Acute exposure to high altitude results in:
(a) Increase arterial $PaCO_2$
(b) Increase arterial in PaO_2
(c) Increase systemic vascular resistance
(d) Increase in cardiac output

1224. The organisms predominating in hospital acquired pneumonia are:

(a) P. aeruginosa

(b) Acinetobacter spp.

(c) MDR enterobacteriaceae

(d) All of the above

1225. The most effective management of catheter related urinary tract infection is:

(a) Removal of the catheter

(b) Systemic antibiotic treatment

(c) Topical metal antimicrobial

(d) Drainage bag disinfectants

1226. The most important treatment of non-alcoholic fatty liver disease is:

(a) Weight loss

(b) UDCA (Ursodeoxycholic aci(d)

(c) Glitazones

(d) Statins

1227. H. pylori is a cofactor in the development of all *except:*

(a) Duodenal or gastric ulcers

(b) Gastric cancer

(c) Gastric mucosa-associated lymphoid-tissue (MALT) lymphoma

(d) Barrett's esophagus

1228. In COPD corticosteroid treatment that is likely to benefit severely symptomatic patients is:

(a) 40 mg of prednisone taken once daily for 10 to 14 days

(b) 40 mg of prednisone taken once daily for upto 8 weeks

(c) 10 mg of prednisone taken once daily for 10 to 14 days

(d) Not beneficial at all

1229. Effective drugs used in treatment of hepatic encephalopathy include all *except:*

(a) Lactulose (b) Rifaximin

(c) Neomycin (d) Vitamin supplementation

1230. The most common cause of Cushing's syndrome is: (a) Secretion of corticotrophin from the pituitary gland:

(a) Adrenal tumours

(b) Iatrogenic administration of exogenous glucocorticoids

(c) Ectopic production of corticotrophin

1231. Asthmatic attacks may be triggered by all of the following *except:*

(a) Viral respiratory infections

(b) Airborne allergens

(c) Cold air

(d) Food

1232. In patients with COPD, prognosis can be improved by all *except:*

(a) Cessation of smoking

(b) Oxygen therapy

(c) Lung volume reduction

(d) Use of mucolytic agents

1233. Lung abscess is a common complication of infection caused by:

(a) Anaerobic bacteria

(b) Influenza virus

(c) Mycoplasma pneumoniae

(d) Legionella pneumophilia

1234. The classic form of HCV-related glomerular disease is:

(a) Membranoproliferative glomerulonephritis

(b) Membranous glomerulonephritis

(c) Fibrillary glomerulonephritis

(d) Focal segmental glomerulosclerosis

1235. Most common is HIV-associated nephropathy is:

(a) Mesangio capillary glomerulonephritis

(b) Collapsing glomerular lesions in the kidney biopsy

(c) Chronic renal failure

(d) Hypertensive nephrosclerosis

1236. In patients who have HIV and HCV co-infection the most appropriate treatment option is:

(a) Combination of pegylated interferon (peginterferon) alfa and weight-based ribavirin for 24 weeks

(b) Combination of pegylated interferon (peginterferon) alfa and weight-based ribavirin for 48 weeks

(c) Use of HAART alone

(d) None of the above

1237. The emergency treatment options for acute stroke within 3-4 hours include:

(a) Intravenous recombinant tissue plasminogen activator (n-PA)

(b) Endovascular interventions
(c) Mechanical embolectomy
(d) Ultra-arterial thrombolysis

1238. Definite indications for initiation of antiretroviral therapy include all *except:*

(a) Acute infection syndrome
(b) Chronic infection with symptoms
(c) Asymptomatic diseases CD4+ T-cell count <350/pL
(d) All of the above

1239. Which one of the following tests measure biosynthetic liver function?

(a) Blood ammonia
(b) AST and ALT
(c) Serum prothrombin time
(d) Serum bilirubin

1240. The duration of treatment, with oral anticoagulants in patients with first episode of' idiopathic of DVT and pulmonary embolism is:

(a) 3-6 months (b) 6-12 months
(c) 12-24 months (d) Lifelong

1241. In nosocomial urinary tract infections, the following are true *except:*

(a) Treatment of candiduria is indicated in obstruction
(b) Recovery of S. aureus in wine culture should be treated with systemic antibiotics
(c) Irrigation of catheters with antimicrobial agents is recommended
(d) In chronic indwelling bladder catheterization, it is necessary to replace the catheter and obtains fresh sample for culture

1242. The most common presentation of primary hyperparathyroidism is:

(a) Peptic ulcer
(b) Proximal limb weakness
(c) Renal stones
(d) Asymptomatic

1243. Oral anticoagulant induced skin necrosis is associated with:

(a) Antithrombin III deficiency
(b) Plasminogen deficiency
(c) Protein C deficiency
(d) Protein S deficiency

1244. Which one of the following is not a high anion 88, gap acidosis?

(a) Ketoacidosis (b) Lactic acidosis
(c) Chronic renal failure (d) Diarrhoea

1245. The severity of beta thalassemia can be ameliorated by:

(a) Co inheritance of alpha thalassemia
(b) Co inheritance of Hb E
(c) Presence of iron deficiency
(d) Presence of iron overload

1246. Polycythemia vera rubra is characterised by:

(a) Splenomegaly
(b) Hyperviscosity symptoms
(c) Presence of JAK 2 mutation
(d) Elevated levels of plasma erythropoietin

1247. Which of the following organisms would be most likely to cause infection in a splenectomised patient?

(a) Streptococcus pneumoniae
(b) Hemophilus influenza
(c) E. coli
(d) Plasmodium vivax

1248. Protein conjugate pneumococcal vaccine rather than capsular polysaccharide vaccine is recommended in:

(a) Adults more than 65 years
(b) Patients with CSF leak
(c) Children less than 2 years
(d) Patients with HIV

1249. In Wernicke's aphasia, which of the following is preserved?

(a) Comprehension
(b) Repetition of spoken language
(c) Naming
(d) Fluency

1250. WHO defines anaemia in women as a hemoglobin level of:

(a) Less than 14 gm/dl (b) Less than 13 gm/dl
(c) Less than 12 gm/dl (d) Less than 11 gm/dl

1251. The following is true of tuberculous arthritis *except:*

(a) It involves large weight bearing joints
(b) Normal chest X-ray
(c) Absence of fever
(d) Coexisting osteomyelitis

1252. Clinical identification of metabolic syndrome does not include:

(a) Waist circumference as indicator of abdominal obesity
(b) LDL cholesterol
(c) Triglyceride level
(d) Fasting blood glucose

1253. Significant action on dopaminergic receptors:

(a) Dobutamine (b) Dopexamine
(c) Vasopressin (d) Epinephrine

1254. Beta blockers are recommended as first line anti-arrhythmic therapy in the following *except:*

(a) Long QT syndrome
(b) RVOF VT
(c) Brugada syndrome
(d) Arrhythmogenic RV dysplasia

1255. Gooseneck deformity in angiography is a feature of: (a) Common atrium (b) Partial AV canal defect (c) Complete AV canal defect:

(a) a, b, c (b) a, b
(c) b, c (d) c, a

1256. Findings in pre-renal azotemia:

(a) Urinary NA< 10 m mol/L and SG > 1.018
(b) Urinary NA > 10 m mol/L and SG < 1.018
(c) Urinary NA < 10 m mol/L and SG < 1.018
(d) Urinary NA < 10 m mol/L and SG > 1.018

1257. Proportionate elevation of blood urea as compared to serum creatinine occurs in:

(a) Acute-tubular necrosis
(b) Pre renal azotemia
(c) None of the above

1258. Contributing to bone disease in chronic renal failure include:

(a) Phosphate retention
(b) Metabolic acidosis
(c) Reduced calcitriol production
(d) All of the above

1259. Bolic abnormalities secondary to chronic renal failure include:

(a) Hyperphosphatemia
(b) Hypophosphatemia
(c) Metabolic alkalosis
(d) None of the above

1260. Diagnosis of chronic failure can be established on the basis of:

(a) Hyperkalemia
(b) Metabolic acid
(c) Neutrally reduced renal size
(d) Presence of hydronephrosis

1261. Symptomatic patient with HIV infection a definite indication for starting anti retroviral should be CD4 count less than:

(a) 200 mm^3 (b) 100 mm^3
(c) 400 mm^3 (d) 500 mm^3

1262. Indication for starting anti retroviral therapy in an asymptomatic patient with HIV a normal CD 4 count would be a viral load above:

(a) 100 copies/ml (b) 1000 copies/ml
(c) 10000 copies/ml (d) 20000 copies/ml

1263. Primary prophylaxis against the following opportunistic infections would be appropriate in a patient with HIV infection and a CD 4 count below 100/mm^3:

(a) Cytomegalovirus infection
(b) Cryptococcal meningitis
(c) PCP
(d) All of the above

1264. Lactic acidosis is a serious complication associated with the use of:

(a) NRTIs (b) NNRTIs
(c) Pls (d) Fusion inhibitors

1265. Ritonavir is best used:

(a) In combination with NNRTIs
(b) As monotherapy
(c) As a pharmacokinetic booster of other Pls
(d) None of the above

1266. Infections mononucleosis is caused by:

(a) Ebstein-Barr virus
(b) Cytomegalovirus
(c) Herpes simplex virus
(d) Toxoplasmosis

1267. Doxycycline is used in the treatment of following disease *except:*

(a) Leptospirosis (b) Q fever

(c) Borreliosis (d) All of the above

1268. The antibiotic of choice for the treatment of leptospirosis is:

(a) Chloramphenicol (b) Penicillin

(c) Co-trimoxazole (d) Ciprofloxacin

1269. The drug used in the treatment of quinolone resistant typhoid is:

(a) Co-trimoxazole (b) Ceftriaxone

(c) Amoxycillin (d) Chloramphenicol

1270. The drug of choice for the treatment of tapeworm infestation is:

(a) Albendazole (b) Metronidazole

(c) Praziquantel (d) Primaquin

1271. In Conn's syndrome there is excess production of hormone:

(a) Testosterone (b) Cortisol

(c) Nor-epinephrine (d) Aldosterone

1272. Diagnosis of spontaneous bacterial peritonitis (SBP) is made when the ascetic fluid neutrophil count is above:

(a) $250/mm^3$ (b) $500/mm^3$

(c) $1000/mm^3$ (d) $100/mm^3$

1273. Bleeding time predicts abnormality of function of:

(a) Coagulation protein (b) Fibrinolysis

(c) Platelets (d) Vessel wall

1274. In iron deficiency anaemia, the total iron binding capacity (TIBC) will be:

(a) Decreased (b) Increased

(c) Unchanged (d) Variable

1275. A single seizure, the risk of subsequent seizures is:

(a) 90% (b) 10%

(c) 40% (d) 100%

1276. Pulmonary fibrosis can be caused by all the following drugs *except:*

(a) Amiodarone (b) Hydralazine

(c) Busulphan (d) Gold

1277. Referred drug used in the treatment of refractory SIADH is:

(a) Lithium (b) Demeclocycline

(c) Ethanol (d) Phenytoin

1278. Treatment of hypothyroidism the efficacy of drug is assessed by testing:

(a) T3 (b) T4

(c) Free T4 (d) TSH

1279. Pretibial myxoedema is seen in:

(a) Graves' disease (b) Hypothyroidism

(c) Addison's disease (d) Cushing's syndrome

1280. Hyperthyroidism is treated with all of the following *except:*

(a) Methimazole (b) Propylthiouracil

(c) Radioactive Iodine (d) Lithium

1281. Drugs that have profound effects on the thyroid function are all of the following *except:*

(a) Amiodarone (b) PAS

(c) Hydralazine (d) Lithium

1282. Café au lait spots are seen in:

(a) Infective edocarditis

(b) Von Recklinghausen's disease

(c) Ulcerative colitis

(d) Hypothyroidism

1283. The 'half and half' nail, with a white proximal and red distal half is seen in patients with:

(a) Chronic renal failure

(b) Infective endocarditis

(c) Cirrhosis liver

(d) Dermatomyositis

1284. Erythema nodosum can be caused by all of the following *except:*

(a) Sarcoidosis (b) Tuberculosis

(c) Behcet's disease (d) Infective endocarditis

1285. The skin test used to differentiate viral lesions of skin from pemphigus is called:

(a) Tzanck test (b) Schilling test

(c) Mantoux test (d) Patch test

1286. In severe aortic stenosis the drug which is contra-indiacted is:

(a) Vasodilators

(b) Beta blockers

(c) Calcuim channel blockers
(d) Diuretics

1287. In infective endocarditis the tender nodules in the pulps of fingers are called:

(a) Aschoff's nodes (b) Osler's nodes
(c) Roth's spots (d) Janeway lesions

1288. The characteristic feature of the pulse in cardiac tamponade is described as:

(a) Pulsus alternans (b) Collapsing pulse
(c) Pulsus paradoxus (d) Pulsus bisferiens

1289. The normal upper limit of Jugular venous pressure above the sterna angle is:

(a) 9 cms (b) 8 cms
(c) 6 cms (d) 4 cms

1290. Kussmaul's sign in Jugular venous pulse is diagnostic of:

(a) Constrictive pericarditis
(b) Aortic stenosis
(c) Cor pulmonale
(d) Cardiomyopathy

1291. Continuous murmurs heard during systole and diastole are caused by:

(a) Co-arctation of aorta
(b) Patent ductus arteriosus
(c) Aortic regurgitation
(d) Aortic stenosis

1292. The following test differentiates intravascular hemolysis from extravascular hemolysis:

(a) Polychromatophilia in peripheral smear
(b) Increased reticulocyte count
(c) Erythroid hyperplasia in bone narrow
(d) Hemosiderin in urine

1293. The syndrome of defective hypothalamic gonadotropins - releasing hormone synthesis is called:

(a) Sheehan's syndrome (b) Kallman syndrome
(c) Cushing's syndrome (d) Fröhlich's syndrome

1294. Drugs causing hypothyroidism are all of the below *except:*

(a) Lithium
(b) Para-aminosalicylic acid
(c) Amiodarone
(d) Rifampicin

1295. Pituitary tumour developing following bilateral total adrenalectomy is called:

(a) Conn's syndrome (b) Nelson's syndrome
(c) Cushing's disease (d) Schmidt's syndrome

1296. According to guidelines of American Heart Association the target LDL valves in diabetic individual without cardiovascular disease should be:

(a) Less than 100 mg/dl (b) Less than 150 mg/dl
(c) Less than 75 mg/dl (d) Less than 200 mg/dl

1297. A third cranial nerve palsy with contralateral hemiplegia is called:

(a) Claudis syndrome (b) Fvilles' syndrome
(c) Weber's syndrome (d) Jackson's syndrome

1298. Dementia can be caused by deficiency of all of the following *except:*

(a) Thiamine (b) Vit B_{12}
(c) Nicotinic acid (d) Folic acid

1299. Motor neuron disease with features of both upper motor neuron and lower motor neuron is called:

(a) Primary lateral sclerosis
(b) Spinal muscular atrophy
(c) Amyotrophic lateral sclerosis
(d) Familial spastic paraplegia

1300. Herpes zoster of geniculate ganglion causing facial palsy is called:

(a) Ramsay Hunt syndrome
(b) Bell's palsy
(c) Heerfordt's syndrome
(d) Sjögren's syndrome

1301. The vascular system first appears in embryos of about:

(a) 3 weeks gestation age
(b) 5 weeks gestation age
(c) 8 weeks gestation age
(d) 12 weeks gestation age

1302. Partitioning of the embryonic heart is accomplished by the formation of:

(a) 3 Septa (b) 5 Septa
(c) 7 Septa (d) 10 Septa

1303. Regarding ethanol which is not true?

(a) It most commonly causes hypertriglyceridemia

(b) Alcoholic cardiomyopathy (Systolic dysfunction) is irreversible
(c) Most common is AF
(d) It is a risk factor for HTN in male

1304. Neurotransmitter in presynaptic receptor during is:
(a) NO (b) Substance P
(c) Acetylcholine (d) Nor adrenaline

1305. Key Hodgkin murmur is:
(a) Severe anemia
(b) LAD stenosis
(c) Retroversion of aortic cusp with AR
(d) Severe acute MR

1306. Cholestrol absorption at intestine decreased by:
(a) Fenofibrate (b) Ezetimibe

1307. 25-OH vit D half life:
(a) 1 week (b) 3 weeks
(c) 6 weeks

1308. Variable matched:
(a) Matching (b) Dependent
(c) Independent

1309. Study retrograde:
(a) Prospective (b) Retrospective
(c) Descriptive

1310. Intracranial bleed is least common in:
(a) Putamen (b) Pons
(c) Thalamus (d) Cerebellum

1311. Effect of intervention in previously treated patient:
(a) Carry over effect

1312. Gene for glucocorticoid remediable HTN:
(a) Chr 6 (b) Chr 8
(c) Chr 11 (d) Chr 22

1313. Preoperative non invasive function assessment done in:
(a) 45 years old, HTN, DM with ruptured appendix for emergency surgery
(b) 65 years old female with CAD with CABG 3 years back now asymptomatic undergoing carotid endarterectomy
(c) 65 years old female with history of previous angina with no CAD posted for hysterectomy
(d) 65 years old female with HTN and recurrent angina on minimal exertion posted for prostatectomy

1314. SLE with pericardial tamponade:
(a) Decreased HR on inspiration
(b) Decreased HR with expiration
(c) Decreased SBP with inspiration
(d) Decreased SBP with expiration

1315. Calcineurin inhibitor without T cell proliferation and differentiation:
(a) Azathiopurine (b) MMF
(c) Tacrolimus (d) Sirolimus

1316. Dyslipidemia with antiretroviral drugs A/E:
(a) Zidovudine (b) Didanosine
(c) Saquinavir (d) Raltegravir

1317. Memory T cell A/E:
(a) SAH
(b) Intermittent LBBB
(c) Posterior ventricular pacing
(d) WPW syndrome with intermittent preexcitation

1318. Approach to conceptualizing components of CVS medicine:
(a) Quality hexagone
(b) Donabedian framework
(c) Dartmouth series
(d) Quality control of Lohr and Shredder

1319. Kviem test:
(a) Amyloidosis (b) Sarcoidosis

1320. Breast milk component that decreases E. coli colonization:
(a) Lactoferrin (b) Lysozyme

1321. Therapy is best assessed by:
(a) Survival rate (b) Case fatality rate
(c) Crude death rate (d) Specific death rate

1322. Incidence of disease among exposed to incidence of disease among non exposed:
(a) Odd's ratio
(b) Relative risk
(c) Attributable risk
(d) Population specific risk

1323. Probiotic true A/E
(a) Derived from human
(b) Increased bacteria in large gut
(c) Secretes antimicrobial substance

1324. Recurrent coma, vomiting on fasting cause is:
(a) IDDM (b) NIDDM
(c) Calcific pancreatitis (d) LCAT deficiency

1325. Hereditary spherocytes A/E:
(a) AD (b) Severe anemia
(c) Fluctuating jaundice (d) Gallstone

1326. CF is scare no includes:
(a) Fever
(b) Culture report (tracheal aspirate)
(c) Previous antibiotic
(d) Chest X-ray finding

1327. Indian guideline for outpatient treatment of pneumonia without comorbidity drug given is:
(a) Levofloxacin
(b) Levofloxacin + azithromycin
(c) Doxycycline
(d) Amoxicillin

1328. Osteoporosis not caused by:
(a) Lithium (b) Tamoxifen
(c) Heparin (d) Thyroxine

1329. Brainstem reflex in death A/E:
(a) Corneal reflex (b) Plantar reflex
(c) Light reflex (d) Gag reflex

1330. Diabetic nephropathy undergoing renal transplant true is:
(a) No I.V. cannula too be put in arms
(b) ACE- I useful in ESRD

1331. DCT is not positive in:
(a) Acute hemolytic reaction after blood transfusion
(b) Delayed hemolytic reaction after blood transfusion
(c) Hereditary spherocytosis

1332. PET not required in:
(a) Cancer staging
(b) For detection of renal function
(c) Prior to going radiotherapy

1333. Fanconi syndrome A/E:
(a) Hypokalemia (b) Hypocalcemia
(c) Hyperuricemia (d) Aminoaciduria

1334. H1N1 True for vaccination:
(a) Vaccination contraindicated in pregnancy
(b) Given after every 2-3 year
(c) Protective immunity after 2-3 week
(d) Protective immunity after 30 weeks

1335. Patient is having reactive airway disease which of the following agent not used for rapid intubation:
(a) Ketamine (b) Propofol
(c) Thiopental sofdium (d) Barbiturates

1336. Hypoglycemia associated with:
(a) TSH (b) Norepinephrine
(c) Thyroxine (d) Cortisone

1337. Insulin sensitivity increased by A/E:
(a) Metformin (b) Thiazolidiones
(c) Glibenclamide (d) IGF-1

1338. Physiological conc. FDG in body present in:
(a) Lung (b) Intestine
(c) Liver (d) Brown adipose tissue

1339. Polyglandular syndrome type II false:
(a) Male predominance (b) Adrenal insufficiency
(c) Graves' disease (d) DM

1340. Not a treatment for uncomplicated vivax infection:
(a) Artesunate
(b) Artesunate + lumefantrine
(c) ACT combination
(d) Artesunate + mefloquine

1341. MDR not seen in:
(a) Home wound care
(b) Hospitalization for 1 day in last 30 days
(c) Previous antibiotic therapy

1342. Patient with MVP after dental extraction having hematuria within 2-3 days true:
(a) Do IgA level
(b) Serum complement decreases
(c) Do ANCA screening

1343. VAP not a treatment:
(a) Ertapenem (b) Levoflox
(c) Tigecycline

1344. Acute pancreatitis false is:
(a) Patient with hypertriglyceridemia have increased amylase level

1345. Oral anticoagulant:
(a) Dabigatran
(b) Apixaban
(c) Bivalirudin

1346. Significant hypomagnesium seen in:
(a) Vincristine therapy
(b) Procarbazine therapy
(c) Post parathyroidectomy
(d) Hypoaldosteronism

1347. Abnormality caused by acetazolamide and diarrhea are differentiated by:
(a) Serum AG (b) Urine AG
(c) Urine PH (d) Potassium conc.

1348. Refeeding syndrome characteristic abnormality:
(a) Hypophosphatemia (b) Hyperkalemia
(c) Hyponatremia (d) Hypophosphatemia

1349. Metabolic acidosis with increased anion gap with increased osmolar gap:
(a) Ethylene glycol poisoning
(b) Propylene poisoning
(c) Mannitol infusion

1350. Lp (a) level decreased by:
(a) Niacin (b) Clofibrate
(c) Fenofibrate (d) Omega 3 fatty acid

1351. Massive blood transfusion reduces A/E:
(a) Leucocyte (b) Platelet
(c) Factor V (d) Factor VIII

1352. Irradiation of blood is done to prevent:
(a) GVHD
(b) Febrile reaction
(c) Acute hemolytic reaction
(d) To prevent CMV infection

1353. After pituitary damage hormone decreased in following manner:
(a) GH> FSH > TSH > ACTH
(b) FSH >TSH >ACTH >GH
(c) TSH >FSH >ACTH > GH
(d) ACTH >FSH >TSH > GH

1354. Mean ± SD =18.1 ± 1.9 persons having value less than 20 are, if total population are 1000:
(a) 68.3 (b) 873

1355. If patient is treated for tubercular lymphadenitis after completing 6 months ATT, his LAP persists, next step:
(a) Do FNAC of node + mycobacterial culture
(b) Counsel the patient that lymph node may persists
(c) Start second dose ATT

1356. F Na > 1.1 seen in:
(a) CHF
(b) Acute glomerlonephritis
(c) ATN
(d) Hypovolemia

1357. Pregnancy change false: (T/F)
(a) RBC mass increases more plasma volume
(b) Increases lower extremity venous pressure
(c) BP reduction starts in first trimester
(d) >50% plasma volume seen in 2nd trimester
(e) Plasma volume starts increasing in 6th week

1358. Diving reflex: (T/F)
(a) Increases sympathetic tone to heart and increases parasympathetic tone to periphery
(b) Can be used for therapy of paroxysmal AF
(c) Increases organ perfusion
(d) Causes autonomic dysfunction (cerebral vasoconstriction)
(e) Hypoxia followed by tachycardia

1359. TH-1, TH-2 cells A/E:
(a) TH-17 is added
(b) Unlike mice, less robust in human
(c) Coding from thymus
(d) TH- 1 delayed hypersensitive, TH-2–atopy

1360. Visceral leismaniasis:
(a) RK-39 Ab sensitive but not specific
(b) LD bodies present extracellularly
(c) Oral miltefosine is 1st line drug in Bihar
(d) TS-2 polarization

1361. Eosinophilic gastroenteritis A/E:
(a) D-xylose abnormal (b) Bronchial asthma
(c) Hyoalbuminemia (d) ↑ IgE

1362. Acute DIC A/E:
(a) Normal reteplase time
(b) ↓ Factor VIII
(c) ↑ Thrombin time
(d) ↑ D-dimer

1363. Hereditary angioedema A/E:
(a) Skin involvement (b) CNS
(c) Upper airway (d) GIT

1364. Clostridium difficle diarrhoea due to A/E:
(a) Oral rifaximin (b) Oral metronidazole
(c) I.V. vancomycin (d) Stool transplantation

1365. Cephalosporin active against MRSA:
(a) Cefuroxime (b) Cefepime
(c) Cefoxitin (d) Ceftaroline

1366. Left diastolic HF best drug:
(a) Nevobilol (b) Spironolactone
(c) Perindopril (d) Digoxin

1367. MRSA nosocomial true:
(a) Pneumonia is common
(b) Skin and soft tissue inf.
(c) Cassette II staphylococcal protein
(d) PLV toxin

1368. Adult Digeorge syndrome:
(a) Basal ganglia calcification
(b) Thin upper lip
(c) Low set ears
(d) Retinal detachment

1369. Anti snake venom indicate:
(a) ARF (b) Acute hypotension
(c) Fang marks (d) Local edema

1370. HUS A/E:
(a) In spite of thrombocytopenia, no purpura
(b) E. Coli O157 H7 treatment with ciprofloxacin
(c) Helmet cell >2% (RBC's)
(d) Acute cortical necrosis causing severe decline in renal function

1371. Serum osmolarity Na=128 meq/dl, K=4 meq/dl, urea=5 mmol/l, creatinine=89 mmol/l, glucose= 13 mmol/l
(a) 269 (b) 279
(c) 282 (d) 288

1372. Hyponatremia with increased serum osmolarity:
(a) Thiazide (b) SIADH
(c) Hypothyroidism (d) Renal failure

1373. Tolvaptan receptors:
(a) V1a (b) V1b
(c) V2 (d) V3

1374. Cisplatin induced nephrotoxicity A/E:
(a) ↑ Mg
(b) Anemia
(c) Fanconi anemia
(d) Thrombotic microangiopathic anemia

1375. Tigecycline not indicated:
(a) Skin and soft tissue infections
(b) VAP
(c) New Delhi metallo B–lactamases variant
(d) Intra-abdominal infections

1376. Ankylosing spondylitis:
(a) Bilateral sacrolitism all patients
(b) HLA B27 in all patients
(c) Hip joint involvement poor prognosis
(d) Complication–anterior uveitis, orchitis and enthesis

1377. False positive PET scan A/E:
(a) Fungal granuloma
(b) Hyperglycemia
(c) Radiation pneumonitis
(d) Rheumatoid nodule

1378. NCCT in stroke not an early sign:
(a) Hyperattenuation of ischemic territory
(b) Loss of insular ribbon
(c) Lentiform nucleus obscuration
(d) Effacement of sulci

1379. Likelihood ratio for positive:
(a) 1- sensitivity/specificity
(b) Sensitivity/1- specificity
(c) 1- specificity/ sensitivity
(d) 1- sensitivity/1- specificity

1380. Transthyretin amyloidosis A/E:
(a) Neuropathy (b) Renal failure
(c) Cardiac amyloidosis (d) Dementia

1381. Diffusion coefficient K_{CO} is not reduced in:
(a) Lung resection (b) Anemia
(c) Fibrosis (d) Emphysema

1382. Autosomal dominant A/E:
(a) Males > females
(b) 50% transmission
(c) All generations involved
(d) If phenotypically normal parents then no transmission

1383. GM 1 gangliosidosis A/E:
(a) Polyneuropathy
(b) Hepatosplenomegaly
(c) Angiokeratoma
(d) Psychomotor retardation

1384. Brainstem death A/E:
(a) Responsiveness (b) Corneal reflex
(c) Pupil size (d) Babinski sign

1385. Drug reducing hospitalization in HF:
(a) Digoxin (b) Furosemide
(c) ACE–I (d) Salt/water restriction

1386. PBC first presentation:
(a) Fatigue (b) Jaundice
(c) Pruritis (d) Xanthelesma

1387. Which is not a function of proximal convulated tubules?
(a) Uric acid secretion (b) H^+ secretion
(c) Na absorption (d) Glucose absorption

1388. Not a risk factor for HCC:
(a) Carrier HBV (b) NASH
(c) Hemochromatosis (d) Statin

1389. Heterotopic gastric mucosa:
(a) Tech- 99 pertechnate
(b) Tech- 99 RBC
(c) Tech- 99 sulphur colloid
(d) Tech- 99 DTPA

1390. Resistant HTN A/E:
(a) Spironolactone
(b) Diuretics
(c) Carotid baroreceptor denervation
(d) Renal denervation

1391. Adult still disease:
(a) Leukopenia (b) Renal involvement
(c) Anti CCP Ab (d) ↑ Sr. Ferritin

1392. Adult overweight, cigarette smoker, teetotaller, no family history of CAD, BP > 130/80, Sr. Cholesterol = 250 mg/dl, next treatment option is:
(a) Reduce BMI to 24 (b) Reduce smoking
(c) Start regular statin (d) Start moderate alcohol

1393. Exenatide side effect most common:
(a) Rash (b) Nausea
(c) Hepatic dysfunction (d) Palpitation

1394. Clindamycin least effective:
(a) Bacteroides (b) Toxoplasma
(c) Enterococci (d) Plasmodium

1395. Falciparum treatment not approved:
(a) Artesunate + lumefantrine
(b) Artesunate + primaquine
(c) Artesunate + mefloquine
(d) Artesunate + atovaqone + proquanil

1396. Anti-synthetase syndrome A/E:
(a) Mechanic hand (b) Myositis
(c) Sclerodactyly (d) Polyarthritis

1397. Mucormycosis DOC:
(a) Caspofungin (b) Voriconazole
(c) Fluconazole (d) Posaconazole

1398. H1 N1 not used:
(a) Adefovir (b) Osletamivir
(c) Zanamivir (d) Peramavir

1399. Adenosine A/E:
(a) Catecholamine induced VT
(b) Atrial fibrillation
(c) Atrial flutter
(d) WPW

1400. Acute hemolytic transfusion reaction:
(a) Extravascular hemolysis
(b) Not a/w ABO incompatibility
(c) IgG induced
(d) IgM induced

1401. Plateau phase on ventilation:
(a) End expiratory (b) End inspiratory
(c) Start of resp. cycle (d) Mid of resp. cycle

1402. Hemodialysis better than peritoneal dialysis A/E:
(a) β2 microglobin (b) Lithium
(c) Phosphate (d) Uric acid

1403. Hemophagocytosis A/E:
(a) Pancytopenia
(b) ↑ TG level
(c) Transfusion > 450 mg/l
(d) Acute liver failure

1404. Cat scratch disease A/E:

(a) B. Hanselae (b) B. Microti

(c) Leptospira

1405. Snake sp. A/E:

(a) Echis carinata

(b) Naja naja

(c) Bungurans caeruleus

(d) Daboi russelli

(e) Hypnale hypnale

1406. Epidemic dropsy A/E: (T/F)

(a) Sanquirine (b) Oubain

(c) Protopine (d) Cdunbamine

1407. Mean of 2 independent variable without normal distribution:

(a) Fischer test (b) Man whitney U test

(c) Wilkins (d) Kruskel

1408. Rheumatoid arthritis A/E:

(a) Anti CCP more specific than RF

(b) Anti CCP more sensitive than RF

(c) Quantitative titre is also important, not only the presence

(d) Combine (RF + Anti CCP) is more sensitive

1409. Zinc deficiency associated with A/E:

(a) Acrodermatitis

(b) Follicular hyperkeratosis

(c) Pigmentation

(d) Scaly dermatitis

1410. ↑ LVEDP in:

(a) AR

(b) ↑ LV compliance

(c) ↑ pulm. Artery pressure

(d) ↓ LV stroke work index

1411. Ventilator associated pneumonia prevented by A/E:

(a) Prone position

(b) Daily withdrawal of sedation

(c) Propped up head position

(d) Selective GI decontamination

1412. Arsenic poisoning A/E:

(a) Non patch pigmentation seen, drop nail, beau nail

(b) Hair and nails for chronic toxicity

(c) Chelating agents are used but not beneficial

(d) May cause chronic cough, cirrhosis and PVD

1413. Sjögren syndrome:

(a) It causes Sicca in eye , oral mucosa and vagina

(b) Ro- LA + in every patients

(c) RA/ANA often present

(d) Histopathology mononuclear cells infiltrates

1414. Hyponatremia A/E:

(a) Diabetes insipidus (b) SIADH

(c) Hypothyroidism (d) Addison disease

1415. Metabolic alkalosis A/E:

(a) Renin secreting tumour

(b) Paraldehyde ingestion

(c) Conn's syndrome

(d) Bartter syndrome

1416. Gerstmann syndrome A/E:

(a) Acalculia (b) Agraphia

(c) Aphasia (d) Finger anomia

1417. Toll like receptors A/E:

(a) It identifies pattern recognition

(b) It is + on cell membrane only

(c) Innate immunity response and found on macrophage and monocytes

(d) Name derived from toll gene on dorsophilla

1418. Obligate carrier of X-linked recessive:

(a) Lady with 2 brother affected

(b) Lady with one brother and one son affected

(c) Lady with maternal uncle and one brother affected

1419. Assisted mechanical ventilation incidence in asthma:

(a) RR > 45/min on room air

(b) PO_2 – 40 mm Hg on room air

(c) PCO_2– 45 mm Hg on room air

(d) FiO_2 – 45% required for normoxic response

1420. All used in HOCM A/E:

(a) Disopyramide (b) NTG

(c) B blocker (d) Verapamil

1421. Acute headache (sudden onset) with bitemporal hemianopia with sixth nerve palsy:

(a) Pituitary apoplexy

(b) Rupture of ophthalmic artery aneurysm

(c) Cavernous sinus thrombosis
(d) Multiple sclerosis

1422. Gouty arthritis:
(a) ↑ uric acid present in > 99% is > 6 mg/dl
(b) Most common joint is knee joint
(c) Uricosuric agents and xanthine oxidase inhibitor is given in all patients
(d) If Rx started targeted S. Uric acid < 6 mg/dl

1423. Spontaneous bacterial peritonitis A/E:
(a) WBC count < 500 in uncomplicated ascitis
(b) WBC can be 1000 in diuretic patient
(c) SAAG > 1.1 is diagnostic of portal HTN
(d) LDH is low in Spon. Bacterial peritonitis

1424. For diagnosis of hepatic cyst, Tc is given (Tc scintigraphy):
(a) Intravenous
(b) Intraperitoneal
(c) Intrapleural
(d) Both I/V and intraperitoneal

1425. Folic acid A/E:
(a) Daily requirement > 400 mg
(b) 5-Formyl THF
(c) FA for only purine and not pyrimidine
(d) Cobalamine def. Anemia will be responsive to folic acid

1426. Ranson criteria A/E:
(a) Amylase > 2 times (b) LDH > 40
(c) AST > 350 (d) Glucose > 220 mg/dl

1427. Non traumatic bleed A/E:
(a) Myomyoma
(b) Cerebral AV malformation
(c) Amyloid angiopathy
(d) Cerebral vein thrombosis

1428. HIV pathogenesis A/E:
(a) Relative C8–T lymphocytosis and correlates with viremia
(b) Decrease Ig production from B cell
(c) Can also involve dendritic and langehans cells of skin
(d) Monocytes act as reservoir

1429. Septic shock–indication for I/V fluid:
(a) RAP ↑ on SLR (straight leg raising test)
(b) CVP ↑ 10 mmHg on SLR
(c) ↑ central venous O_2 saturation more than 10 on SLR
(d) Dry gangrene

1430. 60 years old patients has 3 years history of dyspnea on exertion and in winter he had evaluation which respond to antibiotics. PFT shows obstructive pattern with FEV1 – 68% what should be the initial treatment?
(a) Inhaled formetrol only
(b) Inhaled ipratropium
(c) I/L formeterol + I/L triotropium
(d) I/L formeterol + I/L budesonide

1431. Amp C resistant A/E:
(a) Darepenem
(b) Amikacin
(c) Cefipime + salbactam
(d) Pipericillin tazobactam

1432. Bile salt malabsorption:
(a) Cirrhosis (b) Biliary obstruction
(c) Bacterial overgrowth (d) Chronic pancreatitis

1433. Which is not pierced in LP?
(a) Post longitudinal ligament
(b) Dura mater
(c) Ligamentum flavum
(d) Supraspinous ligament

1434. Barotraumas prevented by:
(a) Low tidal volume
(b) Peak pr. Plateau < 30
(c) Peak pr. Inspiratory > 40 mm Hg

1435. All True *except* in cardiac cycle:
(a) Systole is shown by QT interval
(b) QRS varies according to heart rate
(c) PR interval – 220 ms
(d) RR may vary

1436. Thrombotic cytopenic purpura:
(a) Hemolytic anemia
(b) INR > 1.5
(c) Schistocytes seen in PBF
(d) LDH increased

1437. Familial heterozygotes hypercholesterolemia A/E:
(a) Autosomal recessive
(b) Tendon xanthoma as a clinical feature
(c) If arcus senilis is present < 45 then f-HCL can be present
(d) LDL receptors Chr–19 defect

1438. Drug decreases mortality in Systolic HF A/E:
(a) Bisoprolol (b) Digoxin
(c) Spironolactone (d) Ramipril

1439. Autosomal recessive A/E:
(a) Both parents heterozygotes–25% children affected
(b) Male and female equally affected
(c) Vertical transmission
(d) One homozygous, other heterozygous, children may be homozygous

1440. Alport syndrome A/E:
(a) Thick glomerular BM
(b) Hematuria
(c) Lenticonus
(d) SN hearing loss

1441. SIADH A/E:
(a) Hyperuricemia
(b) ↓ urea
(c) Low serum osmolarity
(d) U Na > 40 meq/l

1442. Diffuse antinuclear Ab seen in:
(a) U1- RNP (b) Histone
(c) Scl-70 (d) PM-1

1443. Criteria for usual interstitial pneumonia:
(a) Intra alveolar opacity on CXR
(b) Nodular opacity on HRCT
(c) Heterogenous appearance on histology
(d) Intra alveolar macrophages

1444. Klinefelter A/E:
(a) 47 XXY
(b) Short stature
(c) MR
(d) Volume loss in temporal lobe

1445. Empty delta sign in:
(a) Cerebral Venous Thrombosis
(b) Chronic hydrocephalous
(c) Thalassemia

1446. Medial Medullary syndrome:
(a) Ipsilateral hemiplegia
(b) Contralateral proprioception loss
(c) Contralateral hearing loss
(d) Ipsilateral cerebellar loss

1447. CPPD A/E:
(a) Small joints of upper and lower limbs
(b) Symmetrical sacroileitis
(c) Sacroileitis asymptomatic
(d) Asymmetrical peripheral arthritis

1448. Papillary calcification of CT abdomen seen in:
(a) Analgesic nephropathy
(b) MSK
(c) Tuberculosis

1449. DOC of stenotrophomonis maltophilia:
(a) Ampicillin (b) Clindamycin
(c) Cotrimoxazole (d) Chloramphenicol

1450. Not a risk factor for cancer:
(a) MSK (b) Neurofibromatosis
(c) VHL (d) FAP

1451. Aliskiren:
(a) Hypokalemia
(b) Angioedema
(c) Increased CV mortality
(d) Decreased non fatal stroke

1452. Pioglitazone A/E:
(a) CCF (b) Fluid retention
(c) Polycythemia (d) Decreased BMD

1453. Palmitronate side effects:
(a) Osteonecrosis (b) CCF
(c) Respiratory failure (d) Hypercalcemia

1454. ph = 7.55, PCO_2=38 mm Hg, HCO_3= 33, Na=140, Cl= 91, K=4, AG=16:
(a) Metabolic alkalosis with respiratory alkalosis
(b) Metabolic alkalosis with respiratory acidosis
(c) Metabolic acidosis with respiratory acidosis
(d) Metabolic acidosis with respiratory alkalosis

1455. Patient presented with persistent vomiting 5 days, urinary finding:
(a) Urine Ph < 5.5 (b) Increased urine K^+
(c) Increased urine Cl (d) Increased urine Na

1456. A. aegypti–not vector in:
(a) Yellow fever (b) Dengue
(c) Rift valley (d) West Nile fever

1457. Cat scratch disease caused in:
(a) B. Hensalae (b) B. Microti

1458. T. pertenue caused by:
(a) Yaws (b) Pinta
(c) Bijel (d) Syphilis

1459. All are live attenuated *except*:
(a) Measles (b) Mumps
(c) Polio (d) Rubella

1460. Echinocandins not useful in:
(a) Candida glabrata (b) Candida albicans
(c) Cryptococcus (d) Aspergillus

1461. Malaria A/E:
(a) Light microscopic–gold standard
(b) RDT with ELISA
(c) LDH and aldolase–target antigen
(d) Stain Wood Giemsa

1462. APLA–all are diagnostic criteria *except*:
(a) Arterial thrombosis (b) Venous thrombosis
(c) VDRL positive (d) β_2–GPL

1463. MRSA–Commonly acquired is:
(a) Skin and soft tissue infection
(b) LRTI
(c) Urinary
(d) Blood stream

1464. Dabigatran monitoring:
(a) No need (b) Anti Xa
(c) APPT

1465. Hypophosphatemia A/E:
(a) Respiratory failure (b) Hypocalciuria
(c) Metabolic encephalopathy

1466. Gittleman syndrome A/E:
(a) High BP (b) Hypomagnesia
(c) Metabolic alkalosis (d) Hypoaldosteronism

1467. Sepsis A/E:
(a) Cold skin (b) Oliguria
(c) AG academia (d) Restlessness

1468. O_2 delivery to peripheral tissue depend in A/E:
(a) Hb conc (b) CO
(c) MVO_2 saturation (d) Arterial O_2 saturation

1469. All are reverse transcriptase inhibitor *except*:
(a) Abacavir (b) Tenofovir
(c) Amprenavir (d) Entracitabine

1470. Atypical antipsychotic A/E:
(a) Haloperidol (b) Resperidone
(c) Olanzepine (d) Clozapine

1471. Wrong match:
(a) Epidemic typhus–louse
(b) RMSF–flea
(c) Scrub typhus–mite
(d) Trench fever–louse

1472. 65 years female with 30 years of biogas use, 6 months of non productive cough with progressive breathlessness, 2 months of wheeze, investigation in series:
(a) Sputum AFB, CXR, Spirometry
(b) CXR, sputum AFB, Spirometry
(c) CXR, Spirometry, sputum AFB
(d) Sputum AFB, Spirometry, CXR

1473. Drug used in scorpion sting:
(a) Prazocin (b) Amlodipine
(c) Atropine (d) Propranolol

1474. Thyroid Ca A/E:
(a) Differentiated Ca–surgery primary treatment
(b) Post operative metastasis–radioiodine should be given
(c) Levothyroxine should be avoided in distant metastasis
(d) Thyroglobulin–marker of choice in post operative further investigation

1475. False negative test:
(a) 1–sensitivity
(b) 1–specificity
(c) 1–false positive
(d) Identify patient without disease

1476. Chylothorax A/E:
(a) TG > 110 mg%
(b) Cholesterol > 250 mg%

(c) Lymphocyte predominant
(d) Sudan stain positive

1477. Shoyhoi fever caused by:
(a) Burdorferi mallei
(b) B. cepeci
(c) Pseudomonas aeruginosa
(d) Franciscella tularensis

1478. Normal PT, APTT, platelet with:
(a) Factor XIII deficiency
(b) Factor VIII deficiency
(c) Severe liver disease
(d) Factor V leiden

1479. Pregnancy A/E:
(a) Continuous murmur
(b) EDM
(c) Exaggerated pulmonary component of S2
(d) Loud S1

1480. ATT drugs A/E:
(a) Rifampicin (b) Aminoglycoside
(c) Ciprofloxacin (d) Amphotericin B

1481. Colistin active agent A/E:
(a) Actinobactericae (b) Pseudomonas
(c) E coli (d) Staph aureus

1482. Aztreonam A/E:
(a) Effect on Gram negative
(b) No effect on anaerobes
(c) No effect on gram positive
(d) Cross sensitive against penicillin

1483. TH1 cell response augmented by:
(a) IL-4 (b) IL-5
(c) IFN α (d) IFN γ

1484. Large vessel vasculitis:
(a) Kawasaki
(b) Temporal arteritis
(c) PAN
(d) Churg Strauss syndrome

1485. IgG deposit in BM:
(a) Goodpasture's disease
(b) Membranous nephritis
(c) Alport-split BM disease
(d) Nail patella syndrome

1486. Pulmonary artery aneurysm in A/E:
(a) Wegener granulomatosis
(b) Behcet's disease
(c) Takayasu arteritis
(d) Giant cell arteritis

1487. Bacillary angiomatosis:
(a) Bartonella
(b) Gardenerella
(c) Mycobacterium
(d) No relation with bacterial infection

1488. Fabry disease A/E:
(a) AR
(b) Thin wall LV
(c) Angiokeratoma
(d) Symptoms more common in female

1489. Kussmaul's sign A/E:
(a) CCP (b) CHF
(c) VSD (d) TS

1490. Calceneurin inhibitor:
(a) Tacrolimus
(b) Sirolimus
(c) Mycophenolate mofetil
(d) Azathioprine

1491. Cryoprecipitate contains A/E:
(a) Fibrinogen (b) VWF
(c) Factor VII (d) Factor VIII

1492. Weight loss with fever A/E:
(a) RCC (b) Thyrotoxicosis
(c) Pheochromocytoma (d) TB

1493. AA amyloidosis seen A/E:
(a) RA (b) Leprosy
(c) Alzheimer's disease (d) FMF

1494. Benzidine test:
(a) Myoglobin (b) Porphobilinogen
(c) Bilirubin (d) Glucose

1495. False +ve guaic test for occult blood A/E:
(a) Red meat
(b) Vit C intake
(c) Fasting and less fluid intake
(d) Vegetables brochioli and red turnip

1496. Pleural fluid eosinophilia seen in:
(a) Microfilaria (b) TB
(c) Bronchogenic Ca (d) Hydropneumothorax
(e) All of the above

1497. Urine Analysis useful A/E:
(a) Barbiturate overdose (b) Choriocarcinoma
(c) Steroid abuse (d) Porphyria (AIP)
(e) All of the above

1498. Interstitial fibrosis all ↓se *except*:
(a) FRC (b) FVC
(c) FEV1 (d) FFV1/FVC

1499. Pulmonary rehabilitation is useful for A/E:
(a) Improved pulmonary function
(b) Dyspnoea desensitization
(c) Motivation ↑se
(d) ↑se mechanical skin

1500. COPD in smokers:
(a) <20% (b) 20-33%
(c) 33-50% (d) >50%

1501. Prion disease:
(a) Fatal familial insomnia
(b) Huntington disease
(c) Pick's disease
(d) Alzeihemer's disease

1502. Sternal angle demarcate:
(a) T2 (b) T3
(c) T4 (d) T1

1503. Not freely excreted in capillary of glomeruli:
(a) Creatinine (b) Thyroxine
(c) Bicarbonate (d) Glucose

1504. Hirsutism seen A/E:
(a) Acromegaly (b) Hyperthyroidism
(c) Cushing (d) Hyper prolactinemia

1505. Which Antibiotic can penetrate respiratory secretion?
(a) Quinolone (b) Newer macrolides
(c) Aminoglycoside (d) Clindamycin

1506. Hepatorenal syndrome A/E:
(a) Urino osmolality < plasma osmolality
(b) Urine Na <10
(c) Sr Na < 130
(d) Proteinuria < 500 mg%

1507. Tumour lysis syndrome A/E:
(a) Hyperkalemia (b) Hypercalcemia
(c) Hyperuricemia (d) Hyperphosphatemia

1508. Unilateral ventricular dilatation with hydrophosphaturia:
(a) Foramen Monro
(b) Foramen Lushka
(c) Foramen Magendie's
(d) SA space

1509. ↑ MCV is A/E:
(a) Sideroblastic (b) Hypothyroidism
(c) MDS (d) Megaloblastic

1510. Sickle cell mutation:
(a) Mis sense (b) Non sense
(c) Polymorphum (d) Deletion

1511. Hydatid cyst-pericyst in lung formed by:
(a) Germinal layer
(b) Blood capsule
(c) Pleura
(d) Compressed atelectatic lung

1512. LAD is characterstic of:
(a) Ebstein Anomaly (b) TA
(c) TOF (d) TAPVC

1513. Tracheobronchial aspiration not associated with swallowing seen in A/E:
(a) Achalasia cardia (b) GERD
(c) Globus hystericus (d) Zenker diverticulum

1514. Pseudotumour cerebri seen in A/E:
(a) Venous sinus thrombous
(b) Hyperthyroidism
(c) Hyper PTH
(d) Hypervitaminosis A

1515. Pulse oximetry false +ve:
(a) Methemoglobinemia (b) HCT < 30%
(c) Fetal Hb (d) Severe jaundice

1516. ↑T3, ↑T4, ↓TSH, ↓se RAIU:
(a) Hashimoto thyroiditis
(b) Subacute thyroiditis
(c) Toxic nodular goitre
(d) Graves' disease

1517. Non modulating essential hypertension A/E:

(a) ACE I correct pathophysiology
(b) Low renin activity
(c) Insulin resistance
(d) More commom in post menopausal

1518. Acute leukemia TLC 200 × 10^9 primary treatment A/E:

(a) Leukopharesis (b) BM examination
(c) Low dose cytarabine (d) Hydroxyurea

1519. CD 13 and CD33 +ve, MPO +ve early treatment A/E:

(a) Steroids (b) Hydration
(c) Low dose cytarabine (d) Allopurinol

1520. ↑T_3 and T_4↓ TSH and radioactive iodine uptake, diagnosis:

(a) Hashimoto (b) Graves
(c) Toxic nodular goiter (d) Subacute thyroiditis

1521. Ph = 7.3, pO_2 = 60, pcO_2= 50, P(A – a) gradient:

(a) 28 (b) 40
(c) 20 (d) 35

1522. D – dimer true about:

(a) High negative predictive value
(b) Useful in pulmonary thromboembolism in hospitalised patient
(c) Estimated by PCR
(d) Increased in acute MI

1523. Pain in pulmonary disease occurs due to:

(a) Visceral pleura (b) Perivascular sheath
(c) Interstitium (d) Alveoli

1524. SVO_2 Max. in which shock?

(a) Septic shock (b) Hypovolemic shock
(c) Neurogenic shock (d) Cardiogenic shock

1525. Relapsing polychondritis characterised by:

(a) Sparing of ear lobes
(b) Eye involvement at presentation
(c) Rapidly progressive renal failure
(d) Bronchiolitis obliterans

1526. Superior vena cava thrombosis, treatment before definite diagnosis:

(a) CT (b) Radiotherapy
(c) CT + Radiotherapy (d) Endovascular stenting

1527. Rituximab best medicine in which lymphoma?

(a) Diffuse large B cell lymphoma
(b) Burkitts
(c) Precursor T cell
(d) Mycosis fungoides

1528. NHL international prognostic index A/E:

(a) B_2 microglobulin
(b) Age > 60
(c) Ann arbour III/IV
(d) More than one extranodal site

1529. Aztreoname A/E:

(a) Active against gram –ve
(b) Inactive against gram +ve
(c) Inactive against anerobes
(d) Cross reactivity with patients sensitive to penicillin

1530. Friedreich's ataxia A/E:

(a) Diabetes insipidus (b) Diabetes mellitus
(c) Cushing (d) ILD

1531. Inhalational anthrax characteristic finding in CXR:

(a) Mediastinal widening and pleural effusion
(b) Interstitial infiltrates and pleural effusion
(c) Bilateral lobar consolidation
(d) Right consolidation and contralateral pleural effusion

1532. Actinomycosis treatment A/E:

(a) Penicillin (b) Amoxicillin
(c) Tetracycline (d) Oxacillin

1533. Arterial thrombosis associated with:

(a) APLA
(b) Protein C deficiency
(c) Prothrombin gene mutation
(d) Factor V leiden

1534. Insulin resistance A/E:

(a) Hirsutism (b) Acne
(c) Central obesity (d) Moon facies

1535. Takayasu arteritis fundus finding A/E:

(a) Venous dilation (b) AV shunt
(c) Papilledema (d) Hard exudates

1536. Ataxia telangiectasia associated with:

(a) Ovarian agenesis

(b) Positive response to live vaccine
(c) Thymus is normal
(d) Pulmonary infection is uncommon

1537. Pulmonary alveolar proteinosis A/E:
(a) BAL may be beneficial
(b) Normal serum surfactant level
(c) Increase LDH
(d) Bat wing appearance bilateral

1538. HCV 2 genotype A/E:
(a) Ribaverin + INF for 24 weeks
(b) Ribaverin + INF for 48 weeks
(c) INF for 24 weeks
(d) INF for 48 weeks

1539. Congenital heart block indication of pacing A/E:
(a) Asymptomatic HR > 60
(b) Cardiomegaly on CXR
(c) CHF
(d) Chronotropic incompetence

1540. Complete heart block associated with:
(a) Endocardial cushion defect
(b) Muscular VSD
(c) Truncus arteriosus
(d) Bicuspid aortic valve

1541. Aortic root dilation A/E:
(a) Bicuspid aortic valve + stenosis
(b) Rheumatic AS
(c) TOF + pulmonary atresia
(d) Marfan

1542. Acute severe AR vs chronic AR A/E:
(a) Loud S_1 (b) LV S_3
(c) LV S_4 (d) Austin flint murmur

1543. LA enlargement absent in:
(a) Lutembacher (b) Secundum ASD
(c) PDA (d) ECD

1544. Renal infarct occurs in:
(a) Candida (b) Coccidioidomycosis
(c) Pneumocystis (d) Apophycomycosis

1545. Peritoneal dialysis not effective in:
(a) Fluid overload (b) Hyperkalemia
(c) Metabolic acidosis (d) Uremic encephalopathy

1546. Overflow proteinuria:
(a) MCD (b) Amyloid
(c) Fanconi (d) Multiple myeloma

1547. MCD A/E:
(a) In adult less response to treatment than children
(b) Relapse rate after remission more common in adult
(c) Steroid dependent patients may be responsive to cyclophosphamide
(d) Adult and children are treated for 6 weeks for first time

1548. Small vessel vasculitis:
(a) PAN
(b) Churg-Strauss syndrome
(c) Takayasu arteritis
(d) Giany cell arteritis

1549. Development upto terminal bronchiole occur in:
(a) 8 weeks (b) 12 weeks
(c) 16 weeks (d) 28 weeks

1550. Surfactant A/E:
(a) Secreted by type II pneumocytes
(b) Bronchial glands also produce it
(c) Secretion after > 28 weeks gestation
(d) Best hopeful agent in ARDS

1551. C4–C8 lesion A/E:
(a) Decreased FEV1/FVC
(b) Decreased FVC
(c) Absent tidal percussion on the side of lesion
(d) Decreased peak inspiratory

1552. Airway resistance primary suggested by:
(a) Forced expiration time
(b) Lung compliance
(c) TLC
(d) Slow vital capacity

1553. Indication of ICD drainage:
(a) Rheumatoid arthritis with ILD–pleural fluid glucose < 30 mg%
(b) Post traumatic hemothorax HCT=30%
(c) Left sided massive pleural effusion with right breast Ca and mediastinal shift
(d) Opaque hemithorax + ipsilateral mediastinal shift

1554. Anemia true A/E:
(a) Western women Hb = 12.5 g%

(b) At birth Hb = 17 g%
(c) Celiac disease–macrocytic anemia
(d) Normocytic normochromic anemia in anemia of chronic disease

1555. Massive splenomegaly A/E:
(a) Chronic myelomonocytic leukemia
(b) Hairy cell leukemia
(c) Sarcoidosis
(d) Gaucher's disease

1556. Microcytic hypochromic anemia A/E:
(a) Sideroblastic anemia (b) Thalassemia
(c) AIHA (d) Celiac disease

1557. Infarction on CT scan all early signs *except*:
(a) Loss of gray/white differentiation
(b) Insular ribbon sign
(c) Sulcal effacement
(d) Hypodensity

1558. Drug induced lupus not seen:
(a) Anti histone Ab common
(b) Serositis
(c) Renal involvement
(d) Anti dsDNA rare

1559. Hemorrhage best seen in MRI:
(a) GRE (b) DWI
(c) T2 Weighted (d) T1 Weighted

1560. Pure motor neuropathy all *except*:
(a) Lead (b) Dapsone
(c) Pyridoxine excess (d) Hypoglycemia

1561. IgA nephropathy is associated with:
(a) Cirrhosis
(b) Gluten hypersensitivity
(c) Purpura fulminans
(d) Dermatitis herpetiformis

1562. All are true about TSS *except*:
(a) Blood culture +ve (b) Fever
(c) Shock (d) Renal failure

1563. Stroke associated with cardiac arrhythmias:
(a) Frontal lobe (b) Occipital lobe
(c) Right midbrain (d) Right insula

1564. HCV genotype all *except*:
(a) Type II–6 months therapy
(b) Type I–6 months treatment
(c) Type I is less responsibe to treatment
(d) Type III–6 months therapy

1565. Status epilepticus can be ppt by:
(a) Sertraline (b) Pantoprazole
(c) Imi-cella (d) Lisinopril HCTZ

1566. Raynaud's phenomenon can be treated by all *except*:
(a) CCB (b) ACE-I
(c) ARB (d) Sildenafil

1567. All the following are D/D of heat stroke:
(a) Viral encephalitis
(b) Benign intracranial HTN
(c) ICH
(d) Valproate toxicity

1568. True about heat stroke:
(a) Classical is common in young male
(b) Exertion HS is common in trained athletes
(c) Classical is seen associated with increased production of heat and exertional is seen associated with decrease dissipation
(d) Classical is seen associated with products of heat and exertional is seen associated with ed dissipation

1569. H5 N1 drug which is used is:
(a) Zanamivir (b) Zidovudine
(c) Nevirapine (d) Efavirenz

1570. Not used in treatment of acute gout:
(a) NSAIDS (b) Probenecid
(c) Colchicine (d) ACTH

1571. Antiepileptic causing depression:
(a) Phenobarbitone (b) Carbamazepine
(c) Valproate (d) Phenytoin

1572. Antiepileptic least/no interaction with OCP:
(a) Oxcarbamazepine (b) Carbamazepine
(c) Valproate (d) Topiramate

1573. Risk factor for NSAID induced mucosal injury *except*:
(a) Male (b) Streptococci
(c) Old age (d) NSAID with CST

1574. CSF shunt infection (Most common organism):
(a) Staph. (b) Strept.
(c) E. coli (d) Pseudomonas

1575. Colistin is not used in treatment of:

(a) Staph aureus (b) Acinetobacter

(c) Pseudomonas (d) E. Coli

1576. Daptomycin is not effective against staph. at which site:

(a) Lung (b) Skin

(c) Subcutaneous tissue (d) Septicemia

1577. Weaning from ventilator (which is not indicator):

(a) Vital capacity > 10l/minute

(b) PEEP < 5

(c) $PO_2 > 60$ on $FiO_2 < 50\%$

(d) Static compliance > 30 cm/H_2O

1578. Post transplant after 6 months which is not a common infection: (T/F)

(a) CMV (b) PCP

(c) Nocardia (d) Aspergillosis

1579. Physical sign indication (not primary poly-cythemia):

(a) Cyanosis (b) Aquatic pruritus

(c) Bruising easy (d) Splenomegaly

1580. Rabies is not associated with bite of:

(a) Rat (b) Raccon

(c) Fox (d) Bat

1581. Microcytic hypochromic anemia is seen in all *except*:

(a) Celiac disease

(b) Sideroblastic

(c) Thalassemia

(d) Anemia of Chronic Disease

1582. Not a protease inhibitor:

(a) Nelfinavir (b) Ritonavir

(c) Lopinavir (d) Tenofovir

1583. Good prognosis in IPF A/E:

(a) Young age

(b) Current smoker

(c) Male sex

(d) Predominant cellular histology

1584. γ-APC is used in cases of:

(a) APACHE > 25

(b) APACHE < 25

(c) Single organ involve

(d) None of the above

1585. Anti centromere antibodies is associated with:

(a) Limited SSC (b) Diffuse SSC

(c) MCTD (d) Overlap syndrome

1586. Calcification on CT least commonly found in:

(a) Meningioma (b) Ependymoma

(c) Oligodendroglioma (d) Craniopharyngioma

1587. Uveitis/arthritis/erythema nodosum:

(a) Lofgren's syndrome (b) Heerford's syndrome

(c) Loffler's syndrome (d) Fowler's syndrome

1588. Male hypogonadism:

(a) Low testosterone is not a risk factor

(b) Waist hip ratio versus BMI–BMI more important

(c) Inverse relation between metabolic syndrome and testosterone

1589. Clinical trials all *except*:

(a) Ethical committee permission not mandatory

1590. A young patient 1 month fever, gross splenomegaly, pancytopenia:

(a) Oral miltefosine (b) IV ciprofloxacin

(c) IV paromomycin (d) Amphotericin B

1591. Patient with fever, petechiae, Hb–5 g%, TLC–9000, Neutrophil–2%, lymphocyte–96%, Which is supportive treatment?

(a) Oral ciprofloxacin (b) IV ciprofloxacin

(c) G-CSF (d) Packed RBC

1592. Hepatorenal syndrome not a diagnostic criteria:

(a) Proteinuria > 500 (b) Low GFR

(c) Absence of shock (d) RBC <50

1593. RA which drug in not used?

(a) Rituximab (b) Methotrexate

(c) Abatacept (d) Interferon α

1594. Prolonged plalelet inhibition (delayed recovery) is found with:

(a) Abciximab (b) Tirofiban

(c) Eptifibatide (d) Infliximab

1595. Systemic antifungal of choice is:

(a) IV AMB (b) Fluconazole

(c) Nystatin

1596. Not a revised ACR criteria for RA:

(a) Morning stiffness for 1 hour
(b) Anti CCP +ve
(c) Anti RA +ve
(d) Rheumatoid nodule

1597. Which is not risk factor for cholelithiasis?

(a) Pregnancy (b) High protein diet
(c) Obesity (d) Hemolytic anaema

1598. Pancreatic cancer true is:

(a) 5 years survival–5%
(b) Mean age of diagnosis–49
(c) At presentation is mostly amenable to surgery
(d) Most common site for adeno Ca is tail

1599. Which is not a recent marker for atherosclerosis?

(a) RA (b) Small dense HDL
(c) Hypofibrinogenemia (d) Lp(a)

1600. Not a feature of relapsing polychondritis:

(a) ILD (b) Aortic root dilatation
(c) Auricular chondritis (d) Nose involvement

1601. Not used in acute gout:

(a) Colchicine (b) Corticosteroids
(c) ACTH (d) Probenecid

1602. Not used in RA:

(a) IFN-α (b) Rituximab
(c) Abatacept (d) Methotrexate

1603. Not a cause for hemoptysis in MI:

(a) Pulmonary venous HT
(b) Pulmonary artery HTN
(c) Resolving pneumonia
(d) Pulmonary edema

1604. IBD (UC) not a feature:

(a) Current smoker
(b) Age 15-30 years
(c) Appendix intact
(d) Fraternal sister not affected

1605. MCHC anemia A/E:

(a) Anemia of chronic disease
(b) Sideroblastic anemia
(c) Thalassemia
(d) Celiac disease

1606. Correlation between two functional status markers is 0.8:

(a) 80% fall on regression line
(b) 64% fall on regression line
(c) 80% variation can be explained by other factor
(d) 64% variation can be explained by other factor

1607. Extracorpuscular hemolysis:

(a) TTP (b) Sickle cell anemia
(c) PNH (d) Elliptocytosis

1608. APC given in:

(a) APACHE > 25
(b) Single organ involvement
(c) APACHE < 25
(d) None of the above

1609. Not a Protease inhibitor:

(a) Indinavir (b) Tenofovir
(c) Nelfinavir (d) Ropinavir

1610. Which does not ↑ renin:

(a) β Blocker (b) ACE-I
(c) α-blocker (d) ECF–contraction

1611. LGBS occurs in HIV in:

(a) Early in course (b) Late HIV
(c) Irrespective of stage (d) Failure of ART

1612. Large fibre neuropathy:

(a) Taxol (b) Cisplatin
(c) Pyridoxine (d) All of the above

1613. Trypanosoma and N. gonorrhoea develops resistance to host by:

(a) Activation of pre-existing genes
(b) Acquiring fertility plasmids by transduction
(c) Acquiring fertility plasmids by conjugation
(d) Mutation in hot spots

1614. Hypercalcemia hypophosphatemia in a patient with left upper lobe mass:

(a) Adeno Ca
(b) Small cell Ca
(c) Squamous cell Ca
(d) Bronchoalveolar carcinoma

1615. Not a feature of hypercalcemia:

(a) Diarrhoea (b) Polyuria
(c) Confusion (d) Nephrolithiasis

1616. S. Protein–9 mg%, Albumin–3.2 mg%, axillary cutaneous Manifestation, cardiac-renal neuropathy diagnosis by:

(a) Fat pad biopsy (b) Bone marrow biopsy
(c) RV catheterisation (d) Renal ultrasound

1617. Anti-centromere antibodies:

(a) Diffuse SSc (b) MCTD
(c) Limited SS (d) Overlap syndrome

1618. PFT in patient of myasthenia gravis:

(a) ↓ TLC, ↑ RV, ↓ MIC, Normal FFV1/FVC
(b) ↓ TLC, ↑ RV, ↓ MIC, ↓ FFV1/FVC
(c) ↑ TLC, ↓ RV, ↓ MIC, Normal FFV1/FVC

1619. Classical sign of foramen magnum herniation:

(a) Ipsilateral pupillary dilatation (3rd Nerve compression)
(b) Locked-in state
(c) Miotic pupil
(d) Respiratory arrest

1620. Subacute thyroiditis:

	T3	T4	TSH	Radioactive I uptake
(a)	↑	↑	↓	↑
(b)	↑	↑	N	↑
(c)	↓	↓	↑	USG mass
(d)	↓	↓	↑	Painful thyroid for 4 months

1621. Heat seizure treatment of Choice:

(a) Clonazepam (b) Valproate
(c) Benzodiazepine (d) Phenytoin

1622. Anorexia nervosa all *except*:

(a) Exercise exclusively
(b) Avoid food related occupation
(c) Distortion of body image
(d) Rarely complain of hunger

1623. Male hypogonadism:

(a) Primary failure–does not have ↑ gonadotrophin
(b) Secondary failure–does not have Normal gonadotrophin
(c) ↓ bone density, obesity, muscle loss, ↑ fat deposit are some of signs
(d) Normal libido

1624. ↑ IgM without involvement of helper T-cell:

(a) Penicillin–BSA complex bovine S. albumin
(b) Toxic shock syndrome Ag
(c) Tetanus toxin
(d) Bacterial polysaccharide

1625. Vit D related ↑ Ca++ all *except:*

(a) Sarcoidosis
(b) Hyperthyroidism
(c) Idiopathic hypercalcemia of infancy
(d) Vit D intoxication

1626. MHC class I and II most appropriate statement:

(a) Activation of complement
(b) Presentation of Ag by macrophage to cause phagocytosis
(c) Stimulation of B cell to cause precipitation and neutralisation
(d) Not specific stimulation of T cell

1627. Absolute indication for IE–Surgery all *except:*

(a) Moderate to severe HF
(b) Vegetation > 10 mm
(c) Myocardial abscess
(d) Relapsed prosthetic valve endocarditis

1628. Good clinical practice A/E:

(a) IRB and ethical committee review is not essential
(b) Informed consent taken
(c) Detail protocols explained
(d) Benefit of patient comes ahead of benefit of trial

1629. OA-75 years old, DM, obese most potent risk factor:

(a) Age (b) Obesity
(c) Gender (d) Previous injury

1630. Polyarthritis, uveitis, erythema nodosum in sarcoidosis:

(a) Loffler's syndrome
(b) Loffgren's syndrome
(c) Heerford's syndrome
(d) Fowler's syndrome

1631. DNA and RNA presents in:

(a) Bacteria (b) Virus
(c) Prion (d) Plasmid

1632. Keith-Wegener classification class III:

(a) AV nipping
(b) Silver wiring
(c) Flame shaped hemorrhage
(d) Papilloedema

1633. Which of following not required for DTR:

(a) α-neuron (b) γ-motor
(c) Pyramidal tract (d) Spinal efferent

1634. Ascitis– differentiating point between SVC obstruction and cirrhosis (intrinic):

(a) Blood flow towards umbilicus
(b) Pulsatile liver
(c) Venous hum at umbilicus
(d) Bulging flanks

1635. NSAID induced mucosal injury risk factor A/E:

(a) Steroids (b) Age
(c) Male gender (d) Severe infection

1636. Headache A/E:

(a) Hypoxia (b) Hypercapnia
(c) Hyperglycemia (d) Hypoglycemia

1637. 72 years old male, smoker, HTN, lytic lesion in lumbar vertebra, backache during lying–relieved on waking up/raised ALP, most likely is:

(a) Non small cell carcinoma
(b) Osteosarcoma
(c) Ca-pancrea
(d) Gastric Ca

1638. Intra corpuscular hemolytic anemia A/E:

(a) Microangiopathic hemolytic anemia
(b) Hemoglobinopathies
(c) Enzyme deficiency
(d) PNH

1639. Ca prostate with hypercalcemia – 12.4 mg% with S. Creat. – 4.2 mg % with altered sensorium with dry tongue treatment A/E:

(a) Fluids (NS)
(b) Furosemide when euvolumia
(c) Pomidronate
(d) Dexamethasone

1640. Peripheral vertigo signifies A/E:

(a) Bidirectional (b) Spin towards fast
(c) Fall towards slow (d) Tinnitis

1641. Trial of portal vein thrombosis with hemolysis and pancytopemia seen in:

(a) PNH
(b) TTP
(c) HUS
(d) Pro-myelocytic leukemia

1642. Palpable purpura A/E:

(a) Ecthyma gangrenosum
(b) Livedoid vasculitis
(c) Leucocytoclastic vasculitis
(d) PAN

1643. Clopidogrel – mech of action:

(a) P2Y12 ADP receptor blockade
(b) Cyclooxygenase blockade

1644. AD in A/E:

(a) Hemochromatosis
(b) Non-polyposis hereditary polyposis coli
(c) Basal cell nevus syndrome

1645. Thrombocytosis (> 6,00,000) in A/E:

(a) IDA (b) Pernicious anemia
(c) MDS (d) CML

1646. Deficiency of which leads to cardiomyopathy:

(a) Selenium (b) Zn
(c) Mn (d) Phosphorous

1647. Influenza vaccination true is:

(a) Intramuscular injection causes GBS–is to be explained to patient
(b) Egg allergy is C/I
(c) A and B strain of influenza made from last year strain
(d) Flu mist is inactivated vaccine

1648. Influenza indicated in A/E:

(a) Age > 65 years
(b) 1st trimester pregnancy
(c) Nursing home personal
(d) Household members of high risk persons

1649. CEA is a marker of A/E:

(a) Colon (b) Lung
(c) Thyroid (d) Pancreas

1650. In I.E. embolic risk maximum in:

(a) 5 mm vegetation on mitral valve
(b) 5 mm vegetation on tricuspid valve
(c) 11 mm vegetation on mitral valve
(d) 11 mm vegetation on aortic valve

1651. Invasive aspergillosis least likely in:
(a) GVHD
(b) HIV
(c) Post solid organ transplant with frequent rejection
(d) Leukemia

1652. HIV surveillance used A/E:
(a) Chronic ulcer with HSV
(b) Extra-pulmonary cryptococeosis
(c) Oropharyngeal candidiasis
(d) M. Tuberculosis

1653. Latent TB should be looked for in all HIV patients because of many reasons *except:*
(a) Drug interaction difficiult to manage
(b) At 6 months, HIV related mortality is increased
(c) ↓ efficacy of anti–TB drugs
(d) Extrapulmonary TB more common

1654. C- ANCA in A/E:
(a) Wegener granulomatosis
(b) Churg-Strauss syndrome
(c) Microscopic polyangitis
(d) PAN

1655. Valsalva maneuver ↑ murmur in:
(a) HOCM (b) MS
(c) MR (d) AR

1656. Kala-azar with symptoms, true is:
(a) Splenic aspirate has highest field
(b) Blood counts can be normal on Peripheral Smear
(c) Cell mediated immunity may be present in this patient
(d) Treatment can be started after confirmation of diognosis

1657. Interstitial nephritis A/E:
(a) Lymphoma (b) Leptospirosis
(c) Sulphonamide (d) Vasculitis

1658. Hepatitis B female patient wants to become pregnant, monogamous relationship, IV drug user, non-alcoholic true is:
(a) 2 doses 1 month apart
(b) C/I in 1st trimester
(c) In this patient, hepatitis serology to be done before vaccinations
(d) Indicated in only high risk patients

1659. AF with risk of stroke A/E:
(a) Spontaneous echo contrast in LA
(b) HTN
(c) LAA velocity > 20 cm/sec
(d) Complex atheroma in aorta

1660. ST ↑ A/E:
(a) Brugada syndrome (b) Prinzmental angina
(c) Hyperthermia (d) Pericarditis (Acute)

1661. Diabetic female with mucormycosis true is:
(a) Immediate biopsy followed by liposomal AMB
(b) Immediate biopsy followed by voriconazole
(c) Biopsy to r/o anthrax
(d) Antibiotics

1662. Cardiac cath ↑ mortality in A/E:
(a) Right coronary disease
(b) Renal failure
(c) Valvular heart disease
(d) Class IV symptoms

1663. Congenital acyanotic disease without a shunt A/E:
(a) MS
(b) PS
(c) ALCAPA
(d) Ruptured sinus of valsalva aneurysm

1664. A 64 years male collapsed suddenly on football ground–monitor s/o ventricular fibriliation true is:
(a) Immediate defibrillate with 300-360 J, if it fails, CPR for 60-90 secs and then repeat
(b) Continuous CPR for 5 min, then defibrillate
(c) IV access and amiodarone
(d) ET intubation followed by defibrillation

1665. Female, 5 mm redness at right nasolabial fold, ↑es to 5 cm with pain followed by–flaccid bulla tender (within 2 days), treatment is:
(a) Penicillin
(b) Penicillin + clindamycin
(c) Clindamycin
(d) Acyclovir

1666. CHD in adults complications A/E:
(a) PHT (b) Eisenmeger
(c) Stroke (d) IE

1667. Past history of TB, presented with abdominal distension with edema, CT s/o pericardial calcification true in:

(a) Rapid descent in JVP (b) Double apical impulse
(c) Opening snap (d) Cannon a wave

1668. Framingham major A/E:

(a) Hepatomegaly
(b) Cardiomegaly
(c) Rales
(d) Neck vein engorgement

1669. Episodic palpitations with headache postural fall of BP in a female best investigation for diagnosis:

(a) Serum catecholamines
(b) 24 hours urine for HIA
(c) 24 hours urine for VMA + metanephrines
(d) Renal vein sampling for renin

1670. Post renal transplant, 1-6 months opportunistic infection A/E:

(a) BK virus (b) Legionella
(c) CMV (d) PCP

1671. Which does not help in differentiating hyperbilirubinemia induced jaundice from other causes?

(a) Greenish discolouration of skin
(b) Present in nasolabial fold
(c) Involves palms and soles
(d) Does not effect non-sun exposed area

1672. MEN I A/E:

(a) Pheochromocytoma (b) Parathyroid adenoma
(c) Lichen amyloidosis (d) Islet cell hyperplasia

1673. GI bleeding –upper GI endoscopy done–which is s/o least risk of bleeding after 3 days?

(a) Clean base ulcer
(b) Adherent clot
(c) Ulcer with AV malformation
(d) Non bleeding vessel seen

1674. Most characteristic symptom of carcinoid:

(a) Flushing (b) Pain
(c) Diarrhoea (d) Asthma

1675. HIV with CD-4 count : 21, Patient on fluconazole, septran and ethambutol rifabutin develop pancreatitis next step is:

(a) Replace clarithromycin with azithromycin
(b) Stop co-trimoxazole
(c) Stop co-trimoxazole replace with dapsone
(d) Replace fluconazole with AMB

1676. Hemophagocytosis syndrome A/E:

(a) Spenomegaly
(b) Pancytopenia
(c) Hypertriglyceridemia
(d) Hyperphosphatemia

1677. VAP-ET aspirate CFU to differentiate between colonization and infection:

(a) 10^2 (b) 10^3
(c) 10^4 (d) 10^5

1678. VAP-decrease incidence:

(a) Close vs open suctioning
(b) Nasopharyngeal vs oropharyngeal intubation
(c) Interruption of sedation for checking respiratory effect
(d) Chlorhexidine 0.2% frequent instillation

1679. Least likely causing gastric ulcer:

(a) Cryptosporidium (b) H. pylori
(c) T. pallidium (d) CMV

1680. Severe malaria–include A/E:

(a) Thrombocytopenia (b) Lactic acidosis
(c) Renal failure (d) Splenomegaly

1681. Earthquake victim – acute injury prevention:

(a) Starting I.V. hydration even when trapped
(b) Soda bicarb
(c) Mannitol
(d) Prophylactic dialysis

1682. Young female DKA, Na^+= 149, K= 5.2, HCO_3=12, glucose= 549 mg%, S. creat.=2.1, urine ketones= 4+ : initial treatment of choice:

(a) ½ NS+ insulin (b) NS+insulin
(c) NS+insulin+HCO_3

1683. 70 years/female with chronic fatigue CD=20+/23+/5+, HCT=38.2, TLC=98,000 DLC=P-45, L-50, M3, E2, treatment:

(a) Observation
(b) Chlorambucil + prednisolone
(c) BMT
(d) Chlorodeoxyadenosone

1684. P. aeroginosa MDR gene:

(a) TEM (b) SHU
(c) AMPc (d) CTM

1685. Imipenem-cilastin combination rationale:

(a) Inhibit renal degrading enzyme of imipenem

1686. APC given in:

(a) APACHE > 25
(b) APACHE<25
(c) Single ogan involvement
(d) None of the above

1687. Renal failure true:

(a) 5% doesn't recover
(b) ↓ mortality of 25% over 20 years
(c) Oliguric have poor prognosis than non-oliguric

1688. Which doesn't rule out prerenal cause of ARF?

(a) Urine Na^+ >20 (b) Osmolality < 200
(c) Erythrocyte cast (d) Absence of oliguria

1689. H1N1 all *except:*

(a) Paramyxoma family
(b) Pregnancy adverse outcome
(c) Spread by droplets
(d) Resistance to amantadine

1690. CJD–True:

(a) It can be inherited
(b) It is retroviral infection
(c) Limited to USA/Europe
(d) Peglated IF-α useful in treatment resistance

1691. Not used in RA:

(a) MTx (b) IF-α
(c) Abtacept (d) Rituximab

1692. Acute sarcoidosis with lymphadenopathy/erythema nodosum:

(a) Lofgren's syndrome (b) Loffler's syndrome
(c) Heerfordt syndrome

1693. Old lady with chronic deforming RA on MTx and NSAIDs, now present with indurated swelling in Elbow; febrile - 37.1°C:

(a) Intraarticular steroids + ↑ NSAIDS
(b) Add 10 mg predinsolone
(c) Diagnostic aspiration to rule out gout and infection
(d) Leflunamide addition

1694. Anticentromere antibody present in:

(a) Limited SS (b) Diffuse SS
(c) MCTD (d) Over lap syndrome

1695. OA A/E:

(a) Oral glucosaamine delay disease progression
(b) BMD is low
(c) Subchondral sclerosis and osteophytes and ↓ joint space
(d) TLC < 2000 in joint aspirate

1696. Microcytic hypochromic anemic:

(a) Celiac disease
(b) Thalassemia
(c) Anemia of chronic disease
(d) Sideroblastic anemia

1697. Which is not likely to cause vitamin B_{12} deficiency?

(a) Ileal malabsorption
(b) Strict vegetarian diet
(c) Oral antibiotic for 10 days
(d) Pancreatic exocrine insufficiency

1698. Dyspepsia with anemia (55 years/male) next line of investigation:

(a) Stool occult blood
(b) Prokinetic and PPI for 1 month
(c) UGI Endoscopy
(d) Sigmoidoscopy

1699. Na^+-120, S. Osmolality–264, urine osmolality–300, cigarette smoker, TFT–normal, mild asthma on albuterol, urine Na >48–Treatment:

(a) 3% NS (b) Fluid restriction
(c) NS infusion (d) Diuretics

1700. HTN+COPD with progressive dyspnea, which is best indicator of LV systolic dysfunction?

(a) Apical murmur grade IV radiating to axilla
(b) Recumbent dyspnea
(c) Pulsus alternans

1701. In patient with gastrinoma, other than octreotide scan, which investigation is sensitive?

(a) Endoscopic US (b) PET scan
(c) CT-abdomen (d) Transabdominal USG

1702. CHF, day 3 develop tachypnea, normal JVP, clean chest, no calf tenderness, next line of management:

(a) D-dimer
(b) CT-angiography
(c) Duplex USG
(d) Pulmonary angiography with cath.

1703. Leptospira – which is true?

(a) Peak during dry winter

(b) ME is uncommon presentation

(c) Case fatality 50-60%

(d) Easily demonstrated on biopsy

1704. OSA: Elderly female, Body Weight-110 kg, apnea index–30 per hour, next line management:

(a) Nasal oxygenation (b) MDPA

(c) Tracheostomy (d) Nasal CPAP

1705. Acute pancreatitis, not severity marker:

(a) S. amylase level

(b) CRP

(c) CT abdomen

(d) Urine trypsinogen level

1706. Not seen in heat stroke:

(a) Piloerection (b) Anhidrosis

(c) Coagulopathy (d) Core temp > 40°C

1707. Which is not seen in heat stroke?

(a) DIC (b) Thrombocytopenia

(c) Leukocytosis (d) Hemophagocytosis

1708. Rhabdomylosis true:

(a) Large volume of crystalloid

(b) Dextrose insulin 6 hourly

(c) Na HCO_3 infusion

1709. Which does not improve with PPD?

(a) Uremic encephalopathy

(b) Fluid overload

(c) ↑ K^+

(d) Metabolic acidosis

1710. Catheter associated UTI true:

(a) Majority develop bacterimia after 2 weeks

(b) Majority are symptomatic

(c) Prophylactic ciprofloxacin

(d) Povidone iodine periurethral

1711. Young hypogonadism true:

(a) Evening testosterone as screening test

(b) Equilibrium dialysis not seen now-a-days

(c) Testosterone can be started after DRE/PSA level

(d) Most testosterone is unbound

1712. Which is not seen in PTE?

(a) LV S3 gallop (b) Bilateral basal rales

(c) Tachypnea (d) Hemoptysis

1713. AVRT:

(a) ↓ during pregnancy

(b) SCD can occur in WPW syndrome due to VF

(c) In AF with WPW–verapamil is used

(d) Ablation is not possible due to AVRT

1714. Endogenous nephrotoxin A/E:

(a) Myoglobin (b) UA

(c) Oxalate (d) Aristocholic acid

1715. CHF trials drug not decreasing mortality:

(a) ACE-I (b) Metoprolol

(c) Spirinolactone (d) Digoxin

1716. Treatment of acute gout A/E:

(a) Colchicine (b) Probenecid

(c) ACTH (d) Steroid

1717. Sarcoid – uveitis + acute polyarthritis + enythema nodosum:

(a) Loeffler's syndrome

(b) Lofgren's syndrome

(c) Heerford's syndrome

(d) Fowler's syndrome

1718. Pulmonary arterial HTN:

(a) > 25 mm Hg at rest and exertion

(b) > 30 mm Hg at rest and exertion

(c) > 25 mm Hg at rest and > 30 mm Hg at exertion

(d) > 20 mm Hg at rest > 25 mm Hg at exertion

1719. See-saw nystagmus:

(a) Cerebeller lesion

(b) Tumour of 3rd ventricle

(c) CV junction anomaly

(d) Multiple sclerosis

1720. Small vessel vasculitis:

(a) Takayasu's arteritis (b) Giant cell arteritis

(c) PAN (d) Churg Strauss arteritis

1721. Activated protein C indicated in:

(a) Single organ involvement

(b) APACHE < 25

(c) APACHE > 25
(d) None of the above

1722. Absolute C/I of thrombolysis A/E:
(a) Trauma < 3 months
(b) Acute pericarditis
(c) Active peptic ulcer
(d) Intracranial hemorrhage

1723. Absolute C/I of stress test A/E:
(a) Myocarditis
(b) Unstable angina
(c) Acute MI < 2 days
(d) Asymptomatic severe AS

1724. Angiotensin gene mutation – HT—treatment:
(a) Clonidine (b) Ramipril
(c) Clinidipine (d) Sotalol

1725. Longest recovery of platelet function after:
(a) Abciximab (b) Eptifibatide
(c) Tirofiban (d) All of the above

1726. MRI acute hemorrhage diagnosis:
(a) Diffuse weighed image
(b) MR spectroscopy
(c) Guided echo
(d) Proton density image

1727. Most common neurological complication of pacli-texal:
(a) Motor neuropathy (b) Sensory neuropathy
(c) Encephalopathy (d) Multiple myoclonus

1728. UC in pregnancy:
(a) Flare up
(b) Abortion
(c) ↑ extracolonic manifestation
(d) Birth defect

1729. Most common organism in CSF shunt infection:
(a) Strept pneumococci
(b) Staph aureus
(c) Pseudomonas aeruginosa
(d) E. Coli

1730. Most common cause of bilateral trigeminal neuralgia:
(a) Vascular compression
(b) Idiopathic
(c) Multiple sclerosis
(d) Schwannoma

1731. Toxic shock syndrome A/E:
(a) Fever
(b) +ve blood culture
(c) Renal failure
(d) Macular desquamating erythroderma

1732. Ataxia telangiectasia true:
(a) Ovarian agenesis
(b) Thymus normal development
(c) +ve response to live vaccine
(d) Pulmonary infection less

1733. Highest risk of CVD at BP___ in 70 years male patient.
(a) 110/90 mm Hg (b) 120/96 mm Hg
(c) 140/80 mm Hg (d) 150/70 mm Hg

1734. Non modulating essential HT A/E:
(a) Low renin
(b) Pathology modulated by ACE-I
(c) More common in female
(d) Insulin resistance

1735. Arterial thrombosis:
(a) Antiphospholipid syndrome
(b) Factor – V mutation
(c) Protein – C deficiency
(d) Protein – C deficiency

1736. Acute leukaemia initial treatment A/E:
(a) Cytarabine low dose (b) BM examination
(c) Hydroxyurea (d) Leukapheresis

1737. Most common cause of venous thrombosis:
(a) Factor – V deficiency
(b) Prothrombin G 2021 A mutation
(c) Protein-C deficiency
(d) Protein-S deficiency

1738. Nephrolithiasis:
(a) Sequinavir (b) Indinavir
(c) Ritonavir (d) Nelfinavir

1739. X-ray picture in anthrax (Characteristic):
(a) Mediastinal widening + bilateral PE
(b) Mediastinal infiltration + pleural effusion
(c) Consolidation + contralateral PE

1740. Non cardiogenic cause of pulmonary edema A/E:
(a) Aspirin (b) Sepsis
(c) Pneumonia (d) Lung re-expansion

1741. Overflow proteinuria:
(a) Fanconi anemia
(b) Amyloidosis
(c) Minimal Change Disease
(d) Multiple myeloma

1742. Drugs used in RA A/E:
(a) Methotrexate (b) Rituximab
(c) IFN-α (d) Abtacept

1743. Most common Ab in Wegener's granulomatosis:
(a) ANA (b) C-ANCA
(c) P-ANCA

1744. Acute renal failure True:
(a) About 5% never recover
(b) Sepsis is less common cause
(c) Mortality far more in oliguric than nonoliguric RF
(d) ↓ed mortality over 25% in last 25 years

1745. Treatment before definitive diagnosis is SVC syndrome:
(a) Radiation
(b) Radiation + chemotherapy
(c) Chemotherapy
(d) Endovascular stent

1746. Alveolar- arterial O_2 difference- PaO_2- 50, $PaCO_2$-60, HCO_3-30 , pH- 7.36:
(a) 20 mm Hg (b) 35 mm Hg
(c) 28 mm Hg (d) 10 mm Hg

1747. Oval retinal hemorrhage with pale centre A/E:
(a) SLE
(b) Severe anemia
(c) Infective Endocarditis
(d) Polycythemia vera

1748. Bacterial endotoxin A/E:
(a) Gram +ve bacteria
(b) Gram –ve bacteria
(c) Lipopolysaccharide
(d) Required for viability of organism

1749. Tumour lysis syndrome:
(a) Hypocalcemia (b) Hypercalcemia
(c) Hyperkalemia (d) Hyperphosphatemia

1750. Normal Blood pH:
(a) 7.36-7.42 (b) 7.36-7.44
(c) 7.38-7.44 (d) 7.38-7.42

1751. Aniline dye ingestion –most appropriate treatment:
(a) O_2
(b) Methylene blue
(c) Exchange transfusion
(d) Hemodialysis

1752. ↑ T4,T3, ↓TSH, ↓Radio active uptake:
(a) Graves' disease
(b) Subacute thyroiditis
(c) Hashimoto's thyroiditis
(d) Toxic nodular goitre

1753. D-dimer true:
(a) High negative predictive valve
(b) Low in MI
(c) Used in hospitalized patient
(d) Diagnosed by PCR

1754. CMV in HIV treatment indication:
(a) CMV Ag in BAL
(b) Cytopathic effect on transbronchial biopsy
(c) IgG in serum

1755. Iron loss in 1 unit of BT:
(a) 200-250 mg
(b) 100-150 mg
(c) Does not reduce iron
(d) 150-200 mg

1756. DOC for idiopathic generalized epilepsy:
(a) Valproate and lamotrigine
(b) Phenytoin
(c) Vigabatrin
(d) Carbamazepine

1757. Refsum disease A/E:
(a) ↓ phytanic acid
(b) Progressive sensorimotor neuropathy
(c) Cerebellar ataxia
(d) Retinitis pigmentosa

1758. Depression occurs in:

(a) Valproate (b) Phenytoin
(c) Carbamazepine (d) Phenobarbitone

1759. Complex partial seizures A/E:

(a) Coma
(b) Automatism
(c) Behavioural arrest
(d) Dissociation from surrounding

1760. EMG in radiation plexopathy:

(a) Myokymia (b) Fasciculation
(c) Normal (d) Myotonia

1761. Intramedullary lesion–more characteristic:

(a) Saddle anaesthesia
(b) Early bladder involvement
(c) Asymmetric weakness
(d) Radiculopathy

1762. Antiepileptic drugs – teratogenic effects most seen in:

(a) First trimester (b) Second trimester
(c) Early third trimester (d) Late third trimester

1763. Celiac disease–not seen is:

(a) Anti-endomysial (b) Anti-gliadin
(c) Anti-gluten (d) Anti-TTG

1764. Tracheo-bronchial aspiration not seen during swallowing A/E:

(a) Achalasia cardia (b) Zenker's diverticulum
(c) GERD (d) Globus hystericus

1765. Tumour lysis syndrome A/E:

(a) Hypo Ca^{2+} (b) Hyper Ca^{2+}
(c) Hyper K^+ (d) Hyper PO_4

1766. High T_3, ↑T_4, TSH ↓Radio-iodine uptake:

(a) Subacute thyroiditis (b) Graves' disease
(c) Hashimoto's disease (d) Toxic nodular goiter

1767. Pernicious anemia A/E:

(a) High incidence of gastric CA
(b) Life long cabalamine therapy
(c) Antibody against NA^+ K^+ ATPase
(d) Hypergastrinema

1768. All are cause of vitamin B_{12} deficiency A/E:

(a) Blind loop syndrome
(b) MTx therapy
(c) Nitrous oxide (N_2O)
(d) Zollinger-Ellison syndrome

1769. Chronic PPI therapy causes A/E:

(a) Hypergastrinemia
(b) ↑ Small bowel bacterial overgrowth
(c) ↓ intrinsic factor release
(d) Decreased release of vitamin B_{12}

1770. Migratory motor complex true:

(a) Occur in fasting
(b) Lasts for <1 min
(c) ↑ mixing of food with digestive enzymes occurs
(d) Causes sweeping movement of colon

1771. Relapsing polychondritis characteristic:

(a) Sparing of ear lobes
(b) Bronchiolitis obliterans

1772. Kidney involvement in Sjögren's syndrome:

(a) Distal RTA
(b) Acute interstitial nephritis
(c) Amyloidosis
(d) Obstructive uropathy

1773. 12/Male presented with genu valgum with muscle weakness with bilateral vesicoureteric reflux, normal GFR true is:

(a) ↓K^+, Normal Cl, ↓blood pH, ↓urine pH
(b) ↓K^+ ↑Cl, ↓blood pH, ↑urine pH
(c) ↑K^+, ↑Cl, ↓blood pH, ↑urine pH
(d) ↑K^+, ↑Cl, ↓blood pH, ↓urine pH

1774. Acute nephritis with ↑ glycosuria, ↑aminoaciduria:

(a) Cystinosis (b) Amyloidosis
(c) IgA nephropathy (d) Minimal change disease

1775. Foix-Cheyne-Marie syndrome:

(a) Spastic paraplegia (b) Pseudobulbar palsy
(c) Peripheral neuropathy

1776. Paniotopolous syndrome A/E:

(a) Autonomic imbalance associated with vomiting + loss of consciousness
(b) Brain imaging normal
(c) EEG-occipital spike during interictal phase
(d) Homonymous hemianopia

1777. MRI better than CT A/E:

(a) Infract (b) Calcification
(c) Dysplasia (d) Demyelination

1778. Survival to childhood is exceptional A/E:

(a) TGA
(b) Ebstein's anomaly
(c) Pulmonary atresia with intact septum
(d) Interrupted aortic arch

1779. Change in fetal circulation of birth immediately:

(a) Anatomical PFO closure
(b) Anatomical PDA closure
(c) ↑ SVR
(d) ↓ pulmonary flow

1780. Congenital heart disease associated with MR:

(a) Ebstein's anomaly (b) ALCAPA
(c) Congenital MS (d) SVC to LA

1781. Fetal circulation physiology is affected by:

(a) Mitral atresia
(b) Tricuspid atresia with restrictive VSD
(c) Ductus arteriosus
(d) Large VSD

1782. Congenital heart discuss with LAD with counter-clockwise rotation A/E:

(a) DORV (b) ECD
(c) TGA (d) Tricuspid atresia

1783. Highest mixed venous oxygen saturation:

(a) Hypovolumic shock (b) Neurogenic shock
(c) Septic shock (d) Cardiogenic shock

1784. pO_2=60, pcO_2=50, ph=7.38 alveolar-oxygen difference:

(a) 10 (b) 28
(c) 35

1785. 40/M with intakes of local alcohol, with sudden loss of vision, ph=7.05, HCO_3=8, treatment of choice:

(a) Hemodialysis
(b) Veno-venous hemofiltration
(c) Forced alkaline diuresis
(d) Peritoneal dialysis

1786. Young adult presenting with fever acute renal dysfunction, renal biopsy–numerous crescents with neutrophil infiltration in glomerular tufts true is:

(a) Anti-GBM
(b) ANCA-related
(c) Churg-Strauss syndrome
(d) Post-infectious crescenteric glomerlonephritis

1787. CAD with stenting on aspirin, ticlopidine, ACE-I, BB develops fever renal dysfunction:

(a) Ticlopidine (b) Aspirin
(c) BB (d) ACE-I

1788. Patient with acute leukemia with 200 × 10^9 with initial treatment A/E:

(a) Hydroxyuria (b) BM examination
(c) Cytarabine (d) Leukopharesis

1789. SVC syndrome before definitive diagnosis, treatment (initial):

(a) Endovascular stent (b) Chemotherapy
(c) Radiotherapy (d) Chemo + radiotherapy

1790. Most serious complication with TPN:

(a) Chronic cholestasis with fibrosis
(b) Chronic cholestasis with bridging necrosis
(c) Chronic cholestasis with hepatocyte necrosis
(d) Chronic cholestasis with portal vein thrombosis

1791. O_2 carried by plasma:

(a) 2.5 ml/l (b) 5 ml/l
(c) 7.5 ml/l (d) 10 ml/l

1792. Most specific test for Fe-deficiency anemia:

(a) PBF-hypochromic microcytic anemia
(b) ↓ S. ferritin
(c) ↓ S. iron
(d) ↓ MCV

1793. Most common cause of venous thrombosis:

(a) Protein S deficiency (b) Protein C deficiency
(c) Factor V deficiency (d) Prothrombin mutation

1794. True about d-dimer:

(a) Useful for diagnosis of PTE in hospitalised people
(b) Detected by PCR
(c) ↓ MI
(d) High NPV for PTE

1795. Congenital hemochromatosis:

(a) Skin depigmentation
(b) Saturation (transferrin) > 45%

(c) Gonadal failure
(d) Diabetes mellitus

1796. MMSE – attention, calculation score:
(a) 1 (b) 2
(c) 3 (d) 5

1797. Metabolic encephalopathy, most specific neurologic sign:
(a) Multifocal myoclonus
(b) Focal neuro deficit
(c) Constricting pupil
(d) Bilateral extensor plantar

1798. Cause of macrocytic anemia A/E:
(a) Aplastic anemia
(b) Sideroblastic anemia
(c) Megaloblastic anemia
(d) MDS

1799. Acute pancreatitis in HIV patient:
(a) Cryptococci (b) MAC
(c) Isospora belli (d) Microsporidia

1800. Hirsutism is a side effect of:
(a) Minoxidil
(b) Cycloserine
(c) Vincristine

1801. CD 13+, CD 10+, CD 33+, CD 19 + leukaemia:
(a) Biphenotypic leukaemia
(b) AML M0
(c) AML M2

1802. Pb toxicity type of anemia A/E:
(a) Protoporphyrinuria (b) Macrocytic anemia
(c) Haemolytic anemia (d) Fanconi anemia

1803. Typical manifestation of CRF:
(a) Impaired glucose tolerence
(b) Severe fasting hyperglycemia
(c) EPO resistant anemia common
(d) Normal BT

1804. Glomerular origin of hematuria:
(a) Gross hematuria (b) Dysmorphic RBCs
(c) Proteinuria

1805. HUS peripheral blood smear:
(a) Schistocytes (b) Microcytes
(c) Spherocytes (d) Normal RBC

1806. Multiple myeloma patient develops jaw pain and ulceration:
(a) Zoledronate (b) Zygomycosis
(c) Tb (d) Amyloidosis

1807. 35 years old male with BP=150/110 mmHg, mono-neuritis multiplex with massive splenomegaly, diagnosis:
(a) Hairy cell leukaemia
(b) CML
(c) Tropical splenomegaly
(d) Kala azar

1808. 20 years old female well developed secondary sexual character with absent pubic and axillary hair:
(a) Androgen insensitivity syndrome
(b) Hypogonadotrophic hypogonadism
(c) Gonadal agenesis
(d) Gonadotropin secreting pituitary tumour

1809. 35 years old female obese with purple straie on abdomen, low dose DST abnormality, high dose DST normal:
(a) Obesity (b) Pituitary tumour
(c) Adrenal neoplasia (d) Lung Ca

1810. Low HDL caused by:
(a) Cholestasis
(b) Estrogen
(c) Chlorinated hydrocarbon
(d) Gaucher's disease

1811. Anemia, osteopenia, neutropenia, impaired myelination, depigmented hair:
(a) Cu deficiency (b) Zn deficiency
(c) Se deficiency (d) Iodine deficiency

1812. Emphysema:
(a) RV normal (b) PEFR normal
(c) FVC decreased (d) Increased PCO_2 always

1813. Restrictive lung disease A/E:
(a) Decreased FVC
(b) Decreased FEV1

(c) Decreased TLC
(d) Decreased FEV1/FVC < 80%

1814. 2nd day PIH, APPT increased, PT and TT normal, factor VIII 10% of normal:
(a) Acquired haemophilia
(b) Inherited haemophilia A
(c) Anti cardiolipin
(d) Lupus anticoagulant

1815. Bilateral DVT, 1 episode of PTE, frequent joint pain with fever:
(a) Protein C deficiency (b) Protein S deficiency
(c) Lupus anticoagulant (d) Increased AT III

1816. Weight loss with fever A/E:
(a) TB (b) Thyrotoxicosis
(c) Pheochromocytoma (d) RCC

1817. CCP:
(a) Kussmaul's sign (b) RA collapse
(c) LVS3 (d) Pulsus paradoxus

1818. BMV suitable in A/E:
(a) LVS3 (b) Loud S1
(c) Loud OS (d) Widened A2-OS gap

1819. QRS and QT increased:
(a) Quinidine toxicity (b) SAH
(c) TCA overdose (d) Hypothermia

1820. Peripheral cyanosis seen in:
(a) Cold exposure
(b) Methemoglobulinemia
(c) Pulmonary AV fistula
(d) High altitude

1821. PSVT all used *except:*
(a) Lidocaine (b) Verapamil
(c) Adenosine (d) Propranolol

1822. Pseudolymphoma:
(a) Sjögren's syndrome (b) MCTD
(c) Behcet's disease (d) Systemic sclerosis

1823. Pulsus alternans seen in:
(a) LVH
(b) Severe LV systolic dysfunction
(c) Digitalis

1824. Electrical alternans seen in:
(a) Large pericardial effusion
(b) PTE
(c) CCP

1825. Oliguria defined as urine output less than —— ml/day.
(a) 1000 (b) 50
(c) 400 (d) 100

1826. Oxalate crystals in urine seen in:
(a) Ethylene glycol (b) Methanol

1827. Earliest manifestation of autonomic neuropathy in DM:
(a) Postural hypotension
(b) Erectile dysfunction
(c) Cystopathy
(d) Diarrhoea

1828. Vasculitis affecting large arteries:
(a) PAN (b) Takayasu arteritis
(c) Kawasaki disease (d) Churg-Struass disease

1829. Chronic alcoholism with anemia A/E:
(a) Macrocytic (b) Fe deficiency
(c) Sideroblastic anemia (d) ALD

1830. Bleeding due to platelet disorder A/E:
(a) Superficial bleeding usual
(b) Controlled by local measures
(c) Hematoma and hemoarthrosis common
(d) Bleeding is immediately after injury

1831. Cardiopulmonary stress testing in favour of respiratory cause:
(a) Hypotension (b) > 85% of THR
(c) Decreased SaO_2 (d) Decreased MVO_2

1832. Cirrhosis liver with raised PT (25/12) and APTT (60/35), platelet count 2 lacs, TT (15/15):
(a) Normal D-dimer
(b) Fibrinogen conc. < 100
(c) Increased protein C
(d) Increased AT III

1833. 20 years old female with Hb A2–40%, Hb–10.5 g% mild microcytic anemia:

(a) α- thalassemia trait

(b) β- thalassemia major

(c) β- thalassemia trait heterozygous

(d) Sideroblastic anemia

1834. 20 years old female MCV–65, MCH–27, RDW–17, Hb–9 g%, RBC–5.2 million, diagnosis:

(a) Fe deficiency anemia (b) Sideroblastic anemia

(c) β- thallasemia minor (d) AIHA

1835. Acute onset jaundice with anemia Hb–6 g%, TLC–15,400, platelet–2 lac, 10000, retic count–24% A/E:

(a) Increased serum hepatoglobulin

(b) Hemosiderinuria

(c) BM hyperplasia

1836. Drugs in CML A/E:

(a) Imatinib (b) Dasatinib

(c) Nilotinib (d) Tipsfranib

1837. Acute leukemia with markers CD10+, CD19+, CD33+, CD13+:

(a) Biphenotypic (b) L2

(c) M0 (d) M2

1838. Therapeutic hemopheresis contraindicated in:

(a) Renal failure (b) Hepatic failure

(c) ACE -I therapy (d) Paraquat poisoning

1839. ROC:

(a) Sensitivity versus 1-specificity

(b) Specificity versus 1-sensitivity

(c) Senstivity versus 1-sensitivity

(d) Specificity versus 1-specificity

1840. Blood plasma without erythrocytes O2/L blood:

(a) 2.5 (b) 5

(c) 7.5 (d) 10

1841. Visceral leishmaniasis in HIV characteristic:

(a) GI (b) Renal

(c) CNS (d) Skin

1842. TPN most serious complication:

(a) Cholestasis with fibrosis

(b) Cholestasis with hepatic necrosis

(c) Cholestasis with bridging necrosis

(d) Cholestasis with portal vein thrombosis

1843. Tumor lysis syndrome A/E:

(a) ↓ Ca (b) ↑ Ca

(c) ↑ PO4 (d) ↑ K

1844. 10 years old female prepuberty, menorrhagic, PTT ↑, PT Normal, TT Normal, vWD factor VIII 10% of normal:

(a) Hemiphilia A

(b) Hemophilia B

(c) Von Willebrand disease

(d) Glanzmann's thrombocytopenia

1845. HUS caused by:

(a) Cyclosporine (b) Allopurinol

(c) Azathiopine

1846. pH of blood:

(a) 7.36-7.44 (b) 7.38-7.42

(c) 7.38-7.44 (d) 7.36-7.42

1847. Miliary shadow:

(a) Hepatoma (b) Broncho alveolar Ca

(c) Endometrial Ca (d) Melanoma

1848. Zoledromic acid in:

(a) Myeloma (b) Hg poisoning

(c) Renal failure (d) ↓ Mg

1849. DVT patient with 4 mg warf, PT-16/12, ISI-1:

(a) Appropriate dose (b) Underdose

(c) Mild overdose (d) Gross overdose

1850. Cirrhosis patient platelet- 2 lac, APPT↑, PT↑, TT Normal:

(a) D-dimer Normal (b) AT III↑

(c) Protein C↑ (d) Fibrinogen < 100 mg

1851. Anemia with ↑ MCV A/E:

(a) Megaloblastic anemia

(b) Sideroblastic anemia

(c) Hypothyrod

(d) MDS

1852. Most common cause of venous thrombosis:

(a) Factor V deficiency

(b) Prothrombin mutation

(c) Protein C deficiency

(d) Protein S deficiency

1853. 25 years male with recurrent jaundice, anemia, moderate splenomegaly, family history of gall stones:

(a) Hereditary spheroyctosis
(b) α-thalasemia trait
(c) β-thalasemia heterozgyous
(d) G6PD deficiency

1854. Male with 18 gm Hb on 3 occasions, best test:

(a) Red cell mass (b) Hct
(c) TLC

1855. 5 days neonate with sepsis, bleeding and venepuncture bleeding A/E:

(a) Schistocytes on smear
(b) PT ↑
(c) Fibrinogen ↑
(d) D-dimer ↑

1856. Stress ulcer prevention in ICU:

(a) H2 blocker (b) Sucralfate
(c) Pantop (d) Antacid

1857. Vasopressor in septic shock:

(a) Epinephrine (b) Norepinephrine
(c) Dopamine (d) Dobutamine

1858. Most common manifestation of parvo B_{19} virus infection in adults:

(a) Erythema infectiosum
(b) Arthropathy
(c) Pure red cell aplasia
(d) Bone morrow aplasia

1859. Rat bite treatment:

(a) TT/Antibiotic/Cleaning
(b) TT
(c) Antibiotic
(d) TT/Antibiotic

1860. 40 years with acute leukemic with WBC 200 × 10^9 not to be done:

(a) BM exam
(b) Cytarabine
(c) Hydroxyurea
(d) Leukopheresis

1861. SVC syndrome without definite diagnosis what can be done?

(a) RT (b) CT
(c) RT+CT (d) Endovascular stenting

1862. Acute GVHD A/E:

(a) Diarrhoea (b) Jaundice
(c) Pneumonitis (d) Rash

1863. Drug for ESBL:

(a) Imipenem (b) Ceftazidine
(c) Taxim (d) Cefoperazone

1864. Wegener's granulomatosis–ANCA against:

(a) Proteinase 3 (b) MPO

1865. HIV with CMV infection should be treated when:

(a) BAL with Ag +
(b) Transbronchial with intranuclear inclusion
(c) CT– Interstitial pneumonitis
(d) Ig G +

1866. Celiac disease all antibodies *except:*

(a) Anti–gliadin (b) Anti–TTG
(c) Anti–endomysial (d) Anti–gluten

1867. Pregnancy with UC:

(a) Flare up
(b) Abortion
(c) Fetal malformations
(d) Extra–intestinal manifestations increased

1868. Hemorrhage in retina with pale centre A/E:

(a) Severe anemia (b) SLE
(c) Polycythemia vera (d) IE

1869. Large vegetation with culture negative:

(a) H. parainfluenzae

1870. 50 years male with S1Q3T3 with dyspnea, normal echo treatment:

(a) tPA (b) STK
(c) Heparin (d) Warfarin

1871. Water deficit in 60 kg man, Na–154:

(a) 2.2 l (b) 3.6 l
(c) 4.2 l (d) 7.6 l

1872. Aniline poisoning with cyanosis treatment:

(a) Methylene blue IV (b) O_2
(c) Hemodialysis

1873. Endotoxin A/E:

(a) Gram +ve (b) Gram –ve
(c) Essential for viability (d) Lipopolysaccharides

1874. Contrast nephropathy prevention:
(a) $NaHCO_3$ (b) Potassium chloride
(c) $MgCl_2$ (d) $CaCl_2$

1875. 80 years female with < 8% plasma cells, monoclonal spike IgG 1.5 gm/dl asymptomatic:
(a) Myeloma (b) MGUS
(c) Waldenstrom (d) Indolent myeloma

1876. Most significant marker for predicting CAD:
(a) Hs CRP (b) Fibrinogen
(c) Homocysteine (d) Lp-a

1877. 48 hours storage of blood leads to deficiency of A/E:
(a) Platelets (b) WBC
(c) Factor V (d) Factor VII

1878. Rituximab most useful in:
(a) Diffuse large cell lymphoma
(b) Mycosis fungoides
(c) Burkitt lymphoma
(d) Precursor B cell lymphoma

1879. HCV 2 treatment is:
(a) Peg IFNα 2a + ribavarin × 48 weeks
(b) Peg IFNγ 2a × 24 weeks
(c) Peg IFNα 2a + ribavarin × 24 weeks
(d) Peg IFNγ 2a × 48 weeks

1880. Non modulating HTN A/E:
(a) Low renin
(b) ACE I alters the pathophysiology
(c) Insulin resistant
(d) More common in post menopausal women and among men

1881. Goal of HTN in DM:
(a) < 130/80 mm Hg (b) < 130/85 mm Hg
(c) 120/80 mm Hg

1882. Insulin resistance seen A/E:
(a) Moon facies (b) Acne
(c) Central obesity (d) Hirsuitism

1883. Lipodystrophy associated with:
(a) FSGN (b) MCD
(c) Membranos GN (d) MPGN

1884. Hb carries A/E:
(a) O_2 (b) CO_2
(c) Nitrous oxide (d) SO_2

1885. Virchows triad A/E:
(a) Epithelial injury
(b) Endothelial injury
(c) Imbalance between procoagulant and anticoagulant
(d) Slow flow

1886. ATN true is:
(a) Muddy brown cast (b) RF index < 1
(c) FENa <1 (d) Urine Na < 20

1887. 30 years old male breathing spontaneously, pH – 7.36, PaO_2- 60 mm Hg, $PaCO_2$-50, HCO_3- 30, A-a gradient is:
(a) 10 (b) 20
(c) 28 (d) 35

1888. Pulmonary alveolar proteinosis true A/E:
(a) BAL helpful in some patient
(b) Serum surfactant normal
(c) Bat wing appearance
(d) Raised LDH

1889. CXR finding in inhalational anthrax:
(a) Mediastinal widening with pleural effusion
(b) Bilateral consolidation
(c) Lobar consolidation with contralateral pleural effusion
(d) Interstitial infiltration with effusion

1890. Nephrolithiasis caused by:
(a) Indinavir (b) Nelfinavir
(c) Squanavir (d) Nevirapine

1891. Most common infection in 7 years old male with febrile neutropenia on chemotherapy for AML with no history of previous infection:
(a) Aspergillus (b) Gram positive bacteria
(c) HSV (d) Oral candidiasis

1892. IPI A/E:
(a) Beta 2 microglobulin
(b) >1 extranodal site
(c) Age > 60 years
(d) Ann arbour stage III- IV
(e) Serum LDH raised
(f) Performance status ≥ 2 ECOG or ≤ 70 karnofsky

1893. Arterial thrombosis caused by:
(a) APLA syndrome
(b) Factor V leiden
(c) Prothrombin gene mutation
(d) Protein C deficiency

1894. Acquired haemophilia test abnormal is:
(a) Raised PT (b) Raised APPT
(c) INR (d) TT

1895. Cirrhosis of liver cause of thrombocytopenia A/E:
(a) Hepatorenal syndrome
(b) Hypersplenism
(c) Thrombopoietin deficiency
(d) DIC

1896. True, D-dimer:
(a) Highest NPV
(b) Helpful in diagnosis of PE in hospitalised patient
(c) Assay by PCR

1897. Characteristic finding of relapsing polychondritis at presentation:
(a) Ear lobe sparing
(b) Early eye involvement
(c) Bronchiolitis obliterans
(d) Rapid progression of renal dysfunction

1898. Drugs to be avoided in actinomycosis:
(a) Penicillin G (b) Amoxicillin
(c) Oxacillin (d) Tetracycline

1899. Aztreonam true A/E:
(a) Effective against gram negative
(b) Not effective in anaerobes
(c) Not effective in gram positive
(d) Cross reacts immediate hypersensitivity in penicillin allergic patients

1900. 40 years old male acute leukaemia with TLC – 200 × 10^9 /l, initial management A/E:
(a) BM examination (b) Cytarabine
(c) Hydroxyurea (d) Leukopheresis

1901. Best imaging modality for hemopoietic tissue in BM:
(a) CT (b) MRI
(c) 3D USG (d) 4D USG

1902. Extramedullary hematopoiesis means:
(a) Hematopoiesis in BM, liver, spleen
(b) Hematopoiesis in BM and liver
(c) Hematopoiesis in BM and spleen
(d) Hematopoiesis in liver and spleen

1903. GVHD A/E:
(a) Autologous BMT
(b) Allogenic BMT
(c) Blood transfusion
(d) Umbilical cord stem cell transplant

1904. Hematopoietic GF are:
(a) Glycoprotein (b) Carbopoietin
(c) Carbohydrates (d) Proteins

1905. Highest venous O_2 saturation:
(a) Cardiogenic shock (b) Septic shock
(c) Neurogenic shock (d) Hypovolumic shock

1906. Long term hematopoietic growth:
(a) CD34+ and CD138+ (b) CD34+ and CD138-
(c) CD34+ and CD38- (d) CD34+ and CD38+

1907. Fundus finding in takayasu A/E:
(a) Venous dilatation (b) AV shunt
(c) Papilledema (d) Hard exudates

1908. SVC syndrome before definitive diagnosis treatment:
(a) Stenting (b) Chemotherapy
(c) CT + RT (d) RT

1909. Bile acid diarrhoea A/E:
(a) Good response to cholestyramine
(b) Limited ileal disease
(c) Bile pool decreased
(d) Decrease bile absorption in ileum

1910. Friedreich ataxia is associated with:
(a) DM (b) DI
(c) Cushing's syndrome

1911. Ataxia telangiectasia:
(a) Ovarian agenesis
(b) Pulmonary infection uncommon
(c) Early response to live vaccine
(d) Thymus is normal

1912. Patient had stenting on beta blocker, nitrate, ticlopidine, aspirin, ACE-I develops fever, renal dysfunction, PBS-schisocytes, which drug is responsile?

(a) Ticlopdipine (b) Beta blocker
(c) Nitrates (d) Aspirin

1913. Raised T3, raised T4, decreased TSH, decreased Radioiodine uptake diagnosis is:

(a) Toxic nodular goitre
(b) Hashimoto's thyroiditis
(c) Graves' disease
(d) Subacute thyroiditis

1914. Paraeoplastic cerebellar degeneration:

(a) Anti – Yo (b) Anti – Hu
(c) Anti –ACK (d) Anti –Tr

1915. Male patient 1 unit blood donation, iron loss:

(a) 150-200 mg (b) 100-150 mg
(c) 200-250 mg (d) No iron loss

1916. HLA B-72 all *except:*

(a) Psoriasis vulgaris
(b) Anterior acute uveitis
(c) Anyklosing spondylitis
(d) Reiter's syndrome

1917. Carpel tunnel syndrome:

(a) Haemodialysis (b) Haemochromatosis
(c) Vincristine (d) Fabry's disease

1918. CPPD crystal seen in all *except:*

(a) Posterior meniscus (b) Haemochromatosis
(c) Hypomagnesia (d) Hyperphosphatemia

1919. Aeromons septicaemia DOC:

(a) Ciprofloxacin (b) Clindamycin
(c) Clarithromycin (d) Chloramphenicol

1920. Drugs used in CML A/E:

(a) Hemoharringtone (b) Herbamycin A
(c) Fludaribine (d) STI-571

1921. Bortezomab used in:

(a) Multiple myeloma (b) NHL
(c) ALL (d) Hodgkin's lymphoma

1922. Prognostic marker in multiple myeloma:

(a) Beta 2 microglobulin (b) Alkaline phosphatase

1923. Most common renal manifestations of Sjögren's disease:

(a) Membraneous GN
(b) MPGN
(c) AIN
(d) Tubulointerstitial nephritis

1924. Most common cause of PUO:

(a) TB (b) Enteric fever
(c) Malaria (d) SLE

1925. Dependent variable in CPAP A/E:

(a) FiO_2 (b) I:E ratio
(c) Airway pressure (d) Tidal volume

1926. Ventilation for ARDS all used *except:*

(a) High tidal volume
(b) FiO_2 >0.6
(c) Prone position
(d) Inspiratory pressure < 30 cm H_2O

1927. Vasculitis not due to infection:

(a) PAN
(b) EMC
(c) Hypersensitivity vasculitis
(d) Wegener's granulomatosis

1928. Properdin D – infection seen:

(a) Pyogenic
(b) Neisseria
(c) Immune complex disease
(d) HUS

1929. Cytokine involved in apoptosis:

(a) IL-2 (b) IL-6
(c) IL-10 (d) Caspases

1930. 8 years old girl beta thalassemia no requirement of BT A/E:

(a) α thalassemia trait (b) Sideroblastic
(c) Beta thalassemia trait (d) Beta thalassemia major

1931. Sickle cell anemia Hb fall from 9 to 5 g% A/E:

(a) Aplastic anemia (b) Sickle cell crisis
(c) Megaloblastic (d) Extravascular hemolysis

1932. Young female with mild microcytic anemia, Hb=10.2 g%, Hb A2=40%, diagnosis:
(a) Beta thalassemia trait heterozygous
(b) Beta thalassemia major homozygous
(c) Sideroblastic anemia
(d) α thalassemia

1933. α coma on EEG:
(a) Hepatic coma
(b) Sedative overdose
(c) Pontine haemorrhage
(d) Hyponatremia

1934. Macrovesicular steatosis seen in A/E:
(a) Alcohol (b) Lipodystrophy
(c) TPN (d) Reye's syndrome

1935. Thrombocytopenia due to destruction A/E:
(a) SLE (b) TTP
(c) ITP (d) Thiazide

1936. Hyperkalemia when GFR decreases:
(a) 50 ml/min (b) 25 ml/min
(c) 15 ml/min (d) 40 ml/min

1937. Deoxycoformycin acid:
(a) Antimetabolite (b) Alkylating agent
(c) Antimitotic (d) Anti tumour antibiotic

1938. Ifosfamide induced encephalopathy treatment:
(a) Dilantin (b) Valproic acid
(c) Methylene blue (d) Vitamin C

1939. Calcium pyrophosphate deposits seen in A/E:
(a) Hyperparathyroidism
(b) Hemochromatosis
(c) Hypermagnesemia
(d) Post meniscectomy

1940. Foscarnet used in:
(a) CMV retinitis (b) Lymphoma
(c) Herpetic (d) Keratitis in AIDS

1941. CRF dermatological manifestation:
(a) Calciphylaxis (b) Purpura
(c) Ecchymosis (d) Blue nail

1942. Proximal RTA characterized by A/E:
(a) HCO_3 flitered < 15%
(b) Minimum urine pH < 5.5
(c) Normal serum anion gap
(d) Increased urinary anion gap

1943. Cold agglutinin seen in:
(a) Mycoplasma (b) Lymphoma
(c) Penicillin (d) CLL

1944. Itraconazole used in A/E:
(a) Candidiasis (b) Mucormycosis
(c) Dermatophytosis (d) Aspergillosis

1945. Most important step in cardiopulmonary resuscitation:
(a) Mouth to mouth respiration
(b) Endotracheal intubation
(c) Cardiac massage
(d) Defibrillation

1946. BP=80/60, ST depression in anterior leads, Echo–normal LV function, RV dilated and dysfunction, CXR– normal, acute breathlessness:
(a) IV NTG (b) IV heparin
(c) IV STK (d) IV morphine

1947. Endogenous angiogenesis inhibitor:
(a) Endostatin (b) IL-8
(c) TNF- α

1948. Warfarin in protein C deficiency:
(a) Skin necrosis (b) Thrombosis

1949. ACE gene polymorphism associated with A/E:
(a) Diabetic nephropathy
(b) HTN retinopathy
(c) LVH
(d) IgA nephropathy

1950. Hypomagnesemia is caused by A/E:
(a) Diuretic-thiazide (b) Hypoaldosteronism
(c) Acute pancreatitis (d) Small bowel bypass

1951. Villonodular synovitis– synovial fluid:
(a) Hemorrhagic (b) Clear
(c) Turbid (d) Yellow

1952. Biliary sludge is caused by:
(a) Ceftriaxone (b) Cefoperazone
(c) Cefipime

1953. PAN not involved is:
(a) Lung (b) Liver
(c) GIT (d) Kidney

1954. Hb =6.7 g%, platelet count = 2 lac, reticulocyte–24%, WBC–15,000, A/E:

(a) Increased hepatoglobin
(b) Direct antiglobulin test positive
(c) Hemosiderin in urine
(d) BM hyperplasia

1955. Hanta virus reservoir is:

(a) Mouse (b) Cat
(c) Dog (d) Pig

1956. ATN characterized by:

(a) Muddy brown cast
(b) Specific gravity > 1.020
(c) Urinary sodium < 10
(d) Urine creatinine/plasma BUN > 40

1957. 80 years old asymptomatic female with monoclonal spike of IgG and 8% plasma cells on BM biopsy, diagnosis:

(a) Indolent myeloma (b) Multiple myeloma
(c) MGUS (d) Tuberculosis

1958. Acute leukemia with immunophenotype (CD 19+, 10+, 33+, 13+) most likely has which variety?

(a) Biphenotypic leukemia
(b) AML-M0
(c) ALL-L 2
(d) AML-M2

1959. Young female with Hb of 10.5 g% and HbA2 of 40% on Hb electrophoresis has:

(a) α thalassemia trait
(b) Heterozygous β-thalassemia trait
(c) β-thalassemia major
(d) Sideroblastic anemia

1960. Young female presents with acute anemia and jaundice Hb of 6.5 g%, retic count of 24% will have all of the following *except:*

(a) Increased serum haptoglobulin
(b) Positive direct antiglobin test
(c) BM hyperplasia
(d) Hemosiderin in urine

1961. Postpartum haemorrhage in a primiparous lady with increased APTT, factor VIII levels < 10% and normal BT, PT and TT has:

(a) Inherited haemophilia A
(b) Acquired haemophilia A
(c) DIC
(d) Lupus anticoagulant

1962. The chromosome affected in Wilson's disease is:

(a) 21 (b) X
(c) 10 (d) 13

1963. Acanthocytosis is seen in:

(a) Ataxia telangiectasia
(b) Refsum's disease
(c) Basen Kurnzweing's syndrome
(d) Tangier's disease

1964. Incidence of thymoma in MG:

(a) <10% (b) 10-15%
(c) 20-25% (d) >40%

1965. Akathasia means:

(a) Increased rigidity (b) Restlessness
(c) Abnormal posturing (d) Decreased movements

1966. All are seen in MND *except*:

(a) Fasciculations (b) Numbness
(c) Weakness (d) Atrophy

1967. Target goals for LDL in a diabetic are:

(a) < 70 mg% (b) 70-100 mg%
(c) 100-130 mg% (d) > 130 mg%

1968. All are true about anaplastic large cell lymphoma *except:*

(a) High grade
(b) 5 years survival rate > 80%
(c) CD 30+
(d) Mimics Hodgkin's disease

1969. Scorpion sting is managed with:

(a) Captopril (b) Lignocaine
(c) Bretylium (d) Prazosin

1970. Suboptimal antibiotic in plaque:

(a) Gentamicin (b) Chloramphenicol
(c) Cefotaxime (d) Prazosin

1971. Thalidomide is used in:

(a) AML (b) ALL
(c) Multiple myeloma (d) Hairy cell leukemia

1972. Which is an angiogenesis inhibitor:

(a) Endostatin (b) Leptin
(c) TNF α (d) IL-8

1973. Culture negative afebrile indolent I.E. caused by:

(a) HACEK (b) Coxiella burnetti
(c) T. Whippeli (d) Bartonella

1974. Meningoencephalitis in an immunocompetent adult caused by which protozoa:

(a) Entamoeba histolytica
(b) Acanthamoeba
(c) Balamuthia
(d) Cysticercosis

1975. Eye movement towards upwards and left by:

(a) Right inferior oblique muscle
(b) Right superior oblique muscle
(c) Left superior oblique muscle
(d) Left inferior oblique muscle

1976. G-CSF is used for:

(a) Autologous BM transplantation
(b) Afebrile neutropenic patients
(c) Priming in cancer chemotherapy
(d) Increased intensity of chemotherapy

1977. Diminished ability to respond to an attack of TB bacilli:

(a) Repeated tubercular testing
(b) BCG vaccination
(c) Previous attack of TB
(d) Live vaccine administration of measles

1978. High probability of PE in VQ scan:

(a) Large lobar defect with normal ventilation
(b) Multiple segmental defects with normal ventilation
(c) Multiple subsegmental defects with matched
(d) Large wedge shaped perfusion defects

1979. Safest ATT in first trimester pregnancy:

(a) INH (b) Streptomycin
(c) Ethambutol (d) Thiaacetazone

1980. Transpulmonary pressure gradient means pressure between mouth and:

(a) Alveolus (b) Airway
(c) Chest wall (d) Pleural cavity

1981. High AG acidosis is seen in all *except:*

(a) Ethylene glycol poisoning
(b) CO poisoning
(c) CRF
(d) RTA (distal)

1982. Vasodilatation is caused by:

(a) Prostacyclin (b) Renin
(c) Endothelin (d) Norepinephrine

1983. Free oxygen radical induced cardiac injury is caused by:

(a) Cisplatin (b) Mitoxantrone
(c) 5-FU (d) Bleomycin

1984. Vaccine not to be given to HIV positive patients:

(a) OPV
(b) Hepatitis B vaccine
(c) Influenza
(d) Pneumococcal polyvalent vaccine

1985. Infections in neutropenic patients are A/E:

(a) Aspergillus (b) Pneumocystis
(c) Staph. Aureus (d) Klebsiella

1986. Microangiopathic haemolytic anemia is caused by:

(a) Malignant HTN (b) HSP
(c) Crescentic GN (d) Venous thrombosis

1987. Pitressin resistant DI is caused by:

(a) Sarcoidosis (b) Nephrogenic DI
(c) Histiocytosis (d) CRF

1988. Type of anemia in Pb poisoning A/E:

(a) Macrocytic (b) Haemolytic
(c) Protoporphyrinuria (d) Fanconi's like anemia

1989. Asterixis is caused by A/E:

(a) Hypoxic encephalopathy
(b) Organophosphorus poisoning
(c) Metabolic encephalopathy
(d) Upper midbrain lesion

1990. Common cause of RVT is:

(a) Minimal change disease
(b) Membranous GN
(c) Lupus nephritis
(d) Diabetic nephropathy

1991. Treatment of promyelocytic leukaemia:

(a) ATRA + chemotherapy
(b) High induction chemotherapy
(c) Supportive therapy
(d) BMT as initial therapy

1992. JVP in cardiac tamponade:

(a) Prominent X, y descent

(b) Prominent X, prominent y

(c) X descent, prominent y

(d) X descent, y descent

1993. Cold sore is caused by:

(a) Mycobacterium (b) Treponema pallidum

(c) Leishmania tropica (d) Herpes

1994. Metabolic alkalosis is caused by:

(a) K^+ depletion (b) Hypokalemia

(c) Septicaemia (d) Lactic acidosis

1995. Prion disease:

(a) Familial fatal insomnia

(b) SSPE

(c) PML

1996. Anemia, osteopenia, hair depigmentation, impaired myelination is caused by:

(a) Zn deficiency

(b) Se deficiency

(c) Chromium deficiency

(d) Copper deficiency

1997. 25 years old with lower limb DVT, platelet count 50,000/cumm, right MCA territory stroke, probable diagnosis, PTTK 7 sec:

(a) APLA

(b) TTP

(c) Dysfibrinogenemia

(d) Antithrombin deficiency

1998. Free radical induced cardiotoxicity:

(a) Bleomycin (b) Cytosine arbinoside

(c) Fludarabine (d) Doxorubicin

1999. Hyperglycemia:

(a) AZT (b) Stavudine

(c) Nevirapine (d) Nelfinavir

2000. Warfarin induced skin necrosis:

(a) Homozygous protein C deficiency

(b) Homozygous protein S deficiency

(c) Antithrombin III deficiency

2001. T-lymphocyte function A/E:

(a) Phytohemagglutnin

(b) Cancavalin-A

(c) NBT

(d) Mixed lymphocyte culture

2002. Thalidomide is used in A/E:

(a) MDS (b) Chronic phase of CML

(c) Multiple myeloma (d) Chronic GVD

2003. IFN α used in A/E:

(a) Sezary syndrome (b) CML

(c) Multiple sclerosis (d) GVHD

2004. Streptococcal sore throat, least effective is:

(a) Ciprofloxacin (b) Cefuroxime

(c) Amoxicillin (d) Azithromycin

2005. G-6PD deficiency with typhoid fever C/I is:

(a) Ciprofloxacin (b) Aztreonam

(c) Ceftriaxone (d) Ampicillin

2006. Watery diarrhoea due to clindamycin, oral drug to be given:

(a) Vancomycin (b) Fluconazole

(c) Ciprofloxacin (d) Cotrimoxazole

2007. Prognosis not altered by following in severe falciparum malaria:

(a) IV dexamethasone (b) Exchange pheresis

(c) Red cell phresis (d) PCV transfusion

2008. Hospital undergoing construction, incidence of which fungus infection is increased:

(a) Zygomycosis (b) Aspergillosis

(c) Pneumocystis (d) Cryptococcus

2009. Amenorrhoea, galactorrhoea, inability to conceive in 25 years old female:

(a) Estrogen

(b) Estrogen and progesterone

(c) Bromocriptine

2010. HRT all have been seen *except*:

(a) Increased incidence of Ca breast

(b) Increased incidence of venous thrombosis

(c) Decreased non traumatic fracture

(d) Impaired cognition

2011. Haloperidol induced fever, muscle rigidity with labile HTN, treatment is:

(a) Pacitane

(b) Phenergen

(c) Dandrolene

(d) Bromcriptine

2012. Phenytoin toxicity is caused by due to decreased metabolism:

(a) Warfarin (b) Clopidogrel
(c) Amoxicillin (d) Allopurinol

2013. Profuse painless large volume diarrhoea persists on fasting:

(a) IBS (b) Celiac disease
(c) Lactase deficiency (d) Carcinoid syndrome

2014. CRF with secondary pigmentation all can be given *except:*

(a) Oral alendronate (b) Calcium CO_3
(c) Oral calcitriol (d) Low phosphate diet

2015. Venous and arterial thrombosis occur in:

(a) MTHFR deficiency
(b) Factor V leiden mutation
(c) Prothrombin gene mutation
(d) Antithrombin III deficiency

2016. Photosensitivity seen in *except:*

(a) AIP (b) PKU
(c) Niacin deficiency (d) Carcinoid syndrome

2017. Multiple gene affect causing single disease diagnosed by:

(a) Real time PCR (b) Southern blot test
(c) Western blot test (d) DNA microarray test

2018. Patient with nystagmus, altered sensorium treatment is:

(a) Vitamin B_1 (b) Vitamin B_{12}
(c) Nicotinic acid

2019. Which of following is cofactor in fatty acid synthesis favouring rise to synthetic malonyl COA, involving acyl COA carboxylase is:

(a) Riboflavin (b) Biotin
(c) Niacin

2020. Patient of CRF on iron and EPO develops sudden anemia with decreased erythroid precursors on BM:

(a) Al toxicity
(b) PRCA induced by anti EPO Ab
(c) Blood loss
(d) Vitamin B_{12} deficiency

2021. Increased correct reticulocytic count is seen in:

(a) Thrombotic angiopathy
(b) Polycythemia rubra
(c) Pernicious anemia

2022. Following is positive in MCTD:

(a) Anti U1 RNP (b) Anti SS DNA
(c) RA factor (d) Anti RNA polymerase

2023. 13 years old boy with stunted growth, ataxia, ageusia, acrodermatitis and hyperpigmentation:

(a) Zinc (b) Vitamin E
(c) Vitamn A (d) Selenium

2024. Hyperpigmentation, SOB with knee pain, hyperglycemia in middle age man:

(a) D-penicillamine (b) S. cerloplasmin
(c) Weekly phlebotomy (d) Vitamin B_{12} deficiency

2025. Young female on OCP with abdominal pain and quadriparesis, enzyme deficiency:

(a) Uro decarboxylase
(b) ALA – dehydrogenase
(c) Porphobilinogen deaminase
(d) Ferrochelatase

2026. Closed chest tube drainage is indicated in:

(a) Ph > 7.2
(b) Pressure of pus
(c) Presence of bacteria on gram stain
(d) WBC > 1000

2027. Hypokalemia least likely in:

(a) Amphotericin B (b) Rhabdomyolysis
(c) Villous adenoma (d) Hypoaldosteronism

2028. Metabolic alkalosis occur in:

(a) Mineralocorticoid excess
(b) Septicemia
(c) Hypoxemia
(d) CRF

2029. PH < 7.2, HCO_3 =10 mmol/l, Na= 136 meq/dl, Cl= 100 meg/dl, pCO_2= 25 with crystalluria in urine:

(a) Ethylene glycol (b) Salicylates
(c) Lactic acidosis (d) Methanol poisoning

2030. Hereditary spherocytosis patient with aplastic crisis, most probable cause:

(a) CMV (b) Pravo virus
(c) HIV (d) HSV-8

2031. FEV1/FVC is normal with decreased VC is seen in:

(a) Emphysema due to α1- antitrypsin deficiency
(b) Idiopathic pulmonary fibrosis
(c) Asthma
(d) Pulmonary embolism

2032. T-tube drainage with biliary surgery on antibiotic develop coagulopathy all of the following are not likely to be cause:

(a) Prothrombin deficiency
(b) Factor VII deficiency
(c) Factor VIII deficiency
(d) Fibrinogen deficiency

2033. Incidence of GVHD can be minimized by:

(a) Blood irradiation
(b) PCV transfusion
(c) First degree relative blood transfusion
(d) Autotransfusion

2034. ACE-I C/I in:

(a) Pregnancy
(b) Unilateral RAS
(c) DM with microalbuminuria

2035. Accelerated HTN A/E:

(a) Cocaine (b) Amphetamine
(c) MAO-B inhibitor (d) Ferrous sulphate

2036. 40 years old male with hypotension, RV dilatation ECG showing ST depression in anterior leads, TOC:

(a) IV heparin (b) IV streptokinase
(c) IV NTG (d) beta blocker

2037. Beta thalassemia major not transfused possibility is:

(a) Concomitant α thalassemia
(b) Associated E thalassemia
(c) X Mn mutation
(d) Splice Gs mutation

2038. Beta thalassemia clinically normal, no requirement of blood transfusion:

(a) α thalassemia trait
(b) Sideroblastic
(c) Beta thalassemia trait
(d) Beta thalassemia major

2039. Sickle cell anemia acute drop in Hb:

(a) Extravascular hemolysis
(b) Sickle cell crisis
(c) Megaloblastic anemia
(d) Aplastic anemia

2040. Hemolytic anemia all *except:*

(a) Increased hemosiderin in urine
(b) Increased haptoglobulin
(c) Increased direct antiglobulin test

2041. Cold Ab haemolytic anemia seen in:

(a) SLE (b) Mycoplasma
(c) NHL (d) CLL

2042. Multiple myeloma prognostic factor:

(a) Beta 2 microglobulin
(b) Alkaline phosphatase
(c) Osteocalcin

2043. Bortezomib definitely used in:

(a) MM (b) Hodgkin lymphoma
(c) NHL

2044. CML all used *except:*

(a) Hemoharrington (b) Herbimycin A
(c) ST 1571 (d) Fludarabine

2045. Foscarnet used in:

(a) CMV retinitis
(b) Cryptococcal meningitis

2046. Itraconazole all *except:*

(a) Aspergillosis (b) Mucormycosis
(c) Candidiasis (d) Dermatophytosis

2047. DOC for aeromonas septicemia:

(a) Ciprofloxacin (b) Ceftriaxone
(c) Clindamycin (d) Clarithromycin

2048. Most common cause for PUO in India:

(a) Tb (b) SLE
(c) Malaria (d) Enteric fever

2049. Hanta virus reservoir:

(a) Mouse (b) Dog
(c) Cat (d) Pig

2050. Biliary sludge occur with:

(a) Ceftriaxone (b) Cefoperazone
(c) Cefotaxime (d) Cefipime

2051. CRF–dermatological feature:

(a) Purpura (b) Ecchymosis
(c) Calciphylaxis (d) Blue nail

2052. ATN feature:

(a) Muddy brown cast (b) Hyaline cast

2053. K^+ increases at which GFR level?

(a) 50 ml/min (b) 40 ml/min
(c) 25 ml/min (d) 15 ml/min

2054. Kidney in Sjögren's syndrome biopsy feature

(a) MPGN (b) MGN
(c) Tubulointerstitial (d) Amyloidosis

2055. RTA A/E:

(a) Bicarbonate < 15
(b) Normal AG acidosis
(c) Increased urinary AG
(d) Urine ph < 5.5

2056. CPPD causes *except:*

(a) Hyper PTH (b) Hypermagnesia
(c) Post menisectomy (d) Hemochromatosis

2057. Hypomagnesia seen in A/E:

(a) Thiazide
(b) Hypoaldosteronism
(c) Small bowel byass surgery
(d) Acute pancreatitis

2058. Mechanical ventilation in ARDS A/E:

(a) High TV
(b) Inspiratory pressure > 30 mm Hg
(c) $FiO_2 < 0.6$
(d) Prone position

2059. All dependent variable in CPAP *except:*

(a) TV
(b) FiO_2
(c) Intra-airway pressure
(d) I/E ratio

2060. Which is not infection related vasculitis?

(a) PAN
(b) EMC
(c) Hypersensitive vasculitis
(d) Wegener's granulomatosis

2061. α- coma on ECG:

(a) Hepatic failure
(b) Sedative poisoning
(c) Pontine damage
(d) Hyponatremia

2062. PAN involves A/E:

(a) Lung (b) Liver
(c) Kidney (d) Gastrointestinal tract

2063. HLA–B 27 is all associated *except:*

(a) Ankylosing spondylitis
(b) Psoriasis vulgaris
(c) Acute anterior uveitis
(d) Reiter's syndrome

2064. Properdin deficiency is associated with:

(a) Neisseria infection
(b) Pyogenic infection
(c) Immunocompromised patient

2065. Programmed cell death pathway:

(a) Caspases (b) IL-2
(c) IL-6 (d) IL-10

2066. ACE gene polymorphism seen in A/E:

(a) Diabetic nephropathy
(b) IgA nephropathy
(c) LVH
(d) HTN retinopathy

2067. Deoxycoformycin:

(a) Alkylating agent
(b) Antimetabolites
(c) Antitumour antibiotic
(d) Antimiotic

2068. Which is endogenous inhibitor of angiogenesis:

(a) Endostatin (b) Leptin
(c) IL-6 (d) TNF–α

2069. All are macrovesicular liver disease *except:*

(a) TPN (b) Reye's syndrome
(c) Alcohol (d) Lipodystrophy

2070. Which inflammatory marker not used in drug trial?

(a) Evoculomab (b) Trikaneb

2071. Optimal dose of drug decided in which phase of drug RCT?

(a) I (b) II
(c) III (d) IV

2072. Sarcoidosis true A/E:

(a) Commonly presents with biventricular failure
(b) Mitral regurgitation common

2073. Intention to treat analysis RCT cover all of the following *except*:

(a) Type II error (b) Non compliance
(c) Cross over

2074. Spinal muscular atrophy A/E:

(a) VSD is most common
(b) Type I and II CHD
(c) Most common arrhythmias atrial standstill, AF, block
(d) III- DCM

2075. Iridodonesis:

(a) EDS
(b) Marfan syndrome
(c) Osteogenesis imperfecta
(d) Down syndrome

2076. Not to be given in angle closure glaucoma:

(a) Propafenone (b) Disopyramide
(c) Mexiletine (d) Quinidine

2077. Mental retardation seen with A/E:

(a) Marfan syndrome
(b) Mucopolysaccharidosis
(c) Trisomy 18
(d) Cri du chat syndrome

2078. RA A/E:

(a) Fibrinous pericarditis
(b) Sterile endocarditis
(c) CCP
(d) Cardiac tamponade

2079. Dose of atropine in pediatric heart block:

(a) 0.01 - 0.03 (b) 0.1 - 0.5
(c) 0.75 - 1 (d) 1 - 1.5

2080. GFR in a 40 years old male, 60 kg with plasma creatinine–2 mg%:

(a) 41 (b) 70
(c) 50 (d) 60

2081. Following statement is true regarding cardio-vascular deaths in adults:

(a) Approximately 50% of these are sudden death
(b) Approximately 25% of these are sudden death
(c) Approximately 10% of these are sudden death
(d) Approximately 5% of these are sudden death

2082. Following statement is true regarding cardio-vascular diseases in men compared to women:

(a) The percentage of all deaths secondary to cardio-vascular disease is higher among women Than among men
(b) Coronary artery disease is more frequently associated with dysfunction of the coronary microcirculation in man than in woman
(c) Exercise ECG has higher diagnostic accuracy in the prediction of epicardial obstruction in woman than in man
(d) The absolute number of deaths secondary to cardiovascular disease has declined over the past decades in women.

2083. Organophosphorus poisoning: (T/F)

(a) Irreversibly inhibit acetylcholinestearse
(b) Atropine DOC
(c) Pralidoxime reverse CNS effect
(d) Muscarinic effect—sweating diarrhea salivation
(e) Slowly excreted by kidney

2084. T/F:

(a) Fludaribine inhibits nucleoside
(b) MMF inhibit IMP dehydrogenase
(c) Allopurinol inhibits adenosine deaminase
(d) Azathiopurine inhibits purine nucleosidase
(e) Adenosine deaminase carnitine dehydrogenase

2085. MALTOMA: (T/F)

(a) Stomach most common site
(b) T 11: 18 q 22-q 21 common
(c) CD 20/CD 5
(d) Treatment of H pylori–regression in 75% cases
(e) Survival > 60% at 5 years

2086. Chronic diarrhea: (T/F)

(a) Small bowel diarrhea–few and large
(b) Fasting donot decrease malabsorption
(c) Rectum–tenesmus
(d) D xylose–in small intestine mucosal disease
(e) Steatorrhoea in pancreatic deficiency

2087. Hypothyroidism: (T/F)

(a) Most common goiterous—Hashimoto hypo-thyroidism
(b) TSH can differentiate primary and secondary hypothyroidism
(c) Small age group start with increased dose
(d) Levothyroxine given empty stomach
(e) Start with high dose to prevent myxedema

2088. T/F:

(a) TPO–Hashimoto disease
(b) LES
(c) Limited sclerosis–topoisomerase
(d) Myositis–aminoacyl tRNA
(e) Autoimmune hepatitis–cyto P450

2089. Carpel tunnel syndrome: (T/F)

(a) Median nerve proximal flexor reticulum
(b) USG – gold standard
(c) Shoulder pain
(d) Nocturnal pain classic
(e) May present in thyrotoxicosis

2090. Malaria: (T/F)

(a) Exoerythrocytic in P. vivax
(b) 2 or more in P. vivax
(c) Artesunate + pyrimethamine–DOC for P. falciparum
(d) Antigen detection test–gold standard

2091. T/F:

(a) Impetigo–staphylococcus
(b) Slapped cheek–rubella
(c) Koplik spot–precede skin rash
(d) Erysipelas–streptococcus cellulitis of face
(e) Clostridium perfringens–most comon in gas gangrene

2092. Hepatitis A vaccine: (T/F)

(a) Sub unit vaccine
(b) Given intramuscular
(c) Not effective when given post exposure
(d) Two doses
(e) Given after 6 months of age

2093. T/F:

(a) Diphtheria–toxoid
(b) OPV–two strain
(c) Hepatitis B–killed vaccine
(d) Influenza–toxoid
(e) MMR– live attenuated

2094. Daily requirement: (T/F)

(a) Vitamin B_{12}– 2-4 mg
(b) Thiamine–1-1.5 mg
(c) Oleic acid–essential fatty acid
(d) Vitamin C–hydroxylate connective tissue
(e) Cu deficiency–microhypochromic anemia

2095. Innate immunity: (T/F)

(a) Plasmocystoid dendritic cells secrete TNF–α has antiviral activity
(b) Inflasome is intracellular and releases TNF–α
(c) TOLL only on cell receptors surface
(d) CRP help in opsonize
(e) NK Cell bind HLA II

2096. PSGN: (T/F)

(a) After 1-2 weeks of skin infection
(b) Immunosuppressive treatment can delay renal failure
(c) C3/C4 ratio decreases
(d) Oliguria/HTN/edema

2097. T/F:

(a) Fluoxitine better than sertaline
(b) SSRI increases suicidal risk in children
(c) TCA–xerostomia
(d) MAO and SSRI can be given together
(e) Sertaline given in morning

2098. T/F:

(a) FTSD present with widespread pain
(b) Panic disorder peak in 10 min
(c) Autonomic hyperactive in generalized anxiety disorder
(d) Social phobia–present

2099. T/F:

(a) CML–9: 22 Mutation present
(b) XYY–Inheritable
(c) FISH–specific for trisomy
(d) Trisomy 21–AML

2100. T/F:

(a) Fathery brown eyes–dominant
(b) Mother blue eyes– recessive has children (3 girls) all have brown eyes
(c) Mother blue eyes– recessive has children (3 girls) all have one boy with blue eyes

2101. Father homozygous mother homozygous–X linked: (T/F)

(a) 50% chances of next male child having disease
(b) 50% chances of next female child having disease

2102. CROSS over TRIAL: (T/F)
(a) Small number of patient in companion to other trial
(b) 2 weeks not required to persist over effect
(c) Longitudinal study

2103. Statistics: (T/F)
(a) Chi square test (b) Paired t test
(c) Log rank test (d) Mcwitney test

2104. Most sensitive marker of myositis:
(a) Aldolase (b) Creatinine Kinase
(c) SGOT (d) SGPT

2105. Statistics: (T/F)
(a) 1 SD–69.2%
(b) NNT– 100/ ARR
(c) Mathematical risk is defined by people having risk factor from not having risk factor
(d) C.I. – .83 Statistically significant but clinically insignificant
(e) Probability data occurring by chance

2106. SLE involvement: (T/F)
(a) Most common – pericarditis > 60%
(b) IHD – Most common cause is coronary arteritis
(c) Mother with SLE – child with CHB
(d) Valvular involvement > 50%
(e) Tamponade is rare

2107. Sleep apnea: (T/F)
(a) > 10 secs is definition of sleep apnea
(b) Central sleep apnea no respiratory effort
(c) More in elderly male
(d) Hypothyroidism and acromegaly
(e) Predisposes to OSA

2108. Phlebotomy indication: (T/F)
(a) Non cardiac surgery and Hct > 65%
(b) Microcytosis with hyperviscosity
(c) It ↓es pulm vascular resistance in cor pulmonale
(d) Ac cor pulmonale – can be used
(e) Long term O_2 therapy ↑ es polycythemia

2109. True or False:
(a) At birth mean PAP 50 mm Hg can be normal
(b) At high altitude 3.5 – 4.5 wood unit PVR is normal
(c) At high altitude PA systolic pressure 50 mm Hg is normal
(d) Indexed PVR more than non-indexed PVR

2110. Cytotoxic diarrhea in:
(a) S. typhi (b) B. cereus
(c) Giardia (d) Cl. Difficile

2111. Amsel criteria for:
(a) Syphilis (b) Chancroid
(c) Bacterial vaginosis (d) Trichomoniasis

2112. Portal HTN pressure more than:
(a) 5 mm Hg (b) 10 mm Hg
(c) 15 mm Hg (d) 20 mm Hg

2113. DM nephropathy A/E:
(a) Microalbuminemia associated with HTN
(b) Retinopathy seen almost always
(c) Reversible microalbuminemia if strict glycemic control

2114. DM true *except*:
(a) Decrease protein kinase activity
(b) Increased tyrosine kinase activity
(c) Decreased mitochondrial oxidation capacity
(d) Fat stored in red muscle

2115. Rose spot:
(a) Within 2 weeks (b) < 30%
(c) Culture < 10% (d) Chest and trunk

2116. Maltoma skin by:
(a) Borrelia (b) H. pylori
(c) HHV-8 (d) EBV

2117. Struvite stone by:
(a) Proteus (b) E.coli
(c) Klebsiella

2118. ATT prodrug:
(a) Isoniazid (b) Rifampicin
(c) Pyrazinamide (d) Ethambutol

2119. POEMS A/E:
(a) Lymphadenopathy (b) Osteolytic bony lesions
(c) Thrombocytopenia (d) Increased VEGF

2120. Lymphedema A/E:
(a) Klinefelter syndrome (b) Yellow Nail syndrome
(c) Down syndrome (d) Turner syndrome

2121. Psoriasis lesions increased by all *except:*
(a) Amiodarone (b) Lithium
(c) Beta blocker (d) Antimalarial

2122. Keratoderma blenorrhagia:
(a) Lupus dermatitis (b) Reactive arthritis
(c) Secondary syphilis

2123. AKI A/E:
(a) 20% O_2 consumption by kidney
(b) Can be with only ischemia
(c) Tubuloglomerular feedback in proximal kidney
(d) Glomerulus early susceptible

2124. Fabry's disease A/E:
(a) Zebra bodies seen
(b) Biopsy – FSGN
(c) Female can be involved
(d) Post transplantation graft poor survival

2125. Dohle bodies formed by:
(a) Nuclear membrane
(b) Endoplasmic reticulum

2126. Corynebacterium in neutropenia and malignancy:
(a) C. jeikeium (b) C. pseudotuberculosis
(c) C. ulcerans (d) C. urealyticum

2127. Post splenectomy sepsis by:
(a) Streptococci (b) Staph
(c) Babesio microti

2128. Hot tub folliculitis by:
(a) Pseudomonas (b) Staphylococci
(c) Streptococci

2129. Hypersplenism A/E:
(a) BM suppression
(b) Cytopenia
(c) Respond to splenectomy
(d) Splenomegaly

2130. Most medial structure:
(a) Ventral spinothalamic tract
(b) Fascicular cuneatus
(c) Anterior corticospinal tract
(d) Rubrospinal

2131. Hypomagnesia cause A/E:
(a) Hyperparathyroidism

2132. Iodine requirement:
(a) 15 μg/day (b) 40 μg/day
(c) 150 μg/day (d) 400 μg/day

2133. Hypothyroidism associated with:
(a) Selenium (b) Zinc
(c) Chromium (d) Copper

2134. GFR – stage V:
(a) < 15 ml/min (b) 15-30 ml/min
(c) 30-60 ml/min (d) 60-90 ml/min

2135. DHF true:
(a) Type 2 most dangerous
(b) Female are less affected
(c) Malnutrition is protective
(d) Chances of susceptibility decreases after age of 12 years

2136. Isolated microscopic hematuria A/E:
(a) Familial (b) IgA nephropathy
(c) MPGN

2137. Spirometry not helpful in:
(a) FRC (b) VC
(c) IRV (d) IC

2138. At FRC:
(a) Pleural pressure is zero
(b) Lung tissue shows maximum compliance
(c) Alveolar pressure = atm. Pressure
(d) Inspiratory muscle work balanced by expiratory muscle

2139. Parkinsonism risk in:
(a) REM (b) Bruxism
(c) Dystonia

2140. Addison disease least common:
(a) Mucosal pigmentation
(b) Weakness
(c) Weight loss

2141. Earliest in tuberous sclerosis:
(a) Ash leaf spot (b) Shagreen patch
(c) Adenoma sebaceum

2142. SNHL seen in:
(a) Paclitaxel (b) Irinotecan
(c) Cisplatin (d) Anthracycline

2143. Least nephrotoxic:
(a) Streptomycin (b) Tobramycin
(c) Gentamicin

2144. CSF in bacterial meningitis true:
(a) Lymphocyte and neutrophil dominance
(b) Culture positive in < 10%
(c) PCR not helpful
(d) Prior to LP– glucose infusion will cause spurious increase of glucose

2145. Genes remain together:
(a) Cross over (b) Imprinting
(c) Linkage

2146. Hemolytic anemia true:
(a) Reticulocytosis characteristic
(b) Bilirubin > 4-5 mg/dl
(c) OT can be increased

2147. Desmopressin A/E:
(a) Causes hyponatremia
(b) Used in severe hemophilia
(c) Increases factor VIII 2-3 fold

2148. Cyroprecipitate A/E:
(a) Factor I (b) Factor VIII
(c) Factor IX (d) vwF

2149. Complement convergence:
(a) C1 (b) C2
(c) C3 (d) C4

2150. GBS true:
(a) Pain common
(b) Early bladder involvement
(c) IVIG + plasmapheresis better than earlier
(d) Fever help in diagnosis

2151. Adenocarcinoma:
(a) Female common
(b) Common in non smoker
(c) Young
(d) Centrally located

2152. Sarcoidosis true:
(a) Ranges from solitary nodule to diffuse disease
(b) CD8/CD4 > 3.5 in BAL sample

2153. Cystic fibrosis:
(a) 90% males are sterile
(b) Decrease sweat from childhood
(c) Predisposes to Tb
(d) Hypertonic saline used in treatment

2154. ABG-arterial O_2 saturation difference not seen in:
(a) CO poisoning (b) Sulfhemoglobin
(c) Meth Hb (d) CN poisoning

2155. Kronsky algorithm used for tumour size regression after:
(a) Radiotherapy (b) Chemotherapy
(c) Surgical ablation (d) All of the above

2156. Cell cycle Go is followed by:
(a) G2 S G1 M (b) G1 S G2 M
(c) M G1 S G2

2157. 30 years female, recurrent pneumothorax, chylous Pleural Effusion and obstructive PFT?
(a) Lymphangioleiomyomatosis
(b) Langerhan's cell histiocytosis
(c) PAP
(d) Pulmonary-histoplasmosis

2158. Behcet's triad A/E:
(a) Oral ulcers (b) Genital ulcers
(c) Uveitis (d) Glomerulonephritis

2159. Na$^+$: 140, Kt: 3.0, 0: 95, HCO_3: 25, PCO_3: 40 PH: 7.42 most likely:
(a) COPD with diuretics
(b) Uraemia with vomiting
(c) Gram -ve sepsis
(d) Diarrhea with mild lactic acidosis

2160. Stimulating auto Ab seen in:
(a) Wegener's (b) Pernicious
(c) Hashimoto's (d) M. Gravis

2161. Iron deficiency anemia:
(a) Serum iron–24 (b) Ferritin–10
(c) TIBC–400 (d) Transferrin–8
(e) All of the above

2162. Highest risk of thrombosis:
(a) Homozygous factor V
(b) Protein S deficiency
(c) Protein C deficiency
(d) Homozygous prothrombin deficiency

2163. P-value suggests:
(a) Clinical significance
(b) Suggest the result is just by pure chance
(c) Shows associated with casual factor
(d) None of the above

2164. Most common cause of adrenal hypertension:
(a) Desoxycorticosterone
(b) Aldosterone
(c) Catecholamines
(d) Cortisol

2165. MEN-1 all *except:*
(a) Pancreas (b) Pituitary
(c) Parathyroid (d) Adrenal

2166. Necrotizing fasciitis is by:
(a) Staph (b) St repto
(c) Pseudomonas (d) E. Coli

2167. Polyploidy normal in:
(a) Megakaryocytes (b) Giant cell
(c) Germ Cell (d) Stem cell

2168. Cyclosporine least toxicity:
(a) B.M. suppression (b) Nephrotoxicity
(c) Hypenuticemia (d) Hyperlipidemia

2169. Neonatal screening to exclude metabolic disorders includes:
(a) Phenylketonuria
(b) Congenital adrenal disorder
(c) Thyroid disorder
(d) All of the above

2170. All *except* hairy cell leukemia:
(a) Predisposes 2° infections
(b) Pancytopenia
(c) Hypercellular marrow
(d) Good response to chemotherapy

2171. PT does not evaluate:
(a) V (b) IX
(c) VII (d) X

2172. Structure which does not come in medulla:
(a) Vasa recta
(b) Terminal collecting duct
(c) Loop of Henle
(d) DCT

2173. Who → filaria elimination in non-Endemic countries single dose therapy?
(a) DEC + doxycyline
(b) DEC + Albendazole
(c) Albendazole + ivermectin
(d) Albendazole

2174. Most common congenital bleeding disorder:
(a) VWD
(b) Glazamann thromboasthenia
(c) Hemophilia
(d) Bernard Soulier disease

2175. Vitamin levels least in bone:
(a) Vitamin C (b) Vitamin B1
(c) Vitamin A (d) Vitamin E

2176. Energy to Brain in Starvation:
(a) Glucose (b) 13-hydroxybutyric acid
(c) Fatty Acids (d) Glycerol

2177. Acyclovir A/E:
(a) CMV (b) HSV
(c) VZV (d) EBV

2178. Lactic acidosis least in:
(a) Zidovudine (b) Stavudine
(c) Zalcitabine (d) Lamivudine

2179. Dorsum of foot A/E:
(a) L4 (b) 1.5
(c) S1 (d) S2

2180. ACE increased in A/E:
(a) Sarcoidosis (b) Miliary TB
(c) Leprosy (d) Lymphoma

2181. NREM phase 3 and 4 A/E:
(a) Slow wave sleep
(b) Constitute 40-50% of total sleep in young adults
(c) Progressively less with increasing age
(d) Predominant in first 1/3rd of sleep

2182. Insulin secretion-sensiting trace mineral:
(a) Zinc (b) Selenium
(c) Chromium (d) Copper

2183. All are true about leptospirosis *except:*
(a) Vaculitis is most common cause of major manifestation

(b) Fulminant hapatitis recovery is characterstic
(c) Renal failure may be due to interstitial nephritis and ATN
(d) Altered capillary permeability may cause renal failure

2184. All *except* Weil's syndrome:
(a) Most common site of hemorrhage is lung
(b) Renal failure oligouric/Non-oligouric
(c) Hepatocellular necrosis and lung parenchymal inflammation characteristics
(d) Myocarditis can occur

2185. False regarding primary pulmonary TB:
(a) 50% of cases have clinical illness
(b) Affects mid and lower zones
(c) Primary focus peripheral
(d) Majority have hilar /Paratracheal lymphadenopathy

2186. A patient of scleroderma with malignant hypertension with microagiopathic hemolytic anemia with renal failure, DOC:
(a) ACE-I (b) ARB
(c) Diuretics (d) Nitroprusside

2187. Migratory annular erythema A/E:
(a) Secondary syphilis (b) Malignancies
(c) Lyme Disease (d) RF

2188. True regarding Primary chancre:
(a) Painless papule (b) Multiple papule
(c) Non-indurated (d) Hard

2189. True regarding cardiovascular syphilis:
(a) Linear calcification of ascending aorta in CXR suggest syphilis
(b) Most common involves abdominal aorta
(c) Can cause aortic dissection and SCD
(d) Cause fusiform aneurysm in ascending aorta

2190. All/Except for S. typhi:
(a) Cefixime (b) Azithromycin
(c) Ofloxacin (d) Amikacin

2191. HIV mucous membrane transmission:
(a) 0.03% (b) 0.09%
(c) 0.3% (d) 0.9%

2192. Multiple myeloma A/E:
(a) Hypercalcemia
(b) Hyper gammaglobulinemia
(c) Cryoglobulinemia
(d) Hyper viscosity

2193. Multiple myeloma A/E:
(a) Bone pain most common symptoms
(b) Most common site–back or ribs
(c) Night pain characteristics
(d) Pain worsen with movement

2194. 50 years male, migratory polyarthritis, diarrhea, PAS +ve inclusions on intestinal biopsy:
(a) Chronic antibiotics (b) IVIg
(c) Steroids (d) Sulfasalaziline

2195. RF in RA true statement:
(a) Good screening test
(b) This and Severity do not correlate
(c) Uniformly present in patients with subcutaneous nodules/vasculitis
(d) Good predictive value for diagnosis

2196. Gottron's papule -+ Diagnosis:
(a) Polymyositis (b) Dermatomyositis
(c) Scleroderma (d) Sjögren's syndrome

2197. All are seen in seronegative spondyloarthrisis *except:*
(a) Serositis (b) Sacroilitis
(c) Sinusitis (d) HLA B27 positivity

2198. Petechiae/mucosal bleeding in which malaria?
(a) Vivax (b) Falciparum
(c) Ovale (d) Malariae

2199. Earliest features of I.V. hemolysis:
(a) Hemoglobinemia (b) Hemoglobinuria
(c) Hemosidenuria (d) Less Haptoglobin

2200. Sickle cell trait A/E:
(a) Asymptomatic
(b) Painless hematuria
(c) Isothenuria
(d) Anemia and bone pain are common

2201. Genetic Counselling A/E:
(a) Mother > 35 years
(b) Father > 45 years
(c) Consanguity
(d) Family history of genetic disorder

2202. Most common mechanism of antibiotic associated diarrhoea:
(a) Led colonic short chain fatty acid
(b) Pseudomembranouscolitis
(c) Enterotoxin mediated secretary diarrhoea
(d) Micro Villous flattening

2203. Most common cause of ectopic ACTH:
(a) SCLC (b) Thyroid ca
(c) Adrenal

2204. Oncogenic osteomalacia A/E:
(a) Normal PTH
(b) Decreased Ca^{2+}
(c) Decreased Phosphate
(d) ↓ 1,25 (OH)2 vitamin D

2205. Wilson disease copper level:
(a) 250 µg/gm of liver (b) 2.5 mg/g of liver
(c) 800 µg/g of liver (d) 80 mg/g of liver

2206. Hypokalemia/Normal BP/ ↑ urinary Cl:
(a) Gittlemen syndrome
(b) Liddle's syndrome
(c) 11 α hydroxylase deficiency
(d) 17 (OH) deficiency

2207. Haemophilia A A/E:
(a) < 1% severe hemophilia
(b) Most common presentation < 1 year of age (90%)
(c) Ankle joint most common involved in infancy
(d) Since it crosses placenta it never present before 3-6 months

2208. Central DI treatment A/E:
(a) Fluid therapy
(b) Thiazide
(c) Desmopressin
(d) Vasopressin synthetic preparation

2209. Pseudolymphoma:
(a) Phenytoin (b) Thioridazone
(c) Warfarin

2210. Non scaring alopecia caused by:
(a) Cutaneous lupus (b) Metastatic
(c) Secondary syphilis (d) Folliculitis decalavan's

2211. Piokiloderma:
(a) Sarcoidosis (b) CREST
(c) Dermatomyositis (d) GVHD

2212. Creatinine and creatinine clearance A/E:
(a) S. creatinine level not affected by diet and exercise
(b) Overestimate GFR
(c) CRCL < 10 ml/min – Indication for dialysis
(d) Not reliable in chronic glucocorticoid therapy

2213. Tubercular lymphadenitis A/E:
(a) Painless
(b) Most common by M. tuberculosis
(c) Uncommon in HIV
(d) AFB in 50% cases

2214. Ab when react with heterologous serum is known as:
(a) Allotype (b) Idiotype
(c) Isotype (d) None of the above

2215. Cause of infective arthritis in young adult:
(a) Gonococcal (b) Staph. aureus
(c) Borrelia burgdorferi (d) M. Tuberculi

2216. Child pug score A/E:
(a) APTT (b) Ascites
(c) Albumin (d) Bilirubin

2217. Crohn's disease common feature A/E:
(a) Recurrence after surgery
(b) ANCA positive rarely
(c) Cobblestone appearance on endoscopy
(d) SI obstruction

2218. Prolactionoma A/E:
(a) > 100 pg/ml indicate macroadenoma
(b) More in female (microadenoma)
(c) Large size in female than male
(d) Microadenoma changes to macroadenoma in 5%

2219. Suspected hypothyroidism with normal TSH, normal Free T4, next step:
(a) Free T3 (b) No further test
(c) TPO (d) Pituitary function

2220. Micropathy in DM A/E:
(a) CAD
(b) Diabetic nephropathy
(c) Autonomic nephropathy
(d) Macular edema

2221. Hypomagnesium A/E:
(a) Gittleman's syndrome
(b) Hyper Ca^{2+}
(c) Bartter's syndrome
(d) Hypoaldosteronism

2222. 1st line antiepileptic for GTCS A/E:
(a) Lamotrignine (b) Topiramate
(c) Phenytoin (d) Valproic acid

2223. True about F. ataxia A/E:
(a) 90% cardiac involvement
(b) Usually presentation after 25 years
(c) DM common
(d) AR

2224. Tumour lysis syndrome:
(a) Hypocalcemia (b) Hypophosphatemia
(c) Hypouricemia (d) Hypokalemia

2225. Niacin induced flushing prevented by A/E:
(a) Aspirin
(b) Brufen
(c) Laropiprant
(d) Chlorphenarmine maleate

2226. DPP IV inhibitor A/E:
(a) ↑ insulin (b) ↓ glucagon
(c) ↓ incretin

2227. Novobiocin MOA:
(a) Protein synthesis inhibition
(b) DNA gyrase inhibition
(c) Act on wall synthesis
(d) Inhibits RNA synthase

2228. Cornabacterium jeikeium treatment:
(a) Levofloxacin (b) Ciprofloxacin
(c) Vancomycin (d) Penicillin G

2229. CMP caused by:
(a) Trastuzomab (b) Rituximab
(c) Bacilituzomab (d) Desilizumab

2230. Carbegoline:
(a) D1 agonist (b) D1 antagonist
(c) D2 antagonist (d) D2 agonist

2231. HIV nephropathy:
(a) FSGN
(b) MCD
(c) Diffuse membranous GN
(d) IgA nephropathy

2232. Dabigatran:
(a) 20 mg bd (b) 40 mg bd
(c) 75 mg bd (d) 150 mg bd

2233. Batwing appearance of alveolar type seen in:
(a) PAP (b) LCH
(c) COP (d) BOOP

2234. Antibiotic with cell membrane depolarization:
(a) Daptomycin (b) Streptogramin
(c) Metronidazole (d) Ertopenam

2235. Sporadic porphyria most common:
(a) AIP
(b) VP
(c) PCT
(d) Erythropoietic porphyria

2236. Both venous + arterial thrombosis A/E:
(a) Dysfibrinognemia
(b) Essential thrombocytopenia
(c) AT III deficiency
(d) PNH
(e) HIT

2237. Arthritis of RA A/E:
(a) Anti CCP poor screening test
(b) Morning stiffness differentiate it from other non infectious arthritis
(c) Bone erosion poor prognosis
(d) RA factor negative is 30%

2238. Adult onset still disease A/E:
(a) Rash (b) RA factor negative
(c) ↑ S. ferritin level (d) ANA positive
(e) Lymphadenopathy

2239. Earliest marker of iron deficiency anemia:
(a) TIBC
(b) Free erythropoietic protophorphyrin
(c) S. iron level
(d) Sideroblast in marrow increases
(e) Transferrin saturation

2240. Immune complex vasculitis A/E:
(a) PAN

(b) HSP
(c) Churg-Strauss syndrome
(d) SLE

2241. Tuberculosis A/E:
(a) HIV infected are less more infection than non HIV
(b) Cavitatory lesion more infection
(c) Extra pulmonary virtually non infectious
(d) Skin contact/placental transmission are epidemiological non significant

2242. Urease producing/Renal calculi/UTI causing organisms:
(a) Enterobacter (b) Proteus
(c) Klebsiella (d) S. saprophyticus

2243. Diagnosis of GERD most sensitive test:
(a) Barium swallow
(b) 24 hours ambulatory pH monitoring
(c) Endoscopy
(d) Endoscopic USG

2244. Amyloidosis protein A/E:
(a) Light chain (b) P-glycoprotein
(c) B_2 microglobulin (d) Transferrin
(e) Protein A

2245. Nucleotide repeat A/E:
(a) Kent Sayre syndrome (b) F. ataxia
(c) Myotonic dystrophy (d) Huntington chorea

2246. PHT with pregnancy vasodilator C/I:
(a) Epoprostenol (b) Nifedipine
(c) Sildenafil (d) Bosentan

2247. Unsafe method of diagnosis of CAD in pregnancy:
(a) CT angio (b) MR angio (plain)
(c) PET (d) Radionuclide scanning

2248. Plasmodium vivax stage in mosquito:
(a) Zygote (b) Hypnozygote
(c) Merozoite (d) Schzinzoite

2249. Stroke least ↓ by which intervention?
(a) Tight glycemic control
(b) HT
(c) Smoking
(d) Hyperlipidemia

2250. Connective tissue disorder least eye involvement:
(a) RA
(b) Psoriatic arthritis
(c) Ankylosing spondylitis
(d) Enteropathy spondylitis

2251. Salt restriction effective in A/E:
(a) Pheochromocytoma (b) Conn's syndrome
(c) ACE-I therapy (d) Essential HT

2252. Steroid used in treatment of which HT?
(a) 11-B hydroxylase deficiency
(b) Liddle syndrome
(c) 21 beta OH deficiency
(d) Bartter's syndrome

2253. Prostaglandin infusion causes A/E:
(a) Ductal aneurysm (b) Fever
(c) Apnea (d) Pyloris stenosis

2254. Sonicated albumin for:
(a) Plaque rupture and characteristic of stability
(b) LV contour and perfusion
(c) Valve anatomy
(d) Coronary anatomy

2255. Factor V leiden mutation A/E:
(a) Life time risk only 5-10% of thrombosis
(b) AR
(c) Most common hereditary cause
(d) APC resistance for lab diagnosis in 90% of cases

2256. HIV primary malignancy of heart:
(a) Kaposi sarcoma (b) NHL
(c) Leiomyosarcoma (d) Spindle cell carcinoma

2257. Hyperhomocysteinemia treatment is:
(a) Cyanocobalamin (b) Retinoic acid
(c) α-tocopherol (d) Ascorbic acid

2258. Palpable purpura seen in:
(a) HSP
(b) Essential thrombocytopenia
(c) TTP
(d) HIT

2259. Diet treatment successful in first disease:
(a) Phenyl ketonurea (b) DM
(c) Pompe's disease (d) Leisch-Nyhan disease

2260. CHF, DM, skin pigmentation, ↓ libido, diagnosis:
(a) Hemochromatosis (b) Amyloidosis
(c) Carcinoid syndrome (d) MVP

2261. Drug used in HIV causing crystalluria and renal stone:
(a) Indinavir (b) Septran
(c) Acyclovir

2262. Tegmentum pontine lesion causes:
(a) Downbeat nystagmus
(b) Upbeat nystagmus
(c) Gaze evoke nystagmus
(d) Opsoclonus

2263. Least elevated in obstructive jaundice:
(a) AST and ALT
(b) 5 nucleotidase
(c) Alkaline phosphatase
(d) GGT

2264. TN/TN + FP:
(a) Sensitivity (b) Specificity
(c) PPV (d) NPV

2265. Rifabutin A/E:
(a) Orange pigmentation of skin
(b) Pseudojaundice
(c) Increased ICT
(d) Skin pigmentation

2266. ATT A/E:
(a) Linezolid (b) Ofloxacin
(c) Amoxyclav (d) Lincomycin

2267. Portal circulation normal in:
(a) Adrenal (b) Heart
(c) Kidney (d) All
(e) None of the above

2268. HIVAN A/E:
(a) HTN is rare
(b) Due to direct effect of HIV
(c) Kidney biopsy normal in majority
(d) Boteairio is hallmark

2269. Normal cortisol secretion:
(a) 10-30 mg/d (b) 300-400 mg/d
(c) 100-300 mg/d (d) 1-2 mg/d

2270. PPAR against:
(a) Telmisartan (b) Rosiglitazone
(c) Folic acid derivative (d) All
(e) None of the above

2271. Hepatorenal syndrome:
(a) Biopsy shows tubular necrosis
(b) Na retention
(c) Normal urinalysis
(d) Intense renal vasoconstriction can be the cause

2272. Insulin Secretogauge:
(a) Meglitinide (b) Rosiglitazone
(c) Biguanide (d) All
(e) None of the above

2273. HLA B27 A/E:
(a) Psoriasis (b) AS
(c) Reiter's syndrome (d) SLE

2274. Age > 50 years male with testicular swelling most common tumour:
(a) Seminoma
(b) Epidermoid yolk sac tumours
(c) Teratoma
(d) Lymphoma

2275. PSA valve suggestive of Ca prostate:
(a) > 15 ng/ml (b) > 1.5 ng/ml
(c) > 4 ng/ml (d) 0.1-0.5 ng/ml

2276. Reactive arthritis most common after:
(a) Shigella boydi (b) Shigella shiga
(c) Shigella Flexneri (d) Shigella Dysenteriae

2277. SLE A/E:
(a) Anti ds DNA (b) Anti centromere
(c) Anti RNP (d) Anti Smith

2278. Intramural coronary thickening typical of:
(a) Scleroderma
(b) MCTD
(c) Ankylosing spondylitis
(d) RA

2279. Risk factor for thyroid Ca in nodule A/E:
(a) Radiotherapy to head and neck
(b) Increase in size
(c) Hyper functioning nodule
(d) Vocal cord paralysis

2280. Hydroxyurea used in:

(a) α-thalassemia (b) β-thalassemia
(c) Sickle cell anemia (d) PCH

2281. Thrombocytopenia A/E:

(a) TTP (b) HUS
(c) DIC (d) Prosthetic aortic valve

2282. Diffuse foot process effacement characteristic of:

(a) Membranous GN
(b) MCD
(c) MPGN
(d) Menangioproliferative GN

2283. Prerenal azotemia A/E:

(a) BUN/Plasma creatinine > 20:1
(b) Urine creatinine/serum creatinine < 40:1
(c) FE Na < 1%
(d) Urine osmolality > 500

2284. Urine concentration in DCT is always irrespective of final urine concentration:

(a) Hypo osmolar (b) Iso osmolar
(c) Hyper osmolar (d) Iso osmolar to urine

2285. Aδ unmyelinated fibres carry:

(a) Pain (b) Temp
(c) Proprioception (d) Touch and pressure

2286. 30 years hypoxic male with hypercapnia with AV O_2 difference > 40 mm Hg and no improvement with O_2 therapy then diagnosis:

(a) High altitude (b) Neuromuscular
(c) ILD (d) Atelectasis

2287. Hypertension with hypokalemic alkalosis, decreased PRA and absent aldosterone level, treatment:

(a) Amiloride (b) Spironolactone
(c) NSAID (d) ↑ salt intake

2288. Intra erythrocytic bacilli:

(a) Bartonella (b) Babesia microtic
(c) Borrelia (d) Malaria

2289. H. pylori true A/E:

(a) 14 days treatment better than 10 days
(b) Triple drug better than double drug
(c) Should not be treated after 1 episode peptic ulcer
(d) MALT is reduced post treatment

2290. H. pylori:

(a) Gram positive Flagellate bacilli
(b) MALT is reduced post treatment
(c) Present in 30-60% of GU
(d) Present in 70% of DU

2291. Post splenectomy:

(a) Increased risk of unencapsulated organism infection
(b) Babesia microtic septicemia
(c) Splenic rupture common indication
(d) Vaccine pneumococcal given post splenectomy

2292. Hereditary angioneurotic edema A/E:

(a) Epinephrine is not effective
(b) Intestinal obstruction is common
(c) Laryngeal edema is common
(d) All of the above

2293. TH -1 cells secretes:

(a) IL-2 (b) IFN-γ
(c) Both of the above (d) None of the above

2294. Resident doctor treating MAC patient develops fever with chills with pulmonary nodule Mantoux test >12 mm, then X-ray chest showing hilar lymphadenopathy with infiltrates. Next to be done:

(a) HIV status
(b) Gastric lavage and culture
(c) Directly start HIV treatment
(d) INH for 1 year at 300 mg

2295. Immunocompromised patient most common mycobacterial infection:

(a) M.Tb (b) MAC
(c) M scrofulacium (d) M. hansei

2296. Characteristic of myopathy A/E:

(a) Relative preservation of muscle mass
(b) Reflexes preserved
(c) Fasciculation
(d) Proximal muscle involvement more

2297. Follow up of 15 years of patients of gestational DM, incidence of DM:

(a) 25 (b) 33
(c) 50 (d) 60

2298. Typical organochlorine compound poisoning endocrinal manifestation:

(a) SIADH (b) Diabetes insipidus
(c) Infertility (d) Hematuria

2299. Allergy angitis and Churg-Strauss caused by:

(a) Methotrexate
(b) Glucocorticoids
(c) Normal saline infusion
(d) Leukotriene modifiers

2300. Window period of HBV, marker for an acute infection:

(a) IgM anti HBc (b) IgM anti HBe
(c) IgG anti HBc (d) IgG anti HBe

2301. In acute MI, sequence of event in perfusion is: (1) Perfusion abnormal (2) RWMN (3) Systolic dysfunction (4) Diastolic dysfunction.

(a) 1→4→3→2 (b) 1→2→3→4
(c) 4→1→3→2 (d) 4→1→2→3

2302. All used for chronic HBV A/E:

(a) Zidovudine (b) Lamivudine
(c) IFN α (d) Adefovir

2303. Long acting peakless analogue of insulin:

(a) Glargine (b) Aspartate
(c) Lispro (d) All of the above

2304. 50 years patient had ASD closure at 30 years comes for dental procedure, I.E. prophylaxis is required:

(a) Amoxicillin 2 g 1 hour before surgery
(b) Clindamycin 500 mg 1 hour before surgery
(c) Amoxicillin 2 g before and 6 hours after surgery
(d) No prophylaxis required

2305. Most common presentation of Wilson's disease:

(a) Jaundice (b) Anemia
(c) Dysarthria (d) Tremor

2306. Feco-oral route:

(a) Hepatitis E (b) Hepatitis B
(c) Hepatitis C (d) Hepatitis G

2307. False about hepatitis D:

(a) HDV is a DNA virus
(b) 20% have fulminant course
(c) Transmitted by parenteral route
(d) Require infection by hepatitis B virus

2308. True about gastrointestinal tumour:

(a) 90% in body of pancreas
(b) 50% in MEN-1
(c) Associated with hyperplastic gastritis
(d) Peptic ulcer
(e) Diarrhea due to increased HCl in duodenum

2309. ZE syndrome increased secretion of:

(a) Gastrin (b) Cholecystokinin
(c) VIP (d) Somatostatin

2310. Hypercalcemia A/E:

(a) Addison's disease
(b) Thyrotoxcosis
(c) Hyperparathyroidism
(d) Vitamin D intoxication

2311. Hypokalemia A/E:

(a) Conn's syndrome
(b) Hyporeninemic hypoaldosteronism
(c) Bartter's syndrome
(d) Cushing's syndrome
(e) Renal tubular acidosis

2312. HIV true A/E:

(a) Due to lenti virus group of retro virus
(b) P-24 antigen positive after infection 6 months
(c) Glycoprotein identifies CD-4 on T cell surface
(d) Subgroup M and O

2313. All nucleoside analogue *except:*

(a) Acyclovir (b) Oseltamavir
(c) Vidarabine (d) Valacyclovir

2314. DNA found out by:

(a) Western blot (b) Northern blot
(c) Southern blot

2315. PAS positive biopsy diagnostic of:

(a) Celiac sprue (b) Tropical sprue
(c) Whipple's disease

2316. H. pyloric true A/E:

(a) 90-95% in duodenal ulcer
(b) 70% in stomach asymptomatic
(c) Due to gram positive spiral bacilli
(d) Causes various gastritis syndrome

2317. Weil's disease true A/E:

(a) Caused by leptospira interrogans

(b) Infect through intact skin and mucous membrane
(c) Cause renal failure, liver failure, meningitis
(d) Treatment with penicillin, ampicillin and clindamycin
(e) Lymphopenia

2318. Nuclear protein is:
(a) Dystrophin (b) Emerin
(c) Cavectin (d) Calepcin

2319. Lymph node on either side of diaphragm, grading in Ann Arbor:
(a) I (b) II
(c) III (d) IV

2320. USA, trop positive– treatment A/E:
(a) Aspirin (b) Clopidogrel
(c) Tirofiban (d) Eptifibatide
(e) Abciximab

2321. Diagnosis of uremic ventilator insufficiency on ABG:
(a) CO_2 ↑, normal pH, ↑ HCO_3
(b) CO_2 ↑, acidosis, ↓ HCO_3
(c) CO_2 ↓, alkalosis, ↓ HCO_3
(d) CO_2↓, normal pH, ↑ HCO_3

2322. Patient with ostium primum ASD, all true *except:*
(a) RBBB with RAD
(b) Wide fixed S2
(c) ESM at LPS area
(d) Diastolic murmur at apex

2323. Wrong match:
(a) TOF–BT shunt
(b) TGA with ASD–Sennings
(c) Single ventricle with PAH–cavopulmonary shunt
(d) AS–Ross

2324. Linked autosomal inheritance A/E:
(a) Incidence in females twice of males
(b) Expression in females variable
(c) Hypophosphatemic rickets is an example
(d) Transmitted in all daughters and half sons

2325. NSAID's causes:
(a) MGN (b) FSGN
(c) MPGN (d) MCD

2326. ARDS true A/E:
(a) Acute onset
(b) Bilateral pulmonary infilterate
(c) $PaO_2/FiO_2 < 100$
(d) PA pressure < 10 mm Hg

2327. True about MPGN A/E:
(a) HBV causes it
(b) Complement low
(c) Mesangial proliferation
(d) BP and GFR are abnormal

2328. Distribution in a normal population A/E:
(a) Skewed to right
(b) Mean and median same

2329. Cannot be detected by mean ± S.D.:
(a) No. of visits by stable angina patient over 2 years
(b) Stages of retinopathy in HTN patients on treatment
(c) Money spent by 30 hospitals

2330. Not involved in aorta arteritis:
(a) Femoral artery (b) Carotid artery
(c) Pulmonary artery (d) Coronary artery
(e) Renal artery

2331. Blue toe syndrome seen in:
(a) Scleroderma (b) Atheroebolism
(c) Warfarin

2332. Budd-Chiari syndrome true A/E:
(a) Sinusoidal obstruction
(b) Ascitis main presentation
(c) Hepatic vein pressure increases
(d) Portal HTN

2333. Erythema marginatum true:
(a) Acute rheumatic fever
(b) Sepsis
(c) GN
(d) All of the above

2334. Brain abscess due to CHD A/E:
(a) TOF most common cause
(b) Right to left shunt present
(c) I.E. not required
(d) Multiple
(e) High mortality

2335. Normal anion gap acidosis seen in:
(a) RTA
(b) DKA
(c) Lactic acidosis
(d) Ethylene glycol poisoning

2336. Klinefelter's syndrome:
(a) Most common cause of gonadal ambiguity
(b) Azoospermia
(c) Decrease gonadotropin secretion
(d) Gynaecomastia

2337. Biphasic shock better than monophasic:
(a) DC C/I in patients on pacemaker
(b) Non synchronized shock if rhythm is irregular

2338. Conjugated hyperbilirubinemia A/E:
(a) Dubin Johnson's syndrome
(b) Gilbert's syndrome
(c) OCP
(d) Parenteral nutrition

2339. True in CLL A/E:
(a) Cell mediated immunity normal
(b) Warm Ab hemolytic anemia
(c) Cold Ab
(d) Increase Ig

2340. All are myeloproliferative disease *except:*
(a) Polycythemia vera
(b) Myeloid metaplasia
(c) Essential thrombocytosis
(d) Hairy cell luekaemia
(e) CML

2341. Myocyte regeneration due to stem cell can be by:
(a) Skeletal myocyte
(b) Hemopoietic stem cell
(c) Mesodermal stem cell
(d) All of the above

2342. True about apoptosis A/E:
(a) Energy dependent process
(b) Inflammatory exudates absent
(c) Cells take up water and burst
(d) Nuclear degeneration

2343. Apoptosis inhibited by:
(a) Insulin like growth factor
(b) Caspases
(c) Ischemia
(d) Dobutamine

2344. True about TAPVC A/E:
(a) Equal O_2 saturation in all 4 chambers
(b) Figure of 8 in CXR in infradiaphragmatic type
(c) Wide fixed S2
(d) Continuous murmur

2345. Polygenic inheritance A/E:
(a) Cystic fibrosis (b) HTN
(c) SLE

2346. Stem cell transplantation effective in A/E:
(a) ADA deficiency
(b) Cystic fibrosis
(c) Hypercholesterolemia
(d) Retinitis pigmentosa

2347. India ink staining in cryptococcal meningitis sensitivity:
(a) 10-20% (b) 30-50%
(c) 50-60% (d) 80-90%
(e) 100%

2348. All in ECG of 72 hours old neonate *except:*
(a) T upright in V_1 and inverted in V_6
(b) P wave axis + 60
(c) QRS axis +90
(d) R/S ratio in V1 >1 and in V6 <1

2349. True about tricyclic antidepressant A/E:
(a) Bradycardia (b) Constipation
(c) Urinary retention (d) Blurring of vision
(e) Weight gain

2350. Best tolerated in pregnancy:
(a) Eisenmenger (b) Marfan with AR
(c) Severe MS (d) Severe MR

2351. Operation indication for A/E:
(a) Small ASD with shunt > 2:1
(b) Mild Ebstein's
(c) Small PDA
(d) Mild TOF

2352. PDA closure true A/E:

(a) Small PDA by coil and large PDA with device
(b) Anticoagulation for 6 months after closure
(c) Hemolytic anemia can occur
(d) PDA narrowest at the pulmonary end

2353. Myocardial O_2 consumption dependent on A/E:

(a) HR
(b) Inotropic state
(c) Wall tension
(d) O_2 carrying capacity of blood

2354. Hypothyroidism true A/E:

(a) Pretibial myxedema (b) T3 may be normal
(c) Galactorrhoea (d) Constipation

2355. Splenectemised patient to be given vaccine A/E:

(a) Pneumococcus (b) Meningococci
(c) H. influenza (d) Streptococci

2356. Lauric acid is:

(a) Saturated fatty acid (b) Trans fatty acid
(c) Monosaturated fats (d) PUFA
(e) Omega 3 fatty acids

2357. Differentiate prerenal from renal azotemia:

(a) Fractional excretion of Na <1
(b) Na excretion >40
(c) Plasma BUN/creatinine >40
(d) Osmolality > 500

2358. Bronchiectasis A/E:

(a) Tb (b) ABPA
(c) Measles (d) Pertussis
(e) Varicella

2359. High glycemic index A/E:

(a) Legumes (b) Wheat
(c) Rice (d) Sugar

2360. PDA A/E:

(a) Surgery for calcified PDA and patent with device
(b) Diastolic flow at apex significant shunt
(c) Both are true

2361. AVR with Chitra valve, history of TIA with INR–2.3, valve on echo–normal next management:

(a) Aspirin 325 mg/d
(b) Increase warfarin, target INR=3-4
(c) Increase warfarin, target INR=4-5
(d) Aspirin 75 mg/d with INR=3-3.5

2362. Which one of the following statement regarding the pleura is false?

(a) The source of blood supply to the pleura depends on its thickness
(b) Both parietal and visceral pleura are lined with multilayered stratified mesothelial cells
(c) Microvilli are present diffusely and are most abundant on the inferior aspect of visceral pleura
(d) Mesothelial cells are active structures and sensitive to various stimuli

2363. Pseudogout associated with:

(a) Calcium pyrophosphate
(b) Hydroxyapatite
(c) Na urate crystals
(d) Cholesterol crystals

2364. Calcium metabolism A/E:

(a) 98% in bones
(b) Concentrations of serum protein is an important determinant of calcium ion concentration
(c) Stored in cytosol as insoluble complexes
(d) Max. absorption in distal small intestine

2365. Café-au-lait spots associated with:

(a) Neurofibromatosis (b) SLE
(c) Enteric fever (d) Bacterial endocarditis

2366. Rubella syndrome A/E:

(a) Hydrocephalus (b) PDA
(c) Atypical coarctation (d) PS

2367. HSP associated with A/E:

(a) Extremely low platelet count
(b) Intracranial bleeding
(c) Palpable purpura
(d) Commonly involves face and upper extremities

2368. 1st carpo metacarpal involvement with DIP and sparing of MCP, wrist and ankle:

(a) Psoriatic (b) Rheumatoid arthritis
(c) Tubercular (d) OA

2369. Fat embolism associated with A/E:

(a) Thrombocytopenia (b) Hypoxia
(c) Arrhythmia (d) Cognitive dysfunction

2370. Lung CA most common associated with endocrine abnormality:

(a) Squamous cell carcinoma
(b) Oat cell carcinoma
(c) Adeno carcinoma
(d) Alveolar cell carcinoma

2371. S/E characteristic seen of cyclophosphamide is:

(a) Cardiotoxicity
(b) Hemorrhagic cystitis
(c) Pneumonia like symptoms
(d) Neurotoxicity

2372. Posterior mediastinal tumour most common:

(a) Bronchogenic cyst (b) Neurogenic cyst
(c) Fibroma (d) Oesophageal cyst

2373. Spastic paraplegia A/E :

(a) Vitamin B_{12} deficiency
(b) Chronic lead poisoning
(c) Cervical spondylosis
(d) MND

2374. CMT usual feature:

(a) LL hyperreflexia
(b) LL hyporeflexia
(c) Asymmetric muscle weakness
(d) No sensory involvement

2375. Massive proteinuria A/E:

(a) Renal vein thrombosis
(b) PAN
(c) Polycystic kidney disease
(d) Amyloidosis

2376. All of the following antimicrobials may cause thrombocytopenia *except:*

(a) Meropenem (b) Cefoperazone
(c) Tiecoplanin (d) Linezolid

2377. Calcified subcutaneous nodule with seizures most likely cause:

(a) TB
(b) Cysticercosis
(c) Hyperparathyroidism
(d) Excess vitamin D

2378. Hyperchloremic acidosis A/E:

(a) Renal tubular acidosis
(b) Ureterosigmoidostomy
(c) Chronic pyelonephritis
(d) Lactic acidosis

2379. Chickenpox A/E:

(a) Rarely involves mucosa
(b) All lesions at same time
(c) All lesions of smallpox seen but at rapid rate
(d) Peripheral in distribution, being more involves extremities and face

2380. Pregnancy lung function changes A/E:

(a) Vital capacity remains same
(b) FRC ↑ed
(c) ↓ed residual volume
(d) Expiratory reserve volume ↓ed

2381. Myaesthenia gravis associated with:

(a) Thymoma
(b) Thyroid adenoma
(c) Pheochromocytoma
(d) Sarcoidosis

2382. Wilson's seen:

(a) ↑ed urinary copper excretion
(b) ↑ed plasma copper
(c) ↑ed ceruloplasmin levels
(d) ↓ed copper deposition in brain

2383. Immune reconstitution inflammatory syndrome (IRIS):

(a) Seen after 6 weeks after starting treatment
(b) Continuation of HAART will ↓se symptoms
(c) Associated with fever and leucocytosis
(d) Occurs due to recovery of pathogen specific immune response

2384. Looser's zone associated with:

(a) Osteomalacia
(b) Osteoporosis
(c) Hyperparathyroidism
(d) Skeletal fluorosis

2385. Pseudo fracture of long bone associated with:

(a) Osteomalacia
(b) Hyperparathyroidism
(c) Pseudohypoparathyroidism
(d) Hypoparathyroidism

2386. Erosive arthritis A/E:
(a) SLE (b) RA
(c) Gout (d) OA

2387. Hypercapnic acidosis manifestations A/E:
(a) Papilloedema (b) Warm extremities
(c) Kussmaul breathing (d) Collapsing pulse

2388. Neutropenia prone to infection with:
(a) Pseudomonas (b) Pneumocystis
(c) CMV (d) M tuberculosis

2389. Invasive aspergillosis A/E:
(a) Amphotericin B (b) Fluconazole
(c) Variconazole (d) Caspofungin

2390. Tumour markers A/E:
(a) α-fetoprotein (b) CEA
(c) β-HCG (c) β2-Microglobulin

2391. Renal vein thrombosis A/E:
(a) Trauma (b) Toxemia of pregnancy
(c) Nephrotic syndrome (d) Renal cell Ca

2392. Alveolar-arterial gradient not ↑ed in:
(a) Central hypoventilation syndrome
(b) IPF
(c) ARDS
(d) Bronchiectasis

2393. Gynecomastia caused by A/E:
(a) Hypothyroidism (b) Renal failure
(c) Digoxin (d) Cyclosporine

2394. Particles of following size are deposited in lower respiratory tract:
(a) 10–50 μ (b) 50–100 μ
(c) 0.01–0.2 μ (d) 0.2–5.0 μ

2395. All of the following are contraindication for the use of non-invasive ventilation *except:*
(a) Upper airway obstruction
(b) Facial surgery
(c) Hemodynamic instability
(d) Acute respiratory failure

2396. Glycemic control of last few weeks is determined by:
(a) Glycated Hb (b) PPBS
(c) Urine acetone (d) Serum lipids

2397. Which statement regarding Asbestosis is false?
(a) Disease is related to intensity as well as duration of exposure
(b) Spirometry reveals a restrictive pattern
(c) Pleural involvement is common
(d) Lung cancer usually occurs within 10 years of diagnosis

2398. HIV–neurologic manifestation A/E:
(a) Mononeuritis multiplex
(b) Myopathy
(c) Autonomic dysfunction
(d) Myelopathy

2399. Which is not a paraneoplastic manifestations of bronchogenic carcinoma?
(a) Neuropathy (b) Hyponatremia
(c) Hypocalcemia (d) Cushing syndrome

2400. Hemophilia:
(a) ↑ APTT (b) Normal PT
(c) Factor VIII normal (d) ↑ factor IX

2401. All of the follwing conditions can cause gynaecomastia *except*:
(a) Hypothyroidism (b) Renal failure
(c) Lung cancer (d) Viral orchitis

2402. Austin flint murmur vs MS:
(a) Valsalva (b) Amyl nitrate
(c) Isometric handgrip (d) Leg raising

2403. Pseudogout associated with:
(a) Calcium pyrophosphate
(b) Hydroxyapatite
(c) Na urate crystals
(d) Cholesterol crystals

2404. Calcium metabolism A/E :
(a) 98% in bones
(b) Concentrations of serum protein is an important determinant of calcium ion concentration
(c) Stored in cytosol as insoluble complexes
(d) Max. absorption in distal small intestine

2405. Café au lait spots associated with:
(a) Neurofibromatosis (b) SLE
(c) Enteric fever (d) Bacterial endocarditis

2406. Rubella syndrome A/E:
(a) Hydrocephalus (b) PDA
(c) Atypical coarctation (d) PS

2407. HSP associated with A/E:
(a) Extremely low platelet count
(b) Intracranial bleeding
(c) Palpable purpura
(d) Commonly involves face and upper extremities

2408. 1st carpo metacarpal involvement with DIP and sparing of MCP, wrist and ankle:
(a) Psoriatic (b) Rheumatoid arthritis
(c) Tubercular (d) OA

2409. Fat embolism associated with A/E:
(a) Thrombocytopenia (b) Hypoxia
(c) Arrhythmia (d) Cognitive dysfunction

2410. Lung CA most common associated with endocrine abnormality:
(a) Squamous cell carcinoma
(b) Oat cell carcinoma
(c) Adeno carcinoma
(d) Alveolar cell carcinoma

2411. S/E characteristic seen of cyclophosphamide is:
(a) Cardiotoxicity
(b) Hemorrhagic cystitis
(c) Pneumonia like symptoms
(d) Neurotoxicity

2412. Posterior mediastinal tumour most common:
(a) Bronchogenic cyst (b) Neurogenic cyst
(c) Fibroma (d) Oesophageal cyst

2413. Spastic paraplegia A/E:
(a) Vitamin B_{12} deficiency
(b) Chronic lead poisoning
(c) Cervical spondylosis
(d) MND

2414. CMT usual feature:
(a) LL hyperreflexia
(b) LL hyporeflexia
(c) Asymmetric muscle weakness
(d) No sensory involvement

2415. Massive proteinuria A/E:
(a) Renal vein thrombosis
(b) PAN
(c) Polycystic kidney disease
(d) Amyloidosis

2416. Carcinoid syndrome A/E:
(a) Coronary spasm
(b) PS
(c) High output cardiac failure
(d) ↑ QT interval

2417. Calcified subcutaneous nodule with seizures most likely cause:
(a) TB
(b) Cysticercosis
(c) Hyperparathyroidism
(d) Excess vitamin D

2418. Hyperchloremic acidosis A/E:
(a) Renal tubular acidosis
(b) Ureterosigmoidostomy
(c) Chronic pyelonephritis
(d) Lactic acidosis

2419. Chickenpox A/E:
(a) Rarely involves mucosa
(b) All lesions at same time
(c) All lesions of smallpox seen but at rapid rate
(d) Peripheral in distribution, being more involves extremities and face

2420. Pregnancy lung function changes A/E:
(a) Vital capacity remains same
(b) FRC ↑ed
(c) ↓ed residual volume
(d) Expiratory reserve volume ↓ed

2421. Myaesthenia gravis associated with:
(a) Thymoma
(b) Thyroid adenoma
(c) Pheochromocytoma
(d) Sarcoidosis

2422. Wilson's seen:
(a) ↑ed urinary copper excretion
(b) ↑ed plasma copper
(c) ↑ed ceruloplasmin levels
(d) ↓ed copper deposition in brain

2423. Immune reconstitution inflammatory syndrome (IRIS):

(a) Seen after 6 weeks after starting treatment
(b) Continuation of HAART will ↓se symptoms
(c) Associated with fever and leucocytosis
(d) Occur due to recovery of pathogen specific immune response

2424. Looser's zone associated with:

(a) Osteomalacia
(b) Osteoporosis
(c) Hyperparathyroidism
(d) Skeletal fluorosis

2425. Pseudo fracture of long bone associated with:

(a) Osteomalacia
(b) Hyperparathyroidism
(c) Pseudohypoparathyroidism
(d) Hypoparathyroidism

2426. Erosive arthritis A/E:

(a) SLE (b) RA
(c) Gout (d) OA

2427. Hypercapnic acidosis manifestations A/E:

(a) Papilloedema (b) Warm extremities
(c) Kussmaul breathing (d) Collapsing pulse

2428. Neutropenia prone to infection with:

(a) Pseudomonas (b) Pneumocystis
(c) CMV (d) M tuberculosis

2429. Invasive aspergillosis A/E:

(a) Amphotericin B (b) Fluconazole
(c) Variconazole (d) Caspofungin

2430. Tumour markers A/E:

(a) α-fetoprotein (b) CEA
(c) β-HCG (d) β2-Microglobulin

2431. Renal vein thrombosis A/E:

(a) Trauma (b) Toxemia of pregnancy
(c) Nephrotic syndrome (d) Renal cell Ca

2432. Alveolar-arterial gradient not ↑ed in:

(a) Central hypoventilation syndrome
(b) IPF
(c) ARDS
(d) Bronchiectasis

2433. Gynecomastia caused by A/E:

(a) Hypothyroidism (b) Renal failure
(c) Digoxin (d) Cyclosporine

2434. Pulm edema without cardiomegaly:

(a) AR (b) MR
(c) ASD (d) Pure MS

2435. CPVT is characterized by:

(a) Bidirectional VT
(b) Sinus tachycardia at rest
(c) Adult onset
(d) ICD is TOC

2436. Glycemic control of last few weeks is determined by:

(a) Glycated Hb (b) PPBS
(c) Urine acetone (d) Serum lipids

2437. All ↓es with age *except:*

(a) Closing volume (b) PaO_2
(c) Vital capacity (d) FEV_1

2438. HIV – neurologic manifestation A/E:

(a) Mononeuritis multiplex
(b) Myopathy
(c) Autonomic dysfunction
(d) Myelopathy

2439. Which is not a paraneoplastic manifestations of bronchogenic carcinoma?

(a) Neuropathy (b) Hyponatremia
(c) Hypocalcemia (d) Cushing syndrome

2440. Hemophilia:

(a) ↑ APTT (b) Normal PT
(c) Factor VIII normal (d) ↑ factor IX

2441. All of the following conditions can cause gynaecomastia *except:*

(a) Hypothyroidism (b) Renal failure
(c) Lung cancer (c) Viral orchitis

2442. Tall 'T' wave short QT?

(a) Hyperkalemia, ↑ Ca
(b) ↓ K, ↑ Ca
(c) ↓ K, ↑ Ca

2443. ↑ ICT – Most common Nerve involved ....
(a) III (b) IV
(c) VI (d) VII

2444. Impact factor role
(a) Journal (b) Article
(c) Publication house (d) Trial

2445. Normal level of proteinuria:
(a) < 150 (b) < 250
(c) < 350 (d) < 450

2446. Confidence interval shows:
(a) Denotes point
(b) Interval in which mean lies of population
(c) Internal in which mean lies of study
(d) Significance

2447. Diarrhoea positive HUS:
(a) Salmonella (b) E coli
(c) C. Jejuni

2448. SPPS used in:
(a) Statistics (b) Laboratory

2449. GERD (Prevalence):
(a) 10% (b) 30%
(c) 50% (d) 2%

2450. Tetanus most common nerve:
(a) VI (b) VII
(c) VIII (d) IX

2451. 60 years old male meningitis treatment:
(a) Xone + gentamicin
(b) Xone + Vanco + ampicillin
(c) Ampi + Vanco
(d) Ampi + gentamicin

2452. Live vaccine A/E:
(a) Measles (b) Hepatitis B
(c) OPV (d) BCG

2453. Nephrotic syndrome good prognosis A/E:
(a) Normal cholesterol (b) H/O HTN
(c) Age 2-10 years (d) Response to steroids

2454. Most common accidental poisoning:
(a) Aspirin (b) Dhatura
(c) Kerosene (d) OPC

2455. ITP A/E:
(a) Hematuria
(b) Hemarthrosis
(c) BM–megakaryocytes

2456. SIADH A/E:
(a) Plasma osmolality > 270
(b) Plasma osmolality < 150
(c) Urinary Na > 130
(d) Serum Na < 130

2457. Generalized anxiety disorder true is:
(a) Worry for 2 months
(b) SSRI in refractory cases
(c) Short acting BZD are used
(d) Alcohol addiction and substance abuse may cause GAD

2458. ORS–WHO–sodium:
(a) 50 (b) 75
(c) 80 (d) 90

2459. BCG vaccine normal response:
(a) Papule within 24 hours
(b) Papule within 7 days
(c) Papule within 3 weeks
(d) Ulcer within 7 days

2460. 17 years old male Marathon → SCD → CPR fail. No family H/O SCD cause of SCD:
(a) IHD
(b) HOCM
(c) Anomalous coronary artery origin

2461. COPD patient on salbutamol recurrent episode in past 9 months (>3 episodes) SPo2 – 94% therapy to reduce exacerbation:
(a) Long term oxygen therapy
(b) Pneumococcal vaccine
(c) Low dose steroid
(d) Tiotropium bromide

2462. Prematurity syndrome AIE:
(a) Meconium aspiration
(b) IVH
(c) HMD
(d) Hypothermia

2463. Apoptosis–definition:
(a) Programmed cell death

2464. AD inheritance true:
(a) 50% irrespective of gender
(b) 25% irrespective of gender

2465. Down syndrome:
(a) 18 chr (b) 13 chr
(c) 21 chr

2466. Hypothermia definition:
(a) 31 (b) 30
(c) 34 (d) 35

2467. Linezolid is:
(a) Antimicrobial (b) Antiseptic

2468. Indication for intubation A/E:
(a) Respiratory arrest or < 8 /min
(b) Tachypnoea
(c) $PCO_2 > 40$
(d) $PO_2 < 70$

2469. AFP A/E:
(a) HCC
(b) Medullary thyroid CA
(c) Testicular teratoma
(d) Non-seminomatous ovarian GCT

2470. Sister Mary Joseph nodule:
(a) Breast (b) Ovary
(c) Cervix (d) Lung

2471. JVP A/E:
(a) Raised in hyponatremia
(b) PTE
(c) Increase in cardiac failure

2472. PUO definition (duration):
(a) 2 weeks (b) 3 weeks
(c) 4 weeks (d) 6 weeks

2473. Leishmaniasis spread by:
(a) Sand fly (b) Mosquito
(c) Flea (d) Tick

2474. Prolactinoma 1st line treatment:
(a) RT (b) Surgery
(c) Dopamine agonist (d) No treatment

2475. Cysticercosis caused by:
(a) T-solium (d) T-saginata
(c) Echinococcus

2476. Oliguria definition:
(a) < 500 ml/day (b) < 400 ml/day
(c) < 300 ml/day (d) < 100 ml /day

2477. Sarcoidosis seen A/E:
(a) Lymphocytosis
(b) Parotid enlargement
(c) Bilateral hilar enlargement
(d) Lupus pernio
(e) All of the above

2478. Thyrotoxic crisis mortality:
(a) 30% (b) 10%
(c) 5% (d) 20%

2479. Right lung involvement A/E:
(a) Pleural effusion (b) Nodules
(c) Pneumonia (d) Fibrosis

2480. Amiodarone has structural resemblance:
(a) T_3 (b) T_4
(c) TSH (d) ACTH

2481. Not secreted by stomach:
(a) Gastrin (b) Cholecystokinin
(c) Somatostatin (d) Ghrelin

2482. Fabry's disease due to deficiency of:
(a) Hexosaminidase I and II
(b) α-galactosidase
(c) Glucocerebrosidase

2483. Palpable purpura seen in:
(a) Warfarin
(b) Scurvy
(c) Fat embolism
(d) Disseminated gonococci

2484. ZES A/E:
(a) ↑ somatostatin
(b) ↑ acid level
(c) Severe gastric ulcer
(d) Non beta cell pancreatic tumour

2485. H1N1 patient 5 days of oseltamivir given still symptomatic, next (CDC guideline):
(a) Zoltemivir (b) Continue 5 days more
(c) Stop (d) PCR H1N1

2486. Rhabdomyolysis first treatment:
(a) Crystalloid (b) Diuretic
(c) Bicarbonate (d) Mannitol

2487. Class I evidence definition:
(a) Cohort (b) Metanalysis
(c) Case control (d) Expert opinion

2488. Recurrent bacterial meninigitis A/E:

(a) Dural tear
(b) Complement deficiency
(c) HIV infection
(d) CSF rhinorrhoea

2489. Labourer female 39 years old polyarthritis not involving DIP, X-ray–multiple nodules:

(a) Sarcoidosis (b) Caplan syndrome
(c) Felty syndrome

2490. 100 ml milk (buffalo), protein:

(a) 1.0 (b) 0.5
(c) 3 (d) 4.3

2491. Bronchiolitis most common cause:

(a) RSV (b) Adenovirus
(c) Polio

2492. Cavernous sinus thrombosis A/E:

(a) Papilloedema (b) Proptosis
(c) Facial palsy (d) Headache

2493. FLACC score is used for:

(a) Pain (b) Acute kidney injury
(c) Acute lung injury (d) Osteo arthritis

2494. Atrial natriuretic peptide causes:

(a) Increased GFR (b) Increased rennin
(c) Hypervolumia (d) Increased ECF

2495. Most effective therapy for nocturnal enuresis is:

(a) Alarm therapy (b) Oxyloutinin
(c) Imipramine (d) Demopressin

2496. All are true about Fragile X syndrome *except:*

(a) Most common cause of inherited mental retardation in males
(b) Abnormality of long arm of chromosome X
(c) Microorchidism
(d) Stereotyped behavior

2497. Uniparental diasomy causing Prader-Willi syndrome is due to abnormality of which chromosome?

(a) 6 (b) 7
(c) 14 (d) 15

2498. Other than bone mineral density which is most important risk factor for fracture?

(a) Previous fragility fracture
(b) Risk of frequent falling
(c) Silent vertebral fracture
(d) Traumatic fracture

2499. Treatment of hypernatremic dehydration:

(a) 0.9% normal saline
(b) 0.45% normal saline
(c) 5% glucose
(d) 0.45% normal saline + 5% glucose

2500. Low osmolarity condition compensatory mechanisms increasing urine by:

(a) Inhibits ADH
(b) Increases intraglomerular hydrostatic pressure
(c) Increase GFR

2501. H^+ is transported across the parietal cell in stomach. What other ion is transported concomitantly?

(a) HCl (b) K
(c) Na (d) Cl

2502. Long standing untreated type 2 DM. Which of the following is not seen?

(a) Positive nitrogen balance
(b) Ketonemia
(c) Ketonuria
(d) Low with peptide concentration

2503. Most common cause of acid production in body:

(a) Protein catabolism
(b) Carbohydrate catabolism
(c) Triglyceride catabolism
(d) Oxidative metabolism

2504. All are true about hyperaldosteronism *except:*

(a) Volume overload (b) Hypernatremia
(c) Hyperkalemia (d) Metabolic alkalosis

2505. Podocin mutation is seen in:

(a) Minimal change disease
(b) FSGN
(c) MPGN
(d) Membranous GN

2506. Volume of air in the lung after maximal inspiration is:

(a) Total lung capacity
(b) Vital capacity
(c) Inspiratory residual volume
(d) Functional respiratory capacity

2507. Instrument which correctly the thing that it is supposed to measure indicate:

(a) Sensitivity (b) Validity
(c) Effectiveness (d) Internal consistency

2508. Green line in gum is seen in which poisoning?

(a) Lead (b) Copper
(c) Mercury (d) Arsenic

2509. Mechanisms of anti-inflammatory action of gluco-corticoids is by:

(a) Increased capillary permeability
(b) Prevention of release of pyrogens from leucocytes
(c) Increase in macrocortin

2510. Difference between GLP-1 and GIP is:

(a) Beta cell mass expansion
(b) Glucose mediated insulin secretion
(c) Extrapancreatic glucose lowering action
(d) Superior glucagon secretion

2511. 1 kg increase in weight in the population increase the risk of diabetes by:

(a) 10.5% (b) 8.5%
(c) 6.5% (d) 4.5%

2512. According to NCEP and IDF, the percentage of obese patients in Indian diabetes is:

(a) 20-40% (b) 40-60%
(c) 60-80% (d) 50-70%

2513. Incidence of carotid sinus hypersensitivity in elderly is:

(a) 1% (b) 10%
(c) 20% (d) 30–70%

2514. Rate of chest compression as per ACLS is:

(a) 40/min (b) 60/min
(c) 80/min (d) 100/min

2515. DOC in PEA according to PALS is:

(a) Adenosine (b) Epinephrine
(c) Atropine (d) Lignocaine

2516. DOC to prevent autonomic storm in scorpion bite is:

(a) Prazosin (b) Nifedipine
(c) Atropine

2517. Verbal paraphasic speech indicates:

(a) Replacement of one correct word for another
(b) Fluent meaning less speech

2518. Short term memory is tested by recollection of:

(a) Three objects after 10 min
(b) Three objects after 5 min
(c) Five objects after 3 minutes
(d) Five objects after 5 min

2519. Silofiller's disease is due to:

(a) NO_2 (b) SO_2
(c) HCN (d) NH_3

2520. Total birth rate/1000 population is:

(a) Crude birth rate
(b) Age specific fertility rate
(c) Total fertility rate

2521. Tic doloreaux is:

(a) Trigeminal neuralgia
(b) Amayurosis fugax

2522. High frequency jet ventilation use the principle of:

(a) High inspiratory pressure
(b) High PEEP
(c) Mean airway pressure
(d) Maximum inspiratory pressure

2523. Linear correlation of age and SBP for HTN is calculated by:

(a) Correlation coefficient
(b) Coefficient of variation
(c) Standard deviation
(d) T-test

2524. 95% confidence limit in S.D. is:

(a) Mean ± S.D. (b) Mean ± 2 S.D.
(c) Mean ± 3 S.D. (d) Mean ± 4 S.D.

2525. 100 mg IFA is given to pregnant lady before and after a test. Best method:

(a) T–test (b) Paired t test
(c) Chi-square

2526. If the maximum depolarization is -30 mv in the ECG, maximum QRS voltage will be in which lead?

(a) I (b) avL
(c) II (d) avR

2527. Most important drug used in the treatment of malignant hypertension:
(a) Dandrolene (b) Succinylcholine
(c) Chlorpromazine

2528. Benzodiazepines causes A/E:
(a) Anxiolytics (b) Analgesics
(c) Amnesia (d) Antiplatelet

2529. Best investigation to diagnose a pancreatic tumour < 2 cm size:
(a) MDCT
(b) Double contrast enhanced CT
(c) Multiplaner CT with 3D reconstruction
(d) Dynamic CECT

2530. Atrial infarction all true *except*:
(a) LA more common than RA
(b) Commonly associated with LV – MI
(c) Associated with supraventricular tachycardia
(d) Atrial rupture can be fatal

2531. Medical negligence IPC:
(a) 304 (b) 304 A
(c) 306 (d) 309

2532. In salicylate poisoning, pH should be maintained between:
(a) 7.10 – 7.2 (b) 7.2 – 7.35
(c) 7.35 – 7.45 (d) 7.45 – 7.55

2533. Epidemic dropsy is caused by:
(a) Castor oil (b) Lathyrus sativus
(c) Argemone oil

2534. Cardiac index is:
(a) CO/BSA (b) CO/BMI
(c) HR X EF

2535. Which is true regarding warfarin?
(a) Enhances epoxide reductase
(b) Increases protein C and S
(c) Inhibits vit K dependent clotting factors II, VII, IX and X
(d) African resistant and Asian American sensitive

2536. Pulse oximeter measure:
(a) Oxygen content of arterial blood
(b) Oxygen content of venous blood
(c) Oxygen saturation in arterial blood
(d) Oxygen saturation of venous blood

2537. Variable of linear regression:
(a) Nominal (b) Ordinal
(c) Continuous (d) Dichotomous

2538. Dupuytren contracture least commonly involves:
(a) Little finger (b) Middle finger
(c) Index finger (d) Ring finger

2539. Mumps is most infectious during:
(a) Incubation period
(b) Prodromal period
(c) After swelling appear
(d) Before swelling

2540. OMINOUS OCTET in A/E:
(a) Brain (b) Kidney
(c) Alpha cell (d) Endothelium

2541. Xenobiotic is A/E:
(a) Molasses
(b) Occupational chemicals
(c) Corn oil
(d) Environmental pollutants

2542. Total energy expenditure is:
(a) BMR + Activity factor
(b) BMR × Activity factor
(c) BMR to the power activity

2543. Feature of IFN α induced destructive thyrotoxicosis:
(a) TSH ↓, anti TSH ab ↓, T3 ↓, T4 ↓

2544. SIMV in mechanical ventilation stands for:
(a) Synchronized intermittent mandatory ventilation
(b) Synchronized intermediate mandatory ventilation

2545. Shrinking lung syndrome:
(a) SLE (b) RA
(c) Sarcoidosis (d) Scleroderma

2546. Cushing syndrome A/E:
(a) Central obesity (b) Easy bruising
(c) Impaired IGT (d) Proximal myopathy

2547. SILO Filer:
(a) Nitrogen dioxide (b) H_2S
(c) Hcn (d) Cl

2548. Autism A/E:
(a) < 3 years of age
(b) ↓ brain volume

(c) ↓ eye contraction
(d) Communication impairment

2549. Broca's aphasia:
(a) Fluent
(b) Non fluent
(c) Comprehension impairment
(d) Repetition impairment

2550. Glasgowcomascale—eyeopening,incomprehensible sound, withdrawl to pain:
(a) 9 (b) 8
(c) 7 (d) 6

2551. MMS – Short term memory:
(a) 3 in 5 min (b) 5 in 5 min
(c) 3 in 10 min (d) 5 in 10 min

2552. Most common pituitary tumour:
(a) Prolactinoma
(b) Corticotrophin producing tumour
(c) Gonadotrophin producing tumour

2553. Inappropriate serum TSH A/E:
(a) Sheehan syndrome
(b) Drug induced hypothyroid
(c) TSH secretory adenoma

2554. Peripheral eosinophilia A/E:
(a) T cell malignancy
(b) Acute eosinophilic pneumonia
(c) Hyper eosinophilic pneumonia
(d) CSS

2555. Burkitt lymphoma associated with chromosome:
(a) CD 15 and 30 (b) CD 20 and 30
(c) CD 15 and 20

2556. Intracellular organisms more common in:
(a) AML (b) CLL
(c) Multiple myeloma (d) Hodgkin lymphoma

2557. Female, normal stature, normal breast, amenorrhea, blind vagina sac, absent pubic hair and axillary hair:
(a) 45 XO (b) 46 XY
(c) 46 XX (d) 47 XXY

2558. Male, polyuria, polydipsia, serum osmolality <270, urine osmolality < 280, cause:
(a) Central diabetes insipidus
(b) Diabetes mellitus
(c) Nephrogenic DI
(d) Psychogenic polydipsia

2559. Hypocalcemia associated with:
(a) Increased QT (b) Short QT
(c) Increased ST (d) Decreased ST

2560. ST elevation associated with:
(a) Hypocalcemia (b) Hypothermia
(c) Acute pericarditis (d) DC shock

2561. After pulseless activity which will give:
(a) Atropine sulphate (b) Epinephrine
(c) I/V lignocaine (d) Amiodarone

2562. CO poisoning, O_2 dissociation curve shift to:
(a) Left (b) Right
(c) Down (d) Up

2563. NPH associated with A/E:
(a) Dementia (b) Unstable gait
(c) Urinary incontinence (d) Aphasia

2564. Myotonic dystrophy A/E:
(a) Proximal muscle disease
(b) CTG repeat
(c) Phenytoin treatment of choice
(d) Myotonia

2565. Podocin mutation cause all *except:*
(a) Minimal change disease
(b) FSGN
(c) MPGN

2566. CKD cast:
(a) Granular (b) Broad
(c) Epithelial (d) Hyaline

2567. Investigation of choice in ILD:
(a) CXR
(b) MRI
(c) HRCT
(d) Gadulinium enhancing scan

2568. ATT (Isoniazid) induced hepatitis, asymptomatic patient, level of ALT for stopping ATT:
(a) 2 times increase (b) 3 times increase
(c) 4 times increase (d) 5 times increase

2569. Traveller diarrhea:
(a) Invasive E. coli
(b) Enteropathogenic E. coli
(c) Enterohemorrhaic E. coli
(d) Enterotoxigenic E. coli

2570. Definition of orthostatic hypotension:
(a) SBP decrease > 10 mm Hg
(b) SBP decrease > 20 mm Hg
(c) SBP decrease > 5 mm Hg
(d) SBP decrease > 25 mm Hg

2571. Dukes criteria, major A/E:
(a) Fever
(b) Culture positive
(c) New valvular regurgitation
(d) New dehiscence

2572. Jones criteria, major A/E:
(a) Carditis
(b) Chorea
(c) Subcutaneous nodules
(d) Polyarthralgia

2573. Primaquine causes hemolysis:
(a) G6PD deficiency
(b) Hexokinase deficiency

2574. Intravascular hemolysis A/E:
(a) Increased hepatoglobin
(b) Hemoglobinuria
(c) Increased LDH
(d) Hemosiderinuria

2575. Microcytic anemia A/E:
(a) Lead poisoning (b) IDA
(c) Thalassemia (d) Fanconi anemia

2576. Hereditary spherocytosis A/E:
(a) Increased MHC
(b) Increased MCHC
(c) Increased osmotic fragility
(d) Reticulocytosis

2577. Microcytosis definition:
(a) 80 (b) 76
(c) 86 (d) 60

2578. Rheumatic fever, penicillin sensitive all drug given A/E:
(a) Clindamycin (b) Azithromycin
(c) Clarithromycin (d) Tetracycline

2579. For bed wetting most effective treatment:
(a) Bed alarm (b) Desmopressin
(c) Imipramine

2580. Lighter than all:
(a) Methane (b) Ethane
(c) Ethylene (d) Nitrogen

2581. Dyspepsia alarming sign A/E:
(a) Abdomen mass (b) Hemetemesis
(c) Dysphagia (d) Nausea

2582. Acute pancreatitis most common complication:
(a) Pleural effusion (b) Peritonitis
(c) Pseudocyst pancreas (d) Abscess

2583. Gait aprasia seen:
(a) Frontal lobe lesion (b) Parietal lobe lesion
(c) Occipital lobe lesion (d) Cerebellar lobe lesion

2584. Graham Steel murmur:
(a) TS (b) TR
(c) PR (d) PS

2585. High frequency ventilation depend on:
(a) PEEP
(b) FiO_2
(c) Peak inspiratory pressure
(d) Mean airway pressure

2586. Parkinsonism involve:
(a) Red nucleus (b) Occipital lobe
(c) Frontal lobe (d) Substantia nigra

2587. Which antibody seen in hepatitis D:
(a) LKM1 (b) LKM3
(c) ANA (d) SLA

2588. Following HLA cross matching and decreased incidence of:
(a) Hyperacute rejection
(b) Acute vascular reaction
(c) Acute cellular reaction
(d) Chronic GVD

2589. Vitamin K depends on factor A/E:
(a) Factor V (b) Factor X
(c) Factor IX (d) Factor VII

2590. Dengue, WHO A/E:

(a) Dengue fever
(b) Dengue with warning sign
(c) Dengue HF
(d) Severe dengue

2591. DOC in PSVT:

(a) Adenosine (b) Metoprolol
(c) Verapamil

2592. Mononeuritis multiplex:

(a) LL (b) BL
(c) TL (d) None of the above

2593. Cockroft gault formula used for:

(a) GFR
(b) CO
(c) Iron estimation for correction of anemia

2594. SSPE caused by:

(a) Measles (b) Herpes
(c) Mumps

2595. DOC for status epilepticus:

(a) Lorazepam (b) Diazepam
(c) Topiramate

2596. Bcr gene location:

(a) 22q11 (b) 9q34
(c) 9q35 (d) 11q22

2597. Ecthyma gangrenosum A/E:

(a) Staphylococcus (b) Pseudomonas
(c) Aspergillus (d) Mucormycosis

2598. DOC for PCP:

(a) Cotrimoxazole (b) Pentamidine
(c) Dapsone (d) Leucovorin

2599. Folic acid deficiency most common cause:

(a) Nutritional (b) Malabsorption
(c) Increased utilization (d) Alcohol

2600. HIV–ELISA negative, window period, next investigation:

(a) p 20 Ag (b) p 24 Ab
(c) Gp 120 Ag (d) Gp 120 Ab

2601. Dysphagia associated with:

(a) Cranial nerve involvement
(b) Cerebellum involvement
(c) Cortical and subcortical involvement
(d) Brainstem

2602. Extreme obesity BMI:

(a) > 40 (b) > 36
(c) > 42 (d) > 44

2603. Austin flint murmur is A/W:

(a) AR (b) MR
(c) PR (d) TR

2604. 9-year-old boy with polyuria and polydypsia S. OSM-275, U.OSM 285, diagnosis:

(a) DM
(b) DI
(c) Neph DI
(d) Psychogenic polydipsic

2605. Clubbing A/W A/E:

(a) Chromic bronchitis
(b) Central bronchiectasis
(c) Cryptogenic fibrosing alveolitis
(d) Primary biliary cirrhosis

2606. Central cyanosis A/W A/E:

(a) CHF
(b) Alveolar hypoventilation
(c) Congenital PS
(d) Chronic severe asthma

2607. Mycoplasma pneumoriac treatment of choice:

(a) Penicillin (b) Cefuroxine
(c) Tetracycline (d) Erythromycin

2608. Patient presents with polyuria, polydipsia N/V, short QT on ECG, likely diagnosis:

(a) Hypokalemia (b) Hypercalcemia
(c) Hypocalcemia (d) Hypomagnesemia

2609. Vancouver system, *et al.* used it authors more than:

(a) 4 (b) 5
(c) 6 (d) 7

2610. Vancouver system–reference:

(a) Asterisk and mentioned at bottom of page
(b) Parenthesis with full citation
(c) No. and mentioned at end
(d) Full name of author

2611. Child with recurrent sinopulmonary infections and eczema, has thrombocytopenia with small platelets:

(a) Wiskott Aldrich syndrome

(b) Job disease
(c) Bernard Soulier syndrome

2612. A 10 years old boy with hemophilia recurrent VIII factor transfusions develops bleeding not controlled by factor VIII, appropriate treatment:
(a) Cryoppt. (b) FFP
(c) Factor IX (d) Achievated factor VII

2613. APLA syndrome A/E:
(a) Venous thrombosis (b) Recurrent abortion
(c) Pancytopenia (d) Pulm HTN

2614. Aschcoff's nodules characterizes:
(a) Rheumatic carditis (b) SABE

2615. Only agent approved for thrombolysis of stroke:
(a) STK (b) Urokinase
(c) Alteplase

2616. Amiodarone A/E:
(a) ↑ toxicity of digoxin
(b) ↓es action of warfarin
(c) 40% iodine, so causes hypo as well as hyperthyroidism
(d) Corneal deposit occur commonly after long term treatment

2617. Peripheral eosinophilia A/E:
(a) Churg Strauss syndrome
(b) ABPA
(c) Pulm eosinophilic granuloma
(d) Loffler's syndrome

2618. Patient with ↑ neutrophils, basophils, platelets, eosinophils likely diagnosis:
(a) AML (b) CML
(c) ALL (d) MDS

2619. Most common site of extrapulmonary TB:
(a) LN (b) Pleura
(c) Liver (d) Skin

2620. For central cyanosis reduced Hb should be more than:
(a) 4 (b) 3
(c) 5 (d) 6

2621. Antibiotic that causes pyloric stenosis in infants is:
(a) Linezolid (b) Erythromycin
(c) Cefuroxime (d) Azithromycin

2622. Essential amino acid in children:
(a) Methionine (b) Arginine
(c) Taurine (d) Choline

2623. Sarcoidosis A/E:
(a) DI (b) Osteomalacia
(c) Hypercalemia (d) Addison disease

2624. Z-score indicate:
(a) Standard deviation
(b) Difference of actual valve and mean
(c) Range
(d) Mean

2625. 1 standard deviation from mean covers:
(a) 68% (b) 95%
(c) 99% (d) 34%

2626. Quadruple test to screen for fetal anomalies which fourth test was added:
(a) Estriol (b) B-HCG
(c) α-fetoprotein (d) Inhibin-A

2627. 6-year-boy with fever, N/V, malaise, maculopapulor red rash, tourniquets test +ve, PCV-36%, platelets-54,000. According to classification:
(a) DHF (b) Severe dengue
(c) Dengue with warning sign

2628. Viral infection mosquito A/E:
(a) H1N1 (b) Dengue
(c) Chikungunia (d) IE

2629. Snake bite, recent guideline:
(a) Immobilization (b) Incision
(c) Suction (d) Tourniquet

2630. Reversible dementia A/E:
(a) Huntington's disease
(b) NPH
(c) Brain tumor
(d) Vitamin B_{12} deficiency

2631. 38-year-male, thunderclap headache, 3rd nerve palsy and altered sensorium, diagnosis:
(a) SAH (b) ICH
(c) SDH (d) Hemiplegic migraine

2632. Primary amenorrhea in female, no axillary/pubic hair, breast developed N, vagina blind-ended, karyotype?
(a) 45X0 (b) 46XY
(c) 46XX (d) 47XXY

2633. Best test to differentiate anemia of iron deficiency from that of chronic disease:

(a) S-transferrin (b) S-ferritin
(c) MCV (d) Transferrin saturation

2634. Post hip surgery on day 6, breathlessness, CXR N, Echo shows RV hypokinesia with ↓ flow through TV, diagnosis:

(a) RVMI (b) Pulm embolism

2635. Digitalis toxicity, A/E:

(a) A. flutter (b) Atrial tachycardia
(c) Bigeminy (d) Junctional tachycardia

2636. Prognosis in acute pancreatitis A/E:

(a) Serum amylase (b) Calcium
(c) Trypsinogen (d) AST

2637. Blood sugar nil, urine sugar +:

(a) Renal glycosuria (b) Alimentary glycosuria

2638. Drug – approved in MND:

(a) Rilazole (b) Danazol

2639. Status – epilepticus – all given *except:*

(a) Phenobarbitone (b) Levitiracetam
(c) Carbamazepine (d) Valproate

2640. COPD A/E:

(a) ↓ FEV 1 (b) ↓ PEFR
(c) ↑ RV (d) ↓ diffusion capacity

2641. Compensation of metabolic alkalosis by respiration:

(a) ↑ CO_2 by 0.5-08 per I meq HCO_3
(b) ↑CO_2 by 1 per 1 meq HCO_3
(c) ↑CO_2 by 2 per meq HCO_3
(d) ↓CO_2

2642. Split-fixed S2 caused by A/E:

(a) LBBB (b) ASD
(c) PS

2643. Syncope Inv. A/E:

(a) Holter ECG (b) Implanted monitor
(c) Tilt table (d) FDG PET

2644. Protein-losing enteropathy, diagnosis by fecal:

(a) α1- AT (b) Chymotrypsin
(c) Gliadin

2645. 1½ years child with history of–febrile seizure and from last 6 months–non febrile GTCS and myoclonus diagnosis:

(a) Lennoxl-Gastaert syndrome
(b) Status epilepticus

2646. RAS A/E:

(a) PAN (b) Atherosclerosis
(c) FMD (d) Takayasu arteritis

2647. RAS criteria for intervention A/E:

(a) Pulmonary oedema
(b) Resistant HTN
(c) Persistent ↑ in serum creatinine
(d) Renal index > 0.8

2648. Lateral medullary syn A/E:

(a) Vertebral artery
(b) PICA
(c) Superior cerebellar artery
(d) Medial medullary artery

2649. Most common congenital heart disease:

(a) ASD (b) VSD
(c) PDA (d) TOF

2650. Child with absent femoral pulse in 5 days develops CHF at 7 days bluish discoloration of both feet immediate treatment:

(a) PGE1 drip
(b) Ibubrufen
(c) Atrial septotomy

2651. Causes of clubbing A/E:

(a) Chronic bronchitis (b) Bronchiectasis
(c) PAP (d) PBC

2652. D dimer used in:

(a) PE (b) Pericardial effusion
(c) PPH

2653. Type II error:

(a) False +ve (b) False –ve
(c) Double –ve (d) Double +ve

2654. Extraneous variable that depends independent variable and effects dependent variable called:

(a) Confounding
(b) Moderator variable
(c) Independent variable

2655. Multiple regression uses how many variables?

(a) 1 (b) 2
(c) 3 (d) >3

2656. Regression equation: y = 0.5 X1 + 10 X2 + 25; (X1 = 10 X2 = 5) =:

(a) 80 (b) 68
(c) 100

2657. Likerts scale also known as:

(a) Interview protocol (b) Summation scale

2658. Non overlapping intervals also known as:

(a) Exclusive (b) Exhaustive
(c) (a) and (b) (d) Inclusive

2659. Hyperkalemia all used in treatment *except:*

(a) Digoxin (b) Insulin
(c) Glucose (d) Dialysis

2660. Hypokalemia ppt toxicity of:

(a) Digoxin (b) Furosemide
(c) Insulin (d) Warf

2661. GFR measurement best by:

(a) DMSA (b) DTPA
(c) MAG 3 (d) IVP

2662. Hornone levels measured by all *except:*

(a) Mass spectroscopy
(b) Radioimmuno assay
(c) Chromatographic assay
(d) Electrophorasis

2663. Unexplained cyanotic spell in newborn most common cause:

(a) H fistula (b) CVS malformations
(c) Lung cyst (d) Intestinal atresia

2664. Apple peeling or Christmas tree seen in intestinal atresia:

(a) Type I (b) II
(c) III (d) IV

2665. Most common HCV genotype in India:

(a) 1 (b) 2
(c) 3 (d) 4

2666. ADA level in pericardial effusion (TB):

(a) 15 (b) 20
(c) 25 (d) 30

2667. Highest transmission rate with blood transfusion:

(a) HIV (b) Hep-B
(c) Hep-C (d) Malaria

2668. Translocation Burkitt lymphoma:

(a) 8, 14 (b) 14, 18
(c) 12, 14

2669. Lung maturity L/S ratio:

(a) 3: 1 (b) 2:1
(c) 4:1 (d) 5:1

2670. Height protein binding:

(a) Propranolol (b) Metoprolol
(c) Atenolol (d) Bisoprolol

2671. Bosentan:

(a) Endothelin antagonist
(b) Prostacycline inhibitor
(c) PDE inhibitor

2672. Mirror image movement:

(a) Kallman (b) Turner
(c) Klinfelter (d) Cretinism

2673. HCC ascitis best treatment:

(a) Spironolactone (b) Furosemide
(c) Hydroclorthiazide (d) Mannitol

2674. Adrenomedullin secreted by A/E:

(a) Hypothalamus (b) Leukocytes
(c) Kidney (d) Adrenal gland

2675. Fasting hyperglycemia:

(a) Impaired glucose tolerence
(b) ↑ insulin resistance in liver
(c) ↑ insulin resistance in adepose tissue
(d) ↓ secret of insulin from B-cell

2676. Thiamine deficiency in A/E:

(a) Homocystinuria (b) Chronic alcohol
(c) CHF on diuretic (d) Food faddist

2677. DIC Vs TTP:

(a) aPTT (b) ↓ APC
(c) RBC lysis (d) Renal failure

2678. Tumorlysis syndrome A/E:

(a) LDH > 1500
(b) Allopurinol 300 $mg/m^2/day$

(c) ARF less when UA < 10
(d) ↑ Ca^{+2}, ↑ K^+, ↓pH

2679. HRT ↓ risk of:
(a) Ca breast (b) Ca ovary
(c) Ca colon (d) Ca endometrial

2680. ↑ Pa O_2, ↓ Pa CO_2, ↓H+ will cause:
(a) Hypoventilation (b) Hyperventilation
(c) Hypercapnea (d) Hypoxia

2681. Endocanabinoids secreted by:
(a) Presynaptic neuron (b) Postsynaptic neuron
(c) Dentrites (d) Nodes of ranvier

2682. Human genome size:
(a) 5000 gene (b) 40000 gene
(c) 3 bp/46 chromosome (d) 1bp/23 chromosome

2683. Term limbic system termed by:
(a) Paul Mclean

2684. Protein secreted out of cell by:
(a) Endocytosis
(b) Exocytosis
(c) Packed by Golgi apparatus
(d) Synthesis in Mitochondria

2685. Sum of all chemical reaction in body:
(a) Metabolism (b) Homeostasis
(c) Physiology (d) Dynamic reaction

2686. 1 gene from mother, 1 from father:
(a) Genomic imprinting (b) Inheritance

2687. Alcohol black out at level:
(a) 30-80 mg/dl (b) 80-200
(c) 200-300 (d) 300-400

2688. Neonatal hypoglycemia definition RBS <:
(a) 40 (b) 60
(c) 100

2689. NMS by:
(a) Domperidone (b) Succinylcholine
(c) Amphetamine (d) Anticholinergic

2690. Pancytopemia with cellular marrow A/E:
(a) G 6 PD def (b) PNH
(c) Myelodysplasia (d) Megaloblastic

2691. Hb not seen in sickle cell anaemia is:
(a) HbA (b) Hb A2
(c) HbS (d) HbF

2692. CxR showing pneumatocele:
(a) Staph aureus (b) S pneumonia

2693. T 1/2 of carboxy Hb:
(a) 30 min (b) 1 hour
(c) 4 hours (d) 1 day

2694. Hemoglobinuria in A/E:
(a) $CuSO_4$
(b) Snakebite
(c) Thalassemia
(d) Blood transfusion mismatch

2695. Advanced HIV and TB A/E:
(a) Sputum +ve TB
(b) Lymphadenopathy intrathoracic
(c) Diffuse pulmonary infilterates
(d) Cavitatory lesion not seen

2696. Autism A/E:
(a) ↑ Serotonin
(b) ↓ Brain size
(c) Altered normal cytoarchitecture
(d) Inability to recognize fusiform facial region

2697. Asymptomatic bacteriuria treatment indicated in A/E:
(a) Pregnant women
(b) Elderly
(c) Obstruction uropathy
(d) Neutropenia

2698. Ambulatory BP in A/E:
(a) Newly diagnosed HT (b) Autonomic failure
(c) Resistant HT (d) White coat HT

2699. Kangaroo care for:
(a) Hypothermia (b) Hyperthermia
(c) Hypoglycemia

2700. Most common enzyme deficiency in adrenogenital syndrome:
(a) 21 β-OH def (b) 11 β-OH def
(c) 17-α OH def

2701. Multiple disease causing alleles when inherited together, chance of disease is more than additive effect called:

(a) Epistasis (b) Epistaxis
(c) Inheritance (d) Heritability

2702. ↑ S. Fe, ↑ ferritin, ↑ transferritin %, diagnosis is:

(a) Hemochromatosis
(b) Anemia of chronic disease
(c) IDA

2703. High frequency mechanical ventilation:

(a) TV $\geq$ 2 dead space, f–150
(b) TV = dead space, f–1000
(c) TV < dead space, f–150
(d) TV –

2704. Snakebite recent guideline:

(a) Immobilize (b) Torniquet
(c) Suction (d) Incision

2705. Hyperkalemia treatment A/E:

(a) Glucose infusion (b) Insulin
(c) Dialysis (d) Digoxin

2706. High plasma protein binding:

(a) Propranolol (b) Atenolol
(c) Metoprolol

2707. Hyperkalemia treatment not given:

(a) Insulin (b) Digoxin
(c) Glucose (d) Hemodialysis

2708. Adrenomedullin is present in high conc. A/E:

(a) Basophil (b) Leucocyte
(c) Renal adrenal gland (d) Kidney
(e) Hypothalamus

2709. Klinefelter's syndrome most characteristic:

(a) Increased breast cancer
(b) Normal sec. sexual character
(c) Aggressive behaviour
(d) Precocious puberty
(e) Aortic dissection

2710. P53 true:

(a) Chr 13p17.1
(b) Inhibits apoptosis
(c) Inhibit entry of cell into S phase
(d) Early deletion of P53 in colorectal CA progression
(e) Not associated with familial breast CA

2711. Not associated with exclusive deletion:

(a) Patau syndrome
(b) Edward
(c) Cri-du-chat syndrome
(d) Marfan syndrome
(e) CML

2712. Repeat sequence *except:*

(a) Myotonic (b) Ataxia telangiectasia
(c) Fredreich ataxia (d) Huntington chorea
(e) Muscular dystrophy

2713. Pure sensory neuropathy:

(a) Porphyria
(b) Cisplatin
(c) Lead
(d) Organophosphorus poisoning
(e) Diphtheria

2714. β thalassemia most common abnormality:

(a) Intron 22 deletion (b) Intron 1 inversion
(c) 3.2 (d) 4.7
(e) 649

2715. Acute phase reactants A/E:

(a) Fibrinogen (b) CRP
(c) SAA (d) Haemosiderin
(e) IL-1

2716. VAP if carbepenemase producing then DOC:

(a) Colistin
(b) Ampicillin + sulbactam
(c) Tobramycin
(d) Levoflox
(e) Meropenem

2717. Leptin true:

(a) ↓ in obese (b) Cross BBB
(c) Suppress appetite (d) Stimulate appetite
(e) Secreted by hypothalamus

2718. ANP:

(a) Vasoconstriction (b) Hypervolumia ↑ ANP
(c) Secreted by JG cell (d) Cause HTN
(e) Retain Na from renal

2719. Protein C activates:

(a) Va (b) VIIIa
(c) Va and VIIIa (d) IX
(e) Plasmin

2720. Amiodarone S/E A/E:
(a) Lupus like syndrome
(b) Photosensitivity
(c) Hyperthyroidism
(d) Pulmonary fibrosis
(e) Peripheral neuropathy

2721. SIADH:
(a) ↑ urinary specific gravity
(b) ↓ Sr. osmolality
(c) Hyponatremia
(d) Excess Na excretion
(e) ↑ S. uric acid

2722. Regression equation Y= 25 + 0.5 X_1 + 10X_2 X_1=10, X_2=5 predict the result:
(a) 80 (b) 35
(c) 40 (d) 42

2723. Type II error:
(a) False positive
(b) False negative
(c) Positive predictive value
(d) Negative predictive value
(e) None of the above

2724. Extraneous variable–systemically vary with independent variable–influence the dependent variable known as:
(a) Confounding variable
(b) Dependent variable
(c) Variate analysis

2725. Hypoglycemia true is:
(a) C peptide level ↑ in factitious insulin
(b) ↓proinsulin/insulin in insulinoma
(c) Epinephrine most important counterregulatory hormone
(d) Symptoms occur < 70 mg%
(e) Octreotide is used as treatment

2726. Middle age male with acromegaly and 1.7 cm pituitary growth:
(a) Transsphenoid surgery
(b) Bromocriptine
(c) Octreotide
(d) Cobalt therapy
(e) Yitrium imlant

2727. Plasmaphresis A/E:
(a) TTP (b) HUS
(c) M. gravis (d) GB syndrome
(e) Goodpasture syndrome

2728. Legionella pneumonia diagnosed best by:
(a) Acute serology (b) Blood culture
(c) Urine antigen testing (d) CT lung
(e) Yttrium implant

2729. Miliary TB:
(a) CXR may be normal
(b) 80% sputum negative
(c) Mantoux negative
(d) May be associated with hypokalemia
(e) TBM uncommon

2730. Campylobacter jejuni A/E:
(a) GB syndrome (b) Diarrhea
(c) Cholecystitis (d) Peptic ulcer
(e) Reactive arthritis

2731. Most specific test for RA:
(a) Anti CCP (b) RA factor
(c) IgM Ab (d) IgG Ab
(e) IgA Ab

2732. Parvo B_{19} true is:
(a) Infect mature RBC
(b) Erythema infectiosa
(c) RNA virus
(d) Persistent anemia in adult
(e) Most common cause of diarrhea in children

2733. H1N1 in pregnancy 2009 criteria includes:
(a) Neurological complications
(b) Cardiac disease
(c) CRF
(d) Immunosuppression
(e) Chronic lung disease

2734. TNF α:
(a) Secreted by bronchogenic CA
(b) Suppress other i/f mediaters
(c) Causes cachexia
(d) TOC in RA
(e) ↓ thermoset

2735. IL-1:
(a) Infusion causes hypotension
(b) Indicates severity of RA
(c) Antagonized by TNF-α
(d) Only secreted by leucocyte

2736. B-cell A/E:
(a) Burkitt
(b) Anaplastic large cell CA
(c) Follicular
(d) Hairy cell CA
(e) Mantle cell CA

2737. Nephrocalcinosis A/E:
(a) Medullary cystic disease
(b) Distal RTA
(c) Milk alkali syndrome
(d) Hypervitaminosis A
(e) Sarcoidosis

2738. High anion gap A/E:
(a) Distal RTA (b) Ethylene glycol
(c) DKA (d) Methanol
(e) Toluene

2739. In DM life threatening A/E:
(a) Emphysematous pyelonephritis
(b) Emphysematous appendicitis
(c) DKA
(d) Rhino mucormycosis
(e) Malignant otitis externa

2740. Congronous hemianopia due to lesion at:
(a) Optic tract (b) Optic chiasma
(c) Optic nerve (d) Optic radiation
(e) Occipital cortex

2741. If author more than _________ in citation then *et al.* is used.
(a) 2 (b) 3
(c) 4 (d) 5
(e) 6

2742. After heavy meal, patients collapse. CXR showing shadow in left lower lung:
(a) Boerrhave syndrome
(b) Mallory Weiss syndrome
(c) C tamponade
(d) MI
(e) Gastritis

2743. Narcolepsy A/E:
(a) Cataplexy
(b) Sleep paralysis
(c) Hypnogogic hallucinosis
(d) ↑ tone in EMG REM sleep
(e) Day time sleepiness

2744. CPAP not responding to treatment, most common cause:
(a) Non compliance
(b) Drug induced
(c) Structural CNS damage
(d) Depression
(e) Sleep disorder

2745. Hypokalemia ppt toxicity in:
(a) Digoxin (b) Insulin
(c) Warfarin

2746. Antigen presenting cell to T Cell in initial stage A/E:
(a) Eosinophil (b) CD 8+ T cell
(c) Neutrophil (d) Macrocyte
(e) Dendritic cell

2747. CKD target for anemia:
(a) Hb > 13
(b) Transferring saturation 30-40%
(c) Hb < 10 g%
(d) Erythropoietin level 10 Miu /ml
(e) Ferritin < 100

2748. Pulmonary embolism inv. of choice:
(a) Pulmonary angiography
(b) V. P. mismatch
(c) Multidetector CT chest
(d) D Dimer
(e) Echo

2749. Multiple myeloma cause A/E:
(a) Anemia (b) Hyperviscosity
(c) Hypercalcemia (d) ↑ ESR
(e) ↑ ALP

2750. Pulmonary hypertension used A/E:
(a) CCB
(b) B blockers
(c) Phosphodiesterase inhibitors
(d) Anticoagulant
(e) Lung transplant

2751. Oxygen Hb dissociation curve, shift to right side A/E:
(a) ↑ pH (b) ↑H^+
(c) ↑ temp. (d) ↑ 2,3- DPG
(e) ↑ CO_2

2752. Aromatase inhibitor causes:
(a) Endometrial CA (b) Pancreatic CA
(c) Hepatoma (d) Thromboembolism
(e) Osteoporosis

2753. Drugs nucleosidase inhibitors A/E:
(a) Didanosine (b) Tenofovir
(c) Squanavir (d) Dilaviridine
(e) Lamivudine

2754. Drug resistance in gram negative:
(a) ↑ efflux pump inhibitors
(b) ↑ β lactamase activity
(c) Mutation in porine channel
(d) Lipopolysaccharide mutation

2755. Lithium causes:
(a) Ebstein anomaly (b) VSD
(c) PDA (d) COA

2756. Hypercalcemia by A/E:
(a) Anticonvulsants (b) Thiazide
(c) Hypervitaminosis A (d) Vit. D intoxication
(e) Lithium

2757. Class Ib AAD:
(a) Phenytoin (b) Metoprolol
(c) Sotalol (d) Amiodarone
(e) Bertylium

2758. Very LBW defined as:
(a) 2.5-1.6 (b) > 2.5
(c) 1.5-1.0 (d) < 0.5
(e) 0.5-1.0

2759. Most common cause of pancreatitis in children:
(a) Trauma (b) Viral infection
(c) Valproate (d) Alcohol
(e) Cholelithiasis

2760. Adrenaline in LA solution (1:2,00,000):
(a) 20 μg/ml (b) 5 μg/ml
(c) 2.5 μg/ml (d) 10 μg/ml
(e) 12.5 μg/ml

2761. Kangaroo mother care for:
(a) Hypothermia (b) Hypoglycemia
(c) Hypokalemia

2762. Cystic hygroma most common site:
(a) Posterior triangle of neck
(b) Anterior triangle of neck
(c) Axilla
(d) Mediastinum

2763. Modified bone criteria:
(a) Neonatal sepsis
(b) Diaphragmatic eventration
(c) TEF
(d) MI

2764. Bartter's disease A/E:
(a) ↓ K^+ (b) Met alkalosis
(c) ↓ Ca^+ (d) ↑ Mg^+

2765. Digitalis toxicity:
(a) ↓ K^+ (b) ↑ K^+
(c) ↓ Ca^+ (d) ↑ Ca^+

2766. High altitude pulmonary edema:
(a) Nifedipine (b) Frusemide
(c) Salbutamol (d) Acetylsalicylic acid

2767. KAL gene responsible for:
(a) Gonadal dysgenesis
(b) Precocious puberty
(c) Tall stature
(d) Hypogonado hypogonadism

2768. Non-dominant parietal lobe lesion:
(a) Alexia
(b) Gerstman syndrome
(c) Ideomotor apraxia
(d) Topographical memory loss

2769. NE causes vasoconstriction is all vascular bed, *except:*
(a) Skin (b) Heart
(c) Muscle (d) Liver

2770. Vit K dependent factor A/E:
(a) II (b) VII
(c) V (d) X

2771. Duchenne's muscular dystrophy A/E:
(a) Intellectual impairment
(b) DCM
(c) X-linked recessive
(d) Present early infancy

2772. Down beat nystagmus, cerebellar sign, post column sign + small ms of hand atrophy:

(a) Chiari malformation + syringomyelia

(b) Basilar invagination with attanto –axial discolation

(c) Intra medullary tumor C7 – T1

(d) 4th ventricular ependymoma

2773. Shunt meningitis caused by:

(a) E coli (b) Pseudomonas

(c) Staph epidermidis (d) Pneumococci

2774. Not present in NCEP definition of metabolic syndrome:

(a) ↓ HDL (b) ↑ TG

(c) HTN (d) Micro albuminuria

2775. RV-failure in COPD cause A/E:

(a) Alveolar hypoventilation

(b) Respiratory acidosis

(c) Muscular stenosis in RVOT

(d) ↑ Pa CO_2

2776. EEG in occipital region 8–12 hz:

(a) α (b) β

(c) Delta (d) Theta

2777. DM bladder involvement due to (Peripheral+ autonomic) reason–earlier sensory afferent neuron. (T/F)

2778. S-Hb A1c indicates tissue hyperglycemia:

R–RBC no nucleus. (T/F)

2779. RFLP- DNA marker and affected gene are inherited together. (T/F)

R-DNA marker and gene are so closed that during meiosis can't be separated. (T/F)

2780. Kappa statistics–true:

(a) To compare population mean

(b) To compare population median

(c) Observes variation proportion

2781. Human genome project A/E:

(a) Purpose to clone human and body parts

(b) To investigation social, ethical genetic implication

(c) DNA mapping at all human beings

2782. R. DNA is based on:

(a) C- DNA

(b) Plasmid

(c) Restriction endonucleases

(d) PCR

2783. NH4 detoxified in brain as:

(a) Glutamine (b) GABA

(c) Urea (d) Uric acid

2784. Degeneracy of genetic code:

(a) Contains 2 base

(b) Multiple codons for single aminoacid

(c) Non coding gene

(d) Over expression of base

2785. Mosaicism:

(a) Germ line mosaicism not cause reccurrence

(b) More than 2 cell line

(c) Meiotic non-dysfunction

(d) Single cell line

2786. Nerve biopsy indication:

(a) Vascultic neuropathy (b) DM

(c) Toxic (d) GB syndrome

2787. Acromegaly with normal pituitary:

(a) Pituitary apoplexy

(b) GnRH-secreting carcinoid

(c) Hypothalamic hamartoma

(d) Most common Cune-Albright

2788. Headache in acromegaly:

(a) ↑ opioid tension

(b) Vascular compression

(c) Relaxation of periosteal

(d) None of the above

2789. Asymmetric septal hypertrophy

(a) Amyl nitrate ↓ murmur

(b) Autosomal dominance full penetrance

(c) Syncope not related to gradient

(d) Bifid carotid pulse, triple apex beat

2790. Most common site of athescloretic aneurysm:

(a) Ascending (b) Arch of AO

(c) Abdominal (d) Thoracic

2791. Fructose marker of:

(a) Prostate (b) Epididymis
(c) Testis (d) Seminal vesicle

2792. 1st child thalassemia major, chance in next child:

(a) 25 (b) 50
(c) 100 (d) <10

2793. RBC volume calculated by:

(a) 51 chromium (b) 60 cobalt
(c) 131 Iodine (d) Phosphorus

2794. Female, short stature, wide spaced nipple, primary amenorrhea genotype:

(a) 47 XXX (b) 47 XXY
(c) 45 X (d) 46 XX

2795. Peripheral signs of AR:

(a) Roth spot (b) Splinter hemorrhage
(c) Hill's sign (d) Osler node

2796. Sample–means:

(a) Subset of population (b) Mimature population
(c) Smaller units of population

2797. Scattered diagram:

(a) Associated with two variables
(b) Shows frequency
(c) Shows trend of pie chart
(d) Time trend

2798. Chi-square enjoys:

(a) Repetitive (b) Additive
(c) Multiplicative (d) Divisive

2799. Type II error:

(a) Accepting true null hypothesis
(b) Accepting false null hypothesis
(c) Rejecting false null hypothesis
(d) Rejecting true null hypothesis

2800. Cholesterol measured before and after MI in 60 people, means:

(a) Paired t
(b) Unpaired t
(c) Chi-square

2801. Categorical data changed to numerical data, number signifies:

(a) Interval (b) Ratio
(c) Ordinal (d) Nominal

2802. Area covered under 1 SD of N curve:

(a) 66% (b) 95%
(c) 82% (d) 75%

2803. Mitral valve how many leaflet?

(a) 4 (b) 3
(c) 2 (d) 5

2804. O_2 dissociation curve:

(a) Straight line (b) Sigmoid curve
(c) Hyperbola (d) Scattered line

2805. Contraindication of C-mitral valvatomy:

(a) Calcification (b) TR
(c) AF (d) Sev PAH

2806. Ribozyme:

(a) Enzyme of RNA
(b) Small ribonucleic protein
(c) Used in processing of m-RNA

2807. Intracranial volume is:

(a) 80% brain, 15% CSF, 5% blood
(b) 70% brain, 15% CSF, 15% blood
(c) 90% brain, 5% CSF, 5% blood
(d) 5% brain, 15% CSF, 80% blood

2808. Down's with balanced translocation 21-21, chance of transmission in next offspring's:

(a) 100 (b) 0
(c) 50 (d) 25

2809. Phosphaturia:

(a) Most common of cloudy urine
(b) Clears with alkalization
(c) Can occur after heavy consumption of milk
(d) Amorphous crystals on microscopy

2810. Urinary pH:

(a) N is 9.5-8
(b) Alkaline is 6.5-8
(c) Cystine stores associated with acidic urine
(d) RTA pH < 5.5 can be done with acid load

2811. Hematuria True A/E:

(a) Urinary dipstick detects hematuria in > 30%
(b) > 1000 RBC/ml normal
(c) Hematuria of nephrogenic origin occur without proteinuria
(d) Dysmorphic RBC in glomerular origin

2812. Persistent ↓ C_3 in A/E:
(a) PSGN (b) Shunt GN
(c) Active lupus (d) MPGN

2813. Most common cause of pulmonary embolism:
(a) ASD (b) Pyelonephritis
(c) Septic abortion (d) ST

2814. Methotrexate antagonism:
(a) Niacin (b) Folate
(c) Riboflavin

2815. Primaquine cause hemolytic in:
(a) G6PD def (b) NADP def

2816. Statin used in:
(a) PAD (b) Renal art aneurysm
(c) Mod calcific PS (d) AF

2817. Type 2 DM:
(a) Only insulin resistance
(b) Insulin def. and resistance + glucagon excess
(c) ↑ glucagon
(d) ↓ resistance

2818. Paraneoplastic A/E:
(a) Pleural effusion
(b) ↑ Ca
(c) Neuropathy
(d) Pulmonary osteoarthropathy

2819. Non-restrictive large VSD A/E:
(a) Tachycardia
(b) Tachypnea
(c) Growth retardation
(d) Present in 1st year of life

2820. Operon:
(a) Acts as an operator (b) Present in eukaryote

2821. Severity of MS:
(a) OS-A2 interval (b) OS – P2
(c) Loud S1 (d) Diast murmur

2822. Mid systolic click:
(a) MVP (b) PS
(c) MS (d) AS

2823. Strict glycemic control necessary:
(a) Brittle diabetes
(b) All pregnant women
(c) Infant with diabetes
(d) Elderly with recent diagnosis

2824. Cord blood stem all used A/E:
(a) AML
(b) Gaucher's
(c) Cirrhosis
(d) Stem transplant after burn

2825. Best stimulus of ADH secretion:
(a) ↓ volume (b) ↑ OSM
(c) ↑ Na^+

2826. Cushing's A/E:
(a) ↑ K^+ (b) Alkalosis
(c) Thin skin (d) Wide purple striae

2827. Father–hemophilic:
(a) All girls carrier (b) 50% girls carrier
(c) 50% son affected

2828. Rituximab acts on:
(a) CD3 (b) CD4
(c) CD20 (d) CD40

2829. HOCM A/E:
(a) Bela blockers decrease the risk of sudden cardiac death
(b) Dual chamber pacing in symptomatic patients
(c) Alcohol ablation of the septum is a good option
(d) Intra cardiac defibrillator to be implanted in patients with history of cardiac arrest

2830. Squatting decreases the murmur of:
(a) AS (b) MVP
(c) MS (d) VSD

2831. Treatment of HACEK endocarditis:
(a) Imipenam (b) Ciplox
(c) Ceftriaxone (d) Penicillin

2832. Rat bite treatment is:
(a) Cleaning
(b) Cleaning+antibiotic+washing+TT
(c) Cleaning+antibiotic+washing+TT+Anti-rabies
(d) Cleaning+antibiotic+washing+TT+Anti-rabies+Ig

2833. Clindamycin is drug of choice for:
(a) Giardia (b) Babebiosis
(c) Cryptosporidiosis (d) Trypanosomiasis

2834. Quartan malaria nephropathy in:

(a) P. vivax (b) P. falciparum
(c) P. ovale (d) P. malariae

2835. Renal papillary necrosis in:

(a) IV heroine abuse (b) Gold
(c) Penicillin (d) NSAIDS

2836. Metabolic syndrome has all *except:*

(a) Abdominal obesity (b) Increased LDL
(c) Decreased HDL (d) Decreased TG

2837. Feature of zinc deficiency:

(a) Hypoguesia
(b) Impaired glucose tolerance
(c) Heart failure
(d) Muscle weakness

2838. Labourer sleeping outside presented in the morning with flaccid quadriparesis with normal serum biochemistry. Treatment is:

(a) Antivenom
(b) Ivlg
(c) Potassium supplementation
(d) Dextrose

2839. All of the following variables are used to calculate sensitivity *except:*

(a) False positive (b) False negative
(c) True positive (d) True negative

2840. The type of anaemia found in Lesch-Nyhan syndrome is:

(a) Hemolytic (b) Normocytic
(c) MCHC (d) Megaloblastic

2841. Renal involvement seen in LCAT deficiency is:

(a) MCD (b) MPGN
(c) MGN (d) FSGN

2842. Increased T3, increased T4, decreased iodine uptake is seen in:

(a) Subacute thyroiditis (b) Hashimoto's disease
(c) Toxic nodular goiter (d) Multimodular goiter

2843. Limitation of cord – blood stem cell use is:

(a) Less number of nucleated cells
(b) Decreased telomere length
(c) Decreased cell cycle length
(d) Decreased clonogenic growth

2844. Trans fatty acids cause:

(a) Increased risk of CAD
(b) Decrease risk of HTN
(c) Decreased risk of hyperlipidemia

2845. Non invasive ventilation not for:

(a) COPD (b) Sleep apnoea
(c) Pneumonia (d) Non-trained person

2846. APLA associated with all *except:*

(a) Anti-Smith
(b) Anti cardiolipin
(c) Antilupus anticoagulant
(d) Anti beta$_2$ microglobulin

2847. Patient with HTN, pain abdomen and testicular pain has:

(a) PAN (b) Takayasu
(c) Wegener's (d) Churg-Strauss

2848. Bortezomib is used in:

(a) Multiple myeloma (b) ALL
(c) AML (d) Harry cell leukemia

2849. Use of the following leads to increase in HDL:

(a) Niacin (b) Exercise
(c) Fenofibrate (d) Reosvastatin

2850. Duration of insulin glargine action is:

(a) 4 hours (b) 6 hours
(c) 12 hours (d) 24 hours

2851. Treatment of HCV genotype l:

(a) Ribavarin
(b) Ribavarin + Peg II N-alpha for 12 weeks
(c) Ribavarin + Peg II N-alpha for 24 weeks
(d) Ribavarin + Peg II N for 48 weeks

2852. Metabolic abnormality seen in unilateral renal artery stenosis:

(a) Decreases Na (b) Decreased K
(c) Decrease Ca (d) Decrease Mg

2853. Best treatment for unilateral limb swelling with pulmonary embolism:

(a) Heparin (b) STK
(c) IV ceftriaxone (d) Filter

2854. Atheroembolic renal disease presents with:

(a) Red cell casts
(b) Heavy proteinuria

(c) Eosinophilia
(d) Clinical evidence of pulmonary embolism

2855. Colon carcinoma in ulcerative colitis:
(a) Arises from adenomatous polyp
(b) Multiple synchronous cancers associated in 1%
(c) Mean age = 60 years
(d) Uniform involvement of whole colon

2856. Whipple's disease D/E:
(a) Dementia is late
(b) T whipelli is the cause
(c) Migratory large joint polyarthritis
(d) TMT + SMX for 14 days

2857. Free water defiant in a 50 kg man when serum Na is 160 meq/1:
(a) 1.91 (b) 2.91
(c) 3.91 (d) 4.91

2858. pH= 6.43, PO_2=40, PCO_2=50, HCO_3=6:
(a) DKA
(b) Cardiorespiratory arrest
(c) Salicylate poisoming
(d) CO_2 narcosis

2859. Anti-D in TTP:
(a) Immediate increase in platelets
(b) Anemia
(c) Neutrophilia

2860. HUS caused by:
(a) Vincristine (b) Cyclophosphamide
(c) Rituximab (d) Mitomycin-C

2861. Treatment of orthostatic hypotension:
(a) Fludrocortisone (b) Epinephrine
(c) B-blockers

2862. Glucocorticoid remediable aldosteronism:
(a) Increase in aldosterone on standing
(b) Family history
(c) Onset in middle age
(d) Increased renal angiotensin

2863. Eaton Lambert has all *except:*
(a) Ptosis
(b) Normal reflexes
(c) Decremental response
(d) Limbs not involved

2864. Brain metastasis is most common with:
(a) Ca lung (b) Ca Breast
(c) Melanoma (d) Prostate carcinoma

2865. Urinary Ph normal range:
(a) 2 (b) 5
(c) 10 (d) 7

2866. Most urgent non specific marker for neonatal sepsis:
(a) TLC
(b) Neutrophils
(c) Immature: mature ratio
(d) Band forms

2867. Normotensive PR:
(a) < 40 mm Hg (b) > 55
(c) > 40

2868. JNC 7 stage I hypertension A/E:
(a) Life style modification
(b) Diuretics
(c) B blockers
(d) Moderation of alcohol intake

2869. 20-year-old male, urethral discharge treated with IV ceftriaxone, discharge persists but culture negative:
(a) HSV
(b) Gonococcus
(c) Chlamydia psittaci
(d) Chlamydia trachomatis

2870. CPR A/E:
(a) Cardiac arrest has 3 phases – electrical, mechanical and metabolic
(b) AED part of advanced life support
(c) 2.0 J/kg in a child
(d) Adult sized paddles used in a child > 10 kg

2871. Bronchiectasis occur in A/E:
(a) Mycoplasma
(b) ABPA
(c) Kartagener
(d) Endobronchial carcinoids

2872. Alopecia with preserved hair follicle:
(a) Propranolol (b) Lithium
(c) Isotretinion (d) Daunorubicin

2873. Schistosoma mansoni with liver involvement most common findings:

(a) Esophageal varices (b) Jaundice
(c) Ascitis (d) Gynaecomastia

2874. Most infectious TB:

(a) Child of mother with sputum negative but culture +ve
(b) HIV negative spouse of HIV + ve TB patients
(c) Co-worker of a patient with laryngeal TB in a crowded work place
(d) Spouse of patients with miliary TB

2875. About giardiasis in AIDS, true is all *except:*

(a) Common cause of malabsorption in India
(b) Nifurtimox is given
(c) Can cause fatal disease in AIDS
(d) Antigen detection in stool is as sensitive as detection of microorganism in stool

2876. Gubler's sign is seen in:

(a) Arsenic (b) Lead
(c) Cobalt (d) Cadmium

2877. Drug induced myopathy seen A/E:

(a) Zidovudine (b) CCB
(c) Chloroquine (d) Cyclosporine

2878. Osmotic diuresis is said to be present when urinary osmolality is more than:

(a) 360 (b) 400
(c) 600 (d) 750

2879. Tract of Lissauer's is for:

(a) Pain (b) Motor
(c) Proprioception (d) Efferent spindle

2880. Nephrogenic DI is caused by all *except:*

(a) Lithium (b) Amphotericin
(c) Hypokalemia (d) Hypoxia

2881. After transaction at C5 level, spasticity with increased reflexes appear at:

(a) 1-3 days (b) 3 days – 3 weeks
(c) 1-3 months (d) 2-4 months

2882. Fluid used in the treatment of metabolic alkalosis is:

(a) Ringer lactate (b) 5% NS
(c) Saline (d) 5% dextrose

2883. Criteria for diagnosis of ABPA includes all *except:*

(a) Bronchial asthma
(b) Increased IgA in serum
(c) Peripheral eosinophilia > 1500
(d) Pulmonary infiltrates

2884. Diagnostic criteria for ulcerative colitis includes all *except:*

(a) 6 stools/day (b) Tachycardia > 90
(c) Bleeding (d) Fever > 37° C

2885. Poor prognosis in pancreatitis includes all *except:*

(a) Pulse > 130/min (b) Ranson < 3
(c) Apache II > 8 (d) GI bleed

2886. Bulemia nervosa includes all *except:*

(a) Hyponatremia
(b) Hypokalemia
(c) Hypochloremic alkalosis
(d) Normal renal function

2887. Cause of symptomatic trigeminal neuralgia include all *except:*

(a) Schwannoma/acoustic neuroma
(b) Basilar artery aneurysm
(c) Posterior fossa meningioma
(d) Tolosa Hunt syndrome

2888. Root valve of 1st dorsal interossei is:

(a) 3C5-6 (b) C6-7
(c) C8-TI (d) TI-2

2889. Most common vision defect in classic migraine is:

(a) Homonymous hemianopia
(b) Centrocaecal scotoma
(c) C shaped scotoma
(d) Bi temporal

2890. Ascariasis all *except:*

(a) Transmission via percutaneous route
(b) Eggs are infective
(c) 15-20 cm in length
(d) Mostly found in jejunum

2891. Side effects of imatinib mesylate include all *except:*

(a) Peripheral neuropathy
(b) Edema

(c) Licheniform eruptions
(d) Hepatotoxicity

2892. AVF lead criteria in LVH (r wave):
(a) 15 (b) 20
(c) 30 (d) 35

2893. TB in AIDS, all are true *except:*
(a) Meningitis and tuberculomas are common
(b) Extra pulmonary manifestations 40-60%
(c) Cavitatory lesions common in late stages
(d) Sputum negativity is common

2894. Chronic HVC therapy:
(a) IFN-alpha
(b) IFN-alpha+lamivudine
(c) IFN-alpha (peg) + ribavirin
(d) Ribavirin

2895. Anti-malarial drug that is gametocidal:
(a) Chloroquine (b) Mefloquine
(c) Halofantrin (d) Primaquine

2896. Splenomgealy in malaria, all are true *except:*
(a) Sickle cell trait is protective in P. vivax
(b) There is year round infection with stable transmission
(c) Raised IgM
(d) Unstable low erratic and focal

2897. For Wegener's granulomatosis all are true *except:*
(a) ANCA is helpful in diagnosis
(b) Renal involvement lung involvement
(c) Chronic necrotizing vasculitis (i.e. vessel biopsy) is diagnostic
(d) Staph aureus infection is recurrent in it

2898. ESR varies with:
(a) Weight (b) Age
(c) Both of the above (d) None of the above

2899. In SLE, poor prognostic sign in A/E:
(a) Proteinuria < 2.5 g/day
(b) Creatinine > 1.5
(c) Hb < 12.4
(d) Hypocomplimentemia

2900. In Hodgkin's lymphoma, most common infection is:
(a) Streptococcus (b) P. carinii
(c) Staphylococcus (d) Listeria

2901. Cause of OPCA is:
(a) Hereditary (b) Neurotoxin
(c) Post encephalitis (d) Hypoxia

2902. Treatment of type – I lepra reaction is:
(a) Glucocorticoid
(b) Thalidomide
(c) Clofazimine
(d) Glucocorticoid+ thalidomide

2903. Pheochromocytoma A/E:
(a) Incidence 0.12% of all cases of HTN
(b) 10% are malignant
(c) Size usually < 10 cm
(d) 10% are familial

2904. All cause hyperprolactinemia *except:*
(a) Metaclopramide (b) Chlorpromazine
(c) Mozapride (d) Fluoxetine

2905. For toxoplasmosis all are true *except:*
(a) All cells affected except RBC's
(b) Prophylaxis in AIDS with CD_4 count < 100
(c) Congenital infections are usually asymptomatic but can cause choriotertinitis
(d) Not transmitted by organ transplantation

2906. ACE inhibitors cause hyperkalemia in all *except:*
(a) DM
(b) Bilateral renal artery stenosis
(c) Unilateral renal artery stenosis
(d) Decreased arterial volume

2907. Amiodarone induced in initial stage:
(a) Increased T3 (b) Decreased T3
(c) Increased T4 (d) Decreased T4

2908. Urinary bladder in MS:
(a) Frequent voiding and small
(b) Large residual volume bladder
(c) Small maximum
(d) Loss of voluntary control

2909. Rheumatoid arthritis can cause:
(a) CLL (b) AML
(c) T cell lymphoma (d) B cell lymphoma

2910. True about risk of stroke in atrial fibrillation is all *except:*
(a) < 65 cause of age
(b) CHF

(c) HTN
(d) Previous history of stroke

2911. All are caused to reduce proteinuria *except:*
(a) ACE inhibitor
(b) Ca^{+} channel blockers
(c) NSAIDs
(d) Angiotensin receptor blocker

2912. For Gilles de la Tourette's syndrome, all are true *except:*
(a) Motor and vocal tics
(b) Foul utterance
(c) Paranoid delusions and hallucinations
(d) Disease persists after 1 year

2913. For amoebiasis all are true *except:*
(a) Most commonly by Entamoeba histolytica
(b) IgG is protective against recurrent infections
(c) 10% of world population is infected by E hist
(d) Instestinal invasion protection by IgA

2914. For sarcoidosis true is:
(a) Increased ACE levels in 2/3rd of patients
(b) Kveim test is diagnostic
(c) Facial palsy occurs rarely
(d) Erythema nodosum is rare

2915. Whipple disease false:
(a) Dementia is late
(b) T. whippli causative
(c) Migratory large joints polyarthritis
(d) TMP + SMX for 14 days

2916. Bortezomib used in:
(a) Multiple myeloma (b) ALL
(c) AML (d) Hairy cell leukemia

2917. ↑ HDL:
(a) Niacin (b) Exercise
(c) Fenofibrate (d) Rosvastatin

2918. Duration of action of insulin glargine:
(a) 4 hours (b) 6
(c) 12 (d) 24

2919. HUS caused by:
(a) Vincristine
(b) Cyclophosphamide
(c) Rituximab
(d) Mitomycin C

2920. Free water deficit when 160 meq/l Na in 50 kg man:
(a) 1.9 (b) 2.9
(c) 3.9 (d) 4.9

2921. SLE prognostic factor A/E:
(a) Hypocomplementemia
(b) Hb < 12 g%
(c) Proteinuria > 2.5 g
(d) Serum creatinine > 1.5

2922. Amyloidosis with cardiac disease, best diagnosed by:
(a) Endomyocardial biopsy
(b) Abdominal fat aspirate
(c) Rectal biopsy
(d) Colon biopsy

2923. Cell nucleus was discovered by:
(a) Robert Brown

2924. Guardian of human genome is:
(a) P53 gene (b) ATP
(c) Topoisomerase (d) Endonuclease

2925. Best indicator of recent malnutrition is:
(a) Fibronectin
(b) Albumin
(c) Pre albumin
(d) Retinal binding protein

2926. Hypokalemia has all *except:*
(a) QT prolongation (b) Tall T

2927. A patient receive vaccination for HBV she has in her serum:
(a) HbsAg +ve (b) Anti HBc IgM
(c) Anti HBe IgM (d) Anti HBs IgM

2928. Gene therapy has been established for:
(a) SCID (b) Thalassemia major
(c) Gaucher's disease (d) Hemophilia

2929. For common variable immunodeficiency true is:
(a) All patients affected
(b) Symptomatic in childhood

(c) Give normal schedule of immunization
(d) Causes diarrhea and recurrent bronchitis

2930. Most common site of osteoporosis fractures:
(a) Hip (b) Wrist
(c) Leg (d) Vertebrae

2931. A lady with nocturnal paresthesias in two and a half fingers on radial side with wasting:
(a) Carpal tunnel syndrome
(b) de Quervain syndrome

2932. Most common cause of shunt infection is:
(a) Staph. epidermidis (b) Staph. aureus
(c) Enterobacteriaceae (d) Streptococcus

2933. All cause metastasis to brain *except:*
(a) Ovary (b) Breast
(c) Lung (d) Melanoma

2934. All are metastasis to liver *except:*
(a) Lung (b) Breast
(c) Prostate (d) Colon

2935. All are vitamin K dependent factors *except:*
(a) VII (b) VIII
(c) IX (d) Protein-C

2936. A diabetic female on OCPs dies after consuming 3 beer bottles. She had LDL levels > 1000. Cause of death was:
(a) Acute pancreatitis (b) Sudden cardiac death
(c) DVT

2937. OCPs are beneficial for all *except:*
(a) Cardiac events (b) Vasomotor symptoms
(c) Osteoporosis (d) Decrease LDL

2938. Bad prognostic factor in pancreatitis:
(a) Increase amylase (b) Increased lipase
(c) WBC >20,000 (d) Diastolic BP >90

2939. All are causes of bronchiectasis in a 45 years old man *except:*
(a) Kartagener's syndrome
(b) Endobronchial carcinoid
(c) ABPA
(d) Mycoplasmal infection

2940. All are causes of thoracic aortic aneurysm:
(a) Osteogenesis imperfecta
(b) Ankylosing spondylitis
(c) PAN
(d) Takayasu

2941. Schistosoma japonicum presents with:
(a) Esophageal varices (b) Jaundice
(c) Ascitis (d) Gynaecomastia

2942. Which of the following leads to shaft loss with preserved hair follicle?
(a) Doxorubicin (b) Beta blocker
(c) Lithium (d) Retinoic acid

2943. All are true for IDA *except:*
(a) Decreased TIBC
(b) Decreased serum ferritin
(c) Increased reticulocyte response

2944. In case of anaphylaxis, first step of treatment is:
(a) Epinephrine (b) Dexamethasone
(c) Antihistaminic (d) Anti-venom

2945. Most common disease making patients land in a dialysis unit:
(a) DM (b) HTN
(c) CGN

2946. All are criteria for nephrotic syndrome *except:*
(a) Hyperlipidemia
(b) Urine protein > 3 g/day
(c) HTN
(d) Edema

2947. No response in culture negative urethral discharge, after receiving certriaxone:
(a) N. gonorrhoea
(b) Chlamydia trachomatis
(c) Chlamydia psittacosis
(d) Herpes

2948. Reiter's triad (urethritis, conjunctivitis, arthritis) has all *except:*
(a) Early GIT involvement
(b) ANA is likely to be +
(c) Organism is Neisseria
(d) Rheumatoid factor +

2949. Heparin does not lead to:
(a) Factor V increase
(b) Osteoporosis
(c) Thrombocytopenia
(d) Prolongation of a PTT

2950. Treatment for pulmonary embolism with RV dysfunction with normal BP:

(a) Thrombolysis (b) Surgery

2951. Atherosclerosis involves all *except:*

(a) MCA (b) Proximal LAD
(c) Carotid bifurcation (d) Proximal renal artery

2952. Maximum chance of infection in TB is when:

(a) Child of smear –ve culture +ve parent
(b) Laryngeal TB in a closed office
(c) HIV –ve partner of HIV +ve patient with TB
(d) Spouse of patient with military TB

2953. Legionnaire disease A/E:

(a) Hyponatremia (b) Lymphocytosis
(c) Normal PMN (d) DIC

2954. SSRI due to:

(a) ↑ stores of monoamines
(b) Presynaptic accumulation of amines
(c) Both 1 and 2
(d) Depletion of stores

2955. Kurtosis seen in:

(a) Tail (b) Hump
(c) Front (d) All of the above

2956. Biomedical liquid waste disposal:

(a) 5 (b) 7
(c) 8 (d) 10

2957. Lower level scapula:

(a) T 3 (b) T 7
(c) T 5 (d) T 9

2958. Lead poisoning in urine (μg/l):

(a) 0.7 (b) 0.8
(c) 0.9 (d) 1.0

2959. Hypoosmolar hyponatremia A/E:

(a) Burns (b) Diarrhea
(c) Osmotic diuresis (d) Mannitol

2960. Characteristic of type III hyperlipidemia:

(a) Xanthelesma
(b) Palmer crease xanthoma
(c) Tuberoeruptive

2961. Retina is extension of:

(a) Mesencephalon (b) Diencephalon
(c) Metecephalon (d) Myelencephalon

2962. Micronodular cirrhosis:

(a) Acute viral hepatitis
(b) Wilson disease
(c) Drugs
(d) Glycogen storage disease

2963. Couinaud classification of liver:

(a) Hepatic Vein + Portal Vein
(b) Hepatic Vein + bile duct
(c) Portal Vein + bile duct
(d) Portal Vein + hepatic duct

2964. Purkinje cells of cerebellum:

(a) Ends on excitatory synapse
(b) Ends on cerebellar nuclei
(c) Main efferent output
(d) Synapse on spinal cord

2965. Weight lowering of elbow joint:

(a) Active shortening of forearm flexor
(b) Active shortening of forearm extensor
(c) Passive shortening of forearm flexor
(d) Passive shortening of forearm extensor

2966. Homocysteinuria A/E:

(a) Dislocation of lens
(b) Thromboembolic episodes
(c) Deficiency of cystathione ligase
(d) Deficiency of cystathione synthetase

2967. Drug prolonging repolarization:

(a) Sotalol (b) Verapamil
(c) Lignocaine (d) Flecainide

2968. Primary amoebic encephalitis caused by:

(a) Naegleria Floweri
(b) Entamoeba hartmanni
(c) Entamoeba Coli
(d) Entamoeba histolytica

2969. Pneumocystis Carnii Pneumonia A/E:

(a) Common CD4 < 400
(b) Cannot be cultured
(c) Fluorescent antibody technique is available for it
(d) Can be seen in giemsa

2970. Fluoroquinolones active against:

(a) Gram negative only
(b) Gram positive only

(c) Only against mycoplasma, chlamydia
(d) Both gram positive and gram negative

2971. Acute gastroenteritis, E. Coli–0157: H7 (haemorrhagic colitis) diagnosed by:
(a) Sorbital MacConkey agar
(b) Blood agar
(c) TCBS
(d) Ether agarose

2972. Deoxyribonuclease affect which:
(a) Conjugation (b) Transformation
(c) Transduction (d) Transfection

2973. Mycoplasma pneumonia true is:
(a) Inhibited by Penicillin G
(b) Contain both DNA/RNA
(c) Can grow extracellularly in vivo
(d) Can grow in cell free medium

2974. New drug introduced for treatment of disease, other factors are not changed:
(a) Incidence no change
(b) Prevalence no change
(c) Both will change
(d) Both will not change

2975. Bainbridge reflex involves:
(a) Tachycardia
(b) Increased peripheral Vascular Resistance
(c) Increased vasopressin
(d) Increased Na excretion

2976. Rate limiting enzyme in polyamine synthesis:
(a) S-Adenosyl Methionine synthetase
(b) Ornithine decarboxylase
(c) Superoxide synthase

2977. Non disjunction causes:
(a) Trisomy
(b) Monosomy
(c) Loss of Y chromosome
(d) All of the above

2978. Conjunctival and corneal reflexes–afferent is:
(a) Trigeminal (ophthalmic division)
(b) Abducent nerve
(c) Facial nerve
(d) Optic nerve

2979. Tip of nose supplied by:
(a) Ophthalmic nerve (b) Maxillary
(c) Upper buccal (d) Lower buccal

2980. Poor prognosis in AML A/E:
(a) Age > 60 (b) Inversion of chr. 16
(c) Deletion 5q (d) Complex karyotype

2981. Thymus false A/E:
(a) Behind trachea
(b) Regress soon after birth
(c) Lymphocyte rich
(d) Arises from fourth pharyngeal arch

2982. Membrane digestion of carbohydrate:
(a) Isomaltase (b) Amylase
(c) Glucoamylase (d) Sucrose

2983. Intravenous immunoglobin–MOA:
(a) Blocks Fc receptors
(b) CD3 Inhibition
(c) Calcineurin Inhibition
(d) Complement mediated reduction of lymphocytes

2984. Physiological insulin antagonist:
(a) Glucagon (b) Adrenaline
(c) Adrenal steroid (d) All of the above

2985. Riboflavin activity assessed by:
(a) RBC transketolase
(b) G6PD
(c) Glutathione synthase
(d) Glutathione reductase

2986. Pellagra like:
(a) Hartnup disease (b) Carcinoid syndrome
(c) Polished rice (d) Sorghum

2987. Glycated Hb decreased in:
(a) DM
(b) Renal failure
(c) Iron deficiency anemia
(d) AIHA

2988. Alkaline phosphatases marker of:
(a) Bile secretion
(b) Hepatic metabolism
(c) Hepatocyte membrane integrity
(d) Hepatic excretion

2989. Connexins:
(a) Made up of 6 subunits
(b) Found in liver
(c) Can conduct electrical activity
(d) < 10 KDA sized particles allowed

2990. Brain edema A/E:
(a) Glutamate increases in brain
(b) Increase entry of sodium followed by water
(c) Neuroglial cell swelling
(d) All nerve fibre with axons are swollen

2991. Absolute Refractory Period:
(a) No action potential can be generated
(b) Start with depolarization and end at half of repolarization
(c) Time dependent pacemaker
(d) Indicate ST segment

2992. Secular trend:
(a) Periodic fluctuation (b) Seasonal trend
(c) Long term change (d) Short term change

2993. Best correlation between two variable for direction and magnitude:
(a) Fried test (b) Correlation coefficient
(c) Chi-square test (d) Wilkoxon paired t test

2994. Persistent low C3:
(a) PSGN (b) Lupus
(c) SABE (d) MPGN

2995. Common between influenza and corona virus:
(a) Segmented genome
(b) Both contain infectious RNA
(c) Both are negative sense
(d) High rate of genetic reassortment during replication

2996. LS surge:
(a) Puberty (b) Adolescence
(c) Before ovulation (d) Menopause

2997. All are falsely elevated in blood sample (hemolysed):
(a) K^+ (b) Na^+
(c) AST (d) Urea

2998. Radioactive iodine emits:
(a) Gamma rays (b) Beta rays
(c) Both of the above (d) None of the above

2999. Vitamin D_3 supplementation:
(a) Paget's disease (b) Osteomalacia
(c) Hypocalcemia (d) Hyophosphatemia

3000. IUGR with maternal smoking:
(a) Case control study
(b) Prospective study
(c) Cross-sectional study
(d) Clinical trial

3001. Acute MI pathology <4 hours chest pain succumbs to death <24 hours, autopsy shows hemorrhagic infarct. light. Microscopy shows:
(a) Waviness of fibres
(b) Myocyte necrosis with neutrophil infiltration
(c) Coagulation necrosis + granulation tissue
(d) Hemosiderin deposition with macrophage

3002. Sporotrichosis:
(a) Dimorphic fungus
(b) Usually seen in immunocompromised patients
(c) Etiology not known

3003. MS with oligogonal band seen in:
(a) CSF electrophoresis
(b) Serum electrophoresis
(c) CSF + serum electrophoresis
(d) Serum immunophoresis

3004. Phase 2 denotes:
(a) End of QRS (b) Isoelectric ST
(c) T wave

3005. Infection causing cardiac conduction defect:
(a) Lyme's disease
(b) Chagas disease
(c) Tuberculous pneumonia
(d) Diphtheria myocarditis

3006. Not a single gene defect:
(a) Long QT (b) HOCM
(c) Marfan's syndrome (d) RAS

3007. Not a Mendelian inheritance caused by single gene defect:
(a) SCD due to LQTS (b) Premature CAD
(c) Marfan's syndrome

3008. Which is not T-Cell inhibitor:
(a) Azathioprine (b) Mycophenolate
(c) Sirolimus (d) Cyclosporine

3009. 5th stage transition in epidemiology of cardiovascular disease:

(a) Increasing CHF, stroke and CAD cause most of death
(b) Increase in CAD and HTN
(c) Reversal of decreased mortality with increasing age
(d) Increase prevalence of RHD

3010. AV Node artery is a branch:

(a) Anterior Atrial branch of RCA
(b) Post atrial branch of RCA
(c) Post descending branch of RCA
(d) LCA

3011. EBV most commonly producing resembling:

(a) IL-1 (b) IL-2
(c) IL-9 (d) IL-10

3012. Th-2 cells stimulated by:

(a) IL-1 (b) IL-2
(c) IL-4 (d) IL-8

3013. Baby diarrhea with oral but normal with intravenous. Which channel of intestine affected?

(a) Na-K (b) SGLT-1
(c) NeF- 3 (d) H^+K^+

3014. Fanconi's anemia is:

(a) Haemolytic anemia (b) IDA
(c) Aplastic anemia (d) Megaloblastic anemia

3015. Classical complement starts by

(a) Activation of C1
(b) C3 converter
(c) Cleavage of C4 and C1
(d) NAC

3016. Intracellular receptor complex A/E:

(a) Norepinephrine (b) Steroid
(c) Vit D_3 (d) Retinoic acid

3017. Post translational modification of protein by:

(a) Vitamin E (b) Vitamin K
(c) Vitamin A (d) Retinoic acid

3018. Spongiform cells of kajoj cell seen with:

(a) Lichen planus (b) Seborrheic dermatitis
(c) SLE (d) Psoriasis

3019. Bacteria which acts by inhibiting fusion of phagosome and cytosome:

(a) Yersinea
(b) Mycoplasma
(c) Chlamydia
(d) Legionella pneumophilia

3020. Intracytoplamic basophilic inclusion with perinuclear halo seen in:

(a) EBV (b) HPV
(c) CMV (d) HBV

3021. N K ATPase is inhibited by:

(a) Insulin (b) Thyroxine
(c) Dopamine (d) Aldosterone

3022. Benzodiazepine with more hangover:

(a) Lorazepam (b) Oxazepam
(c) Clonazepam (d) Etilozepam

3023. Benzodiazepine which would not have cumulative effect:

(a) Clonazepam (b) Lorazepam
(c) Etizolam (d) Alprazolam

3024. Ca lung has high fatality rate which is true?

(a) High incidence rate
(b) High mortality rate
(c) Mortality and incidence rate same in a year
(d) Can't be commented

3025. Insulin receptor has following dormant activity of:

(a) Tyrosine kinase (b) $Na^+ K^+$ ATPase

3026. Requirement ↑ed in lactation > pregnancy A/E:

(a) Iron (b) Vitamin C
(c) Vitamin A (d) Energy requirement

3027. Energy is breast milk in 1st month:

(a) 640-720 kcal (b) 320-450 kcal
(c) 850 kcal (d) None of the above

3028. CMT due to defect in:

(a) Connexins (b) Cadherins
(c) Myelin

3029. MAO-A inhibitor:

(a) Metabolises NE, serotonins and tyramine
(b) Metabolises dopamine specifically
(c) Metabolises serotonin and dopamine
(d) Epinephrine and dopamine

3030. TCA's have which effect?

(a) Antimuscarinic effect

(b) Antihistaminic

(c) α-blocker

(d) All of the above

3031. Coronary vasodilation by sympathetic stimulation via:

(a) α-receptor stimulation

(b) β receptor stimulation

(c) Metabolic production

(d) Sympathetic cholinergic activities

3032. Antiarrhythmic drug used in neuropathic pain:

(a) Lignocaine (topically) with mexilitine

(b) Quinidine

(c) Amiodarone

3033. Myelination A/E:

(a) Starts with cervical and runs caudally, starts with motor and progresses to sensory

(b) Caused by oligodendrocytes

(c) Maximum speed soon after delivery to 6 months and continues upto puberty

(d) Soon after delivery upto 5 years

3034. EPO A/E:

(a) Produced by J-G apparatus in kidney

(b) Produced in brain

(c) Produced in liver

(d) Recombinant EPO available

3035. Malondialdehyde react with:

(a) Sulfuric acid (b) Mercapto ethanol

(c) Ferric chloride (d) Thiobarburic acid

3036. Klinefelter inheritance pathology:

(a) Non disjunction in spermatogenesis in father

(b) Non disjunction in blastocyst formation in mother

(c) Anaphase lag in mother

(d) Anaphase lag in father

3037. Lymph node histopathology:

(a) Primary follicles contain both B and T cells

(b) Follicular B-cell, parafollicular T cell

(c) Bounded by cell processes and collagen

(d) A criminal centre has lymphoblast

3038. Lymph Node drainage Forehead:

(a) Submandibular Lymph Node

(b) Preauricular Lymph Node

(c) Cervical Lymph Node

3039. Association both 2 variable influenced by 3rd variable indirectly:

(a) Confounding (b) Bias

(c) Chance

3040. Most common side effect of citalopram:

(a) Headache (b) Prolonged QT

(c) Bradycardia (d) Tachycardia

3041. 60 years old male with renal failure with pericardial rub, the type of pericarditis is:

(a) Fibrinous (b) Serous

(c) Hemorrhagic (d) Purulent

3042. What of the following is not suggestive of exudative pleural effusion?

(a) Plasma glucose < 60 mg/dl

(b) Plasma LDH/Serum LDH <0.6

(c) Pleural fluid protein/serum protein < 0.6

(d) None of the above

3043. Pneumonia (CAP) to be given empirically:

(a) Doxycycline (b) Macrolides

(c) Quinolones (d) Any of the above

3044. Carpal Tunnel syndrome all *except:*

(a) Adductor following paralysis

(b) Opponens pollicis palsy

(c) Lateral 3 finger sensory palsy

(d) 1st and 2nd lumbrical palsy

3045. Regarding hand true all *except:*

(a) Both radial ulnar bursa above 2.5 cm in flexor retinaculum

(b) Sensory supply – C7

(c) C8-T1 for small muscle

(d) Artery and nerve cross superficial to metacarpal ligament

3046. Pro drug:

(a) Gemifloxacin (b) Prulifloxacin

(c) Pancuronium (d) Lisinopril

3047. True about multiple sclerosis:

(a) Disease of Grey matter
(b) Disease of PNS (chronic remitting) relapsing disease
(c) Infectious disease
(d) Optic Nerve/cerebellum are most common site

3048. Most common side effect of lithium:

(a) Diabetes insipidus (b) Tremor
(c) Odema (d) Sick sinus syndrome

3049. Purine synthesis' substrate required:

(a) Ribose PO (b) PPRP
(c) Thymidine (d) Arc b

3050. MOTT true:

(a) Not cause pulmonary disease immunocompetent individual
(b) Rifampicin usually active
(c) Sensitive to clarithromycin

3051. Leptospira diagnostic test (most sensitive):

(a) CFT (b) ELISA
(c) MAT

3052. HbA Ic indicates:

(a) 6-12 weeks (b) 8-12 weeks
(c) 6-8 weeks

3053. New drug in India after license takes:

(a) 3 years (b) 5 years
(c) 10 years (d) 7 years

3054. Most common cause of embolic CVA:

(a) AF (b) Prosthetic valve
(c) DCMP (d) IE

3055. Mycotic aneurysm:

(a) TE (b) Atherosclerosis
(c) Marfan's (d) None of the above

3056. CCP echo feature:

(a) Thickened pericardium
(b) Multi-phasic hepatic vein flow
(c) Excessive respiratory variation in AV inflow velocities
(d) Notching in pulmonary valve in M mode in systole

3057. True about anatomy all *except:*

(a) IVS 45 to sagittal plane
(b) Right AV valve almost vertical axis
(c) FtA is anterior inferior to right of LA
(d) Anterosuperior leaflet of tricuspid valve is largest and attached to IVS through anterior and papillary muscles

3058. Causal relation best determined by:

(a) RCT (b) Prospective cohort
(c) Retrospective cohort (d) Case control

3059. In well fed state the enzyme increased in fatty tissue:

(a) Glycerol kinase
(b) Glycogen synthase
(c) G POose
(d) Glycogen phosphorylase

3060. Prevalence increase by:

(a) In migration of susceptible
(b) Moving out causes decrease incidence
(c) Decrease incidence
(d) Migration of healthy individual

3061. Swine Flu (Influenza A):

(a) MI 16 H cause swine infection
(b) All 9 N cause bird infector
(c) Genetic resortment cause pandemic
(d) RT PCR is diagnostic

3062. REM sleep LS due to:

(a) Adrinergic (b) Cholinergic
(c) Serotonergic (d) PGE2

3063. Most common cause of embolic CVA:

(a) AF (b) Prosthetic valve
(c) DCMP (d) IE

3064. Gibbus at T6 spinal cord segment compress:

(a) T6 (b) T7
(c) T8 (d) T9

3065. Cytogentic abnormality in leukemia all *except:*

(a) CML 9 : 22 (b) AML 15 : 17
(c) ALL 9 : 20 (d) Burkitt 18 : 14

3066. Apoptosis mediated:

(a) GMP (b) AMP
(c) Cyt c. (d) No synthetase

3067. CSF storage in pyogenic meningitis for few hours:

(a) -20°C (b) 4
(c) 10 (d) 37°C

3068. Most common site for cerebral haemorrhage:

(a) Ext. capsule/Putamen
(b) Pons
(c) Ventricle

3069. Thyroid anatomy:

(a) Isthmus opposite to 4-6 ring
(b) Literal lobe derived from 4th branchial arch
(c) Thyrocalcitonin release cause hype Ca^{++}
(d) L drainage to jugulo digastric nodes

3070. A-V shunt of skin:

(a) Not sensitive to circulating epinephrine
(b) Depends on metabolic need
(c) Respond to autoregulation

3071. Cholinergic drug causing latent TB reactivation:

(a) Nitozoxinide (b) Tomoxifen
(c) Leflunomide (d) Cedolovir

3072. Niacin side effect all *except:*

(a) Hyperuricemia (b) Hyperglycemia
(c) Hypercalcemia (d) Ilepatotoxicity

3073. Regarding anatomy of kidney true are all *except:*

(a) DCT cell more eosinophilic than PCf
(b) Macula densa cell are non-striated muscle
(c) Since supplied symp N the renal disease may present as large bowl obstruction

3074. Hirsutism caused by:

(a) Cyclosporine (b) Methyl dopa
(c) Hydroxyurea (d) Vincristine

3075. Psychosis with peripheral neuropathy:

(a) Cycloserine (b) Ethionomide
(c) Rifampicin (d) PZA

3076. Mitochondrial myopathy caused by:

(a) Alcohol (b) Pencillamine
(c) Zidovudine (d) Glucocorticoid

3077. Avian influenza caused by:

(a) H5N1 (b) H1N5
(c) H3N (d) H

3078. Vitamin deficient in most strict carnivorus:

(a) Thiamine (b) Vitamin B12
(c) Niacin (d) Vitamin C

3079. Intracellular cholesterol accumulation in:

(a) Neimann Pick disease type C
(b) Gaucher disease
(c) Pick's disease
(d) Alzheimer

3080. Spongiform pustules of Kajoj:

(a) Psoriasis (b) Lichen planus
(c) SLE (d) Seborrheic dermatitis

3081. Case control study all *except:*

(a) Incidence can be measured
(b) No risk to subject
(c) No attrition
(d) Few subject required for study

3082. Most common cranial N. involved in intracranial aneurysm:

(a) 3rd (b) 6th
(c) 7th (d) 8th

3083. Luteolysis caused by all *except:*

(a) PGF2α (b) Oxytocin
(c) PGE2 (d) ET 1

3084. RMP most commonly affected by changes in intra-cellular concentration of:

(a) Na (b) K
(c) Cl (d) HCO_3

3085. In the presence of ADH, most of the water reabsorbed:

(a) DCT (b) LOH
(c) Medullary CD (d) Cortical CD

3086. "Diaphragm" disease associated with:

(a) Unilateral phrenic nerve palsy
(b) NSAIDS
(c) Whipple disease
(d) Abdominal pelvic diaphragm developmental abnormality

3087. Patient with Rheumatoid Arthritis on long term aspirin develop strongly positive urine test for proteinuria. Renal Biopsy will show:

(a) Papillary necrosis
(b) Interstitial nephritis
(c) MCD
(d) Light chain deposition

3088. Strong correlation with colorectal Ca:
(a) FAP
(b) Peutz-Jeghers
(c) Juvenile polyposis
(d) Hyperplastic polyps

3089. Reactions are divided into catabolic and anabolic, which is characteristically amphibolic:
(a) Glycolysis
(b) Beta Oxidation Fatty Acids
(c) TCA
(d) Lipolysis

3090. In TCA cycle, following is recycled and hence has catabolic:
(a) OAA (b) Citrate
(c) Succinate (d) Acetyl COA

3091. Glucagon function is:
(a) Gluconeogenesis (b) Pentose PO_4
(c) TCA (d) Glycolysis shunt

3092. ATP generation is less in muscles and brain with glucose molecule as compared to kidney liver because:
(a) Diff. shuttle much are used
(b) Less mitochondria
(c) Less ATP generation enzyme
(d) Less requirement of ATP

3093. X-linked sideroblastic anemia, true:
(a) Less common in male
(b) Pallor and weakness in infancy
(c) Polychromasia is infrequent
(d) Intravascular hemolysis is uncommon

3094. G6PD all true *except:*
(a) Autosplenectomy seen
(b) Intermittent hemolysis
(c) Heinz bodies may be seen
(d) Bite cell seen

3095. Autosomal dominant:
(a) Familial combined hyperlipidemia
(b) α1 antitrypsin deficiency
(c) Cystic fibrosis
(d) Phenyl ketonuria

3096. Intravascular hemolysis all true *except:*
(a) ↓ Haptoglobin
(b) Hyperbilirubinemia
(c) Absence of urobilinogen in faeces and urine
(d) ↑ in methemoglobinemia

3097. Golgi tendon organs supplied by:
(a) Ia (b) Ib
(c) II (d) III

3098. Unilateral RAS associated with:
(a) Hyponatremia (b) Hypokalemia
(c) ↓ Ca (d) Hypouricemia

3099. Human specific Ig given in all *except:*
(a) Chicken pox (b) Measles
(c) Hepatitis B virus (d) Rabies

3100. Drug having primary anaerobic infection action:
(a) Meropenem (b) Cefoperazone
(c) Clindamycin (d) Ampicillin

3101. Follicular lymphoma:
(a) T-14, 18 (b) T-9, 22
(c) T4, 11

3102. Most important measure with CPR:
(a) Defibrillation
(b) Endotrachial intubations
(c) I/V adrenaline
(d) I/V soda bicarb

3103. In treatment of PCP, which of drug is given aerosol in sulfonamide allergy?
(a) Dapsone (b) Pentamidine
(c) Ciprofloxacin (d) Azithromycin

3104. Cylosporine toxicity precipitated by all *except:*
(a) Grape fruit juice (b) Diltiazem
(c) Erythromycin (d) Metoprolol

3105. Ewing sarcoma true:
(a) T (11 : 22) (b) T (8: 14)
(c) T (4:11)

3106. Intracellular cholesterol deposition seen in:
(a) Gaucher disease (b) Neimann Pick disease
(c) Pick's disease (d) Alzheimer

3107. Asialoglycoprotein in hepatocytes absorbed by:

(a) Receptor mediated endocytosis
(b) Facilitated deposition
(c) Active transport
(d) Passive diffusion

3108. CCK-PZ acts through:

(a) K^+ channel opening in basolateral membrane
(b) Ca^{++} dependent K channel opening in basolateral membrane
(c) $H^+ K^+$ ATPase in basolateral membrane
(d) None of the above

3109. Ubiquinilated protein degraded by:

(a) Proteosome (b) Endosome
(c) Lysosome (d) Ribosome

3110. True about macrophage *except:*

(a) Secretes IL-1
(b) Secretes IL-2
(c) Antigen presenting cell
(d) Phagocytosis

3111. Angiotensin II causes vasoconstriction through:

(a) Endothelin- A (b) AT-1
(c) AT-2 (d) All of the above

3112. Botulism toxin:

(a) It inhibits Ach release
(b) Achase is present in RBC
(c) Butyryl cholinestrase is dominant degrader of Ach
(d) Remifentanyl

3113. NO:

(a) Arginine (b) Citrulline
(c) Ornithine

3114. Pyridoxal deficiency leads to defective metabolism of:

(a) Tryptophan (b) Tyrosine
(c) Histidine (d) Phenylalanine

3115. Zn deficiency A/E:

(a) Growth retardation (b) Parasthesia
(c) Diarrhea (d) Gonadal atrophy

3116. HBsAg negative, HBV DNA positive means:

(a) Non existent
(b) Non progressive
(c) Precore mutant
(d) Good response to treatment

3117. Silk associated with:

(a) α-helix (b) Beta – sheet
(c) Triple helix (d) Random

3118. Blood passing through systemic capillaries all seen *except:*

(a) Increased hematocrit
(b) Increased protein
(c) Left shift of oxygen dissociation
(d) Decreased pH

3119. William associated tumour A/E:

(a) WAGR
(b) Denny's Drash syndrome
(c) Von Hippel disease
(d) Bechmann with syndrome

3120. Live vaccine C/I in:

(a) Actinomycin D (b) Doxorubicin
(c) Vincristine (d) Cytrabine

3121. Chemotherapy induced nausea and vomiting–drug given:

(a) Apomorphine (b) Aprepitant
(c) Hydrocortisone (d) Midazolam

3122. Which is catecholamines?

(a) Dopamine (b) Dopexamine
(c) Fenoldapam (d) Mephentramine

3123. Free radical scavenger A/E:

(a) Catalase
(b) Flutathione peroxidase
(c) Phosphorylase
(d) Superoxidase dismutase

3124. Most sensitive for bronchospasm:

(a) Fixed static compliance
(b) Dynamic compliance
(c) Vital capacity decreased
(d) Fixed specific compliance

3125. Hyperglycemia, lipid abnormality, lipodystrophy, central obesity:

(a) Protease inhibitor (b) Beta blocker

3126. Heidenhain patch A/E:

(a) Gastric mucosal epithelial pouch

(b) To measure gastric acid secretion

(c) Increase acid in response to neuronal stimuli

(d) Increase acid in response to hormonal stimuli

3127. Cyanide inhibits at which step of respiratory chain?

(a) Step I (b) Step II

(c) Step III (d) Step IV

3128. HDL with antiatherosclerotic property:

(a) I (b) II

(c) III (d) IV

3129. Patient with unilateral limb swelling with dyspnea, hypotension sudden onset, treatment is:

(a) T-PA (b) Furosemide

3130. Patient comes with scleroderma like thickening of skin with dysphagia and eosinophilia, cause is:

(a) L-tryptophan ingestion

(b) Botulism

3131. Tumour lysis syndrome A/E:

(a) Hypercalcemia (b) Hypocalcemia

(c) Hyperuricemia (d) Hyperkalemia

3132. Calciphylaxis seen in:

(a) Multiple myeloma (b) CRF

(c) Anaphylaxis

3133. Large vegetation in I.E.:

(a) Staph. Aureus (b) Enterococcus

(c) Pneumococcal (d) Streptococci

3134. Stone in ulcerative colitis:

(a) Oxalate (b) Cysteine

(c) Xanthine (d) Calcium

3135. Which is not a phase I reaction?

(a) Conjugation (b) Oxidation

(c) Reduction (d) Hydrolysis

3136. Non genetic disease is:

(a) ARVD (b) CPVT

(c) Brugada syndrome (d) LQTS

3137. Treatment of scorpion bite:

(a) α-methyl dopa (b) Propranolol

(c) Captopril (d) Prazosin

3138. Vincristine intrathecal used in:

(a) ALL

(b) AML

(c) Primary CNS lymphoma

(d) Intrathecal is lethal

3139. Eosinophilia is seen in A/E:

(a) Lobar pneumonia

(b) Worm infestation

(c) Dermatitis herpetiformis

(d) Bronchial asthma

3140. All are derived from bone marrow *except:*

(a) Kupffer cell (b) Langherhans cell

(c) Osteoblast (d) RBC

3141. Massive splenomegaly A/E:

(a) Sickle cell anemia (b) Sarcoidosis

(c) Lymphoma (d) CML

3142. Hypersplenism criteria A/E:

(a) Thrombocytopenia (b) BM hypoplasia

(c) Neutropenia

3143. Insulin action:

(a) Glucose absorption in intestine

3144. Alcohol chronic intake A/E:

(a) MES system decreases

(b) Increase uric acid excretion

(c) Increase gluconeogenesis

(d) Increase lactate

3145. Uric acid stone:

(a) Oxalate (b) Urate

3146. Maximum volume of blood:

(a) Isovolumic contraction

(b) Diastasis

(c) Isovolumic relaxation

3147. Ecthyma gangrenosum caused by:

(a) Pseudomonas

(b) Streptococci

(c) Staphylococci

3148. Metabolic encephalopathy A/E:

(a) Focal neurodeficit (b) Extensor planter

3149. Distal RTA caused by:

(a) Amphotericin B (b) Sulphonamide

3150. Erythropoietin secreted by:

(a) Interstitial cells

(b) Peritubular capillary tissue

3151. Maximum volume of blood in:

(a) Capillaries (b) Vein

(c) Artery

3152. Carotid sinus stimulation causes:

(a) Increase HR, decrease central aortic pressure

(b) Decrease HR, increase central aortic pressure

3153. ATN – urinary cast:

(a) Muddy brown (b) Hyaline cast

3154. HUS- PBF:

(a) Schistocytes

(b) Decreased platelet count

3155. Extrapyramidal symptoms least with:

(a) Thioridazine

3156. Fluoxetine acts on:

(a) Serotonin receptors

3157. Cardiomyopathy by:

(a) Selenium deficiency

3158. Asplenia – infections more seen:

(a) Streptococci pneumococci

3159. Dengue A/E:

(a) Type I is most dangerous

3160. Intracellular receptors:

(a) Thyroid receptors (b) Guanyl cyclase C

3161. Pseudohyponatremia:

(a) Hyperlipidemia

3162. Porphyria photosensitivity A/E:

(a) AIP (b) Protoporphyria

3163. Afterload decrease maximum seen in:

(a) Captopril

3164. Rickets:

(a) Unmineralized

(b) Increased osteoid matrix

3165. Gynaecomastia A/E:

(a) Testicular tumour

3166. All neurotransmitter associated with adverse effects:

(a) Glutamate (b) Valine

(c) Glycine (d) Leucine

3167. In a randomized trial, primary end point is seen in 9% patients on experimental drug versus 11% patients on placebo treatment. The number needed to prevent one such primary event (NNT) using experimental drug will be:

(a) 2 (b) 20

(c) 50 (d) 98

3168. All are involved in the pathogenesis of clubbing *except:*

(a) Prostaglandin dehydrogenase gene mutation

(b) Hyposia

(c) Vagal stimulation

(d) Vascular endothelial growth factor

3169. Which of the following is a Class I indication of pacing as per ACC/AHA guidelines?

(a) Patient with inferior wall MI and complete heart block lasting 7 days

(b) An asymptomatic 18-year-old female with congenital CHB and escape rate of 50/min

(c) Recurrent syncope of undetermined etiology with LBBB

(d) Symptomatic chronotropic incompetence

3170. The most common CNS complication of mumps is:

(a) Encephalitis

(b) Aseptic meningitis

(c) Guillain-Barré syndrome

(d) Cerebellar ataxia

3171. The gender of human fetus is distinguishable at gestational age:

(a) 8 weeks (b) 10 weeks

(c) 12 weeks (d) 16 weeks

3172. An infant starts staring at their own hand at:

(a) 2 months (b) 3 months

(c) 4 months (d) 6 months

3173. Endomorphic somatotype of physical pattern is characterized by:

(a) Stocky built and abundant soft tissue

(b) Stocky built and abundant bony tissue

(c) Stocky built and less muscle mass

(d) Light bone structure and small body mass

3174. Congenital varicella syndrome can occur if mother gets chickenpox at:

(a) 7-20 weeks of gestation
(b) 22-26 weeks of gestation
(c) 28-32 weeks of gestation
(d) 36-40 weeks of gestation

3175. True statement for Pneumocystis Jeruvecci:

(a) Is an obligate intracellular organism
(b) Can cause disease outside respiratory system
(c) Can have normal chest X-ray with prominent clinical signs
(d) May be usually diagnosed by serology

3176. A couple brings their 7 years old daughter to clinic concerned about her development. She has a history speech, ataxia with a broadbased gait and also has been diagnosed with epilepsy. She has a strange affect characterized by inappropriate laughter. Her karyotype is normal. What is the most likely diagnosis in this patient?

(a) Alice in Wonderland syndrome
(b) Angelman syndrome
(c) Asperger's syndrome
(d) Prader-Willi syndrome

3177. Causes of dilated pupils include:

(a) Argyll Robertson pupil
(b) Ethylene glycol poisoning
(c) Myotonic dystrophy
(d) Organophosphate poisoning

3178. Which of the following statements regarding phenylketonuria is correct?

(a) Serum tyrosine levels are typically low
(b) Urinary phenylalanine metabolites are typically high
(c) Mental retardation does not occur in the patient who adheres to a phenylalanine free diet
(d) Inheritance is X-linked recessive

3179. A 2 years old child weighing 8 kg presents with pallor and poor appetite. His Hb is 6 gm/dl, MCV is 65, RDW is 12% and RBC count is 6 million/cumm. P/S shows microcytic hypochromic blood picture. What is the most likely diagnosis?

(a) Beta thalassemia trait
(b) Sideroblastic anemia
(c) Iron deficiency anemia
(d) Lead toxicity

3180. A well breast fed baby at 36 hours of life has been found to have jaundice. His serum bilirubin level is 16 mg/dl, the blood group of mother and baby are O-negative and A-negative. The blood peripheral smear shows spherocytes and reticulocytes. What is the likely diagnosis?

(a) Hereditary spherocytosis
(b) ABO incompatibility
(c) Breast milk associated jaundice
(d) Alpha thalassemia

3181. A 2 weeks old neonate presented with hypotonia, lethargy and poor feeding. He was born at term with 3 kg weight and had no feeding problem till 5 days. On admission: he was found to be severely hypotonic, lethargic with poor neonatal reflexes and needed mechanical ventilation. His Hb was 12 gm, WBC count 12,000/cumm, platelets normal, blood glucose 75 mgdl. Lactate 206 mmol/I, CSF lactate and ammonia normal. MRI head was normal but the EEG showed epileptic encephalopathy. What is the likely diagnosis?

(a) Non ketotic hyperglycinemia
(b) Paroxysmal disorders
(c) Organic acidemia
(d) Fatty acid oxidation disorders

3182. The minimum bed strength of a special care newborn unit in a district hospital with 3000 deliveries per year and for referral admission of outborn babies under Government of India's facility based newborn care program is:

(a) 9 (b) 12
(c) 15 (d) 20

3183. Which of the following vaccine is developed by reverse vaccinology technique?

(a) Human papilloma virus vaccine
(b) Meningococcal B vaccine
(c) Varicella Zoster vaccine
(d) Dengue vaccine

3184. Which of the following statement is correct regarding prevention of parent to child transmission of HIV in highly endemic states of India as per NACO guidelines?

(a) One dose of Nevirapine to mother at the onset of labour and one dose of Nevirapine to newborn
(b) Mothers should be treated with Zidovudine and Nevirapine from 14 weeks of pregnancy till delivery
(c) Mother should be treated with three drug ART starting from 14 weeks till mother to child risk period

(d) Treat mother with triple drug ART starting from 14 weeks and continue till the risk period of mother to child transmission with Nevirapine for 6 weeks to baby if on exclusive breast feed

3185. Critical level of sound pressure level in neonatal intensive care unit should not exceed:

(a) 30 db (b) 35 db
(c) 40 db (d) 45 db

3186. WHO treatment formula "F-100" for treatment of hospitalized patients with severe acute malnutrition has protein of gm/100 ml:

(a) 0.9 (b) 1.5
(c) 2.0 (d) 2.9

3187. An atrioventricular septal defect is different from an ostium secondum atrial septal defect because the atrio ventricular septal defect:

(a) Does not manifest heart failure
(b) Does not create volume overload
(c) Has the same ECG findings
(d) Produces an early tendency for pulmonary hypertension

3188. Excess of Vitamin D can cause:

(a) Neuropathy (b) Pseudotumour cerebri
(c) Oxaluria (d) Hypercalcemia

3189. The length of the "tip to the vocal cord guide" of an endotracheal tube size of 3 is:

(a) 2.0 mm (b) 2.2 mm
(c) 2.4 mm (d) 2.6 mm

3190. Myocardial contractility is mainly determined by:

(a) Extracellular ca^{++} in resting state
(b) Fast inward current through L-type ca^{++} channels
(c) Absolute quantity of ca^{++} crossing sarcolemma
(d) Induced ca^{++} release from sarcoplasma reticulum

3191. Loud P_2 is best defined as:

(a) P_2 heard in mitral area
(b) P_2 heard in left parasternal area in end inspiration
(c) P_2 heard in right 2nd intercostal space
(d) P_2 heard in left parasternal area in end expiration

3192. On ECG left main coronary artery disease is denoted by:

(a) Inferior ST depression, ST elevation in avR>V1
(b) Anterior ST depression, ST elevation in V1>avR
(c) Anterior ST depression, ST elevation in avR>V1
(d) Inferior ST depression, ST elevation in V1>avR

3193. Restrictive diastolic filling pattern on echo is denoted by:

(a) E/A > 1.5, ↑ deceleration time, ↑ LAP
(b) E/A < 1, ↓ deceleration time, ↑ LAP
(c) E/A > 1.5, ↓ deceleration time, ↑ LAP
(d) E/A > 1.5, ↑ deceleration time, ↓ LAP

3194. Drug of choice for wide complex tachyarrhythmia of unknown origin is:

(a) Quinidine (b) Flecainide
(c) Sotalol (d) Procainamide

3195. Retractory hypertension in a middle aged woman may be controlled by addition of:

(a) Clonidine (b) Torsemide
(c) Clonidipine (d) Spironolactone

3196. In cases of atherosclerotic renal artery stenosis response to vascular repair is best indicated by:

(a) Gadolinium contrast MRA showing proximal renal artery stenosis
(b) Presence of collateral vessels to the ischaemic kidney on angiography
(c) Lateralizing renal vein renin ratio of > 1.5
(d) Significant pressure gradient across the renal artery lesion

3197. Treatment of obstructive sleep apnoea is useful when Epworth sleepiness score is:

(a) > 8 (b) > 10
(c) > 12 (d) > 15

3198. In ventilation associated pneumonia the most sensitive component of improvement in CPIS is:

(a) Leucocytosis reduction
(b) Fever below 38.9°C
(c) Chest radiography clearing
(d) Improvement in oxygenation (PaO_2/FiO_2>250)

3199. Shadows in upper lobes on X-ray chest are not seen in:

(a) Sarcoidosis
(b) Nonspecific interstitial pneumonia (NSIP)
(c) Silicosis
(d) ABPA

3200. Steroid resistant asthma is defined as failure to respond to:

(a) 40 mg/day oral prednisolone for 2 weeks

(b) 60 mg/day oral prednisolone for 1 week
(c) 12 mg/day oral dexamethasone for 2 weeks
(d) 400 mg/day oral hydrocortisone for 1 week

3201. Mixed acid based disorder on ABG is not denoted by:
(a) PCO_2 and HCO_3- moving in opposite directions
(b) Respiratory disorder with HCO_3– < 15 mmol/L or > 35 mmol/L
(c) Metabolic disorder with maximum compensation having last 2 digits of PH not equal to PCO_2
(d) Metabolic disorder with HCO_3– < 15 mmol/L or > 35 mmol/L

3202. Lung volumes can be normal in the following ILD on X-ray chest:
(a) Sarcoidosis
(b) BOOP
(c) Desquamative interstitial pneumonia
(d) Berylliosis

3203. Urinary antigen is useful in diagnosis of:
(a) Legionella pneumonia
(b) Mycoplasma pneumonia
(c) Coxiella burnetii pneumonia
(d) Burkholderia pseudomallei pneumonia

3204. Type III respiratory failure is treated by all *except:*
(a) Invasive high pressure support ventilation
(b) Non-invasive positive pressure support ventilation
(c) Frequent changes of posture
(d) Control of abdominal/incisional pain

3205. In spontaneous breathing trial of mechanically ventilated patients which of the following is not true:
(a) CPAP of 5 cm H_2O can be used
(b) Open T-piece breathing system can be used
(c) Trial can be given for 30-120 mins
(d) Should be done when PEEP is < 10 cm H_2O

3206. Mortality in ARDS can be predicted by:
(a) Extent of hypoxemia
(b) Level of PEEP used in mechanical ventilation
(c) Extent of alveolar infiltrates on chest X-ray
(d) Age > 60 years and sepsis

3207. ICU admission by severe community acquired pneumonia score (SCAP) is determined by one of the following alone:
(a) PaO_2 <54 or PaO_2/FiO < 250 mm Hg
(b) Arterial PH < 7.3
(c) Confusion
(d) Respiratory rate > 30/min

3208. Pleural fluid eosinophilia is rarely seen in:
(a) Benign asbestosis (b) Pulmonary embolism
(c) Hodgkin's lymphoma (d) Sarcoid pleurisy

3209. Zollinger-Ellison syndrome is diagnosed by all *except:*
(a) Fasting gastrin levels of 75-150 pg/ml
(b) Duodenal ulcer in second part of duodenum
(c) Diarrhoea with acid peptic disease
(d) Gastrinomas of duodenal wall

3210. Type B gastritis in characterized by all *except:*
(a) Malt lymphoma
(b) Parietal cell antibody
(c) H pylori dependent
(d) Present almost universally in > 70 years age

3211. Collagenous colitis is characterized by all *except:*
(a) Female to male ratio 9:1
(b) Association with rheumatoid arthritis
(c) Association with celiac disease
(d) Intra epithelial lymphocytes

3212. Co-infection with hepatitis B and hepatitis C virus can have all *except:*
(a) Prolonged HBSAg antigenemia
(b) Lower peak serum transaminase levels
(c) Increased risk of fulminant hepatic failure
(d) Higher rate of cirrhosis

3213. Early virological response to treatment of chronic HCV infection is defined as:
(a) 12 weeks HCV RNA fall by 2-$\log_{10}$ drop
(b) 6 weeks HCV RNA fall by 2-$\log_{10}$ drop
(c) 4 weeks HCV RNA fall by 2-$\log_{10}$ drop
(d) 6 weeks HCV RNA fall to undetectable levels

3214. Which of the following is not true for porphyria cutanea tarda?
(a) 40% have gene for haemochromatosis

(b) 50% have associated hepatitis C

(c) May be associated with estrogen medication

(d) Hyper pigmentation of trunk and arms

3215. An exclusive feature of type I renal tubular acidosis is:

(a) Short stature

(b) Urinary potassium wasting

(c) Hypercalciuria

(d) Osteomalacia

3216. Treatment for class V lupus nephritis is:

(a) Steroids + pulse cyclophosphamide

(b) Steroids + Azathioprine

(c) Mycophenolate mofetil with/without steroids

(d) Tacrolimus + cyclophosphamide

3217. Hepatorenal syndrome is diagnosed by:

(a) S creatinine > 2.5 mg with liver disease

(b) ↑BUN and urinary sodium of < 10 mmol/L

(c) ↑S creatinine and urinary sodium of > 10 mmol/L

(d) Creatinine clearance of < 40 ml/min and urinary sodium of < 10 mmol/L

3218. IgA nephropathy is not seen in:

(a) Chronic liver disease with cirrhosis

(b) Dermatitis herpetiformis

(c) Sjögren's syndrome

(d) Microscopic polyangiitis

3219. Pathology of HIV nephropathy is usually:

(a) Membranous glomerulonephritis

(b) Focal segmental glomerulosclerosis

(c) Mesangioproliferative glomerulonephritis

(d) Membranoproliferative glomerulonephritis

3220. Truncal sensory loss in 'bathing trunk' distribution is a feature of:

(a) Tangier's disease

(b) Familial amyloid neuropathy

(c) Refsum disease

(d) Porphyric neuropathy

3221. Macular sparing hemianopia is a feature of lesions of:

(a) Optic peduncle

(b) Meyer's loop in temporal lobe

(c) Fibres in lateral geniculate body

(d) Anterior visual cortex

3222. Internuclear ophthalmoplegia is characterized by all *except:*

(a) Failure of adducting movements of eye on attempted lateral gaze to opposite side

(b) Lesions of medial longitudinal fasciculus on the same side

(c) Lesion of medial longitudinal fasciculus and or abducens nucleus on opposite side

(d) Adduction of eye is normal during convergence gaze

3223. Lambert Eaton myasthemic syndrome is not characterized by:

(a) Proximal myopathy of lower limbs

(b) Absent deep tendon reflexes

(c) Decremental response on repetitive stimulation on EMG

(d) Can antedate small cell carcinoma of lung

3224. Diabetic third nerve cranial palsy is characterized by all *except:*

(a) Dilated pupil with sluggish light reflex

(b) Diplopia

(c) Unilateral ptosis

(d) Intense retro orbital pain

3225. Drug induced hallucinations is usually a feature of:

(a) Dementia with lewy body

(b) Frontotemporal dementia

(c) Cruetzfield Jakob dementia

(d) Vascular dementia

3226. Hypercapnic respiratory failure with increased dead space can be seen in all *except:*

(a) Asthma (b) Cystic fibrosis

(c) Myxedema (d) Pulmonary fibrosis

3227. Features of BiPAP ventilation includes all *except:*

(a) Inspiratory support decreases work of breathing

(b) Inspiratory support prevents alveolar collapse

(c) Can be successfully used in COPD

(d) PSv level of 5-10 cm H_2O and CPAP of 3-5 cm H_2O should be used initially

3228. Main goal of PEEP during mechanical ventilation is to keep:

(a) PaO_2 > 90 mm Hg with FiO_2 < 50%

(b) PaO_2 > 70 mm Hg with FiO_2 < 60%

(c) PaO_2 > 55-60 mm Hg with FiO_2 < 60%

(d) PaO_2 > 55-60 mm Hg with FiO_2 > 60%

3229. The best biochemical marker of hepatic fibrogenesis is:

(a) Hyaluronan (b) Apo Lipoprotein A1

(c) α-2 Macroglobulin (d) Haptoglobin

3230. In ascites due to portal hypertension, a falsely low SAAG could be seen in all *except:*

(a) Very low serum albumin

(b) Systemic hypotension

(c) Chylous ascites

(d) Very high serum globulin

3231. Treatment of choice for lamivudine resistant chronic HBV infection:

(a) Tenofovir alone

(b) Entecavir alone

(c) Lamivudine + Tenofovir

(d) Lamivudine + Entecavir

3232. True about celiac disease all *except:*

(a) Spontaneous remission occurs during the 2nd decade of life which may be permanent in some

(b) Absence of DQ2/DQ8 excludes the diagnosis

(c) A small intestinal biopsy is required to establish the diagnosis

(d) Anti EMA and anti tTg antibodies are linked to the pathogenesis and histopathological changes characteristic of the disease

3233. All the following are common movement disorders in Wilson's disease *except:*

(a) Myoclonus (b) Tremor

(c) Dystonia (d) Incoordination

3234. Breast milk to serum concentration ratio of the following anti-epileptic drug (AED) is maximum:

(a) Valproate (b) Levetiracetam

(c) Carbamazepine (d) Ethosuximide

3235. Most common cause of seizures in a patient with HIV infection is:

(a) Cerebral toxoplasmosis

(b) Primary CNS lymphoma

(c) Cryptococcal meningitis

(d) Progressive multifocal leukoencephalopathy

3236. Following markers are used to assess disease activity in SLE *except:*

(a) Anti-ds DNA (b) Complement C3

(c) Anti-Ro (d) NGAL

3237. Regarding the anti CCP antibody in rheumatoid arthritis the following statements are true *except:*

(a) It is included in the new 2010 ACR-EULAR criteria

(b) May be detected in sera long before clinical disease

(c) It has a specificity of 60-70%

(d) It has important prognostic significance

3238. Beside β2 microglobulin the following parameter is also used by the international staging system for multiple myeloma:

(a) Serum globulin

(b) Serum albumin

(c) Circulating plasma cells

(d) M-protein in serum

3239. The best investigation to establish the diagnosis of polycythemia vera is:

(a) JAK 2 mutation

(b) Serum erythropoietin

(c) Bone marrow cytology

(d) Red cell distribution width

3240. True about disseminated intravascular coagulation (DIC) are all *except:*

(a) Most sensitive test is FDP

(b) Schistocytes are common in the peripheral smear

(c) Fibrinogen levels falls acutely in all cases

(d) PT and APTT may be normal in chronic DIC

3241. The most important indication of ICT drain in parapneumonic effusion is:

(a) Pus is aspirated on pleurocentesis

(b) Loculated effusion is present

(c) Pleural fluid culture is positive for Klebsiella

(d) If fluid separates the lung from the chest wall by > 10 mm on lateral decubitus X-ray

3242. Contrast induced nephropathy is characterized by all *except:*

(a) Diabetics are more susceptible

(b) Serum creatinine peaks in 3-5 days

(c) Active urinary sediments

(d) Resolve within a week

3243. Waxy casts are seen in:

(a) Chronic renal failure (b) Nephrotic syndrome
(c) Interstitial nephritis (d) Transplant rejection

3244. One of the following situations is not associated with high trans tubular K^+ gradient (TTKG):

(a) Loop diuretics (b) Osmotic diuresis
(c) Liquorice use (d) Distal RTA

3245. True about Vasopressin antagonists all *except:*

(a) Conivaptan also has action on the VIA receptor
(b) They are not approved for use in acute hyponatremia
(c) Strict fluid restriction is an essential component of management
(d) Can lead to rapid correction of hyponatremia with consequent ODS

3246. Decrease in the anion gap (AG) is associated with all *except:*

(a) Lithium intoxication
(b) Cation exchange resins
(c) Plasma cell dyscrasias
(d) Nephrotic syndrome

3247. Fall in serum albumin by 1g/dl from the normal value (4.5 g/dl) alters the Anion Gap as follows:

(a) AG decrease by 2.5 meq/L
(b) AG increase by 2.5 meq/L
(c) AG fall by 1.5 meq/L
(d) Does not change the AG at all

3248. The ABG of a patient with DKA have PH 6.90 and HCO_3 10 meq/L, what would be the most appropriate respiratory compensation ($PaCO_2$) in the absence of any mixed acid base disturbance?

(a) 21-25 mm Hg (b) 26-30 mm Hg
(c) 30-34 mm Hg (b) 34-38 mm Hg

3249. Pyridoxine is used as an antidote for all *except:*

(a) Isoniazid
(b) Wernicke's encephalopathy
(c) Hydralazine
(d) Fungus (Gyromitra esculenta)

3250. Whole grains contain:

(a) Bran (b) Germ
(c) Endosperm (d) All of the above

3251. Descriptive study–False:

(a) Causal association
(b) Hypothesis formation
(c) Epidemiological trends
(d) Project trends and make a location of resources

3252. Sensitivity:

(a) High PPV (b) High NPV
(c) High prevalence (d) High likelihood ratio

3253. Sensitivity:

(a) Useful to rule out disease
(b) Not useful in screening
(c) Useful when positive

3254. Short bowel syndrome–A/E:

(a) Increase renal Ca Oxalate stone
(b) Increase risk of CAD
(c) Steatorrhoea
(d) Cholesterol gallstone

3255. Meningitis – total patient–112:

Test under study positive–75
Gold standard positive–63
Both positive–60
Specificity

(a) 69.3% (b) 59.4%
(c) 81% (d) 92%

3256. Snake bite:

(a) Splint (b) Ice
(c) Cut and core (d) Tourniquet

3257. CPR rise of chest compressions:

(a) 100–120 (b) 100 – 150
(c) 120–140 (d) 60–80

3258. Which is incorrect?

(a) Occam's razor
(b) Sutton law
(c) Anchoring heuristic
(d) Representative heuristic

3259. ABG ph-7.5, PO_2-60 pCO_2-30 HCO_3-23 BE=0 all true *except*:

(a) Primary disorder is respiratory alkalosis
(b) (A-a) gradient is normal
(c) HCO_3 value is according to adequate compensation
(d) Hyperventilation

3260. CT abdomen, which can be expected in peripherals serum?

(a) Lymphoblast (b) Howell Jolly bodies
(c) Skull cells (d) Spherocytes

3261. Grey literature:

(a) Constraint analysis
(b) RCT
(c) Case control study
(d) Disertation – abstract case reports, conference discussion

3262. Case control study:

(a) Effect to cause (b) Cause to effect
(c) Effect to effect (d) Cause to cause

3263. Polycythemia vera: (T/F)

(a) Erythropoietin level rules out DX
(b) Thrombocytosis increases risk of thrombotic event
(c) Commonly leads to ———
(d) Aspirin given to all to present thrombosis

3264. Longest t½:

(a) Digoxin
(b) Cardarone
(c) Lignocaine

3265. Hepatotoxicity (Direct):

(a) Chlorpromazine (b) Halothane
(c) Phenytoin (d) Acetaminophen

3266. Sildenafil + Nitrate:

(a) Massive Hypotension
(b) Vent. Arrhythmia

3267. A 60 years diabetic dyspnea on walking while walking – NYHA class:

(a) II (b) II
(c) IV (d) IV

3268. Longest acting insulin:

(a) Lispro (b) Degludec
(c) Glulisine (d) Detemir

3269. Non erosive arthritis:

(a) SLE (b) RA
(c) PA (d) Psoriatic arthritis

3270. Earliest clinical presentation of RA?

(a) Soft tissue swelling
(b) Juxta articular osteopenia
(c) No abnormality
(d) Subchondral ossification

3271. Poorly controlled Ulcerative colitis, Hb–7, Ferritin – 150, MCV reduced diagnosis:

(a) IDA (b) Folate deficiency
(c) Hemochromatosis (d) Chronic inflammation

3272. 54 years old female joint involvement, recently diagnosed diabetes, previously no history of diabetes, USG suggestive of hepatomegaly–diagnosis:

(a) Hemochromotosis (b) Wilson disease
(c) Porphyria (d) Addison disease

3273. Not required for Diagnosis of Behcet's disease:

(a) Large vessel vasculitis
(b) Pathergy test
(c) Uveitis
(d) Recurrent oral ulceration

3274. Wilson's true:

(a) AD
(b) S.Cu 2-3 times normal
(c) Most common involves liver and brain
(d) Early DX is indicated because of effective treatment

3275. Recurrent hypoglycemia, increase pigmentation, BP=80/60, K+ = 6.3, Na+ = 121:

(a) CKD
(b) Insulinoma
(c) Cushing's with Dexamethasone injection
(d) Addison disease

3276. Lung abscess–DOC:

(a) Clindamycin (b) Metronidazole
(c) Cotrimoxazole (d) Penicillin

3277. Cryoglobulin with 34 years male with cutaneous vasculitis and renal dysfunction diagnosis:

(a) HBsAg (b) PCR for HCV
(c) C-ANCA

3278. 60 years male, gustatory hallucination, delirium, not following command – only oriented to person. CSF – 32 cells, all lymphocytes, Protein – 60:

(a) Herpes (b) EBV
(c) Varicella (d) West nite

3279. Intramural Hematoma – ECHO – Not seen:

(a) Intimal flap
(b) Radiolucency in aortic wall
(c) Eccentric calcification

3280. DKA – all *except*:
(a) Normal Anion gap acidosis
(b) K^+ – 3.3, do not give insulin
(c) Most common cause of death – cerebral edema
(d) Type I DM – commonly

3281. Creatinine clearance – True:
(a) Cockroft gault equation includes age, weight and creatinine to calculate GFR
(b) Average of urea and creat. is better to cal. GFR
(c) 24 hours urine collection to under estimate GFR
(d) 52 years diabetic, with Normal creat. has creat clearance decreased by 25%

3282. Severe hypovolemic shock with blood loss:
(a) 10–20% (b) 20–30%
(c) 30–40% (d) > 40%

3283. 285 patients, 190 positive by test, culture positive 165, Both positive – 146, PPV ____.
(a) 81 (b) 76

3284. Healthy man–trial done:
(a) Quality of life (b) Therapeutic
(c) Diagnostic (d) Preventive

3285. Polymyositis:
(a) Gottron's rash
(b) Prox. muscle involvement
(c) Pharyngeal muscle involvement
(d) Limb pain

3286. Pre-renal ARF *except*:
(a) FeNa < 1% (b) Uri. osmolality > 500
(c) Uri. Na^+ > 40 (d) Improve with IV fluids

3287. Not used in ovulation:
(a) HCG (b) HMG
(c) Danazol (d) Clomiphene

3288. Epicardial hyperenhancement in cardiac MRI is not seen in:
(a) Sarcoidosis
(b) Andersen Fabry disease
(c) Amyloidosis
(d) Chagas disease

3289. Which of the following is incorrect match?
(a) VERITAS – Tezosentan
(b) PROTECT – Rolofylline
(c) ASCEND HF – Milrinone
(d) CARRESS-HF – Ultrafiltration

3290. All are common manifestations of Von Willebrand disease *except*:
(a) Epistaxis (b) Menorrhagia
(c) Hemarthrosis (d) Angiodysplasia

3291. In which stage of sleep, somnambulism and night terrors occur:
(a) Stage 1 (b) Stage 2
(c) REM (d) Slow wave sleep

3292. Abscopal effect is seen in which tumour?
(a) CLL (b) CML
(c) Hodgkin lymphoma (d) Melanoma

3293. Which of the following is not method of percussion of spleen?
(a) Nixon (b) Castella
(c) Traube (d) Middleton

3294. Aplastic anemia is associated with all of the following *except*:
(a) NSAID
(b) Kostmann syndrome
(c) Seronegative hepatitis
(d) Carbimazole

3295. Thymoma is associated with all of the following *except*:
(a) Erythrocytosis (b) Red cell aplasia
(c) Mysthenia gravis (d) Addison disease

3296. Which of the following cancer is least likely to metastatize to bone?
(a) Lung (b) Breast
(c) Kidney (d) Colon

3297. Which of the following disease does not cause hypercalcemia?
(a) Sarcoidosis
(b) Hyperthyroidism
(c) Adrenal insufficiency
(d) Activating CASR mutation

3298. Which of the following is not a risk factor for Legionella pneumonia?
(a) Steroid use (b) HIV
(c) Neutropenia (d) Smoking

3299. Which of the following fungi are dimorphic?
(a) Aspergillus fumigatus

(b) Candida glabrata

(c) Histoplasma

(d) Rhizopus

3300. Dose of dialysis currently defined as:

(a) Counter current flow rate of dialysate

(b) Fractional urea clearance

(c) Hours per week of dialysis

(d) Number of sessions per month

3301. B_{12} malabsorption is less commonly seen in:

(a) Bacterial overgrowth syndrome

(b) Severe pancreatitis

(c) Ulcerative colitis

(d) Crohn's disease

3302. How many percentage of HLA B27 patients develop ankylosing spondylitis?

(a) 60% (b) 15%

(c) 30% (d) 90%

3303. Relapsing polychondritis is associated with all of the following *except*:

(a) Primary biliary cirrhosis

(b) Myelodysplasia

(c) Scleroderma

(d) Rheumatoid arthritis

3304. Which of the following is not much useful in Sarcoidosis?

(a) Infliximab (b) Etanercept

(c) Methotrexate (d) Prednisolone

3305. All are associated with increased levels of total T_4 with normal free T_4 *except*:

(a) Cirrhosis

(b) Pregnancy

(c) Sick euthyroid

(d) Familial dysalbumenic hyperthyroxinemia

3306. Alteration of which of the following hormone levels is first defence in hypoglycemia?

(a) Glucagon (b) Cortisol

(c) Decreased insulin (d) IGF

3307. All of the following cause increased LDL *except:*

(a) Anorexia nervosa (b) Cirrhosis

(c) Hypothyroidism (d) Thiazides

3308. All have reduced atheroembolic stroke in primary and secondary prevention *except*:

(a) Aspirin (b) Warfarin

(c) Statins (d) Clopidogrel

3309. Which of the following is not common initial manifestation of mutiple sclerosis?

(a) Sensory loss (b) Weakness

(c) Optic neuritis (d) Dementia

3310. First test to become positive in hemochromatosis is:

(a) Decreased serum iron

(b) Increased ferritin

(c) Increased transferrin saturation

(d) Decreased TFBC

3311. Periungual telangiectasias are seen in all *except*:

(a) SLE

(b) Scleroderma

(c) Mixed connective tissue disorder

(d) Dermatomyositis

3312. Which of the following drug is not used for squamous cell carcinoma of lung?

(a) Cisplatin (b) Bevacizumab

(c) Gemcitabine (d) Pemetrexed

3313. Most common mutation seen in hereditary spherocytosis:

(a) Ankyrin (b) Band 3

(c) Band 4 (d) Spectrin

3314. All of the following are favourable prognostic markers in AML *except*:

(a) t(8 : 21) (b) FLT 3 – ITD

(c) CEBPA mutation (d) NPM 1 mutation

3315. Which of the following drug is effective against T3151 mutation in CML?

(a) DASATINIB (b) NILOTINIB

(c) BOSUTINIB (d) PONATINIB

3316. Which of the following is not included in CPIS Score?

(a) Age (b) Chest X-ray

(c) Tracheal aspirate (d) Fever

3317. Which of the following drug is not used in plague prophylaxis?

(a) Doxycycline (b) Ciprofloxacin

(c) Septran (d) Erythromycin

3318. Which of the following atypical mycobacteria closely resembles TB?

(a) M. kansasi (b) M. marinum
(c) MAC (d) M. gordonae

3319. HIV associated nephropathy most commonly associated with:

(a) MPGN
(b) FSGS
(c) DPGN
(d) Minimal change disease

3320. Treatment of choice for disseminated strongyloidosis:

(a) Ivermectin (b) Albandazole
(c) Mebandazole (d) Suramin

3321. Which of the following US grading for echinococcal cysts is inactive?

(a) CE 1 (b) CE 4
(c) CE 3 (d) CL

3322. All are true about hypersensitivity pneumonitis *except*:

(a) Decreased risk in smokers
(b) Mycobacteria may be associated
(c) Lung bases are frequently involved
(d) Antigen avoidance is the first line of treatment

3323. Upper lobe involvement of lung is seen in:

(a) Post radiation fibrosis
(b) MAC infection
(c) Aspiration
(d) Hypogammaglobulinemia

3324. Erythropoietin is raised in all of the following conditions *except*:

(a) High altitude (b) Polycythemia vera
(c) Smoking (d) C.O.P.D.

3325. Which of the following drug inhibits JAK?

(a) Tofacitinib (b) Ipilimumab
(c) Omacetaxin (d) Adalimumab

3326. All of the following conditions are associated with diffuse specific changes in small intestinal mucosal biopsy *except*:

(a) Whipple's disease
(b) Agammaglobulinemia
(c) Abetalipoproteinemia
(d) Eosinophilic gastroenteritis

3327. Which of the following statement is not appropriate?

(a) HUS is due to defect in alternate complement pathway
(b) Pneumococcal infections can cause atypical HUS
(c) Plasma exchange is treatment of choice in HUS
(d) Plasma infusion can be used in Upshaw Schulmann disease

3328. Strongest association of clinical risk factor in epidemiological studies and calcific aortic valve disease is found in:

(a) Age (b) Male sex
(c) Body mass index (d) Dyslipidemia

3329. Which of the following is not a criterion for trial of spontaneous respiration in mechanically ventilated patients?

(a) PaO_2/FIO_2 (partial pressure of oxygen/fraction of inspired oxygen) > 200
(b) PEEP ≥ 8 cm H_2O
(c) Cough and airway reflexes are intact
(d) No vasopressor agents or sedatives are being administered

3330. REWIND trial include:

(a) EMPAGLIFLOZIN (b) CANAGLIFLOZIN
(c) DULAGLUTIDE (d) SITAGLIPTIN

3331. All statements regarding cardiovascular pharmacogenetics are true, *except*:

(a) A prerequisite for pharmacogenetics is heterogeneity in drug response
(b) Genetic variants in the hepatic transporter, SLCO1B1, influence the risk of adverse events
(c) Carriers of 5 variant of SLCO1B1 leads to higher plasma statin concentrations
(d) Risk for myopathy with *5 variant of SLCO1B1 depends on the statin type: the risk is greatest for fluvastatin

3332. Which of the following statement regarding Receiver Operating Characteristic Curves is true?

(a) Obtained by plotting a test's true positive rate (sensitivity) against its false positive rate (100 minus specificity)
(b) A test that discriminates perfectly between the presence and absence of disease would have an ROC curve that passes exactly through the centre
(c) The closer the curve is to the lower right corner, the higher the overall accuracy of the test

(d) A completely random test would have an ROC curve that passes through the upper left corner

3333. Which of the following is not true about omega 3 fatty acids?

(a) High dose omega 3 fatty acids have shown modest but significant reduction in BP
(b) DHA more effective than EPA in BP reduction
(c) Diastolic BP is reduced by about 6–8 mm Hg
(d) May lead to decreased secretion of aldosterone

3334. The micro RNAs (miRNAs) play a role in several diseases and are advancing to clinical application in acute coronary syndromes, acute myocardial infarction, cardiomyopathies, type 2 diabetes, hypertension and heart failure. Which statement is true about miRNAs?

(a) miRNAs interfere with transcription through degradation of the message RNA
(b) miRNAs are usually 2–10 nucleotides in length
(c) miRNAs are also known as small interfering RNAs
(d) miRNA act through a silencing complex and inhibit gene expression by binding to complementary 32 untranslated regions of target mRNA

3335. Each of the following statements regarding Genome Wide Association Studies (GWASs) is true, *except*:

(a) These studies provide information on common DNA variants associated with complex phenotypes
(b) The total number of loci for coronary artery disease now exceeds 46
(c) Together, these variants accounts for 90% of the heritability of CAD
(d) Region on chromosome 9 near the genes CDKN2A/CDKN2B—represent truly novel risk variants

3336. All are true regarding SPRINT TRIAL *except*:

(a) Involved diabetic patients
(b) Target blood pressure level in intensive treatment group is systolic <120 mm Hg
(c) Target blood pressure level in standard treatment group is systolic <140 mm Hg
(d) Incidence of AKI was higher in intensive treatment group

3337. Association is done by ___ in case control.

(a) Odd's ratio (b) Risk rate
(c) Rate ratio (d) Hazard ratio

3338. Measure of dispersion all *except*:

(a) Mean (b) SD
(c) Variance (d) Range

3339. Randomization done in:

(a) Experimental
(b) Case control
(c) Cohort
(d) Observational analytical

3340. A study between alcoholic and non alcoholic shows RR of 1.31 P value 0.03 is evaluate of MI. Now the subgroup analysis between smoker and non- smoker the RR in smoker 0.98, P value 0.87. Non- smoker RR 0.97, P value 0.63. Reason:

(a) Confounding
(b) Calculate error
(c) Cause modification
(d) Recall bias

3341. Drug recently approved for weight reduction:

(a) Sibutramine (b) Orlistat
(c) Lorcaserin (d) Phenetermine

3342. FMD all are T/E:

(a) Common in females
(b) Otherwise normal vessels
(c) Involves ostial arteries
(d) Renal angioplasty is helpful

3343. Preoperative discontinuation advised:

(a) BB (b) CCB
(c) ACEI (d) Diuretics

3344. About hypomagnesemia what is false?

(a) Tetany (b) Perioral numbness
(c) Chovstek sign (d) Sr. Mg – 2.8 mg/dl

3345. A patient with hypereosinophilic syndrome (HES) presented with progressive pedal edema and ascites. Echo showed S/O restrictive ventricular pattern. Endomyocardial biopsy will show:

(a) Endomyocardial infiltration of eosinophils
(b) Amyloid deposition
(c) Hypertrophied myocytes
(d) Fibrosis

3346. Hb of patients with SD of 4, mean–12. How many will have Hb between 8 and 16?

(a) 50% (b) 95%
(c) 99% (d) 68%

3347. Medical study looking at the prevalence of cancer amongst a certain population is:

(a) Cohort study (b) Case control study
(c) Prospective study (d) Cross-sectional study

3348. A new intervention shows a promising 30% reduction in mortality. How many patients will be saved if intervention is done on 40 patients?

(a) 12 (b) 6
(c) 4 (d) Insufficient data

3349. An exponential distribution has a skewness of:

(a) 2 (b) 1
(c) 0 (d) 3

3350. About CPR all are T/E:

(a) Chest compression depth 5 cm
(b) Compression rate 120/min
(c) Respiration 30.2
(d) In 2 breaths if one breath doesn't expands the chest its normal

3351. Which drug is not diabetogenic?

(a) HCTZ (b) Atorvastatin
(c) Ranolazine (d) Atenolol

3352. Type I error is:

(a) False positive (b) False negative
(c) True negative (d) True positive

3353. Not a high risk criteria in noncardiac surgery:

(a) Type II DM on insulin
(b) TIA
(c) Pancreaticoduodenectomy
(d) LVEF–40%

3354. Hemorrhagic stroke risk A/E:

(a) Dyslipidemia (b) Age/Alcohol
(c) Smoking (d) Hypertension

3355. Lead poisoning A/E:

(a) Hepatic fibrosis (b) Hypertension
(c) Tremors (d) Increased uric acid

3356. Primary hyperaldosteronism true:

(a) LVH is disproportionate to degree of HTN compared to essential HTN
(b) Mild metabolic acidosis is seen
(c) Adrenal adenoma is most common cause
(d) Pedal edema is seen

3357. All true *except*:

(a) Stochastic effect–DNA damage in a single value
(b) Deterministic–Dose dependent
(c) Sievert–Effective dose
(d) ALARA–As low as radiation achievable

3358. Duplication of chromosome is seen in:

(a) Angelman syndrome
(b) Prader Willi syndrome
(c) William syndrome
(d) Charcot-Marie tooth syndrome

3359. ABG of patient–pH–7.18, PCO_2–78%, PO_2–62%, SPO_2–80%:

Diagnosis can be A/E:

(a) Flail chest (b) CHF
(c) Narcotic overdose (d) GBS

3360. Acid base disorders true A/E:

(a) 10 mm Hg increase in PCO_2– increases 1 mmol in HCO_3 acutely
(b) 10 mm Hg increase in PCO_2– increase 4 mmol in HCO_3 chronically
(c) 10 mm Hg decrease in PCO_2 – decrease 4 mmol HCO_3 chronically
(d) 10 mm Hg decrease in PCO_2– increases pH by 0.2

3361. Nicotine causes:

(a) Increase in HR and BP
(b) Increase in HDL
(c) Increase in DM and IGT
(d) Vasoconstriction
(e) Increase in LDL

3362. True of ACLS:

(a) Pulse less VT best treated by synchronized cardioversion
(b) Pulseless VT best treated by defibrillation
(c) VT with pulse best treated by synchronized cardioversion
(d) VT with pulse best treated by direct DC cardioversion

3363. CPR:

(a) ACB to CAB
(b) 30 : 2
(c) Single rescuer should do both compression and breathing

(d) VF is more common
(e) 1.5 – 2 inch to 1 inch compression

3364. Hypercalcemia:
(a) Sinus tachycardia (b) Short QTc interval
(c) Long QTc interval (d) Prominent U wave
(e) Sine wave pattern

3365. Air pollution causes:
(a) Accelerated atherosclerosis
(b) Decreased fibrinogen
(c) Increased heart rate variability
(d) Cardiac dysrhythmias are common
(e) Acute vascular dysfunction, plaque instability are seen

3366. What is NNT if a drug reduces the risk of a bad outcome from 50 per cent to 30 per cent?
(a) 2 (b) 3
(c) 4 (d) 5

3367. 10 g Hb is equal to how much volume of O_2?
(a) 12 (b) 13
(c) 15 (d) 16

3368. pH–7.1, $PaCO_2$–34, PaO_2–90, HCO_3–12:
(a) Metabolic acidosis, compensated
(b) Metabolic acidosis with respiratory acidosis
(c) Metabolic acidosis with respiratory alkalosis
(d) Metabolic alkalosis

3369. pH–7.48, pCO_2–53, pO_2–92, HCO_3–31, BE –+7:
(a) Metabolic alkalosis, compensated
(b) Metabolic alkalosis with respiratory acidosis
(c) Metabolic alkalosis with respiratory alkalosis
(d) Metabolic acidosis

3370. ICH–all are used *except*:
(a) Urapidil (b) Nicardipine
(c) Nitroprusside (d) Labetalol

3371. Adverse drug event includes:
(a) Medication errors
(b) Adverse drug reactions
(c) Allergic reactions
(d) All of the above

3372. Disposal of waste all are T/E:
(a) Used gloves in red bag
(b) Chemical waste in red bag
(c) Antibiotic vials in blue bag
(d) Paper and tissues in green bag

3373. Sphingomyelinase deficiency causes:
(a) Nieman-Pick (b) Gaucher
(c) Fabry (d) Hunter

3374. Recurrent infection with immune defect and giant leukocytic granules are seen in:
(a) Chronic granulomatous disease
(b) Chediak Higashi syndrome
(c) Griscelli disease
(d) Elejalde disease

3375. Cyclic AMP as secondary messenger in A/E:
(a) LH (b) FSH
(c) Insulin (d) TSH

3376. Glycoprotein hormone:
(a) Testosterone (b) Estrogen
(c) Insulin (d) FSH

3377. Hypertriglyceridemia and steatorrhea:
(a) Lipoprotein lipase deficiency
(b) Phospholipase deficiency
(c) Pancreatic lipase deficiency
(d) All of the above

3378. Adverse drug reactions all T/E:
(a) Cisplatin–liver failure
(b) Bleomycin–pulmonary fibrosis
(c) Cyclophosphamide–hemorrhagic cystitis
(d) Doxorubicin–cardiomyopathy

3379. Treatment of long QT syndrome:
(a) CCB (b) Beta blockers
(c) Lidocaine (d) Digoxin

3380. ANCA associated vasculitis:
(a) SLE
(b) RA
(c) Churg-Strauss syndrome
(d) Henoch-Schönlein purpura

3381. Henoch-Schönlein purpura biopsy:
(a) IgG deposits (b) IgD deposits
(c) IgE deposits (d) IgA deposits

3382. Gemcitabine is:
(a) Antimetabolite
(b) Topoisomerase II inhibitor
(c) Alkylating agent
(d) None of the above

3383. DVT, pancytopenia, hemolysis:
(a) APLA (b) AIHA
(c) PNH (d) PV

3384. PNH definitive diagnosis by:
(a) LAP score (b) Bone marrow
(c) FLAER (d) Peripheral smear

3385. Marker of HCC and germ cell tumor:
(a) CEA (b) AFP
(c) PSA (d) CA 19-9

3386. Extracellular buffer:
(a) Phosphate buffer (b) Bicarbonate buffer
(c) Protein buffer (d) Hb buffer

3387. Familial Hypercholesterolemia occurs due to deficiency of:
(a) Lipoprotein A (b) Lipoprotein D
(c) Lipoprotein C (d) LDL receptor

3388. Burkitt lymphoma due:
(a) Point mutation (b) Translocation
(c) Amplification (d) Deletion

3389. Tumor lysis syndrome true is:
(a) Hyperuricemia, hyperkalemia, hyperphosphatemia, hypocalcemia
(b) Hyperuricemia, hypokalemia, hyperphosphatemia, hypocalcemia
(c) Hyperuricemia, hyperkalemia, hyperphosphatemia, hypercalcemia
(d) Hyperuricemia, hyperkalemia, hypophosphatemia, hypocalcemia

3390. Corkscrew appearance is seen in:
(a) Achalasia
(b) Stricture
(c) Diffuse esophageal spasm
(d) Esophagitis

3391. Juvenile hemochromatosis:
(a) Ferroportin (b) Hemojuvelin
(c) HEF (d) Ferritin

3392. Chemical adrenalectomy:
(a) Metyrapone (b) Cabergoline
(c) Conazole (d) Steroids

3393. Direct inhibitor of ACTH in Conn's syndrome:
(a) Pegvisomant (b) Cartisone
(c) Ketaconazole (d) Eptide

3394. Approved drug for type I DM:
(a) Pramlintide (b) GLP analogue
(c) Acarbose (d) MF

3395. FDA approved drug for sickle cell anemia:
(a) Hydroxyurea (b) Glutamine
(c) Daunorubicin (d) None of the above

3396. Extracorpuscular hemolytic anemia:
(a) HS (b) PNH
(c) HE (d) TTP

3397. Bite cells are seen in:
(a) G6PD deficiency (b) PNH
(c) TIP (d) HUS

3398. Hemolysis all can be seen *except*:
(a) Increased LDH
(b) Increased heptoglobin
(c) Increased reticulocyte
(d) Increased bilirubin

3399. Lytic lesions are seen in A/E:
(a) Multiple myeloma (b) CLL
(c) LCH (d) Metastasis

3400. Gum hypertrophy seen in:
(a) AML
(b) AMML (myelomonoblastic)
(c) CML
(d) MDS

3401. HUS caused by:
(a) E. Coli (b) Chlamydia
(c) Salmonella (d) Campylobacter

3402. ALL initial workup A/E:
(a) Flow cytometry (b) PET/CT
(c) Plasma viscosity (d) Metabolic workup

3403. Snake poisoning causing rhabdomylosis, flaccid paralysis:
(a) Pit viper (b) Sea snake
(c) Rat viper (d) Cobra

3404. Seizure caused by A/E:
(a) Hypocalcemia
(b) Hypokalemia
(c) Hyponatremia
(d) Posterior encephalopathy syndrome

3405. Recurrent abortion due to deficiency of:
(a) Factor 7 (b) 8
(c) 11 (d) 13

3406. Bernard-Soulier syndrome:
(a) Does not bind collagen
(b) Giant platelets
(c) Due to defect in IIb/IIIa
(d) All of the above

3407. Shortest half life clotting factor:
(a) Factor 5 (b) 7
(c) 9 (d) 12

3408. HHV8 causes A/E:
(a) PEL (b) KS
(c) Castleman (d) Nasopharyngeal Ca

3409. Pure red cell aplasia A/E:
(a) Anterior mediastinal mass
(b) Parvovirus B_{19}
(c) Low erythropoietin
(d) Giant pronormoblast

3410. Most common inherited prothrombotic state:
(a) APC resistance
(b) Protein C deficiency
(c) Antithrombin III deficiency
(d) Factor VIII deficiency

3411. Binet scoring is used for:
(a) CLL (b) T cell lymphoma
(c) MDS (d) AML

3412. In denaturation:
(a) Primary structure preserved
(b) Secondary structure preserved
(c) Quaternary structure preserved

3413. Amniotic fluid erythropoietin is derived from:
(a) Fetal liver
(b) Fetal endothelial cells
(c) Decidua
(d) Fetal urine

3414. BRAF mutations are seen in:
(a) Melanoma (b) Lung cancer
(c) Stomach cancer (d) Uterine cancer

3415. Metal associated with cancer true is:
(a) Cadmium— lung cancer
(b) Mercury—liver cancer
(c) Lead— stomach cancer
(d) Arsenic — lung cancer

3416. All are vitamin K dependent proteins *except*:
(a) Protein C (b) Factor II
(c) Factor VIII (d) Factor X

3417. Most common test used for thiamine deficiency:
(a) RBC transketolase assay
(b) Serum thiamine level
(c) Aldolase assay
(d) RBC aldolase assay

3418. Most common used fungal stain:
(a) Grams (b) Giemsa
(c) PAS (d) AFB

3419. Vemurafenib is used for:
(a) Thymoma
(b) Metastatic melanoma
(c) Metastatic lung cancer
(d) Gut cancer

3420. Osteogenesis imperfecta:
(a) Brittle bone
(b) Type I is most severe
(c) Type II is mild form
(d) Most patients have mutation in type II collagen

3421. ALK gene is seen in:
(a) Breast cancer (b) Blood cancer
(c) Lung cancer (d) Skin cancer

3422. Niacin toxicity:
(a) Skin hyper pigmentation
(b) Lung fibrosis
(c) Fulminant hepatitis
(d) Renal failure

3423. Thiamine deficiency affects:
(a) Transketolase (b) Aldolase
(c) Hydroxylase (d) Oxidase

3424. Drug causing centrilobular necrosis in hepatocytes:
(a) Isoniazid (b) Acetaminophen
(c) Digoxin (d) Ciplox

3425. Components of Meniere's disease A/E:
(a) Episodes of vertigo
(b) High frequency sensorineural hearing loss
(c) Tinnitus
(d) No better diagnosis

3426. 20 years female with fever, asymmetric swelling in oral cavity, uvula shifted to opposite side:
(a) Parapharyngeal abscess
(b) Retropharyngeal abscess
(c) Peritonsillar abscess
(d) Tonsillitis

3427. Best for renal clearance calculation:
(a) Inulin (b) Creatinine
(c) Creatine (d) Albumin

3428. Renal tubular acidosis IV all T/E:
(a) Hyperkalemia is proportionate to reduction in GFR
(b) Seen DM, obstructive uropathy
(c) Urinary ammonium excretion is depressed
(d) Generalized distal RTA

3429. Pleural effusion of acute pancreatitis:
(a) Left sided (b) Right sided
(c) Bilateral (d) No predilection

3430. Emery dreifuss muscular dystrophy mode of inheritance:
(a) AD (b) AR
(c) X-linked recessive (d) X-linked dominant

3431. Investigation for definitive diagnosis of hereditary spherocytosis:
(a) Osmotic fragility
(b) Acid glycerol lysis test
(c) SDS-gel electrophoresis
(d) Molecular studies

3432. Hemorrhagic cystitis caused by:
(a) Irinotecan (b) Ifosfamide
(c) Paclitaxel (d) Imatinib

3433. Treatment of acute severe asthma:
(a) Steroids
(b) Increase steroid inhaler
(c) Increase short acting beta agonists
(d) Increase long acting beta agonists

3434. Exercise induced asthma:
(a) Mechanism is hypoventilation
(b) Typically begins with the thought of exercise
(c) Worse in hot, humid conditions
(d) Best prevented by regular treatment with ICS

3435. Salmon patch:
(a) Relatively uncommon
(b) Also known as nevus simplex
(c) Persist throughout life
(d) Red macules

3436. Vitamin C toxicity:
(a) Renal stones (b) Skin cancer
(c) Hepatitis (d) Iron efficiency

3437. Snake bite leading to pituitary insufficiency:
(a) Pit viper (b) Sea snake
(c) Russel Viper (d) Cobra

3438. Medial medullary syndrome components A/E:
(a) Occlusion of lower basilar artery
(b) Ipsilateral twelfth nerve
(c) Contralateral pyramidal tract
(d) Ipsilateral medial lemniscus

3439. Dravet syndrome A/E:
(a) Seizures (b) First year of life
(c) Self limiting (d) Febrile seizures

3440. Components of juvenile myoclonic epilepsy:
(a) Weak genetic background

(b) Myoclonic jerks are more common in evening
(c) Generalized tonic clonic seizures are not seen
(d) Sodium valproate is the DOC

3441. Gerstmann syndrome A/E:
(a) Dysgraphia (b) Acalculia
(c) Finger agnosia (d) Prosopagnosia

3442. Autoantigen involved in myoclonus and opsoclonus:
(a) Hu proteins (b) Ri proteins
(c) Recoverin (d) Yo protein

3443. MSA all T/E:
(a) Atypical parkinsonism
(b) Orthostatic hypotension
(c) Degeneration of Inferior olivary nucleus
(d) No cerebellar signs

3444. PSP all T/E:
(a) Slow ocular saccades
(b) Eyelid apraxia
(c) Restricted vertical eye movements
(d) Pontine hot cross bun sign is seen

3445. Normal pressure hydrocephalus all are T/E:
(a) Apractic gait
(b) Dementia
(c) Urinary urgency
(d) Enlarged lateral ventricles with cortical atrophy

3446. All are components of dermatomyositis *except*:
(a) Heliotrope rash
(b) Gottron papules
(c) Proximal greater than distal weakness
(d) Skin lesions and muscle weakness occur together

3447. Brown-Sequard's syndrome true is:
(a) Ipsilateral loss of proprioception
(b) Ipsilateral loss of pain and temperature
(c) Contralateral loss of motor and vibration
(d) Memory loss

3448. Other methods of eliciting babinski sign include A/E:
(a) Chaddock's sign (b) Oppenheim's reflex
(c) Gordon's sign (d) Hoffmann's sign

3449. Multiple sclerosis MRI features include A/E:
(a) Black holes are markers of reversible demyelination
(b) MS plaques are visible as areas of hyper-intensity on T2 weighted imaging
(c) Dawson's fingers
(d) Lesions more than 6 mm in corpus callosum are helpful

3450. GBS CSF changes:
(a) Elevated protein without pleocytosis
(b) CSF is abnormal within 48 hours of presentation
(c) Transient pleocytosis is always seen
(d) Cell count goes upto -1000/uL

3451. Sl nerve root localization:
(a) Medial part of thigh
(b) Lateral part of calf
(c) Lateral part of thigh
(d) Medial part of calf

3452. L2 nerve involving movement occurs at:
(a) Ilioinguinal (b) Femoral
(c) Obturator (d) Tibial

3453. Huntington disease area of brain affected are A/E:
(a) Head of the caudate nucleus
(b) Putamen
(c) Striatum
(d) Pons

3454. MLF lesion causes A/E:
(a) Nystagmus
(b) INO
(c) Cannot adduct eye ipsilaterally
(d) Medial rectus will not contract with convergence

3455. Lacunar infarct stroke syndrome:
(a) Pure sensory can be seen
(b) Due to major vessel involvement
(c) Perforators are never affected
(d) Dysarthria–clumsy hand is due to MCA involvement

3456. Deposits in dermatitis herpetiformis are:
(a) IgA subendothelial

(b) IgA papillary dermis only

(c) IgA in papillary dermis and along epidermal basement membrane zone

(d) IgG deposits

3457. EBV causes A/E:

(a) Nasopharyngeal Ca

(b) Infectious mononucleosis

(c) Burkitt's lymphoma

(d) T cell lymphoma

3458. Congenital thyroid resistance in child:

(a) Mental status good (b) Mental status low

(c) Thyroid size normal (d) Thyroid size large

3459. TSH-B receptors are present in:

(a) Thyroid (b) RBC

(c) Muscle (d) Brain

3460. Thyroid Ca with lateral lymph node staging according to AJCC:

(a) Stage I (b) Stage II

(c) Stage III (d) Stage IVa

3461. MEN 1 most common tumor:

(a) Pancreas (b) Thyroid

(c) Parathyroid (d) Pituitary

3462. Nodular adrenal hyperplasia most common mutation:

(a) ARMC5 (b) PRKAR1A

(c) GNAS1 (d) HSD2

3463. Medullary thyroid Ca what is incorrect?

(a) Accounts for about 5% of thyroid cancers

(b) MTC is more aggressive in MEN2A than in MEN2B

(c) Elevated serum calcitonin

(d) Surgery is treatment

3464. Cyclic AMP mediated action:

(a) ACTH (b) GH

(c) GHRH (d) Prolactin

3465. Most common Cain thyroglossal cyst:

(a) Follicular (b) Papillary

(c) Medullary (d) Anaplastic

3466. Most common hormone affected in cranial irradiation:

(a) GHRH (b) GH

(c) LH (d) Prolactin

3467. Lymphocytic hypophysitis of pituitary what is not true?

(a) Sheets of lymphocytes present

(b) Pituitary not enlarged

(c) Increased ICP

(d) Headache

3468. Rathkes cyst true is:

(a) Can cause seizures

(b) Raised ICP

(c) Visual disturbances

(d) Hypopituitarism

3469. Serum calcium is 6.5, albumin is I, what is corrected calcium?

(a) 9.62 mg/dl (b) 8.6

(c) 7.6 (d) 10

3470. ATP7A mutation is seen in:

(a) Wilson (b) Menkes

(c) CF (d) Oxyluria

3471. Hypothalamus affection will not lead to:

(a) Adipsia (b) Depression

(c) Temperature change (d) Apathy

3472. Autoimmune diabetes with destruction of islets is:

(a) Type 1 (b) Type 2

(c) Type 3 (d) Type 4

3473. Primary adrenal insufficiency which is not the cause?

(a) Steroid (b) TB

(c) Bilateral infarcts (d) Lymphomas

3474. APS 2 what is not present?

(a) Type 1 DM

(b) Hypothyroidism

(c) Adrenal insufficiency

(d) Hypoparathyroidism

3475. Pseudohypoparathyroidism what is not seen?

(a) High PAH (b) Low PAH

(c) Hypocalcemia (d) Skeletal defects

3476. Adult with growth hormone deficiency, what is not the side effect of GH?

(a) Depression (b) Hyperglycemia

(c) HTN (d) Increase in HDL

3477. Centrally acting anti obesity drug that can be given for long term:
(a) Lorcaserin (b) Topiramate
(c) Bupropion (d) Liraglutide

3478. Acromegaly DOC:
(a) Somatostatin analogues
(b) Pegvisomant
(c) A+B
(d) Cabergoline

3479. Choreoathetosis with congenital hypothyroidism which mutation?
(a) TTF2 (b) TTFl
(c) PAX8 (d) NKX2.5

3480. Gynecomastia, small testis, tall male. Investigations include A/E:
(a) Serum testosterone (b) hCG beta
(c) FSH (d) TSH

3481. Mutation in testicular dysgenesis:
(a) SRY gene (b) INSL3
(c) KML gene (d) MYC gene

3482. Sudden attack without loss of consciousness is seen in A/E:
(a) Vertibrobasilar insufficiency
(b) Anterior MCA infarct
(c) SAH
(d) TIA of carotid origin

3483. Transudative pleural effusion seen in:
(a) Drug induced
(b) Peritoneal dialysis
(c) Post liver transplant
(d) Iatrogenic injury

3484. Drug causing pleural effusion:
(a) Amiodarone (b) Methotrexate
(c) Phenytoin (d) All of the above

3485. Haemorrhagic cystitis present in:
(a) Mycophenolate mefetil
(b) Cyclophosphamide
(c) Metotrexate
(d) Rifampicin

3486. Kussmaul's breathing:
(a) Hyperventilation with metabolic acidosis in renal failure
(b) Hyperventilation with metabolic alkalosis in renal failure
(c) Hypoventilation with metabolic acidosis in renal failure
(d) Hypoventilation with metabolic alkalosis in renal failure

3487. Disease caused due to ATP 7A defect:
(a) Cystic fibrosis
(b) A-1- antitrypsin deficiency
(c) Wilson's syndrome
(d) Menke's disease

3488. Alagille syndrome component is:
(a) Pulmonary hypoplasia
(b) Osteolytic lesions
(c) PDA
(d) None of the above

3489. SAPHO syndrome components are A/E:
(a) Hyperostosis
(b) Acne
(c) Synovitis
(d) Organomegaly

3490. Fish eye disease is due to deficiency of:
(a) ApoA (b) LCAT
(c) Acyl transferase (d) None of the above

3491. In Wilson's disease hepatic copper concentration in specimen should be:
(a) > 50 ug/dl (b) > 100 ug/dl
(c) > 200 ug/dl (d) > 250 ug/dl

3492. CD 56 is a marker of:
(a) B-cell (b) T-cell
(c) NK-cell (d) All of the above

3493. B-cell marker among the following:
(a) CD-19 (b) IL-6
(c) CD-45 (d) All of the above

3494. IgG variant predominantly found in serum of normal person:
(a) G1 (b) G2
(c) G3 (d) G4

3495. Acrodermatitis enteropathica is caused due to deficiency of:

(a) Selenium (b) Zinc
(c) Magnesium (d) None of the above

3496. Acrodermatitis enteropathica like skin eruptions is caused due to toxicity of:

(a) Cadmium (b) Manganese
(c) Chromium

3497. Which supplementation is used in Rx of sideroblastic anemia?

(a) B_6 (b) B_{12}
(c) Vit C (d) Vit A

3498. Supplement used in Chediak-Higashi syndrome:

(a) Vit C (b) Vit B_{12}
(c) Vit B_6 (d) All of the above

3499. Electrolyte abundantly seen in gastric secretion:

(a) Cl (b) H
(c) Na (d) K

3500. Hormone that stimulates satiety centre:

(a) Y neuropeptide (b) Orexin
(c) Cortisol (d) GH

3501. Inhibition of emesis done by:

(a) Dl receptors (b) Muscarinic
(c) Serotonin (d) Adrenaline

3502. Most common serotype of HBV in India:

(a) A (b) B
(c) C (d) D

3503. Feline esophagitis:

(a) Achalasia
(b) Gastric carcinoma
(c) Eosinophilic esophagitis
(d) GERD

3504. Bombesin test:

(a) Achlorhydria
(b) Intestinal peristalsis
(c) Pancreatic exocrine function
(d) None of the above

3505. Dieulafoy's Lesion:

(a) Pancreas (b) Stomach
(c) Intestine (d) Liver

3506. ATP 7B disease is:

(a) Wilson's (b) Rotor
(c) Menke (d) None of the above

3507. A 30 years female with elevated liver enzymes with hemolysis and thrombocytopenia, amenorrhoea:

(a) Hemolytic anemia (b) DIC
(c) HELLP syndrome (d) FLP

3508. In chronic cor pulmonale lower limb edema is present secondary to:

(a) Hypoxia (b) Hypercarbia
(c) Neurohumoral (d) All of the above

3509. Chronic bronchitis and asthma are differentiated by:

(a) X-ray (b) Atopy
(c) Auscultation (d) Spirometry

3510. Articular disorders characterized by A/E:

(a) Swelling
(b) Deep pain
(c) Deformities
(d) Pain aggravated on active movement but not in passive movement

3511. Sausage like pancreas seen in:

(a) Autoimmune pancreatitis
(b) Alcohol related pancreatitis
(c) Malignancy of pancreas
(d) None of the above

3512. Complication of orthotopic liver transplantation:

(a) Bleeding intra-abdominal
(b) Failure of biliary tree
(c) Deranged LFf
(d) All of the above

3513. Drug of choice for IBD-D:

(a) Alosetron (b) Cellulose
(c) Loperamide (d) All of the above

3514. Diagnosis of GERD:

(a) Manometry (b) 24 hrs pH monitoring
(c) Endoscopy (d) Histology

3515. In endoscopy for visualization of rebleeding risk, stage IIB refer to:

(a) Advanced clot
(b) Non-bleeding visible vessel
(c) Visible bleeding vessel
(d) None of the above

3516. In Forrest classification lesion without bleeding refers to:
(a) Type I (b) Type II
(c) Type III (d) None of the above

3517. Parasite causing portal venous hypertension:
(a) Wuchereria (b) Schistosomiasis
(c) Ancylostoma (d) All of the above

3518. Crohn's disease differentiating feature from ulcerative colitis:
(a) Rectosigmoidal sparing
(b) Perianal fistula
(c) Transmural involvement
(d) All of the above

3519. Drug that is cytoprotective and radioprotective:
(a) Sucralfate (b) Magnesium sulphate
(c) Bismuth (d) None of the above

3520. Best method for GFR calculation:
(a) Creatinine clearance (b) Inulin clearance
(c) Creatine clearance (d) All of the above

3521. Nephrotic syndrome related peritonitis caused by:
(a) Staphylococcus (b) H. influenza
(c) Listeria (d) E. coli

3522. Familial adenomatous polyposis with medulloblastoma seen in:
(a) Gardner's variant (b) Turcot variant
(c) Classical FAP (d) None of the above

3523. Most common position of appendix:
(a) Retrocecal (b) 2 O'clock
(c) 6 O'clock (d) 9 O'clock

3524. Nicotinamide is mixed with laropiprant to avoid:
(a) Hepatotoxicity (b) Hyperglycemia
(c) Vomiting (d) Flushing

3525. Hemolytic uremic syndrome A/E:
(a) Idiopathic thrombocytopenic purpura
(b) Hemolytic anemia
(c) Stroke
(d) Renal failure

3526. Trypsinogen is activated to trypsin by:
(a) Pepsinogen (b) Lipase
(c) Enterokinase (d) None of the above

3527. PTH dependent hypercalcemia occurs in:
(a) Familial hypocalciuric hypercalcemia
(b) X-linked hypocalciuric hypercalcemia
(c) Idiopathic hypercalcemia of infancy
(d) None of the above

3528. CFTR mutation is inherited as:
(a) Autosomal recessive (b) Autosomal dominant
(c) X-linked recessive (d) None of the above

3529. Maintenance of hygiene provides protection from:
(a) UTI (b) PSGN
(c) Cresentic GN (d) All of the above

3530. Common infection post-splenectomy:
(a) Cryptococcus (b) Pneumococcus
(c) Staph (d) E. coli

3531. Left sided portal hypertension Rx of choice:
(a) Portocaval shunt (b) Splenorenal shunt
(c) Both of the above (d) None of the above

3532. Usual interstitial pneumonia:
(a) Interstitial fibrosis (b) BIL hilar opacities
(c) Nodular changes (d) Bat wing appearance

3533. Drug to be used in IPF for survival benefit:
(a) NAC (b) Pirfenidone
(c) Steroid (d) Cyclophosphamide

3534. Diarrhea, dermatitis, dementia in deficiency of:
(a) B_1 (b) B_3
(c) B_{12} (d) Vit A

3535. Most common complication of diverticulosis:
(a) Abscess (b) Stricture
(c) Perforation (d) None of the above

3536. Aromatic androgen is:
(a) Testosterone (b) Androstendione
(c) Estradiol (d) Progesterone

3537. Hepatic carcinogen (angiosarcoma):
(a) Hep B virus (b) Alcohol
(c) Smoking (d) Vinyl chloride

3538. Afferent pain carried by:
(a) A beta and C (b) A delta and C
(c) Norepinephrine (d) None of the above

3539. Keshan disease due to deficiency of:

(a) Boron (b) Manganese
(c) Selenium (d) Aluminium

3540. Factor not synthesized by liver:

(a) II (b) V
(c) VII (d) X

3541. Murphy's sign:

(a) Hepatitis (b) Cholecystitis
(c) Pancreatitis (d) None of the above

3542. Amylase not increased in pleural effusion of:

(a) Esophageal rupture
(b) Malignancy
(c) Pneumonia
(d) Pancreatic pleural effusion

3543. Clinical staging of HIV:

(a) Category A – Recurrent pneumonia
(b) Category B – Peripheral neuropathy
(c) Category C – Asymptomatic

3544. Tubular proteinuria:

(a) LMW protein (b) Albumin
(c) Hb (d) None of the above

3545. Alpert syndrome A/E:

(a) Rezal failure
(b) Sensorineural hearing loss
(c) Tall stature
(d) Ocular abnormalities

3546. Neonatal scurvy A/E:

(a) Moeller-Barlow disease
(b) Deficiency of vitamin C (ascorbic acid)
(c) Hypothyroidism
(d) Corner sign

3547. Bisphosphonate used in Rx of:

(a) Osteoporosis (b) Metastasis
(c) Paget's disease (d) All of the above

3548. Most common relapse in ALL:

(a) Testis (b) CNS
(c) Bone marrow (d) Lymph node

3549. Most common type of choledochal cyst:

(a) I (b) II
(c) III (d) IV

3550. Bloom syndrome:

(a) Autosomal recessive disorder
(b) Growth deficiency
(c) Photosensitive skin changes
(d) All of the above

3551. Charcoat pentad:

(a) Fever (b) Abdominal pain
(c) Jaundice (d) All of the above

3552. Saint Louis triad:

(a) Gallstones (b) Diverticulosis
(c) Hiatus hernia (d) All of the above

3553. AML with gum bleed:

(a) M1 (b) M2
(c) M3 (d) M4

3554. Transient LOC is possible in A/E:

(a) ACA ischemia
(b) SAH
(c) Vertibrobasilar insufficiency
(d) Syncope

3555. ADA recommends screening for DM:

(a) >45 years and 3 yearly
(b) >40 and 3
(c) >50
(d) >60

3556. DOC for dyslipedemia in diabetes:

(a) Statins (b) Ezetimibe
(c) Finofibrate (d) Niacin

3557. Most common site of lodging of foreign body in esophagus:

(a) Upper (b) Middle
(c) Lower (d) Same

3558. Causes of odynophagia

(a) Pill esophagitis (b) CMV esophagitis
(c) Behcet (d) All of the above

3559. A 70 years old presented with frequent back fall, down gaze palsy:

(a) PSP (b) Shy dragger
(c) Wilson (d) None of the above

3560. Dunhill procedure is done in:

(a) Parathyroid (b) Ca prostate
(c) Ca stomach (d) Thyroid

3561. POEM syndrome:

(a) Polyneuropathy (b) Splenomegaly
(c) Papilledema (d) All of the above

3562. Beck's triad comprises:

(a) Hypotension, muffled heart sounds, absent y and deep x on NP
(b) Hypotension, pulsus paradoxus, raised NP with absent y and deep x
(c) Pulsus paradoxus, muffled heart sounds, raised NP
(d) Hypotension, muffled heart sound, absent y, pulsus paradoxus

3563. All are true regarding mechanism of levosimendan, *except*:

(a) K channel opener
(b) Ca channel sensitizer
(c) Decreases AF and hypotension incidence compared to dopamine
(d) Acts on vascular K-ATP channel

3564. Continuous murmur is present in A/E:

(a) ALCAPA (b) ASD with MS
(c) VSD with AR (d) Peripheral PS

3565. Drug contraindicated in Prinzmetal angina:

(a) CCB (b) Beta blockers
(c) Aspirin (d) Nitrates

3566. Irreversible P_2Y_{12} inhibitor:

(a) Prasugrel (b) Ticagrelor
(c) Dipyridamole (d) Aspirin

3567. True regarding tricuspid stenosis:

(a) Gradient of >5 mm Hg is required to diagnose
(b) Increase of murmur on Muller maneuver
(c) Easily heard
(d) All of the above

3568. True regarding STEM A/E:

(a) Prognosis of rupture of IVS is worse in anterior wall MI than IWMI
(b) Rupture of VS is most common in AWMI than IWMI
(c) IWMI associated with CHB
(d) Free wall rupture is most common in absence of collaterals

3569. Antibodies seen in primary biliary cirrhosis are:

(a) ANA (b) AMA
(c) Anti-LKM (d) D2DNA

3570. Fulminant hepatic failure is caused by A/E:

(a) Hepatitis D (b) Lassa fever
(c) CMC (d) None of the above

3571. Common gene in the pathogenesis of ALD with NASH:

(a) PNPLA3 (b) Aldolase
(c) PRP (d) All of the above

3572. Rate limiting step in the bilirubin metabolism:

(a) Formation of bilirubin preproducers
(b) Transfer of bilirubin into bile canaliculus
(c) Excretion of bile into cannaliculus
(d) All of the above

3573. Platypnea-orthdeoxia syndrome in A/E:

(a) Hepatopulmonary syndrome
(b) Portopulmonary syndrome
(c) Chronic kidney disease
(d) A-V pulmonary fistula

3574. Mild conjugated hyperbilirubinemia is associated with:

(a) Gilbert syndrome
(b) Crigler-Najjar I
(c) Crigler-Najjar II
(d) Dubin Johnson syndrome

3575. Esophageal manometry showed hypertensive LES:

(a) Diffuse esophageal spasm
(b) Achalasia cardia
(c) Scleroderma
(d) Nut cracker esophagus

3576. Acute fatty liver of pregnancy is associated with which trimester?

(a) 1st (b) 2nd
(c) 3rd (d) Postpartum

3577. GIST arises from:

(a) Parietal cells
(b) Interstitial cells of Cajal
(c) Oxytocic cells
(d) None of the above

3578. Most common disorder associated with chorea:

(a) SLE (b) Wilson
(c) HIV (d) MCTD

3579. Bilateral lesion in fusiform gyrus causes:

(a) Prosopagnosia (b) Hemianopia
(c) Achromatopsia (d) None of the above

3580. Argyll Robertson pupil is caused by lesion of:

(a) Pretectal nuclei in midbrain
(b) Post ganglionic fibres of parasympathetic innervations of eye
(c) Afferent defect at the level of optic nerve/retina
(d) None of the above

3581. Treatment of ICH A/E:

(a) Mannitol (b) Glycerol
(c) Craniotomy (d) Hypoventilation

3582. Mitochondrial disorder without lactic acidosis:

(a) NARP (b) Lebers
(c) MELAS (d) MERRF

3583. Anton's syndrome is caused due to:

(a) Bilateral PCA territory occlusion
(b) Due to infarct of watershed areas between PCA and MCA
(c) Vertebral artery occlusion
(d) MCA territory infarct

3584. A 70 years male with recent memory loss, feels other is replaced by imposter, diagnosis:

(a) Pick's (b) Alzheimer's
(c) DLB (d) Parkinsonism

3585. Ataxia with deafness is associated with:

(a) Mitochondrial disorder
(b) SCA3
(c) Freidrich's ataxia
(d) Ataxia telangiectasia

3586. Neuropathic joint disease is associated with A/E:

(a) TB (b) Syringomyelia
(c) DM (d) Syphilis

3587. BODE index includes:

(a) Dyspnea grading
(b) Measurement of FVC
(c) Less than 2 is associated with mortality of less than 10% in 2 years
(d) All of the above

3588. Difference between chronic bronchitis and emphysema can be done with:

(a) DLCO
(b) Residual volume
(c) Increased compliance
(d) All of the above

3589. Tracheostomy is indicated in A/E:

(a) Weaning from mechanical ventilation
(b) Foreign body in lung
(c) Therapy in OSA
(d) HIE

3590. Indication of long term O_2 therapy in COPD:

(a) PaO_2–50-55 mm Hg with polycythemia
(b) SpO_2–88-90% with polycythemia
(c) SpO_2–50-55% with polycythemia
(d) PaO_2–68 mm Hg

3591. Indication of omalizumab in bronchial asthma:

(a) Severe asthma when total dose of steroids >400 mg/month
(b) Severe asthma when total dose of steroids >600 mg/month
(c) Severe asthma when total dose of steroids >800 mg/month
(d) None of the above

3592. Lung volume reduction surgery:

(a) Upper lobe with low exercise capacity has more benefit
(b) Lower lobe with high exercise capacity has more benefit
(c) Upper lobe with high exercise capacity has more benefit
(d) All of the above

3593. Asthma with COPD is seen in:

(a) Old age (b) Young
(c) Mechanical workers (d) All of the above

3594. Disease which causes both exudative and transudative pleural effusion?

(a) Myxedema
(b) Parapneumonic effusion
(c) TB
(d) Malignancy

3595. Aldosterone acts on:

(a) DCT (b) PCT
(c) Collecting ducts (d) Loop of Henle

3596. Assessment of GFR:
(a) Inulin clearance (b) DTPA
(c) DMSA (d) Dextrose

3597. Cause of increased dead space in COPD is due to:
(a) Increased ventilation and decreased perfusion
(b) Decreased ventilation and increased perfusion
(c) Decreased ventilation and decreased perfusion
(d) Increased ventilation and increased perfusion

3598. Toll like receptors:
(a) PRR (pattern recognition receptors)
(b) IL-2
(c) Help in infection
(d) None of the above

3599. Beta-klotho is associated with A/E:
(a) Bile acid diarrhea (b) Aging
(c) Bone loss (d) Alcohol consumption

3600. Cancer becomes detectable at cell count of:
(a) 106 (b) 109
(c) 1012 (d) 1015

3601. Transdifferentiation means:
(a) Cells pose the capacity to differentiate into cell type outside their lineage restriction
(b) Cells pose the capacity to differentiate into cell type within their lineage restriction
(c) Both of the above
(d) None of the above

3602. Tumor calcinosis is characteristic of:
(a) Hypercalcemia (b) Hyperphosphatemia
(c) Increased FGF-23 (d) All of the above

3603. Ferrous iron is oxidized to ferric by:
(a) Hepcidin (b) DMT
(c) Hephaestin (d) All of the above

3604. Polyps in Peutz-Jeghers syndrome:
(a) Hamartomatous polyp
(b) Dysplasia
(c) Sessile
(d) Adenomatous

3605. Recruitment of TH2 helper T cells:
(a) Mast cells (b) Eosinophils
(c) Neutrophils (d) RBC

3606. Frozen shoulder is most common with:
(a) OA (b) DM
(c) Scleroderma (d) SLE

3607. Most common joint involved in pigmented villonodular synovitis:
(a) Knee (b) Ankle
(c) Shoulder (d) Hip

3608. DOC for HCV infection type 3 in a patient of Child Pugh C grade is:
(a) Ledipasvir + Sofosbuvir + IFN alpha
(b) Ledipasvir + Sofosbuvir + Ribavirin
(c) Ritonavir + Sofosbuvir + IFN alpha
(d) None of the above

3609. DOC for Strongyloides:
(a) Albendazole (b) Mebendazole
(c) Ivermectin (d) Praziquantel

3610. Kaposi sarcoma in HIV patient, polymorphic nodular lesion, hyperpigmented caused by:
(a) HHV-8 (b) EBV
(c) HSV (d) None of the above

3611. Mantoux test units of PPD used is:
(a) 5U (b) 1OU
(c) 15U (d) 1U

3612. Best investigational test for giardiasis:
(a) Ileal string test
(b) Duodenal aspirate
(c) Stool examination for ova or cyst
(d) Biopsy of rectum

3613. All can be used in drug resistant TB *except*:
(a) PAS (b) Clofazamine
(c) Ethambutol (d) Ethionamide

3614. Mechanism of SSPE in measles:
(a) Reactivation of virus
(b) Immune mediated
(c) Persistent virus infection
(d) All of the above

3615. Allosensitization in pregnancy:
(a) IgG (b) IgD
(c) IgM (d) IgA

3616. Multiple ring enhancing lesion in brain in a patient of HIV indicates:

(a) Cryptococcosis (b) Primary lymphoma
(c) Toxoplasmosis (d) None of the above

3617. Magnesium deficiency is associated with A/E:

(a) Alcoholic liver disease (b) CKD
(c) Malnutrition (d) Hypothyroidism

3618. Causes of early secondary hyperparathyroidism in a patient of CKD A/E:

(a) Low vit D levels (b) Hypercalcemia
(c) FGF-23 (d) Hyperphosphatemia

3619. Gene associated with AR rickets:

(a) SLCA-43 (b) FGF-23
(c) DMPl (d) All of the above

3620. Most common type of vitamin D dependent rickets:

(a) X-Linked hypophosphatemic rickets
(b) AD hypophosphetemic rickets
(c) Vit D resistant rickets
(d) All of the above

3621. Early anosmia is a feature of:

(a) Idiopathic Parkinson disease
(b) PSP
(c) Alzheimer
(d) PARK2 associated Parkinsonism

3622. A 16 years boy C/o severe headache, ptosis, miosis, hemiplegia diagnosis:

(a) Carotid dissection
(b) CVT
(c) Cavernous sinus thrombosis
(d) Aortic dissection

3623. All are true regarding Parkinsonism *except*:

(a) Anosmia is a finding
(b) Hypophonia can be seen
(c) Levodopa prevents freezing and falls
(d) None of the above

3624. Pancytopenia with cellular bone marrow:

(a) Brucellosis (b) Q-fever
(c) TB (d) Leptospira

3625. Early prosthetic valve endocarditis is caused by:

(a) Streptococcus
(b) Staph. Aureus
(c) Coagulase negative staph
(d) None of the above

3626. Drug not excreted by renal excretion is:

(a) Dabigatron (b) Apixaban
(c) Bivalirudin (d) Argatroban

3627. Phenomenon present in HOCM in which disease is variable in parents and children is due to:

(a) Allelic heterogeneity (b) Incomplete penetrance
(c) Parental dominancy (d) Variable expressivity

3628. Treatment of MAT in a patient of COPD:

(a) CCB (b) BB
(c) ACEI (d) Digoxin

3629. In a patient with no previous history of heart disease AF of 36 hours duration, next line:

(a) Beta blockers (b) DC version
(c) Lanoxin (d) O_2 therapy

3630. Patient with cardiac arrest and VT after 3 minutes Rx is:

(a) DC shock (b) IV amiodarone
(c) CPR (d) Calcium gluconate

3631. Anemia, Hb-11.3 gm, MCV-80.2, TIBC decreased, ferritin-150, normocytic normochromic:

(a) Iron deficiency (b) Renal disease
(c) Inflammation (d) Hypometabolic state

3632. Clotting factor with shortest T l/2:

(a) Factor II (b) Factor VII
(c) Factor XIII (d) FactorY

3633. Donath Landsteiner antibody is associated with:

(a) PNH
(b) Paroxysmal cold hemoglobinuria
(c) CL
(d) All of the above

3634. Test used to differentiate IBS and Crohn disease:

(a) Fecal cellulose (b) Fecal calprotectin
(c) Fecal aldolase (d) All of the above

3635. Management of acute pancreatitis:

(a) Vigorous resuscitation and IV fluids
(b) IV antibiotics
(c) Debulking
(d) Surgery

3636. Treatment of hypoproteinemia in intestinal lymphangiectasia:
(a) High fat diet
(b) Infusion of albumin
(c) High protein diet
(d) Medium-chain triglyceride

3637. Secretin infusion in ZES causes:
(a) Increases gastrin levels
(b) Decreases gastrin levels
(c) No change
(d) None of the above

3638. CT angiography is helpful in:
(a) Zenker diverticulum (b) Meckel's diverticulum
(c) Bile acid diarrhea (d) Steatorrhea

3639. Diabetic patient with fever and red swollen leg:
(a) DVT (b) Thrombophlebitis
(c) Cellulitis (d) Scar

3640. Patient presenting with head injury, urine osmolarity –100, Na–150:
(a) Pituitary DI (b) Nephrogenic DI
(c) Primary polydepsia (d) All of the above

3641. Treatment of hypervolemic hyponatremia
(a) Diuretics (b) Vaptans
(c) Fluid restriction (d) Saline

3642. Diabetic patient with urine proteinuria >3 gm/d, increased LDL, increased cholesterol. All done *except*:
(a) Increase statin dose
(b) Increase ramipril dose
(c) Continue aspirin
(d) All of the above

3643. Rx of pheochromocytoma before surgery:
(a) Alpha blockers (b) Beta blockers
(c) CCB (d) Diuretics

3644. Nephropathy associated with Sjögren syndrome:
(a) Type 2 RTA (b) Type 1 RTA
(c) Type 3 RTA (d) Type 4 RTA

3645. Double contour sign in knee ultrasound:
(a) Pseudogout (b) Gout
(c) OA (d) RA

3646. Investigation of choice in early sacroiliitis is:
(a) MRI (b) CT
(c) USG (d) X-ray

3647. Bouchard nodes:
(a) DIP in OA (b) PIP in OA
(c) DIP in RA (d) PIP in RA

3648. Most common joint involved in hemochromatosis is:
(a) Knee
(b) Ankle
(c) Hip
(d) 2nd and 3rd metacarpophalangeal joints

3649. Male patient with temporal headache and jaw claudication while eating:
(a) Takayasu (b) Giant cell A
(c) Wegener (d) PAN

3650. Vasculitis associated with ANCA:
(a) Wegener (b) GCA
(c) Takayasu (d) PAN

3651. Antibodies positive in drug induced SLE:
(a) Anti ds DNA (b) Anti histone
(c) ANA (d) RNA

3652. Difference between PAN with HBV and without HBV is:
(a) Worse prognosis if both together
(b) ANCA is common
(c) Good prognosis
(d) All of the above

3653. Hemodynamic changes in sepsis, A/E:
(a) Decreased peripheral resistance
(b) Normal sensorium
(c) Hypotension
(d) Tachycardia

3654. Mechanism of action of activated protein C is A/E:
(a) Anti-infective (b) Anti-inflammatory
(c) Anticoagulative (d) Profibrinolytic

3655. Moderate to severe fluorosis is not associated with:
(a) Dental caries
(b) Ligamental calcification
(c) Osteosclerosis
(d) Osteoporosis

3656. ISIS-2 trial was done for:

(a) Clopidogrel (b) Aspirin
(c) Prasugrel (d) Ticagrelor

3657. Patient with pulmonary embolism, normal ECG. Next investigation of choice:

(a) MRI (b) Perfusion scan
(c) CT angio (d) Cardiac cath

3658. Treatment of ITP in splenectomized patients include A/E:

(a) Eculizumab (b) IVIg
(c) Anti Rho-D (d) Platelets

3659. Pooled sample analysis is done for which hormone?

(a) Insulin (b) PTH
(c) Vit D (d) Prolactin

3660. Patient with prosthetic AV on warfarin INR-2.5, planning for EGD:

(a) Continue warf
(b) Stop warf and no bridging with LMWH
(c) Bridging with LMWH
(d) None of the above

3661. Most reactive system after ABO and Rh is:

(a) Kell (b) Duffy
(c) M (d) None of the above

3662. NAPH, metabolite of procainamide is associated with:

(a) Asystole (b) AF
(c) TdP (d) VT

3663. ECG shows ST elevation in A/E:

(a) Hypercalcemia (b) Hyperkalemia
(c) Hypothermia (d) Hypocalcemia

3664. Mortality in MI in males vs female false is:

(a) Females have high mortality than males in acute MI
(b) Females have less mortality in NSTEMI at 35 days
(c) Plaque rupture is most common in female than male
(d) Females present with atypical symptoms

3665. Gold standard for diagnosis of celiac disease:

(a) Anti TTG
(b) Anti endomysial antibodies
(c) Intestinal biopsy
(d) All of the above

3666. MELD score includes A/E:

(a) S. bilirubin (b) S. creatinine
(c) INR (d) Albumin

3667. Viral conjunctivitis pharyngitis encephalitis caused by:

(a) EBV (b) Adenovirus
(c) Coxsakievirus (d) Yellow fever

3668. Liquid gas chromatography acting on small chain fatty acid used for:

(a) C difficile (b) Candida
(c) Acinobacter (d) Pneumocystis

3669. Vaccine CI in a patient on cancer chemotherapy:

(a) Pneumococcal vaccine
(b) Meningococcal vaccine
(c) DPT
(d) Varicella

3670. Antigen associated with P. vivax malaria:

(a) Duffy (b) Kelly
(c) Rh (d) ABO

3671. Normal anion gap metabolic acidosis in:

(a) DKA (b) RTA
(c) Salicylate poisoning (d) Alcohol intoxication

3672. Renal transplant rejection in first week of transplant is due to:

(a) Cell mediated
(b) Antigen mediated
(c) Antibody mediated hyperacute rejection
(d) None of the above

3673. CMV infection after renal transplant usually occurs:

(a) Less than 1 month (b) 1-6 months
(c) More than 6 months (d) More than 12 months

3674. Drug not used in long term prophylaxis of UTI in females:

(a) Norflox (b) TMP-SMX
(c) Hippurate (d) Mitomicin-C

3675. Patient with abdominal mass, Conn's syndrome. IOC:

(a) CT scan (b) ARR ratio
(c) MRI (d) Sr. aldosterone levels

3676. Insulin induced hypokalemia is seen in:
(a) Malnutrition (b) Alcoholism
(c) DKA (d) All of the above

3677. BUN more than Sr. creatinine is seen in A/E:
(a) GI bleed (b) Steroid use
(c) High protein diet (d) Aminoglycoside use

3678. Hyperkalemia is associated with A/E:
(a) Obstructive uropathy
(b) Contrast nephropathy
(c) Aminoglycoside use
(d) Digoxin

3679. Effect of hypothyroidism on kidney vasculature A/E:
(a) Increased blood flow (b) Decreased rennin
(c) Increased creatinine (d) All of the above

3680. First manifestation of optic nerve compression:
(a) Tunnel vision
(b) Bitemporal hemianopia
(c) Loss of color vision
(d) Superior temporal quadrantinopia

3681. Corpus callosum lesions do not affect:
(a) Sequential task (b) Movements
(c) Speech (d) All of the above

3682. Drug used in migraine prophylaxis A/E:
(a) Oxibotulinum toxin (b) CBZ
(c) Topiramate (d) None of the above

3683. Dissociative apraxia:
(a) Inability to comprehend
(b) Inability to repeat
(c) Inability to pantomime to command
(d) All of the above

3684. Rx of meningitis true A/E:
(a) Recurrent epidemics in 8-9 years
(b) Steroid increase the permeability of vancomycin
(c) Pneumococcal most common cause of meningitis more than 20 years
(d) All of the above

3685. True about Huntington's disease:
(a) AR
(b) Progress to rigidity
(c) No behavioral changes
(d) CTG repeats

3686. RCT avoids error:
(a) Recall bias
(b) Dropouts are included
(c) No one is blinded
(d) All of the above

3687. True about Di-George syndrome are A/E:
(a) Hypercalcemia (b) CHD defects
(c) CNS defects (d) AD

3688. Female with absent vagina, normal breast development, absent pubic hair. Diagnosis:
(a) Gonadal dysgenesis
(b) Androgen insensitivity syndrome
(c) Normal variant
(d) None of the above

3689. In renal gluconeogenesis amino acid used is:
(a) Glycine (b) Glutamine
(c) Alanine (d) Histamine

3690. Forearm with scaly lesion wickham striae hyperkeratosis:
(a) Lichen planus (b) Psoriasis
(c) Candidacies (d) All of the above

3691. Upper chest urticaria after eating strawberry Rx:
(a) Aspirin (b) Steroids
(c) Antihistamines (d) All of the above

3692. Hypopigmented lesions of both the legs seen in:
(a) Vitiligo (b) Leprosy
(c) Both of the above (d) None of the above

3693. First pass metabolism means:
(a) Intestinal epithelium + liver
(b) Liver
(c) Intestinal epithelium
(d) None of the above

3694. High risk factor in drug toxicity:
(a) Single route of elimination
(b) Volume of distribution
(c) Narrow therapeutic range
(d) None of the above

3695. Speed ball:
(a) Cocaine + Amphetamine
(b) Cocaine + Alcohol

(c) Cocaine + Heroin
(d) None of the above

3696. Alpha heavy chain disease is associated with A/E:
(a) CLL (b) MALT
(c) IPSID (d) All of the above

3697. Steatorrhea occurs when pancreatic damage occurs more than:
(a) 50% (b) 70%
(c) 90% (d) 100%

3698. Osteomalacia is associated with:
(a) Lamivudine (b) Ritonavir
(c) Didanosine (d) Tenofovir

3699. Measurement of stool pancreatic elastase is done in:
(a) Gastritis
(b) Chronic pancreatitis
(c) Bile acid malabsorption
(d) All of the above

3700. Glomerulonephritis in APLA:
(a) MPGN (b) FSGN
(c) MGN (d) PSGN

3701. An 8 years boy with MCD diagnosed 1 year back on renal biopsy now presents with steroid resistant nephrotic syndrome. All true *except*:
(a) Renal biopsy to look for FSGN
(b) Start rituximab for resistance
(c) Nutritional support
(d) All of the above

3702. APLA nephropathy histology shows A/E:
(a) Cortical atrophy
(b) Thrombotic microangiopathy
(c) Fibrous intimal hyperplasia
(d) Thinned gap

3703. Crystals/stones formed in alkaline urine are:
(a) Calcium oxalate
(b) Ca phosphate
(c) Cysteine
(d) Uric acid

3704. True regarding ADPKD are A/E:
(a) Truncated mutation has better prognosis
(b) 15% have no family history
(c) Aneurysm screening should begin at the age of 30 years
(d) 50% progress to ESRD

3705. Spur calls with stomatocytes are seen in:
(a) CKD (b) CLD
(c) Hemolysis (d) All of the above

3706. Prolonged PT/aPTT with bleeding time:
(a) Hemophilia A (b) Hemophilia B
(c) DIC (d) TTP

3707. Janus kinase mutation is associated with:
(a) CML (b) PV
(c) Myelofibrosis (d) AML

3708. Hemighosts, Heinz bodies, Bite cells are seen in:
(a) Sickle cell anemia (b) PNH
(c) HS (d) G6PD deficiency

3709. Most common site for NHL:
(a) Liver (b) Lung
(c) Stomach (d) Brain

3710. HbF is increased in:
(a) Sickle cell disease (b) Alpha thalassaemia
(c) Both of the above (d) None of the above

3711. Fetal Hb changes to adult form by:
(a) 24 weeks (b) 28 weeks
(c) 32 weeks (d) 36 weeks

3712. Most common reaction occurring after blood transfusion is:
(a) Allergic reaction
(b) TRALI
(c) Febrile nonhemolytic reaction
(d) None of the above

3713. Adenovirus gene therapy is used in which disease?
(a) SCID
(b) Alpha 1 antitripsin deficiency
(c) Lipoprotein lipase deficiency
(d) All of the above

3714. Neurogenic claudication is due to:
(a) Ischemia of the nerve root
(b) Impingement of nerve root into foramina
(c) Nerve compression at peripheral site
(d) All of the above

3715. Drugs used in HIV esophagitis are A/E:
(a) Itraconazole (b) Thalidomide
(c) Sucralfate (d) Dexamethasone

3716. True about inhibin is:
(a) Increases LH secretion
(b) Up regulates FSH secretion, secreted by sertoli cells
(c) Down regulates FSH secretion, secreted by sertoli cells
(d) None of the above

3717. Grape fruit juice inhibits:
(a) CYP2D6 (b) CYP3A4
(c) P-glycoprotein (d) All of the above

3718. Abetalipoproteinemia is associated with:
(a) Apo E (b) Apo D
(c) Apo B (d) Apo A

3719. Toxic metabolite of alcohol:
(a) Formic acid (b) Acetaldehyde
(c) Acetone (d) All of the above

3720. False about multiple sclerosis:
(a) CSF is clear and colorless
(b) CSF peocytosis >75 cells/mm^3
(c) CSF protein is normal
(d) All of the above

3721. Laryngomalacia definition:
(a) Soft, immature cartilage of the upper larynx collapses inward during inhalation, causing airway obstruction
(b) Bony loss of larynx
(c) Infection of cricoid cartilage
(d) None of the above

3722. Disease with restrictive pattern:
(a) COPD
(b) Asthma
(c) Bronchitis
(d) Protein alveolar proteinosis

3723. Alpha 1 antitrypsin deficiency cause:
(a) Panacinar emphysema
(b) Centrilobular emphysema
(c) Both of the above
(d) None of the above

3724. Alcoholic patient presents to emergency with paracetamol overdose. Finding which is in favor of paracetamol poisoning:
(a) Increase in PT/INR
(b) Increase in ALT more than AST
(c) Liver injury
(d) All of the above

3725. HUS is caused by:
(a) E. coli (b) Shigella
(c) Chlamydia (d) All of the above

3726. True about HIT is:
(a) Thrombotic events are common
(b) M>F
(c) Bleeding common
(d) None of the above

3727. Renal transplant in CKD A/E:
(a) Transplant as the answer of uremia
(b) Diabetic with ESRD
(c) ESRD due to PCKD
(d) All of the above

3728. Ticagrelor most common side effect:
(a) Dyspnea (b) Block
(c) Bleeding (d) Gastritis

3729. Which organism doesn't cause atypical pneumonia?
(a) PCP (b) Legionella
(c) Nocardia (d) Mycoplasma

3730. All are features of ARDS *except*:
(a) Increased PCO_2 (b) Decreased PO
(c) Increase in PCW (d) None of the above

3731. Cystic fibrosis:
(a) AD (b) AR
(c) XR (d) XD

3732. NIV is not used in:
(a) Pulmonary edema
(b) When secretions present in trachea and pharynx
(c) COPD
(d) Sleep apnea

3733. RNA virus coated with lipid core:

(a) Dengue (b) Hep E
(c) Rotavirus (d) Hep D

3734. Crystal seen in ethylene glycol poisoning:

(a) Ca oxalate (b) Ca phosphate
(c) Uric acid (d) None of the above

3735. Eosinophilia with bronchitis seen in:

(a) Cystic fibrosis (b) ABPA
(c) PAP (d) Chronic bronchitis

3736. Prodrug is:

(a) Apixaban (b) Rivaroxaban
(c) Dabigatran (d) Aspirin

3737. Antibody to antiphospholipid A2 causes:

(a) FSGN (b) MPGN
(c) MGN (d) MCD

3738. Exercise induced palpitations Rx by:

(a) Amiodarone (b) CCB
(c) ICD (d) Beta blockers

3739. Tacrolimus interferes with fruit interaction:

(a) Guava (b) Tomato
(c) Grapes (d) Citrus fruit

3740. Mineral dust bronchiolitis:

(a) Proliferative bronchiolitis
(b) Restrictive bronchiolitis
(c) Obliterative bronchiolitis
(d) All of the above

3741. FEF50/FIF50 is 1 in:

(a) Variable intrathoracic obstruction
(b) Variable extrathoracic obstruction
(c) Fixed intrathoracic obstruction
(d) Fixed extrathoracic obstruction

3742. Female with normal LFT, HbeAg +ve, HBV DNA –2500, stage:

(a) Immune tolerance phase of chronic hepatitis B
(b) Immune reactive phase of chronic hepatitis B
(c) Carrier hepatitis B
(d) None of the above

3743. Prospective study:

(a) Ecological study
(b) Cross sectional study
(c) Cohort study
(d) None of the above

3744. Marble bone disease:

(a) Dent's disease (b) Osteopetrosis
(c) Type II RTA (d) All of the above

3745. Albumin creatinine ratio A/E:

(a) Useful in renal disease
(b) Can diagnose prerenal vs renal disease
(c) Doesn't depend on bone and muscle mass of patient
(d) None of the above

3746. Hep C with CLD, gradually progressive breathlessness, N ECG, low DLCO–next step:

(a) CT angio (b) Cardiac angio
(c) O_2 inhalation (d) Echo

3747. Koplik spots are seen in:

(a) Measles (b) Rubella
(c) Mumps (d) Yellow fever

3748. Drug causing tendinitis:

(a) Penicillin (b) Cyclosporine
(c) Statins (d) All of the above

3749. False is:

(a) Rhabdomyoma is most common cardiac tumor in children
(b) Myxoma most common cardiac tumor in adults
(c) Carney complex is AR
(d) All of the above

3750. Warfarin metabolizes through:

(a) VKOR1C (b) CYP2A4
(c) CYP2C9 (d) All of the above

3751. Wrong about air pollution is:

(a) Reach alveoli
(b) NCR PM 2.5 is less than 12
(c) PM 2.5 means particle size less than 2.5 u
(d) PM 2.5 of more than 55 is unhealthy

3752. 3rd hand smoking is:

(a) Chemical residual of tobacco smoke contamination that clings to clothing, wall, furniture, carpet, cushions, hair, skin

(b) Smoking E-cigarette
(c) Breathing the smoke from bystanders cigarette
(d) None of the above

3753. PAN false is:
(a) Males 3 times more common than females
(b) Affects medium and small sized arteries
(c) Causes aneurysm in mesenteric and renal arteries
(d) HBV/HCV associated with PAN

3754. Gallbladder not associated with:
(a) Mucus secretion (b) Calcium salt secretion
(c) Concentration of bile (d) Bile reservoir

3755. Methylene blue used as a treatment for:
(a) CO_2 narcosis (b) COHb poisoning
(c) MetHb poisoning (d) All of the above

3756. Not a treatment of methemoglobinemia:
(a) Plasmapheresis (b) Methylene blue
(c) $CuSO_4$ (d) Vit C

3757. Dengue:
(a) Platelet decrease by 7-10 days of fever
(b) Bone marrow suppression not seen
(c) Platelets decrease due to increased sequestration only
(d) Autoantibodies against platelets are seen

3758. RL composition A/E:
(a) pH–6.5 (b) Na–140
(c) K–4 (d) Cl–109

3759. Hypokalemia A/E:
(a) Addison disease (b) Diarrhea
(c) ATN (d) Amphotericin B

3760. Urine Na less than 20:
(a) Acute diarrhea (b) Hyperglycemia
(c) SIADH (d) Hypothyroidism

3761. Efferent of light reflex:
(a) Optic nerve (b) Optic tract
(c) Oculomotor (d) Trigeminal

3762. Drug that can be given in pregnancy:
(a) Ketoconazole (b) Itraconazole
(c) Griseofulvin (d) Terbinafine

3763. Cytokine mediated hyperthermia:
(a) Lymphoma
(b) Heat stroke
(c) Malignant hyperthermia
(d) All of the above

3764. Osteolysis is caused by:
(a) IL-2 (b) IL-6, TNF
(c) IL-2, TGF (d) TGF only

3765. POSCO Act is related to:
(a) Dowry
(b) Murder
(c) Criminal negligence
(d) Child sex abuse

3766. Anterior abdominal wall nerve supply:
(a) T7-T12, Ll (b) T9-12, Ll
(c) T7-12,Ll-3 (d) T9-12, Ll

3767. OCP cause:
(a) Hepatoma (b) FNH
(c) HCC (d) All of the above

3768. 2nd most common cause of upper GI bleeding:
(a) Varices (b) Peptic ulcer
(c) Gastritis/duodenitis (d) Mallory-Weiss tear

3769. Terlipressin in EVL:
(a) No terlipressin after EVL
(b) 1 day terlipressin after EVL
(c) 4 days terlipressin after EVL
(d) None of the above

3770. Deep sulcus sign:
(a) Pleural effusion (b) Pneumomediastinum
(c) Mass (d) Pneumothorax

3771. Most potent breathing stimulus:
(a) Hypoxemia (b) Acidosis
(c) Low CO_2 (d) Alkalosis

3772. 10 g Hb is equal to how much volume of O_2?
(a) 12 (b) 13
(c) 15 (d) 16

3773. Spontaneous bacterial peritonitis:
(a) Recurrence with in 1 year is 25%
(b) Antibiotic given regardless of symptoms
(c) Lymphocytic predominant fluid
(d) All are correct

3774. Anorexia nervosa A/E:
(a) Sinus tachycardia (b) Sinus bradycardia
(c) Increased QTc (d) Hypotension

3775. True statement is:
(a) High prevalence = low predictive value
(b) High prevalence = high sensitivity
(c) Two screening test in series increases specificity
(d) Two screening test in parallel increases specificity

3776. Splenectomy A/E:
(a) Howell Jolley bodies (b) Thrombocytosis
(c) Increases RBC mass (d) Leucopenia

3777. Thiazolidinediones causing bladder cancer:
(a) It's a class effect
(b) It's not a class effect
(c) Doesn't cause bladder cancer
(d) None of the above

3778. Secretion of renin is stimulated by:
(a) PCT (b) DCT
(c) Macula densa (d) All of the above

3779. Thiazide diuretics:
(a) Block ENaC
(b) Doesn't work in kidney disease
(c) Decreases renal blood flow
(d) Causes TdP when given with quinidine

3780. Clinical signal:
(a) Side effect if its proven reporting
(b) Side effect even unproven needs reporting
(c) Reporting is beneficial
(d) Reporting is not beneficial

3781. Microscopy of urine test–heat is used:
(a) To adjust specific gravity
(b) Amorphous urate dissolved
(c) Specific gravity increased
(d) RBC lysis

3782. Theophylline clearance is increased by:
(a) Barbecued meat
(b) Allopurinol
(c) High carbohydrate diet
(d) Pneumonia

3783. Vitamin B12 deficiency causes A/E:
(a) Hyperpigmentation of hands
(b) Megaloblastic anemia
(c) Neuropathy
(d) Roth spot

3784. Hypervitaminosis A:
(a) Hirsutism
(b) Hyperostosis
(c) Liver and splenomegaly
(d) Desquamation

3785. Pellagra seen in A/E:
(a) Niacin deficiency (b) Hartnup
(c) Carcinoid (d) Tryptophan excess

3786. Repeat plateletpheresis can be safely done on the same donor after:
(a) 24 hours (b) 72 hours
(c) 7 days (d) 5 days

3787. INR 2-3 indicated in A/E:
(a) AVR (b) MVR
(c) Pulmonary embolism (d) AF

3788. Transmural corrosive injury grading:
(a) I (b) II
(c) III (d) IV

3789. Fat cerebral embolism syndrome is associated with A/E:
(a) Symptoms develop within 96 hours
(b) Tachycardia
(c) Somnolence
(d) Petechial rash

3790. UV radiation causes mutation by:
(a) Formation of thymidine dimmers
(b) Methylation
(c) Acetylation
(d) All of the above

3791. Chromosomal abnormality associated with promyelocytic leukemia:

(a) 9:22 (b) 15:17

(c) Deletion 4 (d) All of the above

3792. SLE patient C/O chest pain, ECG S/O diffuse ST elevation, diagnosis is:

(a) Pericardial effusion (b) STEMI

(c) Pericarditis (d) Myocarditis

3793. Dialysis associated amyloidosis due to accumulation of:

(a) Beta 1 microglobulin (b) Beta 2 microglobulin

(c) Carotenes (d) None of the above

3794. Tick bite is associated with A/E:

(a) Anaplasmosis (b) Tularemia

(c) Lymes disease (d) Epidemic typhus

3795. Neuroexcitation toxin is associated with A/E:

(a) Wasp (b) Jelly fish

(c) Octopus (d) Tick

3796. VAP pneumonia is associated with A/E:

(a) Antibiotic use within 90 days

(b) Associated with acute heart failure at presentation

(c) Associated with septicemia at presentation

(d) Poor immunity

3797. MRCP uses visualization of biliary tract by:

(a) Contrast (b) Tissue interface

(c) Bile pigment (d) Water

3798. Percutaneous transhepatic biliary drainage:

(a) Subxipoid approach is easier

(b) Least complication with mid axillary approach

(c) 15-20% of biliary drainage is desirable

(d) Less contrast through biliary reflex

3799. Extravascular lung volume is normally around:

(a) 1-3 ml/Kg (b) 3-7 ml/Kg

(c) 7-10 ml/Kg (d) 10-15 ml/Kg

3800. Beta blocker prophylaxis for variceal bleeding is used in A/E:

(a) Procalcitonin levels < 6U

(b) Serum sodium < 122 meq/L

(c) Serum creatinine > 1.5 mg/dl

(d) MAP < 82 mm Hg

3801. Hormone not used in brain dead:

(a) Vasopressin (b) GH

(c) Thyroxine (d) Steroids

3802. Transducer used in transthoracic echocardiography:

(a) 1-2 MHz (b) 3-5 MHz

(c) 5-7 MHz (d) 7-10 MHz

3803. True regarding influenza:

(a) Maximum mortality associated with H 3 NZ

(b) HA assay is the only measure of protective immunity

(c) Vaccine has an efficacy of 60%

(d) Neuraminidase antibody is protective

3804. Webbed neck, increased hairline, small metacarpal, increased carrying angle seen in:

(a) Downs syndrome (b) Turner

(c) Wilson (d) Prader Willi

3805. SLE activity index consists of:

(a) Vasculitis

(b) Kyphosis

(c) Endothelial proliferation

(d) Wire loop lesion

3806. TB infection is associated with deficiency of:

(a) IFN-alpha (b) IFN-beta

(c) INF-gamma (d) INF-delta

3807. APACE-II consists of A/E:

(a) PaO_2, FiO_2 (b) GCS

(c) Age (d) Lactate

3808. Primary lung Eosinophilic disease A/E:

(a) ABPA

(b) Idiopathic Eosinophilic syndrome

(c) Chronic Eosinophilic pneumonia

(d) Loeffler's syndrome

3809. Most common joint involved in RA is:

(a) Wrist (b) Hip

(c) Knee (d) Shoulder

3810. Mumps true:

(a) Frequently causes mortality

(b) No infectivity before parotitis

(c) Only infects parotid glands

(d) Meningoencephalitis can precede parotitis

3811. Most infectious virus:

(a) CMV (b) HIV
(c) EBV (d) HBsAg

3812. Leptospirosis true:

(a) Ceftriaxone is the antibiotic of choice
(b) MAT is positive at the end of 1st week
(c) Endothelial dysfunction
(d) Direct microscopy cork screw morphology

3813. ALL–WBC–2 lac, Hb–7.0 gm, platelet count–10 lac, treatment to do:

(a) Induction of chemotherapy
(b) Radiotherapy
(c) Bone marrow transplantation
(d) Added chemotherapy

3814. HLA on short arm of chromosome:

(a) 4 (b) 6
(c) 8 (d) 11

3815. Leucocyte reduction transfusion decreases A/E:

(a) CMV rate (b) Febrile illness
(c) GVHD (d) All of the above

3816. Primary sclerosing cholangitis A/E:

(a) A/W IBD
(b) A/W 20% case of IG4
(c) GB Ca can occur
(d) Small bile duct involvement has better prognosis

3817. Negative acute phase reactant:

(a) Transferrin (b) Porphyrin
(c) Ceruloplasmin (d) CRP

3818. Delirium in medical disease features are A/E:

(a) Progressive symptomatology
(b) Altered consciousness
(c) Psychomotor depression
(d) Elation

ANSWERS KEY

1.	(a)	2.	(a)	3.	(a,b)	4.	(a)	5.	(a)	6.	(c)	7.	(c)	8.	(b)
9.	(d)	10.	(a)	11.	(a)	12.	(a)	13.	(a)	14.	(d)	15.	(a)	16.	(b)
17.	(b)	18.	(c)	219.	(b)	20.	(b)	21.	(b)	22.	(c)	23.	(d)	24.	(b)
25.	(b)	26.	(c)	27.	(b)	28.	(b)	29.	(b)	30.	(b)	31.	(c)	32.	(a)
33.	(d)	34.	(b)	35.	(b)	36.	(c)	37.	(d)	38.	T	39.	T	40.	(?)
41.	F	42.	(b)	43.	(c)	44.	(d)	45.	(a)	46.	(a)	47.	(c)	48.	(b)
49.	(c)	50.	(c)	51.	(c)	52.	(c)	53.	(a)	54.	(a)	55.	(b)	56.	(c)
57.	(a)	58.	(c)	59.	(d)	60.	(c)	61.	(b)	62.	(a)	63.	(b)	64.	(a)
65.	(d)	66.	(a)	67.	(c)	68.	(a)	69.	(c)	70.	(a)	71.	(a)	72.	(c)
73.	(d)	74.	(d)	75.	(a)	76.	(c)	77.	(d)	78.	(a)	79.	(c)	80.	(b)
81.	TFTTF	82.	TTTTF	83.	FFTFT	84.	TFTTT	85.	T?TTT	86.	FTTFT	87.	TFTTT	88.	TFTTT
89.	FFFTT	90.	FTFFT	91.	TTFTT	92.	FFTFT	93.	TFFTF	94.	FFTFT	95.	FTTFT	96.	FTTFT
97.	TFFTT	98.	TFFFT	99.	TTTTF	100.	TTFFT	101.	TFTTF	102.	TFTTF	103.	TTFTT	104.	TTFTF
105.	TFFFT	106.	FFTFT	107.	FFTF	108.	TTFT	109.	TFFTF	110.	TTTT	111.	FTTTF	112.	FTTTF
113.	FFFTF	114.	TTTFT	115.	TTFTT	116.	FTTTT	117.	TFFT	118.	TTFFF	119.	TFFFF	120.	TTT
121.	TFTFT	122.	FTTTT	123.	FTTTT	124.	(d)	125.	(b)	126.	(b)	127.	(c)	128.	(b)
129.	(d)	130.	(c)	131.	(b)	132.	(b)	133.	(b)	134.	(a)	135.	(d)	136.	(b)
137.	(b)	138.	(b)	139.	(b)	140.	(a)	141.	(a)	142.	(c)	143.	(a)	144.	(d)
145.	(a)	146.	(c)	147.	(a)	148.	(d)	149.	(c)	150.	(c)	151.	(b)	152.	(d)
153.	(a)	154.	(b)	155.	(a)	156.	(b)	157.	(a)	158.	(b)	159.	(a)	160.	(a)
161.	(d)	162.	(a)	163.	(d)	164.	(b)	165.	(c)	166.	(a)	167.	(d)	168.	(d)
169.	(d)	170.	(a)	171.	(b)	172.	(c)	173.	(a)	174.	(a)	175.	(b)	176.	(c)
177.	(b)	178.	(a,b)	179.	(d)	180.	(d)	181.	(b)	182.	(b)	183.	(c)	184.	(d)
185.	(a)	186.	(b)	187.	(a)	188.	(d)	189.	(a)	190.	(b)	191.	(c)	192.	(b)
193.	(c)	194.	(c)	195.	(d)	196.	TTTT	197.	(a)	198.	(a)	199.	(a)	200.	(d)
201.	(c)	202.	(a)	203.	(d)	204.	(b)	205.	(c)	206.	(d)	207.	(d)	208.	(a)
209.	(a)	210.	(a,c)	211.	(a)	212.	(d)	213.	(c)	214.	(c)	215.	(c)	216.	(b)
217.	(a)	218.	(d)	219.	(d)	220.	(a,b)	221.	(b)	222.	(b)	223.	(b)	224.	(b)
225.	(b)	226.	(c)	227.	(a)	228.	(c)	229.	(c)	230.	(b)	231.	(a)	232.	(a)
233.	(c)	234.	(a)	235.	(b)	236.	(c)	237.	(a)	238.	(b)	239.	(a)	240.	(a)
241.	(a)	242.	(c)	243.	(c)	244.	(d)	245.	(a)	246.	(b)	247.	(a)	248.	(d)
249.	(c)	250.	(a)	251.	(a)	252.	(a)	253.	(a)	254.	(b)	255.	(a)	256.	(b)
257.	(b)	258.	(d)	259.	(b)	260.	(b)	261.	(d)	262.	(b)	263.	(c)	264.	(a)
265.	(b)	266.	(c)	267.	(a)	268.	(d)	269.	(a)	270.	(a)	271.	(a)	272.	(b)
273.	(b)	274.	(c)	275.	(c)	276.	(b)	277.	(a)	278.	(b)	279.	(a)	280.	(a)
281.	(b)	282.	(a)	283.	(b)	284.	(a)	285.	(a)	286.	(a)	287.	(a)	288.	(a)
289.	(b)	290.	(d)	291.	(a)	292.	(b)	293.	(c)	294.	(a)	295.	(b)	296.	(d)
297.	(a)	298.	(c)	299.	(c)	300.	(a)	301.	(c)	302.	(b)	303.	(a)	304.	(a)
305.	(b)	306.	(a)	307.	(a)	308.	(a)	309.	(b)	310.	(e)	311.	(a)	312.	(a)

313.	(a)	314.	(a)	315.	(a)	316.	(a)	317.	(a)	318.	(a)	319.	(d)	320.	(b)
321.	(c)	322.	(a)	323.	(b)	324.	(b)	325.	(a)	326.	(a)	327.	(a)	328.	(a)
329.	(b)	330.	(c,d)	331.	(a)	332.	(b)	333.	(d)	334.	(a)	335.	(a)	336.	(b)
337.	(a)	338.	(a)	339.	(a)	340.	(a)	341.	(a)	342.	(a)	343.	(a)	344.	(a)
345.	(b)	346.	(b)	347.	(a)	348.	(a)	349.	(a)	350.	(c)	351.	(b)	352.	(a)
353.	(c)	354.	(a)	355.	(a)	356.	(c)	357.	(a)	358.	(c)	359.	(a)	360.	(a)
361.	(b)	362.	(a)	363.	(d)	364.	(a)	365.	(d)	366.	(a)	367.	(a)	368.	(a)
369.	(a)	370.	(a)	371.	(a)	372.	(a)	373.	(a)	374.	(a)	375.	(b)	376.	(a)
377.	(d)	378.	(a)	379.	(a)	380.	(a)	381.	(a)	382.	(d)	383.	(b)	384.	(c)
385.	(b)	386.	(a)	387.	(b)	388.	(c)	389.	(c)	390.	(c)	391.	(d)	392.	(b)
393.	(a)	394.	(d)	395.	(a)	396.	(b)	397.	(a)	398.	(a)	399.	(c)	400.	(c)
401.	(a)	402.	(a)	403.	(a)	404.	(a)	405.	(b)	406.	(d)	407.	(c)	408.	(c)
409.	(c)	410.	(c)	411.	(a)	412.	(b)	413.	(e)	414.	(a)	415.	(a)	416.	(a)
417.	(b)	418.	(a)	419.	(a)	420.	(e)	421.	(b)	422.	(a)	423.	(a)	424.	(a)
425.	(d)	426.	(a)	427.	(b)	428.	(a)	429.	(a)	430.	(a)	431.	(a)	432.	(a)
433.	(b)	434.	(b)	435.	(b)	436.	(a)	437.	(c)	438.	(a)	439.	(a)	440.	(a)
441.	(c)	442.	(a)	443.	(a)	444.	(a)	445.	(a)	446.	(a)	447.	(a)	448.	(b)
449.	(a)	450.	(a)	451.	(a)	452.	(a)	453.	(a)	454.	(c)	455.	(a)	456.	(a)
457.	(a)	458.	(a)	459.	(a)	460.	(a)	461.	(a)	462.	(a)	463.	(a)	464.	(a)
465.	(a)	466.	(a)	467.	(c)	468.	(a)	469.	(d)	470.	(a)	471.	(c)	472.	(a)
473.	(b)	474.	(a)	475.	(a)	476.	(b)	477.	(c)	478.	(c)	479.	(a)	480.	(b)
481.	(b)	482.	(b)	483.	(c)	484.	(d)	485.	(a)	486.	(c)	487.	(b)	488.	(b)
489.	(c)	490.	TTFT	491.	FFT	492.	(a)	493.	(c)	494.	(a)	495.	(d)	496.	(a)
497.	(a)	498.	(a)	499.	(c)	500.	(a)	501.	(a)	502.	(c)	503.	(a)	504.	(b)
505.	(d)	506.	(a)	507.	(a)	508.	(c)	509.	(a)	510.	(a)	511.	(a)	512.	(b)
513.	(a)	514.	(a)	515.	(a,d)	516.	(c)	517.	(a)	518.	(a)	519.	(a)	520.	(a)
521.	(b)	522.	(a)	523.	(a)	524.	(d)	525.	(a)	526.	(d)	527.	(c)	528.	(c)
529.	(a)	530.	(a)	531.	(a)	532.	(b)	533.	(d)	534.	(c)	535.	(b)	536.	(b)
537.	(a)	538.	(b)	539.	(c)	540.	(a)	541.	(a)	542.	(b)	543.	(b)	544.	(a)
545.	(b)	546.	(a)	547.	(a)	548.	(c)	549.	(a)	550.	(b)	551.	(b)	552.	(a)
553.	(d)	554.	(a)	555.	(d)	556.	(a)	557.	(c)	558.	(c)	559.	(c)	560.	(b)
561.	(b)	562.	(a)	563.	(a)	564.	(b)	565.	(b)	566.	(a)	567.	(a)	568.	(a)
569.	(b)	570.	(b)	571.	(a)	572.	(d)	573.	(a)	574.	(d)	575.	(c)	576.	(a)
577.	(d)	578.	(a)	579.	(a)	580.	(c)	581.	(a)	582.	(c)	583.	(d)	584.	(c)
585.	(a)	586.	(a)	587.	(b)	588.	(d)	589.	(d)	590.	(b)	591.	(d)	592.	(b)
593.	(d)	594.	(a)	595.	(a)	596.	(b)	597.	(b)	598.	(c)	599.	(b)	600.	(c)
601.	(a)	602.	(d)	603.	(a)	604.	(a)	605.	(c)	606.	(d)	607.	(d)	608.	(d)
609.	(d)	610.	(c)	611.	(b)	612.	(c)	613.	(a)	614.	(b)	615.	(d)	616.	(c)
617.	(c)	618.	(c)	619.	(d)	620.	(c)	621.	(a)	622.	(c)	623.	(d)	624.	(a)
625.	(a)	626.	(b)	627.	(a)	628.	(c)	629.	(b)	630.	(a)	631.	(b)	632.	(a)
633.	(c)	634.	(d)	635.	(a)	636.	(c)	637.	(b)	638.	(c)	639.	(a)	640.	(b)
641.	(c)	642.	(b)	643.	(a)	644.	(a)	645.	(b)	646.	(a)	647.	(b)	648.	(d)
649.	(a)	650.	(b)	651.	(c)	652.	(a)	653.	(d)	654.	(a)	655.	(a)	656.	(b)

657. (d)	658. (a)	659. (c)	660. (a)	661. (b)	662. (a)	663. (a)	664. (c)
665. (a)	666. (c)	667. (c)	668. (a)	669. (a)	670. (a)	671. (a)	672. (c)
673. (c)	674. (a)	675. (b)	676. (a)	677. (a)	678. (a)	679. (a)	680. (a)
681. (a)	682. (a)	683. (a)	684. (a)	685. (b)	686. (a)	687. (c)	688. (b)
689. (a)	690. (a)	691. (b)	692. (a)	693. (c)	694. (a)	695. (a)	696. (a)
697. (a)	698. (c)	699. (d)	700. (b)	701. (a)	702. (a)	703. (d)	704. (b)
705. (b)	706. (a)	707. (a)	708. (b)	709. (a)	710. (a)	711. (d)	712. (b)
713. (a)	714. (b)	715. (a)	716. (a)	717. (a)	718. (a)	719. (c)	720. (a)
721. (b)	722. (c)	723. (b)	724. (d)	725. (a)	726. (a)	727. (d)	728. (b)
729. (b)	730. (d)	731. (a)	732. (b)	733. (a)	734. (d)	735. (a)	736. (d)
737. (a)	738. (b)	739. (b)	740. (a)	741. (a)	742. (a)	743. (a)	744. (c)
745. (a)	746. (b)	747. (a)	748. (a)	749. (a)	750. (b)	751. (d)	752. (c)
753. (a)	754. (c)	755. (d)	756. (b)	757. (a)	758. (b)	759. (a)	760. (a)
761. (c)	762. (a)	763. (a)	764. (a)	765. (a)	766. (b)	767. (c)	768. (d)
769. (b)	770. (a)	771. (c)	772. (a)	773. (c)	774. (b)	775. (a)	776. (a)
777. (a)	778. (a)	779. (c)	780. (c)	781. (b)	782. (d)	783. (b)	784. (d)
785. (a)	786. (c)	787. (a)	788. (c)	789. (a)	790. (a)	791. (a)	792. (b)
793. (c)	794. (c)	795. (b)	796. (d)	797. (c)	798. (b)	799. (b)	800. (a)
801. (a)	802. (b)	803. (a)	804. (a)	805. (b)	806. (a)	807. (b)	808. (a)
809. (c)	810. (a)	811. (d)	812. (c)	813. (d)	814. (a)	815. (a)	816. (b)
817. (d)	818. (d)	819. (b)	820. (a)	821. (c)	822. (a)	823. (d)	824. (a)
825. (b)	826. (a)	827. (a)	828. (a)	829. (a)	830. (b)	831. (d)	832. (a)
833. (a)	834. (c)	835. (a)	836. (c)	837. (b)	838. (b)	839. (d)	840. (c)
841. (d)	842. (a)	843. (b)	844. (d)	845. (c)	846. (b)	847. (d)	848. (a)
849. (b)	850. (b)	851. (a)	852. (c)	853. (a)	854. (a)	855. (a)	856. (b)
857. (a)	858. (d)	859. (a)	860. (c)	861. (a)	862. (a)	863. (a)	864. (b)
865. (a)	866. (a)	867. (b)	868. (b)	869. (a)	870. (b)	871. (c)	872. (b)
873. (a)	874. (b)	875. (a)	876. (a)	877. (a)	878. (a)	879. (b)	880. (a)
881. (c)	882. (b)	883. (a)	884. (a)	885. (a)	886. (a)	887. (b)	888. (b)
889. (a)	890. (b)	891. (a)	892. (a)	893. (d)	894. (b)	895. (a)	896. (a)
897. (a)	898. (a)	899. (c)	900. (a)	901. (d)	902. (c)	903. (a)	904. (a)
905. (a)	906. (a)	907. (a)	908. (a)	909. (b)	910. (a)	911. (a)	912. (b)
913. (a)	914. (b)	915. (a)	916. (a)	917. (a)	918. (d)	919. (d)	920. (d)
921. (a)	922. (a)	923. (a)	924. (d)	925. (b)	926. (a)	927. (b)	928. (b)
929. (d)	930. (a)	931. (c)	932. (c)	933. (b)	934. (b)	935. (c)	936. (b)
937. (c)	938. (b)	939. (b)	940. (a)	941. (d)	942. (c)	943. (d)	944. (d)
945. (a)	946. (a)	947. (a)	948. (d)	949. (c)	950. (a)	951. (c)	952. (a)
953. (c)	954. (a)	955. (a)	956. (a)	957. (a)	958. (a)	959. (b)	960. (b)
961. (b)	962. (d)	963. (a)	964. (c)	965. (a)	966. (d)	967. (a)	968. (b)
969. (a)	970. (c)	971. (c)	972. (b)	973. (c)	974. (a)	975. (c)	976. (c)
977. (d)	978. (d)	979. (b)	980. (c)	981. (b)	982. (d)	983. (a)	984. (a)
985. (b)	986. (a)	987. (c)	988. (a)	989. (c)	990. (d)	991. (b)	992. (c)
993. (d)	994. (b)	995. (b)	996. (a)	997. (d)	998. (b)	999. (a)	1000. (a)
1001. (a)	1002. (c)	1003. (a)	1004. (d)	1005. (d)	1006. (b)	1007. (b)	1008. (c)
1009. (c)	1010. (a)	1011. (a)	1012. (a)	1013. (a)	1014. (b)	1015. (a)	1016. (b)
1017. (c)	1018. (d)	1019. (d)	1020. (a)	1021. (c)	1022. (c)	1023. (c)	1024. (d)

1025.	(c)	1026.	(d)	1027.	(d)	1028.	(a)	1029.	(a)	1030.	(b)	1031.	(a)
1032.	(a)	1033.	(b,c)	1034.	(a)	1035.	(b)	1036.	(a)	1037.	(c)	1038.	(b)
1039.	(b)	1040.	(c)	1041.	(c)	1042.	(a)	1043.	(b)	1044.	(c)	1045.	(a)
1046.	(a)	1047.	(c)	1048.	(b)	1049.	(b)	1050.	(a)	1051.	(c)	1052.	(b)
1053.	(b)	1054	(a)	1055.	(a)	1056.	(a)	1057.	(a)	1058.	(b)	1059.	(a)
1060.	(a)	1061.	(a)	1062.	(a)	1063.	(d)	1064.	(d)	1065.	(b)	1066.	(c)
1067.	(a)	1068.	(a)	1069.	(a)	1070.	(a)	1071.	(c)	1072.	(c)	1073.	(a)
1074.	(a)	1075.	(a)	1076.	(b)	1077.	(c)	1078.	(d)	1079.	(c)	1080.	(c)
1081.	(c)	1082.	(a)	1083.	(b)	1084.	(b)	1085.	(a)	1086.	(d)	1087.	(a)
1088.	(a)	1089.	(a)	1090.	(b)	1091.	(c)	1092.	(a)	1093.	(b)	1094.	(c)
1095.	(e)	1096.	(b)	1097.	(c)	1098.	(a)	1099.	(b,c)	1100.	(a)	1101.	(a)
1102.	(a)	1103.	(a)	1104.	(b)	1105.	(a)	1106.	(a)	1107.	(c)	1108.	(a)
1109.	(c)	1110.	(a)	1111.	(d)	1112.	(a)	1113.	(c)	1114.	(b)	1115.	(c)
1116.	(a)	1117.	(d)	1118.	(c)	1119.	(d)	1120.	(c)	1121.	(b)	1122.	(b)
1123.	(a)	1124.	(d)	1125.	(a)	1126.	(d)	1127.	(b)	1128.	(b)	1129.	(d)
1130.	(c)	1131.	(d)	1132.	(d)	1133.	(d)	1134.	(d)	1135.	(c)	1136.	(d)
1137.	(a)	1138.	(d)	1139.	(c)	1140.	(b)	1141.	(c)	1142.	(c)	1143.	(c)
1144.	(d)	1145.	(c)	1146.	(d)	1147.	(c)	1148.	(b)	1149.	(d)	1150.	(d)
1151.	(c)	1152.	(d)	1153.	(a)	1154.	(a)	1155.	(a)	1156.	(d)	1157.	(b)
1158.	(d)	1159.	(d)	1160.	(c)	1161.	(c)	1162.	(d)	1163.	(b)	1164.	(a)
1165.	(a)	1166.	(b)	1167.	(b)	1168.	(d)	1169.	(a)	1170.	(d)	1171.	(a)
1172.	(a)	1173.	(b)	1174.	(c)	1175.	(c)	1176.	(c)	1177.	(c)	1178.	(a)
1179.	(d)	1180.	(b)	1181.	(d)	1182.	(b)	1183.	(a)	1184.	(c)	1185.	(d)
1186.	(a)	1187.	(a)	1188.	(b)	1189.	(b)	1190.	(d)	1191.	(b)	1192.	(a)
1193.	(a)	1194.	(a)	1195.	(c)	1196.	(d)	1197.	(d)	1198.	(c)	1199.	(d)
1200.	(d)	1201.	(d)	1202.	(b)	1203.	(a)	1204.	(c)	1205.	(a)	1206.	(a)
1207.	(d)	1208.	(d)	1209.	(b)	1210.	(c)	1211.	(b)	1212.	(b)	1213.	(a)
1214.	(a)	1215.	(a)	1216.	(d)	1217.	(c)	1218.	(a)	1219.	(b)	1220.	(a)
1221.	(c)	1222.	(b)	1223.	(d)	1224.	(d)	1225.	(a)	1226.	(a)	1227.	(d)
1228.	(a)	1229.	(d)	1230.	(c)	1231.	(d)	1232.	(d)	1233.	(a)	1234.	(b)
1235.	(b)	1236.	(b)	1237.	(a)	1238.	(d)	1239.	(c)	1240.	(d)	1241.	(c)
1242.	(d)	1243.	(c)	1244.	(d)	1245.	(a)	1246.	(d)	1247.	(a)	1248.	(c)
1249.	(d)	1250.	(c)	1251.	(c)	1252.	(b)	1253.	(b)	1254.	(c)	1255.	(a)
1256.	(a)	1257.	(b)	1258.	(d)	1259.	(a)	1260.	(c)	1261.	(a)	1262.	(d)
1263.	(d)	1264.	(a)	1265.	(a)	1266.	(a)	1267.	(d)	1268.	(b)	1269.	(b)
1270.	(c)	1271.	(d)	1272.	(a)	1273.	(c)	1274.	(b)	1275.	(c)	1276.	(b)
1277.	(b)	1278.	(d)	1279.	(a)	1280.	(a)	1281.	(c)	1282.	(b)	1283.	(a)
1284.	(d)	1285.	(a)	1286.	(a)	1287.	(b)	1288.	(c)	1289.	(b)	1290.	(a)
1291.	(b)	1292.	(d)	1293.	(b)	1294.	(b)	1295.	(b)	1296.	(a)	1297.	(c)
1298.	(d)	1299.	(a)	1300.	(a)	1301.	(a)	1302.	(b)	1303.	(b)	1304.	(c)
1305.	(c)	1306.	(b)	1307.	(b)	1308.	(a)	1309.	(b)	1310.	(d)	1311.	(a)
1312.	(b)	1313.	(d)	1314.	(c)	1315.	(b)	1316.	(d)	1317.	(a)	1318.	(b)
1319.	(b)	1320.	(a)	1321.	(a)	1322.	(b)	1323.	(a)	1324.	(a)	1325.	(b)
1326.	(b)	1327.	(d)	1328.	(b)	1329.	(b)	1330.	(b)	1331.	(c)	1332.	(b)
1333.	(c)	1334	(c)	1335.	(d)	1336.	(a)	1337.	(d)	1338.	(a)	1339.	(a)
1340.	(d)	1341.	(b)	1342.	(b)	1343.	(c)	1344.	(a)	1345.	(a)	1346.	(d)
1347.	(a)	1348.	(a)	1349.	(a)	1350.	(a)	1351.	(d)	1352.	(a)	1353.	(a)

1354. (a)	1355. (a)	1356. (c)	1357. FTTTT	1358. FTTFF	1359. (a)	1360. (d)
1361. (a)	1362. (a)	1363. (b)	1364. (c)	1365. (d)	1366. (a)	1367. (c)
1368. (d)	1369. (d)	1370. (a)	1371. (b)	1372. (d)	1373. (c)	1374. (a)
1375. (b)	1376. (c)	1377. (d)	1378. (a)	1379. (b)	1380. (b)	1381. (d)
1382. (a)	1383. (c)	1384. (d)	1385. (a)	1386. (c)	1387. (b)	1388. (d)
1389. (a)	1390. (c)	1391. (d)	1392. (b)	1393. (b)	1394. (c)	1395. (b)
1396. (c)	1397. (d)	1398. (a)	1399. (a)	1400. (c)	1401. (b)	1402. (a)
1403. (c)	1404. (a)	1405. (d)	1406. TFFF	1407. (?)	1408. (b)	1409. (b)
1410. (a)	1411. (a)	1412. (c)	1413. (b)	1414. (a)	1415. (b)	1416. (c)
1417. (b)	1418. (b)	1419. (b)	1420. (b)	1421. (c)	1422. (d)	1423. (a)
1424. (d)	1425. (b)	1426. (a)	1427. (d)	1428. (d)	1429. (a)	1430. (d)
1431. (b)	1432. (b)	1433. (a)	1434. (c)	1435. (b)	1436. (b)	1437. (a)
1438. (d)	1439. (c)	1440. (a)	1441. (a)	1442. (a)	1443. (c)	1444. (b)
1445. (a)	1446. (b)	1447. (b)	1448. (a)	1449. (c)	1450. (a)	1451. (d)
1452. (c)	1453. (a)	1454. (a)	1455. (c)	1456. (c)	1457. (a)	1458. (a)
1459. (c)	1460. (c)	1461. (b)	1462. (c)	1463. (a)	1464. (a)	1465. (b)
1466. (a)	1467. (a)	1468. (c)	1469. (d)	1470. (b)	1471. (b)	1472. (c)
1473. (a)	1474. (c)	1475. (a)	1476. (b)	1477. (c)	1478. (a)	1479. (b)
1480. (d)	1481. (d)	1482. (d)	1483. (d)	1484. (b)	1485. (a)	1486. (a)
1487. (a)	1488. (a)	1489. (c)	1490. (a)	1491. (c)	1492. (c)	1493. (c)
1494. (a)	1495. (b)	1496. (e)	1497. (e)	1498. (d)	1499. (a)	1500. (a)
1501. (a)	1502. (c)	1503. (b)	1504. (b)	1505. (b)	1506. (a)	1507. (b)
1508. (a)	1509. (a)	1510. (a)	1511. (d)	1512. (b)	1513. (c)	1514. (c)
1515. (d)	1516. (b)	1517. (b)	1518. (b)	1519. (c)	1520. (d)	1521. (a)
1522. (a)	1523. (b)	1524. (a)	1525. (a)	1526. (d)	1527. (a)	1528. (a)
1529. (d)	1530. (b)	1531. (a)	1532. (d)	1533. (a)	1534. (d)	1535. (c)
1536. (a)	1537. (b)	1538. (a)	1539. (a)	1540. (a)	1541. (b)	1542. (a)
1543. (b)	1544. (d)	1545. (b)	1546. (d)	1547. (b)	1548. (b)	1549. (c)
1550. (d)	1551. (a)	1552. (a)	1553. (a)	1554. (c)	1555. (a)	1556. (c)
1557. (d)	1558. (c)	1559. (d)	1560. (c)	1561. (d)	1562. (a)	1563. (d)
1564. (b)	1565. (c)	1566. (b)	1567. (b)	1568. (c)	1569. (a)	1570. (b)
1571. (a)	1572. (d)	1573. (a)	1574. (a)	1575. (d)	1576. (a)	1577. (a)
1578. FTTT	1579. (a)	1580. (a)	1581. (d)	1582. (d)	1583. (b)	1584. (a)
1585. (a)	1586. (b)	1587. (a)	1588. (c)	1589. (a)	1590. (b)	1591. (b)
1592. (a)	1593. (d)	1594. (a)	1595. (a)	1596. (b)	1597. (b)	1598. (a)
1599. (b)	1600. (a)	1601. (d)	1602. (a)	1603. (b)	1604. (a)	1605. (a)
1606. (b)	1607. (a)	1608. (a)	1609. (b)	1610. (a)	1611. (a)	1612. (d)
1613. (c)	1614. (c)	1615. (a)	1616. (b)	1617. (c)	1618. (a)	1619. (d)
1620. (d)	1621. (c)	1622. (b)	1623. (c)	1624. (?)	1625. (b)	1626. (d)
1627. (b)	1628. (a)	1629. (a)	1630. (b)	1631. (a)	1632. (b)	1633. (c)
1634. (b)	1635. (c)	1636. (c)	1637. (a)	1638. (a)	1639. (d)	1640. (a)
1641. (a)	1642. (b)	1643. (a)	1644. (a)	1645 (b)	1646. (a)	1647. (b)
1648. (b)	1649. (c)	1650. (c)	1651. (b)	1652. (c)	1653. (c)	1654. (d)
1655. (a)	1656. (a)	1657. (d)	1658. (a)	1659. (c)	1660. (c)	1661. (a)
1662. (a)	1663. (d)	1664. (a)	1665. (a)	1666. (c)	1667. (a)	1668. (a)
1669. (c)	1670. (a)	1671. (d)	1672. (c)	1673. (a)	1674. (c)	1675. (c)
1676. (d)	1677. (d)	1678. (c)	1679. (a)	1680. (d)	1681. (a)	1682. (b)

1683. (a)	1684. (c)	1685. (a)	1686. (a)	1687. (c)	1688. (d)	1689. (b)
1690. (c)	1691. (b)	1692. (a)	1693. (c)	1694. (a)	1695. (a)	1696. (c)
1697. (d)	1698. (a)	1699. (d)	1700. (c)	1701. (b)	1702. (d)	1703. (b)
1704. (d)	1705. (a)	1706. (a)	1707. (a)	1708. (c)	1709 (b)	1710. (d)
1711. (c)	1712. (b)	1713. (b)	1714. (d)	1715. (d)	1716. (b)	1717. (b)
1718. (c)	1719. (b)	1720. (d)	1721. (c)	1722. (b)	1723. (d)	1724. (c)
1725. (a)	1726. (d)	1727. (b)	1728. (a)	1729. (b)	1730. (c)	1731. (b)
1732. (a)	1733. (b)	1734. (a)	1735. (a)	1736. (a)	1737. (b)	1738. (b)
1739. (a)	1740. (d)	1741. (d)	1742. (c)	1743. (b)	1744. (c)	1745. (d)
1746. (c)	1747. (d)	1748. (a)	1749. (b)	1750. (b)	1751. (b)	1752. (b)
1753. (a)	1754. (a)	1755. (a)	1756. (a)	1757. (a)	1758. (d)	1759. (a)
1760. (a)	1761. (b)	1762. (a)	1763. (c)	1764. (d)	1765. (b)	1766. (a)
1767. (c)	1768. (b)	1769. (c)	1770. (a)	1771. (a)	1772. (a)	1773. (d)
1774. (a)	1775. (b)	1776. (d)	1777. (b)	1778. (b)	1779. (c)	1780. (b)
1781. (c)	1782. (c)	1783. (c)	1784. (b)	1785. (a)	1786. (d)	1787. (a)
1788. (b)	1789. (a)	1790. (a)	1791. (a)	1792. (b)	1793. (d)	1794. (d)
1795. (a)	1796. (d)	1797. (a)	1798. (b)	1799. (b)	1800. (a)	1801. (a)
1802. (a)	1803. (a)	1804. (b)	1805. (a)	1806. (a)	1807. (a)	1808. (a)
1809. (b)	1810. (d)	1811. (a)	1812. (c)	1813. (d)	1814. (a)	1815. (c)
1816. (c)	1817. (a)	1818. (a)	1819. (a)	1820. (a)	1821. (a)	1822. (a)
1823. (b)	1824. (a)	1825. (c)	1826. (a)	1827. (b)	1828. (b)	1829. (c)
1830. (c)	1831. (c)	1832. (a)	1833. (c)	1834. (d)	1835. (a)	1836. (b)
1837. (a)	1838. (c)	1839. (a)	1840. (a)	1841. (a)	1842. (d)	1843. (b)
1844. (c)	1845. (a)	1846. (a)	1847. (b)	1848. (a)	1849. (b)	1850. (a)
1851. (b)	1852. (a)	1853. (a)	1854. (a)	1855. (c)	1856. (c)	1857. (b)
1858. (b)	1859. (a)	1860. (a)	1861. (d)	1862. (c)	1863. (a)	1864. (a)
1865. (a)	1866. (d)	1867. (b)	1868. (b)	1869. (a)	1870. (c)	1871. (b)
1872. (a)	1873. (a)	1874. (a)	1875. (b)	1876. (a)	1877. (a)	1878. (a)
1879. (c)	1880. (a)	1881. (a)	1882. (a)	1883. (d)	1884. (d)	1885. (a)
1886. (a)	1887. (c)	1888. (b)	1889. (a)	1890. (a)	1891. (b)	1892. (a)
1893. (a)	1894. (b)	1895. (a)	1896. (a)	1897. (a)	1898. (c)	1899. (d)
1900. (a)	1901. (b)	1902. (d)	1903. (a)	1904. (a)	1905. (b)	1906. (c)
1907. (c)	1908. (a)	1909. (c)	1910. (a)	1911. (a)	1912. (a)	1913. (d)
1914. (a)	1915. (c)	1916. (a)	1917. (a)	1918. (d)	1919. (a)	1920. (c)
1921. (a)	1922. (a)	1923. (d)	1924. (a)	1925. (a)	1926. (a)	1927. (d)
1928. (b)	1929. (d)	1930. (a)	1931. (d)	1932. (a)	1933. (c)	1934. (d)
1935. (a)	1936. (c)	1937. (a)	1938. (c)	1939. (c)	1940. (a)	1941. (a)
1942. (a)	1943. (a)	1944. (b)	1945. (d)	1946. (c)	1947. (a)	1948. (a)
1949. (b)	1950. (b)	1951. (a)	1952. (a)	1953. (a)	1954. (a)	1955. (a)
1956. (a)	1957. (c)	1958. (a)	1959. (c)	1960. (a)	1961. (b)	1962. (d)
1963. (c)	1964. (b)	1965. (b)	1966. (b)	1967. (b)	1968. (b)	1969. (d)
1970. (c)	1971. (c)	1972. (a)	1973. (c)	1974. (c)	1975. (c)	1976. (a)
1977. (d)	1978. (b)	1979. (a)	1980. (d)	1981. (d)	1982. (a)	1983. (b)
1984. (a)	1985. (b)	1986. (a)	1987. (b)	1988. (a)	1989. (b)	1990. (b)
1991. (a)	1992. (a)	1993. (d)	1994. (a)	1995. (a)	1996. (d)	1997. (a)
1998. (d)	1999. (d)	2000. (a)	2001. (c)	2002. (b)	2003. (c)	2004. (a)
2005. (a)	2006. (a)	2007. (a)	2008. (b)	2009. (c)	2010. (d)	2011. (d)
2012. (a)	2013. (d)	2014. (a)	2015. (a)	2016. (a)	2017. (d)	2018. (a)

2019.	(b)	2020.	(b)	2021.	(a)	2022.	(a)	2023.	(a)	2024.	(c)	2025.	(c)
2026.	(b)	2027.	(d)	2028.	(a)	2029.	(a)	2030.	(b)	2031.	(b)	2032.	(c)
2033.	(a)	2034.	(a)	2035.	(d)	2036.	(b)	2037.	(b)	2038.	(c)	2039.	(a)
2040.	(b)	2041.	(b)	2042.	(a)	2043.	(a)	2044.	(d)	2045.	(a)	2046.	(b)
2047.	(a)	2048.	(a)	2049.	(a)	2050.	(a)	2051.	(c)	2052.	(a)	2053.	(d)
2054.	(c)	2055.	(d)	2056.	(b)	2057.	(b)	2058.	(a)	2059.	(c)	2060.	(d)
2061.	(c)	2062.	(a)	2063.	(b)	2064.	(a)	2065.	(a)	2066.	(d)	2067.	(b)
2068.	(a)	2069.	(b)	2070.	(b)	2071.	(a)	2072.	(a)	2073.	(b)	2074.	(a)
2075.	(b)	2076.	(b)	2077.	(a)	2078.	(b)	2079.	(a)	2080.	(a)	2081.	(b)
2082.	(a)	2083.	TTTTT	2084.	TTTTF	2085.	TFFTF	2086.	FFTTT	2087.	FTFTF	2088.	T?FFT
2089.	TFFTF	2090.	TTTT	2091.	TFTTT	2092.	TTFTT	2093.	TTFFT	2094.	TTTTT	2095.	TFTFT
2096.	TTTT	2097.	TTTFF	2098.	TTTT	2099.	TTTT	2100.	???	2101.	TT	2102.	TTF
2103.	TTTT	2104.	(b)	2105.	FTFTT	2106.	TFTTT	2107.	TTTTT	2108.	TTTTF	2109.	FTFF
2110.	(d)	2111.	(c)	2112.	(b)	2113.	(a)	2114.	(b)	2115.	(c)	2116.	(a)
2117.	(a)	2118.	(c)	2119.	(b)	2120.	(a)	2121.	(a)	2122.	(b)	2123.	(b)
2124.	(d)	2125.	(b)	2126.	(a)	2127.	(c)	2128.	(a)	2129.	(a)	2130.	(c)
2131.	(a)	2132.	(c)	2133.	(a)	2134.	(a)	2135.	(a)	2136.	(c)	2137.	(a)
2138.	(c)	2139.	(a)	2140.	(a)	2141.	(a)	2142.	(c)	2143.	(a)	2144.	(b)
2145.	(c)	2146.	(a)	2147.	(b)	2148.	(c)	2149.	(c)	2150.	(c)	2151.	(d)
2152.	(a, b)	2153.	(d)	2154.	(d)	2155.	(d)	2156.	(b)	2157.	(a)	2158.	(d)
2159.	(b)	2160.	(a)	2161.	(e)	2162.	(a)	2163.	(a)	2164.	(b)	2165.	(d)
2166.	(b)	2167.	(a)	2168.	(a)	2169.	(d)	2170.	(c)	2171.	(a)	2172.	(d)
2173.	(b)	2174.	(a)	2175.	(a)	2176.	(d)	2177.	(a)	2178.	(c)	2179.	(b)
2180.	(d)	2181.	(b)	2182.	(d)	2183.	(b)	2184.	(a)	2185.	(a)	2186.	(a)
2187.	(d)	2188.	(a)	2189.	(a)	2190.	(d)	2191.	(c)	2192.	(c)	2193.	(c)
2194.	(a)	2195.	(d)	2196.	(b)	2197.	(c)	2198.	(b)	2199.	(d)	2200.	(d)
2201.	(b)	2202.	(a)	2203.	(a)	2204.	(b)	2205.	(a)	2206.	(a)	2207.	(d)
2208.	(d)	2209.	(a)	2210.	(c)	2211.	(c)	2212.	(a)	2213.	(c)	2214.	(b)
2215.	(a)	2216.	(a)	2217.	(b)	2218.	(c)	2219.	(b)	2220.	(a)	2221.	(d)
2222.	(c)	2223.	(b)	2224.	(a)	2225.	(d)	2226.	(c)	2227.	(b)	2228.	(c)
2229.	(a)	2230.	(d)	2231.	(a)	2232.	(d)	2233.	(a)	2234.	(a)	2235.	(c)
2236.	(c)	2237.	(a)	2238.	(d)	2239.	(a)	2240.	(d)	2241.	(a)	2242.	(b)
2243.	(b)	2244.	(b)	2245.	(a)	2246.	(b)	2247.	(a,c)	2248.	(a)	2249.	(a)
2250.	(b)	2251.	(a)	2252.	(a)	2253.	(d)	2254.	(b)	2255.	(b)	2256.	(b)
2257.	(a)	2258.	(a)	2259.	(a)	2260.	(a)	2261.	(a)	2262.	(b)	2263.	(a)
2264.	(b)	2265.	(c)	2266.	(c)	2267.	(e)	2268.	(d)	2269.	(a)	2270.	(d)
2271.	(a)	2272.	(a)	2273.	(d)	2274.	(d)	2275.	(c)	2276.	(c)	2277.	(b)
2278.	(a)	2279.	(c)	2280.	(c)	2281.	(b)	2282.	(b)	2283.	(b)	2284.	(a)
2285.	(a)	2286.	(d)	2287.	(a)	2288.	(b)	2289.	(c)	2290.	(d)	2291.	(b)
2292.	(a)	2293.	(c)	2294.	(d)	2295.	(a)	2296.	(c)	2297.	(c)	2298.	(b)
2299.	(b)	2300.	(a)	2301.	(a)	2302.	(a)	2303.	(d)	2304.	(d)	2305.	(a)
2306.	(a)	2307.	(a)	2308.	(b)	2309.	(a)	2310.	(a)	2311.	(b)	2312.	(b)
2313.	(c)	2314.	(c)	2315.	(c)	2316.	(c)	2317.	(b)	2318.	(b)	2319.	(c)
2320.	(e)	2321.	(a)	2322.	(a)	2323.	(c)	2324.	(a)	2325.	(d)	2326.	(d)
2327.	(d)	2328.	(a)	2329.	(b)	2330.	(a)	2331.	(b)	2332.	(a)	2333.	(a)
2334.	(b)	2335.	(a)	2336.	(c)	2337.	(?)	2338.	(b)	2339.	(c)	2340.	(b)
2341.	(d)	2342.	(c)	2343.	(a)	2344.	(b)	2345.	(c)	2346.	(d)	2347.	(d)
2348.	(a)	2349.	(a)	2350.	(d)	2351.	(b)	2352.	(a)	2353.	(d)	2354.	(a)

2355. (d)	2356. (a)	2357. (a)	2358. (e)	2359. (a)	2360. (c)	2361. (d)
2362. (c)	2363. (a)	2364. (d)	2365. (a)	2366. (a)	2367. (a)	2368. (d)
2369. (c)	2370. (b)	2371. (b)	2372. (b)	2373. (b)	2374. (b)	2375. (c)
2376. (b)	2377. (b)	2378. (d)	2379. (d)	2380. (b)	2381. (a)	2382. (a)
2383. (a)	2384. (a)	2385. (a)	2386. (a)	2387. (c)	2388. (a)	2389. (b)
2390. (c)	2391. (b)	2392. (a)	2393. (a)	2394. (d)	2395. (d)	2396. (a)
2397. (d)	2398. (c)	2399. (c)	2400. (d)	2401. (a)	2402. (b)	2403. (a)
2404. (d)	2405. (a)	2406. (a)	2407. (a)	2408. (d)	2409. (c)	2410. (b)
2411. (b)	2412. (b)	2413. (b)	2414. (b)	2415. (c)	2416. (d)	2417. (b)
2418. (d)	2419. (d)	2420. (b)	2421. (a)	2422. (a)	2423. (a)	2424. (a)
2425. (a)	2426. (a)	2427. (c)	2428. (a)	2429. (b)	2430. (d)	2431. (b)
2432. (a)	2433. (a)	2434. (d)	2435. (a)	2436. (a)	2437. (a)	2438. (c)
2439. (c)	2440. (d)	2441. (a)	2442. (a)	2443. (c)	2444. (a)	2445. (a)
2446. (a)	2447. (b)	2448. (a)	2449. (a)	2450. (b)	2451. (a)	2452. (b)
2453. (b)	2454. (c)	2455. (a)	2456. (a)	2457. (d)	2458. (d)	2459. (c)
2460. (b)	2461. (b)	2462. (a)	2463. (a)	2464. (a)	2465. (c)	2466. (d)
2467. (a)	2468. (c)	2469. (b)	2470. (b)	2471. (a)	2472. (b)	2473. (a)
2474. (c)	2475. (a)	2476. (b)	2477. (e)	2478. (b)	2479. (?)	2480. (b)
2481. (c)	2482. (b)	2483. (d)	2484. (a)	2485. (b)	2486. (a)	2487. (b)
2488. (a)	2489. (c)	2490. (c)	2491. (a)	2492. (a)	2493. (a)	2494. (a)
2495. (a)	2496. (c)	2497. (d)	2498. (a)	2499. (d)	2500. (a)	2501. (b)
2502. (a)	2503. (b)	2504. (c)	2505. (b)	2506. (a)	2507. (b)	2508. (b)
2509. (b)	2510. (d)	2511. (d)	2512. (c)	2513. (d)	2514. (d)	2515. (b)
2516. (a)	2517. (a)	2518. (b)	2519. (a)	2520. (a)	2521. (a)	2522. (d)
2523. (a)	2524. (b)	2525. (b)	2526. (b)	2527. (a)	2528. (b)	2529. (b)
2530. (a)	2531. (b)	2532. (d)	2533. (c)	2534. (a)	2535. (c)	2536. (c)
2537. (c)	2538. (c)	2539. (a)	2540. (d)	2541. (d)	2542. (b)	2543. (a)
2544. (a)	2545. (a)	2546. (c)	2547. (a)	2548. (b)	2549. (b)	2550. (b)
2551. (a)	2552. (a)	2553. (a)	2554. (a)	2555. (a)	2556. (c)	2557. (b)
2558. (d)	2559. (a)	2560. (c)	2561. (b)	2562. (a)	2563. (d)	2564. (a)
2565. (b)	2566. (b)	2567. (c)	2568. (d)	2569. (d)	2570. (b)	2571. (a)
2572. (d)	2573. (a)	2574. (a)	2575. (d)	2576. (a)	2577. (a)	2578. (d)
2579. (a)	2580. (a)	2581. (d)	2582. (c)	2583. (a)	2584. (c)	2585. (d)
2586. (d)	2587. (b)	2588. (a)	2589. (a)	2590. (c)	2591. (a)	2592. (b)
2593. (a)	2594. (a)	2595. (a)	2596. (a)	2597. (c)	2598. (a)	2599. (a)
2600. (a)	2601. (a)	2602. (a)	2603. (a)	2604. (d)	2605. (a)	2606. (a)
2607. (d)	2608. (b)	2609. (c)	2610. (c)	2611. (a)	2612. (d)	2613. (c)
2614. (a)	2615. (c)	2616. (b)	2617. (c)	2618. (b)	2619. (a)	2620. (c)
2621. (d)	2622. (b)	2623. (b)	2624. (a)	2625. (a)	2626. (d)	2627. (c)
2628. (a)	2629. (a)	2630. (a)	2631. (a)	2632. (b)	2633. (b)	2634. (b)
2635. (a)	2636. (a)	2637. (a)	2638. (a)	2639. (b)	2640. (d)	2641. (a)
2642. (a)	2643. (d)	2644. (a)	2645. (a)	2646. (a)	2647. (d)	2648. (c)
2649. (a)	2650. (c)	2651. (a)	2652. (a)	2653. (b)	2654. (a)	2655. (a)
2656. (a)	2657. (b)	2658. (b,c)	2659. (a)	2660. (a)	2661. (b)	2662. (d)
2663. (a)	2664. (c)	2665. (c)	2666. (d)	2667. (b)	2668. (a)	2669. (a)
2670. (a)	2671. (a)	2672. (a)	2673. (a)	2674. (b)	2675. (b)	2676. (a)
2677. (a)	2678. (d)	2679. (c)	2680. (a)	2681. (b)	2682. (b)	2683. (a)
2684. (c)	2685. (a)	2686. (b)	2687. (c)	2688. (a)	2689. (a)	2690. (a)

2691. (a)	2692. (a)	2693. (c)	2694. (c)	2695. (a)	2696. (d)	2697. (b)
2698. (a)	2699. (a)	2700. (a)	2701. (a)	2702. (a)	2703. (c)	2704. (a)
2705. (d)	2706. (a)	2707. (b)	2708. (a)	2709. (a)	2710. (d)	2711. (c)
2712. (b)	2713. (b)	2714. (b)	2715. (d)	2716. (a)	2717. (c)	2718. (b)
2719. (c)	2720. (a)	2721. (c)	2722. (a)	2723. (b)	2724. (a)	2725. (d)
2726. (a)	2727. (b)	2728. (c)	2729. (c)	2730. (d)	2731. (a)	2732. (b)
2733. (e)	2734. (c)	2735. (a)	2736. (b)	2737. (a)	2738. (a)	2739. (b)
2740. (d)	2741. (e)	2742. (a)	2743. (d)	2744. (a)	2745. (a)	2746. (b)
2747. (a)	2748. (c)	2749. (e)	2750. (b)	2751. (a)	2752. (e)	2753. (d)
2754. (a)	2755. (a)	2756. (a)	2757. (a)	2758. (c)	2759. (a)	2760. (b)
2761. (a)	2762. (a)	2763. (a)	2764. (d)	2765. (a)	2766. (c)	2767. (d)
2768. (d)	2769. (a)	2770. (c)	2771. (d)	2772. (a)	2773. (c)	2774. (d)
2775. (c)	2776. (a)	2777. T	2778. F	2779. T	2780. (a)	2781. (c)
2782. (a)	2783. (a)	2784. (b)	2785. (b)	2786. (a)	2787. (d)	2788. (b)
2789. (d)	2790. (c)	2791. (b)	2792. (b)	2793. (a)	2794. (c)	2795. (c)
2796. (b)	2797. (a)	2798. (b)	2799. (b)	2800. (a)	2801. (b)	2802. (a)
2803. (c)	2804. (b)	2805. (a)	2806. (c)	2807. (a)	2808. (a)	2809. (c)
2810. (a)	2811. (d)	2812. (a)	2813. (c)	2814. (b)	2815. (a)	2816. (a)
2817. (b)	2818. (a)	2819. (d)	2820. (a)	2821. (a)	2822. (a)	2823. (b)
2824. (b)	2825. (b)	2826. (a)	2827. (a)	2828. (c)	2829. (b)	2830. (b)
2831. (c)	2832. (b)	2833. (b)	2834. (d)	2835. (d)	2836. (b)	2837. (a)
2838. (a)	2839. (d)	2840. (b)	2841. (b)	2842. (a)	2843. (a)	2844. (a)
2845. (d)	2846. (a)	2847. (a)	2848. (a)	2849. (a)	2850. (d)	2851. (d)
2852. (b)	2853. (a)	2854. (c)	2855. (d)	2856. (d)	2857. (c)	2858. (b)
2859. (a)	2860. (d)	2861. (a)	2862. (b)	2863. (c)	2864. (a)	2865. (d)
2866. (c)	2867. (c)	2868. (d)	2869. (a)	2870. (b)	2871. (a)	2872. (d)
2873. (a)	2874. (c)	2875. (b)	2876. (b)	2877. (b)	2878. (d)	2879. (c)
2880. (d)	2881. (b)	2882. (c)	2883. (b)	2884. (a)	2885. (b)	2886. (a)
2887. (c)	2888. (c)	2889. (c)	2890. (a)	2891. (a)	2892. (b)	2893. (c)
2894. (c)	2895. (d)	2896. (a)	2897. (b)	2898. (d)	2899. (a)	2900. (d)
2901. (a)	2902. (a)	2903. (d)	2904. (c)	2905. (d)	2906. (c)	2907. (d)
2908. (a)	2909. (d)	2910. (a)	2911. (c)	2912. (d)	2913. (b)	2914. (a)
2915. (d)	2916. (a)	2917. (a)	2918. (d)	2919. (d)	2920. (c)	2921. (c)
2922. (b)	2923. (a)	2924. (a)	2925. (a)	2926. (a)	2927. (d)	2928. (c)
2929. (d)	2930. (d)	2931. (a)	2932. (a)	2933. (a)	2934. (c)	2935. (b)
2936. (a)	2937. (a)	2938. (c)	2939. (d)	2940. (c)	2941. (a)	2942. (a)
2943. (a)	2944. (a)	2945. (a)	2946. (c)	2947. (d)	2948. (c)	2949. (a)
2950. (a)	2951. (a)	2952. (b)	2953. (c)	2954. (d)	2955. (a)	2956. (c)
2957. (b)	2958. (d)	2959. (d)	2960. (b)	2961. (b)	2962. (a)	2963. (a)
2964. (b)	2965. (d)	2966. (c)	2967. (a)	2968. (a)	2969. (a)	2970. (d)
2971. (a)	2972. (b)	2973. (a)	2974. (a)	2975. (a)	2976. (b)	2977. (d)
2978. (a)	2979. (a)	2980. (b)	2981. (c)	2982. (b)	2983. (a)	2984. (d)
2985. (a)	2986. (a)	2987. (d)	2988. (b)	2989. (a)	2990. (a)	2991. (c)
2992. (c)	2993. (b)	2994. (b)	2995. (a)	2996. (c)	2997. (a)	2998. (c)
2999. (d)	3000. (b)	3001. (b)	3002. (a)	3003. (c)	3004. (b)	3005. (b)
3006. (d)	3007. (b)	3008. (b)	3009. (a)	3010. (c)	3011. (b)	3012. (a)
3013. (b)	3014. (c)	3015. (a)	3016. (a)	3017. (b)	3018. (d)	3019. (d)
3020. (b)	3021. (c)	3022. (c)	3023. (c)	3024. (c)	3025. (a)	3026. (b)

3027. (b)	3028. (c)	3029. (c)	3030. (d)	3031. (b)	3032. (a)	3033. (c)
3034. (b)	3035. (d)	3036. (a)	3037. (a)	3038. (b)	3039. (a)	3040. (a)
3041. (a)	3042. (a)	3043. (b)	3044. (a)	3045. (a)	3046. (b)	3047. (d)
3048. (b)	3049. (a)	3050. (c)	3051. (c)	3052. (b)	3053. (b)	3054. (a)
3055. (a)	3056. (c)	3057. (b)	3058. (a)	3059. (b)	3060. (a)	3061. (d)
3062. (b)	3063. (a)	3064. (c)	3065. (c)	3066. (c)	3067. (b)	3068. (a)
3069. (a)	3070. (a)	3071. (c)	3072. (c)	3073. (a)	3074. (a)	3075. (a)
3076. (c)	3077. (a)	3078. (d)	3079. (a)	3080. (a)	3081. (a)	3082. (a)
3083. (c)	3084. (b)	3085. (d)	3086. (b)	3087. (a)	3088. (a)	3089. (c)
3090. (b)	3091. (a)	3092. (c)	3093. (c)	3094. (a)	3095. (a)	3096. (c)
3097. (b)	3098. (b)	3099. (a)	3100. (c)	3101. (a)	3102. (a)	3103. (b)
3104. (a)	3105. (a)	3106. (a)	3107. (a)	3108. (b)	3109. (a)	3110. (b)
3111. (b)	3112. (a)	3113. (a)	3114. (a)	3115. (b)	3116. (a)	3117. (b)
3118. (c)	3119. (c)	3120. (b)	3121. (c)	3122. (a)	3123. (c)	3124. (b)
3125. (a)	3126. (b)	3127. (d)	3128. (b)	3129. (a)	3130. (a)	3131. (a)
3132. (b)	3133. (a)	3134. (a)	3135. (a)	3136. (a)	3137. (d)	3138. (d)
3139. (a)	3140. (c)	3141. (a)	3142. (b)	3143. (a)	3144. (b)	3145. (b)
3146. (b)	3147. (a)	3148. (a)	3149. (a)	3150. (a)	3151. (a)	3152. (b)
3153. (a)	3154 (a)	3155. (a)	3156. (a)	3157. (a)	3158. (a)	3159. (a)
3160. (a)	3161. (a)	3162. (a)	3163. (a)	3164. (a)	3165. (a)	3166. (a)
3167. (c)	3168. (c)	3169. (d)	3170. (b)	3171. (c)	3172. (b)	3173. (a)
3174. (a)	3175. (b)	3176. (b)	3177. (b)	3178. (b)	3179. (a)	3180. (b)
3181. (a)	3182. (b)	3183. (b)	3184. (d)	3185. (d)	3186. (d)	3187. (d)
3188. (d)	3189. (c)	3190. (d)	3191. (b)	3192. (a)	3193. (c)	3194. (d)
3195. (d)	3196. (c)	3197. (c)	3198. (d)	3199. (b)	3200. (a)	3201. (d)
3202. (b)	3203. (a)	3204. (a)	3205. (d)	3206. (d)	3207. (b)	3208. (d)
3209. (a)	3210. (b)	3211. (c)	3212. (a)	3213. (a)	3214. (d)	3215. (b)
3216. (c)	3217. (d)	3218. (d)	3219. (b)	3220. (d)	3221. (d)	3222. (c)
3223. (c)	3224. (a)	3225. (a)	3226. (c)	3227. (b)	3228. (c)	3229. (a)
3230. (c)	3231. (c)	3232. (d)	3233. (a)	3234. (b)	3235. (a)	3236. (c)
3237. (c)	3238. (b)	3239. (a)	3240. (c)	3241. (a)	3242. (c)	3243. (b)
3244. (b)	3245. (c)	3246. (b)	3247. (a)	3248. (a)	3249. (b)	3250. (d)
3251. (d)	3252. (b)	3253. (a)	3254. (b)	3255. (a)	3256. (d)	3257. (a)
3258. (d)	3259. (b)	3260. (b)	3261. (d)	3262. (b)	3263. TTFT	3264. (b)
3265. (b)	3266. (a)	3267. (b)	3268. (b)	3269. (a)	3270. (b)	3271. (d)
3272. (a)	3273. (a)	3274. (c)	3275. (b)	3276. (a)	3277. (c)	3278. (a)
3279. (a)	3280. (b)	3281. (a)	3282. (d)	3283. (b)	3284. (d)	3285. (c)
3286. (c)	3287. (b)	3288. (c)	3289. (c)	3290. (d)	3291. (d)	3292. (d)
3293. (d)	3294. (b)	3295. (a)	3296. (d)	3297. (d)	3298. (d)	3299. (d)
3300. (b)	3301. (b)	3302. (c)	3303. (d)	3304. (c)	3305. (d)	3306. (c)
3307. (b)	3308. (d)	3309. (d)	3310. (c)	3311. (c)	3312. (b)	3313. (a)
3314. (b)	3315. (d)	3316. (a)	3317. (d)	3318. (b)	3319. (b)	3320. (a)
3321. (b)	3322. (b)	3323. (c)	3324. (d)	3325. (a)	3326. (b)	3327. (d)
3328. (a)	3329. (b)	3330. (c)	3331. (d)	3332. (a)	3333. (c)	3334. (d)
3335. (c)	3336. (a)	3337. (a)	3338. (a)	3339. (a)	3340. (c)	3341. (c)
3342. (c)	3343. (c)	3344. (d)	3345. (a)	3346. (d)	3347. (d)	3348. (d)
3349. (a)	3350. (d)	3351. (c)	3352. (a)	3353. (c)	3354. (a)	3355. (a)
3356. (c)	3357. (d)	3358. (d)	3359. (c)	3360. (c)	3361. (a,c,d,e)	3362. (b,c)
3363. (a,b,d)	3364. (a,b)	3365. (a,d,e)	3366. (d)	3367. (b)	3368. (b)	3369. (a)

3370. (c)	3371. (d)	3372. (b)	3373. (a)	3374. (b)	3375. (c)	3376. (d)
3377. (a)	3378. (a)	3379. (b)	3380. (c)	3381. (d)	3382. (a)	3383. (c)
3384. (c)	3385. (b)	3386. (b)	3387. (d)	3388. (b)	3389. (a)	3390. (c)
3391. (b)	3392. (a)	3393. (c)	3394. (a)	3395. (b)	3396. (d)	3397. (a)
3398. (b)	3399. (b)	3400. (b)	3401. (a)	3402. (d)	3403. (b)	3404. (b)
3405. (d)	3406. (b)	3407. (b)	3408. (d)	3409. (c)	3410. (a)	3411. (a)
3412. (a)	3413. (d)	3414. (a)	3415. (d)	3416. (c)	3417. (a)	3418. (c)
3419. (b)	3420. (a)	3421. (c)	3422. (c)	3423. (a)	3424. (b)	3425. (b)
3426. (c)	3427. (a)	3428. (a)	3429. (a)	3430. (c)	3431. (d)	3432. (b)
3433. (c)	3434. (d)	3435. (b)	3436. (a)	3437. (c)	3438. (d)	3439. (c)
3440. (d)	3441. (d)	3442. (b)	3443. (d)	3444. (d)	3445. (d)	3446. (d)
3447. (a)	3448. (d)	3449. (a)	3450. (a)	3451. (b)	3452. (a)	3453. (d)
3454. (d)	3455. (a)	3456. (c)	3457. (d)	3458. (d)	3459. (a)	3460. (d)
3461. (c)	3462. (a)	3463. (b)	3464. (a)	3465. (b)	3466. (b)	3467. (b)
3468. (a)	3469. (a)	3470. (b)	3471. (a)	3472. (a)	3473. (a)	3474. (d)
3475. (b)	3476. (a)	3477. (d)	3478. (c)	3479. (b)	3480. (d)	3481. (a)
3482. (a)	3483. (b)	3484. (a)	3485. (b)	3486. (a)	3487. (d)	3488. (a)
3489. (d)	3490. (b)	3491. (c)	3492. (c)	3493. (a)	3494. (a)	3495. (b)
3496. (?)	3497. (a)	3498. (a)	3499. (a)	3500. (?)	3501. (c)	3502. (d)
3503. (d)	3504. (c)	3505. (b)	3506. (a)	3507. (c)	3508. (d)	3509. (d)
3510. (d)	3511. (a)	3512. (d)	3513. (c)	3514. (b)	3515. (a)	3516. (b)
3517. (b)	3518. (d)	3519. (a)	3520. (b)	3521. (a)	3522. (b)	3523. (a)
3524. (d)	3525. (c)	3526. (c)	3527. (a)	3528. (a)	3529. (a)	3530. (b)
3531. (b)	3532. (a)	3533. (b)	3534. (b)	3535. (a)	3536. (c)	3537. (d)
3538. (b)	3539. (c)	3540. (a)	3541. (b)	3542. (c)	3543. (b)	3544. (a)
3545. (c)	3546. (c)	3547. (d)	3548. (c)	3549. (a)	3550. (d)	3551. (d)
3552. (d)	3553. (c)	3554. (a)	3555. (a)	3556. (a)	3557. (a)	3558. (d)
3559. (a)	3560. (d)	3561. (d)	3562. (a)	3563. (c)	3564. (a)	3565. (b)
3566. (a)	3567. (b)	3568. (a)	3569. (b)	3570. (b)	3571. (a)	3572. (b)
3573. (c)	3574. (d)	3575. (b)	3576. (c)	3577. (b)	3578. (a)	3579. (a)
3580. (a)	3581. (d)	3582. (b)	3583. (a)	3584. (b)	3585. (a)	3586. (a)
3587. (a)	3588. (d)	3589. (a)	3590. (a)	3591. (c)	3592. (a)	3593. (c)
3594. (d)	3595. (a)	3596. (a)	3597. (a)	3598. (a)	3599. (a)	3600. (b)
3601. (a)	3602. (b)	3603. (c)	3604. (a)	3605. (a)	3606. (c)	3607. (a)
3608. (b)	3609. (c)	3610. (a)	3611. (a)	3612. (c)	3613. (c)	3614. (c)
3615. (a)	3616. (c)	3617. (d)	3618. (b)	3619. (b)	3620. (a)	3621. (a)
3622. (c)	3623. (c)	3624. (b)	3625. (c)	3626. (d)	3627. (d)	3628. (a)
3629. (b)	3630. (a)	3631. (c)	3632. (b)	3633. (b)	3634. (b)	3635. (a)
3636. (d)	3637. (a)	3638. (b)	3639. (c)	3640. (a)	3641. (c)	3642. (c)
3643. (a)	3644. (b)	3645. (b)	3646. (a)	3647. (b)	3648. (d)	3649. (b)
3650. (a)	3651. (b)	3652. (a)	3653. (b)	3654. (a)	3655. (d)	3656. (b)
3657. (c)	3658. (a)	3659. (d)	3660. (c)	3661. (a)	3662. (c)	3663. (d)
3664. (c)	3665. (c)	3666. (d)	3667. (c)	3668. (a)	3669. (d)	3670. (a)
3671. (b)	3672. (c)	3673. (b)	3674. (d)	3675. (b)	3676. (c)	3677. (d)
3678. (c)	3679. (a)	3680. (c)	3681. (a)	3682. (b)	3683. (c)	3684. (b)
3685. (b)	3686. (a)	3687. (a)	3688. (b)	3689. (b)	3690. (a)	3691. (c)
3692. (c)	3693. (a)	3694. (c)	3695. (c)	3696. (a)	3697. (c)	3698. (d)
3699. (b)	3700. (c)	3701. (a)	3702. (d)	3703. (b)	3704. (a)	3705. (b)

3706. (c)	3707. (b)	3708. (d)	3709. (a)	3710. (a)	3711. (a)	3712. (c)
3713. (b)	3714. (b)	3715. (a)	3716. (c)	3717. (b)	3718. (c)	3719. (b)
3720. (b)	3721. (a)	3722. (d)	3723. (a)	3724. (b)	3725. (a)	3726. (a)
3727. (a)	3728. (a)	3729. (a)	3730. (c)	3731. (b)	3732. (b)	3733. (d)
3734. (a)	3735. (b)	3736. (c)	3737. (c)	3738. (d)	3739. (c)	3740. (b)
3741. (c)	3742. (a)	3743. (c)	3744. (b)	3745. (c)	3746. (d)	3747. (a)
3748. (c)	3749. (c)	3750. (c)	3751. (b)	3752. (a)	3753. (a)	3754. (b)
3755. (c)	3756. (c)	3757. (d)	3758. (b)	3759. (a)	3760. (a)	3761. (c)
3762. (d)	3763. (a)	3764. (b)	3765. (d)	3766. (a)	3767. (a)	3768. (a)
3769. (c)	3770. (d)	3771. (c)	3772. (b)	3773. (c)	3774. (a)	3775. (c)
3776. (d)	3777. (d)	3778. (c)	3779. (d)	3780. (a)	3781. (b)	3782. (a)
3783. (d)	3784. (a)	3785. (d)	3786. (b)	3787. (b)	3788. (c)	3789. (a)
3790. (a)	3791. (b)	3792. (c)	3793. (b)	3794. (d)	3795. (b)	3796. (b)
3797. (c)	3798. (a)	3799. (b)	3800. (d)	3801. (b)	3802. (b)	3803. (c)
3804. (b)	3805. (b)	3806. (c)	3807. (d)	3808. (d)	3809. (a)	3810. (d)
3811. (a)	3812. (b)	3813. (a)	3814. (b)	3815. (c)	3816. (c)	3817. (a)
3818. (c)						

CHAPTER ELEVEN

MISCELLANEOUS

1. **Angiogram showing LAD and RCA aneurysm in 5 years old child after 5 months of fever and skin rash:**
   (a) Methotrexate (b) Aspirin
   (c) Steroid (d) IFN α

2. **ECG—showing bidirectional VT A/E:**
   (a) Long QT (b) Digoxin
   (c) Anderson syndrome (d) Aconite

3. **CXR showing pneumothorax after PPI, clinical feature:**
   (a) Syncope (b) Dyspnoea
   (c) Anemia

4. **ECG showing wide QRS tachycardia true:**
   (a) Anteroseptal MI
   (b) Left accessory pathway
   (c) Ectopic atrial tachycardia
   (d) Balhasen's syndrome

5. **ECG showing STEIWMI with CHB true:**
   (a) IWMI with block (b) Brugada

6. **Lead in RA-CXR:**
   (a) Ryle tube dislocation (b) CVP dislocated
   (c) PPI (d) Artifact

7. **PFT- FEV1/FVC- 88%, DLCO- 38%:**
   (a) Asthma
   (b) COPD with emphysema
   (c) Restrictive lung physiology

8. **LV angiography Figure:**
   (a) AV canal defect
   (b) HOCM
   (c) LV diverticulum

9. **Lung scan true:**
   (a) Normal
   (b) Breast artifact
   (c) Goodpasture syndrome
   (d) PTE

10. **Pressure cath data: LV- aorta:**
    (a) HOCM (b) Severe AS
    (c) Apical ballooning (d) AS + AR

11. **Figure showing external cardiac defibrillator. Who invented it?**
    (a) Microski (b) Grossmann

12. **Dextrocardia + situs inversus in infertility true**
    (a) AD (b) Recurrent sinusitis
    (c) Increased risk of congenital heart disease

13. **Epsilon wave on ECG. Next Investigation of choice:**
    (a) EPS (b) MRI
    (c) Perfusion scanning (d) Provocative testing

14. **Extended matching:**
    (a) Pheochromocytoma (b) COA
    (c) RAS (d) Atherosclerosis
    (e) Mineralocorticoid excess
    (1) Spironolactone responsive
    (2) 34 years adult with normal routine checkup at 1 month back, presents with sweating and episode of palpitations
    (3) Upper limb BP higher than lower limb BP
    (4) 70 years male presents with HTN
    (5) Patient of HTN on diuretics, beta blockers and CCB with creatinine–1.1 mg%, after adding enalapril 2.6 mg% in a week

Extended matching:

Options (a) pulmonary pruning (b) widening of carina (c) water fall (d) egg on side (e) snow man (f) oligemic lung fields (g) shimtes (h) ↑ PBF (i) flask shaped. (15-19)

15. **30 years old postpartum women BP–Normal, HR–100, edema and dyspnea.**

16. **2 years old cyanotic mild cyanosis right infraclavicular continuous murmur, tachypnea, tachycardia, feeding difficulties.**

17. **Young male JVP ↑, fever with dyspnea, BP–80 mm Hg, pulse–120/min, Heart sounds distant.**

18. **7-year-old child recurrent chest infection with continuous murmur in left ICS.**

19. **34 years female DOE, fatique, syncope.**

Extended matching:

Options: (a) unstable angina (b) prinz metal angina (c) walking through angina (d) atypical chest pain (e) post MI angina (f) angina equivalent (g) CCS I (h) CCS II (i) CCS III (j) CCCS IV. (20-24)

20. **36 years female with Raynaud phenomenon recurrent chest pain, on Holter ST ↑ II, III, Avf at 3 AM.**

21. **2 months prior MI with chest pain (new onset).**

22. **1 year back MI, pain on walking for 5 minutes but could not walk for 40 minutes.**

23. **Truck driver chest pain on lifting rice rack.**

24. **40 years old smoker had chest pain on walking 2 flights of stairs.**

Extended matching–AF:

(a) Vernakalant (b) Dronedone (c) Dabigatran (d) Pacemaker (e) Pacemaker with b blocker (f) AFFIRM study (g) DC shock (h) I.V. digoxin (i) I.V. dilzem. (25-29)

25. **Rate control is equivalent to rhythm control.**

26. **Cardioversion, patient not willing for DC shock.**

27. **HTN, DM, LV dysfunction drug to be given.**

28. **Recurrent syncope, on Holter HR > 180 bpn and intermittent pauses > 4 sec treatment.**

29. **Drug not be given in severe LV dysfunction:**

Case series–Cath data

RA-18 mmHg, PA-100/48, mean 63 mm Hg, RV-100/18 mm Hg, PCWP-9, Cardiac index- 2 l/min/m²

Extended matching:

Options: (a) RSOV (b) PS (c) hypertrophic subaortic stenosis (d) PDA (e) MR (f) ASD (g) AR. (30-34)

30. **Continuous murmur, peaking at 2nd heart sound.**

31. **Continuous murmur ↑ in diastole grade VI.**

32. **ESM extending after A2.**

33. **EDM.**

34. **↑ murmur ESM on valsalva**

35. **Look ahead trial:**

(a) ASA no role in idiopathic DCMP
(b) In DM, weight loss and diet not helpful
(c) In CKD, ASA not helpful without CVD
(d) In DM without CAD, ASA helpful

4 hours chest pain, ↑ JVP, clear lung field, shock. (36-38)

36. **Diagnosis:**

(a) RVMI (b) IWMI

37. **Management:**

(a) Fluid (b) Thrombolysis
(c) PCI

38. **Artery involved:**

(a) Prox RCA (b) LCx
(c) LAD

39. **Prolonged episode of AF terminated by cardioversion:**

(a) Pure (b) Prolonged
(c) Paroxysmal (d) Persistent

40. **Diagnosis:**

(a) RVMI (b) IWMI

41. **Management:**

(a) Fluid (b) Thrombolysis
(c) PCI

42. **Artery involved:**

(a) Prox RCA (b) LCx
(c) LAD

Case series–Cath data RA-18 mmHg, PA-100/48, mean 63 mm Hg, RV-100/18 mm Hg, PCWP-9 Cardiac index-2 l/min/m². (43-45)

43. **PVR index:**
 (a) 27 (b) 37
 (c) 47

44. **Transpulmonary gradient is:**
 (a) 54 (b) 60
 (c) 64

45. **Likely diagnosis:**
 (a) ASD (b) VSD
 (c) PDA (d) Veno occlusive disease
 (e) PPH

46. *Extended matching - Rheumatic fever:*
 Options: chorea, subcutaneous nodule, erythema marginatum, polyarthritis, carditis, low grade carditis, acute phase reactants, fever. (46-47)
 (a) 1992 Jone's criterna revision added chorea and______
 (b) Earliest manifestation which is variable in severity and self limiting
 (c) Most specific finding
 (d) Feature corelate with carditis (moderate to severe) appears within weeks and disappear by 1-2 months
 (e) Correlate with disease activity

47. **Admixture physiology:**
 (a) Tricuspid atresia (b) TOF
 (c) Ebstein's anomaly (d) Truncus arteriosus

Extended matching–AF

Options–(a) Vernakalent (b) Dronedarone (c) Dabigatran (d) Pacemaker (e) Pacemaker with beta blocker (f) AFFIRM study (g) DC shock (h) I/V digoxin (i) I/V dilzem. (48-52)

48. **Rate control is equivalent to rhythm control.**

49. **Cardioversion, patient not willing for DC shock.**

50. **HTN, DM, LV dysfunction drug to be given.**

51. **Recurrent syncope on Holter HR> 180/min and intermittent pauses > 4 secs treatment.**

52. **Drug not to be given in severe LV dysfunction.**

Extended matching–55 years old male diabetic with 4 hours chest pain and come to emergency:

Options: (a) Dual antiplatelet (b) Clopidogrel without aspirin (c) High dose statin (d) Standard statin dose (e) Primary PCI (f) Thrombolysis (g) haemorrhage stroke (h) Ischemic stroke. (53-56)

53. **Initial treatment.**

54. **Absolute C/I for thrombolysis.**

55. **Drugs to be given for first year minimum even if no intervention done or not.**

56. **Loading dose after initial investigation to be given.**

Extended matching:

Options: (a) AR (b) MVP (c) HOCM (d) Supra valvular AS (e) Valvular AS. (57-62)

57. **40 years males with PS systolic murmur in second IC space radiating to carotids.**

58. **Double peaking with radiation to left 3rd and 4th ICS.**

59. **Paget's disease with another murmur at apex.**

60. **Multiple clicks with murmur with apex.**

61. **Thrill with radiation only to carotids with BP difference in two arms.**

62. **Pulsus parvus et tardus with thrill in carotids.**

63. **Criteria for LVH all** ***except:***
 (a) Skolon (b) Cornell
 (c) Tablott (d) Bazzett
 (e) Romhilt

64. **Claudication at 100 metres:**
 (a) Fontan IIa (b) IIb
 (c) III (d) I

Case series–45 years old male, 1 month fever with gradual onset BLN, pansystolic apical murmur (3/6), absent left radial and right dorsal pedis, cardiomegaly present.

65. **Diagnosis:**
 (a) SABE (b) Takayasu
 (c) Buerger

66. **Common organism:**
 (a) Strept viridans (b) G A streptococci
 (c) Fungi (d) HACEK

67. **Most common additional finding:**
(a) Massive splenomegaly
(b) Microscopic hematuria
(c) Proteinuria

68. **Management:**
(a) 3 cultures with empirical cefazolin + amikacin at high fever
(b) 3 cultures irrespective of fever with Crystalline Penicillin + gentamicin
(c) Steroid + antibiotic

Case series–30 years with progressive dry cough and progressive breathlessness, joint pain erythema nodosum, red eye, X-ray=reticulonodular shadow with hilar LN. (69-71)

69. **Diagnosis:**
(a) Sarcoidosis (b) RA
(c) Pulmonary koch

70. **Best PFT:**
(a) FVC (b) FEV_1
(c) PEFR (d) DLCO
(e) FEV_3

71. **Additional most common finding:**
(a) Parotid enlargement
(b) Neuropathy
(c) Splenomegaly
(d) Anemia

Case series–30 years male with severe sudden chest pain maximum at onset radiating to neck and back. BP Right arm–90/70, Left–140/90, murmur of early diastolic, ST elevation in inferior and depression on ant leads. (72-74)

72. **Diagnosis:**
(a) Type-A
(b) Type-B
(c) MI
(d) Rupture of Asc. aneurysm

73. **Management:**
(a) Thrombolysis (b) Surgery
(c) Angioplasty (d) Medical

74. **Most appropriate initial investigation when patient unstable:**
(a) Aortogram (b) TTE
(c) TEE (d) CT
(e) MRI

Extended matching:

Options: (a) Sildenafil, (b) Bosentan, (c) Milrinone, (d) Epoprostenol, (e) Iloprost, (f) Vasopressin, (g) Epinephrine, (h) Lisnopril. (75-86)

75. **Methydopa.**

76. **ACE I.**

77. **Non specific ET antagonist with 125 mg BD.**

78. **Inhalational.**

79. **IV cannulation.**

80. **cGMP enhancer 20 mg TDS.**

81. **High doses of drug and waited for response:**

82. **Vasodilation with inotropy.**

83. **In shock, not effective due to depletor of NE stores.**

84. **Effective in place of epinephrine, cause vasoconstriction without tachycardia.**

85. **Used in shock and anaphylaxis, but causes B2 stimulation and hyperglycemia.**

86. **Endoyeous $\alpha 1$ agonist.**

Extended matching:

Options: (a) Atherosclerosis, (b) Cushing, (c) Addison, (d) RAS, (e) Thyrotoxicosis, (f) Pheochromocytoma, (g) Mineralocorticoid excess. (87-90)

87. **Young female on 3 antihypertensive not responding but controlled with spironolactone alone.**

88. **80 female with normal exam with bilateral osteoarthritis and BP of 220/90 mm Hg.**

89. **Young male with normal exam, suddenly ↑ in creat. from 1.2 to 2.5 on ACE I.**

90. **Young female normal 1 month back, presented with sudden palpitations, headache, raised BP.**

91. **Brugada syndrome: (T/F)**
(a) Not seen in young is SE Asian
(b) SCN5-A
(c) LBBB morphology common
(d) RBBB morphology common

92. Brugada syndrome: (T/F)
(a) Familial
(b) Common in young female
(c) Na channel late recovery defect

93. WBC in acute MI: (T/F)
(a) Peak in 2-5 days (b) Can be > 20,000
(c) Good prognostic (d) Starts in 2 hours
(e) Band forms absent

94. Primary prevention in CAD: (T/F)
(a) LDL < 160 (b) HDL > 40 in male
(c) HDL > 60 in female (d) TG < 200
(e) LP (a) < 30

95. VSR is MI: (T/F)
(a) IWMI with basoseptal better prognosis
(b) More in female
(c) Fibrinolysis increase incidence
(d) AWMI > IWMI
(e) Max in 24 hours and 3-5 days

96. Cat I for CAD: (T/F)
(a) Diabetes (b) Obesity
(c) HTN (d) Smoking
(e) Lp (a)

97. True or False:
(a) Disopyramide used in glaucoma

98. Kussmaul sign:
(a) Most common cause is RV failure
(b) Pericarditis can cause
(c) On inspiration JVP ↓

99. LVH criteria–R in I + S in III:
(a) 11 mm (b) 20 mm
(c) 25 mm (d) None of the above

100. E/A ratio diagnostic for diastolic HF according to ECS:
(a) < 1.5 (b) < 1
(c) 0.5 (d) None of the above

101. Imaging of choice in patient with LBBB:
(a) Bicycle ergometry
(b) Exercise ECG
(c) Pharmacological perfusion
(d) Exercise nuclear

102. CT Ca^{++} scoring:
(a) Low specificity
(b) Low sensitivity
(c) Additive to clinical evaluation
(d) Corelates with degree of stenosis
(e) Don't corelates with extensive atherosclerosis

Case series–Obese male BMI 32, BP-180/100, collides with tree while driving, history of recurrent automobile accidents. (103-105)

103. Diagnosis is:
(a) OSA (b) Stokes Adams

104. ECG changes/cardiac findings:
(a) RVH (b) ST ↓ V_{1-4}
(c) Sinus bradycardia with AV block

105. TOC:
(a) CPAP
(b) DDD pacemaker
(c) Weight reduction with antihypertensives including diuretics

106. ECG changes: (T/F)
(a) Hypothermia–convex J
(b) Flattening of T with U (Prominent)–hypokalemia
(c) Small QT with T wave notching–hypercalcemia
(d) T ↓ V_1-V_4 sinus tachycardia, RBBB–pulmonary embolism
(e) P-QRS-T–Alternans–pericardial effusion
(f) All are true

107. Endopeptidase inhibition:
(a) Potentiate natriuretic peptide
(b) ↓ ANP
(c) ↑es RAS
(d) None

108. Thrombolysis is acute pulmonary embolism can be done within:
(a) 2 weeks of symptom onset
(b) 2 days of symptom onset
(c) 2 hours of symptom onset
(d) Six hours of symptom onset

109. During induced polymorphic VT can be treated by:
(a) Propafenone (b) Digoxin
(c) Ventricular pacing (d) Adenosine

110. Severe coronary artery disease in stress myocardial perfusion scan is suggested by all *except*:

(a) Multiple large areas of ischemia
(b) Transient left ventricular dilatation
(c) Increased lung uptake of tracer
(d) Regional thinning in SPECT

111. Small cardiac silhouette in chest X-ray occurs in:

(a) Addison disease
(b) Conn Syndrome
(c) Hyperparathyroidism
(d) Chronic constrictive pericarditis

112. Absolute contraindication to pregnancy:

(a) Severe aortic stenosis (b) Severe AR
(c) VSD (d) ASD

113. Unequal radial pulse is caused by all *except*:

(a) Supravalvular aortic stenosis
(b) Aortoarteritis
(c) Supravalvular aortic stenosis
(d) Embolic occlusion of unilateral radial artery

114. In penetrating trauma which structure is most commonly involved?

(a) Right ventricle (b) Pulmonary
(c) Mitral valve (d) Aorta

115. In cardiac sarcoidosis, most common part involved:

(a) LV apex (b) IVS
(c) RV inflow (d) RVOT

116. True about Eprotirome:

(a) Lowers LDL level
(b) Elevates HDL Level
(c) Acts through TR a receptors
(d) It acts on intestinal mucosa

117. Which of the following is correct for U wave?

(a) Amplitude of U wave is usually more than 0.1 mv
(b) It has same polarity as the preceding T wave
(c) It is smallest in V_1, and V_2 leads
(d) It may be caused by early repolarization of purkinje fibres

118. Which of the following is false about cardiac tumor?

(a) Myxoma accounts for > than 50% of primary cardiac tumors in adults
(b) Most common valvular tumor is fibroelastoma
(c) Microscopically sporadic and familial myxoma are similar
(d) None of the above

119. ZEBRA STRIPE circumferential pattern of LGE on MRI is characteristic of:

(a) Sarcoidosis
(b) Amyloidosis
(c) Iron over cardiomyopathy
(d) ARVD

120. A wave is equal to v wave in JVP in all except:

(a) Tamponade
(b) Hypervolemia
(c) Hypovolemia
(d) Constrictive pericardial disease

121. Which is wrong about MYOCARDIAL BRIDGING?

(a) It occurs in 2-5% of the population on autopsy
(b) Usually confined to LAD artery
(c) Myocardial bridging has been associated angina, arrhythmia and, sudden cardiac death
(d) Diastolic flow abnormality may be present on Doppler study

122. Which is not true about endothelin?

(a) The three ET peptide ET-1, ET-2, and ET-3 all are strong vasoconstrictor
(b) Endothelin dysregulation can lead to different types of cancers
(c) Endothelin is primarily synthesized by cardiac myocytes
(d) ET (B) receptors are involved in release of NO and prostacyclin

123. Which combination is false?

(a) ADHERE TRIAL–Enoximone
(b) Revive-II TRIAL–Levosimendan
(c) SURVIVE TRIAL–Levosimendan
(d) Everest Trial–Tolvaptan

124. Which of the following is not a minor Framingham Criteria?

(a) Dyspnea on exertion (b) Neck vein distension
(c) Tachycardia (d) Night cough

125. Which of the following is not correct in HFpTF?

(a) More than 50% of patients with HF have HFpTF
(b) Prevalence of HF increasing with age

(c) HF syndrome much more common in female than male iin younger age
(d) Prevalence of HFpTF appears to be increasing

126. Which of the following is not a characteristic feature of TRUE aneurysm?
(a) Wide base
(b) Wall composed of myocardium
(c) High risk of rupture
(d) Low risk of rupture

127. Which of the following is ranolazine trial?
(a) MARISA (b) TERISA
(c) CARISA (d) All of the above

128. Which of the following is false for troponins?
(a) Elevated levels are associated with adverse outcome
(b) All elevations are ischemic in origin
(c) Troponin T binds to Tropomyosin, Interlocking to form Troponin Tropomyosin Complex
(d) Can be elevated in blunt chest injury

129. Thrombolytic agent with least incident of intracranial haemorrhage:
(a) STK (b) TNK
(c) TPA (d) Reteplase

130. Benefit from thrombus aspiration was seen in which trial?
(a) TASTE (b) TAPAS
(c) HORIZON AMI (d) REPLACE 2

131. Which is a false statement for Post MI free wall rupture?
(a) More common in older patients
(b) More common in hypertensive patients
(c) Usually occurs near junction of infarct and normal muscle
(d) Usually occurs in RCA territory

132. Primary PCI via radial route has shown mortality benefit over femoral route in:
(a) RIVAL Trial (b) RIFLE STEAC Trial
(c) Both (d) None

133. Angioplasty of non-infarct related artery in Primary PCI was tested in:
(a) RIFLE trial (b) RIVAL trial
(c) PACT trial (d) PRAMI trial

134. Renal angioplasty did not show benefit over medical treatment in which trial:
(a) PRAMI (b) CORAL
(c) DRASTIC (d) ISAR

135. Platelet life span is:
(a) 24 hours (b) 48-72 hours
(c) 7-10 days (d) 15-30 days

136. All of the following are primary prevention trials *except*:
(a) JUPITER (b) WOSCOPS
(c) ASCOT-LLA (d) TNT

137. Antiplatelet agent causing bradycardia is:
(a) Ticlopidine (b) Prasugrel
(c) Ticagrelor (d) Clopidogrel

138. All are used in Heart failure except:
(a) Cinaciguat (b) Ularitide
(c) Tezosentan (d) Ealectine

139. ABG: pH-7.33, pCO_2-65, HCO_3-31 suggestive of:
(a) Chronic respiratory acidosis compensated
(b) Chronic metabolic acidosis
(c) Chronic respiratory alkalosis

140. Kawasaki disease all *except*:
(a) Coronary aneurysm in 20%
(b) Steroid ineffective
(c) Pericarditis
(d) Rare in India

141. TR velocity 4 m/sec, RVSP:
(a) 64 mm Hg + RA pr (b) 85 + RAP

142. EM biopsy shows atypical lymphocytes severe necrosis, mitotic figures immunoblastic picture:
(a) Post transplant lymphoproliferative disorder
(b) Acute rejection
(c) Myocarditis
(d) Chronic carditis

143. Which of the following is considered an absolute contraindication to hyperbaric oxygen therapy?
(a) Carbon monoxide poisoning
(b) History of high altitude pulmonary edema

(c) Radiation proctitis
(d) Untreated pneumothorax

144. LV was stress peaks in:
(a) Early systole (b) Mid systole
(c) End systole (d) End diastole

145. Percutaneous intervention effective in: (T/F)
(a) Degenerative prosthetic valve
(b) AS calcific
(c) Degenerative RVOT conduit in TOF
(d) HOCM
(e) Paravalvular leak

146. Pulse: (T/F)
(a) Bisferiens–brachial
(b) Bigeminy–two peaks
(c) Alternans–regularly irregular
(d) Reverse pulsus paradoxus in HCM

147. True or false:
(a) Cannon wave seen in pacemaker syndrome
(b) Lead in coronary sinus in LV pacing

148. Stroke: (T/F)
(a) Infarct MCA–conduction aphasia
(b) Posterior cerebral A–spatial discrimination
(c) Cerebral edema common on 10th day
(d) Thrombolysis effective in 6 hours
(e) Haemorrhage maximum deficit early

149. HIV India: (T/F)
(a) 5 million
(b) 27% prevalence
(c) 7% children
(d) In pregnancy lifelong ART irrespective of CD4 count
(e) ¼ death due to TB

150. Bronchial asthma: (T/F)
(a) Nocturnal cough
(b) PEFR good for follow up
(c) Acute attack PCO_2 normal–good prognosis
(d) Reversible decrease in FEV1 and FEV1/FVC

151. Heart failure: (T/F)
(a) DOE is minor
(b) Circulation time > 2 sec–minor
(c) Same survival in HFr EF and HF p EF
(d) Ace-I improves survival

152. T/F:
(a) Penicillamine–neuropathy
(b) Cyclosporine–hypokalemia
(c) Ceftriaxone–gallstone
(d) Metronidazole–peripheral motor neuropathy
(e) Captopril–chronic cough

153. T/F:
(a) PROSPECT trial– QRS > 120 ms
(b) QRS > 150 ms – dysynchrony
(c) If QRS > 120 ms is marker of dysynchrony irrespective of EF

154. T/F:
(a) EF= EDV- ESV / ESV

155. PAD: (T/F)
(a) ABI < 0.5 – critical ischemia
(b) 10% ↓se in ABI – correlation with clinical symptoms
(c) >90% obstruction area S/O gradient
(d) ABI correlates with claudication distance and speed
(e) > 20 difference in successive cuff – S/O PAD in upper limb

156. Septal ablation: (T/F)
(a) LBBB
(b) Complete RBBB
(c) Severe LV dysfunction
(d) VSD
(e) ↑ CPK MB

157. CFR Normal valve seen in (coronary flow reserve): (T/F)
(a) 39 years old female with strong family history of CAD
(b) 58 years male with 80% prox LAD
(c) 75 years with HTN with LVH
(d) 60% mid LAD
(e) 75 for female with TVD

158. MVO_2 requirement detected by: (T/F)
(a) Contractility (b) RR interval
(c) EDP (d) LV dimension/vol
(e) Diastolic relaxation

159. Pulsus alternans: (T/F)

(a) Brachial best seen
(b) Most common in HF with MR
(c) Due to variation in recovery of myocyte function
(d) For several beats following SVT in Normal person
(e) When the respiratory rate is half the pulse rate

160. ECG: (T/F)

(a) 1901–Einthoven discovered
(b) Wilson central terminal of precordial leads – negative terminal is formed by 2 limb leads
(c) V_9- left spinal
(d) Einthoven law = 1 = II + III
(e) Augmented lead = –ve pole formed by other 2 limb leads

161. False positive perfusion stress test: (T/F)

(a) Elderly female with high likelihood
(b) Elderly male with significant disease
(c) Eldely male with single RCA > 80%
(d) Pulmonary HTN on theophylline with COPD
(e) Obese female with angina

162. True or false:

(a) Congenital left sided obstructive lesions common in females

163. RVH A/E:

(a) Ebstein anomaly (b) Mitral atresia
(c) Simple TGA (d) TAPVC

164. Malaria–CDC guidelines:

(a) Rpt smear twice in 12-24 hours
(b) Rpt rapid kit twice in 12-24 hours
(c) Rpt smear thrice 12-24 hours
(d) Rpt smear 4 times in 12-24 hours

165. Fluorosis:

(a) Inter osseos calcification
(b) Loser's zone
(c) Picture frame
(d) Ivory vertebra

166. Septic shock–definition:

(a) < hypotension
(b) Mean BP <110 after ½ hr fluid treatment but < 40 from Normal BP
(c) < 80 after 1 hour fluid treatment
(d) < 90 after 1 hour fluid treatment, MAP <70

167. Weber syndrome A/E:

(a) Ipsilateral 3rd nerve palsy
(b) Contralateral hemiplegia
(c) Dorsal midbrain
(d) Anterior cerebral peduncle

168. C-protein synthesized by:

(a) Liver (b) Spleen
(c) Thymus (d) Bone marrow

169. Parkinsonism A/E:

(a) Essential tremor
(b) Bradykinesia
(c) Loss of postural reflexes
(d) Rigidity

170. 1st gen sulphonylurea:

(a) Glibenclamide
(b) Glipizide
(c) Chlorpropamide

171. S-Genomic imprinting does not follow Mendelian rule:

R-Phenotypic expression is different when comes from mother or father (T/F)

172. Plateau phase of action potential:

(a) K+ moves out, Ca in
(b) Na/Ca moves in
(c) Na moves out
(d) Ca/K out

173. Which is false about absolute refactory period?

(a) Twice the ST segment length
(b) Time dependent in pacemaker tissue
(c) No action potential can be generated
(d) Depolarization and half of repolarization

174. Rubella A/E:

(a) Most common abnormal hearing and heart defect
(b) IgG persist > 6 months
(c) IgM at birth
(d) Most common chances of infection if infection > 16 weeks

175. Which is true in AV reentry:

(a) Type α- fast pathway

(b) Type β- slow and β has longer ERP

(c) Type α- long refractory period

(d) None

176. Scleroderma A/E:

(a) PHT

(b) Proteinuria

(c) Peripheral neuropathy

(d) Telangiectasia

177. q wave in V5-V6, I, avL with T wave inversion in 3 weeks old child irritable during breastfeeding and sweating: (T/F)

(a) ALCAPA

(b) Congenital myocarditis

(c) LV non-compaction

(d) Aorta to LV tunnel

178. Newborn with HTN A/E:

(a) COA

(b) RAS

(c) Renal parenchymal disease

(d) Bronchopulmonary dysplasia

179. A 45-year-old patient presents to medical emergency with chest pain and hypotension. CT angiography of the patient is shown below. The urgent treatment of this patient should include:

(a) Aortic root replacement

(b) Thrombolytic therapy with tenecteplase

(c) Chest tube drainage

(d) Percutaneous coronary intervention

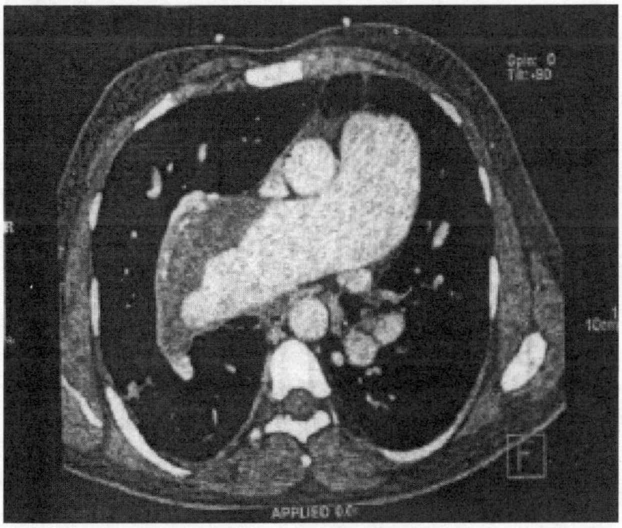

180. A 43-year-old patient presents with sudden onset palpitation and hypotension. The likely diagnosis based on the ECG as shown below is:

(a) Polymorphic ventricular tachycardia

(b) Atrial fibrillation with antidromic AVRT

(c) Persistent junctional reciprocating tachycardia (PJRT)

(d) PSVT with aberrant conduction

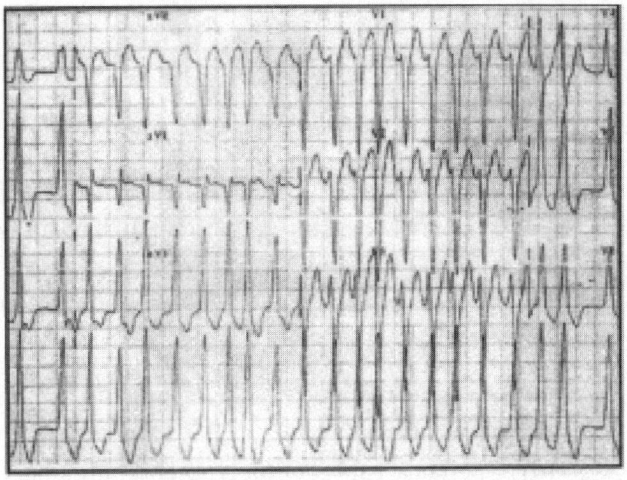

181. A 15-year-old child has history of increasing cyanosis since childhood. The X-ray chest is shown below. The likely diagnosis is:

(a) ASD with Eisenmenger syndrome

(b) d-transposition of great arteries (d-TGA)

(c) Ebstein's anomaly

(d) Tricuspid atresia

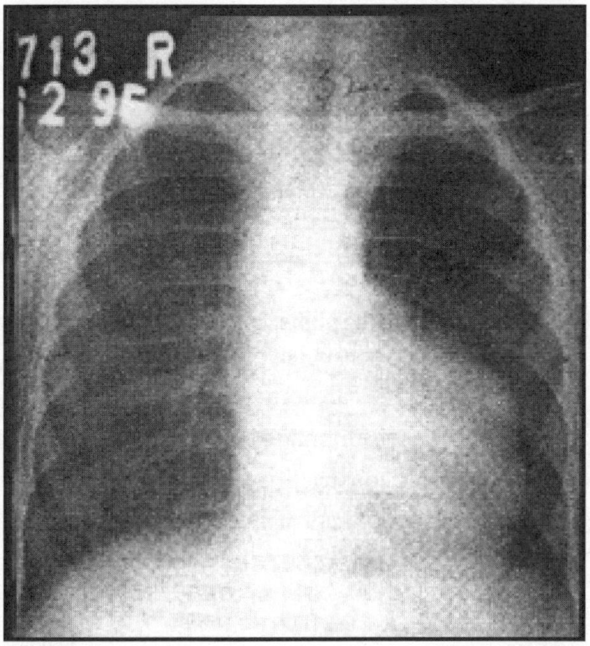

182. The likely management of a 45-year-old female patient having the oximetry and hemodynamic data as shown below should be:

Chamber	O_2 Saturation	Pressure
SVC	65	–
IVC	60	
RA	82	a 16, v 16, m 14
RV	80	60, ed 16
PA	80	60/24, m 36
PCW	98	a 15, v 16, m 14
LA	98	a 16, v 16, m 14
LV	98	100, ed 16
FA	98	100/68, m 77

(a) Medical treatment with Sildenafil and Bosentan
(b) Open heart surgery for ASD
(c) Open heart surgery for ASD and mitral valvotomy
(d) Open heart surgery for ASD and pulmonary valvotomy

183. The pull-back pressure recording from left ventricle apex to aorta of a 36-year-old patient is shown below. The likely treatment should be:

(a) Aortic root replacement
(b) Alcohol septal ablation
(c) Aortic valve balloon dilatation
(d) Aortic valve replacement

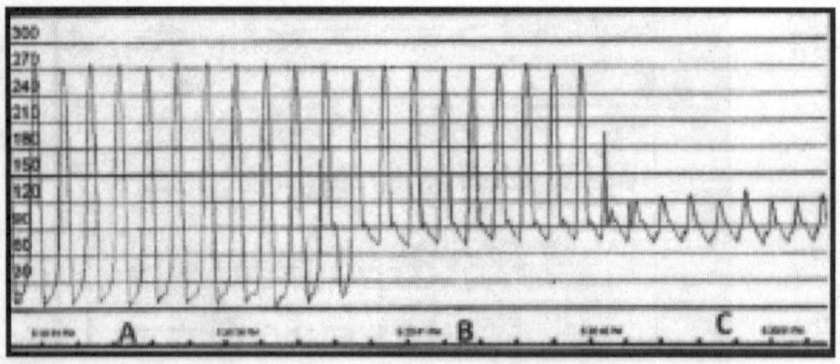

184. The likely diagnosis based on the hemodynamic trace shown below is:

(a) Restrictive cardiomyopathy
(b) Cardiac tamponade
(c) Chronic constrictive pericarditis
(d) Hypertrophic obstructive cardiomyopathy

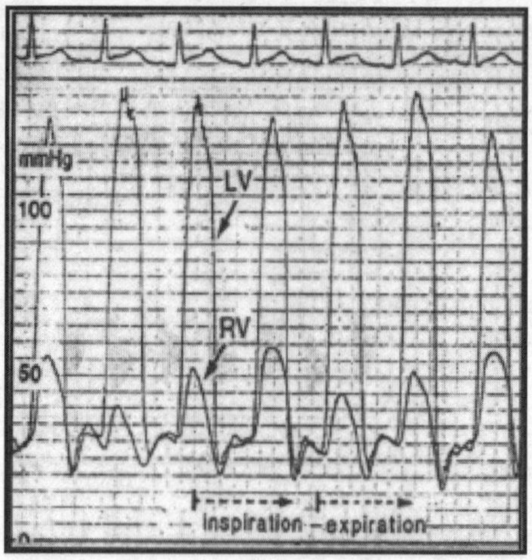

185. A 45-year-old patient presents to the emergency with severe chest pain. The 12-lead ECG done at the time of presentation is shown below. The likely diagnosis is:

(a) Acute pulmonary embolism
(b) Acute pericarditis
(c) STEMI (left main coronary artery occlusion)
(d) STEMI (distal LAD occlusion)

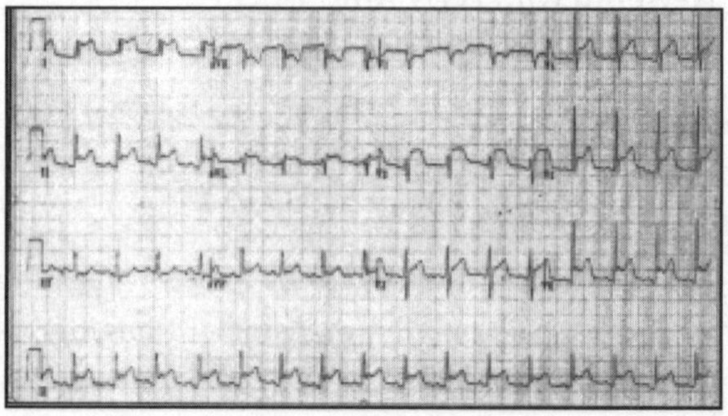

186. A 10-year-old child has history of palpitation. The ECG at the time of symptoms is shown below. The likely anatomical site of origin of ventricular premature contraction is:

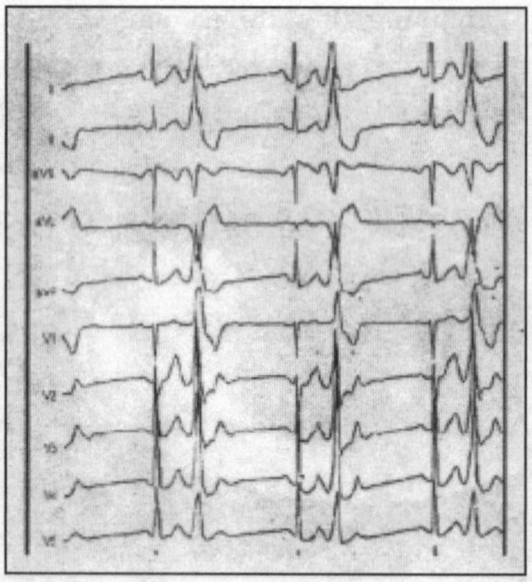

(a) Right ventricle outflow tract
(b) Right ventricle apex
(c) Left ventricular outflow tract
(d) Interventricular septum

187. Increased lung uptake, all *except*:
(a) Rapid transit in pulmonary circulation
(b) Multivessal disease
(c) LV dysfunction
(d) ↑ PCWP

188. All are true about Ajmaline *except*:
(a) Inhibits platelet activity more potently than aspirin
(b) Can cause torsade de pointes
(c) Ajmaline infusion is useful in establishing diagnosis of WPW syndrome occult Chagasic cardiomyopathy and Brugada syndrome
(d) Can cause a decrease in defibrillation threshold

189. All of the following pairs are matched, *except:*
(a) Ezetimibe–epithelial cell Niemann - Pick Cl-like protein
(b) Mipomersen–antisense oligonucleotide that targets apoB-100 mRNA
(c) Eprotirome and sobetirome–Thyroid mimetics
(d) Lomitapide–HDL- bound enzyme cholesterol ester transfer protein inhibitor

Extended matching:

Options: (a) Scleroderma, (b) Pulmonary embolism, (c) Viral Pericarditis, (d) Hypoglycemia, (e) Atherosclerosis, (f) RAS, (g) Pheochromocytoma. (190-206)

190. Middle aged female, rash, finger pain gradual onset breathlessness.

191. Old female, was taking OCP, sudden onset breathlessness.

192. Chronic smoker 35 pack years, L/o wheezing, bout of coughing v/b progressive breathlessness chest pain.

193. Young male, fall in fever state 2 days back, now presents with breathlessness, chest pain, pain increasing on inspiration.

194. 62 > old diabetes presents with sweating, altered sensonium, no focal deficits.

195. 85-year-old lady, BP 200/90 mm Hg, has osteoarthritis, taking NSAIDs, cause of HTN?

196. Middle age female, histor of family HTN, not responding to conventional antihypertensives, subsequently responded to spironolactone alane.

197. 28-year-old male, presents with palpitation, pounding headache sweating.

198. Hypertensive patient poorly responding to bendrofluonethiazide creatinine worsened from 1.5 ng/dl to 2.5 ng/dl after enalapril what is the D?

199. HOCM + Asthma patient.

200. Thyrotoxicosis, 26 years female.

201. AF with fast ventricular rate, BP 120/80 mm Hg.

202. Diabetic patient, MYHA class 4 LV dysfunction.

203. P wave negative in aVR. Positive in 1.2 aVF.

204. Macrore entry in right atrium.

205. Initial P wave of tachycardia is different from subsequent p waves.

206. Automaticity, triggered and reentry, all three are machanism in.

207. Ebola virus: (T/F)
(a) Route of transmission is airborne
(b) Easily destroyed by heat and disinfectants
(c) Convalescent serum beneficial
(d) Replicate well in virtually all cell types
(e) Viral replication is associated with cellular necrosis only in vivo

208. Hemolytic anemia: (T/F)
(a) Anemia is usually normocytic in HS
(b) Refactory cases of HUS→Splenectomy done
(c) Serum haptoglobin in increased
(d) Heinz bodies characteristic in HS
(e) HS–Feature is an increase in MCHC

209. Peripheral neuropathy: (T/F)
(a) Polyradiculopathy is self limiting
(b) Autonomic symptom is sweating
(c) Symmetrically decreased reflexes is plexopathy
(d) Cisplatin neuropathy sensory neuropathy
(e) Gabapentin can be used in neuropathy

210. Vesoreactivity in PAH – desired responses include: (T/F)
(a) mPAP fall by > 20 mm Hg to value less than 40 mm Hg
(b) 50% reduction in pulmonary vascular resistance
(c) Increased cardiac output because of HR
(d) Increased pulmonary arterial saturation
(e) PCWP increased

211. Coagulation factors: (T/F)
(a) -PT. -aPTT suggests factor 5 deficiency
(b) Prothrombin is a vitamin K dependent factor
(c) DDAVP useful in Rx of mild hemophilia A
(d) Factor XII-AD
(e) Repeated dosing of DDAVP results in tachyphylaxis

212. Reduction of periprocedural MI: (T/F)
(a) Intracoronary urokinase
(b) Statins started before procedure
(c) Edoxaban pretreatment
(d) Dual antiplatelet therapy
(e) Abciximab reduces periprocedural CK-MB elevations

213. Regarding cardiac anatomy: (T/F)
(a) Septal leaflet of tricuspid valve is larger high mobile
(b) Anterior papillary muscle has dual blood supply from LCA
(c) RV is less trabeculated
(d) Normal aortic valve has three leaflets of equal size is 80% cases
(e) Dilatation of the mitral valve annulus primarily affects the posterior leaflet

214. Severe patient prosthetic measurements for aortic prosthetic is indicated positive area less than:
(a) 0.55 cm^2/m^2 (b) 0.65 cm^2/m^2
(c) 0.75 cm^2/m^2 (d) 0.85 cm^2/m^2

215. On statin C/I:
(a) Gemfibrozil (b) Clopidogrel
(c) Aspirin (d) Diclofenac

216. Pregnancy with maximum mortality:
(a) Eisenmenger (b) Severe AS
(c) Severe MS (d) IPAH
(e) COA

217. Cilastazol all *except:*
(a) PDE III inhibitor
(b) Vasodilator
(c) Anti-platelet
(d) Not well tolerated

ANSWERS KEY

1. (b)	2. (a)	3. (b)	4. (b)	5. (a)	6. (c)	7. (c)	8. (a)
9. (a)	10. (a)	11. (a)	12. (b)	13. (b)	14. (e,a,b,a,c)	15. (b)	16. (e)
17. (a)	18. (h)	19. (i)	20. (b)	21. (a)	22. (c)	23. (i)	24. (h)
25. (f)	26. (a)	27. (h)	28. (e)	29. (b)	30. (d)	31. (a)	32. (b)
33. (g)	34. (c)	35. (b)	36. (a)	37. (a)	38. (a)	39. (b)	40. (a)
41. (a)	42. (a}	43. (b)	44. (a)	45. (a)	46. (d)	47. (a)	48. (f)
49. (a)	50. (h)	51. (e)	52. (b)	53. (e)	54. (g)	55. (a)	56. (c)
57. (b)	58. (c)	59. (a)	60. (b)	61. (d)	62. (e)	63. (d)	64. (b)
65. (a)	66. (a)	67. (b)	68. (b)	69. (a)	70. (d)	71. (d)	72. (a)
73. (b)	74. (c)	75. (?)	76. (?)	77. (b)	78. (e)	79. (d)	80. (a)
81. (f)	82. (h)	83. (?)	84. (?)	85. (?)	86. (?)	87. (d)	88. (a)
89. (d)	90. (e)	91. FTFT	92. TFF	93. TTFTF	94. FTFFT	95. FTTTT	96. FFTTF
97. F	98. (a)	99. (d)	100. (b)	101. (c)	102. (a,c)	103. (a)	104. (c)
105. (a)	106. (f)	107. (a)	108. (a)	109. (c)	110. (d)	111. (a)	112. (a)
113. (a)	114. (a)	115. (b)	116. (a)	117. (b)	118. (d)	119. (b)	120. (c)
121. (a)	122. (c)	123. (a)	124. (b)	125. (c)	126. (c)	127. (d)	128. (b)
129. (a)	130. (b)	131. (d)	132. (c)	133. (d)	134. (b)	135. (c)	136. (d)
137. (c)	138. (d)	139. (a)	140. (c)	141. (a)	142. (b)	143. (d)	144. (a)
145. FFFTF	146. TTTT	147. TT	148. FTFFT	149. TTTTT	150. TTTT	151. TTTT	152. TFTFT
153. FTT	154. (a)	155. TTTTF	156. TTTTF	157. TFFFF	158. TTTTF	159. FFTTT	160. TFTFT
161. FFFTF	162. F	163. (a)	164. (a)	165. (a)	166. (d)	167. (d)	168. (a)
169. (a)	170. (c)	171. T	172. (a)	173. (b)	174. (d)	175. (d)	176. (b)
177. TFFT	178. (c)	179. (b)	180. (b)	181. (d)	182. (b)	183. (a)	184. (c)
185. (b)	186. (c)	187. (a)	188. (d)	189. (d)	190. (a)	191. (b)	192. (?)
193. (c)	194. (d)	195. (e)	196. (f)	197. (g)	198. (f)	199. (?)	200. (?)
201. (?)	202. (?)	203. (?)	204. (?)	205. (?)	206. (?)	207. TFTTT	208. TFFFT
209. FTFTT	210. FFFFF	211. TTTFT	212. FTFTF	213. FTFFT	214. (b)	215. (a)	216. (a,d)
217. (d)							